POCKET COMPANION

to **Robbins and Cotran**

Pathologic Basis of Disease

FIRST SOUTH ASIA EDITION

POCKET COMPANION to Robbins and Cotran Pathologic Basis of Disease

Richard N. Mitchell, MD, PhD
Lawrence J. Henderson Professor of Pathology and Health Sciences and Technology
Department of Pathology
Harvard Medical School
Staff Pathologist
Brigham and Women's Hospital
Boston, Massachusetts

Vinay Kumar, MBBS, MD, FRCPath
Donald N. Pritzker Professor and Chairman
Department of Pathology
Biologic Sciences Division and the Pritzker School of Medicine
The University of Chicago
Chicago, Illinois

Abul K. Abbas, MBBS
Distinguished Professor and Chair
Department of Pathology
University of California San Francisco
San Francisco, California

Jon C. Aster, MD, PhD
Professor of Pathology
Harvard Medical School
Brigham and Women's Hospital
Boston, Massachusetts

With illustrations by James A. Perkins, MS, MFA

ELSEVIER

ELSEVIER

RELX India Pvt. Ltd.
Registered Office: 818, Indraprakash Building, 8thFloor, 21, Barakhamba Road,
New Delhi - 110001
Corporate Office: 14th Floor, Building No. 10B, DLF Cyber City, Phase II, Gurgaon-122 002, Haryana, India

Pocket Companion to Robbins and Cotran Pathologic Basis of Disease, 9e, Richard N. Mitchell, Vinay Kumar, Abul K. Abbas, Jon C. Aster

ISBN: 978-1-4557-5416-8

This adapted reprint of Pocket Companion to Robbins and Cotran Pathologic Basis of Disease, 9e, by Richard N. Mitchell, Vinay Kumar, Abul K. Abbas, Jon C. Aster was undertaken by RELX India Private Limited and is published by arrangement with Elsevier Inc.

Pocket Companion to Robbins and Cotran Pathologic Basis of Disease, First South Asia Edition, Richard N. Mitchell, Vinay Kumar, Abul K. Abbas, Jon C. Aster

Adapted Reprint ISBN: 978-81-312-4706-8

Notice

Knowledge and best practice in this field are constantly changing. As new research and experience broaden our understanding, changes in research methods, professional practices, or medical treatment may become necessary.

Practitioners and researchers must always rely on their own experience and knowledge in evaluating and using any information, methods, compounds, or experiments described herein. In using such information or methods they should be mindful of their own safety and the safety of others, including parties for whom they have a professional responsibility.

With respect to any drug or pharmaceutical products identified, readers are advised to check the most current information provided (i) on procedures featured or (ii) by the manufacturer of each product to be administered, to verify the recommended dose or formula, the method and duration of administration, and contraindications. It is the responsibility of practitioners, relying on their own experience and knowledge of their patients, to make diagnoses, to determine dosages and the best treatment for each individual patient, and to take all appropriate safety precautions.

To the fullest extent of the law, neither the Publisher nor the authors, contributors, or editors, assume any liability for any injury and/or damage to persons or property as a matter of product liability, negligence or otherwise, or from any use or operation of any methods, products, instructions, or ideas contained in the material herein.

Although all advertising material is expected to conform to ethical (medical) standards, inclusion in this publication does not constitute a guarantee or endorsement of the quality or value of such product or of the claims made of it by its manufacturer.

This publication is licensed for sale in India, Bangladesh, Bhutan, Maldives, Nepal, Pakistan and Sri Lanka only. Circulation of this version outside these territories is unauthorized and illegal.

Content Strategist: Dikshita Khanduja
Sr Project Manager—Education Solutions: Shabina Nasim
Content Development Specialist: Shravan Kumar
Project Manager: Nayagi Athmanathan

Printed in India by Thomson Press India Ltd.

Contributors

Charles E. Alpers, MD
Professor and Vice-Chair, Department of Pathology, University of Washington School of Medicine; Pathologist, University of Washington Medical Center, Seattle, Washington
The Kidney

Douglas C. Anthony, MD, PhD
Professor, Pathology and Laboratory Medicine, Warren Alpert Medical School of Brown University; Chief of Pathology, Lifespan Academic Medical Center, Providence, Rhode Island
Peripheral Nerves and Skeletal Muscles; The Central Nervous System

Anthony Chang, MD
Associate Professor of Pathology, Director of Renal Pathology, Department of Pathology, The University of Chicago, Chicago, Illinois
The Kidney

Umberto De Girolami, MD
Professor of Pathology, Harvard Medical School; Neuropathologist, Brigham and Women's Hospital, Boston, Massachusetts
The Central Nervous System

Lora Hedrick Ellenson, MD
Professor and Director of Gynecologic Pathology, Department of Pathology and Laboratory Medicine, New York Presbyterian Hospital-Weill Cornell Medical College; Attending Pathologist, New York Presbyterian Hospital, New York, New York
The Female Genital Tract

Jonathan I. Epstein, MD
Professor of Pathology, Urology, and Oncology, The Reinhard Professor of Urologic Pathology, The Johns Hopkins University School of Medicine; Director of Surgical Pathology, The Johns Hopkins Hospital, Baltimore, Maryland
The Lower Urinary Tract and Male Genital System

Robert Folberg, MD
Founding Dean and Professor of Biomedical Sciences, Pathology, and Ophthalmology, Oakland University William Beaumont School of Medicine, Rochester, Michigan; Chief Academic Officer, Beaumont Hospitals, Royal Oak, Michigan
The Eye

Matthew P. Frosch, MD, PhD
Lawrence J. Henderson Associate Professor of Pathology and Health Sciences and Technology, Harvard Medical School; Director, C.S. Kubik Laboratory of Neuropathology, Massachusetts General Hospital, Boston, Massachusetts
The Central Nervous System

Andrew Horvai, MD, PhD
Professor, Department of Pathology, Associate Director of Surgical Pathology, University of California San Francisco, San Francisco, California
Bones, Joints, and Soft Tissue Tumors

Ralph H. Hruban, MD
Professor of Pathology and Oncology, Director of the Sol Goldman Pancreatic Cancer Research Center, The Johns Hopkins University School of Medicine, Baltimore, Maryland
The Pancreas

Aliya N. Husain, MBBS
Professor, Department of Pathology, Director of Pulmonary, Pediatric and Cardiac Pathology, Pritzker School of Medicine, The University of Chicago, Chicago, Illinois
The Lung

Christine A. Iacobuzio-Donahue, MD, PhD
Attending Physician, Department of Pathology; Associate Director for Translational Research, Center for Pancreatic Cancer Research, Memorial Sloan Kettering Cancer Center, New York, New York
The Pancreas

Raminder Kumar, MBBS, MD
Chicago, Illinois
Clinical Editor for Diseases of the Heart, Lung, Gastrointestinal Tract, Liver, and Kidneys

Alexander J.F. Lazar, MD, PhD
Associate Professor, Departments of Pathology and Dermatology, Sarcoma Research Center, University of Texas M.D. Anderson Cancer Center, Houston, Texas
The Skin

Susan C. Lester, MD, PhD
Assistant Professor of Pathology, Harvard Medical School; Chief, Breast Pathology, Brigham and Women's Hospital, Boston, Massachusetts
The Breast

Mark W. Lingen, DDS, PhD, PRCPath
Professor, Department of Pathology, Director of Oral Pathology, Pritzker School of Medicine, The University of Chicago, Chicago, Illinois
Head and Neck

Tamara L. Lotan, MD
Associate Professor of Pathology and Oncology, The Johns Hopkins Hospital, Baltimore, Maryland
The Lower Urinary Tract and Male Genital System

Anirban Maitra, MBBS
Professor of Pathology and Translational Molecular Pathology, University of Texas M.D. Anderson Cancer Center, Houston, Texas
Diseases of Infancy and Childhood; The Endocrine System

Alexander J. McAdam, MD, PhD
Vice Chair, Department of Laboratory Medicine, Medical Director, Infectious Diseases Diagnostic Laboratory, Boston Children's Hospital; Associate Professor of Pathology, Harvard Medical School, Boston, Massachusetts
Infectious Diseases

Danny A. Milner, MD, MSc, FCAP
Assistant Professor of Pathology, Assistant Medical Director, Microbiology, Harvard Medical School, Boston, Massachusetts
Infectious Diseases

Richard N. Mitchell, MD, PhD
Lawrence J. Henderson Professor of Pathology and Health Sciences and Technology, Department of Pathology, Harvard Medical School; Staff Pathologist, Brigham and Women's Hospital, Boston, Massachusetts
The Cell as a Unit of Health and Disease; Blood Vessels; The Heart

George F. Murphy, MD
Professor of Pathology, Harvard Medical School; Director of Dermatopathology, Brigham and Women's Hospital, Boston, Massachusetts
The Skin

Edyta C. Pirog, MD
Associate Professor of Clinical Pathology and Laboratory Medicine, New York Presbyterian Hospital-Weill Medical College of Cornell University; Associate Attending Pathologist, New York Presbyterian Hospital, New York, New York
The Female Genital Tract

Peter Pytel, MD
Associate Professor, Director of Neuropathology, Department of Pathology, University of Chicago School of Medicine, Chicago, Illinois
Peripheral Nerves and Skeletal Muscles

Frederick J. Schoen, MD, PhD
Professor of Pathology and Health Sciences and Technology, Harvard Medical School; Director, Cardiac Pathology, Executive Vice Chairman, Department of Pathology, Brigham and Women's Hospital, Boston, Massachusetts
The Heart

Arlene H. Sharpe, MD, PhD
Professor of Pathology, Co-Director of Harvard Institute of Translational Immunology, Harvard Medical School; Department of Pathology, Brigham and Women's Hospital, Boston, Massachusetts
Infectious Diseases

Neil Theise, MD
Departments of Pathology and Medicine, Mount Sinai Beth Israel, Icahn School of Medicine at Mount Sinai, New York, New York
Liver and Gallbladder

Jerrold R. Turner, MD, PhD
Sara and Harold Lincoln Thompson Professor, Associate Chair, Department of Pathology, Pritzker School of Medicine, The University of Chicago, Chicago, Illinois
The Gastrointestinal Tract

Foreword

It is indeed a privilege to write foreword to this first South Asia edition of *Pocket Companion to Robbins and Cotran Pathologic Basis of Disease*.

The main book, *Robbins and Cotran Pathologic Basis of Disease*, has been the standard textbook of pathology for undergraduates and postgraduates. Over the last several decades, it has gained wide acceptance by students and teachers of not only pathology but other allied specialties also. This speaks volumes of its high caliber. However, the book is detailed and sometimes difficult to comprehend by the students in totality. A student who is new to pathology may be intimidated by its vastness.

There is thus a need for a simple and concise book, especially for the undergraduate students. The *Pocket Companion to Robbins and Cotran Pathologic Basis of Disease* fulfills that need and provides the same updated information on various aspects of diseases in a more comprehensive and concise form. The students can easily comprehend the essential facts quickly, which is a boon, while revising the topics especially prior to examination. It is truly a student friendly book.

It follows the same pattern as the "big book" and enables the student to have a focused and complete coverage of the curriculum in a short span of time. As the book is clearly organized, it provides a convenient, easily navigable synopsis of pathology. Most of the figures have been recapitulated as in the main book, further facilitating understanding of the subject.

The book will be of immense help to doctors appearing for the postgraduate entrance examinations and will enable them to revise pathology in limited period of time.

The book lives up to its name of Pocket Companion not only financially but also by virtue of its size and allows the student to carry it easily anywhere virtually providing pathology on the go.

Meera Sikka MD
Director Professor & Head
Department of Pathology
UCMS & GTB Hospital
Delhi

Preface

The dramatic revolution in molecular biology, coupled with the computational ability to make sense of terabytes of data, is changing the face of medicine. With each passing year (indeed with almost every passing *hour*) there is an explosion of new information that requires digestion, comprehension, and assimilation—all of it potentially impacting disease diagnosis and therapy. Integrating and making sense of all the new knowledge is a challenging proposition—even for seasoned physicians and scientists who already enjoy a reasonable (and semi-organized) understanding of pathobiology. However, for the novice student—experiencing the amazing depth and breadth of human disease for the first (or second or third) time—the thirst for knowledge can easily get drowned by a fire hose of information. *Robbins and Cotran Pathologic Basis of Disease* (AKA: the Big Book) has long been the fundamental pathology text for students of medicine, organizing the occasionally bewildering flood of facts and concepts into a comprehensive yet manageable, beautifully illustrated, and eminently readable entrée into the universe of pathobiology. And yet, at more than 1300 pages (and weighing in at 7 pounds in its dead tree form), the Big Book is still a daunting tome.

Enter the *Pocket Companion.* Initially an offspring of the fourth edition of the Big Book in 1991, the Pocket Companion was born of the recognition that the immense wealth of knowledge about human disease could somehow be succinctly organized and made even more accessible for the overwhelmed medical student and harried house officer. In addition, students and educators alike are increasingly reluctant to make a substantial financial commitment to an opus that is constantly being rewritten, keeping up with the ever-changing landscape of modern medicine. Thus the Pocket Companion meets several important needs, being practical and frugal, yet also immensely (and densely) useful—substantially more than a simple topical outline or the "Key Concepts" boxes that are now a prominent feature of the Big Book. In assembling this update, four major objectives have guided the writing:

- Make the detailed expositions in *Robbins and Cotran Pathologic Basis of Disease* easier to digest by providing a condensed overview and also retaining the most helpful figures and tables.
- Facilitate the use of the Big Book by providing the relevant cross-referenced page numbers.
- Help readers identify the core material that requires their primary attention.
- Serve as a handy tool for quick review of a large body of information.

This edition of the Pocket Companion has been rewritten from front to back, reflecting all the innovations and new knowledge encompassed in the Big Book. Illustrative tables and figures also reduce the verbiage, although as before, the beautiful gross and histologic images of the parent volume are not reproduced. Pains have also been taken to present all the material with the same stylistic voice; the organization of the material and level of detail is considerably more uniform between chapters than in previous editions. In doing so we hope that the Pocket Companion retains the flavor and excitement of the Big Book—just in a more bite-size format—and truly is a suitable "companion."

In closing, the authors specifically wish to acknowledge the invaluable assistance and editing skills (and infinite patience) of Rebecca Mitchell and Becca Gruliow; without their help and collaboration, this edition of the Pocket Companion might still be in gestation.

Rick Mitchell
Vinay Kumar
Abul Abbas
Jon Aster

Contents

General Pathology

Systemic Pathology: Diseases of Organ Systems

General Pathology

1

The Cell as a Unit of Health and Disease

Disease pathogenesis is best understood in the context of *normal* cellular structure and function and how that can be deranged; this chapter is a survey of basic principles and recent advances in cell biology as they apply to the rest of the book.

The Genome (p. 1)

Noncoding DNA (p. 1)

The human genome encodes approximately 20,000 proteins, but the sequences involved in coding such genes comprise only 1.5% of the total 3.2 billion DNA base pairs. Up to 80% of the remaining DNA is functional in that it can bind proteins or otherwise regulate gene expression. Major classes of functional nonprotein coding sequences include the following (Fig. 1-1):

- *Promoter* and *enhancer* regions providing binding sites for transcription factors.
- Binding sites for factors that maintain higher-order *chromatin structures.*
- *Noncoding regulatory RNAs.* More than 60% of the genome is transcribed into RNAs that are never translated into protein but that still regulate gene expression (e.g., microRNAs [miRNAs] and long noncoding RNAs) (see later discussion).
- *Mobile genetic elements* (e.g., *transposons*). One third of the genome is composed of such "jumping genes" that are implicated in gene regulation and chromatin organization.
- Special structural regions of DNA (e.g., *telomeres* [chromosome ends] and *centromeres* [chromosome "tethers"]).

Any two individuals share greater than 99.5% of their DNA sequences; thus person-to-person variation, including disease susceptibility and responses to environmental stimuli, is encoded in less than 0.5% of total cellular DNA (15 million base pairs). The two most common forms of DNA variation are as follows:

- *Single-nucleotide polymorphisms (SNPs):* These are variants at single nucleotide positions identified through genome sequencing; they number approximately 6 million. SNPs occur across the genome—within exons, introns, and intergenic regions. Only 1% of these occur in coding regions; SNPs located in noncoding regions may impact gene expression by influencing regulatory elements. Even SNPs that are "neutral" (no effect on gene function or expression) can be useful markers if they are coinherited with a disease-associated gene as a result of physical proximity (*linkage* disequilibrium). In most cases any given SNP has a relatively minimal influence on disease; however, combinations of SNPs may predict risk for complex multigenic disorders (e.g., hypertension).

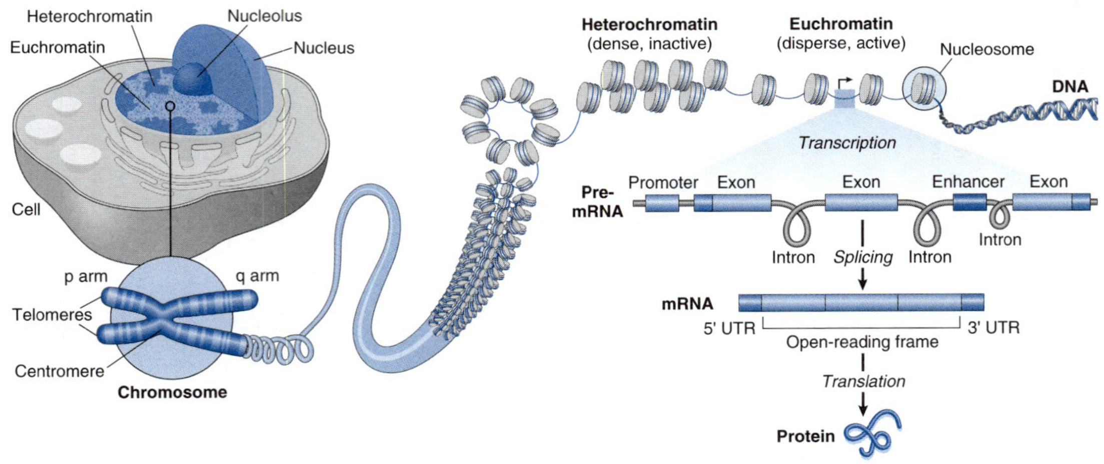

Figure 1-1 **The organization of nuclear DNA.** At the light microscopic level the nuclear genetic material is organized into dispersed, transcriptionally active *euchromatin* or densely packed, transcriptionally inactive *heterochromatin;* chromatin can also be mechanically connected with the nuclear membrane, and nuclear membrane perturbation can thus influence transcription. Chromosomes (as shown) can only be visualized by light microscopy during cell division. During mitosis, they are organized into paired chromatids connected at *centromeres;* the centromeres act as the locus for the formation of a *kinetochore* protein complex that regulates chromosome segregation at metaphase. The *telomeres* are repetitive nucleotide sequences that cap the termini of chromatids and permit repeated chromosomal replication without loss of DNA at the chromosome ends. The chromatids are organized into short "P" ("petite") and long "Q" ("next letter in the alphabet") arms. The characteristic banding pattern of chromatids has been attributed to relative GC content (less GC content in bands relative to interbands), with genes tending to localize to interband regions. Individual chromatin fibers comprise a string of nucleosomes—DNA wound around octameric histone cores—with the nucleosomes connected via DNA linkers. Promoters are noncoding regions of DNA that initiate gene transcription; they are on the same strand and upstream of their associated gene. Enhancers are regulatory elements that can modulate gene expression over distances of 100 kB or more by looping back onto promoters and recruiting additional factors that are needed to drive the expression of pre-mRNA species. The intronic sequences are subsequently spliced out of the pre-mRNA to produce the definitive message that is translated into protein—without the 3′ and 5′ untranslated regions (UTRs). In addition to the enhancer, promoter, and UTR sequences, noncoding elements are found throughout the genome; these include short repeats, regulatory factor binding regions, noncoding regulatory RNAs, and transposons.

- *Copy number variations (CNVs):* These represent different numbers of repeated sequences of DNA—up to millions of base pairs in length. Approximately half of CNVs involve gene-coding sequences; thus CNVs may underlie a large portion of human phenotypic diversity.
- *Epigenetics*—heritable changes in gene expression that are not caused by primary variation in DNA sequence—is also important in generating genetic diversity (see the following section).

Histone Organization (p. 3)

Although all cells have the same genetic material, terminally differentiated cells have distinct structures and functions; these are determined by lineage-specific programs of gene expression driven by *epigenetic factors* (Fig. 1-2):

- *Histones and histone-modifying factors. Nucleosomes* are 147 base pair segments wrapped around a core of *histones;* DNA-histone complexes are joined through DNA linkers and packed together to form *chromatin.* Chromatin exists in two basic forms: (1) cytochemically dense and transcriptionally inactive *heterochromatin* and (2) cytochemically dispersed and transcriptionally active *euchromatin* (Fig. 1-1). Histones are dynamic structures:
    - *Chromatin-remodeling complexes* reposition nucleosomes on DNA, exposing (or obscuring) gene regulatory elements, such as promoters.
    - *Chromatin writer complexes* make chemical modifications *(marks)* on amino acids that include methylation, acetylation, or phosphorylation. Actively transcribed genes have histone marks that render DNA accessible to RNA polymerases; inactive genes have histone marks that enable DNA compaction into heterochromatin.
    - *Chromatin erasers* remove histone marks; *chromatin readers* bind particular marks and thereby regulate gene expression.
    - *Histone acetylation* tends to increase transcription; methylation and phosphorylation can increase or decrease transcription.
- *DNA methylation.* High levels of DNA methylation in gene regulatory elements typically result in transcriptional silencing.
- *Chromatin organizing factors* are proteins that bind to noncoding regions and control long-range looping of DNA to regulating the spatial relationships between gene enhancers and promoters.

MicroRNA and Long Noncoding RNA (p. 4)

miRNA (p. 4) are short RNAs (21 to 30 nucleotides); they do not encode proteins but rather are involved in posttranscriptional silencing of gene expression. miRNA transcription produces a primary miRNA, which is progressively trimmed by the enzyme *DICER,* eventually becoming associated with a multiprotein aggregate called RNA-induced silencing complex (RISC; Fig. 1-3). Subsequent base pairing between the miRNA strand and its target mRNA directs the RISC to either induce mRNA cleavage or repress its translation.

Synthetic *small interfering RNAs (siRNAs)* are short RNA sequences that can be introduced into cells, acting in a manner analogous to endogenous miRNAs. These form the basis for *knockdown* experiments to study gene function and are also being developed as possible therapeutic agents to silence pathogenic genes.

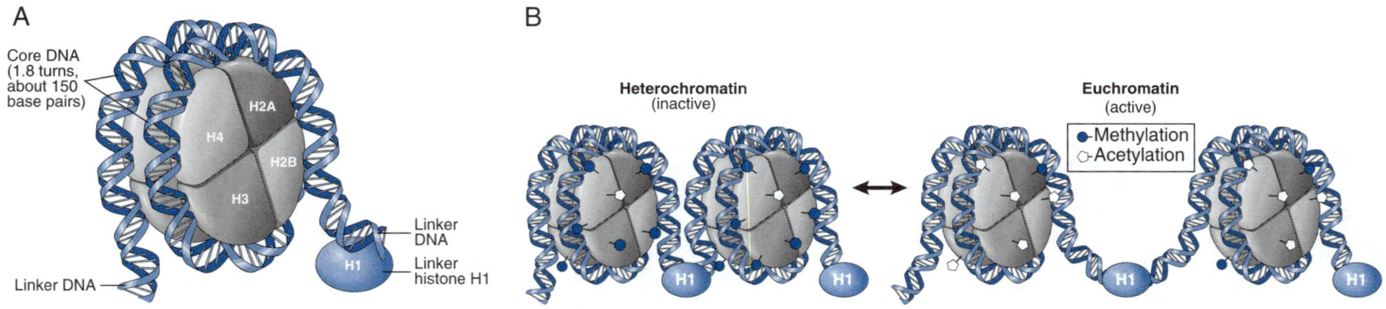

Figure 1-2 Histone organization. A, Nucleosomes are composed of octamers of histone proteins (two each of histone subunits H2A, H2B, H3, and H4) encircled by 1.8 loops of 147 base pairs of DNA; histone H1 sits on the 20- to 80-nucleotide linker DNA between nucleosomes and helps to stabilize the overall chromatin architecture. The histone subunits are positively charged, thus allowing the compaction of the negatively charged DNA. **B,** The relative state of DNA unwinding (and thus access for transcription factors) is regulated by histone modification (e.g., by acetylation, methylation, and/or phosphorylation [so-called "marks"]); marks are dynamically written and erased. Certain marks, such as histone acetylation, "open up" the chromatin structure, whereas others, such as methylation of particular histone residues, tend to condense the DNA and lead to gene silencing. DNA itself can also be also be methylated, a modification that is associated with transcriptional inactivation.

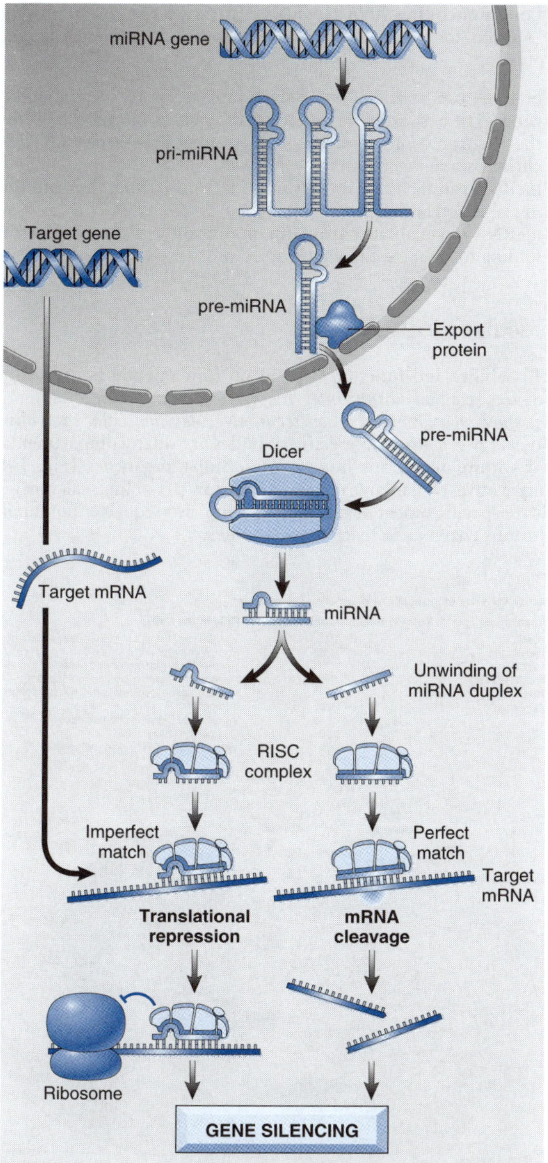

Figure 1-3 Generation of microRNAs (miRNAs) and their mode of action in regulating gene function. miRNA genes are transcribed to produce a primary miRNA *(pri-miRNA)*, which is processed within the nucleus to form *pre-miRNA* composed of a single RNA strand with secondary hairpin loop structures that form stretches of double-stranded RNA. After this pre-miRNA is exported out of the nucleus via specific transporter proteins, the cytoplasmic *Dicer enzyme* trims the pre-miRNA to generate mature double-stranded miRNAs of 21 to 30 nucleotides. The miRNA subsequently unwinds, and the resulting single strands are incorporated into the multiprotein *RISC.* Base pairing between the single-stranded miRNA and its target mRNA directs RISC to either cleave the mRNA target or repress its translation. In either case the target mRNA gene is silenced posttranscriptionally.

Long noncoding RNA (lncRNA) (p. 5) exceed coding mRNAs by tenfold to twentyfold and are involved in modulating gene expression:

- lncRNA can restrict RNA polymerase access to specific coding genes. The best example involves XIST, which is transcribed from the X chromosome and plays an essential role in physiologic X chromosome inactivation.
- lncRNA can facilitate transcription factor binding, thus promoting gene activation.
- lncRNA can facilitate chromatin modification or provide the scaffolding to stabilize chromatin structure.

Cellular Housekeeping (p. 6)

Cell viability and function depend on fundamental housekeeping activities (e.g., *membrane integrity, nutrient acquisition, communication, movement, renewal of senescent molecules, molecular catabolism,* and *energy generation*). Specific activities are often compartmentalized within membrane-bound intracellular organelles (Fig. 1-4); unique intracellular environments (e.g., low pH or high calcium) facilitate specific biochemical pathways and also sequester potentially injurious enzymes or reactive metabolites.

Relative volumes of intracellular organelles (hepatocyte)

Compartment	% Total Volume	Number/Cell	Role in the Cell
Cytosol	54%	1	Metabolism, transport, protein translation
Mitochondria	22%	1700	Energy generation, apoptosis
Rough ER	9%	1*	Synthesis of membrane and secreted proteins
Smooth ER, Golgi	6%	1*	Protein modification, sorting, catabolism
Nucleus	6%	1	Cell regulation, proliferation, DNA transcription
Endosomes	1%	200	Intracellular transport and export, ingestion of extracellular substances
Lysosomes	1%	300	Cellular catabolism
Peroxisomes	1%	400	Very long chain fatty acid metabolism

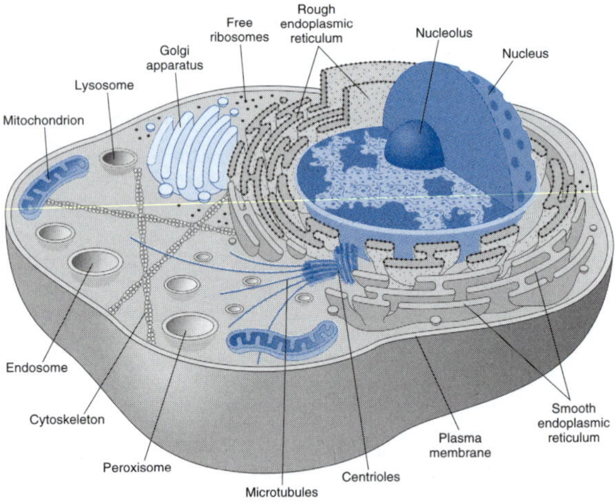

Figure 1-4 Basic subcellular constituents of cells. The table presents the number of the various organelles within a typical hepatocyte, as well as their volume within the cell. The figure shows geographic relationships but is not intended to be accurate to scale. *(Adapted from Weibel ER, Stäubli W, Gnägi HR, et al: Correlated morphometric and biochemical studies on the liver cell. I. Morphometric model, stereologic methods, and normal morphometric data for rat liver.* J Cell Biol *42:68, 1969.)*

Plasma Membrane: Protection and Nutrient Acquisition (p. 7)

Plasma and organellar membranes are fluid bilayers of amphipathic phospholipids with hydrophilic head groups that face the aqueous environment and hydrophobic lipid tails that interact to form a barrier to passive diffusion (Fig. 1-5). Membrane components are distributed heterogeneously and asymmetrically:

- *Phosphatidylinositol* on the inner membrane leaflet can be a phosphorylated scaffold for intracellular proteins, whereas polyphosphoinositides can be hydrolyzed by phospholipase C to generate intracellular second signals, such as diacylglycerol and inositol trisphosphate.
- *Phosphatidylserine* on the inner face provides a negative charge for protein interactions; on the extracellular face (in cells undergoing programmed cell death), it is an "eat me" signal for phagocytes.
- *Glycolipids* and *sphingomyelin* are preferentially expressed on the extracellular face; glycolipids are important in cell-cell and cell-matrix interactions.
- Some membrane components tend to self-associate to form discrete domains known as "lipid rafts."

Membrane proteins associate with lipid membranes by one of several interactions:

- *Transmembrane proteins* have one or more relatively hydrophobic α-helical segments that traverse the lipid bilayer.
- Posttranslational attachment to prenyl groups (e.g., farnesyl) or fatty acids (e.g., palmitic acid) that insert into the plasma membrane.
- Posttranslation glycosylphosphatidylinositol (GPI) modification allow anchorage on the extracellular face of the membrane.
- Peripheral membrane proteins may noncovalently associate with true transmembrane proteins.
- Many plasma membrane proteins function together as large complexes; these may be primarily assembled in the rough endoplasmic reticulum (RER) or form by lateral diffusion in the plasma membrane; the latter is characteristic of many receptors that dimerize in the presence of ligand to form functional signaling units.

Although membranes are laterally fluid, proteins within them can be confined to discrete domains. Thus inserted proteins have different intrinsic solubilities in various lipid domains and can accumulate in different areas (e.g., lipid rafts). Nonrandom protein distributions can also be achieved through intercellular protein-protein interactions (e.g., at *tight junctions*) that establish discrete boundaries; this strategy is used to maintain *cell polarity* (e.g., top/apical versus bottom/basolateral) in epithelial layers. Unique membrane domains can also be generated by the interaction of proteins with cytoskeletal molecules or extracellular matrix (ECM). The resulting nonrandom distribution of lipids and membrane proteins is relevant to cell-cell and cell-matrix interactions, as well as secretory and endocytic pathways.

The extracellular face of the plasma membrane is studded with carbohydrates on glycoproteins and glycolipids, as well as by polysaccharide chains attached to integral membrane proteoglycans. This *glycocalyx* functions as a chemical and mechanical barrier and mediates cell-cell and cell-matrix interactions.

Passive Membrane Diffusion (p. 9)

Small, nonpolar molecules (O_2 and CO_2) and hydrophobic molecules (e.g., steroid-based molecules such as estradiol or vitamin D)

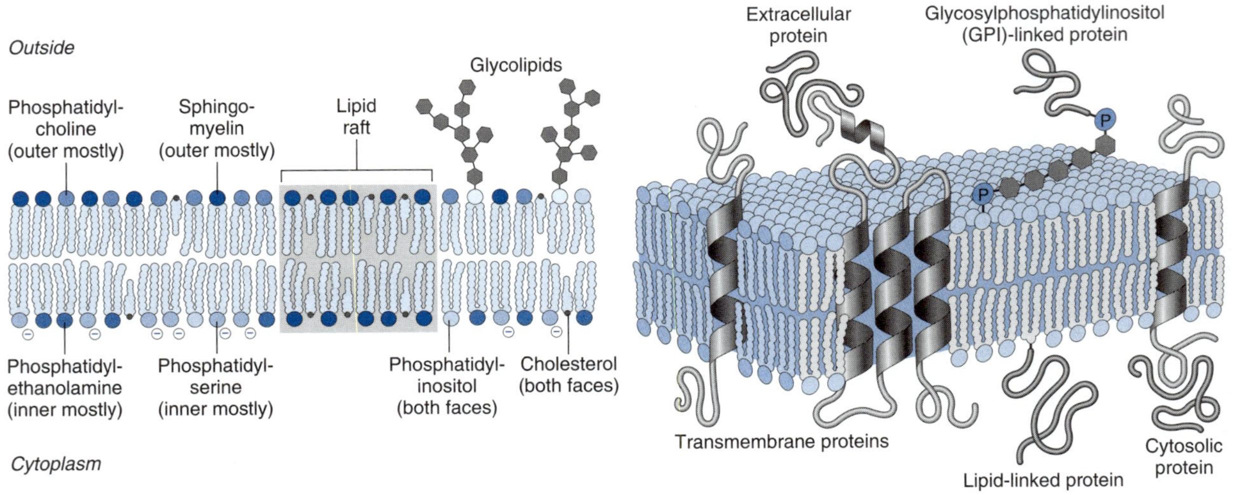

Figure 1-5 Plasma membrane organization and asymmetry. The plasma membrane is a bilayer of phospholipids, cholesterol, and associated proteins. The phospholipid distribution within the membrane is asymmetric due to the activity of *flippases; phosphatidylcholine* and *sphingomyelin* are overrepresented in the outer leaflet, and *phosphatidylserine* (negative charge) and *phosphatidylethanolamine* are predominantly found on the inner leaflet; glycolipids occur only on the outer face, where they contribute to the extracellular glycocalyx. Although the membrane is laterally fluid and the various constituents can diffuse randomly, specific domains—*lipid rafts*—can also stably develop. Membrane-associated proteins may traverse the membrane (singly or multiply) via α-helical hydrophobic amino acid sequences; depending on the membrane lipid content and the hydrophobicity of protein domains, such proteins may have nonrandom distributions within the membrane. Proteins on the cytosolic face may associate with membranes through posttranslational modifications (e.g., farnesylation or addition of palmitic acid). Proteins on the extracytoplasmic face may associate with the membrane via glycosylphosphatidylinositol linkages. In addition to protein-protein interactions within the membrane, membrane proteins can also associate with extracellular and/or intracytoplasmic proteins to generate large, relatively stable complexes (e.g., the *focal adhesion complex*). Transmembrane proteins can translate mechanical forces (e.g., from the cytoskeleton or ECM) as well as chemical signals across the membrane. Similar organizations of lipids and associated proteins occur within the various organellar membranes.

rapidly diffuse across lipid bilayers moving down their concentration gradients. Small, polar molecules (e.g., water, ethanol, and urea) can also cross membranes relatively easily, although large-volume water transport (e.g., renal tubular epithelium) requires *aquaporin* proteins.

Carriers and Channels *(p. 9)*

Polar molecules >75 daltons (e.g., sugars and nucleotides) and all ions require specialized protein transporters to cross cell membranes (plasma or organellar); each solute typically has a highly specific transporter (e.g., a given protein will transport glucose but not galactose) (Fig. 1-6).

- *Channel proteins* create hydrophilic pores, which, when open, permit rapid movement of solutes (restricted by size and charge). Concentration and/or electrical gradients drive the solute movement; plasma membranes typically have an electrical potential difference across them, with the inside negative relative to the outside.
- *Carrier proteins* bind their specific solute and undergo a conformational change to transfer the ligand across the membrane. *Active transport* of certain solutes *against* a concentration gradient can thus be accomplished by carrier molecules (not channels) using energy released by *adenosine triphosphate (ATP)* hydrolysis or a coupled ion gradient.

Because membranes are freely permeable to small polar molecules, water will move across membranes following the relative solute concentrations. Thus extracellular salt in excess of that in the cytosol *(hypertonicity)* causes a net movement of water out of cells, whereas *hypotonicity* causes a net movement of water into cells. Because the cytosol is rich in charged metabolites and protein species that attract a large number of counterions that tend to increase the intracellular osmolarity, cells need to constantly pump out small inorganic ions (e.g., Na^+ and Cl^-) to prevent overhydration. This is accomplished through the activity of the membrane sodium-potassium ATPase; thus loss of the ability to generate energy (e.g., in a cell injured by toxins or ischemia) will result in osmotic swelling and eventual rupture of cells. Similar transport mechanisms regulate intracellular and intraorganellar pH; most cytosolic enzymes have pH optima (and therefore work best) around pH 7.4, whereas lysosomal enzymes function best at pH 5 or less.

Receptor-Mediated and Fluid-Phase Uptake *(Fig. 1-6) (p. 9)*

Endocytosis allows the *import* of macromolecules >1000 daltons: Select molecules can be taken up by invaginations of the plasma membrane called *caveolae,* whereas others are internalized via *pinocytic vesicles* after binding to specific cell-surface receptors.

- *Caveolae-mediated endocytosis.* Caveolae ("little caves") are *non-coated* plasma membrane invaginations associated with GPI-linked molecules, cyclic adenosine monophosphate (cAMP) binding proteins, SRC-family kinases, and the folate receptor. Internalization of caveolae with any bound molecules and associated extracellular fluid is called *potocytosis*—literally "cellular sipping." Although caveolae deliver some molecules to the cytosol (e.g., folate), they also regulate transmembrane signaling and/or cellular adhesion by internalizing receptors and integrins.
- *Pinocytosis* ("cellular drinking") is a fluid-phase process in which the plasma membrane invaginates and is pinched off to form a cytoplasmic vesicle; endocytosed vesicles can recycle back to the plasma membrane for another round of ingestion. Pinocytosis

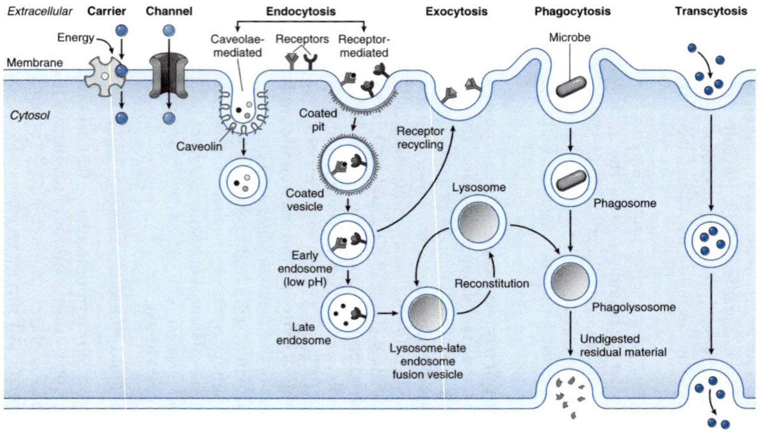

Figure 1-6 Movement of small molecules and larger structures across membranes. The lipid bilayer is relatively impermeable to all but the smallest and/or most hydrophobic molecules. Thus the import or export of charged species requires specific transmembrane transporter proteins; the internalization or externalization of large proteins, complex particles, or even cells requires encircling them with segments of the membrane. Small charged solutes can move across the membrane using either channels or carriers; in general each molecule requires a unique transporter. *Channels* are used when concentration gradients can drive the solute movement. *Carriers* are required when solute is moved *against* a concentration gradient. Receptor-mediated and fluid-phase uptake of material involves membrane-bound vacuoles. *Caveolae* endocytose extracellular fluid, membrane proteins, and some receptor-bound molecules (e.g., folate) in a process driven by caveolin proteins concentrated within lipid rafts *(potocytosis)*. *Pinocytosis* of extracellular fluid and most surface receptor-ligand pairs involves *clathrin-coated pits and vesicles.* After internalization the clathrin dissociates and can be reused, while the resulting vesicle progressively matures and acidifies. In the early and/or late endosome, ligand can be released from its receptor (e.g., iron released from transferrin bound to the transferrin receptor) with receptor recycling to the cell surface for another round. Alternatively, receptor and ligand within endosomes can be targeted to fuse with lysosomes (e.g., epidermal growth factor bound to its receptor); after complete degradation the late endosome-lysosome fusion vesicle can regenerate lysosomes. *Phagocytosis* involves the nonclathrin-mediated membrane invagination of large particles—typically by specialized phagocytes (e.g., macrophages or neutrophils). The resulting phagosomes eventually fuse with lysosomes to facilitate the degradation of the internalized material. *Transcytosis* involves the transcellular endocytotic transport of solute and/or bound ligand from one face of a cell to another. *Exocytosis* is the process by which membrane-bound vesicles fuse with the plasma membrane and discharge their contents to the extracellular space.

and receptor-mediated endocytosis (see later) begin at a specialized region of the plasma membrane called the *clathrin-coated pit,* which invaginates and pinches off to form a *clathrin-coated vesicle;* trapped within the vesicle is a gulp of the extracellular milieu and receptor-bound macromolecules (see later). The vesicles then uncoat and fuse with acidic intracellular structures called *early endosomes* where the contents can be partially digested before further passage to the lysosome.

- Receptor-mediated endocytosis is the major uptake mechanism for certain macromolecules (e.g., transferrin and low-density lipoprotein [LDL]). After binding to receptors localized in clathrin-coated pits, LDL and transferrin are endocytosed in vesicles. In acidic environments LDL and transferrin release their cargo (cholesterol and iron, respectively), which can be discharged into the cytoplasm. The LDL and transferrin receptors are resistant to the degradation, allowing them to be recycled back to the plasma membrane. Defects in receptor-mediated uptake or processing of LDL can be responsible for familial hypercholesterolemia (see Chapter 5).

Cellular *export* of large molecules from cells is called *exocytosis;* proteins synthesized and packaged within the RER and Golgi apparatus are concentrated in secretory vesicles, which then fuse with the plasma membrane to expel their contents. *Transcytosis* is the movement of endocytosed vesicles between the apical and basolateral compartments of cells; this allows transfer of large amounts of intact proteins across epithelial barriers (e.g., ingested antibodies in maternal milk across intestinal epithelia) or for the rapid movement of large volumes of solute.

Cytoskeleton and Cell-Cell Interactions (p. 10)

Cell shape, polarity, intracellular trafficking, and motility depend on intracellular cytoskeleton proteins (Fig. 1-7):

- *Actin microfilaments:* Five- to nine-nanometer-diameter fibrils formed from **g**lobular actin (**G**-actin), the most abundant cytosolic protein; G-actin monomers noncovalently polymerize into **f**ilaments (**F**-actin) forming double-stranded helices with defined polarity; new globular subunits are added (or lost) at the "positive" end of the strand. In nonmuscle cells, actin-binding proteins organize actin into bundles and networks that control cell shape and movement. In muscle cells, contraction occurs through ATP-driven *myosin* ratcheting along actin filaments.
- *Intermediate filaments:* Large and heterogeneous family of 10-nm-diameter fibrils, with characteristic cell- and tissue-specific patterns of expression.
  - *Lamin A, B, and C:* Nuclear lamina of all cells
  - *Vimentin:* Mesenchymal cells (fibroblasts, endothelium)
  - *Desmin:* Scaffold in muscle cells allowing actin and myosin contraction
  - *Neurofilaments:* Axons of neurons, imparting strength and rigidity
  - *Glial fibrillary acidic protein:* Glial cells around neurons
  - *Cytokeratins:* At least 30 distinct varieties, subdivided into acidic (type I) and neutral/basic (type II)

Intermediate filaments exist predominantly in a polymerized form and do not actively reorganize like actin; they are ropelike fibers that bear mechanical stress and form the major structural proteins of skin and hair. Nuclear lamins maintain nuclear morphology and regulate nuclear transcription.

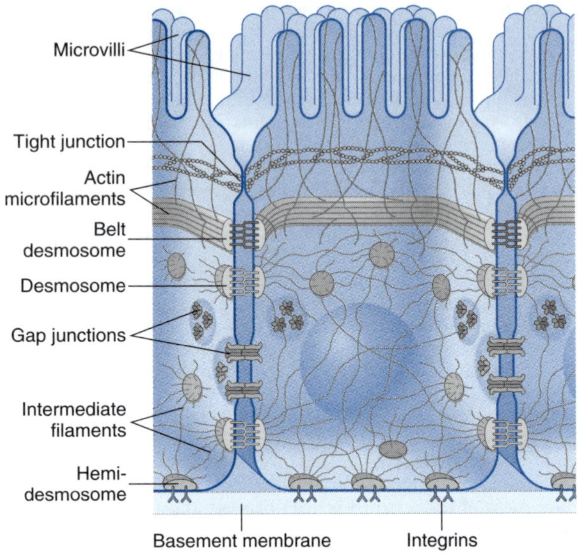

Figure 1-7 Cytoskeletal elements and cell-cell interactions. Interepithelial adhesion involves several different surface protein interactions, including through *tight junctions* and *desmosomes;* adhesion to the ECM involves cellular integrins (and associated proteins) within *hemidesmosomes.*

- *Microtubules:* Twenty-five-nanometer-thick fibrils composed of noncovalently polymerized dimers of α- and β-tubulin. Microtubules are dynamically changing hollow tubes with a defined polarity; the ends are designated "+" or "–"; the "–" end is embedded in a *microtubule-organizing center (MTOC, or centrosome)* near the nucleus associated with paired *centrioles,* whereas the "+" end elongates or recedes by adding or subtracting tubulin dimers. Microtubules are connecting cables that motor proteins "walk" along to move vesicles and organelles around cells: *kinesins* are motor proteins for anterograde (– to +) transport, whereas *dyneins* are for retrograde (+ to –) transport. Microtubules also participate in sister chromatid separation during mitosis and have been adapted to form motile cilia (e.g., in bronchial epithelium) or flagella (in sperm).

Cell-cell interactions (p. 11). Cells interact and communicate via junctional complexes (Fig. 1-7):

- *Occluding junctions (tight junctions)* seal adjacent cells together to create a continuous barrier that restricts the *paracellular* (between cells) movement of ions and other molecules. The junctions are formed from multiple transmembrane proteins, including *occludin, claudin, zonulin,* and *catenin.* In addition to a high-resistance barrier to solute movement, this zone is also the boundary between apical and basolateral domains of cells, helping to maintain cellular polarity. Tight junctions are dynamic structures that can dissociate and reform as required to facilitate epithelial proliferation or inflammatory cell migration.

- *Anchoring junctions (desmosomes)* mechanically attach cells—and their intracellular cytoskeletons—to other cells or to the ECM.
    - *Spot desmosomes (macula adherens)* are small, rivetlike adhesions between cells; similar rivetlike attachments to the ECM are called *hemidesmosomes,* whereas broad intercellular adhesion domains are called *belt desmosomes.*
    - Desmosomes are formed by homotypic association of transmembrane glycoproteins called *cadherins.* In spot desmosomes the cadherins are linked to intracellular intermediate filaments to distribute extracellular forces over multiple cells; in belt desmosomes the cadherins are associated with intracellular actin microfilaments, which can influence cell shape and motility.
    - In hemidesmosomes the transmembrane connector proteins are called *integrins;* these attach to intracellular intermediate filaments, and thus functionally link the cytoskeleton to the ECM.
    - *Focal adhesion complexes* are large (>100 proteins) macromolecular complexes that localize to hemidesmosomes and include proteins that can generate intracellular signals when cells are subjected to mechanical forces (e.g., endothelium in the bloodstream or cardiac myocytes in a failing heart).
- *Communicating junctions (gap junctions)* mediate the passage of chemical or electrical signals between cells. These junctions are dense planar arrays of 1.5- to 2-nm pores (called *connexons*) formed by hexamers of transmembrane proteins called *connexins.* The permeability of gap junctions is reduced by acidic pH or increased intracellular calcium. Gap junctions play a critical role in cell-cell communication; in cardiac myocytes, cell-to-cell calcium fluxes through gap junctions allow the myocardium to behave like a functional syncytium.

Biosynthetic Machinery: Endoplasmic Reticulum and Golgi (p. 12)

All cell constituents are constantly renewed and degraded, although every type of molecule has a distinct half-life.

- *Endoplasmic reticulum (ER).* Membrane proteins and lipids, as well as molecules destined for export, are all synthesized within the *ER.* The ER is composed of distinct domains, distinguished by the *presence* (RER) or *absence* (smooth ER or SER) of ribosomes (Fig. 1-5).
    - *RER:* Membrane-bound ribosomes of the RER translate mRNA into proteins that are extruded into the ER lumen or become integrated into the ER membrane; the process is directed through *signal sequences* on the N-termini of nascent proteins. If proteins lack a signal sequence, translation occurs on free ribosomes in the cytosol, and the vast majority of such proteins remain in the cytoplasm. Proteins inserted into the ER fold and can form polypeptide complexes *(oligomerize);* in addition, disulfide bonds are formed, and *N-linked oligosaccharides* (sugar moieties attached to asparagine residues) are added. *Chaperone molecules* retain proteins in the ER until these modifications are complete and the proper conformation is achieved. If a protein fails to appropriately fold or oligomerize, it is retained and degraded within the ER. Excess misfolded proteins—exceeding the capacity of the ER to edit and degrade them—leads to the *ER stress response* (also called the *unfolded protein response [UPR]*), which triggers cell death through *apoptosis* (see Chapter 2).

- *SER:* The SER in most cells is relatively sparse and primarily exists as the transition zone from RER to transport vesicles moving to the Golgi (see later discussion). However, in cells that synthesize steroid hormones (e.g., in the gonads or adrenals) or that catabolize lipid-soluble molecules (e.g., in the liver), the SER may be abundant. Indeed, repeated exposure to compounds that are metabolized by the SER (e.g., phenobarbital catabolism by the cytochrome P-450 system) can lead to a reactive SER hyperplasia. The SER also sequesters intracellular calcium; subsequent release from the SER into the cytosol can mediate a number of responses to extracellular signals (including apoptotic cell death). In muscle cells, specialized SER called *sarcoplasmic reticulum* is responsible for the cyclical release and sequestration of calcium ions that regulate muscle contraction and relaxation, respectively.

- *Golgi apparatus.* From the RER, proteins and lipids destined for other organelles or for extracellular export are shuttled into the *Golgi apparatus.* This organelle consists of stacked cisternae that progressively modify proteins in an orderly fashion from *cis* (near the ER) to *trans* (near the plasma membrane); macromolecules are shuttled between the various cisternae within membrane-bound vesicles. As molecules move from *cis* to *trans,* the *N-linked oligosaccharides* originally added to proteins in the ER are pruned and further modified in a step-wise fashion; *O-linked oligosaccharides* (sugar moieties linked to serine or threonine) are also appended. Some of this glycosylation is important in directing molecules to lysosomes (via the *mannose-6-phosphate [M6P] receptor*); other glycosylation adducts may be important for cell-cell or cell-matrix interactions or for clearing senescent cells. The *cis-Golgi network* recycles proteins back to the ER, whereas the *trans-Golgi network* sorts proteins and lipids and dispatches them to other organelles (including the plasma membrane) or to secretory vesicles destined for extracellular release.

Waste Disposal: Lysosomes and Proteasomes (p. 13)

Cellular constituent degradation involves lysosomes or proteasomes (Fig. 1-8).

- *Lysosomes* are membrane-bound organelles containing acid hydrolases, including proteases, nucleases, lipases, glycosidases, phosphatases, and sulfatases. Many of these are M6P-modified proteins, which are targeted to lysosomes via binding to M6P receptors on trans-Golgi vesicles. Other macromolecules destined for lysosomes arrive via three pathways (Fig. 1-8):
  - Material internalized by *fluid-phase pinocytosis* or *receptor-mediated endocytosis* passes through various endosomes en route to lysosomes. The early endosome is the first acidic compartment encountered, whereas proteolytic enzymes only begin significant digestion in the late endosome; late endosomes mature into lysosomes. During the maturation process the organelle becomes progressively more acidic.
  - Senescent organelles and large, denatured protein complexes enter lysosomes via *autophagy.* Obsolete organelles are encircled by a double membrane derived from the ER, forming an *autophagosome* that fuses with lysosomes. In addition to facilitating the turnover of aged and defunct structures, autophagy is also used to preserve cell viability during nutrient depletion (see Chapter 2).
  - *Phagocytosis* of microorganisms or large fragments of matrix or debris occurs primarily in professional phagocytes

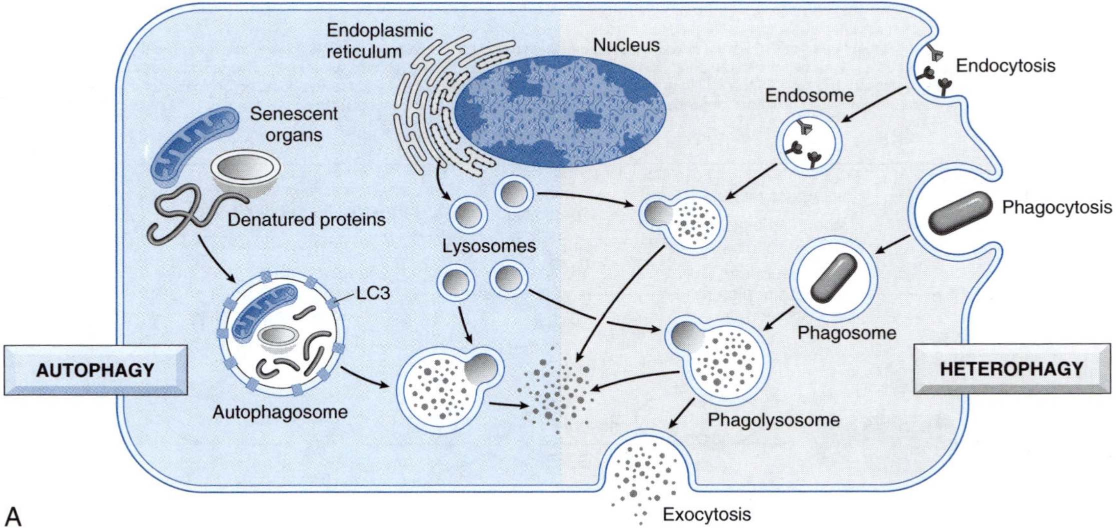

A

Figure 1-8 Intracellular catabolism. A, Lysosomal degradation. In *heterophagy* (right side), lysosomes fuse with endosomes or phagosomes to facilitate the degradation of their internalized contents (Fig. 1-6). The end products may be released into the cytosol for nutrition or discharged into the extracellular space *(exocytosis).* In *autophagy* (left side), senescent organelles or denatured proteins are targeted for lysosome-driven degradation by encircling them with a double membrane derived from the ER and marked by LC3 proteins (microtubule-associated protein 1A/1B-light chain 3). Cell stressors, such as nutrient depletion or certain intracellular infections, can also activate the autophagocytic pathway.

Continued

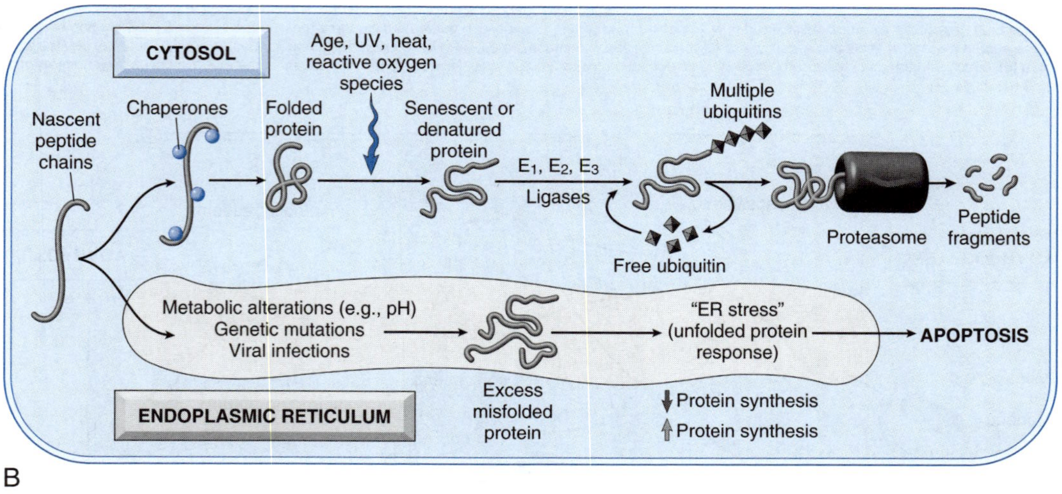

Figure 1-8, cont'd **B,** Proteasome degradation. Cytosolic proteins destined for turnover (e.g., transcription factors or regulatory proteins), senescent proteins, or proteins that have become denatured due to extrinsic mechanical or chemical stresses can be tagged by multiple ubiquitin molecules (through the activity of E_1, E_2, and E_3 ubiquitin ligases). This marks the proteins for degradation by proteasomes, cytosolic multisubunit complexes that degrade proteins to small peptide fragments. High levels of misfolded proteins within the ER trigger a protective *unfolded protein response*—engendering a broad reduction in protein synthesis, but specific increases in chaperone proteins that can facilitate protein refolding. If this is inadequate to cope with the levels of misfolded proteins, apoptosis is induced.

(macrophages or neutrophils). The material is engulfed to form a *phagosome* that subsequently fuses with lysosomes.

- *Proteasomes* are multisubunit protease complexes that degrade cytosolic proteins, including denatured or misfolded proteins, as well as other macromolecules whose lifespan must be regulated (e.g., transcription factors) (Fig. 1-8). Many proteins destined for proteasome destruction are covalently bound to a small protein called *ubiquitin;* polyubiquitinated proteins are then funneled into the proteasome "cylinder of death," where they are digested into small (6 to 12 amino acids) fragments that can further degrade to their constituent amino acids.

Cellular Metabolism and Mitochondrial Function (p. 14)

Mitochondria evolved from ancestral prokaryotes; that origin explains why mitochondria contain their own DNA (1% of total cellular DNA), encoding approximately 1% of total cellular proteins and one fifth of the proteins involved in *oxidative phosphorylation.* The mitochondrial translational machinery is similar to present-day bacteria; mitochondria initiate protein synthesis with *N*-formylmethionine and are sensitive to antibacterial antibiotics. The ovum contributes the vast majority of cytoplasmic organelles to the fertilized zygote; thus mitochondrial DNA is virtually entirely *maternally inherited.* Nevertheless, because the protein constituents of mitochondria derive from both nuclear and mitochondrial genes, mitochondrial disorders can be X-linked, autosomal, or maternally inherited. Mitochondria are constantly turning over, with half-lives ranging from 1 to 10 days.

Each mitochondrion has two separate membranes surrounding a core *matrix* containing most mitochondrial metabolic enzymes (e.g., those involved in the citric acid cycle). The inner membrane contains the enzymes of the respiratory chain folded into *cristae;* the *outer membrane* contains *porin* proteins that form aqueous channels permeable to small (<5000 daltons) molecules. Larger molecules (and even some smaller polar species) require specific transporters. Between these membranes is the *intermembrane space,* which is the site of ATP synthesis. Mitochondria have several roles (Fig. 1-9).

Energy Generation (p. 14)

Most cell energy derives from metabolism in mitochondria; substrates are oxidized to CO_2, transferring the high-energy electrons from the original molecule (e.g., sugar) to molecular oxygen and generating the low-energy electrons of water. The oxidation of various metabolites drives *proton pumps* that transfer H^+ from the core matrix into the intermembrane space. As the H^+ ions flow back down their electrochemical gradient, the energy released is used to synthesize ATP.

Electron transport does not always generate ATP. *Thermogenin,* an inner membrane protein present in high levels in certain tissues (e.g., brown fat), uncouples the process, generating heat instead of ATP. As a natural by-product of substrate oxidation and electron transport, mitochondria are also an important source of reactive oxygen species (e.g., oxygen free radicals, hydrogen peroxide); hypoxia, injury, or even mitochondrial aging can lead to significantly increased levels of intracellular oxidative stress.

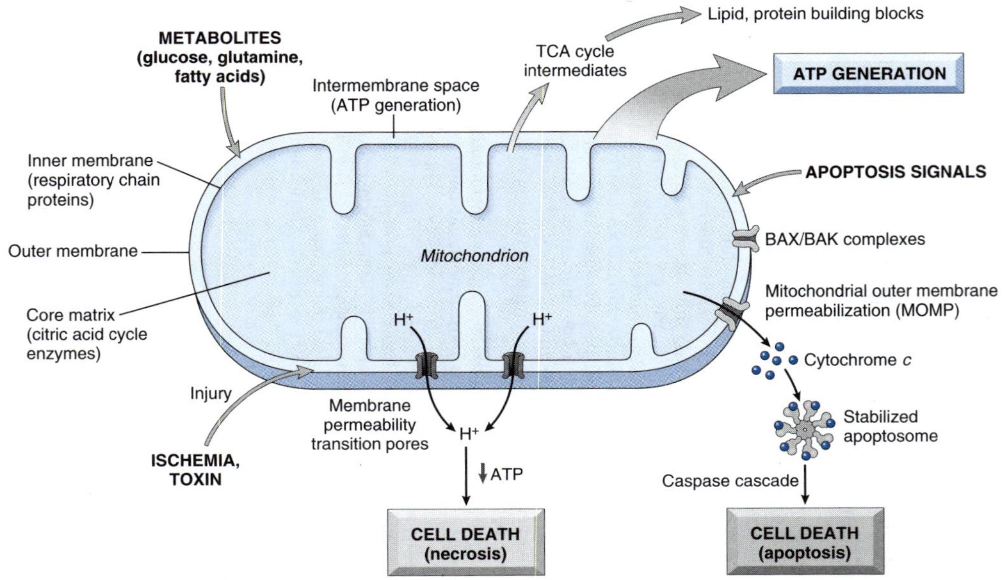

Figure 1-9 Roles of the mitochondria. In addition to the efficient generation of ATP from carbohydrate and fatty acid substrates, mitochondria have an important role in intermediary metabolism, serving as the source of molecules used to synthesize lipids and proteins, and are also centrally involved in cell death pathways.

Intermediate Metabolism (p. 14)

Oxidative phosphorylation produces abundant ATP, but also "burns" glucose to CO_2 and H_2O, leaving no carbon moieties suitable for synthesizing lipids and proteins. Thus rapidly growing cells (both benign and malignant) increase glucose and glutamine uptake and decrease their production of ATP per glucose molecule, a phenomenon called the *Warburg effect* (*aerobic glycolysis;* see Chapter 7). Instead of being used to make ATP, intermediates are "spun-off" to make lipids, nucleic acids, and proteins.

Cell Death (p. 15)

Mitochondria also regulate the balance of cell survival and death. There are two major pathways of cell death (see Chapter 2):

- *Necrosis:* External cellular injury (toxin, ischemia, trauma) can damage mitochondria, causing formation of *mitochondrial permeability transition pores* in the outer membrane that (1) dissipate the proton gradient, (2) prevent ATP generation, and (3) cause cell death.
- *Apoptosis:* Programmed cell death can be triggered by extrinsic signals (including cytotoxic T cells and inflammatory cytokines) or intrinsic pathways (including DNA damage and intracellular stress); mitochondria play a central role in the intrinsic pathway of apoptosis. If mitochondria are damaged or the cell cannot synthesize adequate amounts of survival proteins (because of deficient growth signals), mitochondria leak cytochrome *c* into the cytosol where it forms a complex with other proteins to activate caspases (see Chapter 2).

Cellular Activation (p. 15)

Cell communication controls a variety of functions, including activation, differentiation, and cell death. Loss of effective cellular communication can potentially lead to unregulated growth (cancer) or inappropriate response to stress (shock).

Cell Signaling (p. 15)

Cells can respond to the following extrinsic signals:

- *Pathogens and damage to neighboring cells.* In addition to microbes, cells can sense and respond to damaged cells *(danger signals);* see Chapters 3 and 6.
- *Contact with neighboring cells,* mediated through adhesion molecules and/or gap junctions—the latter through second messenger molecules, such as cAMP.
- *Contact with ECM,* mediated through integrins (see Chapter 3).
- *Secreted molecules,* for example, *growth factors* (see later discussion), *cytokines* (mediators of inflammation and immune responses; see Chapters 3 and 6), and *hormones* (see Chapter 24).

Cell-cell signaling pathways are classified as

- *Paracrine:* Only cells in the immediate vicinity are affected; signaling molecules have minimal diffusion and are rapidly degraded, taken up by other cells, or trapped in the ECM.
- *Autocrine:* When molecules secreted by a cell affect that same cell; this allows entraining groups of cells undergoing synchronous

differentiation (e.g., during development) or can be used to autoamplify or feedback inhibit a response.

- *Synaptic:* Neurons secrete *neurotransmitters* at specialized cell junctions *(synapses)* onto target cells.
- *Endocrine:* Mediator is released into the bloodstream and acts on target cells at a distance.

Signaling molecules *(ligands)* bind their respective receptors and initiate a cascade of intracellular events. Receptors typically have high affinities for their cognate ligands and at physiologic concentrations bind receptors with exquisite specificity. Receptors can be intracellular or on the cell surface (Fig. 1-10):

- *Intracellular receptors* are transcription factors activated by lipid-soluble ligands that readily cross plasma membranes. Such ligands include vitamin D and steroid hormones, which can bind and activate nuclear receptors to drive specific gene transcription. Signaling ligands can also diffuse into adjacent cells; thus nitric oxide produced in one cell (e.g., endothelium) diffuses into neighboring cells (e.g., medial smooth muscle cells) where it activates the enzyme guanylyl cyclase to generate cyclic guanosine monophosphate (GMP), an intracellular second signal for smooth muscle cell relaxation.
- *Cell-surface receptors* are generally transmembrane proteins with extracellular ligand-binding domains. Ligand binding can then (1) open ion channels (e.g., at the synapse between electrically excitable cells), (2) activate an associated guanosine triphosphate (GTP)-binding regulatory protein *(G protein)*, (3) activate an endogenous or associated enzyme, often a tyrosine kinase, or (4) trigger a proteolytic event or a change in protein binding or stability that activates a latent transcription factor.

Signal Transduction Pathways (p. 16)

Ligand binding to surface receptors mediates signaling by inducing clustering of the receptor *(receptor cross-linking)* or by other types of physical perturbations; these trigger intracellular biochemical changes, ultimately activating transcription factors that enter the nucleus to alter gene expression (Fig. 1-10):

- *Receptors associated with kinase activity.* Alterations in receptor geometry elicit intrinsic receptor *protein kinase* activity or promote the enzymatic activity of recruited intracellular kinases—resulting in the addition of charged phosphate residues to target molecules. *Tyrosine kinases* phosphorylate specific tyrosine residues, *serine/threonine kinases* add phosphates to distinct serine or threonine residues, and *lipid kinases* phosphorylate lipid substrates. For example, *receptor tyrosine kinases (RTKs)* are integral membrane proteins that—upon activation—have the capacity to phosphorylate tyrosine residues; these include receptors for insulin, epidermal growth factor, and platelet-derived growth factor. For every phosphorylation event, *phosphatases* exist to remove the phosphate residue and thus modulate signaling.
- Several receptors have no intrinsic catalytic activity (e.g., immune receptors, some cytokine receptors, and integrins). For these, separate intracellular proteins—*nonreceptor tyrosine kinases*—phosphorylate specific motifs on the receptor or other proteins. SRC is the prototype for these; it contains functional domains called *Src-homology 2* (SH2) and *Src-homology 3* (SH3). SH2 domains

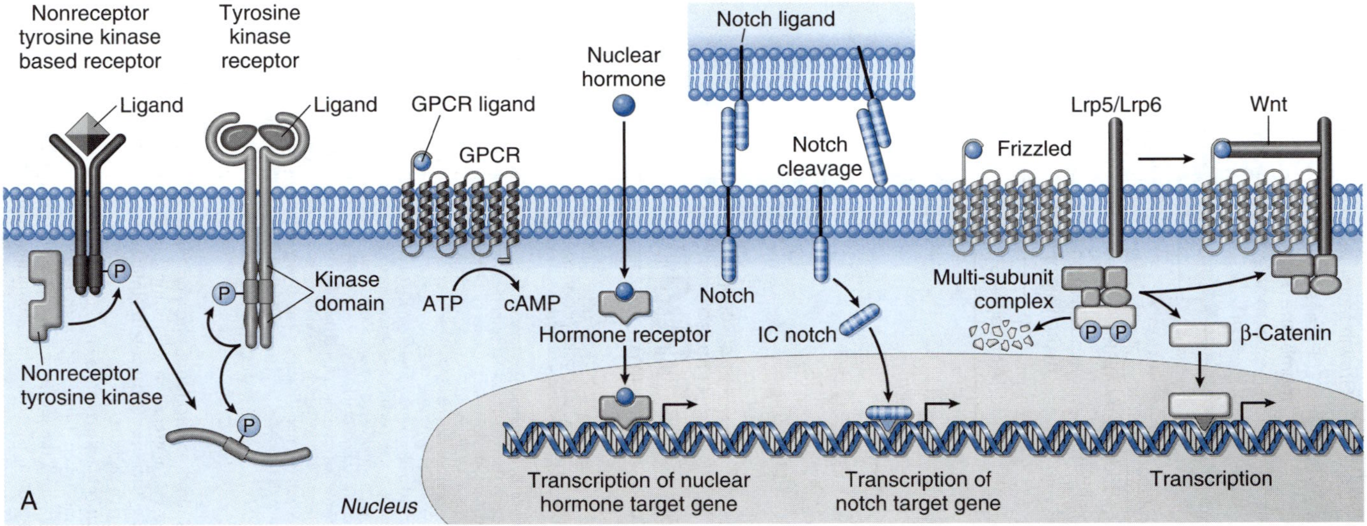

Figure 1-10 Receptor-mediated signaling. A, Categories of signaling receptors: receptors that use a nonreceptor tyrosine kinase; receptor tyrosine kinases; nuclear receptors that bind ligand and influence transcription; a seven-transmembrane receptor linked to heterotrimeric G proteins; *Notch,* which is cleaved yielding an intracellular fragment that enters the nucleus and influences target gene transcription; and Wnt/Frizzled pathway in which activation releases intracellular β-catenin from a protein complex that normally drives its constitutive degradation. The released β-catenin can then migrate to the nucleus and act as a transcription factor. Low-density lipoprotein receptor-related protein 5 (Lrp5) and Lrp6 are homologous coreceptors for Wnt/Frizzled signaling.

Continued

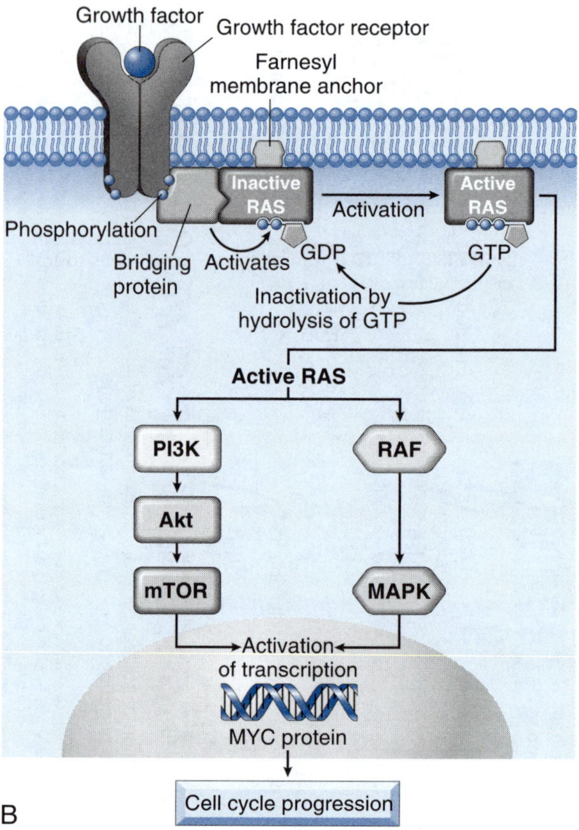

Figure 1-10, cont'd **B,** Signaling downstream of tyrosine kinase receptor-ligand interactions. Ligand binding causes receptor dimerization and autophosphorylation of tyrosine residues. Attachment of adapter (or bridging) proteins couples the receptor to inactive, GDP-bound RAS, allowing the GDP to be displaced in favor of GTP and yielding activated RAS. Activated RAS interacts with and activates RAF (also known as *MAP kinase kinase kinase*). This kinase then phosphorylates mitogen-activated protein kinase (MAPK); in turn, activated MAPK phosphorylates other cytoplasmic proteins and nuclear transcription factors, generating cellular responses. The phosphorylated tyrosine kinase receptor can also bind other components, such as phosphatidyl 3-kinase (PI3 kinase), which activates additional signaling systems. The cascade is turned off when the activated RAS eventually hydrolyzes GTP to GDP, converting RAS to its inactive form. Mutations in RAS that lead to delayed GTP hydrolysis can thus lead to augmented proliferative signaling. *GDP,* Guanosine diphosphate; *GTP,* guanosine triphosphate; *mTOR,* mammalian target of rapamycin.

typically bind to receptors phosphorylated by another kinase, allowing the aggregation of multiple enzymes. SH3 domains mediate other protein-protein interactions, often involving proline-rich regions.

- *G-protein coupled receptors* characteristically traverse the plasma membrane seven times *(seven-transmembrane receptors).* After ligand binding, the receptor associates with an intracellular GTP-binding protein *(G protein)* that contains guanosine diphosphate (GDP). Such G-protein interactions lead to their activation

through the exchange of GDP for GTP, with downstream generation of cAMP and inositol-1,4,5-triphosphate (IP3); the latter releases calcium from the ER.
- Ligand binding to *Notch receptors* leads to proteolytic cleavage of the receptor, with nuclear translocation of the cytoplasmic piece to form a transcription complex.
- *Wnt* protein ligands signal through transmembrane *Frizzled* family receptors to regulate intracellular β-catenin levels. Normally, β-catenin is degraded by proteasomes; however, Wnt binding to Frizzled (and other coreceptors) recruits *Disheveled* proteins that disrupt the degradation-targeting complex. The stabilized pool of β-catenin molecules then translocates to the nucleus to form a transcriptional complex.

Modular Signaling Proteins: Hubs and Nodes (p. 18)

The traditional *linear* view of signaling through an orderly sequence of biochemical intermediates is oversimplified. Any initial signal causes multiple diverging effects, each contributing in varying degrees to the final outcome. Thus even specific phosphorylation of a single protein can allow it to associate with multiple different molecules—with multiple consequences. *Adapter proteins* play a key role in organizing intracellular signaling pathways, functioning as molecular linkers to promote complex assembly. Signal transduction can therefore be visualized as a kind of networking phenomenon with protein-protein complexes forming *nodes* and the biochemical events feeding into or emanating from these nodes being *hubs* (so-called *systems biology*).

Transcription Factors (p. 18)

Most signal transduction pathways ultimately influence cellular function by modulating gene transcription. Conformational changes of transcription factors (e.g., following phosphorylation) can allow their translocation into the nucleus or can expose specific DNA or protein binding motifs. Transcription factors characteristically have distinct binding domains that allow them to bridge select DNA sequences with proteins, such as the RNA polymerase complex, histone-modifying enzymes, and chromatin-remodeling complexes. MYC and JUN are growth-inducing transcription factors, whereas p53 typically leads to growth arrest.

Growth Factors and Receptors (p. 18)

Growth factor activity is mediated through binding to specific receptors, leading to the expression of genes that

- Promote entry into the cell cycle
- Relieve blocks on cell cycle progression
- Prevent apoptosis
- Enhance biosynthesis of cellular constituents
- Drive a host of nongrowth activities, including migration, differentiation, and synthetic capacity

Growth factors are involved in the proliferation of cells at steady state as well as after injury to replace damaged cells. Many growth factor pathway genes are *proto-oncogenes;* uncontrolled proliferation can result when growth factor production is dysregulated or when growth factor signaling pathways become constitutively active. Table 1-1 summarizes selected growth factors; although all these bind to receptors with intrinsic kinase activity, other growth factors can signal through any of the pathways shown in Figure 1-10.

TABLE 1-1 Growth Factors Involved in Regeneration and Repair

Growth Factor	Sources	Functions
Epidermal growth factor (EGF)	Activated macrophages, salivary glands, keratinocytes, and many other cells	Mitogenic for keratinocytes and fibroblasts; stimulates keratinocyte migration; stimulates formation of granulation tissue
Transforming growth factor-α (TGF-α)	Activated macrophages, keratinocytes, many other cell types	Stimulates proliferation of hepatocytes and many other epithelial cells
Hepatocyte growth factor (HGF) (scatter factor)	Fibroblasts, stromal cells in the liver, endothelial cells	Enhances proliferation of hepatocytes and other epithelial cells; increases cell motility
Vascular endothelial growth factor (VEGF)	Mesenchymal cells	Stimulates proliferation of endothelial cells; increases vascular permeability
Platelet-derived growth factor (PDGF)	Platelets, macrophages, endothelial cells, smooth muscle cells, keratinocytes	Chemotactic for neutrophils, macrophages, fibroblasts, and smooth muscle cells; activates and stimulates proliferation of fibroblasts, endothelial, and other cells; stimulates ECM protein synthesis
Fibroblast growth factors (FGFs), including acidic (FGF-1) and basic (FGF-2)	Macrophages, mast cells, endothelial cells, many other cell types	Chemotactic and mitogenic for fibroblasts; stimulates angiogenesis and ECM protein synthesis
Transforming growth factor-β (TGF-β)	Platelets, T lymphocytes, macrophages, endothelial cells, keratinocytes, smooth muscle cells, fibroblasts	Chemotactic for leukocytes and fibroblasts; stimulates ECM protein synthesis; suppresses acute inflammation
Keratinocyte growth factor (KGF) (i.e., FGF-7)	Fibroblasts	Stimulates keratinocyte migration, proliferation, and differentiation

ECM, Extracellular matrix.

Epidermal growth factor (EGF) and transforming growth factor (TGF)-α (p. 19). These both bind to the same receptors, explaining why they share many biologic activities; they are produced by macrophages and epithelial cells and are mitogenic for multiple cell types. The EGF receptor family includes four membrane receptors with intrinsic tyrosine kinase activity. EGFR1 (ERBB1) mutations and/or amplification occur frequently in lung, head and neck, breast, and brain tumors. The ERBB2 receptor (also known as *HER2*) is overexpressed in a subset of breast cancers.

Hepatocyte growth factor (HGF) (p. 19) has mitogenic effects on hepatocytes and most epithelial cells. HGF acts as a *morphogen* in embryonic development (i.e., it influences the pattern of tissue differentiation), promotes cell migration, and enhances hepatocyte survival. HGF is produced by fibroblasts and most mesenchymal cells, endothelium, and nonhepatocyte liver cells. It is synthesized as an inactive precursor (pro-HGF) that is proteolytically activated by serine proteases released at sites of injury. MET is the receptor for HGF; it has intrinsic tyrosine kinase activity and is frequently overexpressed or mutated in tumors, particularly renal and thyroid papillary carcinomas.

Platelet-derived growth factor (PDGF) (p. 19) represents a family of closely related dimeric proteins. Although originally isolated from platelets (hence the name), it is also produced by activated macrophages, endothelium, smooth muscle cells, and a variety of tumors. All PDGF isoforms exert their effects by binding to two cell-surface receptors (PDGFR α and β), both having intrinsic tyrosine kinase activity. PDGF induces fibroblast, endothelial, and smooth muscle cell chemotaxis, proliferation, and matrix synthesis.

Vascular endothelial growth factor (VEGF) (p. 20) comprises a family of homodimeric proteins. VEGF-A is generally referred to simply as VEGF; it is the major *angiogenic* factor after injury and in tumors. VEGF-B and placental growth factor are involved in embryonic vessel development, and VEGF-C and -D stimulate both angiogenesis and lymphatic development *(lymphangiogenesis)*. VEGFs are also involved in the *maintenance* of normal adult endothelium, with the highest expression in epithelial cells adjacent to fenestrated epithelium (e.g., podocytes in the kidney, pigment epithelium in the retina, and choroid plexus in the brain). VEGF induces angiogenesis by promoting endothelial cell migration, proliferation (capillary sprouting), and formation of the vascular lumen; it also induces increased vascular permeability. Hypoxia is the most important inducer of VEGF production (mediated through intracellular hypoxia-inducible factor), in addition to PDGF and TGF-α produced at sites of inflammation or wound healing.

VEGFs bind to a family of RTKs; VEGFR-2 is highly expressed in endothelium and is the most important for angiogenesis. Anti-VEGF antibodies are used to limit angiogenesis in certain malignancies, "wet" age-related macular degeneration, and the retinopathy of prematurity. Anti-VEGF also reduces the leakiness of vessels that causes diabetic macular edema. Increased levels of soluble versions of VEGFR-1 (s-FLT-1) in pregnant women can cause *preeclampsia* (hypertension and proteinuria) by "sopping up" the free VEGF required to maintain normal endothelium.

Fibroblast growth factor (FGF) (p. 20) is a family of >20 growth factors; they associate with heparan sulfate in the ECM, serving as a reservoir for inactive factors that can be released through proteolysis (e.g., at sites of wound healing). FGFs contribute to wound healing responses, hematopoiesis, and development; basic FGF has all the activities necessary for angiogenesis.

Transforming growth factor-β (TGF-β) (p. 20) has three isoforms (β1-β3), each belonging to a family of approximately 30 members that includes bone morphogenetic proteins (BMPs), activins, inhibins, and müllerian inhibiting substance. TGF-β1 (more commonly referred to as TGF-β) has the most widespread distribution; it is a homodimeric protein produced by multiple cell types as a precursor that requires proteolysis to yield the biologically active protein. There are two TGF-β receptors, both with serine/threonine kinase activity that phosphorylate downstream *Smad* transcription factors. TGF-β has multiple and often opposing effects (called *pleiotropic*) depending on the target tissue and concurrent signals. However, primarily TGF-β drives scar formation and applies brakes on the inflammation that accompanies wound healing.

Interaction With the Extracellular Matrix (p. 20)

ECM is a network of interstitial proteins; it is constantly remodeled, with synthesis and degradation accompanying morphogenesis, tissue regeneration and repair, chronic fibrosis, and tumor invasion and metastasis. Cell interactions with ECM are critical for development and healing, as well as for maintaining normal tissue architecture (Fig. 1-11):

- *Mechanical support:* Allowing cell anchorage, cell migration, and maintenance of cell polarity.
- *Control of cell proliferation:* ECM binds growth factors that can be released/activated by proteolysis; ECM can also signal through cell integrins.
- *Scaffolding for tissue renewal:* Integrity of the basement membrane and the stroma of parenchymal cells is critical for the organized regeneration of tissues.
- *Establishment of tissue microenvironments:* Basement membrane is not just a passive support between epithelium and connective tissue; it can also have functionality (e.g., forming part of the filtration apparatus in the kidney).

ECM occurs in two basic forms: interstitial matrix and basement membrane (Fig. 1-12).

- *Interstitial matrix* is synthesized by mesenchymal cells (e.g., fibroblasts); it is present in the spaces between cells in connective tissue and between parenchymal epithelium and the underlying support structures. Its major constituents are fibrillar and nonfibrillar

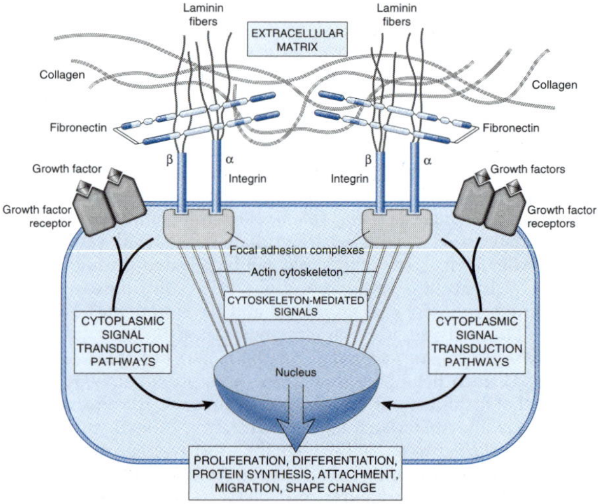

Figure 1-11 Interactions of ECM and growth factor–mediated cell signaling. Cell surface integrins interact with the cytoskeleton at focal adhesion complexes (protein aggregates that include vinculin, α-actinin, and talin). This can initiate the production of intracellular messengers or can directly transduce signals to the nucleus. Cell-surface receptors for growth factors can activate signal transduction pathways that overlap with those mediated through integrins. Signals from ECM components and growth factors can be integrated by the cells to produce a given response, including changes in proliferation, locomotion, and/or differentiation.

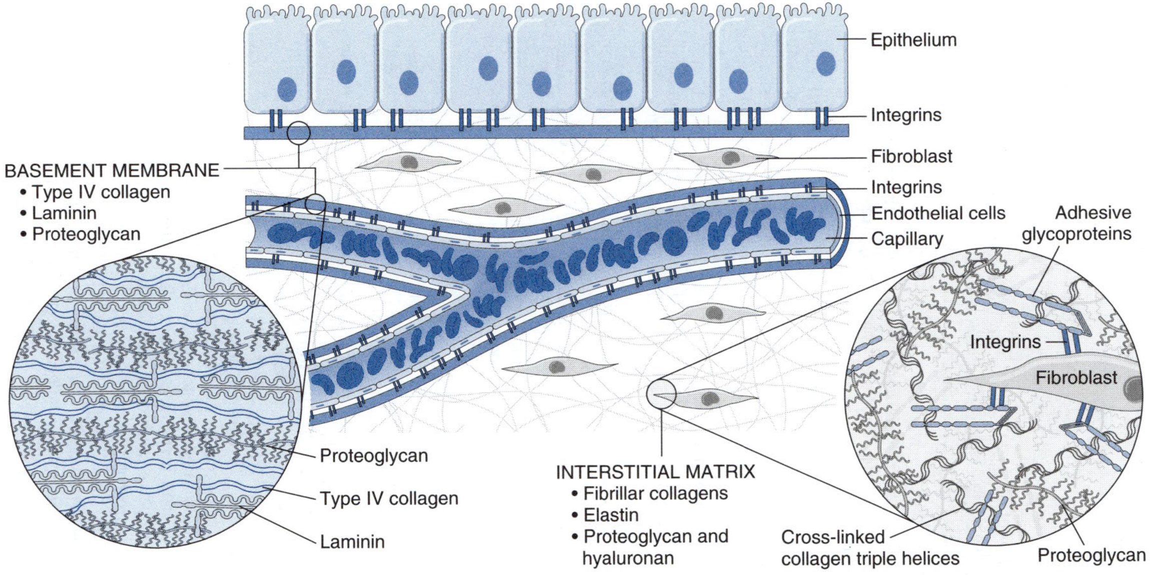

Figure 1-12 Main components of the ECM, including collagens, proteoglycans, and adhesive glycoproteins. Both epithelial and mesenchymal cells (e.g., fibroblasts) interact with ECM via integrins. Basement membranes and interstitial ECM have different architecture and general composition, although certain components are present in both. For the sake of clarity, many ECM components (e.g., elastin, fibrillin, hyaluronan, and syndecan) are not included.

collagens, as well as fibronectin, elastin, proteoglycans, and hyaluronate.
- *Basement membrane* is synthesized from the overlying epithelium and underlying mesenchymal cells, forming a planar mesh (although labeled as a *membrane,* it is quite porous). The major constituents are amorphous nonfibrillar type IV collagen and laminin.

Components of the ECM (p. 21) fall into three groups of proteins:

- *Fibrous structural proteins,* such as collagens and elastins, that confer tensile strength and recoil
- *Water-hydrated gels,* such as proteoglycans and hyaluronan, that permit compressive resistance and lubrication
- *Adhesive glycoproteins* that connect ECM elements to cells and each other

Collagens (p. 23) are composed of three separate polypeptide chains braided into a ropelike triple helix; approximately 30 collagen types have been identified.

- *Fibrillar collagens:* Some collagen types (e.g., types I, II, III, and V) form linear fibrils stabilized by interchain hydrogen bonding; these form a major proportion of the connective tissue in structures such as bone, tendon, cartilage, blood vessels, and skin, as well as in healing wounds and particularly scars. The tensile strength of the fibrillar collagens derives from lateral cross-linking of the triple helices, formed by covalent bonds facilitated by the activity of lysyl oxidase (vitamin C is a necessary cofactor).
- *Nonfibrillar collagens:* These contribute to the structures of planar basement membranes (type IV collagen), help to regulate collagen fibril diameters or collagen-collagen interactions via so-called **f**ibril-**a**ssociated **c**ollagen with **i**nterrupted **t**riple helices (FACITs, such as type IX collagen in cartilage), or provide anchoring fibrils to basement membrane beneath stratified squamous epithelium (type VII collagen).

Elastin (p. 23) allows tissues to recoil and recover their shape after physical deformation; this is especially important in cardiac valves and for large blood vessels (to accommodate pulsatile flow), as well as in the uterus, skin, and ligaments.

Proteoglycans and hyaluronan (p. 23). Proteoglycans form highly hydrated gels that resist compressive forces; in joint cartilage, proteoglycans also provide a layer of lubrication between adjacent bony surfaces. Proteoglycans consist of long polysaccharides called *glycosaminoglycans (GAGs)* attached to a core protein; these are then linked to a long hyaluronic acid polymer called *hyaluronan,* in a manner reminiscent of the bristles on a test tube brush. The negatively charged sulfated sugars of the GAGs attract cations (mostly sodium) that in turn osmotically attract water; the result is a viscous, gelatin-like matrix. In addition to providing compressibility to tissues, proteoglycans also serve as reservoirs for growth factors secreted into the ECM (e.g., FGF and HGF).

Adhesive glycoproteins and adhesion receptors (p. 24) are structurally diverse molecules involved in cell-cell adhesion, cell-ECM, and ECM-ECM interactions (Fig. 1-13). These include:

- *Fibronectin.* A large disulfide-linked heterodimer that exists in tissue and plasma forms; it is synthesized by a variety of cells. Fibronectin has specific domains that can bind to different ECM components (e.g., collagen, fibrin, heparin, and proteoglycans), as well as integrins (Fig. 1-13). In healing wounds, tissue and

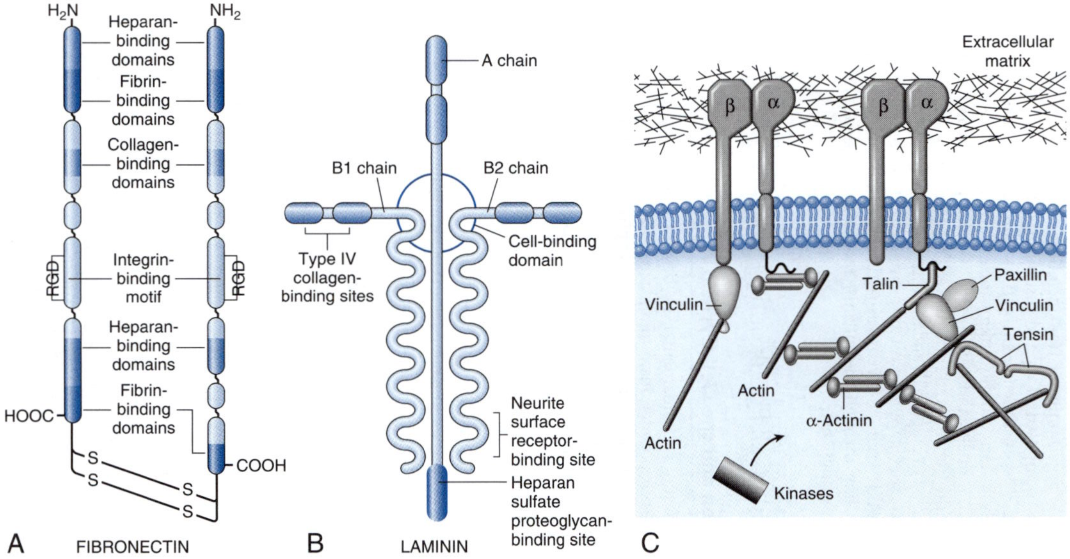

Figure 1-13 Cell and ECM interactions: adhesive glycoproteins and integrin signaling. A, *Fibronectin* consists of a disulfide-linked dimer, with several distinct domains that allow binding to ECM and to integrins, the latter through arginine-glycine-aspartic acid (RGD) motifs. **B,** The cross-shaped *laminin* molecule is one of the major components of basement membranes; its multidomain structure allows interactions between type IV collagen, other ECM components, and cell-surface receptors. **C,** Integrins and integrin-mediated signaling events at focal adhesion complexes. Each α-β heterodimeric integrin receptor is a transmembrane dimer that links ECM and intracellular cytoskeleton. It is also associated with a complex of linking molecules (e.g., vinculin, and talin) that can recruit and activate kinases that ultimately trigger downstream signaling cascades.

plasma fibronectin provide the scaffolding for subsequent ECM deposition, angiogenesis, and re-epithelialization.

- *Laminin.* The most abundant glycoprotein in basement membrane, it is a cross-shaped heterotrimer that connects cells to underlying ECM components such as type IV collagen and heparan sulfate (Fig. 1-13); it can also modulate cell proliferation, differentiation, and motility.
- *Integrins.* A large family of transmembrane heterodimeric glycoproteins (composed of α- and β-subunits) that allow cells to attach to ECM constituents, such as laminin and fibronectin—functionally and structurally linking the intracellular cytoskeleton with the ECM. Integrins on the surface of leukocytes mediate firm adhesion and transmigration across endothelium at sites of inflammation (see Chapter 3), and they play a critical role in platelet aggregation (see Chapter 4). Integrins attach to ECM components via a tripeptide arginine-glycine-aspartic acid motif (abbreviated RGD); binding through the integrin receptors can also trigger signaling cascades (Fig. 1-13).

Maintaining Cell Populations (p. 25)

Proliferation and the Cell Cycle (p. 25)

Cell proliferation is fundamental to development, maintaining steady-state tissue populations, and replacing dead or damaged cells. The key elements that occur during cell cycle proliferation are:

- Accurate DNA replication
- Coordinated synthesis of all other cellular constituents (e.g., organelles)
- Equal apportionment of DNA and other cellular constituents to daughter cells

The cell cycle consists of (Fig. 1-14):

- G_1 (presynthetic *growth*)
- S (DNA *synthesis*)
- G_2 (premitotic *growth*)
- M *(mitotic)* phases

Quiescent cells that are not actively cycling are in the G_0 state; cells can enter G_1 either from the G_0 quiescent cell pool or after completing a round of mitosis (e.g., for continuously replicating cells). Each stage requires completion of the previous step, as well as activation of necessary factors (see later); nonfidelity of DNA replication or cofactor deficiency results in arrest at one of the transition points.

The cell cycle is regulated by activators and inhibitors; progression through the cell cycle is driven by the following (Fig. 1-15):

- Proteins called *cyclins*—named for the cyclic nature of their production and degradation
- Cyclin-associated enzymes called *cyclin-dependent kinases* (CDKs)

CDKs acquire kinase activity (i.e., the ability to phosphorylate protein substrates) by forming complexes with the relevant cyclins. Transiently increased synthesis of a particular cyclin leads to increased kinase activity of its CDK binding partner; as the CDK completes its round of phosphorylation, the associated cyclin is degraded and the CDK activity abates. Thus as cyclin levels rise and fall, the activity of associated CDKs likewise waxes and wanes. Cyclins D, E, A, and B appear sequentially during the cell cycle and bind to one or more CDKs.

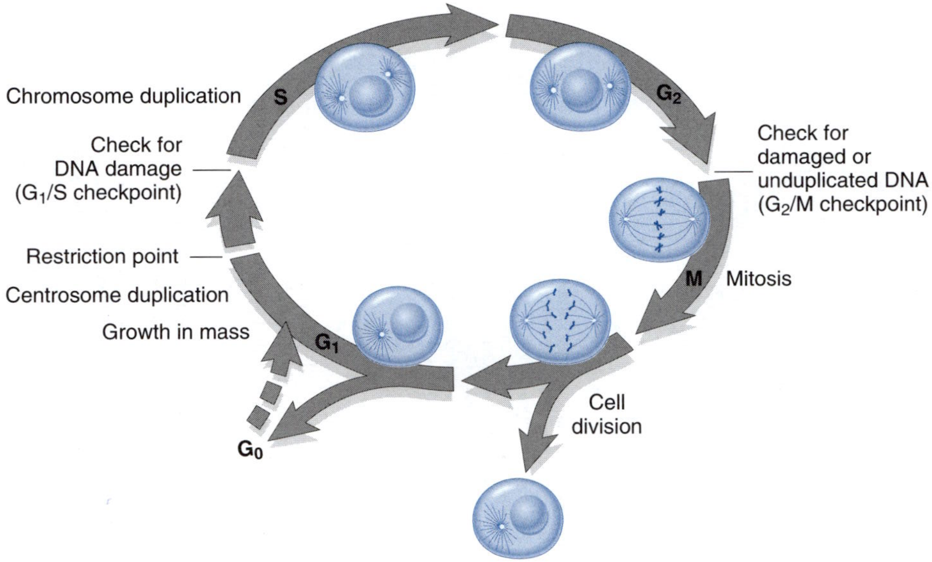

Figure 1-14 Cell cycle showing phases (G_0, G_1, G_2, S, and M), the location of the G_1 restriction point, and the G_1/S and G_2/M cell cycle checkpoints. Cells from labile tissues, such as the epidermis and the gastrointestinal (GI) tract, may cycle continuously; stable cells, such as hepatocytes, are quiescent but can enter the cell cycle; permanent cells, such as neurons and cardiac myocytes, have lost the capacity to proliferate. *(Modified from Pollard TD, Earnshaw WC:* Cell Biology. *Philadelphia, Saunders, 2002.)*

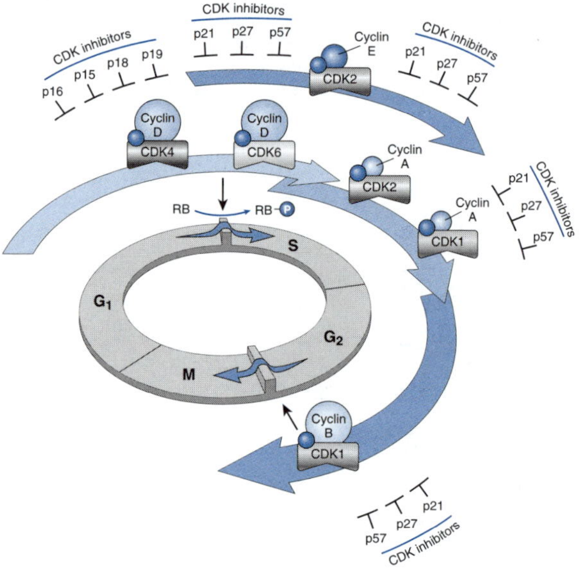

Figure 1-15 Role of cyclins, CDKs, and CDK inhibitors in regulating the cell cycle. The *shaded arrows* represent the phases of the cell cycle during which specific cyclin-CDK complexes are active. As illustrated, cyclin D-CDK4, cyclin D-CDK6, and cyclin E-CDK2 regulate the G_1-to-S transition by phosphorylating the Rb protein (pRb). Cyclin A-CDK2 and cyclin A-CDK1 are active in the S phase. Cyclin B-CDK1 is essential for the G_2-to-M transition. Two families of CDK inhibitors can block activity of CDKs and progression through the cell cycle. The so-called INK4 inhibitors, composed of p16, p15, p18, and p19, act on cyclin D-CDK4 and cyclin D-CDK6. The other family of three inhibitors, p21, p27, and p57, can inhibit all CDKs.

Throughout the cell cycle, surveillance mechanisms assess for DNA damage. These quality controls act at *checkpoints* to ensure that cells with genetic defects do not complete replication.

- The G_1-S checkpoint monitors the integrity of DNA before irreversibly committing cellular resources to DNA replication.
- The G_2-M restriction point ensures that there has been accurate genetic replication before the cell actually divides.

When cells do detect DNA imperfections, checkpoint activation delays cell cycle progression and triggers DNA repair mechanisms. If the genetic derangement is too severe to be repaired, the cells will undergo apoptosis; alternatively, cells can enter a nonreplicative state called *senescence*—primarily through p53-dependent mechanisms (see later).

Enforcing the cell cycle checkpoints is the job of *CDK inhibitors (CDKIs)*; they accomplish this by modulating CDK-cyclin complex activity. There are several different CDKIs:

- One family—composed of three proteins called *p21* (CDKN1A), *p27* (CDKN1B), and *p57* (CDKN1C)—broadly inhibits multiple CDKs.
- The other family of CDKI proteins has selective effects on cyclin CDK4 and cyclin CDK6; these proteins are called *p15* (CDKN2B), *p16* (CDKN2A), *p18* (CDKN2C), and *p19* (CDKN2D).

Defective CDKI checkpoint proteins allow cells with damaged DNA to divide, resulting in mutated daughter cells capable of developing into malignant tumors.

Stem Cells (p. 26)

- During development, *stem cells* give rise to the various differentiated tissues.
- In the adult organism, stem cells replace damaged cells and maintain tissue populations.
- *Stem cells are characterized by two important properties:*
  - *Self-renewal,* which permits stem cells to maintain their numbers.
  - *Asymmetric division,* in which one daughter cell enters a differentiation pathway and gives rise to mature cells, while the other remains undifferentiated and retains its self-renewal capacity.
- There are fundamentally just two varieties of stem cells:
  - *Embryonic stem cells (ES cells)* are the most undifferentiated. Derived from the blastocyst inner cell mass, they have virtually limitless cell renewal capacity and are *totipotent* (i.e., can give rise to every cell in the body) (Fig. 1-16).
  - *Tissue stem cells* (also called *adult stem cells*) have a limited repertoire of differentiation; they can usually only produce cells that are normal constituents of the particular tissue they are found in. Adult stem cells are usually protected within specialized tissue microenvironments called *stem cell niches;* other cells and soluble factors within the niches keep the stem cells quiescent until there is a need for expansion/differentiation.

Hematopoietic stem cells are the best characterized; they continuously replenish all the cellular elements of the blood. Although rare, they can be purified based on cell surface markers and can be used to repopulate marrows depleted after chemotherapy (e.g., for leukemia) or to provide normal precursors to correct various blood cell defects (e.g., sickle cell disease).

The bone marrow (and other tissues such as fat) also contains a population of *mesenchymal stem cells*—multipotent cells that can differentiate into a variety of stromal cells, including chondrocytes (cartilage), osteocytes (bone), adipocytes (fat), and myocytes (muscle).

- *Induced pluripotent stem cells (iPS cells)* can be created in the laboratory by introducing a relative handful of genes into somatic cells (e.g., skin fibroblasts). These genes reprogram the cells to achieve the "stemness" of ES cells, and the resulting iPS cells can then be differentiated into multiple lineages. Researchers also have the capacity to "edit" genetic defects in cells using a Cas9 nuclease and CRISPR guide RNAs. In this way it is hoped that host cells can be rewired and used to replace defective or degenerated tissues—opening up the field of *regenerative medicine* (p. 28).

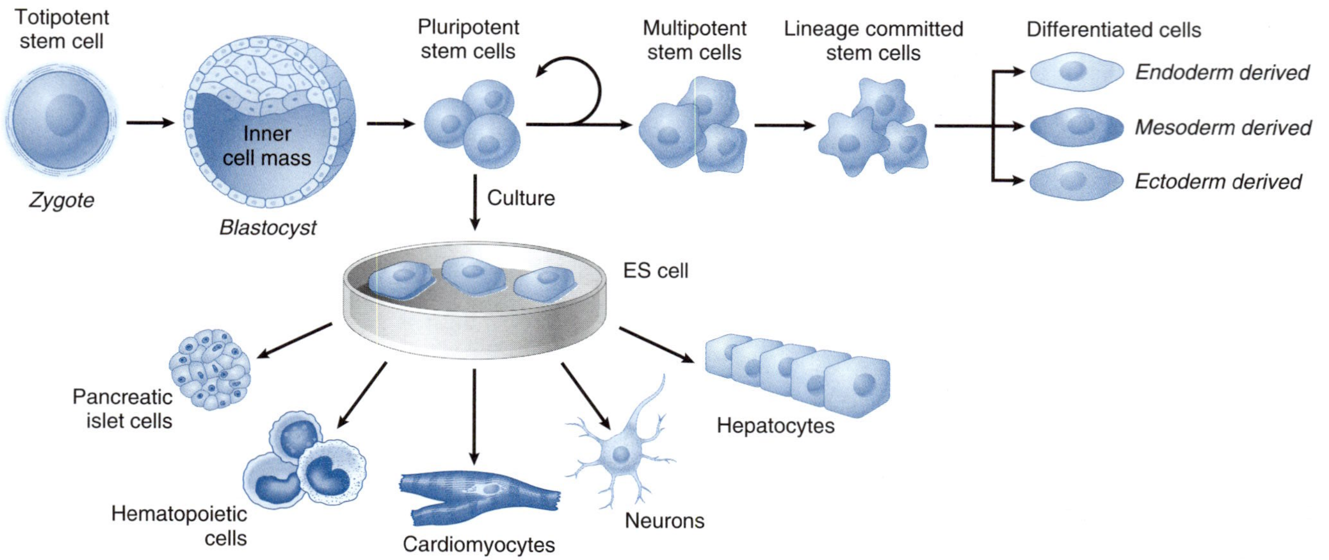

Figure 1-16 Embryonal stem cells. The zygote, formed by the union of sperm and egg, divides to form blastocysts, and the inner cell mass of the blastocyst generates the embryo. The pluripotent cells of the inner cell mass, known as embryonic stem (ES) cells, can be induced to differentiate into cells of multiple lineages. In the embryo, pluripotent stem cells can asymmetrically divide to yield a residual stable pool of ES cells in addition to generating populations that have progressively more restricted developmental capacity, eventually generating stem cells that are committed to just specific lineages. ES cells can be cultured in vitro and be induced to give rise to cells of all three lineages.

Cellular Responses to Stress and Toxic Insults: Adaptation, Injury, and Death

2

Introduction (p. 31)

Pathology is the study of the structural and functional causes of human disease. The four aspects of a disease process that form the core of pathology are as follows:

- The cause of a disease *(etiology)*
- The mechanism(s) of disease development *(pathogenesis)*
- The structural alterations induced in cells and tissues by the disease *(morphologic change)*
- The functional consequences of the morphologic changes *(clinical significance)*

Overview (p. 32)

Normal cell function requires a balance between physiologic demands and the constraints of cell structure and metabolic capacity; the result is a steady state, or *homeostasis.* Cells can alter their functional state in response to modest stress to maintain the steady state. More excessive physiologic stresses, or adverse pathologic stimuli *(injury),* result in (1) adaptation, (2) reversible injury, or (3) irreversible injury and cell death (Fig. 2-1, Table 2-1). These responses may be considered a continuum of progressive impairment of cell structure and function.

- *Adaptation* occurs when physiologic or pathologic stressors induce a new state that changes the cell but otherwise preserves its viability in the face of the exogenous stimuli. These changes include the following:
    - *Hypertrophy* represents increased cell size (p. 34) often in response to increased workload. Induced by growth factors produced in response to mechanical stress or other stimuli; will increase overall organ size as well.
    - *Hyperplasia* is increased cell number (p. 35) often secondary to hormones and other growth factors. Occurs in tissues whose cells are able to divide or contain abundant tissue stem cells.
    - *Atrophy* represents decreased cell size (p. 36); this will also diminish the overall organ size. Can occur secondary to disuse or decreased nutrient supply and is associated with decreased synthesis of cellular building blocks and/or increased breakdown of cellular organelles, involving proteasome degradation or *autophagy.*
    - *Metaplasia* is change from one mature cell type to another (p. 37), often secondary to chronic inflammation. This occurs through an altered differentiation pathway of tissue stem cells and can adversely affect tissue function and/or predispose to malignant transformation.

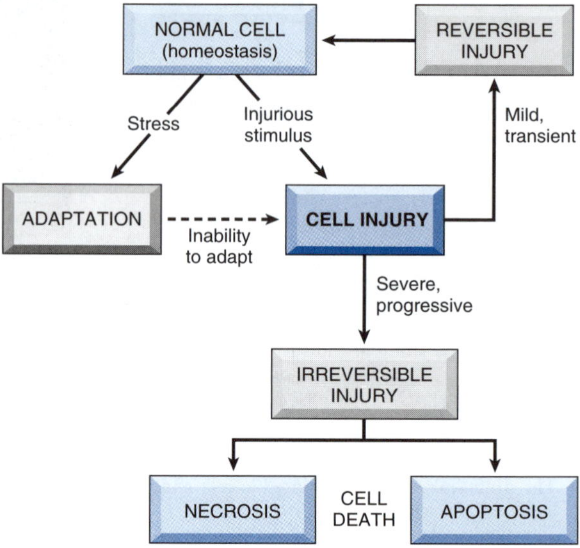

Figure 2-1 Stages of the cellular response to stress and injurious stimuli.

TABLE 2-1 Cellular Responses to Injury

Nature of Injurious Stimulus	Cellular Response
Altered physiologic stimuli; some nonlethal, injurious stimuli	**Cellular adaptations**
Increased demand, increased stimulation (e.g., by growth factors, hormones)	Hyperplasia, hypertrophy
Decreased nutrients, decreased stimulation	Atrophy
Chronic irritation (physical or chemical)	Metaplasia
Reduced oxygen supply; chemical injury; microbial infection	**Cell injury**
Acute and transient	Acute reversible injury, cellular swelling, fatty change Irreversible injury → cell death Necrosis Apoptosis
Metabolic alterations, genetic or acquired; chronic injury	**Intracellular accumulations; calcification**
Cumulative, sublethal injury over long life span	**Cellular aging**

- *Reversible injury* denotes pathologic cell changes that can be restored to normalcy if the stimulus is removed or if the cause of injury is mild.
- *Irreversible injury* occurs when stressors exceed the capacity of the cell to adapt (beyond a *point of no return*) and denotes permanent pathologic changes that cause cell death.
- *Cell death* occurs primarily through two morphologic and mechanistic patterns, *necrosis* and *apoptosis* (Table 2-2). Although necrosis

TABLE 2-2 Features of Necrosis and Apoptosis

Feature	Necrosis	Apoptosis
Cell size	Enlarged (swelling)	Reduced (shrinkage)
Nucleus	Pyknosis → karyorrhexis → karyolysis	Fragmentation into nucleosome-size fragments
Plasma membrane	Disrupted	Intact; altered structure, especially orientation of lipids
Cellular contents	Enzymatic digestion; may leak out of cell	Intact; may be released in apoptotic bodies
Adjacent inflammation	Frequent	No
Physiologic or pathologic role	Invariable pathologic (culmination of irreversible cell injury)	Often physiologic, means of eliminating unwanted cells; may be pathologic after some forms of cell injury, especially DNA damage

always represents a pathologic process, apoptosis may also serve a number of normal functions (e.g., in embryogenesis) and is not necessarily associated with cell injury.

- *Necrosis* is the more common type of cell death, involving severe cell swelling, denaturation and coagulation of proteins, breakdown of cellular organelles, and cell rupture. Usually a large number of cells in the adjoining tissue are affected, and an inflammatory infiltrate is recruited.
- *Apoptosis* occurs when a cell dies by activation of an internal "suicide" program, involving an orchestrated disassembly of cellular components; there is minimal disruption of the surrounding tissue, and there is minimal if any inflammation. Morphologically there is chromatin condensation and fragmentation.

The mechanistic distinction between necrosis and apoptosis is also blurring; in some cases necrosis is also regulated by a series of signaling pathways—a form of programmed cell death called *necroptosis.*

Causes of Cell Injury (p. 39)

- *Oxygen deprivation (hypoxia)* affects aerobic respiration and therefore ability to generate adenosine triphosphate (ATP). This extremely important and common cause of cell injury and death occurs as a result of the following:
  - *Ischemia* (loss of blood supply)
  - Inadequate oxygenation (e.g., cardiorespiratory failure)
  - Loss of oxygen-carrying capacity of the blood (e.g., anemia, carbon monoxide poisoning)
- *Physical agents,* including trauma, heat, cold, radiation, and electric shock (see Chapter 9)
- *Chemical agents and drugs,* including therapeutic drugs, poisons, environmental pollutants, and "social stimuli" (alcohol and narcotics)
- *Infectious agents,* including viruses, bacteria, fungi, and parasites (see Chapter 8)

- *Immunologic reactions,* including autoimmune diseases (see Chapter 6) and cell injury following responses to infection (see Chapter 3)
- *Genetic derangements,* such as chromosomal alterations and specific gene mutations (see Chapter 5)
- *Nutritional imbalances,* including protein-calorie deficiency or lack of specific vitamins, as well as nutritional excesses (see Chapter 9)

Morphologic Alterations in Cell Injury (p. 40)

Injury leads to loss of cell function long before damage is morphologically recognizable. Morphologic changes become apparent only sometime after a critical biochemical system within the cell has been deranged; the interval between injury and morphologic change depends on the method of detection (Fig. 2-2). However, once developed, reversible injury and irreversible injury *(necrosis)* both have characteristic features.

Reversible Injury (p. 40)

- *Cell swelling* appears whenever cells cannot maintain ionic and fluid homeostasis (largely due to loss of activity in plasma membrane, energy-dependent ion pumps).
- *Fatty change* is manifested by cytoplasmic lipid vacuoles, principally encountered in cells involved in or dependent on fat metabolism (e.g., hepatocytes and myocardial cells).

Necrosis (p. 41)

Necrosis is the sum of the morphologic changes that follow cell death in living tissue or organs. Two processes underlie the basic morphologic changes:

- Denaturation of proteins
- Enzymatic digestion of organelles and other cytosolic components

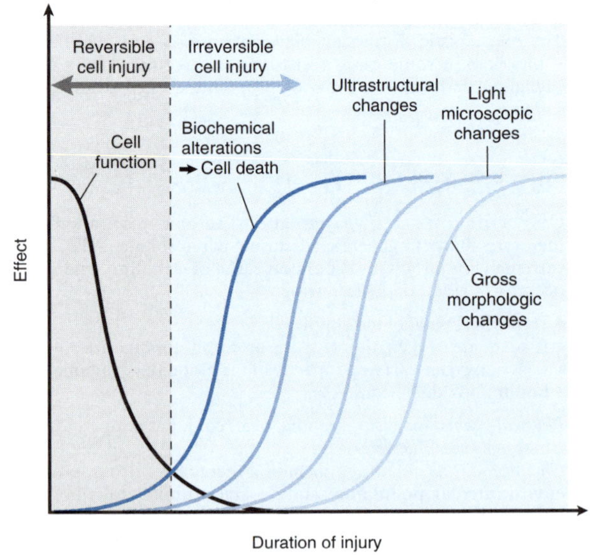

Figure 2-2 Timing of biochemical and morphologic changes in cell injury.

There are several distinctive features: necrotic cells are more *eosinophilic* (pink) than viable cells by standard hematoxylin and eosin (H&E) staining. They appear "glassy," owing to glycogen loss, and may be vacuolated; cell membranes are fragmented. Necrotic cells may attract calcium salts; this is particularly true of necrotic fat cells (forming fatty soaps). Nuclear changes include *pyknosis* (small, dense nucleus), *karyolysis* (faint, dissolved nucleus), and *karyorrhexis* (fragmented nucleus). General tissue patterns of necrosis include the following:

- *Coagulative necrosis* (p. 43) is the most common pattern, predominated by protein denaturation with preservation of the cell and tissue framework. This pattern is characteristic of hypoxic death in all tissues except the brain. Necrotic tissue undergoes either *heterolysis* (digestion by lysosomal enzymes of invading leukocytes) or *autolysis* (digestion by its own lysosomal enzymes).
- *Liquefactive necrosis* (p. 43) occurs when autolysis or heterolysis predominates over protein denaturation. The necrotic area is soft and filled with fluid. This type of necrosis is most frequently seen in localized bacterial infections *(abscesses)* and in the brain.
- *Gangrenous necrosis* (p. 43) is not a specific pattern but is rather just coagulative necrosis as applied to an ischemic limb; superimposed bacterial infection makes for a more liquefactive pattern called *wet gangrene.*
- *Caseous necrosis* (p. 43) is characteristic of tuberculous lesions; it appears grossly as soft, friable, "cheesy" material and microscopically as amorphous eosinophilic material with cell debris.
- *Fat necrosis* (p. 43) is seen in adipose tissue; lipase activation (e.g., from injured pancreatic cells or macrophages) releases fatty acids from triglycerides, which then complex with calcium to create soaps. Grossly these are white, chalky areas *(fat saponification);* histologically there are vague cell outlines and calcium deposition.
- *Fibrinoid necrosis* (p. 44 and Chapter 6) is a pathologic pattern due to antigen-antibody *(immune complex)* deposition in blood vessels. Microscopically there is bright pink amorphous material (protein deposition) in arterial walls, often with associated inflammation and thrombosis.

Mechanisms of Cell Injury (p. 44)

The biochemical pathways in cell injury can be organized around a few general principles:

- Responses to injurious stimuli depend on the type of injury, duration, and severity.
- The consequences of injury depend on the type, state, and adaptability of the injured cell.
- Cell injury results from perturbations in any of five essential cellular elements:
    - ATP production (mostly through effects on mitochondrial *aerobic respiration*)
    - Mitochondrial integrity independent of ATP production
    - Plasma membrane integrity, responsible for ionic and osmotic homeostasis
    - Protein synthesis, folding, degradation, and refolding
    - Integrity of the genetic apparatus

The intracellular mechanisms of cell injury fall into one of six general pathways (Fig. 2-3). Structural and biochemical elements of the cell are so closely interrelated that regardless of the locus of initial injury, secondary effects rapidly propagate through other elements.

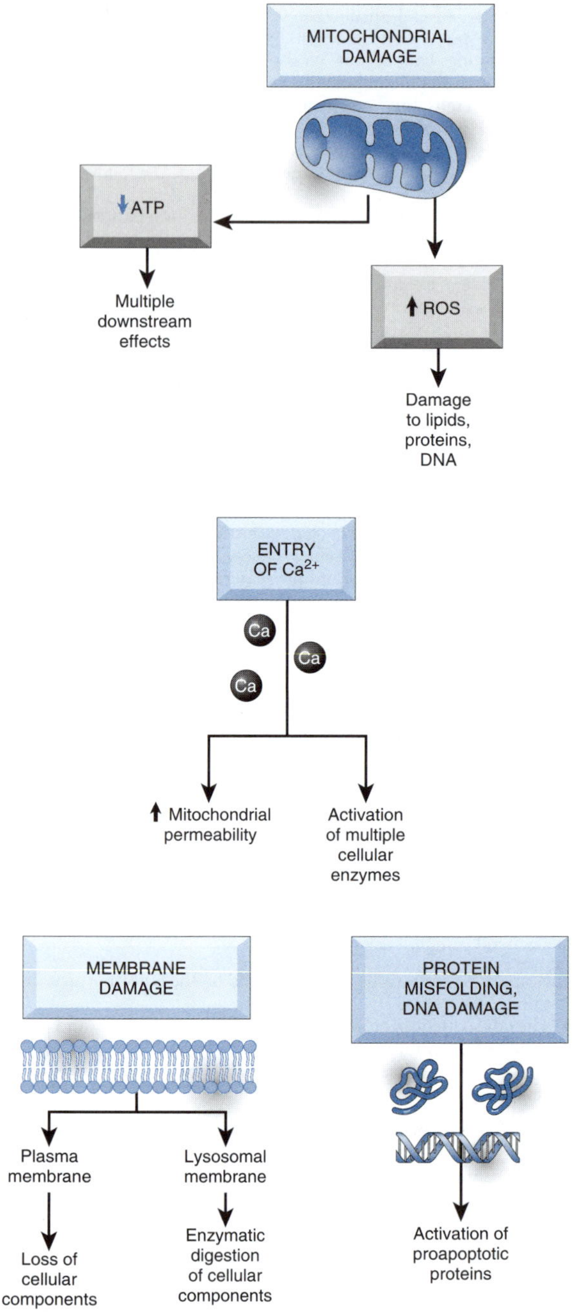

Figure 2-3 Cellular and biochemical sites of damage in cell injury.

Depletion of Adenosine Triphosphate (p. 45)

Decreased ATP synthesis and ATP depletion are common consequences of both ischemic and toxic injury. ATP is generated through glycolysis (anaerobic, inefficient) and oxidative phosphorylation in the mitochondria (aerobic, efficient). Hypoxia will lead to increased anaerobic glycolysis with glycogen depletion, increased lactic acid production, and intracellular acidosis. ATP is critical for membrane transport, maintenance of ionic gradients (particularly Na^+, K^+, and Ca^{2+}), and protein synthesis; reduced ATP synthesis will dramatically impact those pathways.

Mitochondrial Damage (p. 46)

Mitochondrial damage can occur directly due to hypoxia or toxins or as a consequence of increased cytosolic Ca^{2+}, oxidative stress, or phospholipid breakdown. Damage results in formation of a high-conductance channel *(mitochondrial permeability transition pore)* that leaks protons and dissipates the electromotive potential that drives oxidative phosphorylation. Damaged mitochondria also leak cytochrome *c,* which can trigger apoptosis (see later discussion).

Influx of Intracellular Calcium and Loss of Calcium Homeostasis (p. 46)

Cytosolic calcium is maintained at extremely low levels by energy-dependent transport; ischemia and toxins can cause Ca^{2+} influx across the plasma membrane and release of Ca^{2+} from mitochondria and endoplasmic reticulum (ER). Increased cytosolic calcium activates phospholipases that degrade membrane phospholipids; proteases that break down membrane and cytoskeletal proteins; ATPases that hasten ATP depletion; and endonucleases that cause chromatin fragmentation.

Accumulation of Oxygen-Derived Free Radicals (Oxidative Stress) (p. 47)

Free radicals are unstable, partially reduced molecules with unpaired electrons in outer orbitals that make them particularly reactive with other molecules. Although other elements can have free radical forms, oxygen-derived free radicals (also called *reactive oxygen species [ROS]*) are the most common in biologic systems. The major forms are *superoxide anion* ($O_2^{\bar{\cdot}}$, one extra electron), *hydrogen peroxide* (H_2O_2, two extra electrons), *hydroxyl ions* ($OH^{\cdot}$, three extra electrons), and *peroxynitrate ion* ($ONOO^-$; formed by interactions of nitric oxide and $O_2^{\bar{\cdot}}$).

Free radicals readily propagate additional free radical formation with other molecules in an autocatalytic chain reaction that often breaks chemical bonds. Thus free radicals damage lipids (peroxidizing double bonds and causing chain breakage), proteins (oxidizing and fragmenting peptide bonds), and nucleic acids (causing single strand breaks).

Free radical generation occurs by

- Normal metabolic processes, such as the reduction of oxygen to water during respiration; the sequential addition of four electrons leads to small numbers of ROS intermediates.
- Absorption of radiant energy; ionizing radiation (e.g., ultraviolet light and x-rays) can hydrolyze water into hydroxyl ($OH^{\cdot}$) and hydrogen ($H^{\cdot}$) free radicals.
- Production by leukocytes during inflammation to sterilize sites of infection (see Chapter 3).

- Enzymatic metabolism of exogenous chemicals or drugs (e.g., acetaminophen).
- *Transition metals* (e.g., iron and copper) can catalyze free radical formation.
- *Nitric oxide (NO)*, an important chemical mediator (see Chapter 3), can act directly as a free radical or be converted to other highly reactive forms.

Fortunately free radicals are *inherently unstable and generally decay spontaneously.* In addition, several systems contribute to free radical inactivation:

- Antioxidants either block the initiation of free radical formation or scavenge free radicals; these include vitamins E and A, ascorbic acid, and glutathione.
- The levels of transition metals that can participate in free radical formation are minimized by binding to storage and transport proteins (e.g., *transferrin, ferritin, lactoferrin,* and *ceruloplasmin*).
- Free radical scavenging *enzyme* systems catabolize hydrogen peroxide *(catalase, glutathione peroxidase)* and superoxide anion *(superoxide dismutase).*

Defects in Membrane Permeability (p. 49)

- Membranes can be damaged directly by toxins, physical and chemical agents, lytic complement components, and perforins or indirectly as described by the preceding events (e.g., ROS, Ca^{2+} activation of phospholipases). Increased plasma membrane permeability affects intracellular osmolarity as well as enzymatic activity; increased mitochondrial membrane permeability reduces ATP synthesis and can drive apoptosis; altered lysosomal integrity unleashes extremely potent acid hydrolases that can digest proteins, nucleic acids, lipids, and glycogen.

Damage to DNA and Proteins (p. 50)

Damage to DNA that exceeds normal repair capacity (e.g., due to ROS, radiation, or drugs) leads to activation of apoptosis. Similarly, accumulation of large amounts of improperly folded proteins (e.g., due to ROS or heritable mutations) leads to a stress response that also triggers apoptotic pathways.

Within limits, all the changes of cell injury described earlier can be offset, and cells can return to normal after injury abates *(reversible injury)*. However, persistent or excessive injury causes cells to pass a threshold into *irreversible injury* associated with extensive cell membrane damage, lysosomal swelling, and mitochondrial vacuolization with deficient ATP synthesis. Extracellular calcium enters the cell, and intracellular calcium stores are released, leading to activation of enzymes that catabolize membranes, proteins, ATP, and nucleic acids. Proteins, essential coenzymes, and ribonucleic acids are lost from hyperpermeable plasma membranes, and cells leak metabolites vital for the reconstitution of ATP.

The transition from reversible to irreversible injury is difficult to identify, although two phenomena consistently characterize irreversibility:

- *Inability to reverse mitochondrial dysfunction* (lack of ATP generation) even after resolution of the original injury
- Development of profound disturbances in membrane function

Leakage of intracellular enzymes or proteins across abnormally permeable plasma membranes into the bloodstream provides important clinical markers of cell death. Cardiac muscle contains a specific isoform of the enzyme creatine kinase and of the contractile protein troponin; hepatocytes contain transaminases, and hepatic bile duct epithelium contains a temperature-resistant isoform of alkaline phosphatase. Irreversible injury in these tissues is consequently reflected by increased circulating levels of such proteins in the blood.

Examples of Cell Injury and Necrosis (p. 50)

Ischemic and Hypoxic Injury (p. 50)

Ischemia and hypoxic injury are the most common forms of cell injury in clinical medicine. *Hypoxia* is reduced oxygen-carrying capacity; *ischemia* (which also clearly causes hypoxia) is due to reduced blood flow. Hypoxia alone allows continued delivery of substrates for glycolysis and removal of accumulated wastes (e.g., lactic acid); ischemia does neither and therefore tends to injure tissues faster than hypoxia alone.

Hypoxia leads to loss of ATP generation by mitochondria; ATP depletion has multiple, initially **reversible** effects (Fig. 2-4):

- Failure of Na^+/K^+-ATPase membrane transport causes sodium to enter the cell and potassium to exit; there is also increased Ca^{2+} influx as well as release of Ca^{2+} from intracellular stores. The net gain of solute is accompanied by isosmotic gain of water, *cell swelling*, and ER dilation. Cell swelling is also increased owing to the *osmotic load* from accumulation of metabolic breakdown products.
- *Cellular energy metabolism* is altered. With hypoxia, cells use *anaerobic glycolysis* for energy production (metabolism of glucose derived from glycogen). Consequently, *glycogen stores are rapidly depleted*, with lactic acid accumulation and *reduced intracellular pH.*
- Reduced protein synthesis results from detachment of ribosomes from rough ER.

All the aforementioned changes are reversible if oxygenation is restored. If ischemia persists, **irreversible** injury ensues, a transition largely dependent on the extent of *ATP depletion* and *membrane dysfunction,* particularly mitochondrial membranes.

- ATP depletion induces the pore transition change in the mitochondrial membrane; pore formation results in reduced membrane potential and diffusion of solutes.
- ATP depletion also *releases cytochrome c,* a soluble component of the electron transport chain that is a key regulator in driving apoptosis (see later discussion).
- Increased cytosolic calcium activates membrane phospholipases, leading to progressive loss of phospholipids and membrane damage; decreased ATP also leads to diminished phospholipid synthesis.
- Increased cytosolic calcium *activates intracellular proteases,* causing degradation of intermediate cytoskeletal elements, rendering the cell membrane susceptible to stretching and rupture, particularly in the setting of cell swelling.
- Free fatty acids and lysophospholipids accumulate in ischemic cells as a result of phospholipid degradation; these are directly toxic to membranes.

Ischemia-Reperfusion Injury (p. 51)

Restoration of blood flow to ischemic tissues can result in recovery of reversibly injured cells or may not affect the outcome if irreversible damage has occurred. However, depending on the intensity and duration of the ischemic insult, additional cells may die *after* blood flow resumes, involving either necrosis or apoptosis. The process is characteristically associated with neutrophilic infiltrates. The additional damage is designated *reperfusion injury* and is clinically

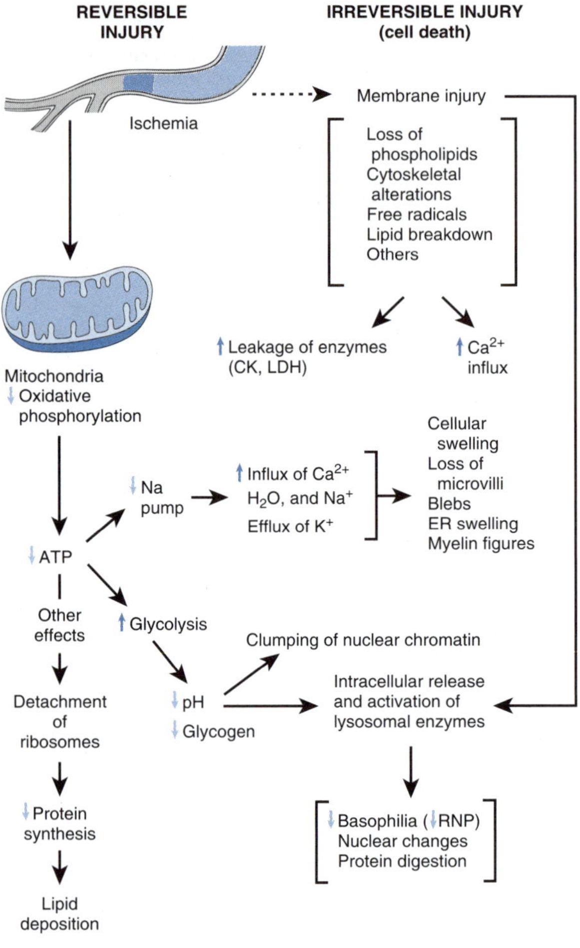

Figure 2-4 Sequence of events in reversible and irreversible ischemic cell injury. Although reduced ATP levels play a central role, ischemia can also cause direct membrane damage. *CK,* Creatine kinase; *ER,* endoplasmic reticulum; *LDH,* lactate dehydrogenase; *RNP,* ribonucleoprotein.

important in myocardial infarction, acute renal failure, and stroke. Several mechanisms potentially underlie reperfusion injury:

- *Oxidative stress:* New damage may occur during reoxygenation by increased generation of ROS from parenchymal and endothelial cells and from infiltrating leukocytes. Superoxide anions produced in reperfused tissue result from incomplete reduction of oxygen by damaged mitochondria or because of the normal action of oxidases from tissue cells or invading inflammatory cells. Antioxidant defense mechanisms may also be compromised, favoring radical accumulation.
- *Intracellular calcium overload:* This occurs due to cell membrane damage and ROS-mediated injury to sarcoplasmic reticulum. Calcium overload drives mitochondrial permeability transition pore opening and subsequent ATP depletion.

- *Inflammation:* Ischemic injury recruits circulating inflammatory cells (see Chapter 3) through enhanced cytokine and adhesion molecule expression by hypoxic parenchymal and endothelial cells. The ensuing inflammation causes additional injury. By restoring blood flow, reperfusion may actually *increase* local inflammatory cell infiltration.
- *Complement activation* (see Chapter 6): Immunoglobulin M (IgM) antibodies can deposit in ischemic tissues; when blood flow is resumed, complement proteins are activated by binding to the antibodies, resulting in further cell injury and inflammation.

Chemical (Toxic) Injury (p. 51)

Chemical injury occurs by two general mechanisms:

- *Directly,* by binding to some critical molecular component (e.g., mercuric chloride binds to cell membrane protein sulfhydryl groups, inhibiting ATPase-dependent transport, and causing increased permeability).
- *Indirectly,* by conversion to reactive toxic metabolites. Toxic metabolites, in turn, cause cellular injury either by direct covalent binding to membrane protein and lipids or more commonly by the formation of reactive free radicals. Two examples are carbon tetrachloride and acetaminophen.

Apoptosis (p. 52)

Programmed cell death *(apoptosis)* occurs when a cell dies through activation of a tightly regulated internal suicide program. The function of apoptosis is to eliminate unwanted cells selectively, with minimal disturbance to surrounding cells and the host. The cell's plasma membrane remains intact, but its structure is altered so that the apoptotic cell fragments and becomes an avid target for phagocytosis. The dead cell is rapidly cleared before its contents have leaked out, and therefore cell death by this pathway does not elicit an inflammatory reaction in the host. Thus apoptosis is fundamentally different from necrosis, which is characterized by loss of membrane integrity, enzymatic digestion of cells, and frequently a host reaction (Table 2-2). Nevertheless, apoptosis and necrosis sometimes coexist, and they may share some common features and mechanisms.

Causes of Apoptosis (p. 52)

Apoptosis can be physiologic or pathologic.

Physiologic Causes *(p. 52)*

- Programmed destruction of cells during embryogenesis
- Hormone-dependent involution of tissues (e.g., endometrium, prostate) in the adult
- Cell deletion in proliferating cell populations (e.g., intestinal epithelium) to maintain a constant cell number
- Death of cells that have served their useful purpose (e.g., neutrophils following an acute inflammatory response)
- Deletion of potentially harmful self-reactive lymphocytes

Pathologic Causes *(p. 53)*

- DNA damage (e.g., due to hypoxia, radiation, or cytotoxic drugs). If repair mechanisms cannot cope with the damage caused, cells will undergo apoptosis rather than risk mutations that could result in malignant transformation. Relatively mild injury may induce apoptosis, whereas larger doses of the same stimuli result in necrosis.

- Accumulation of misfolded proteins (e.g., due to inherited defects or due to free radical damage). This may be the basis of cell loss in a number of neurodegenerative disorders.
- Cell death in certain viral infections (e.g., hepatitis), either caused directly by the infection or by cytotoxic T cells.
- Cytotoxic T cells may also be a cause of apoptotic cell death in tumors and in the rejection of transplanted tissues.
- Pathologic atrophy in parenchymal organs after duct obstruction (e.g., pancreas).

Morphologic and Biochemical Changes in Apoptosis (p. 53)

Morphologic features of apoptosis (Table 2-2) include cell shrinkage, chromatin condensation and fragmentation, cellular blebbing and fragmentation into apoptotic bodies, and phagocytosis of apoptotic bodies by adjacent healthy cells or macrophages. Lack of inflammation makes it difficult to detect apoptosis histologically.

- Protein breakdown occurs through a family of proteases called *caspases* (so-named because they have an active site ***c***ysteine and cleave at ***asp***artate residues).
- Internucleosomal cleavage of DNA into fragments 180 to 200 base pairs in size gives rise to a characteristic ladder pattern of DNA bands on agarose gel electrophoresis.
- Plasma membrane alterations (e.g., flipping of phosphatidylserine from the inner to the outer leaf of the plasma membrane) allow recognition of apoptotic cells for phagocytosis.

Mechanisms of Apoptosis (p. 53) (Fig. 2-5)

Apoptosis is a cascade of molecular events that can be initiated by a variety of triggers. The process of apoptosis is divided into an *initiation phase,* when caspases become active, and an *execution phase,* when the enzymes cause cell death. Initiation of apoptosis occurs through two distinct but convergent pathways: the *intrinsic* mitochondrial pathway, and the *extrinsic* death receptor-mediated pathway.

Intrinsic (Mitochondrial) Pathway (p. 53) (Fig. 2-6)

When mitochondrial permeability is increased, *cytochrome c,* as well as other proapoptotic molecules are released into the cytoplasm; death receptors are not involved. Mitochondrial permeability is regulated by more than 20 proteins of the Bcl family.

- *Antiapoptotic.* Bcl-2 and Bcl-x are the two predominant *antiapoptotic proteins* responsible for reducing mitochondrial leakiness.
- *Proapoptotic.* The two principal proapoptotic proteins are Bax and Bak; these form oligomers that insert into the mitochondrial membrane and create permeability channels.
- *Sensors.* Cellular stressors (e.g., misfolded proteins, DNA damage) or loss of survival signals is sensed by other Bcl members (e.g., Bim, Bid, and Bad); these, in turn, regulate the activity of the proapoptotic and antiapoptotic family members.

The net result of Bax-Bak activation coupled with declining Bcl-2/Bcl-x levels is an increased mitochondrial membrane permeability, leaking out several proteins that can activate caspases. Thus released cytochrome *c* binds to apoptosis activating factor-1 (Apaf-1) to form a large multimeric *apoptosome* complex that triggers caspase-9 (an initiator caspase) activation. *The essence of the intrinsic pathway is a balance between proapoptotic and antiapoptotic molecules that regulate mitochondrial permeability.*

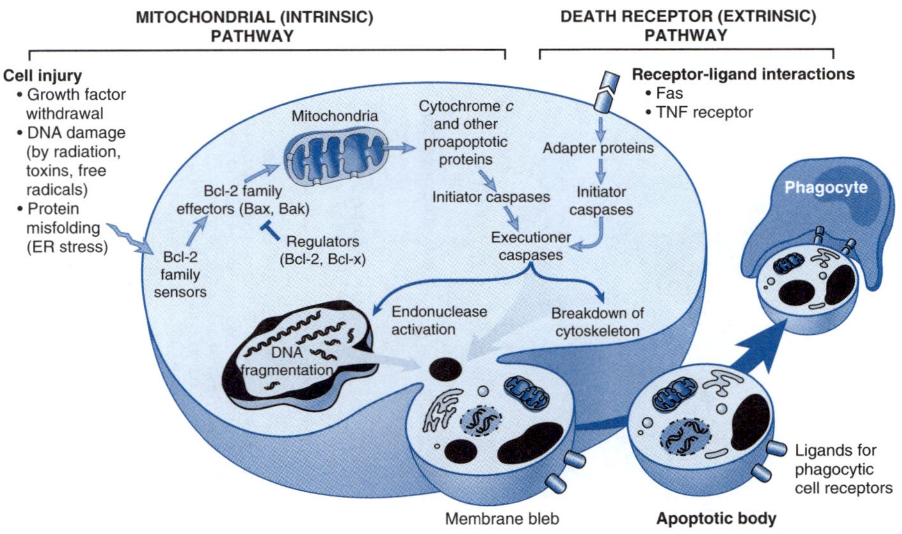

Figure 2-5 Mechanisms of apoptosis. Some of the major inducers of apoptosis include specific death ligands (TNF and FasL), withdrawal of growth factors or hormones, and injurious agents (e.g., radiation). Some stimuli (such as cytotoxic cells) directly activate initiator caspases *(right).* Others act by way of mitochondrial events involving cytochrome *c* and other proapoptotic proteins. The Bcl-2 family of proteins regulate apoptosis by modulating this mitochondrial release. Initiator caspases cleave and activate executioner caspases, which in turn activate latent cytoplasmic endonucleases and proteases that catabolize nuclear and cytoskeletal proteins. This results in a cascade of intracellular degradation, including fragmentation of nuclear chromatin and breakdown of the cytoskeleton. The end result is formation of apoptotic bodies containing intracellular organelles and other cytosolic components; these bodies also express new ligands for binding and uptake by phagocytic cells.

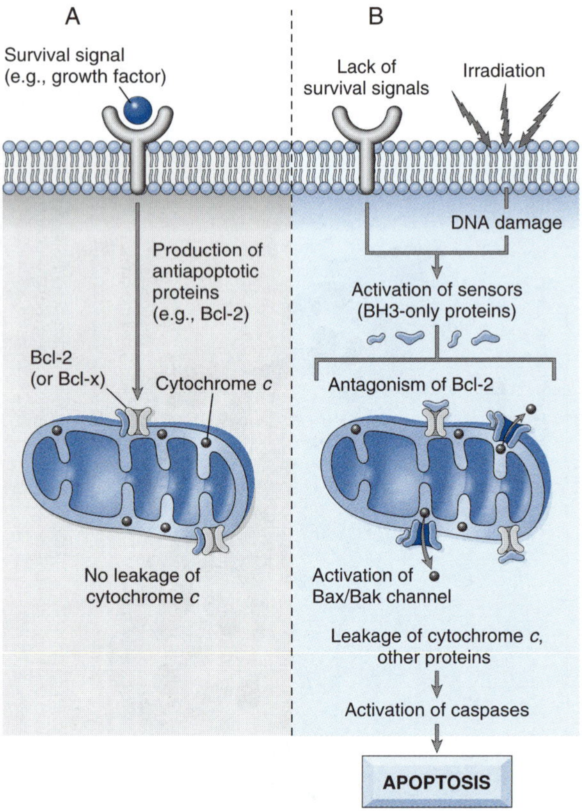

Figure 2-6 The intrinsic (mitochondrial) pathway of apoptosis. A, Cell viability is maintained by the induction of antiapoptotic proteins, such as Bcl-2, by survival signals. These proteins maintain the integrity of mitochondrial membranes and prevent leakage of mitochondrial proteins. **B,** Loss of survival signals, DNA damage, and other insults activate sensors that antagonize the antiapoptotic proteins and activate the proapoptotic proteins Bax and Bak, which form channels in the mitochondrial membrane. The subsequent leakage of cytochrome *c* (and other proteins, not shown) leads to caspase activation and apoptosis.

Extrinsic (Death Receptor-Initiated) Pathway *(p. 56)*

Death receptors are members of the tumor necrosis factor (TNF) receptor family (e.g., type 1 TNF receptor and Fas). They have a cytoplasmic *death domain* involved in protein-protein interactions. Cross-linking of these receptors by external ligands, such as TNF or Fas ligand (FasL) causes them to trimerize to form binding sites for adapter proteins that serve to bring multiple inactive caspase-8 molecules into close proximity. Low-level enzymatic activity of these procaspases eventually cleaves and activates one of the assembled group, rapidly leading to a downstream cascade of caspase activation. This enzymatic pathway can be inhibited by a blocking protein called FLIP; viruses and normal cells can produce FLIP to protect themselves against Fas-mediated death.

Execution Phase (*p. 56*)

Caspases occur as inactive proenzymes that are activated through proteolytic cleavage; the cleavage sites can be hydrolyzed by other caspases or autocatalytically. *Initiator caspases* (e.g., caspase-8 and -9) are activated early in the sequence and induce the cleavage of the *executioner caspases* (e.g., caspase-3 and -6) that do the bulk of the intracellular proteolytic degradation. Once an initiator caspase is activated, the death program is set in motion by rapid and sequential activation of other caspases. Executioner caspases act on many cell components; they cleave cytoskeletal and nuclear matrix proteins, disrupting the cytoskeleton and leading to nuclear breakdown. In the nucleus, caspases cleave proteins involved in transcription, DNA replication, and DNA repair; in particular, caspase-3 activates a cytoplasmic DNAase, resulting in the characteristic internucleosomal cleavage.

Apoptosis in Health and Disease (p. 57)

Growth Factor Deprivation (*p. 57*)

Examples: Hormone-sensitive cells deprived of the relevant hormone, lymphocytes not stimulated by antigens or cytokines, and neurons deprived of nerve growth factor. Apoptosis is triggered by the intrinsic (mitochondrial) pathway due to a relative excess of proapoptotic versus antiapoptotic members of the Bcl family.

DNA Damage (*p. 57*)

DNA damage by any means (e.g., radiation or chemotherapeutic agents) induces apoptosis through accumulation of the tumor-suppressor protein p53. This results in cell cycle arrest at G_1 putatively to allow time for DNA repair (see Chapter 7). If repair cannot take place, p53 then induces apoptosis by increasing the transcription of several proapoptotic members of the Bcl family. Absent or mutated p53 (i.e., in certain cancers) reduces apoptosis and favors cell survival even in the presence significant DNA damage.

Protein Misfolding (*p. 57*)

Accumulation of misfolded proteins—due to oxidative stress, hypoxia, or genetic mutations—leads to the *unfolded protein response*, increasingly recognized as a feature of several neurodegenerative disorders. This response induces increased production of chaperones and increased proteasomal degradation, with decreased protein synthesis. If the adaptive responses cannot keep pace with the accumulating misfolded proteins, caspases are activated and apoptosis results (Fig. 2-7).

TNF Family Receptors (*p. 58*)

Apoptosis induced by Fas-FasL interactions (see preceding discussion) are important for eliminating lymphocytes that recognize self-antigens; mutations in Fas or FasL result in autoimmune diseases (see Chapter 6). TNF is an important mediator of the inflammatory reaction (see Chapter 3) but can also induce apoptosis (as well as *necroptosis*, see later discussion). The major physiologic functions of TNF are mediated through activation of the transcription factor nuclear factor-κB (NF-κB), which in turn promotes cell survival by increasing antiapoptotic members of the Bcl family. Whether TNF induces cell death, promotes cell survival, or drives inflammatory responses depends on which of two TNF receptors it binds, as well as which adapter protein attaches to the receptor.

Cytotoxic T Lymphocytes (*p. 58*)

Cytotoxic T lymphocytes (CTLs) recognize foreign antigens on the surface of infected host cells (see Chapter 6) and secrete *perforin*,

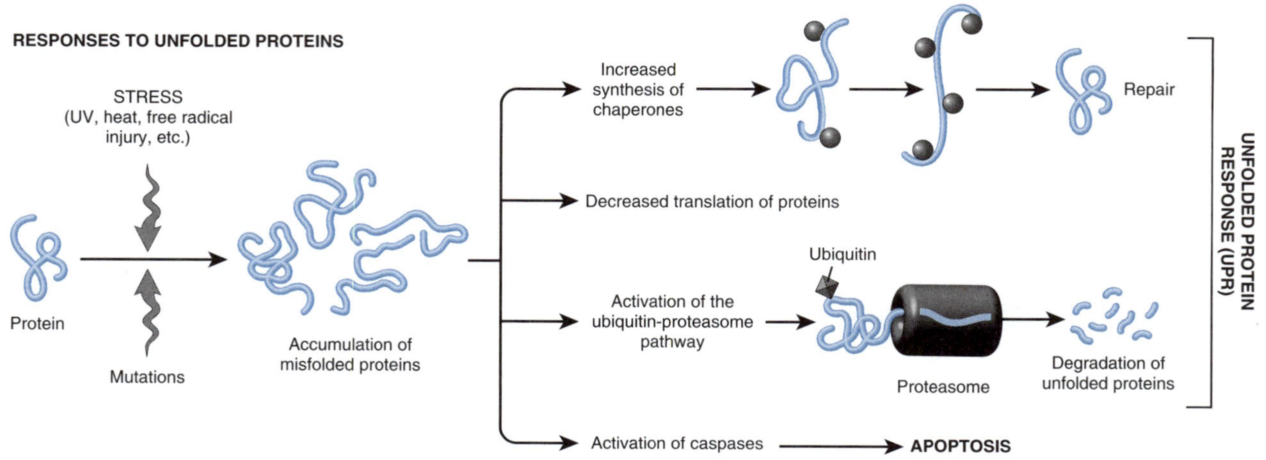

Figure 2-7 Misfolded proteins trigger an unfolded protein response that includes increased chaperone synthesis, decreased protein translation, and activation of proteasome degradation pathways. If these are ineffective in reducing the burden of misfolded proteins, caspase activation and apoptosis ensue.

a transmembrane pore-forming molecule. This allows entry of the CTL-derived serine protease *granzyme B* that in turn activates multiple caspases, thereby directly inducing the effector phase of apoptosis. CTLs also express FasL on their surfaces and can kill target cells by Fas ligation.

Disorders Associated With Dysregulated Apoptosis (p. 58)

Dysregulated ("too little or too much") apoptosis underlies multiple disorders:

- *Disorders with defective apoptosis and increased cell survival.* Insufficient apoptosis may prolong the survival or reduce the turnover of abnormal cells. Such accumulated cells may lead to (1) *cancers,* especially tumors with *p53* mutations, or hormone-dependent tumors, such as breast, prostate, or ovarian cancers (see Chapter 7), and (2) *autoimmune disorders,* when autoreactive lymphocytes are not eliminated (see Chapter 6).
- *Disorders with increased apoptosis and excessive cell death.* Increased cell loss can cause (1) *neurodegenerative diseases,* with dropout of specific sets of neurons (see Chapter 28), (2) *ischemic injury* (e.g., myocardial infarction [see Chapter 12] and stroke [see Chapter 28]), and (3) *death of virus-infected cells* (see Chapter 8).

Necroptosis (p. 58)

Also called "programmed necrosis," necroptosis:

- *Morphologically resembles necrosis* with ATP depletion, cell and organellar swelling, ROS generation, and lysosomal and plasma membrane rupture.
- *Mechanistically resembles apoptosis* in that there are genetically programmed signaling events that result in death; however, it is not caspase-dependent.
- Can be triggered through ligation of cell-surface death receptors and through sensors that detect viral RNA and DNA, as well as genomic injury. These interactions activate *receptor-interacting protein* kinases (aptly named RIP kinases) to form a *necrosome* that drives the intracellular changes leading to cell necrosis (Fig. 2-8).
- Comparable to necrosis, necroptosis also evokes an inflammatory response.

Necroptosis is involved in physiologic events (formation of the mammalian growth plate) as well as pathologic processes (the cell death seen in steatohepatitis, acute pancreatitis, and reperfusion injury). It is also a fail-safe form of cell death for certain viral infections that encode caspase inhibitors (e.g., cytomegalovirus).

Autophagy (p. 60)

Literally translating to "self-eating," autophagy is an evolutionarily conserved mechanism by which cells experiencing nutrient deprivation can survive by cannibalizing themselves and recycling the digested contents. In most cases this involves sequestration and delivery—*via* double membrane-bounded *autophagosomes*—of "gulps" of cytosolic contents (including organelles) to lysosomes for degradation (Fig. 2-9). The process is regulated by several "autophagy-related genes" called *Atgs.* Autophagy is a characteristic feature of atrophy but is also involved in the normal homeostatic turnover of organelles and in clearing intracellular aggregates that occur with aging, cellular stress, and disease states. It also plays a role in host defense by degrading certain intracellular pathogens (e.g., mycobacteria and herpes simplex virus-1). Although autophagy is primarily a survival mechanism, it can also be associated with cell death, as in several neurodegenerative disorders (e.g., Alzheimer disease).

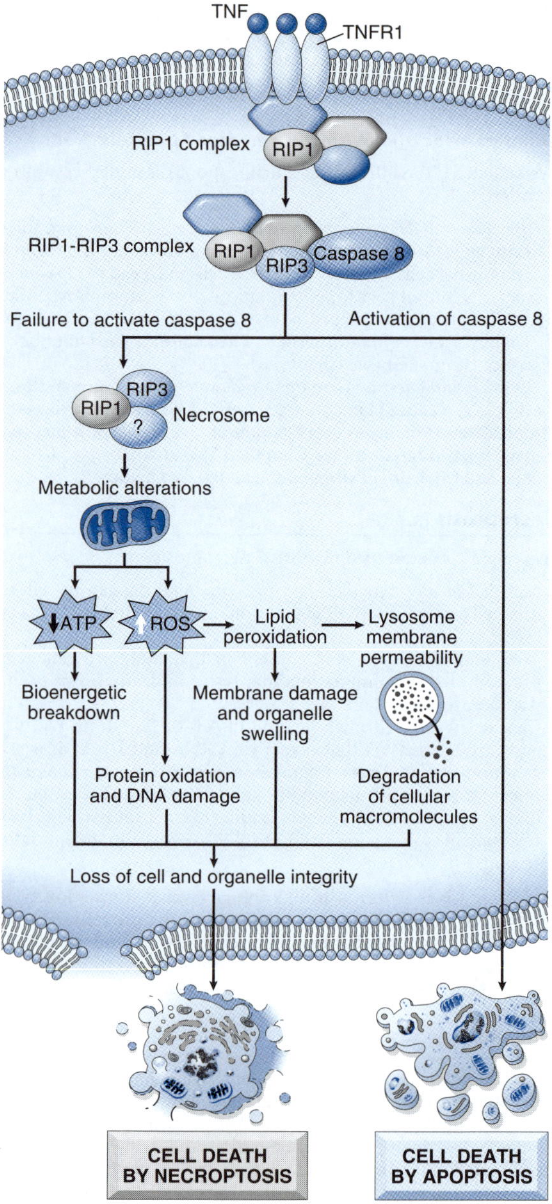

Figure 2-8 Molecular mechanism of TNF-mediated necroptosis. Cross-linking of TNFR1 by TNF causes trimerization and recruitment of a complex that includes TRADD, TRAF 2 and 5, clap, and RIP1. In further steps (not depicted), caspase-8 and RIP3 are recruited to this complex. Caspase inactivates RIP1 and RIP3 and initiates apoptosis. Caspase-8 inactivation leads to the formation of RIP1- and RIP3-containing necrosomes, which in turn interact with mitochondria to reduce ATP and generate ROS, culminating in events that typify necrosis. *(Adapted from Galluzi L, Vanden Berghe T, Vanlangenakker N, et al: Programmed necrosis from molecules to health and disease.* Int Rev Cell Molec Biol *289:1, 2011.)*

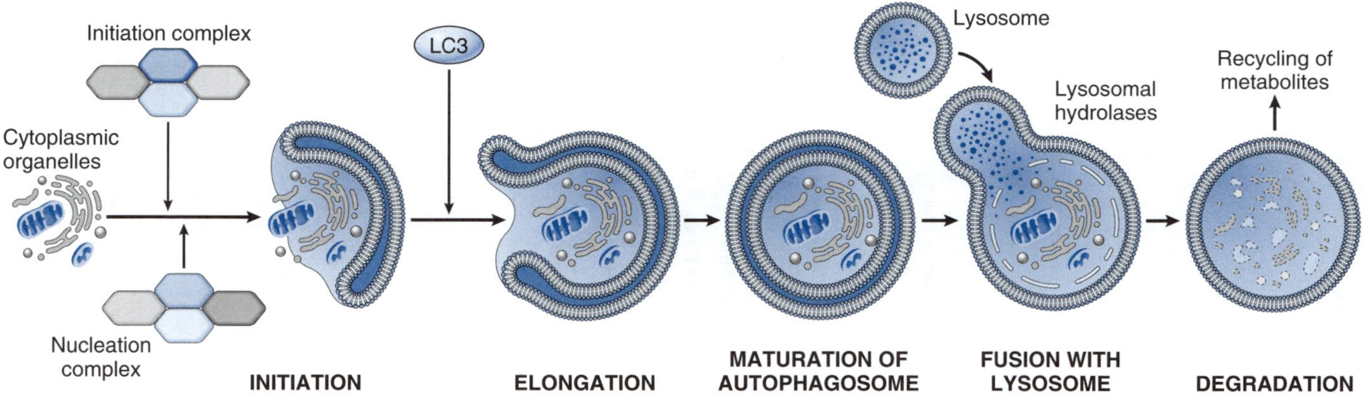

Figure 2-9 Autophagy. Cellular stresses, such as nutrient deprivation, activate autophagy. The pathway proceeds through several phases (initiation, nucleation, and elongation of isolation membrane) and eventually creates double membrane-bound vacuoles (autophagosome) in which cytoplasmic materials, including organelles, are sequestered and then degraded following fusion of the vesicles with lysosomes. In the final stage the digested materials are released for recycling of metabolites. The genes involved and their sites of action are indicated; see text for details. *(Modified from Choi AMK, Ryter S Levine B: Autophagy in human health and disease.* N Engl J Med *368:651, 2013.)*

Intracellular Accumulations (p. 61)

Cells may accumulate abnormal amounts of various substances.

- A *normal* endogenous substance (water, protein, carbohydrate, lipid) is produced at a normal (or even increased) rate, with the metabolic rate inadequate to remove it (e.g., fat accumulation in liver cells).
- An abnormal endogenous substance (product of a mutated gene) accumulates because of defective folding or transport and inadequate degradation (e.g., α_1-antitrypsin disease).
- A *normal* substance accumulates because of genetic or acquired defects in its *metabolism* (e.g., lysososmal storage diseases [see Chapter 5]).
- *Abnormal exogenous substances* may accumulate in normal cells because they lack the machinery to degrade such substances (e.g., macrophages laden with environmental carbon).

Lipids (p. 62)

Triglycerides (the most common), cholesterol and cholesterol esters, and phospholipids can accumulate in cells.

Steatosis (Fatty Change) (p. 62)

The terms describe an abnormal accumulation of triglycerides within parenchymal cells either due to excessive entry or defective metabolism and export. It can occur in heart, muscle, and kidney but is most common in the liver. Hepatic causes include alcohol abuse (most common in the United States), protein malnutrition, diabetes mellitus, obesity, toxins, and anoxia.

Cholesterol and Cholesterol Esters (p. 62)

Cholesterol is normally required for cell membrane or lipid-soluble hormone synthesis; production is tightly regulated but accumulation (seen as intracellular cytoplasmic vacuoles) can be present in a variety of pathologic states:

- *Atherosclerosis:* Cholesterol and cholesterol esters accumulate in arterial wall smooth muscle cells and macrophages (see Chapter 11). Extracellular accumulations appear microscopically as cleft-like cavities formed when cholesterol crystals are dissolved during normal histologic processing.
- *Xanthomas:* In acquired and hereditary *hyperlipidemias,* lipids accumulate in clusters of "foamy" macrophages and mesenchymal cells.
- *Cholesterolosis:* Focal accumulations of cholesterol-laden macrophages occur in the lamina propria of gallbladders.
- *Niemann-Pick disease, type C:* This type of lysosomal storage disease is due to mutation of an enzyme involved in cholesterol catabolism (see Chapter 5).

Proteins (p. 63)

Intracellular protein accumulation may be due to excessive synthesis, absorption, or defects in cellular transport. Morphologically visible accumulations appear as rounded, eosinophilic cytoplasmic droplets. In some disorders (e.g., *amyloidosis* [see Chapter 6]), abnormal proteins deposit primarily in the *extracellular* space.

- *Reabsorption droplets* of proteins accumulate in proximal renal tubules in the setting of chronic proteinuria. The process is reversible; the droplets are metabolized and clear if the proteinuria resolves.

- *Normally secreted proteins* can accumulate if produced in excessive amounts (e.g., immunoglobulin within plasma cells). In that case the ER becomes grossly distended with eosinophilic inclusions called *Russell bodies.*
- *Defective intracellular transport and secretion* (e.g., *α_1-antitrypsin deficiency,* where partially folded intermediates of mutated proteins accumulate in hepatocyte ER). In many cases pathology results not only from the unfolded protein response and apoptosis (see preceding discussion), but also loss of protein function. Thus reduction in secreted α_1-antitrypsin also leads to emphysema (see Chapter 15).
- *Accumulated cytoskeletal proteins.* Excess intermediate filaments (e.g., keratin or certain neurofilaments) are hallmarks of cell injury; thus keratin intermediate filaments coalesce into cytoplasmic eosinophilic inclusions called *alcoholic hyaline* (see Chapter 18), and the *neurofibrillary tangle* in Alzheimer disease contains neurofilaments (see Chapter 28).
- *Aggregates of abnormal proteins.* Aggregation of abnormally folded proteins (e.g., genetic mutations, aging) either intracellular and/or extracellular can cause pathologic change; extracellular amyloid is an example.

Hyaline Change (p. 63)

Hyaline change refers to any deposit that imparts a homogeneous, glassy pink appearance in H&E-stained histologic sections. Examples of *intracellular hyaline change* include proximal tubule epithelial protein droplets, Russell bodies, viral inclusions, and alcoholic hyaline. For example, *extracellular hyaline change* occurs in damaged arterioles (e.g., due to chronic hypertension), presumably due to extravasated proteins.

Glycogen (p. 63)

Glycogen is commonly stored within cells as a ready energy source. *Excessive* intracellular deposits (seen as clear vacuoles) are seen with abnormalities of glycogen storage (so-called *glycogenoses* [see Chapter 5]) and glucose metabolism *(diabetes mellitus).*

Pigments (p. 63)

Pigments are colored substances that can be exogenous (e.g., coal dust) or endogenous, such as melanin or hemosiderin.

- Exogenous pigments include carbon or coal dust (most common); when visibly accumulated within pulmonary macrophages and lymph nodes these deposits are called *anthracosis.* Pigments from *tattooing* are taken up by macrophages and persist for the life of the cell.
- Endogenous pigments include the following:
  - *Lipofuscin,* so-called "wear-and-tear" pigment and usually associated with cellular and tissue atrophy *(brown atrophy).* This is seen microscopically as fine yellow-brown intracytoplasmic granules. The pigment is composed of complex lipids, phospholipids, and protein, probably derived from cell membrane peroxidation.
  - *Melanin,* a normal endogenous brown-black pigment formed by enzymatic oxidation of tyrosine to dihydroxyphenylalanine in melanocytes.
  - *Homogentisic acid* is a black pigment formed in patients with alkaptonuria (lacking homogentisic oxidase) that deposits in skin and connective tissue; the pigmentation is called *ochronosis.*

- *Hemosiderin* is a hemoglobin-derived, golden yellow-brown, granular intracellular pigment composed of aggregated ferritin. Accumulation can be localized (e.g., macrophage-mediated breakdown of blood in a bruise) or systemic (i.e., due to increased dietary iron absorption *[primary hemochromatosis]*), impaired utilization (e.g., thalassemia), hemolysis, or chronic transfusions (see Chapter 18).

Pathologic Calcification (p. 65)

Pathologic calcification—the abnormal tissue deposition of calcium salts—occurs in two forms: *dystrophic calcification* arises in nonviable tissues in the presence of normal calcium serum levels, whereas *metastatic calcification* happens in viable tissues in the setting of hypercalcemia.

Dystrophic Calcification (p. 65)

Although frequently only a marker of prior injury, it can also be a source of significant pathology. Dystrophic calcification occurs in arteries in atherosclerosis, in damaged heart valves, and in areas of necrosis (coagulative, caseous, and liquefactive). Calcium can be intracellular and extracellular. Deposition ultimately involves precipitation of a crystalline calcium phosphate similar to bone hydroxyapatite:

- *Initiation (nucleation)* occurs extracellularly or intracellularly. *Extracellular* initiation occurs on membrane-bound vesicles from dead or dying cells that concentrate calcium due to their content of charged phospholipids; membrane-bound phosphatases then generate phosphates that form calcium-phosphate complexes; the cycle of calcium and phosphate binding is repeated, eventually producing a deposit. Initiation of *intracellular* calcification occurs in mitochondria of dead or dying cells.
- *Propagation* of crystal formation depends on the concentration of calcium and phosphates, the presence of inhibitors, and structural components of the extracellular matrix.

Metastatic Calcification (p. 65)

These calcium deposits occur as amorphous basophilic densities that can be present widely throughout the body. Typically they have no clinical sequelae, although massive deposition can cause renal and lung deficits. Metastatic calcification results from hypercalcemia (four principal causes):

- *Elevated parathyroid hormone* (e.g., hyperparathyroidism due to parathyroid tumors or ectopic parathyroid hormone secreted by other neoplasms)
- *Bone destruction,* as in primary marrow malignancies (e.g., multiple myeloma) or by diffuse skeletal metastasis (e.g., breast cancer), by accelerated bone turnover *(Paget disease),* or immobilization
- *Vitamin D-related disorders,* including vitamin D intoxication and systemic sarcoidosis
- *Renal failure,* causing secondary hyperparathyroidism due to phosphate retention and the resulting hypocalcemia

Cellular Aging (p. 66)

With increasing age, degenerative changes impact the structure and physiologic function of all organ systems. The tempo and severity of such changes in any given individual are influenced by genetic factors, diet, social conditions, and the impact of other comorbidities, such as atherosclerosis, diabetes, and osteoarthritis. *Cellular* aging—reflecting the progressive accumulation of sublethal cellular and molecular damage due to both genetic and exogenous influences—leads to cell death and diminished capacity to respond to injury; it is a critical component of the aging of the entire organism (Fig. 2-10).

Aging—at least in model systems—appears to be a regulated process influenced by a limited number of genes; this, in turn, implies that aging can potentially be parsed into definable mechanistic alterations:

- *Genomic instability* (p. 66). Imperfect DNA repair is an important element of aging. Nuclear and mitochondrial DNA are under constant attack by both exogenous (physical, chemical, and biologic agents) and endogenous (e.g., ROS) agents. Although most damage is successfully repaired, any residual defects become fixed in the primary sequence and will accumulate as cells age.

Premature aging is a feature of disorders associated with abnormal DNA repair (e.g., due to mutations in DNA helicase *[Werner syndrome]*) or defects in the repair of double-strand breaks (*Bloom syndrome* and *ataxia-telangiectasia*).

- *Cellular (replicative) senescence* (p. 67). Cells have a limited capacity for replication; after a fixed number of divisions, cell arrest in a terminally nondividing state. This phenomenon is reflected in the observation that cells from children exhibit more rounds of replication than cells from geriatrics. Cellular senescence is driven by
  - *Telomere attrition* (p. 67). Telomeres are short repeated sequences of DNA that comprise the termini of chromosomes; they ensure complete replication of genes at the ends of chromosomes and also protect the chromosome tips from fusion and degradation. A small segment of telomere is lost with each cell division. Consequently, as somatic cells repeatedly divide, their telomeres progressively shorten until they no longer adequately protect the chromosome tips; this signals a growth checkpoint where cells become senescent. Accelerated telomere shortening has also been associated with diseases such as pulmonary fibrosis and aplastic anemia.

Germ cells, and to a lesser extent stem cells, maintain sufficient telomere length to ensure *unlimited* replication through the activity of *telomerase,* an RNA-protein enzyme complex that uses its own RNA as a template to add nucleotides to the ends of chromosomes. Telomerase is typically undetectable in somatic cells but in cancer cells can become reactivated, allowing telomere stabilization and indefinite proliferation (see Chapter 7).

  - *Activation of tumor suppressor genes* (p. 67). Replicative senescence is also regulated by certain tumor suppressor genes, particularly those at the *INK4a/ARF* locus that regulate G_1 to S phase transition in cell cycling.

- *Defective protein homeostasis* (p. 67). The correct folding of proteins is maintained by *chaperones;* if that mechanism is not adequate to the task, misfolded proteins are degraded through the autophagy-lysosome and/or ubiquitin-proteasome systems. Defects in these systems contribute to aging through effects on replication, cell function, or apoptosis.
- *Deregulated nutrient sensing* (p. 67). *Caloric restriction* increases lifespan, suggesting that aging is also intimately associated with nutritional status and metabolism. The longevity effects of caloric

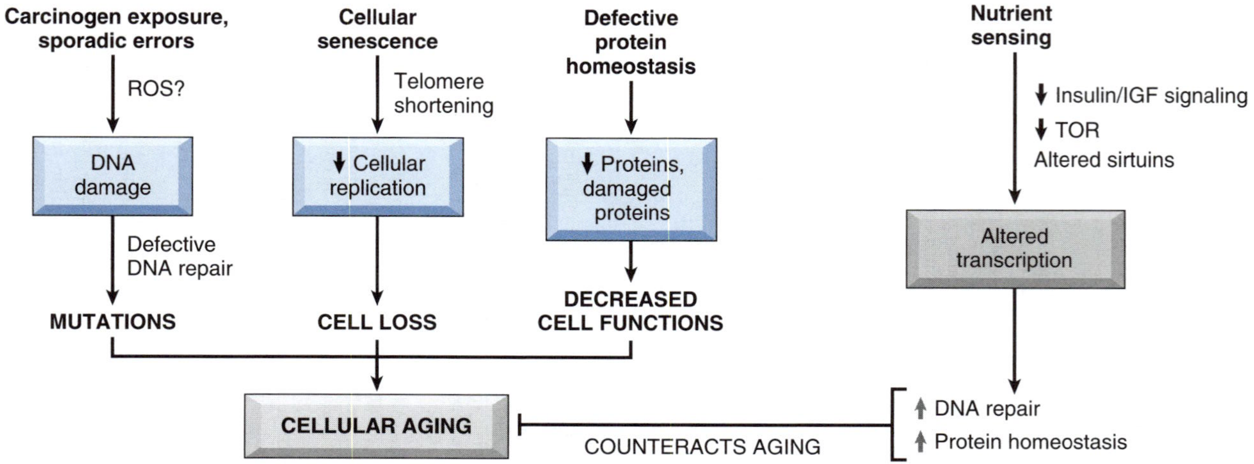

Figure 2-10 Mechanisms that cause and counteract cellular aging. DNA damage, replicative senescence, and decreased and misfolded proteins are among the best described mechanisms of cellular aging. Nutrient sensing exemplified by calorie restriction, counteracts aging by activating various signaling pathways and transcription factors. *IGF,* Insulin-like growth factor; *ROS,* reactive oxygen species; *TOR,* target of rapamycin.

restriction are attributed to the inhibition of the insulin-like growth factor 1 (IGF-1) signaling pathway and by increasing sirtuins:

- *Insulin and IGF-1 signaling pathway* (p. 67). Both mediators signal glucose availability, promoting an anabolic state, as well as cell growth and replication. Among multiple downstream targets, IGF-1 induces mammalian target of rapamycin (mTOR) and Akt (also known as protein kinase B) kinase activities. Notably, some of the beneficial effects of caloric restriction can be mimicked by inhibiting mTOR (e.g., with rapamycin).
- *Sirtuins* (p. 67). These are members of a family of NAD-dependent protein deacetylases that allow cellular adaptation to exogenous stressors, including food deprivation and DNA damage. Sirtuins induce the expression of a variety of genes that cumulatively promote longevity (e.g., by reducing apoptosis, stimulating protein folding, and inhibiting the effects of ROS); they also increase insulin sensitivity and inhibit some metabolic activities.

3 Inflammation and Repair

Overview of Inflammation (p. 69)

Inflammation is the response of vascularized living tissue to injury. It may be evoked by microbial infections, physical agents, chemicals, necrotic tissue, or immune reactions. Inflammation is intended to contain and isolate injury, destroy invading microorganisms and inactivate toxins, and prepare the tissue for healing and repair. Inflammation is characterized by the following:

- Two main components, a vascular wall response and an inflammatory cell response.
- Effects that are mediated by circulating plasma proteins and by factors produced locally by vessel wall or inflammatory cells.
- Local and systemic responses; although the emphasis is on local inflammatory responses to injury, systemic effects also occur (e.g., fever, release of leukocytes from bone marrow, and acute phase responses in liver).
- Termination when the offending agent is eliminated and the secreted mediators are removed; active antiinflammatory mechanisms are also involved.
- Tight association with healing; even as inflammation destroys, dilutes, or otherwise contains injury, it sets into motion events that will ultimately lead to tissue regeneration and/or fibrosis (scarring).
- A fundamentally protective response; however, inflammation can also be harmful (e.g., causing life-threatening hypersensitivity reactions, or relentless and progressive organ damage from chronic inflammation and subsequent fibrosis [e.g., rheumatoid arthritis, atherosclerosis]).
- *Acute* and *chronic* patterns of inflammation with characteristic time of onset, cellular infiltrates, and local and systemic effects (Table 3-1).

Historical Highlights (p. 71)

There are five classic clinical signs of inflammation (most prominent in acute inflammation):

- Warmth (Latin: *calor*), due to vascular dilation
- Erythema (Latin: *rubor*), due to vascular dilation and congestion
- Edema (Latin: *tumor*), due to increased vascular permeability
- Pain (Latin: *dolor*), due to mediator release
- *Loss of function* (Latin: *functio laesa*), due to pain, edema, tissue injury, and/or scar

Causes of Inflammation (p. 71)

Inflammation is triggered by the following:

- Infection: Different types of microorganisms (virus, bacterium, fungus, parasite) elicit different inflammatory responses.

TABLE 3-1 Features of Acute and Chronic Inflammation

Feature	Acute	Chronic
Onset	Fast: minutes or hours	Slow: days
Cellular infiltrate	Mainly neutrophils	Monocytes/macrophages and lymphocytes
Tissue injury, fibrosis	Usually mild and self-limited	Often severe and progressive
Local and systemic signs	Prominent	Less

- Tissue necrosis: Ischemia, trauma, and toxins all elicit inflammation.
- Foreign bodies: These include splinters, dirt, suture, prosthetic devices, urate crystals (gout), and cholesterol esters.
- Immune reactions (hypersensitivity responses) can be directed against self *(autoimmunity)* or exogenous agents *(allergy).*

Recognition of Microbes and Damaged Cells (p. 72)

A variety of cellular receptors can recognize pathogenic stimuli and deliver activating signals (Fig. 3-1).

- *Cellular receptors for microbes* are expressed on a wide variety of cells (epithelial, endothelial, and immune) and can be localized to plasma membranes (for extracellular pathogens), endosomes (ingested microbes), or cytosol (intracellular agents). *Toll-like receptors* (*TLRs;* see Chapter 6) are the best described; binding to the receptors triggers an inflammatory response, including expression of cytokines and endothelial cell adhesion molecules.
- Sensors of cell damage are present in the cytosol of all cells; these recognize molecules that result from cell injury (e.g., uric acid [a product of DNA breakdown], adenosine triphosphate [ATP] [released from damaged mitochondria], reduced intracellular K^+ [reflecting leakage due to plasma membrane injury], and even nonnuclear DNA). The receptors activate a multiprotein complex called the *inflammasome* (see Chapter 6), which generates proinflammatory interleukin-1 (IL-1). Inflammasomes also drive inflammatory reactions to urate crystals (the cause of *gout*), lipids (in metabolic syndrome), cholesterol crystals (in atherosclerosis), and even amyloid deposits in the brain (in Alzheimer disease).
- *Other cellular receptors involved in inflammation* include leukocyte receptors for complement proteins as well as the Fc portion of antibodies. These recognize microbes coated *(opsonized)* with antibodies and complement.

A variety of circulating *proteins* also bind/respond to pathogens and can trigger inflammatory responses. These include the *complement system, mannose-binding lectin* that recognizes microbial sugars, and *collectins.*

Acute Inflammation (p. 73)

Acute inflammation has three major components:

- Vascular dilation leading to increased blood flow
- Structural changes in the microvasculature permitting plasma proteins and leukocytes to leave the circulation
- Leukocyte emigration from blood vessels and accumulation and activation at the site of injury

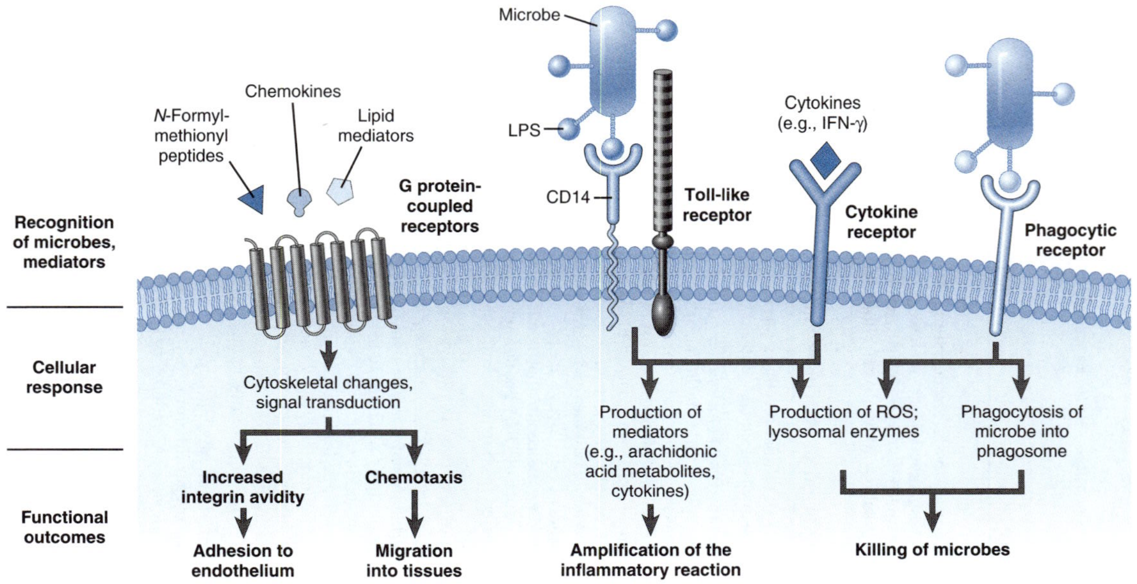

Figure 3-1 Leukocyte activation. Different classes of cell-surface receptors of leukocytes recognize different stimuli. The receptors initiate responses that mediate the functions of the leukocytes. Only a subset of receptors is depicted (see text). Lipopolysaccharide (LPS) first binds to a circulating LPS-binding protein (not shown). *IFN-γ,* Interferon-γ.

Reactions of Blood Vessels in Acute Inflammation (p. 73)

Normal fluid exchange in vascular beds depends on an intact endothelium and is modulated by two opposing forces:

- Hydrostatic pressure causes fluid to move out of the circulation.
- Plasma colloid osmotic pressure causes fluid to move into the capillaries.

Edema is excess fluid in interstitial tissue or body cavities and can be either an exudate or a transudate.

- An *exudate* is an inflammatory extravascular fluid with cellular debris and high protein concentration (high specific gravity); its presence reflects increased vascular permeability.
- A *transudate* is excess extravascular fluid with low protein content (low specific gravity); it is essentially an ultrafiltrate of blood plasma resulting from elevated fluid pressures or diminished plasma osmotic forces.
- *Pus* is a purulent inflammatory exudate rich in neutrophils and cell debris.

Changes in Vascular Flow and Caliber (p. 73)

Beginning immediately after injury, the vascular wall develops changes in caliber and permeability that affect flow; the changes develop at various rates depending on the nature of the injury and its severity.

- Vasodilation increases flow into areas of injury, thus *increasing hydrostatic pressure.*
- Increased vascular permeability causes *exudation* of protein-rich fluid.
- The combination of vascular dilation and fluid loss leads to increased blood viscosity and increased concentration of red blood cells. Slowly moving erythrocytes *(stasis)* grossly manifest as vascular congestion.
- With stasis, leukocytes—mostly neutrophils—accumulate along the endothelium *(marginate)* and are activated by mediators to increase adhesion and migration through the vessel wall.

Increased Vascular Permeability (Vascular Leakage, p.74)

Increased vascular permeability can be induced by the following (Fig. 3-2):

- *Contraction of venule endothelium to form intercellular gaps:*
    - Most common mechanism of increased permeability
    - Elicited by chemical mediators (e.g., histamine, bradykinin, and leukotrienes [LTs])
    - Occurs rapidly after injury and is reversible and transient (15 to 30 minutes), hence the term *immediate transient response*
    - A similar response can occur with mild injury (e.g., sunburn) or inflammatory *cytokines* but is delayed (2 to 12 hours) and protracted (24 hours or more)
- *Direct endothelial injury:*
    - Severe necrotizing injury (e.g., burns) causes endothelial cell necrosis and detachment that affects venules, capillaries, and arterioles.
    - Recruited neutrophils may contribute to the injury (e.g., through reactive oxygen species [ROS]).
    - Immediate and sustained endothelial leakage.

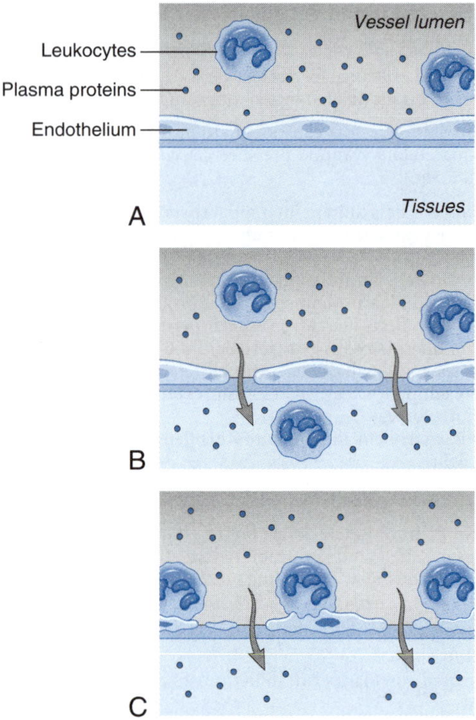

Figure 3-2 Principal mechanisms of increased vascular permeability in inflammation. A, Normal. **B,** Retraction of endothelial cells: (1) induced by histamine, other mediators and (2) rapid and short lived (minutes).
C, Endothelial injury: (1) caused by burns, some microbial toxins and (2) rapid; may be long lived (hours to days).

- *Increased transcytosis:*
  - Transendothelial channels form by interconnection of vesicles derived from the *vesiculovacuolar organelle.*
  - Vascular endothelial growth factor (VEGF) and other factors can induce vascular leakage by increasing the number of these channels.

Responses of Lymphatic Vessels and Lymph Nodes (p. 74)

Lymphatics and lymph nodes filter and "police" extravascular fluids; with the mononuclear phagocyte system, they represent a secondary line of defense when local inflammatory responses cannot contain an infection.

- In inflammation, lymphatic flow is increased to drain edema fluid, leukocytes, and cell debris from the extravascular space.
- In severe injuries, drainage may also transport the offending agent; lymphatics may become inflamed (*lymphangitis,* manifest grossly as red streaks), as may the draining lymph nodes (*lymphadenitis,* manifest as enlarged, painful nodes). The nodal enlargement is usually due to lymphoid follicle and sinusoidal phagocyte hyperplasia (termed *reactive lymphadenitis;* see Chapter 13).

Leukocyte Recruitment to Sites of Inflammation (p. 75)

Leukocytes (especially the phagocytic neutrophils and macrophages) must be recruited to sites of injury, where they recognize invading pathogens and necrotic debris, eliminate them, and produce growth factors to facilitate repair.

The type of leukocyte that emigrates into a site of injury depends on the original stimulus and the duration of the inflammatory response. Bacterial infections tend to initially recruit neutrophils, whereas viral infections recruit lymphocytes, allergic reactions have increased eosinophils, and hypersensitivity reactions induce a mixed infiltrate.

Necrosis will initially induce a neutrophilic recruitment; *neutrophils predominate during the first 6 to 24 hours, then are replaced by monocytes after 24 to 48 hours.* The sequence of recruitment is a function of the successive pattern of expression of specific adhesion molecules and chemokines. After emigration, neutrophils are also short-lived; they undergo apoptosis after 24 to 48 hours, whereas monocytes survive longer.

Leukocytes move from vessel lumen to tissue interstitium in a multistep process (Fig. 3-3):

- Margination, rolling, and adhesion of leukocytes to the endothelium
- Transmigration across the endothelium
- Migration in interstitial tissues toward a chemotactic stimulus

Leukocyte Adhesion to Endothelium (p. 75)

With progressive stasis, leukocytes become distributed along the vessel periphery *(margination)*, where they can *roll* and then *firmly adhere*, before finally crossing the vascular wall. Rolling, adhesion, and transmigration occur by interactions between complementary adhesion molecules on leukocytes and endothelium. Expression of these adhesion molecules is enhanced by secreted proteins called *cytokines*. The major adhesion molecule pairs are listed in Table 3-2:

- Rolling is mediated by *selectins;* these bind via lectin (sugar-binding) domains to oligosaccharides (e.g., sialylated Lewis X [sialyl-Lewis X]) on cell-surface glycoproteins.
- Firm adhesion is mediated by *immunoglobulin family molecules* on endothelial cells that bind *integrins* on leukocytes.
  - The immunoglobulin molecules include intercellular adhesion molecule 1 *(ICAM-1)* and vascular cell adhesion molecule 1 *(VCAM-1)*.
  - *Integrins* are α-β heterodimers; β_2 integrins lymphocyte function associated antigen-1 (LFA-1) and macrophage-1 antigen (Mac-1) (also called CD11a/CD18 and CD11b/CD18) bind ICAM-1; the β_1 integrin very late antigen (VLA)-4 binds to VCAM-1.
- Chemoattractants *(chemokines)* and cytokines affect adhesion and transmigration by modulating the surface expression or avidity of the adhesion molecules:
  - *Redistribution of preformed adhesion molecules to the cell surface.* After histamine exposure, P-selectin is rapidly translocated from the endothelial Weibel-Palade body membranes to the cell surface, where it can bind leukocytes.
  - *Induction of adhesion molecules on endothelium.* IL-1 and tumor necrosis factor (TNF) increase endothelial expression of E-selectin, ICAM-1, and VCAM-1.
  - *Increased avidity of binding.* Integrins are normally present on leukocytes in a low-affinity form; they are converted to high-affinity forms by a variety of chemokines.

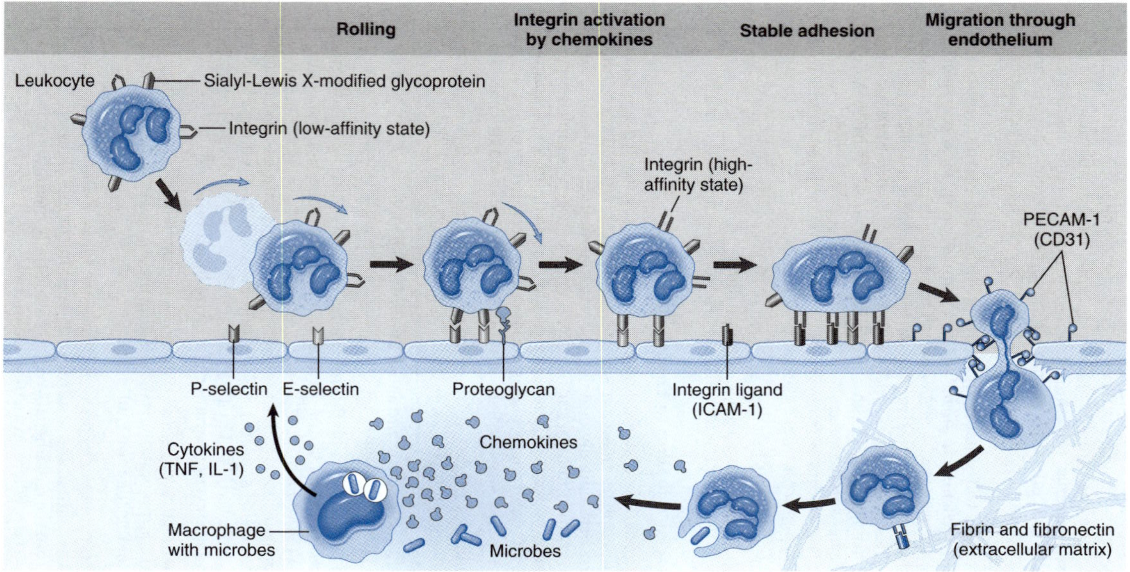

Figure 3-3 Multistep process of leukocyte migration through blood vessels, shown here for neutrophils. The leukocytes first roll (are loosely adherent with intermittent attachment and detachment of receptors), then (in sequence) become activated and firmly adhere to endothelium, transmigrate across the endothelium, pierce the basement membrane, and migrate toward chemoattractants emanating from the source of injury. Different molecules play predominant roles in different steps of this process—selectins in rolling, chemokines in activating the neutrophils to increase avidity of integrins, integrins in firm adhesion, and CD31 (PECAM-1) in transmigration.

TABLE 3-2 Endothelial and Leukocyte Adhesion Molecules

Family	Molecule	Distribution	Ligand
Selectin	L-selectin (CD62L)	Neutrophils, monocytes T cells (naïve and central memory) B cells (naïve)	Sialyl-Lewis X/PNAd on GlyCAM-1, CD34, MAdCAM-1, others; expressed on endothelium (HEV)
	E-selectin (CD62E)	Endothelium activated by cytokines (TNF, IL-1)	Sialyl-Lewis X (e.g., CLA) on glycoproteins; expressed on neutrophils, monocytes, T cells (effector, memory)
	P-selectin (CD62P)	Endothelium activated by cytokines (TNF, IL-1), histamine, or thrombin	Sialyl-Lewis X on PSGL-1 and other glycoproteins; expressed on neutrophils, monocytes, T cells (effector, memory)
Integrin	LFA-1 (CD11aCD18)	Neutrophils, monocytes, T cells (naïve, effector, memory)	ICAM-1 (CD54), ICAM-2 (CD102); expressed on endothelium (upregulated on activated endothelium)
	MAC-1 (CD11bCD18)	Monocytes, DCs	ICAM-1 (CD54), ICAM-2 (CD102); expressed on endothelium (upregulated on activated endothelium)
	VLA-4 (CD49aCD29)	Monocytes T cells (naïve, effector, memory)	VCAM-1 (CD106); expressed on endothelium (upregulated on activated endothelium)
	$\alpha 4\beta 7$ (CD49DCD29)	Monocytes T cells (gut homing naïve effector, memory)	VCAM-1 (CD106), MAdCAM-1; expressed on endothelium in gut and gut-associated lymphoid tissues
Ig	CD31	Endothelial cells, leukocytes	CD31 (homotypic interaction)

CLA, Cutaneous lymphocyte antigen-1; *GlyCAM-1,* glycan-bearing cell adhesion molecule-1; *HEV,* high endothelial venule; *Ig,* immunoglobulin; *MAdCAM-1,* mucosal adhesion cell adhesion molecule-1; *PNAd,* peripheral node addressin; *PSGL-1,* P-selectin glycoprotein ligand-1.

Leukocyte Migration Through Endothelium (p. 76)

Transmigration (also called diapedesis) is mediated by homotypic (like-like) interactions between platelet-endothelial cell adhesion molecule 1 (PECAM-1, CD31) on leukocytes and endothelial cells; it occurs primarily in postcapillary venules.

Chemotaxis of Leukocytes (p. 77)

After emigrating through interendothelial junctions and traversing the basement membrane, leukocytes move toward sites of injury along gradients of chemotactic agents *(chemotaxis)*. For neutrophils these agents include exogenous bacterial products and endogenous mediators (see later), such as complement fragments (particularly C5a), arachidonic acid (AA) metabolites (particularly LT B_4), and chemokines (e.g., interleukin-8).

Chemotactic agents bind to specific leukocyte surface G protein-coupled receptors; these trigger the production of phosphoinositol second messengers, in turn causing increased cytosolic calcium and GTPase activities that polymerize actin and facilitate cell movement. Leukocytes move by extending pseudopods that bind the extracellular matrix (ECM) and then pull the cell forward (front-wheel drive).

Phagocytosis and Clearance of the Offending Agents (p. 78)

Recognition through any of the preceding receptors induces *leukocyte activation* (Fig. 3-1). The most important consequences of activation are enhanced phagocytosis and intracellular killing, along with the release of cytokines, growth factors, and inflammatory mediators (e.g., prostaglandins [PGs]).

Phagocytosis (p. 78)

Phagocytosis involves (1) recognition and attachment of a particle to the leukocyte, (2) engulfment, and (3) killing and degradation of the ingested material (Fig. 3-4).

Phagocytic Receptors (p. 78)

- *Mannose receptors* bind terminal mannose and fucose residues of glycoproteins and glycolipids found on microbial cell walls (mammalian glycoproteins and glycolipids have terminal sialic acid or *N*-acetylgalactosamine).
- *Scavenger receptors* bind and mediate endocytosis of oxidized or acetylated low-density lipoprotein (LDL) particles, as well as a variety of microbes. Macrophage integrins, notably Mac-1 (CD11b/CD18), can also mediate microbial phagocytosis.
- *Opsonins.* Phagocytic efficiency is greatly enhanced when microbes are coated by specific proteins *(opsonized)* for which the phagocytes express high-affinity receptors. The major opsonins are IgG antibodies, the C3b breakdown product of complement, and mannose-binding lectin.

Engulfment (p. 78)

After binding to receptors, cytoplasmic pseudopods enclose the particle and eventually form a *phagosome* vesicle. Subsequent fusion of phagosomes and lysosomes (forming a *phagolysosome*) discharges lysosomal contents into the space around the microbe but can also occasionally dump lysosomal granules into the extracellular space.

Intracellular Destruction of Microbes and Debris (p. 79)

Killing of phagocytosed microbes is accomplished largely by ROS and reactive nitrogen species, mostly from nitric oxide (NO). This is most efficient in activated leukocytes.

***Reactive Oxygen Species** (p. 79).* Phagocytosis stimulates an oxidative burst—a surge of oxygen consumption that produces reactive oxygen metabolites via activation of nicotinamide-adenine dinucleotide phosphate (NADPH) oxidase. The enzyme converts oxygen to superoxide anion (O_2^-), eventually resulting in hydrogen peroxide (H_2O_2). Lysosomal myeloperoxidase (MPO) then converts H_2O_2 and Cl^- into the highly bactericidal HOCl (hypochlorite—the active ingredient in bleach).

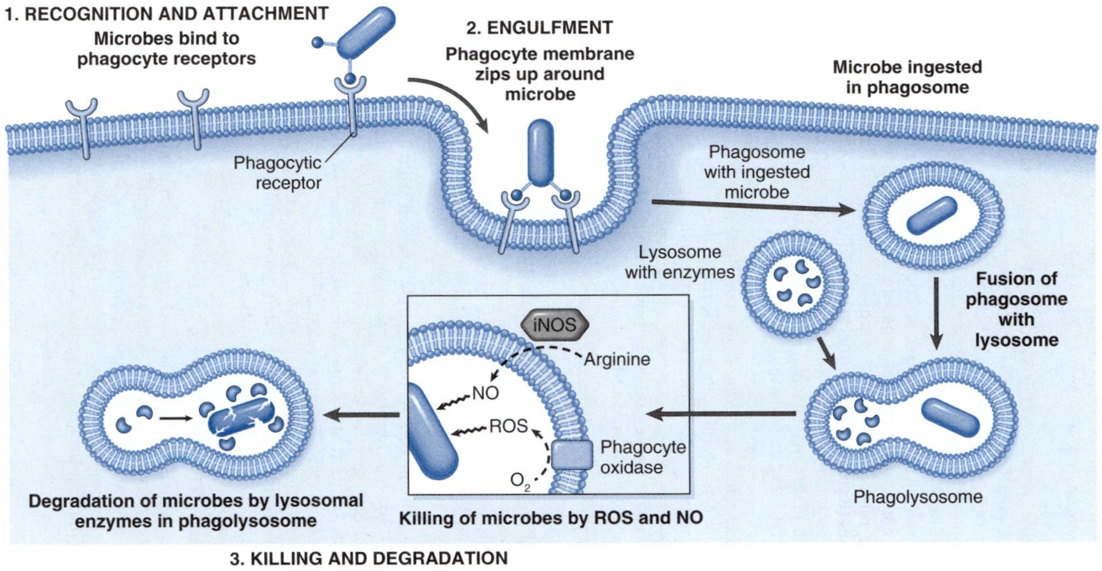

Figure 3-4 Phagocytosis and intracellular destruction of microbes. Phagocytosis of a particle (e.g., a bacterium) involves binding to receptors on the leukocyte membrane, engulfment, and fusion of the phagocytic vacuoles with lysosomes. This is followed by destruction of ingested particles within the phagolysosomes by lysosomal enzymes and by reactive oxygen and nitrogen species. The microbicidal products generated from superoxide (O_2^-) are hypochlorite ($HOCl^-$) and hydroxyl radical (^-OH), and from NO it is peroxynitrite ($OONO^-$). During phagocytosis, granule contents may be released into extracellular tissues (not shown).

Oxygen-derived free radicals (including $O_2^{\bullet-}$, H_2O_2, and hydroxyl radical) can be released extracellularly and cause local tissue damage. Tissues are normally protected from the damaging effects of ROS by multiple pathways (see Chapter 2), including enzymes that degrade them (e.g., superoxide dismutase, catalase, and glutathione peroxidase) and serum proteins that scavenge them. The net effect depends on the balance between production and inactivation.

Nitric Oxide *(p. 80).* NO is synthesized from arginine, molecular oxygen, NADPH, and other cofactors by *nitric oxide synthase* (NOS). Three types of NOS (endothelial [eNOS], neuronal [nNOS], and cytokine inducible [iNOS]) exist, each with distinct expression patterns: (1) eNOS and nNOS are constitutively expressed but are activated with increased cytoplasmic calcium, and (2) iNOS is synthesized by macrophages after exposure to certain cytokines (e.g., IFN-γ).

Nitrogen species, such as peroxynitrite radical ($ONOO^{\bullet}$), derived from NO and superoxide modify lipids, proteins, and nucleic acids and are highly microbicidal. NO also relaxes vascular smooth muscle, promoting vasodilation.

Lysosomal Enzymes and Other Lysosomal Proteins *(p. 80).* Microbes can also be killed via leukocyte granule molecules that increase membrane permeability (e.g., bactericidal permeability increasing protein, cathelicidins, lysozyme, lactoferrin, major basic protein of eosinophils, and defensins). Release of lysosome granules also contributes to the inflammatory response and tissue injury.

- *Neutrophils* have two types of granules:
  - *Azurophil (or primary) granules* contain MPO, bactericidal factors (lysozyme, defensins), acid hydrolases, and a variety of neutral proteases (elastase, cathepsin G, collagenases).
  - *Specific (or secondary) granules* contain lysozyme, collagenase, gelatinase, lactoferrin, plasminogen activator, and histaminase.
- Granule content can be prematurely released from phagocytic vacuoles not yet completely surrounding engulfed material and can be directly secreted or released from dead cells. Although acid proteases are normally active only within phagolysosomes, neutral proteases can function at neutral pH.
- Multiple serum and tissue *antiproteases* (e.g., α_1-antitrypsin inhibits neutrophil elastase) modulate the enzymatic activity; inhibitor deficiencies can result in disease.

Neutrophil Extracellular Traps *(NETs; p. 81)*

NETs are a viscous meshwork of nuclear chromatin that binds and concentrates granule proteins, such as antimicrobial peptides and enzymes; they can also physically trap microbes. NET formation leads to neutrophil death, and NET nuclear chromatin is a likely source of nuclear antigens in systemic autoimmune diseases (see Chapter 6).

Leukocyte-Mediated Tissue Injury *(p. 81)*

During activation and phagocytosis, leukocytes can cause tissue injury by releasing mediators into the extracellular space:

- Normal responses to pathogens cause "collateral damage"; this may be especially important for difficult to eradicate microbes with persistent inflammation (e.g., tuberculosis).

- Responses inappropriately directed against host tissues (*autoimmune disease;* see Chapter 6).
- As an overexuberant response against "harmless" substances (e.g., *allergic reactions*).

The mechanisms underlying the damage inflicted are the same as those involved in antimicrobial defense. The most relevant mediators include the following:

- *Lysosomal enzymes,* regurgitated during *frustrated phagocytosis* (large indigestible materials), premature fusion of lysosomes with forming phagosomes, or when lysosomes are damaged by ingested material (e.g., urate crystals).
- Oxygen- and nitrogen-derived reactive metabolites.

Other Functional Responses of Activated Leukocytes (p. 82)

Activated leukocytes—especially macrophages—produce:

- Cytokines that can amplify or limit inflammatory reactions.
- Growth factors that stimulate endothelial cell and fibroblast proliferation and can drive collagen synthesis.
- Enzymes that remodel connective tissues.

T cells can also contribute to acute inflammation via the production of IL-17 (by so-called T_H17 cells; see Chapter 6); among other activities, IL-17 induces the chemokines that recruit other leukocytes.

Termination of the Acute Inflammatory Response (p. 82)

Inflammation declines in part because mediators are produced only transiently and typically have short half-lives. Inflammation is also regulated by stop signals that are activated. These include the following:

- Switch from proinflammatory arachidonate metabolites *(LTs)* to antiinflammatory forms *(lipoxins)*
- Production of antiinflammatory cytokines, such as transforming growth factor-β (TGF-β) and IL-10
- Synthesis of fatty acid-derived antiinflammatory mediators (*resolvins* and *protectins*)
- Neural impulses that inhibit macrophage TNF production

Mediators of Inflammation (p. 82)

The vascular and cellular events of inflammation are mediated by molecules derived either from plasma or from cells (Table 3-3). Plasma-derived mediators are typically synthesized in the liver and circulate as inactive precursors, which are activated by proteolysis. Cell-derived mediators are either preformed and released by granule exocytosis (leading to immediate activity) or synthesized de novo following a stimulus (with some intrinsic lag time).

- Mediators are produced in response to either microbial products or factors released by necrotic tissues, thus ensuring that inflammation is normally triggered only when and where it is required.
- Most mediators act by binding to specific receptors, although some have direct enzymatic activity (e.g., proteases) or mediate oxidative damage (e.g., ROS).
- Mediators can act in amplifying or regulatory cascades to stimulate the release of other downstream factors.

TABLE 3-3 The Actions of the Principal Mediators of Inflammation

Mediator	Principal Sources	Actions
Cell-Derived		
Histamine	Mast cells, basophils, platelets	Vasodilation, increased vascular permeability, endothelial activation
Serotonin	Platelets	Vasodilation, increased vascular permeability
PGs	Mast cells, leukocytes	Vasodilation, pain, fever
LTs	Mast cells, leukocytes	Increased vascular permeability, chemotaxis, leukocyte adhesion and activation
PAF	Leukocytes, mast cells	Vasodilation, increased vascular permeability, leukocyte adhesion, chemotaxis, degranulation, oxidative burst
ROS	Leukocytes	Killing of microbes, tissue damage
NO	Endothelium, macrophages	Vascular smooth muscle relaxation, killing of microbes
Cytokines (TNF, IL-1)	Macrophages, endothelial cells, mast cells	Local endothelial activation (expression of adhesion molecules), fever/pain/anorexia/hypotension, decreased vascular resistance (shock)
Chemokines	Leukocytes, activated macrophages	Chemotaxis, leukocyte activation
Plasma Protein-Derived		
Complement products (C5a, C3a, C4a)	Plasma (produced in liver)	Leukocyte chemotaxis and activation, vasodilation (mast cell stimulation)
Kinins	Plasma (produced in liver)	Increased vascular permeability, smooth muscle contraction, vasodilation, pain
Protease activated during coagulation	Plasma (produced in liver)	Endothelial activation, leukocyte recruitment

- Once generated, most mediators are short-lived, being degraded by enzymes, subdued by specific inhibitors, scavenged by antioxidants, or just decaying spontaneously.

Vasoactive Amines: Histamine and Serotonin (p. 83)

Released from preformed cellular stores, these are among the first mediators in inflammation; *they cause arteriolar dilation and increased permeability of venules.*

Mast cells are the major source of histamine; basophils and platelets also contribute. Mast cell release is caused by physical agents (e.g., trauma, heat), allergic immune reactions involving IgE (see Chapter 6), complement fragments C3a and C5a *(anaphylatoxins)*, cytokines (e.g., IL-1 and IL-8), neuropeptides (e.g., *substance P*), and leukocyte-derived histamine-releasing factors.

Serotonin (5-hydroxytryptamine) has activities similar to histamine; major sources are platelets and neuroendocrine cells (not mast cells). Platelet release of both histamine and serotonin is stimulated by contact with collagen, thrombin, adenosine diphosphate (ADP), and antigen-antibody complexes, one of several links between clotting and inflammation.

Arachidonic Acid Metabolites (p. 83)

Activated cells release membrane-bound AA through the enzymatic activity of phospholipase A_2. The 20-carbon polyunsaturated AA is then catabolized to generate short-range lipid mediators *(eicosanoids)* through the activities of two major enzyme classes (Fig. 3-5). Eicosanoids bind to membrane G protein-coupled receptors and can mediate almost every aspect of inflammation (Table 3-4).

Prostaglandins (p. 84)

- PGs are produced by a variety of cells including mast cells, macrophages, endothelial cells, and platelets. They are generated by two forms of the enzyme *cyclooxygenase (COX):*
    - COX-1 can be induced by inflammation but is also constitutively expressed in a number of tissues, where it plays a homeostatic role (e.g., fluid and electrolyte balance in the kidneys, cytoprotection in the gastrointestinal [GI] tract).
    - COX-2 is induced by inflammatory stimuli but is low or absent in most normal tissues.
- Different PGs are coded by a letter (e.g., PGD, PGE), with a subscript numeral indicating the number of double bonds; each is derived by the action of a specific enzyme (some with restricted tissue distributions) on a pathway intermediate.
    - Platelets contain the enzyme *thromboxane synthase* that uniquely generates *thromboxane* (TxA_2), a potent platelet-aggregating agent and vasoconstrictor.
    - Endothelium lacks thromboxane synthase but possesses *prostacyclin synthase* and thus uniquely generates *prostacyclin* (PGI_2), a vasodilator and potent inhibitor of platelet aggregation.
    - Mast cells synthesize PGD_2, causing vasodilation, increasing vascular permeability, and recruiting neutrophils. PGE_2, has similar vasodilatory and permeability effects but is synthesized by a wider variety of cells.
    - $PGF_{2\alpha}$ stimulates the contraction of uterine and bronchial smooth muscle and small arterioles.
    - PGs also mediate *pain* and *fever* in inflammation; thus PGE_2 is involved in cytokine-induced fevers and is *hyperalgesic,* rendering the skin hypersensitive to painful stimuli.
- *LTs* (p.85) influence smooth muscle reactivity and help to recruit leukocytes; they are produced by leukocytes and mast cells through the action of *lipoxygenases:*
    - *5-Lipoxygenase* is the major form in neutrophils, generating 5-hydroxyeicosatetraenoic acid (5-HETE), which is chemotactic for neutrophils and the precursor to LTs.
    - LTB_4 is a potent chemotactic agent and activator of neutrophils, causing the generation of ROS and release of lysosomal enzymes.
    - LTC_4, LTD_4, and LTE_4 are cysteinyl-containing LTs; they cause vasoconstriction, bronchospasm (important in asthma), and increased vascular permeability.

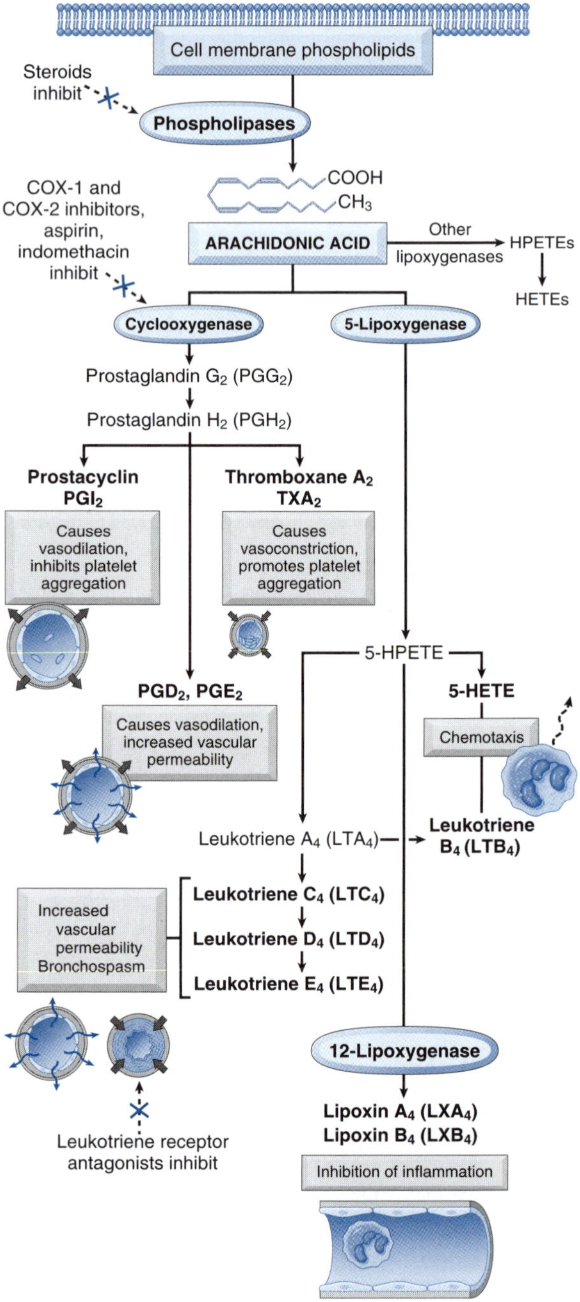

Figure 3-5 Production of AA metabolites and their roles in inflammation. Note the points where pharmacologic inhibitors can block the major pathways (denoted with an X). *COX-1, COX-2,* Cyclooxygenase 1 and 2; *HETE,* hydroxyeicosatetraenoic acid; *HPETE,* hydroperoxyeicosatetraenoic acid.

TABLE 3-4 Principal Inflammatory Actions of Arachidonic Acid Metabolites (Eicosanoids)	
Action	**Eicosanoid**
Vasodilation	PGI_2 (prostacyclin), PGE_1, PGE_2, PGD_2
Vasoconstriction	TxA_2, LTs C_4, D_4, E_4
Increased vascular permeability	LTs C_4, D_4, E_4
Chemotaxis, leukocyte adhesion	LT B_4, HETE

- *Lipoxins* (p. 85) are also generated by the lipoxygenase pathway; however, these AA metabolites inhibit neutrophil adhesion and chemotaxis, thus reducing leukocyte recruitment. They are unusual because two cell populations are required for their synthesis; neutrophils produce precursor molecules that are then converted to lipoxins by platelets.

Pharmacologic Inhibitors of Prostaglandins and Leukotrienes *(p. 85)*

- *COX inhibitors* include aspirin and other nonsteroidal antiinflammatory drugs (NSAIDs); by blocking PG synthesis these reduce pain and fever. Most NSAIDs inhibit both COX isoforms; aspirin irreversibly acetylates the proteins, whereas the other NSAIDs are typically reversible. COX-1 is expressed in a wide variety of tissues, generating PGs that influence not only inflammation but also homeostatic functions, such as fluid and electrolyte balance in the kidneys and gastric cytoprotection. COX-2 has a slightly different pattern of expression and generates PGs primarily involved in only inflammation, thus driving the generation of selective COX-2 inhibitors. However, the distinctions are not absolute; COX-2 also likely plays a role in normal homeostasis. Moreover, selective COX-2 inhibitors appear to increase cardiovascular and cerebrovascular risk; they impair endothelial PGI_2 production while leaving platelet COX-1-mediated TxA_2 production intact.
- *Lipoxygenase and LT receptor antagonists.* 5-Lipoxygenase is not affected by NSAIDs; new agents that do inhibit LT production are useful for treating asthma, as are newer drugs that block LT receptors.
- *Corticosteroids* are broad-spectrum antiinflammatory agents that reduce the transcription of genes encoding COX-2, phospholipase A_2, proinflammatory cytokines (e.g., IL-1 and TNF), and iNOS.
- *Dietary modifications (e.g., certain polyunsaturated fatty acids in fish oil)* can reduce inflammation by conversion to antiinflammatory lipid products rather than proinflammatory PGs and LTs.

Cytokines and Chemokines *(p. 86 and see Chapter 6)*

Cytokines are proteins produced principally by activated lymphocytes and macrophages (but also endothelium, epithelium, and connective tissue cells) that modulate the function of other cell types. *Chemokines* are cytokines that also stimulate leukocyte movement (chemotaxis) (Table 3-5).

Tumor Necrosis Factor and Interleukin-1 (p. 86)

Produced primarily by activated macrophages, these are two of the most important cytokines mediating inflammation. They affect endothelium, leukocyte, and fibroblast activation, as well as induce systemic responses (Fig. 3-6).

TABLE 3-5 Cytokines in Inflammation

Cytokine	Principal Sources	Principal Actions in Inflammation
In Acute Inflammation		
TNF	Macrophages, mast cells, T lymphocytes	Stimulates expression of endothelial adhesion molecules and secretion of other cytokines; systemic effects
IL-1	Macrophages, endothelial cells, some epithelial cells	Similar to TNF; greater role in fever
IL-6	Macrophages, other cells	Systemic effects (acute phase response)
Chemokines	Macrophages, endothelial cells, T lymphocytes, mast cells, other cell types	Recruitment of leukocytes to sites of inflammation; migration of cells in normal tissues
IL-17	T lymphocytes	Recruitment of neutrophils and monocytes
In Chronic Inflammation		
IL-12	Dendritic cells, macrophages	Increased production of IFN-γ
IFN-γ	T lymphocytes, NK cells	Activation of macrophages (increased ability to kill microbes and tumor cells)
IL-17	T lymphocytes	Recruitment of neutrophils and monocytes

The most important cytokines involved in inflammatory reactions are listed. Many other cytokines may play lesser roles in inflammation. There is also considerable overlap between the cytokines involved in acute and chronic inflammation. Specifically, all the cytokines listed under acute inflammation may also contribute to chronic inflammatory reactions.
IFN-γ, Interferon-γ; *NK cells,* natural killer cells.

- Secretion is stimulated by endotoxin, immune complexes, toxins, physical injury, and a variety of inflammatory products.
- Endothelial activation increases the expression of adhesion molecules and chemical mediators (e.g., cytokines, chemokines, growth factors, eicosanoids, and NO), enzymes associated with matrix remodeling, and endothelial thrombogenicity.
- IL-1 and TNF induce systemic *acute-phase responses* associated with infection or injury: fever; anorexia; lethargy; neutrophilia; and release of corticotropin and corticosteroids.
- TNF also *regulates body mass* by promoting lipid and protein mobilization and by suppressing appetite. Sustained elevations in TNF (e.g., due to neoplasm or chronic infections) thus contribute to *cachexia,* a pathologic state characterized by weight loss and anorexia.

Chemokines (p. 87)

Chemokines are a family (>40 known) of small proteins expressed by multiple cell types that act primarily as leukocyte chemoattractants and activators. Chemokines are classified into four major classes, according to the arrangement of conserved cysteine (C) residues:

- *CXC chemokines* have one amino acid residue separating the first two conserved cysteine residues; their major activity involves neutrophil recruitment. IL-8 is typical of this group; it is produced by macrophages and endothelial cells after activation by TNF and IL-1 or microbial products.

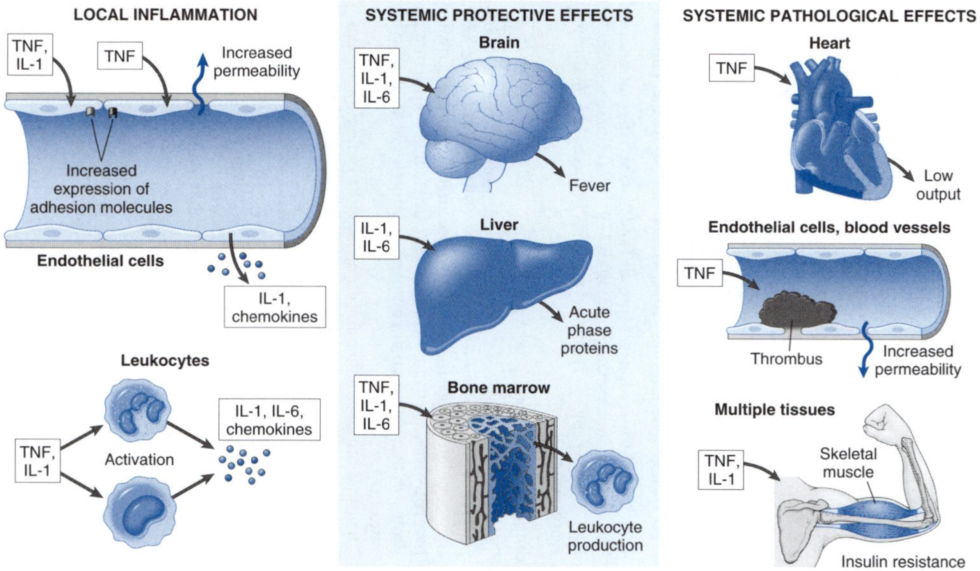

Figure 3-6 Major roles of cytokines in acute inflammation.

- *CC chemokines* have the first two conserved cysteine residues adjacent. CC chemokines (e.g., *monocyte chemoattractant protein-1*) generally recruit monocytes, eosinophils, basophils, and lymphocytes but not neutrophils. Although many chemokines in this class have overlapping properties, *eotaxin* selectively recruits eosinophils.
- *C chemokines* lack two of the four conserved cysteines; these are relatively specific for lymphocytes (e.g., *lymphotactin*).
- The only known *CX_3C chemokine* is *fractalkine.* It exists in two forms: an endothelial surface-bound protein (promotes firm mononuclear cell adhesion) or a soluble form—derived by proteolysis of the membrane-bound form (chemoattractant for mononuclear cells).

Chemokines mediate their activities by binding to G protein-linked receptors (>20 known), designated CXCR for the CXC chemokines and CCR for the CC chemokines. Cells typically express more than one receptor type. There is also receptor-ligand "promiscuity": thus many different chemokine ligands can bind to the same receptor, and multiple receptors can frequently bind the same ligand.

Other Cytokines in Acute Inflammation (p. 88)

The list is long—and growing. However, two of note are the following:

- IL-6: Made by macrophages (mostly) and involved in multiple local and systemic inflammatory responses (e.g., acute phase responses).
- IL-17: Made by T lymphocytes and involved in neutrophil recruitment.

Complement System *(p. 88; Fig. 3-7)*

- The complement system comprises >20 proteins; the most important are numbered C1 through C9. Synthesized by the liver, they circulate in plasma as inactive precursors that are activated by proteolysis. Activated complement fragments are themselves proteases that cleave other complement proteins in an amplifying cascade.
- The most important step for complement's biologic activities is activation of the C3 component. C3 cleavage can occur through three possible mechanisms: the *classical pathway* triggered by C1 binding to antigen-antibody complexes; the *alternative pathway,* triggered—in the absence of antibody—by microbial surface molecules (e.g., endotoxin), complex polysaccharides, or cobra venom; and the *lectin pathway,* in which C1 is activated by microbe carbohydrates interacting with circulating mannose-binding lectins.
- C3 cleavage results in functionally distinct fragments, C3a and C3b. C3a is released, whereas C3b becomes covalently attached to the site where complement is being activated. C3b and other complement fragments combine to cleave C5 into C5a and C5b pieces.
- The biologic functions of complement fall into three general categories: *cell lysis, inflammation,* and *opsonization.*
  - *Cell lysis:* C5b binds the late components (C6 to C9), culminating in the formation of the membrane attack complex (MAC, composed of multiple C9 molecules) that punches holes in cell membranes.
  - Inflammation:
    - C3a and C5a (so-called *anaphylatoxins*) stimulate histamine release from mast cells and thereby increase vascular permeability and vasodilation.

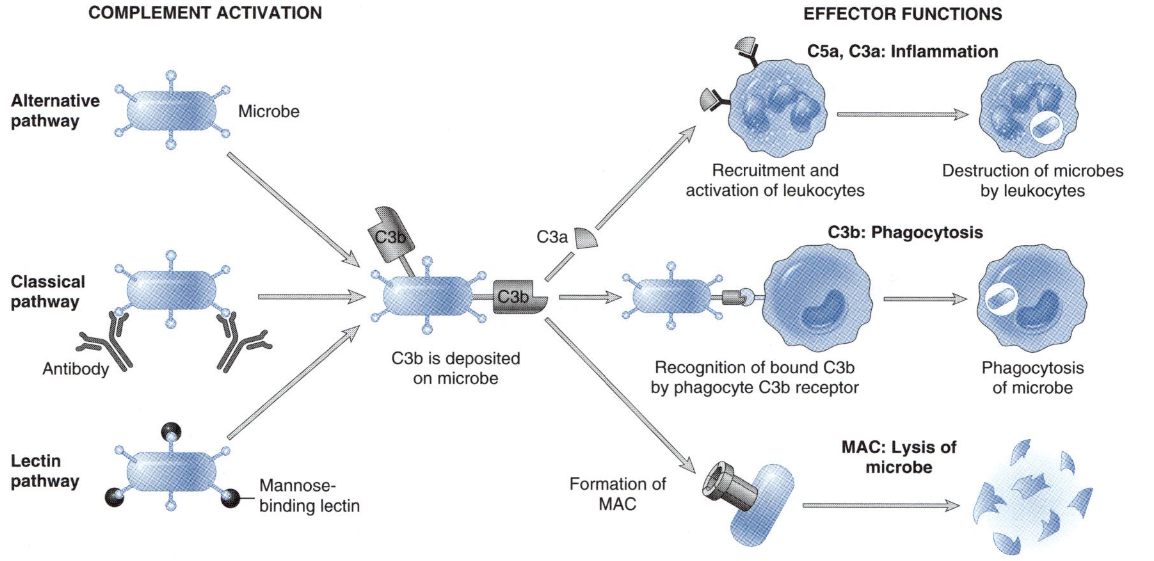

Figure 3-7 Activation and functions of the complement system. Activation of complement by different pathways leads to cleavage of C3. The functions of the complement system are mediated by breakdown products of C3 and other complement proteins and by the MAC.

    - C5a activates the arachidonate metabolism causing additional inflammatory mediator release.
    - C5a is a powerful leukocyte chemoattractant.
  - *Opsonization:* Binding of C3b—or its "inactive" degradation product iC3b—promotes phagocytosis by neutrophils and macrophages through specific C3b receptors.
- Complement activation is tightly regulated by cell-associated and circulating proteins.
  - *C1 inhibitor* blocks C1 activation; deficiency leads to *hereditary angioedema.*
  - Glycophosphatidylinositol (GPI)-linked membrane-anchored proteins:
    - *Decay accelerating factor* (DAF) prevents C3 convertase formation.
    - CD59 inhibits MAC formation.
    - Acquired deficiencies in the enzyme that makes the GPI linker leads to deficient DAF and CD59 expression and excessive complement activation with erythrocyte lysis *(paroxysmal nocturnal hemoglobinuria).*

Other Mediators of Inflammation (p. 89)

Platelet-Activating Factor (p. 89)

Platelet-activating factor (PAF) is a phospholipid-derived mediator produced by mast cells, platelets, leukocytes, and endothelium. In addition to platelet aggregation and granule release (hence its name), PAF can elicit most of the vascular and cellular reactions of inflammation: vasodilation and increased vascular permeability (100 to 10,000 times more potent than histamine), bronchoconstriction, increased leukocyte adhesion, chemotaxis, and the oxidative burst.

Products of Coagulation (p. 89)

Protease-activated receptors (PARs), expressed on platelets and leukocytes, are activated by thrombin (the protease that cleaves fibrinogen to produce fibrin in the coagulation cascade).

Kinins (p. 89)

Kinins are vasoactive peptides derived from plasma protein *kininogens; kallikrein* cleaves *high-molecular-weight kininogen* to produce *bradykinin,* a product that increases vascular permeability, smooth muscle contraction, blood vessel dilation, and pain.

Neuropeptides (p. 89)

Neuropeptides are small peptides (e.g., substance P and neurokinin A) secreted by sensory nerves and various leukocytes; they can initiate and regulate inflammatory responses, including pain transmission.

Morphologic Patterns of Acute Inflammation (p. 90)

Although all acute inflammatory reactions are characterized by vascular changes and leukocyte infiltration, distinctive morphologic changes can be superimposed that suggest a specific underlying cause.

Serous Inflammation (p. 90)

Serous inflammation is marked by fluid transudates, reflecting moderately increased vascular permeability. Such accumulations in the peritoneal, pleural, and pericardial cavities are called *effusions;* serous fluid can also accumulate elsewhere (e.g., burn blisters in skin).

Fibrinous Inflammation (p. 90)

Fibrinous inflammation is a more marked increase in vascular permeability, with exudates containing large amounts of fibrinogen. The fibrinogen is converted to fibrin through coagulation system activation. Involvement of serosal surfaces (e.g., pericardium or pleura) is referred to as *fibrinous pericarditis* or *pleuritis.* Fibrinous exudates can be resolved by fibrinolysis and macrophage clearance of debris. Larger exudates that cannot be cleared will be converted to fibrous scar *(organization)* by the ingrowth of vessels and fibroblasts.

Purulent (Suppurative) Inflammation and Abscess (p. 91)

This pattern is characterized by purulent exudates *(pus)* consisting of neutrophils, necrotic cells, and edema. An *abscess* is a localized collection of purulent inflammation accompanied by liquefactive necrosis, often in the setting of bacterial seeding. With time these may be walled off and then organized into fibrous scar.

Ulcers (p. 91)

Ulcers are local erosions of epithelial surfaces produced by sloughing of inflamed necrotic tissue (e.g., gastric ulcers).

Outcomes of Acute Inflammation (p. 92)

Acute inflammation will be affected by the nature and intensity of injury, the tissue involved, and host responsiveness; the process has one of three general outcomes:

- *Complete resolution,* with regeneration of native cells and restoration to normalcy.
- *Healing by connective tissue replacement (fibrosis)* occurs after substantial tissue destruction, when inflammation occurs in nonregenerating tissues, or in the setting of abundant fibrin exudation (also called *organization*).
- *Progression to chronic inflammation.*

Summary of Acute Inflammation (p. 93)

When encountering an injurious agent (e.g., microbe or dead cells), phagocytes attempt to eliminate these agents and secrete cytokines, PGs, LTs, and other mediators. These act on vascular wall cells to induce vasodilation and on endothelial cells specifically to promote plasma efflux and further leukocyte recruitment. Recruited leukocytes are activated and will phagocytize offending agents, as well as produce additional mediators. As the injurious agent is eliminated, antiinflammatory counter-regulatory mechanisms quench the process, and the host returns to a normal state of health. If the injurious agent cannot be effectively eliminated, the result may be chronic inflammation.

Chronic Inflammation (p. 93)

Chronic inflammation is a prolonged process (weeks or months) in which active inflammation, tissue destruction, and healing all proceed simultaneously. It occurs because of the following:

- After acute inflammation, as part of the normal healing process.
- Due to persistence of an inciting stimulus or repeated bouts of acute inflammation.
- As a low-grade, smoldering response *without* prior acute inflammation.

Causes of Chronic Inflammation (p. 93)

- Persistent infection by intracellular microbes (e.g., tubercle bacilli, viruses) of low direct toxicity but nevertheless capable of evoking immunologic responses
- Hypersensitivity diseases, particularly reactions directed against self (e.g., autoimmune diseases) or abnormally regulated responses to normal host flora (inflammatory bowel disease) or benign environmental substances (allergy) (see Chapter 6)
- Prolonged exposure to potentially toxic exogenous (e.g., silica, causing pulmonary silicosis) or endogenous substances (e.g., lipids, causing atherosclerosis)
- Diseases not conventionally considered inflammatory (e.g., neurodegenerative disorders [Alzheimer disease], metabolic syndrome, and cancers potentially driven by inflammation)

Morphologic Features (p. 93)

In contrast to acute inflammation—characterized by vascular changes, edema, and neutrophilic infiltration—chronic inflammation is typified by the following:

- *Infiltration with mononuclear inflammatory cells,* including macrophages, lymphocytes, and plasma cells
- *Tissue destruction,* induced by persistent injury and/or inflammation
- Attempts at *healing by connective tissue replacement,* accomplished by vascular proliferation *(angiogenesis)* and fibrosis

Cells and Mediators in Chronic Inflammation (p. 94)

Role of Macrophages (p. 94)

Macrophages are the dominant cellular players in chronic inflammation:

- Macrophages derive from circulating monocytes induced to emigrate across the endothelium by chemokines. After reaching the extravascular tissue, monocytes transform into the phagocytic macrophage.
- Macrophages are activated through cytokines produced by immune-activated T cells (especially IFN-γ) or by nonimmune factors (e.g., endotoxin). Depending on the nature of the stimulus (e.g., IFN-γ versus IL-4), macrophages are activated along one of two trajectories:
  - *Classical (M1)* macrophages are induced by microbial products, IFN-γ, or foreign substances including crystals; they secrete proinflammatory cytokines, produce NO and ROS, and upregulate lysosomal enzymes to increase their microbicidal capacity.
  - *Alternative (M2)* macrophages are activated by IL-4 and IL-13 and drive the process of wound repair through production of mediators that cause fibroblast proliferation, connective tissue production, and angiogenesis (Fig. 3-8).

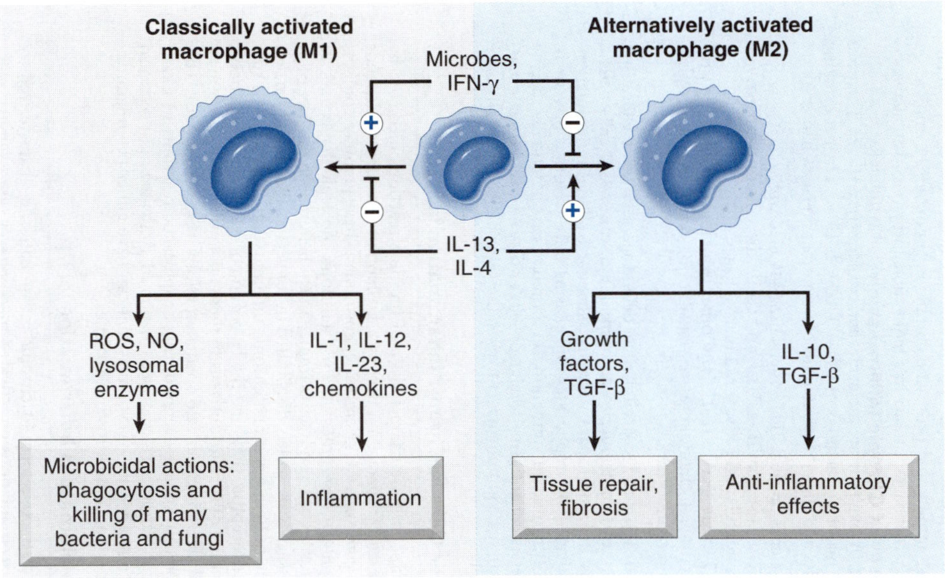

Figure 3-8 Classical and alternative macrophage activation. Different stimuli activate monocytes/macrophages to develop into functionally distinct populations. Classically activated macrophages are induced by microbial products and cytokines, particularly IFN-γ. They phagocytose and destroy microbes and dead tissues and can potentiate inflammatory reactions. Alternatively activated macrophages are induced by other cytokines and are important in tissue repair and the resolution of inflammation.

- Although macrophage products are important for host defense, some mediators induce tissue damage. These include ROS and NO, which are toxic to cells, and proteases that degrade ECM.
- In short-lived inflammation with clearance of the initial stimulus, macrophages relatively quickly die off or exit via lymphatics. In chronic inflammation, macrophage accumulation persists by continued recruitment of monocytes and local proliferation.

Role of Lymphocytes *(p. 96)*

Lymphocytes, activated by microbial and other environmental antigens, amplify and propagate chronic inflammation. Lymphocytes and macrophages interact in a bidirectional way (Fig. 3-9): activated macrophages present antigen to T cells and also influence T cell activation through surface molecules and cytokines (e.g. IL-12). There are three major populations of $CD4^+$ T cells that have distinct cytokine profiles and elicit different kinds of inflammation (see Chapter 6):

- T_H1 cells produce IFN-γ, activating M1 macrophages.
- T_H2 cells secrete IL-4, IL-5, and IL-10; these recruit and activate eosinophils and activate M2 macrophages.
- T_H17 cells secrete IL-17 (and other cytokines), driving the production of chemokines responsible for recruiting neutrophils (and monocytes).

Both T_H1 and T_H17 cells help to defend against many bacteria and viruses and contribute to autoimmune diseases. T_H2 cells defend against helminthic parasites and contribute to allergic inflammation.

Activated B lymphocytes and plasma cells are often present in sites of chronic inflammation; the antibodies are potentially specific for persistent antigens (foreign or self) or may be directed against altered tissue components. However, their specificity and importance is unclear.

Other Cells in Chronic Inflammation (p. 96)

- *Eosinophils* are characteristic of immune reactions mediated by IgE and in parasitic infections. Eosinophil recruitment depends on *eotaxin,* a CC chemokine. Eosinophils have granules containing *major basic protein (MBP),* a cationic molecule that is toxic to parasites but also lyses mammalian epithelium (see Chapter 6).
- *Mast cells* are widely distributed in connective tissues and participate in both acute and chronic inflammation. They express surface receptors that bind the Fc portion of IgE. In acute reactions, binding of specific antigens to these IgE antibodies leads to mast cell degranulation and mediator release (e.g., histamine). This type of response occurs during anaphylactic reactions to foods, insect venom, or drugs (see Chapter 6). Activated mast cells also secrete a wealth of cytokines that can have either proinflammatory or antiinflammatory activities.

Granulomatous Inflammation (p. 97)

This distinctive form of chronic inflammation is characterized by focal accumulations of activated macrophages *(granulomas);* macrophage activation is reflected by enlargement and flattening of the cells (so-called *epithelioid* macrophages).

- Nodules of epithelioid macrophages in granulomatous inflammation are surrounded by a collar of lymphocytes elaborating factors necessary to induce macrophage activation. Activated macrophages may fuse to form multinucleated *giant cells,* and central necrosis may be present in some granulomas (particularly from infectious causes). Older granulomas can be surrounded by a rim of fibrosis.

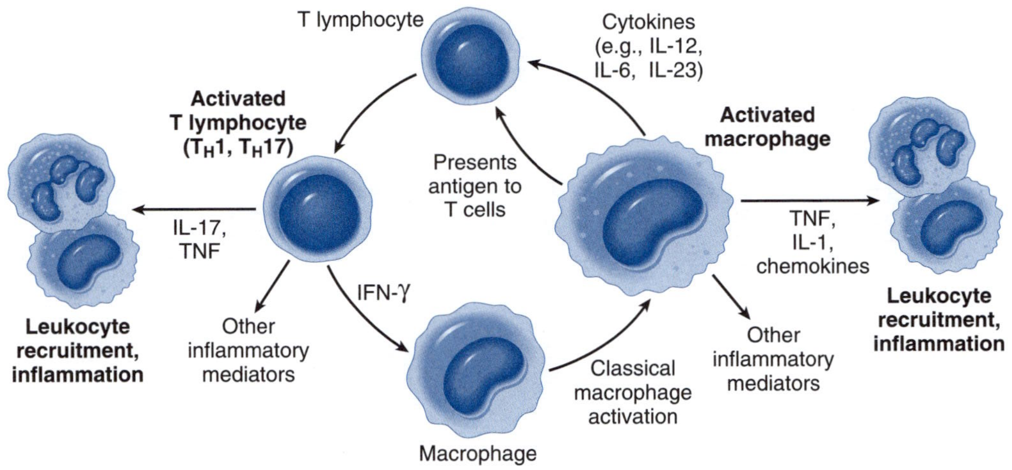

Figure 3-9 Macrophage-lymphocyte interactions in chronic inflammation. Activated T cells produce cytokines that recruit macrophages (TNF, IL-17, chemokines) and others that activate macrophages (IFN-γ). Activated macrophages in turn stimulate T cells by presenting antigens and via cytokines, such as IL-12.

- *Foreign body granulomas* are incited by particles that cannot be readily phagocytosed by a single macrophage but do not elicit a specific immune response (e.g., suture or talc).
- *Immune granulomas* are formed by immune T cell-mediated responses to persistent, poorly degradable antigens. IFN-γ from activated T cells causes the macrophage transformation to epithelioid cells and the formation of multinucleated giant cells. The prototypical immune granuloma is caused by the tuberculosis bacillus; in that setting the granuloma is called a *tubercle* and *classically exhibits central caseous necrosis.*
- *Granulomatous inflammation* is a distinctive inflammatory reaction with relatively few (albeit important) possible causes.
    - Infectious etiologies: Tuberculosis, leprosy, syphilis, cat-scratch disease, schistosomiasis, certain fungal infections
    - Inflammatory causes: Temporal arteritis, Crohn disease, sarcoidosis
    - Inorganic particulates: Silicosis, berylliosis

Systemic Effects of Inflammation (p. 99)

Systemic changes associated with inflammation are collectively called the acute phase response or—in severe cases—the systemic inflammatory response syndrome (SIRS). These represent responses to cytokines produced either by bacterial products (e.g., endotoxin) or by other inflammatory stimuli. The acute phase response consists of several clinical and pathologic changes:

- *Fever:* Temperature elevation (1 to 4° C) occurs in response to *pyrogens*—substances that stimulate PG synthesis in the hypothalamus. For example, endotoxin stimulates leukocyte release of IL-1 and TNF that increase COX production of PGs. In the hypothalamus, PGE_2 stimulates intracellular second signals (e.g., cyclic adenosine monophosphate [cAMP]) that reset the temperature set point. Aspirin reduces fever by inhibiting COX activity to block PG synthesis.
- *Acute-phase proteins* are plasma proteins mostly of hepatic origin; their synthesis increases several hundred-fold in response to inflammatory stimuli (e.g., cytokines, such as IL-6 and TNF). These include C-reactive protein (CRP), fibrinogen, and serum amyloid A (SAA) protein. CRP and SAA bind to microbial cell walls, acting as opsonins and fixing complement; they also help to clear necrotic cell nuclei and mobilize metabolic stores. Elevated fibrinogen leads to increased erythrocyte aggregation (increasing the *erythrocyte sedimentation rate* on ex vivo testing). Hepcidin is another acute-phase reactant responsible for regulating release of intracellular iron stores; chronically elevated hepcidin is responsible for the iron-deficiency anemia associated with chronic inflammation (see Chapter 14).
- *Leukocytosis* (increased white cell number in peripheral blood) is common in inflammatory reactions; there is an accelerated release of bone marrow cells, typically with immature neutrophils in the blood (so-called *shift to the left*). Prolonged infection also induces proliferation of bone marrow precursors due to increased colony-stimulating factor (CSF) production. The leukocyte count usually climbs to 15,000 to 20,000 cells/μL but can reach extraordinarily high levels of 40,000 to 100,000 cells/mL (referred to as a *leukemoid reaction*). Bacterial infections typically increase neutrophil numbers *(neutrophilia);* viral infections increase lymphocyte numbers *(lymphocytosis);* parasitic infestations and allergic disorders are associated with increased eosinophils *(eosinophilia).* Certain infections (typhoid fever, rickettsiae, and some viruses

and protozoans) are associated with decreased circulating white cell numbers *(leukopenia)*.

- *Other manifestations of the acute phase response:* Increased pulse and blood pressure; decreased sweating (due to blood flow diverted from cutaneous to deep vascular beds to limit heat loss); rigors (shivering), chills, anorexia, somnolence, and malaise, all attributed to cytokine effects on the central nervous system (CNS).
- In *sepsis,* organisms and/or endotoxin can stimulate the production of enormous quantities of several cytokines, notably TNF and IL-1. High levels of these cytokines result in a clinical triad of disseminated intravascular coagulation (DIC), metabolic disturbances, and cardiovascular failure described as septic shock (see Chapter 4).

Tissue Repair (p. 100)

Overview of Tissue Repair (p. 100)

Some tissues can be completely reconstituted after injury (e.g., bone after a fracture or epithelium after a superficial skin wound). Such *regeneration* can occur through the proliferation of adjacent surviving cells or through the activity of tissue stem cells.

However, in most cases the restorative capacity is limited, and severe tissue injury that results in extensive damage of parenchyma and/or stromal elements cannot heal by regeneration. In that setting a fibroproliferative response (also called *fibrosis*) deposits collagen and other ECM components *(scar)* that "patch" rather than restore a tissue. Resolution of inflammatory exudates can also lead to fibrosis, a process called *organization.*

In most cases healing is some combination of regeneration and scar; the outcome will be affected by (1) proliferative capacity of the damaged tissue, (2) integrity of the ECM, and (3) the chronicity of the associated inflammation.

Cell and Tissue Regeneration (p. 101)

Cell Proliferation: Signals and Control Mechanisms (p. 101)

Multiple cell types proliferate during tissue repair, including remnant cells of the injured tissue, endothelial cells (*angiogenesis* to provide the nutrients needed for repair), and fibroblasts (source of the scar ECM). The ability of the nonfibroblast and nonendothelial cells to restore normal tissue depends on their intrinsic proliferative capacity:

- *Labile (continuously dividing) tissues:* Such cells are constantly replaced by proliferation of mature cells and/or maturation from tissue stem cells. Examples include marrow hematopoietic cells and most surface epithelia (e.g., skin, oral cavity, ducts draining exocrine organs, GI tract, and urinary tract).
- *Stable tissues:* Such cells are quiescent (in G_0 of the cell cycle) with minimal baseline proliferative activity. However, they can divide after injury or loss of tissue mass. Examples include most solid tissue parenchyma (e.g., liver, kidney, and pancreas, as well as endothelial cells, fibroblasts, and smooth muscle cells).
- *Permanent tissues:* These cells are terminally differentiated and nonproliferative in postnatal life (e.g., cardiomyocytes and most neurons). Although there is limited stem cell replication and differentiation in heart and brain, it is insufficient to produce any significant tissue regeneration. Thus brain or cardiac injury is typically irreversible, resulting in scar. Skeletal muscle is usually also classified as "permanent," but satellite cells attached to the endomysial sheath provide some regenerative capacity for muscle.

Cell proliferation is driven by growth factors (synthesized by macrophages, epithelial, and stromal cells) and signals derived from integrin interactions with the ECM (see Chapter 1); some growth factors even bind to ECM proteins where they can be displayed at high concentrations.

Mechanisms of Tissue Regeneration *(p. 101)*

- In labile tissues, injured cells are rapidly replaced by proliferation of residual cells and differentiation of tissue stem cells—so long as the underlying basement membrane is intact. Loss of blood cells is corrected by proliferation of hematopoietic stem cells, driven by growth factors called CSFs.
- Tissue regeneration in parenchyma composed mostly of stable cell populations is usually limited; pancreas, adrenal, thyroid, and lung have some regenerative capacity, and nephrectomy elicits compensatory hypertrophy and hyperplasia of proximal duct cells in the remaining kidney. The exception is liver, which has extraordinary regenerative capacity (see later).
- Regardless of proliferative capacity, extensive tissue damage leads to incomplete regeneration, accompanied by scarring. Thus a liver abscess will lead to scar formation even though the remaining liver cells have the capacity to regenerate.

Liver Regeneration *(p. 102)*

Liver regeneration occurs by two major mechanisms: proliferation of remaining hepatocytes and repopulation from progenitor cells.

- *Proliferation of hepatocytes following partial hepatectomy:* Resection of up to 90% of the liver can be corrected by residual hepatocyte proliferation triggered by cytokines and polypeptide growth factors (Fig. 3-10).
  - In the priming phase, cytokines, such as IL-6 (from Kupffer cells), make remaining hepatocytes competent to respond to growth factor signals.
  - In the second phase, growth factors, such as hepatocyte growth factor (HGF) and TGF-α, act on primed hepatocytes to stimulate entry into the cell cycle.

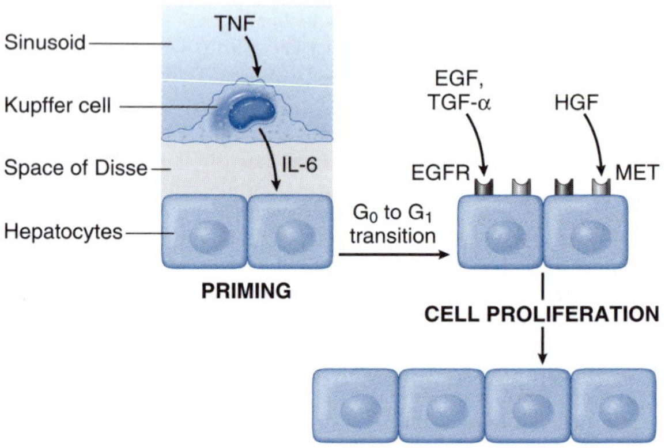

Figure 3-10 Liver regeneration through hepatocyte proliferation. Following partial hepatectomy, the liver regenerates by proliferation of surviving cells. The process occurs in stages, including priming, followed by growth factor-induced proliferation. The main signals involved in these steps are shown. Once the mass of the liver is restored, the proliferation is terminated (not shown). *EGF,* Epidermal growth factor; *EGFR,* epidermal growth factor receptor; *MET,* hepatocyte growth factor receptor.

- The wave of hepatocyte replication is followed by replication of nonparenchymal cells (Kupffer cells, endothelial cells, and stellate cells).
- In the termination phase, hepatocytes return to quiescence; antiproliferative cytokines of the TGF-β family are likely involved.

- *Liver regeneration from progenitor cells:* When hepatocyte proliferative capacity is impaired (chronic liver injury or inflammation), liver progenitor cells (in specialized niches called *canals of Hering*) contribute to repopulation.

Repair by Connective Tissue Deposition (p. 102)

Steps in Scar Formation (*p. 103; Fig. 3-11*)

Macrophages (mostly M2 type) play a central role in repair by clearing offending agents and dead tissue, providing growth factors for

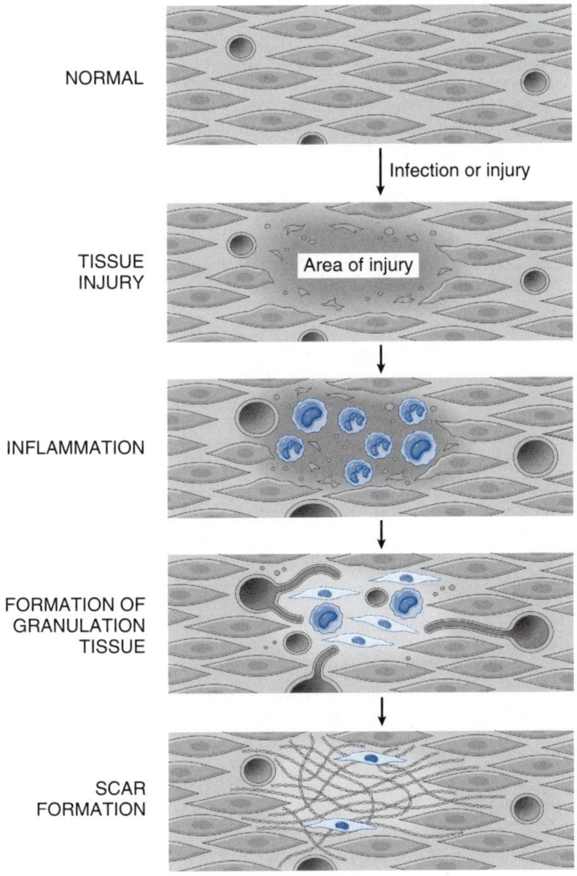

Figure 3-11 Steps in repair by scar formation. Injury to a tissue, such as muscle (which has limited regenerative capacity), first induces inflammation, which clears dead cells and microbes. This is followed by the formation of vascularized *granulation tissue* and then the deposition of ECM to form the scar.

cellular proliferation, and secreting cytokines that stimulate fibroblast proliferation and connective tissue synthesis and deposition. Repair begins within 24 hours of injury; by 3 to 5 days, granulation tissue is apparent:

- *Angiogenesis* is the formation of new blood vessels; these are leaky (accounting for edema in healing wounds) because of incomplete interendothelial junctions and because VEGF increases vascular permeability.
- *Granulation tissue* forms through the migration and proliferation of fibroblasts and deposition of loose connective tissue, combined with the new vessels and interspersed leukocytes. The amount of granulation tissue depends on the size of the tissue deficit created by the wound and the intensity of inflammation.
- *Connective tissue remodeling.* The amount of connective tissue progressively increases in the granulation tissue, forming a scar that can remodel over time.

Angiogenesis *(p. 104)*

Angiogenesis is the process of new blood vessel growth from existing vessels (Fig. 3-12):

- Vasodilation in response to NO and increased permeability in response to VEGF
- Separation of pericytes from the vessel wall and basement membrane breakdown allowing vessel sprouting
- Migration of endothelial cells toward the area of tissue injury
- Proliferation of endothelial cells
- Remodeling into capillary tubes
- Recruitment of periendothelial cells (pericytes for small capillaries and smooth muscle cells for larger vessels)
- Suppression of endothelial proliferation and migration, and redeposition of the basement membrane

Signaling in Angiogenesis

- *VEGF* (mostly VEGF-A) stimulates both migration and proliferation of endothelial cells; fibroblast growth factors (FGFs), mainly FGF-2, also stimulate endothelial cell proliferation, as well as promoting macrophage, epithelial, and fibroblast migration.
- *Angiopoietins 1 and 2* (Ang 1 and Ang 2) drive the structural maturation of new vessels by recruiting pericytes and smooth muscle cells and by driving connective tissue deposition; Ang 1 interacts with a tyrosine kinase receptor on endothelial cells called Tie2. PDGF and TGF-β also participate in the stabilization process.
- *Notch signaling* regulates the sprouting and branching of new vessels, ensuring the proper spacing to effectively supply healing tissues.
- ECM proteins contribute through interactions with integrin receptors in endothelial cells and by providing a mechanical scaffold.
- Matrix metalloproteinases (MMPs) degrade ECM to permit remodeling and extension of the vascular tube.

Deposition of Connective Tissue *(p. 105)*

Deposition of connective tissue occurs through fibroblast migration and proliferation, followed by ECM deposition; PDGF, FGF-2, and TGF-β (mostly from M2 macrophages) all contribute.

TGF-β is most important: it stimulates fibroblast migration and proliferation, increased synthesis of collagen and fibronectin, and decreased degradation of ECM by inhibiting MMPs. Tissue levels are regulated by posttranscriptional activation of latent TGF-β, the rate of secretion of the active molecule, and ECM factors (notably

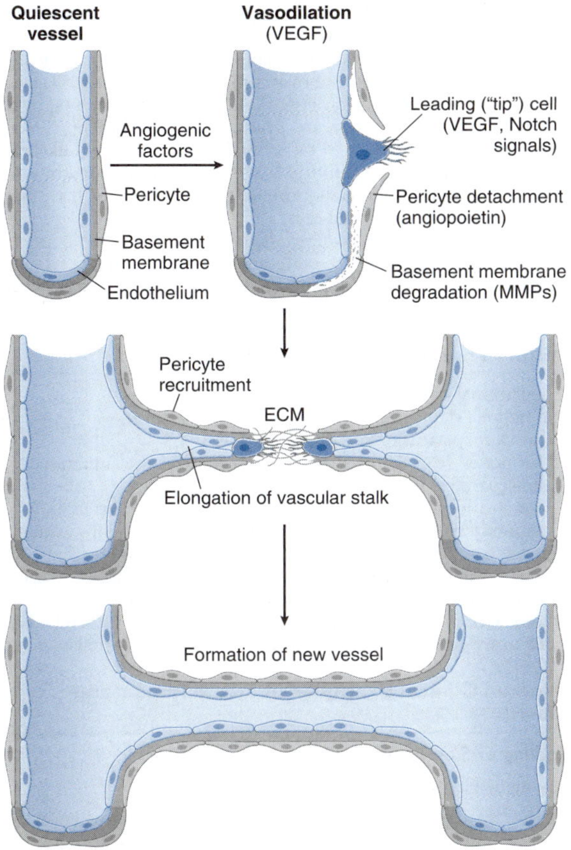

Figure 3-12 Angiogenesis. In tissue repair, angiogenesis occurs mainly by sprouting of new vessels. The steps in the process and the major signals involved are illustrated. The newly formed vessel joins up with other vessels (not shown) to form the new vascular bed.

integrins) that enhance or diminish the cytokine's activity. TGF-β is also an antiinflammatory cytokine that helps to put a brake on inflammatory responses by inhibiting lymphocyte proliferation and curtailing leukocyte activation.

As healing progresses, fibroblasts become progressively less proliferative and more synthetic, increasing the deposition of ECM (collagen is particularly critical to wound strength). Granulation tissue eventually becomes scar composed of largely inactive, spindle-shaped fibroblasts, dense collagen, and other ECM components. There is also progressive vascular regression leading to a largely avascular scar, whereas some fibroblasts develop additional smooth musclelike features (called myofibroblasts) that contribute to scar contraction.

Remodeling of Connective Tissue *(p. 105)*

Remodeling of connective tissue is accomplished by MMPs—distinct from cathepsin G, plasmin, neutrophil elastase, and other serine proteinases that can also degrade ECM. MMPs have zinc at their active site and include *interstitial collagenases* (cleave fibrillar collagen), *gelatinases* (degrade amorphous collagen and fibronectin), and *stromelysins* (catabolize many ECM constituents, including proteoglycans, laminin, fibronectin, and amorphous collagen). MMPs are produced by a variety of cell types, regulated by growth factors and cytokines; they are produced as inactive precursors *(zymogens)* that are activated by proteases (e.g., plasmin) likely to be present only at sites of injury. MMPs are also inhibited by specific tissue inhibitors of metalloproteinases (TIMPs), which are produced by most mesenchymal cells.

ADAMs (a disintegrin and metalloproteinase) are a family of enzymes related to MMPs; these are anchored to the plasma membrane and cleave and release extracellular domains of cell-associated cytokines and growth factors.

Factors That Influence Tissue Repair (p. 105)

- Nutritional status of the host.
- Metabolic status (diabetes mellitus delays healing).
- Circulatory status or vascular adequacy.
- Hormones (e.g., glucocorticoids can impede the inflammatory and reparative process).
- Size and location: Well-vascularized tissues heal faster; inflammation in tissue spaces (e.g., peritoneal cavity) develops exudates that can either *resolve* or undergo *organization.*
- Type of tissue: Labile and stable tissues have better tissue regeneration, whereas permanent tissues form only scar.
- Local factors that delay healing include infections, ischemia, mechanical forces (e.g., motion or wound tension), and foreign bodies.

Selected Clinical Examples of Tissue Repair and Fibrosis (p. 106)

Healing of Skin Wounds (p. 106)

Healing by First Intention (or Primary Union; p. 106)

Healing by first intention (or primary union) occurs when injury involves only the epithelial layer; repair is mainly by epithelial regeneration. In a clean, uninfected surgical incision approximated by surgical sutures there is only focal disruption of the basement membrane and relatively minimal cell death:

- Wounding activates coagulation pathways; the clot (containing fibrin, fibronectin, and complement proteins) stops the bleeding and acts as a scaffold for migrating cells. As dehydration occurs, a scab is formed.
- *Within 24 hours,* neutrophils arrive at the incision margin, releasing proteolytic enzymes that begin to clear the debris. Within 24 to 48 hours, epithelial cells from both edges have migrated and proliferated along the dermis, depositing basement membrane components as they progress.
- *By day 3,* neutrophils have been largely replaced by macrophages, and granulation tissue progressively invades the incision space, with collagen fibers evident at the incision margins.
- *By day 5,* neovascularization reaches its peak with ongoing migration of fibroblasts, which are producing ECM proteins. The epidermis recovers its normal thickness as differentiation of surface cells yields a mature epidermal architecture with surface keratinization.
- *During the second week,* there is continued collagen accumulation and fibroblast proliferation, but leukocyte infiltrate, edema, and vascularity are diminished.

- By 4 weeks, scar is well formed with few inflammatory cells. Although the epidermis is essentially normal, dermal appendages destroyed in the line of the incision are permanently lost.

Healing by Second Intention (or Secondary Union; p. 107)

Healing by second intention (or secondary union) happens when tissue loss is more extensive (e.g., large wounds, abscesses, ulceration, and ischemic necrosis [infarction]); repair involves a combination of regeneration and scarring. The inflammatory reaction is more intense, and there is abundant granulation tissue, with subsequent increased ECM accumulation and formation of a large scar, followed by myofibroblast wound contraction:

- In wounds causing large tissue deficits, inflammation is more intense because large tissue defects have a greater volume of necrotic debris, exudate, and fibrin that must be removed.
- Much larger amounts of granulation tissue are formed.
- The original granulation tissue scaffold is eventually converted into a pale, avascular scar; although the epidermis recovers its normal thickness and architecture, dermal appendages are permanently lost.
- Wound contraction generally occurs in large surface wounds; within 6 weeks, large skin defects can be contracted to 5% to 10% of their original size.

Wound Strength (p. 108)

Carefully sutured wounds have approximately 70% of the strength of normal skin; after suture removal at 1 week, wound strength is approximately 10% of that of unwounded skin. Tensile strength progressively increases through collagen synthesis during the first 2 months of healing, and at later times from structural modifications of collagen fibers (cross-linking, increased fiber size). Wound strength reaches approximately 70% to 80% of normal by 3 months but usually does not substantially improve beyond that point.

Fibrosis in Parenchymal Organs *(p. 109)*

Fibrosis in parenchymal organs is used to denote the excessive deposition of collagen and other ECM components in a tissue. Although *scar* and *fibrosis* are often used interchangeably, *fibrosis* is best used in reference to abnormal deposition of collagen in the setting of chronic (often inflammatory) diseases. The basic mechanisms of fibrosis are the same as those of scar formation (largely driven by TGF-β). Fibrosis can cause substantial organ dysfunction and even organ failure (e.g., liver cirrhosis, systemic sclerosis [scleroderma], fibrosing diseases of the lung [idiopathic pulmonary fibrosis, pneumoconiosis, and drug- or radiation-induced pulmonary fibrosis], end-stage kidney disease, and constrictive pericarditis).

Abnormalities in Tissue Repair (p. 109)

- *Deficient scar formation:* Inadequate granulation tissue or collagen deposition and remodeling can lead to either *wound dehiscence or ulceration.*
- *Excessive repair:* Excessive granulation tissue *(proud flesh)* can protrude above the surrounding skin and block reepithelialization. Excessive collagen accumulation forms a raised *hypertrophic scar;* progression beyond the original area of injury without subsequent regression is termed a *keloid.*
- *Formation of contractures:* Although wound contraction is a normal part of healing, an exaggerated process is designated a *contracture.* It will cause wound deformity (e.g., producing hand *claw* deformities or limit joint mobility).

4 Hemodynamic Disorders, Thromboembolic Disease, and Shock

Disturbances in normal blood flow are major sources of human morbidity and death (35% to 40% of deaths in Western society). These include hemorrhage, clotting, and *embolization* (migration of clots to other sites), as well as extravasation of fluid into the interstitium *(edema)* and blood pressure that is either too low or too high.

Edema and Effusions (p. 113)

The movement of water and solutes between intravascular and interstitial spaces is balanced by the opposing forces of vascular hydrostatic pressure and plasma colloid osmotic pressure. Increased capillary pressure or diminished colloid osmotic pressure results in increased interstitial fluid. If the net movement of water into tissues exceeds lymphatic drainage, fluid will accumulate.

Increased interstitial fluid is called *edema,* whereas fluid in the various body cavities is called *hydrothorax, hydropericardium,* or *hydroperitoneum;* the latter is more commonly called *ascites.* Edema and effusions can have *inflammatory* or *noninflammatory* causes and can be localized (e.g., secondary to isolated venous or lymphatic obstruction) or systemic (as in heart failure); severe systemic edema is called *anasarca.*

Table 4-1 broadly groups edema into *noninflammatory* (yields protein-poor *transudates*) and *inflammatory* (yields protein-rich *exudates;* discussed in Chapter 3).

Noninflammatory causes of edema:

- *Increased hydrostatic pressure* forces fluid out of the vessels. This is most commonly due to impaired venous return; it can be regional (e.g., due to deep venous thrombosis [DVT] in an extremity) or *systemic* (most commonly in the setting of *congestive heart failure* [CHF; see Chapter 12], where compromised right heart function leads to venous blood pooling).
- *Reduced plasma osmotic pressure* (p. 114) occurs with albumin loss (e.g., due to proteinuria in *nephrotic syndrome;* see Chapter 20) or reduced albumin synthesis (e.g., due to cirrhosis [see Chapter 18] or protein malnutrition). Reduced osmotic pressure leads to a net fluid movement into the interstitium with plasma volume contraction. The reduced plasma volume leads to diminished renal perfusion and resultant renin production (and downstream effects on angiotensin and aldosterone), but the subsequent salt and water retention cannot correct the plasma volume due to the underlying protein deficit.
- *Sodium and water retention* (p. 114). Primary salt retention, with obligatory associated water retention, causes *both* increased hydrostatic pressure and reduced osmotic pressure. Sodium retention can occur with any renal dysfunction (see Chapter 20). Primary water retention can occur with release of antidiuretic hormone (ADH) due to increased plasma osmolarity or diminished plasma

TABLE 4-1 Pathophysiologic Categories of Edema

Increased Hydrostatic Pressure
Impaired venous return
Congestive heart failure
Constrictive pericarditis
Ascites (liver cirrhosis)
Venous obstruction or compression
Thrombosis
External pressure (e.g., mass)
Lower extremity inactivity with prolonged dependency
Arteriolar dilation
Heat
Neurohumoral dysregulation
Reduced Plasma Osmotic Pressure (Hypoproteinemia)
Protein-losing glomerulopathies (nephrotic syndrome)
Liver cirrhosis (ascites)
Malnutrition
Protein-losing gastroenteropathy
Lymphatic Obstruction
Inflammatory
Neoplastic
Postsurgical
Postirradiation
Sodium Retention
Excessive salt intake with renal insufficiency
Increased tubular reabsorption of sodium
Renal hypoperfusion
Increased renin-angiotensin-aldosterone secretion
Inflammation
Acute inflammation
Chronic inflammation
Angiogenesis

Data from Leaf A, Cotran RS: *Renal Pathophysiology,* ed 3, New York, 1985, Oxford University Press, p. 146. Used by permission of Oxford Press, Inc.

volume or inappropriately in the setting of malignancy or lung or pituitary pathology.

- *Lymphatic obstruction* (p. 114) blocks removal of interstitial fluid. Obstruction is usually localized and related to inflammation or neoplastic processes.

Morphology (p. 115)

Edema is most easily appreciated grossly; microscopically it manifests only as subtle cell swelling and separation of the extracellular matrix (ECM).

- *Subcutaneous edema* may be diffuse or occur where hydrostatic pressures are greatest (e.g., influenced by gravity, so-called *dependent edema* [legs when standing, sacrum when recumbent]). Finger pressure over substantial subcutaneous edema typically leaves an imprint, so-called *pitting edema.*
- Edema resulting from hypoproteinemia is generally more severe and diffuse; it is most evident in loose connective tissue (e.g., eyelids, causing *periorbital edema*).
- *Pulmonary edema* can result in lungs that are 2 to 3 times their normal weight; sectioning reveals a frothy, blood-tinged mixture of air, edema fluid, and erythrocytes.

- *Brain edema* may be localized to sites of injury (e.g., abscess or neoplasm) or may be generalized (e.g., encephalitis, hypertensive crises, or obstruction to venous outflow). When generalized, the brain is grossly swollen with narrowed sulci and distended gyri flattened against the skull.

Clinical Features (p. 115)

- Subcutaneous edema can impair wound healing or infection clearance.
- Pulmonary edema impedes gas exchange and increases the risk of infection.
- Brain edema within the confined space of the skull can impede cerebral blood flow or cause *herniation,* compromising critical medullary centers.

Hyperemia and Congestion (p. 115)

Both terms mean increased blood volume at a particular site.

- *Hyperemia* is an *active process* due to augmented blood inflow from arteriolar dilation (e.g., skeletal muscle during exercise or at sites of inflammation). Tissues are red *(erythema)* owing to engorgement with oxygenated blood.
- *Congestion* is a *passive process* caused by impaired outflow from a tissue; it can be systemic (e.g., CHF) or local (e.g., an isolated venous obstruction). Tissues are blue-red *(cyanosis)* as worsening congestion leads to accumulated deoxyhemoglobin.
- Long-standing stasis of deoxygenated blood can result in hypoxia severe enough to cause ischemic tissue injury and fibrosis.

Morphology (p. 116)

In *acute congestion,* vessels are distended, and organs are grossly hyperemic; capillary bed congestion is also commonly associated with interstitial edema. In *chronic congestion,* capillary rupture may cause focal hemorrhage; subsequent erythrocyte breakdown results in hemosiderin-laden macrophages. Parenchymal cell atrophy or death (with fibrosis) may also be present. Grossly, tissues appear brown, contracted, and fibrotic. Lungs and liver are commonly affected.

- In *lungs,* capillary engorgement is associated with interstitial edema and airspace transudates. Chronic manifestations include hemosiderin-laden macrophages *(heart failure cells)* and fibrotic septa.
- In *liver,* acute congestion manifests as central vein and sinusoidal distention, occasionally with central hepatocyte degeneration. In chronic congestion the central regions of the hepatic lobules are grossly red-brown and slightly depressed (loss of cells) relative to the surrounding uncongested tan liver (so-called *nutmeg liver*). Microscopically there is *centrilobular necrosis* with hepatocyte dropout and hemorrhage including hemosiderin-laden macrophages. Because the centrilobular area is at the distal end of the hepatic blood supply, it is most subject to necrosis whenever liver perfusion is compromised.

Hemostasis, Hemorrhagic Disorders, and Thrombosis (p. 116)

Hemostasis is the process by which blood clots form at sites of traumatic vascular injury, which prevent or limit the extent of bleeding. In hemorrhagic states, the hemostatic mechanisms are inadequate to prevent abnormal bleeding. Conversely, in thrombotic states, blood clot formation occurs within intact vessels or the heart. In some cases the lines between hemorrhage and thrombosis blur; thus generalized activation of clotting can paradoxically cause bleeding due to consumption of the coagulation factors (disseminated intravascular coagulation [DIC]).

Hemostasis (p. 116)

After injury there is a characteristic hemostatic response (Fig. 4-1):

- Transient reflex neurogenic arteriolar vasoconstriction augmented by endothelin (potent endothelial-derived vasoconstrictor).
- Platelet adhesion and activation (shape change and secretory granule release) by binding to exposed subendothelial ECM. Secreted products recruit other platelets to form a temporary hemostatic plug (primary hemostasis).
- Activation of the coagulation cascade by release of tissue factor (also known as thromboplastin or factor III), a membrane-bound lipoprotein procoagulant factor synthesized by endothelium. Coagulation culminates in thrombin generation and conversion of circulating fibrinogen to insoluble fibrin (see later). Thrombin also induces additional platelet recruitment and granule release. Polymerized fibrin and platelet aggregates together form a solid, permanent plug (secondary hemostasis).
- Activation of counter-regulatory mechanisms (e.g., tissue plasminogen activator [t-PA]) restricts the hemostatic plug to the site of injury.
- The individual components of this hemostatic response are described subsequently.

Platelets (p. 117)

After vascular injury, platelets encounter ECM constituents (collagen, proteoglycans, fibronectin, and other adhesive glycoproteins [Gps]) normally sequestered beneath an intact endothelium. Platelets then undergo *activation* involving adhesion and shape change, secretion (release reaction), and aggregation.

- *Platelet-ECM adhesion* is mediated through von Willebrand factor (vWF), acting as a bridge between platelet receptors (mostly GpIb) and exposed collagen. Genetic deficiencies of vWF *(von Willebrand disease)* or GpIb *(Bernard-Soulier syndrome)* result in bleeding disorders.
- *Platelets change shape* from smooth disks to spiky ovoids with markedly increased surface area; this is accompanied by GpIIb-IIIa changes that increase fibrinogen affinity, as well as by translocation of negatively charged *phospholipid complexes* to the platelet surface, providing a locus for calcium and coagulation factor interactions in the *clotting cascade.*
- *Platelet granule secretion (release reaction)* occurs shortly after adhesion. *Alpha granules* express P-selectin adhesion molecules and contain coagulation and growth factors; *dense bodies* or *delta granules* contain adenosine nucleotides (e.g., adenosine diphosphate [ADP]), calcium, and vasoactive amines (e.g., histamine). ADP is a potent mediator of *platelet aggregation (recruitment),* and calcium is important for the coagulation cascade.
- *Platelet aggregation* (platelets adhering to other platelets) is promoted by ADP and thromboxane A_2 (TxA_2).
- ADP activation changes platelet GpIIb-IIIa receptor conformation to allow fibrinogen binding; fibrinogen bridges multiple platelets forming large aggregates (GpIIb-IIIa deficiencies result in *Glanzmann thrombasthenia* bleeding disorder).

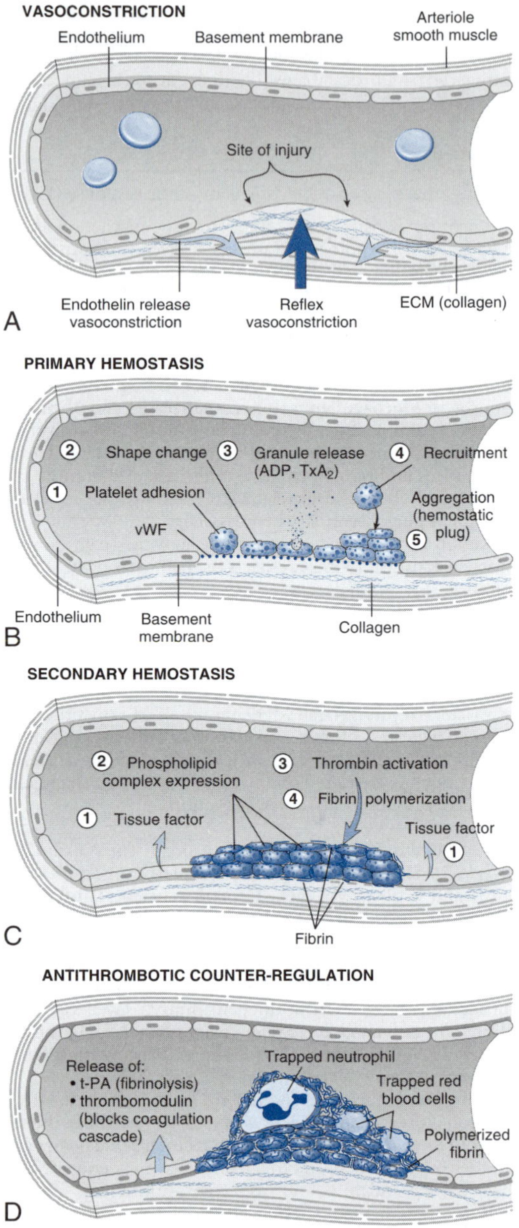

Figure 4-1 Diagrammatic representation of normal hemostasis. A, Vascular injury triggers transient vasoconstriction through local neurohumoral factors. **B,** Platelets adhere to exposed ECM via vWF and are activated, undergoing a shape change and granule release; released ADP and TxA_2 lead to further platelet aggregation to form the primary hemostatic plug. **C,** Local activation of the coagulation cascade (involving tissue factor and platelet phospholipids) results in fibrin polymerization, "cementing" the platelets into a definitive secondary hemostatic plug. **D,** Counter-regulatory mechanisms (e.g., release of t-PA and thrombomodulin) limit the hemostatic process to the site of injury.

- Platelet-derived TxA_2 activates platelet aggregation and is a potent vasoconstrictor (recall that endothelial cell [EC]-derived prostacyclin [PGI_2] inhibits platelet aggregation and is a potent vasodilator).
- Erythrocytes and leukocytes also aggregate in hemostatic plugs; leukocytes adhere to platelets via P-selectin and contribute to the inflammatory response accompanying thrombosis.

Coagulation Cascade *(p. 118)*

This is essentially a sequential conversion of proenzymes into activated enzymes, culminating in the cleavage of insoluble *fibrin* from the soluble plasma protein *fibrinogen.* Coagulation has been traditionally divided into *extrinsic* and *intrinsic* pathways; this distinction is based on the laboratory measurement of clotting (Fig. 4-2). Although different factors induce clot formation in vivo and in vitro, the same general principles apply.

Each step in the cascade involves the following:

- *Enzyme* (activated coagulation factor)
- *Substrate* (inactive proenzyme form of a coagulation factor)
- *Cofactor* (a reaction accelerator)

These are brought together on the negatively charged platelet phospholipid surface. Assembly of the various complexes also requires calcium, which binds to γ-carboxylated glutamic acid residues on factors II, VII, IX, and X. Clotting thus tends to remain localized to sites where assembly can occur (e.g., surfaces of activated platelets or endothelium).

The in vitro measurements include the following:

- *Prothrombin time (PT),* measured after the addition of tissue factor, phospholipids, and calcium; it evaluates the function of extrinsic pathway proteins (VII, X, II, V, and fibrinogen).
- *Partial thromboplastin time (PTT),* measured after the addition of negatively charged particles (e.g., ground glass); it screens for the function of intrinsic pathway proteins (XII, XI, IX, VIII, X, V, II, and fibrinogen).

In vivo, factor VIIa/tissue factor complexes are the important activators of factor IX, and factor IXa/factor VIIIa complexes are the most important activators of factor X (Fig. 4-2, *B*).

In addition to catalyzing the cleavage of fibrinogen to fibrin, thrombin also exerts numerous effects on local vessel wall (promoting *anticoagulation;* see later), platelet activation, and inflammatory cell activation. These effects are mediated through *protease-activated receptors (PARs),* seven-transmembrane spanner proteins.

Factors That Limit Coagulation (p. 120)

Once activated, coagulation must be restricted to sites of vascular injury to prevent clotting of the entire vascular tree:

- Factor activation can only occur at sites of exposed phospholipids. In addition, activated clotting factors are diluted by flow and are cleared by the liver and tissue macrophages.
- Endothelial counter-regulatory activities are extremely important (see later).
- Activation of the coagulation cascade also sets into motion a *fibrinolytic cascade* (Fig. 4-3). *Plasmin* is generated from inactive plasminogen by the activity of factor XIIa or t-PA; plasmin cleaves fibrin and interferes with its polymerization. Plasmin proteolysis is also regulated by α_2-plasmin inhibitors that bind and inhibit plasmin activity. Elevated levels of fibrinogen breakdown products—so-called *fibrin split products,* including *D-dimers* (derived from the proteolysis of cross-linked fibrin)—are good biomarkers of thrombosis.

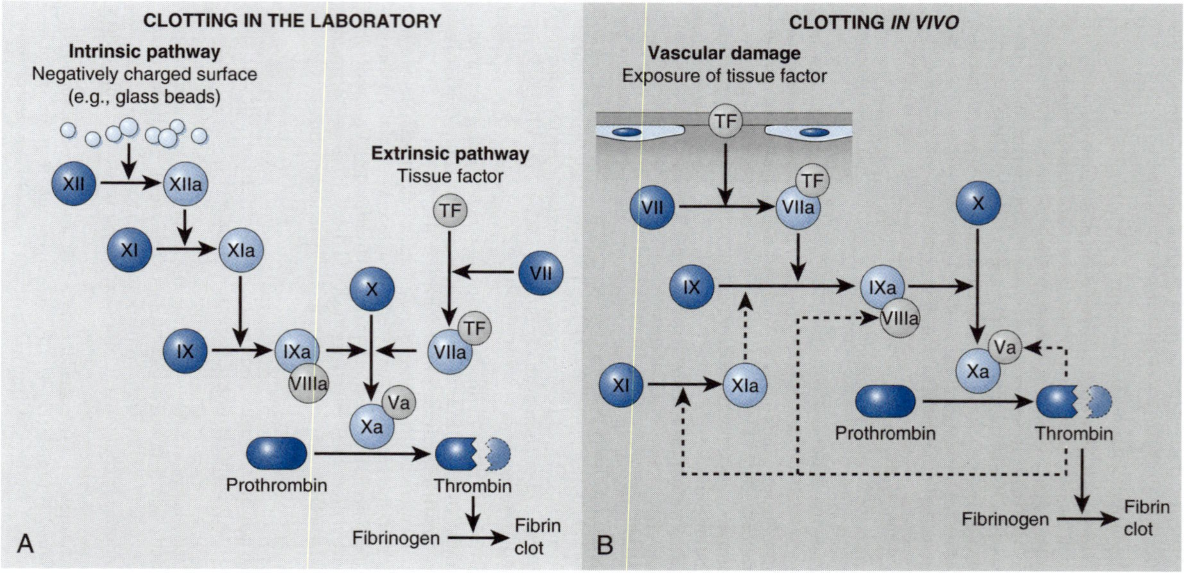

Figure 4-2 The coagulation cascade in vitro and in vivo. A, Clotting is initiated in the laboratory by adding phospholipids, calcium, and either a negatively charged substance such as glass beads *(intrinsic pathway)* or a source of tissue factor *(extrinsic pathway)*. **B,** In vivo, tissue factor is the major initiator of coagulation, which is amplified by feedback loops involving thrombin *(dotted lines)*. The dark blue polypeptides are inactive factors, the light blue polypeptides are active factors, while the gray polypeptides correspond to cofactors. Activated factors are indicated with a lowercase "a."

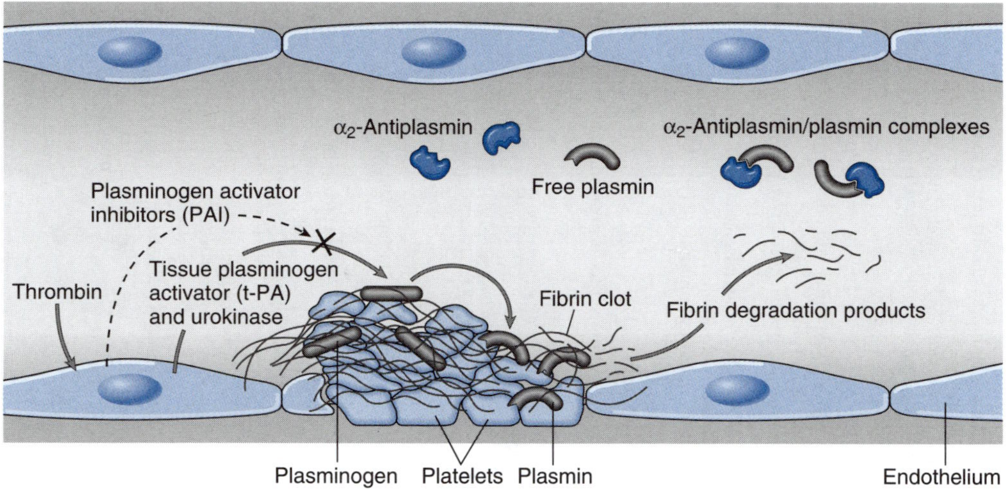

Figure 4-3 The fibrinolytic system, illustrating various plasminogen activators and inhibitors.

Endothelium *(p. 121)*

ECs regulate several, frequently opposing aspects of hemostasis. ECs normally exhibit antiplatelet, anticoagulant, and fibrinolytic properties (Fig. 4-4). However, after injury or activation, ECs exhibit *procoagulant function.* The balance between EC antithrombotic and prothrombotic activities determines whether thrombus formation, propagation, or dissolution occurs.

- *Platelet inhibitory effects* (p. 121)
  - Intact endothelium blocks platelet access to thrombogenic subendothelial matrix.
  - PGI_2 and nitric oxide (NO) inhibit platelet binding.
  - Adenosine diphosphatase degrades ADP, an inducer of platelet aggregation
- *Anticoagulant effects* (p. 121)
  - Membrane-associated thrombomodulin converts thrombin to an anticoagulant protein.
  - Activated protein C/protein S complex potently inhibits factors Va and VIIIa.
  - Heparin-like surface molecules facilitate plasma antithrombin III inactivation of thrombin.
  - Tissue factor pathway inhibitor (TFPI) blocks tissue factor/factor VIIa complexes.
- *Fibrinolytic effects* (p. 121)
  - t-PA cleaves plasminogen to form plasmin, which in turn degrades fibrin.

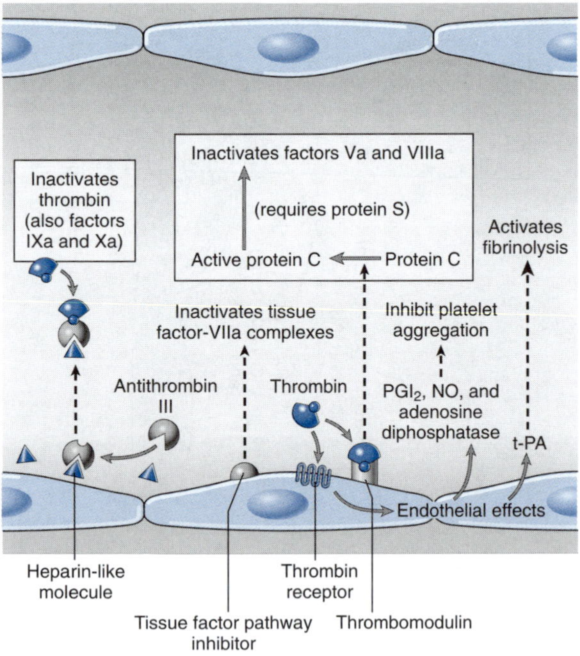

Figure 4-4 Anticoagulant activities of normal endothelium. *NO,* Nitric oxide; *PGI_2,* prostacyclin; *t-PA,* tissue plasminogen activator; *vWF,* von Willebrand factor. The thrombin receptor is also called a PAR.

Hemorrhagic Disorders (p. 121)

Hemorrhage results from disorders of vessel walls, platelets, or coagulation factors. Bleeding can vary from massive (rupture of a major vessel due to trauma or neoplastic erosion) to capillary bleeding in the setting of chronic congestion to subtle defects in clotting that manifest only after physiologic stressors (e.g., pregnancy). The most common etiologies for a mild bleeding tendency are inherited defects in vWF (see Chapter 14), consumption of nonsteroidal antiinflammatory agents (e.g., aspirin), and renal failure (uremia).

- *Defects in primary hemostasis* (p. 121), most commonly due to low platelet counts *(thrombocytopenia),* abnormal platelet function, or von Willebrand disease. These manifest as minute, 1- to 2-mm *petechial hemorrhages* or slightly larger *purpura* in skin, mucous membranes, or serosal surfaces.
- *Defects of secondary hemostasis* (p. 122) involve coagulation factor abnormalities and typically present with bleeding into joints *(hemarthrosis)* or soft tissues.
- *Generalized defects involving small vessels* (p. 122) manifest as >1- to 2-cm subcutaneous *ecchymoses (bruises);* a sufficiently large amount of extravasated blood will generate a palpable mass *(hematoma).* Systematic ecchymoses and palpable purpura can occur secondary to vasculitis or increased vessel fragility (e.g., due to scurvy or amyloid deposition).

The clinical significance of hemorrhage depends on the volume and rate of blood loss. Rapid loss of less than 20% or slow losses of even larger amounts may have little impact; greater losses result in hemorrhagic (hypovolemic) shock. Location is also important: Bleeding that would be inconsequential in subcutaneous tissues may cause death in the brain. Chronic blood loss (e.g., peptic ulcer or menstrual bleeding) can result in iron deficiency anemia.

Thrombosis (p. 122)

Thrombosis is inappropriate activation of blood clotting in uninjured vasculature or thrombotic occlusion of a vessel after relatively minor injury. There are three primary influences on thrombus formation, so-called *Virchow triad:*

1. *Endothelial injury* (p. 122) is dominant and can independently cause thrombosis (e.g., endocarditis or ulcerated atherosclerotic plaque). Injury can be due to hemodynamic stresses (e.g., hypertension or turbulent flow), endotoxin, radiation, or noxious agents (homocystinuria, hypercholesterolemia, or cigarette smoke). Thrombosis results from exposed subendothelial ECM, increased platelet adhesion, elevated procoagulant production (tissue factor, plasminogen activator inhibitor), or reduced anticoagulant activity (PGI_2, thrombomodulin, t-PA).
2. *Alterations in normal blood flow* (p. 123). Normal blood flow is *laminar* (i.e., cellular elements flow centrally in the vessel lumen, separated from endothelium by a plasma clear zone). Stasis and turbulence (the latter forms eddy currents with local pockets of stasis):

   - Disrupt laminar flow and bring platelets into contact with the endothelium.
   - Prevent dilution of activated clotting factors by flowing blood.
   - Retard the inflow of clotting inhibitors.
   - Promote EC activation.

Stasis causes thrombosis in the venous circulation, cardiac chambers, and arterial aneurysms; turbulence causes thrombosis in the arterial circulation as well as endothelial injury. Hyperviscosity syndromes (e.g., polycythemia) or deformed erythrocytes (e.g., sickle cell anemia) result in small vessel stasis and also predispose to thrombosis.

3. *Hypercoagulability* (p. 123) is loosely defined as any alteration of the coagulation pathways that predisposes to thrombosis. It contributes less frequently to thrombosis but is critical in certain conditions (Table 4-2).
   - Heritable hypercoagulable states:
     - Factor V gene mutations are the most common; 2% to 15% of Caucasians (60% of patients with recurrent deep vein thrombosis) carry the so-called Leiden mutation, rendering factor V resistant to protein C inactivation.
     - A single nucleotide change (G20210A) in the 3′ untranslated region of the prothrombin gene (1% to 2% of the population) leads to elevated prothrombin levels and a threefold increased risk of venous thrombosis.
     - Deficiencies of antithrombin III, protein C, or protein S also typically present with venous thrombosis and recurrent thromboembolism.

TABLE 4-2 Hypercoagulable States
Primary (Genetic)
Common
Factor V mutation (Arg to Glu substitution in amino acid residue 506 leading to resistance to activated protein C; factor V Leiden)
Prothrombin mutation (G20210A noncoding sequence variant leading to increased prothrombin levels)
Increased levels of factors VIII, IX, XI, or fibrinogen (genetics unknown)
Rare
Antithrombin III deficiency
Protein C deficiency
Protein S deficiency
Very Rare
Fibrinolysis defects
Homozygous homocystinuria (deficiency of cystathione β-synthetase)
Secondary (Acquired)
High Risk for Thrombosis
Prolonged bed rest or immobilization
Myocardial infarction
Atrial fibrillation
Tissue injury (surgery, fracture, burn)
Cancer
Prosthetic cardiac valves
Disseminated intravascular coagulation
Heparin-induced thrombocytopenia
Antiphospholipid antibody syndrome
Lower Risk for Thrombosis
Cardiomyopathy
Nephrotic syndrome
Hyperestrogenic states (pregnancy and postpartum)
Oral contraceptive use
Sickle cell anemia
Smoking

- Acquired hypercoagulable states:
  - Oral contraceptives or the hyperestrogenic state of pregnancy can cause hypercoagulability via increased hepatic synthesis of coagulation factors and reduced synthesis of antithrombin III.
  - Certain malignancies can release procoagulant products.
- *Heparin-induced thrombocytopenia syndrome* (p. 124) occurs when heparin products induce circulating antibodies that activate platelets and injure ECs.
- *Antiphospholipid antibody syndrome* (p. 124) occurs in patients with antibodies against anionic phospholipids; these activate platelets and/or interfere with protein C activity.

Morphology *(p. 125)*

- Venous thrombi characteristically occur in sites of stasis and are *occlusive.*
- Arterial or cardiac thrombi usually begin at sites of endothelial injury (e.g., atherosclerotic plaque, endocarditis) or turbulence (vessel bifurcation).
  - Aortic or cardiac thrombi are typically *nonocclusive (mural)* due to rapid and high-volume flow in those sites.
  - Smaller arterial thrombi can be *occlusive.*
- Thrombi are generally firmly attached at their site of origin and typically *propagate toward the heart.* Thus arterial thrombi grow retrograde from the attachment point, whereas venous thrombi lengthen in the direction of blood flow. The propagating tail may not be well attached and may fragment to create an *embolus.*
- *Arterial and cardiac mural thrombi* have gross and microscopic laminations *(lines of Zahn)* produced by pale layers of platelets and fibrin alternating with darker erythrocyte-rich layers.
- *Venous thrombi (phlebothrombosis)* typically occur in a relatively static environment, resulting in a fairly uniform cast containing abundant erythrocytes among sparse fibrin strands (*red* or *stasis thrombi*). Phlebothrombosis most commonly affects the veins of the lower extremities (>90% of cases).
- *Valve thrombosis:*
  - *Infective endocarditis:* organisms form large infected thrombotic masses *(vegetations)*, with associated valve damage and systemic infection.
  - *Nonbacterial thrombotic endocarditis:* noninfected, sterile vegetations develop in hypercoagulable states, typically without valve damage.
  - *Verrucous (Libman-Sacks) endocarditis* (sterile vegetations) occurs in systemic lupus erythematosus due to immune complex deposition; inflammation can cause valve scarring.

Fate of the Thrombus *(p. 125)*

If a patient survives the immediate effects of a thrombus, some combination of the following occurs:

- Propagation.
- Embolization: Thrombi dislodge and travel to other sites.
- Dissolution by fibrinolytic activity.
- Organization and recanalization: Ingrowth of ECs, smooth muscle cells, and fibroblasts to create vascular channels or incorporate the thrombus into the vessel wall.
- Rarely, microbial seeding of a thrombus leads to a mycotic aneurysm.

Clinical Features (p. 126)

Thrombi are significant because they (1) *can obstruct vessels* and (2) *can embolize;* the relative importance depends on the site. Thus although venous thrombi can cause distal congestion and edema, embolization is more clinically significant (e.g., from deep leg vein to lung). Conversely, although arterial thrombi can embolize, vascular obstruction (e.g., causing myocardial or cerebral infarctions) is much more important.

Venous Thrombosis (Phlebothrombosis)

Venous thrombosis occurs most commonly in deep or superficial leg veins.

- Superficial thrombi usually occur in varicose saphenous veins, causing local congestion and pain but rarely embolizing. Local edema and impaired venous drainage predispose to skin infections and *varicose ulcers.*
- *Deep thrombi* in larger leg veins above the knee (e.g., popliteal, femoral, and iliac veins) can result in pain and edema, as well as increased risk for embolization. Venous obstruction is usually offset by collateral flow, and deep vein thromboses are asymptomatic in *approximately 50% of patients,* being recognized only after embolization.
- DVT occurs in multiple clinical settings:
  - Advanced age, bed rest, or immobilization, diminishing the milking action of muscles in the lower leg and slowing venous return.
  - CHF.
  - Trauma, surgery, and burns result in reduced physical activity, injury to vessels, release of procoagulant substances from tissues, and reduced t-PA.
  - The puerperal and postpartum states are associated with amniotic fluid embolization (see later) and hypercoagulability.
  - Tumor-associated procoagulant release (*migratory thrombophlebitis* or *Trousseau syndrome*).

Arterial and Cardiac Thrombosis

Atherosclerosis is the major cause of arterial thrombi—due to abnormal flow and endothelial damage. *Myocardial infarction* with dyskinesis and endocardial damage can cause mural thrombi. *Rheumatic valvular disease* resulting in mitral valve scarring and stenosis with left atrial dilation predisposes to atrial thrombus formation; concurrent atrial fibrillation augments the blood stasis and propensity to thrombose. Cardiac and aortic mural thrombi can embolize peripherally; brain, kidneys, and spleen are prime targets.

Disseminated Intravascular Coagulation (p. 127)

DIC is reflected by widespread fibrin microthrombi in the microcirculation. This is caused by disorders ranging from obstetric complications to advanced malignancy. DIC is not a primary disease but rather a complication of any diffuse thrombin activation. Microthrombi can cause diffuse circulatory insufficiency, particularly in the brain, lungs, heart, and kidneys; there is also concurrent consumption of platelets and coagulation factors *(consumption coagulopathy)* with fibrinolytic pathway activation, leading to uncontrollable bleeding. DIC is discussed in greater detail in Chapter 14.

Embolism (p. 127)

Embolism refers to any intravascular solid, liquid, or gaseous mass carried by blood flow to a site distant from its origin. Most (99%)

arise from thrombi, hence the term *thromboembolism.* Rare forms include fat droplets, gas bubbles, atherosclerotic debris *(atheroemboli),* tumor fragments, bone marrow, or foreign bodies (e.g., bullets). Emboli lodge in vessels too small to permit further passage, resulting in partial or complete vascular occlusion and ischemic necrosis *(infarction).*

Pulmonary Embolism (p. 127)

Pulmonary emboli (PE) occur in 0.2% to 0.4% of hospitalized patients and cause approximately 100,000 deaths annually in the United States. Greater than 95% of PE originate from DVT, although DVT are 2 to 3 times more common than PE. PE can occlude the main pulmonary artery, impact across the bifurcation *(saddle embolus),* or pass into smaller arterioles. Multiple emboli can occur, either sequentially or as a shower of small emboli from a single large mass; in general, *one PE puts a patient at risk for more.* Rarely emboli pass through atrial or ventricular defects into the systemic circulation *(paradoxical embolism).*

- Most PE (60% to 80%) are small and clinically silent. They eventually organize and get incorporated into the vessel wall or leave a delicate, bridging fibrous *web.*
- Sudden death, right-sided heart failure *(cor pulmonale),* or cardiovascular collapse occurs when 60% or more of the pulmonary circulation is obstructed with emboli.
- PE in medium-sized arteries can cause pulmonary hemorrhage but usually not pulmonary infarction due to collateral bronchial artery flow. However, with left-sided cardiac failure (and diminished bronchial circulation), infarcts can result.
- PE in small end-arteriolar vessels will typically cause hemorrhage or infarction.
- Multiple emboli over time can cause pulmonary hypertension and right ventricular failure.

Systemic Thromboembolism (p. 127)

Systemic thromboembolism refers to emboli in the arterial circulation. Approximately 80% arise from intracardiac mural thrombi; two thirds are associated with left ventricular wall infarcts, and 25% arise within dilated left atria and fibrillation. Systemic emboli can also originate from aortic aneurysms, thrombi on ulcerated atherosclerotic plaques, or valvular vegetations, and rarely from *paradoxical emboli* (venous emboli that pass through an atrial or ventricular septal defect, including patent foramen ovale); 10% to 15% are of unknown origin. Major sites for arteriolar embolization are the lower extremities (75%) and brain (10%); intestines, kidneys, spleen, and upper extremities are less frequent. The consequences of arterial emboli depend on collateral vascular supply, tissue vulnerability to ischemia, and vessel caliber; most arterial emboli cause tissue infarction.

Fat and Marrow Embolism (p. 128)

Pulmonary embolization of microscopic fat globules (with or without hematopoietic marrow elements) occurs after fractures of long bones or rarely after burns or soft tissue trauma. Fat embolism occurs in 90% of severe skeletal injuries; fewer than 10% have any clinical findings.

Fat embolism syndrome, fatal in approximately 10% of cases, is heralded by sudden pulmonary insufficiency 1 to 3 days after injury; 20% to 50% of patients have a diffuse petechial rash and may have neurologic symptoms (irritability and restlessness) that progress to delirium or coma. Thrombocytopenia and anemia can also occur. The pathogenesis involves mechanical obstruction by neutral fat microemboli, followed by local platelet and erythrocyte aggregation. Subsequent fatty acid release causes toxic injury to endothelium; platelet activation and granulocyte recruitment contribute free radicals, proteases, and eicosanoids.

Edema and hemorrhage (and pulmonary hyaline membranes) can be seen microscopically.

Air Embolism (p. 128)

Air embolism refers to gas bubbles within the circulation obstructing vascular flow and causing ischemia. Small amounts in the coronary or cerebral circulation (introduced by surgery) can be catastrophic. In general in the pulmonary circulation more than 100 cc are required to have a clinical effect; such volumes can be introduced during obstetrical procedures or following chest wall injury.

Decompression sickness is a special form of air embolism caused by sudden changes in atmospheric pressure; deep-sea divers and individuals in unpressurized aircraft in rapid ascent are at risk. Air breathed at high pressure causes increasing amounts of gas (particularly nitrogen) to be dissolved in blood and tissues. Subsequent rapid ascent (depressurization) allows the dissolved gases to expand and bubble out of solution to form gas emboli.

- Formation of gas bubbles in skeletal muscles and joints causes painful *bends.* In lungs, edema, hemorrhage, and focal emphysema lead to respiratory distress, or *chokes.* Gas emboli may also cause focal ischemia in a number of tissues, including brain and heart.
- A more chronic form of decompression sickness is *caisson disease;* persistent gas emboli in poorly vascularized portions of the skeleton (heads of the femurs, tibia, and humeri) lead to ischemic necrosis.

Amniotic Fluid Embolism (p. 129)

Embolization of amniotic fluid into the maternal pulmonary circulation is a serious (mortality rate is approximately >80%) but uncommon (1 in 40,000 deliveries) complication of labor and postpartum period. The syndrome is characterized by sudden severe dyspnea, cyanosis, and hypotensive shock, followed by seizures and coma. Pulmonary edema, *diffuse alveolar damage,* and DIC ensue from release of toxic (fatty acid) and thrombogenic substances in amniotic fluid. Classic histologic findings include fetal squamous cells, mucin, lanugo hair, and fat from vernix caseosa in the maternal pulmonary microcirculation.

Infarction (p. 129)

An infarct is an area of ischemic necrosis caused by occlusion of either the arterial supply or venous drainage in a particular tissue. Almost all infarcts result from thrombotic or embolic events; other causes include vasospasm; extrinsic compression of a vessel by tumor, edema, or entrapment in a hernia sac; and twisting of vessels, such as testicular torsion or bowel volvulus; traumatic vessel rupture is a rare cause. Occluded venous drainage (e.g., venous thrombosis) most often only induces congestion because bypass channels rapidly open to provide outflow. Thus infarcts due to venous thrombosis are more likely in organs with a single venous outflow (e.g., testis or ovary).

Morphology (p. 129)

Infarcts may be either *red (hemorrhagic)* or *white (pale, anemic)* and may be either *septic* or *bland.*

- Red infarcts occur in
  - Venous occlusions (e.g., ovarian torsion)
  - Loose tissues (such as lung)
  - Tissues with dual circulations (e.g., lung and small intestine)
  - Tissues previously congested because of sluggish venous outflow
  - Sites of previous occlusion and necrosis when flow is reestablished
- *White infarcts* occur in solid organs (such as heart, spleen, and kidney) with end-arterial circulations (i.e., few collaterals).
- All infarcts tend to be wedge-shaped; the occluded vessel marks the apex, and the organ periphery forms the base. Lateral margins may be irregular, reflecting the pattern of adjacent vascular supply.
- The dominant histologic feature of infarction in most tissues is *coagulative necrosis,* followed temporally by an inflammatory response (hours to days), and a reparative response (days to weeks) beginning in the preserved margins. Most infarcts are ultimately replaced by scar tissue, although (depending on the tissue) some parenchymal regeneration may occur where the underlying stromal architecture is spared.
- Infarction in the central nervous system results in *liquefactive necrosis.*
- Septic infarctions occur when infected heart valve vegetations embolize or when microbes seed an area of necrosis; the infarct becomes an *abscess.*

Factors that influence development of an infarct (p. 130). The outcomes of vascular occlusion can range from no effect to death of a tissue or person. Major determinants of outcome are as follows:

- *Anatomy of the vascular supply* (i.e., availability of alternative supply). Dual circulations (lung, liver) or anastomosing circulations (radial and ulnar arteries, circle of Willis, small intestine) protect against infarction. Obstruction of end-arterial vessels generally causes infarction (spleen, kidneys).
- *Rate of occlusion.* Slowly developing occlusions less often cause infarction by allowing time to develop alternate perfusion pathways (e.g., collateral coronary circulation).
- *Tissue vulnerability to hypoxia.* Neurons undergo irreversible damage after 3 to 4 minutes of ischemia; myocardial cells die after only 20 to 30 minutes. In contrast, fibroblasts within ischemic myocardium are viable even after many hours.
- *Hypoxemia.* Anemia, cyanosis, or CHF (with hypoxia) can cause infarction in an otherwise inconsequential blockage.

Shock (p. 131)

Shock is systemic hypoperfusion and cellular hypoxia resulting from reduction in either cardiac output or the effective circulating blood volume (hypotension). Shock is the final common pathway for many lethal events, including severe hemorrhage, extensive trauma, large myocardial infarction, massive pulmonary embolism, and sepsis.

Shock is grouped into three major categories:

- *Cardiogenic shock:* Low cardiac output due to outflow obstruction (PE) or myocardial pump failure (e.g., myocardial infarction, arrhythmia, or tamponade).

- *Hypovolemic shock:* low cardiac output due to hemorrhage or fluid loss (i.e., burn).
- *Septic shock* results from vasodilation and peripheral blood pooling caused by microbial infection (and the host immune response); it has a complicated pathogenesis (see later).

Rarer causes of shock are *neurogenic,* with loss of vascular tone and peripheral pooling (anesthetic accident or spinal cord injury), and *anaphylactic,* with systemic vasodilation and increased vascular permeability (IgE-mediated hypersensitivity; see Chapter 6).

Pathogenesis of Septic Shock (p. 131)

With a 20% mortality rate and 200,000 deaths annually in the United States, septic shock ranks first among the causes of death in intensive care units. The incidence is increasing as a result of improved life support for high-risk patients, increasing use of invasive procedures, and greater numbers of immunocompromised individuals.

- Most cases of septic shock are now caused by gram-positive bacteria, followed by gram-negative bacteria and fungi.
- *Superantigens*—a class of secreted bacterial products—can also cause a similar syndrome (e.g., *toxic shock syndrome*) by inducing polyclonal T-cell activation and the systemic release of high levels of proinflammatory cytokines.
- Morbidity and mortality in sepsis are consequences of tissue hypoperfusion and multiorgan dysfunction despite initially preserved or even increased cardiac output. This is due to systemic vasodilation accompanied by widespread EC activation and injury, leading to a hypercoagulable state and DIC. There are also systemic metabolic changes that suppress normal cellular function.
- A similar widespread inflammatory response—*systemic inflammatory response syndrome*—can be triggered after extensive trauma or burn injury, in the absence of any infection.
- The pathogenesis of sepsis is a combination of direct microbial injury and activation of host inflammatory responses (Fig. 4-5):
    - *Inflammatory and counterinflammatory responses* (p. 131). Microbial cell wall components activate leukocytes and EC via Toll-like receptors and other receptors of innate immunity. Activation triggers release of inflammatory cytokines, prostaglandins, reactive oxygen species, and platelet-activating factor (PAF). Coagulation and complement cascades are also directly activated, which can in turn drive additional inflammatory responses (see Chapter 2).
    - *Endothelial activation and injury* (p. 132). Inflammatory cytokine elaboration leads to markedly increased vascular permeability, with associated interstitial edema. Activated EC also produce NO and other vasoactive mediators (e.g., complement fragments and PAF) that cause smooth muscle relaxation and contribute to the systemic hypotension.
    - *Induction of a procoagulant state* (p. 133). EC activation leads to an adhesive, procoagulant EC phenotype with markedly increased thrombotic tendencies (DIC in up to 50% of cases).
    - *Metabolic abnormalities* (p. 133). Insulin resistance and hyperglycemia are characteristic of the septic state, attributable to inflammatory cytokines and the early production of stress-induced hormones, such as glucagon, growth hormone, and cortisol. With time, adrenal insufficiency may supervene.
    - *Organ dysfunction.* Hypotension, edema, and small vessel thrombosis all reduce oxygen and nutrient delivery to tissues; the cellular metabolism in various tissues is also deranged due

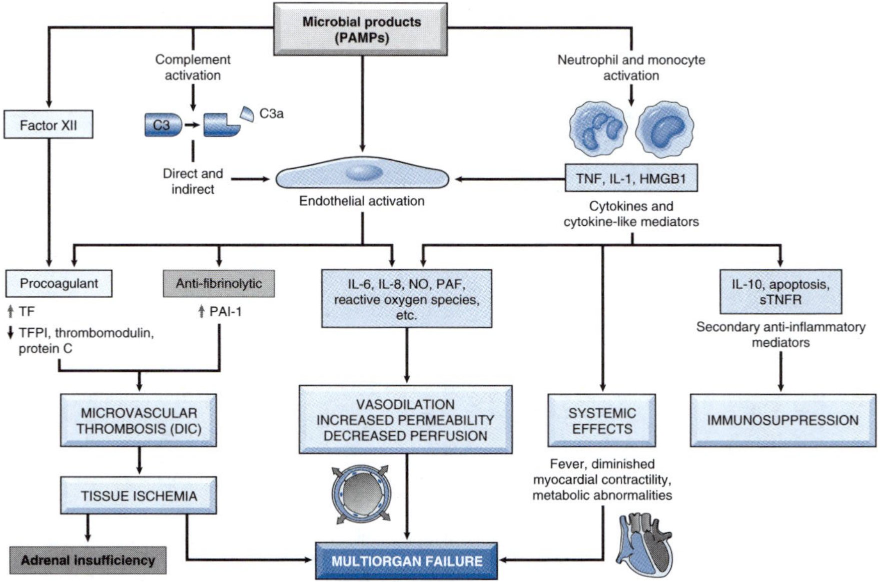

Figure 4-5 Major pathogenic pathways in septic shock. Microbial products (pathogen-associated molecular patterns [PAMPs]) activate ECs and cellular and humoral elements of the innate immune system, initiating a cascade of events that lead to end-stage multiorgan failure. *DIC,* Disseminated intravascular coagulation; *HMGB1,* high mobility group box 1 protein; *IL,* interleukin; *NO,* nitric oxide; *PAF,* platelet activating factor; *PAI-1,* plasminogen activator inhibitor 1; *sTNFR,* soluble tumor necrosis factor receptor; *TF,* tissue factor; *TFPI,* tissue factor pathway inhibitor; *TNF,* tumor necrosis factor.

to insulin resistance. Myocardial contractility may be directly impacted, and endothelial damage underlies the development of *adult respiratory distress syndrome* (see Chapter 15).

The severity and outcome of sepsis are dependent on the extent and virulence of the infection, the immune status of the host, other comorbidities, and the pattern and level of host mediator production. Therapy involves antibiotics, insulin administration, fluid resuscitation, and adequate exogenous steroids to correct adrenal insufficiency; approaches blocking specific inflammatory mediators have not generally been successful.

Stages of Shock (p. 133)

Shock is a progressive disorder often culminating in death. In *septic shock* the patient's demise results from multiorgan failure (as outlined previously). Unless the initial insult is massive and rapidly lethal (e.g., exsanguination), *hypovolemic* or *cardiogenic shock* tends to evolve through three phases:

- *Nonprogressive phase,* in which reflex neurohumoral compensatory mechanisms are activated (catechols, sympathetic stimulation, ADH, renin-angiotensin axis, etc.) and perfusion of vital organs is maintained.
- *Progressive phase,* characterized by tissue hypoperfusion and worsening circulatory and metabolic abnormalities, including lactic acidosis due to anaerobic glycolysis. The acidosis also blunts the vasomotor response causing vasodilation.
- *Irreversible phase,* in which damage is so severe that even if perfusion is restored, survival is not possible. Renal shutdown due to *acute tubular necrosis* and ischemic bowel leaking microbes into the bloodstream *(sepsis)* can be terminal events.

Morphology (p. 134)

Shock of any form causes nonspecific cell and tissue changes largely reflecting hypoxic injury; brain, heart, lungs, kidneys, adrenals, and gastrointestinal tract are particularly affected. The *kidneys* develop extensive tubular ischemic injury (*acute tubular necrosis;* see Chapter 20), causing oliguria, anuria, and electrolyte disturbances. The *lungs* are seldom affected in pure hypovolemic shock; however, *diffuse alveolar damage* (*shock lung;* see Chapter 15) can occur in septic or traumatic shock. Outside of neuron and myocyte loss, virtually all tissues can recover if the patient survives.

Clinical Consequences (p. 134)

Clinical consequences depend on the precipitating insult:

- In hypovolemic and cardiogenic shock there is hypotension with a weak, rapid pulse, tachypnea, and cool, clammy, cyanotic skin. In septic shock the skin may initially be warm and flushed, owing to peripheral vasodilation.
- Cardiac, cerebral, and pulmonary changes secondary to the shock state worsen the situation.
- Patients surviving the initial complications enter *a second phase dominated by renal insufficiency* and marked by a progressive fall in urine output, as well as severe fluid and electrolyte imbalances.
- Prognosis varies with the origin and duration of shock. Thus 90% of young, otherwise healthy patients with hypovolemic shock survive with appropriate management, whereas cardiogenic or septic shock carries markedly worse mortality rates.

5

Genetic Disorders

Genes and Human Diseases (p. 137)

The architecture of the human genome was discussed previously (see Chapter 1).

Genetic disorders are extremely common, with an estimated lifetime frequency of 67%; this includes not only "classic" genetic disorders but also cancer and cardiovascular diseases with complex, multigenic contributions. If one counts all concept uses, the actual frequency is probably greater because 50% of early spontaneous abortions have a demonstrable chromosomal abnormality; the vast majority of genetic disorders do not result in a viable birth. Even so, approximately 1% of newborns have a gross chromosomal abnormality, and 5% of individuals under age 25 have a serious disease with a significant genetic component.

Causes of genetic disorders can be classified as follows:

- *Mutations in single genes.* These are usually *highly penetrant* (i.e., mutation typically results in disease) and follow classical Mendelian inheritance patterns.
- *Chromosomal (cytogenetic) disorders.* These arise from structural (e.g., breaks) or numerical alterations in chromosomes; they are usually highly penetrant.
- *Multigenic disorders.* These are the most common cause of genetic disorders and are caused by the complex interactions of multiple *variant* (not mutant) forms of genes *(polymorphisms)* and environmental factors. Independently, each polymorphism has only a small effect and is of low penetrance. Progress in genomics and bioinformatics has allowed *genome-wide association studies (GWAS)* to begin to identify the various genetic risk factors and contributions.

Mutations (p. 138)

A mutation is a permanent change in the DNA; mutations in germ cells are transmitted to progeny (and cause heritable disease), whereas mutations in somatic cells are not transmissible but can affect cell behavior (e.g., malignant transformation). Mutations can involve changes in coding or noncoding regions of the genome and can affect just one or a few nucleotides or cause complete deletion of a gene.

Point Mutations in Coding Sequences

- *Missense mutation.* Single nucleotide substitutions can change the triplet base code and yield a different amino acid in the final protein product. This can be a *conservative* mutation if the new amino acid is not significantly different from the original, with minimal (if any) consequences. However, *nonconservative* mutations (e.g., substituting amino acids of different size or charge) can lead to loss of function, misfolding, and degradation of the protein or even gain of function.
- *Nonsense mutation.* Single nucleotide substitutions can potentially result in the formation of an inappropriate "stop"

codon; the resulting protein may then be truncated with loss of normal activity.

Mutations Within Noncoding Regions

- Point mutations or deletions in enhancer or promoter regions can significantly affect the regulation or level of gene transcription.
- Point mutations can lead to defective splicing and thus failure to form mature mRNA species.

Frameshift Mutations

Loss of one or more nucleotides can alter the reading frame of the DNA. Insertions or deletions of multiples of three nucleotides may have no effect other than adding or deleting an amino acid; frameshifts of other numbers of nucleotides lead to defective protein products (missense or nonsense).

Trinucleotide Repeat Mutations

This special category of mutations is characterized by amplification of triple-nucleotide sequences (e.g., fragile X syndrome or Huntington disease). Trinucleotide repeats are a common feature of many normal genetic sequences; however, mutations involving these repeats can see a 10- to 200-fold amplification of the normal number, leading to abnormal gene expression. This type of mutation is also dynamic, with the length of the trinucleotide repeat sequences frequently expanding during gametogenesis.

Mendelian Disorders (p. 140)

Mendelian disorders result from mutations in single genes that have a large effect. Every individual is a carrier of five to eight potentially deleterious mutations; 80% will be inherited *(familial),* whereas the remainder represent de novo mutations.

- Whether a given mutation will have an adverse outcome is influenced by compensatory genes and environmental factors.
- Some autosomal mutations produce partial expression in heterozygotes and full expression only in homozygotes (e.g., sickle cell disease).
- Mendelian traits can be dominant, recessive, or *codominant,* the latter referring to full expression of both alleles in a heterozygote.
- *Penetrance* refers to the percentage of individuals who carry a particular gene and also express the trait.
- *Variable expressivity:* Variation in the effect caused by a particular mutation (e.g., manifestations of neurofibromatosis type I range from brown macules to skin tumors to skeletal deformities).
- *Pleiotropism:* Multiple possible end effects of a single mutant gene (e.g., in sickle cell disease, the mutant hemoglobin causes hemolysis and anemia, as well as vascular occlusion leading to splenic infarction and bone necrosis).
- *Genetic heterogeneity:* Multiple different mutations leading to the same outcome (e.g., different autosomal recessive mutations can cause childhood deafness).

Transmission Patterns of Single-Gene Disorders (p. 140)

Autosomal Dominant Disorders *(p. 140) (Table 5-1)*

Autosomal dominant disorders manifest in the heterozygous state and have the following general features:

- Disease is usually also present in a parent. When both parents of an affected individual are normal, a de novo germ cell mutation

TABLE 5-1 Autosomal Dominant Disorders

System	Disorder
Nervous	Huntington disease Neurofibromatosis Myotonic dystrophy Tuberous sclerosis
Urinary	Polycystic kidney disease
Gastrointestinal	Familial polyposis coli
Hematopoietic	Hereditary spherocytosis von Willebrand disease
Skeletal	Marfan syndrome* EDS (some variants)* Osteogenesis imperfecta Achondroplasia
Metabolic	Familial hypercholesterolemia* Acute intermittent porphyria

*Discussed in this chapter. Other disorders listed are discussed in appropriate chapters in the book.

is suggested; this happens more commonly in the sperm of older fathers.

- Clinical features are modified by penetrance and expressivity.
- Clinical onset is often later than in autosomal recessive disorders.
- Most autosomal dominant mutations are *loss-of-function* (i.e., they result in either reduced production of a gene product or reduced activity of a protein).
    - Mutations in a key structural protein (e.g., collagen)—especially if it is part of a multimer—can interfere with the function of the normal gene product (i.e., by affecting folding) leading to *dominant negative* effects.
    - Mutations of components in complex metabolic pathways subject to feedback inhibition (e.g., the low-density lipoprotein [LDL] receptor) are often autosomal dominant.
    - Mutations in enzymes are usually not autosomal dominant because even loss of 50% activity can be compensated.
- *Gain-of-function* autosomal dominant mutations are less common; they cause disease by endowing a gene product with toxic properties or by increasing a normal activity.

Autosomal Recessive Disorders *(p. 141) (Table 5-2)*

Autosomal recessive disorders include most inborn errors of metabolism. In contrast to autosomal dominant disorders, the following features generally apply:

- The expression of the disease features tends to be more uniform.
- Complete penetrance is common.
- Onset is frequently early in life.
- de novo mutations are rarely detected clinically until several generations have passed and a heterozygote-heterozygote mating has occurred.
- Enzymes—rather than structural proteins—are more commonly affected.

X-Linked Disorders *(p. 142) (Table 5-3)*

All sex-linked disorders are X-linked, and most are recessive. They are fully expressed in males because mutant genes on the

TABLE 5-2 Autosomal Recessive Disorders	
System	**Disorder**
Metabolic	Cystic fibrosis Phenylketonuria Galactosemia Homocystinuria Lysosomal storage diseases* α_1-Antitrypsin deficiency Wilson disease Hemochromatosis Glycogen storage diseases*
Hematopoietic	Sickle cell anemia Thalassemias
Endocrine	Congenital adrenal hyperplasia
Skeletal	EDS (some variants)* Alkaptonuria*
Nervous	Neurogenic muscular atrophies Friedreich ataxia Spinal muscular atrophy

*Discussed in this chapter. Many others are discussed elsewhere in the text.

TABLE 5-3 X-Linked Recessive Disorders	
System	**Disease**
Musculoskeletal	Duchenne muscular dystrophy
Blood	Hemophilia A and B Chronic granulomatous disease Glucose-6-phosphate dehydrogenase deficiency
Immune	Agammaglobulinemia Wiskott-Aldrich syndrome
Metabolic	Diabetes insipidus Lesch-Nyhan syndrome
Nervous	Fragile X syndrome*

*Discussed in this chapter. Others are discussed in appropriate chapters in the text.

X chromosome do not have a Y chromosome counterpart (affected males are *hemizygous* for the X-linked mutant gene). Heterozygote females usually do not express the disease due to a paired normal X allele. However, random X inactivation in a population of cells can lead to a variable phenotype. X-linked dominant conditions are rare; affected women will express the disease and transmit it to 50% of their sons *and* daughters, whereas affected men will express the disease and transmit it to 100% of their daughters and none of their sons.

Biochemical and Molecular Basis of Single-Gene (Mendelian) Disorders (p. 142)

Single-gene mutations can cause disease by changing the production of a specific gene or by the formation of an abnormal protein; this can involve enzymes, substrates, receptors, and structural proteins (Table 5-4).

TABLE 5-4 Biochemical and Molecular Basis of Some Mendelian Disorders

Protein Type/Function	Example	Molecular Lesion	Disease
Enzyme	Phenylalanine hydroxylase	Splice-site mutation: reduced amount	Phenylketonuria
	Hexosaminidase	Splice-site mutation or frameshift mutation with stop codon: reduced amount	Tay-Sachs disease
	Adenosine deaminase	Point mutations: abnormal protein with reduced activity	Severe combined immunodeficiency
Enzyme inhibitor	α_1-Antitrypsin	Missense mutations: impaired secretion from liver to serum	Emphysema and liver disease
Receptor	LDL receptor	Deletions, point mutations: reduction of synthesis, transport to cell surface, or binding to LDL	Familial hypercholesterolemia
	Vitamin D receptor	Point mutation: failure of normal signaling	Vitamin D-resistant rickets
Transport			
Oxygen	Hemoglobin	Deletions: reduced amount	α-Thalassemia
		Defective mRNA processing: reduced amount	β-Thalassemia
		Point mutations: abnormal structure	Sickle cell anemia
Ion channels	Cystic fibrosis transmembrane conductance regulator	Deletions and other mutations: nonfunctional or misfolded proteins	Cystic fibrosis

Continued

TABLE 5-4 Biochemical and Molecular Basis of Some Mendelian Disorders—cont'd

Protein Type/Function	Example	Molecular Lesion	Disease
Structural			
Extracellular	Collagen	Deletions or point mutations cause reduced amount of normal collagen or normal amounts of defective collagen	Osteogenesis imperfecta; EDSs
	Fibrillin	Missense mutations	Marfan syndrome
Cell membrane	Dystrophin	Deletion with reduced synthesis	Duchenne/Becker muscular dystrophy
	Spectrin, ankyrin, or protein 4.1	Heterogeneous	Hereditary spherocytosis
Hemostasis	Factor VIII	Deletions, insertions, nonsense mutations, and others: reduced synthesis or abnormal factor VIII	Hemophilia A
Growth regulation	Rb protein	Deletions	Hereditary retinoblastoma
	Neurofibromin	Heterogeneous	Neurofibromatosis type 1

Enzyme Defects and Their Consequences (p. 142)

Mutations can result in the synthesis of a defective enzyme (reduced activity) or reduced synthesis of a normal enzyme. The outcome is a metabolic block with the following:

- Accumulation of a substrate that is toxic (e.g., phenylalanine in *phenylketonuria*).
- Decreased amount of an end product necessary for normal function (e.g., melanin in *albinism*).
- Decreased metabolism of a tissue-damaging substrate (e.g., neutrophil elastase in *α_1-antitrypsin deficiency*).

Defects in Receptors and Transport Systems (p. 143)

Defects can affect the intracellular accumulation of an important precursor (e.g., LDL in *familial hypercholesterolemia*) or export of a metabolite necessary for normal tissue homeostasis (e.g., chloride in *cystic fibrosis*).

Alterations in Structure, Function, or Quantity of Nonenzyme Proteins (p. 144)

Examples include the hemoglobinopathies (e.g., sickle cell disease, thalassemia) or *osteogenesis imperfecta* due to defective collagen.

Genetically Determined Adverse Reactions to Drugs (p. 144)

These otherwise clinically silent mutations are “unmasked” when specific compounds/substrates are administered that lead to toxic intermediates or cannot be appropriately catabolized.

Disorders Associated With Defects in Structural Proteins (p. 144)

Marfan Syndrome (p. 144)

Marfan syndrome is an autosomal dominant disorder resulting from 1 of 600 different (mostly missense) mutations in the *fibrillin-1* gene mapping to 15q21.1. Fibrillin is a glycoprotein component of microfibrils that provides a scaffold for the deposition of elastin; it is especially abundant in the connective tissues of the aorta, ligaments, and ciliary zonules that support the eye lens. The disorder therefore mostly affects the *skeletal, ocular,* and *cardiovascular systems.* Abnormal fibrillin results in defective microfibril assembly resulting in reduced elasticity, as well as reduced sequestration of transforming growth factor-β (TGF-β); excess TGF-β reduces normal vascular smooth muscle development and matrix production.

Morphology (p. 145)

Skeletal changes are as follows:

- Tall stature with exceptionally long extremities
- Long, tapering fingers and toes *(arachnodactyly)*
- Laxity of joint ligaments, producing hyperextensibility
- *Dolichocephaly* (long-headed) with frontal bossing and prominent supraorbital ridges
- Spinal deformities (e.g., kyphosis and scoliosis)

Ocular changes are as follows:

- Bilateral dislocation of lenses (ectopia lentis)
- Increased axial length of the globe, giving rise to retinal detachments

Cardiovascular lesions are as follows:

- Mitral valve prolapse

- Aortic cystic medial degeneration causing aortic ring dilation and valvular incompetence. This is likely exacerbated by the excess TGF-β signaling.

Cutaneous change:

- Striae

Clinical Features (p. 145)

There is great variability in the clinical expression, so that clinical diagnosis requires major involvement of two out of four systems (cardiovascular, skeletal, ocular, and cutaneous), and minor involvement of one other. Mitral valve prolapse is most common, although not life threatening; affected valves are floppy and associated with mitral regurgitation. Cystic medial degeneration of the aorta is less common but clinically more important; the medial degeneration predisposes to medial dissections, often resulting in aortic rupture, a cause of death in 30% to 45% of affected patients.

Ehlers-Danlos Syndrome *(p. 145)*

Ehlers-Danlos syndrome (EDS) is a clinically and genetically heterogeneous group of disorders caused by defects in collagen synthesis; major manifestations involve the following:

- *Skin:* Hyperextensible, extremely fragile, and vulnerable to trauma; wound healing is markedly impaired owing to defective collagen synthesis.
- *Joints:* Hypermobile and prone to dislocation.
- *Visceral complications:* Manifestations include rupture of the colon and large arteries; ocular fragility with corneal rupture and retinal detachment; and diaphragmatic hernias.

EDS are divided into six variants on the basis of predominant clinical manifestations and patterns of inheritance (Table 5-5):

- Reduced activity of lysyl hydroxylase, an enzyme essential for collagen cross-linking.

TABLE 5-5 Classification of Ehlers-Danlos Syndromes

EDS Type*	Clinical Findings	Inheritance	Gene Defects
Classical (I/II)	Skin and joint hypermobility, atrophic scars, easy bruising	Autosomal dominant	*COL5A1, COL5A2*
Hypermobility (III)	Joint hypermobility, pain, dislocations	Autosomal dominant	Unknown
Vascular (IV)	Thin skin, arterial or uterine rupture, bruising, small joint hyperextensibility	Autosomal dominant	*COL3A1*
Kyphoscoliosis (VI)	Hypotonia, joint laxity, congenital scoliosis, ocular fragility	Autosomal recessive	Lysyl hydroxylase
Arthrochalasia (VIIa,b)	Severe joint hypermobility, skin changes mild, scoliosis, bruising	Autosomal dominant	*COL1A1, COL1A2*
Dermatosparaxis (VIIc)	Severe skin fragility, cutis laxa, bruising	Autosomal recessive	Procollagen *N*-peptidase

*EDS were previously classified by Roman numerals. Parentheses show previous numerical equivalents.

- Mutations in type III collagen. Because a structural rather than an enzyme protein is affected, the pattern of inheritance is autosomal dominant. Blood vessels and intestines are especially rich in collagen type III and are therefore most susceptible.
- Mutant procollagen chains that resist cleavage of N-terminal peptides and thus result in defective conversion of type I procollagen to mature collagen. This mutation has a *dominant negative* effect.

Disorders Associated With Defects in Receptor Proteins (p. 147)

Familial Hypercholesterolemia (p. 147)

Familial hypercholesterolemia results from mutations in the gene encoding the receptor for LDL. Mutations affecting other aspects of LDL uptake, metabolism, and regulation can cause a similar phenotype.

Normal Cholesterol Transport and Metabolism (Fig. 5-1)

- LDL is the major transport form of cholesterol in plasma.
- Although most cells possess high-affinity receptors for LDL apoprotein B-100, 70% of plasma LDL is cleared by the liver; uptake by other cells, especially mononuclear phagocytes, can occur

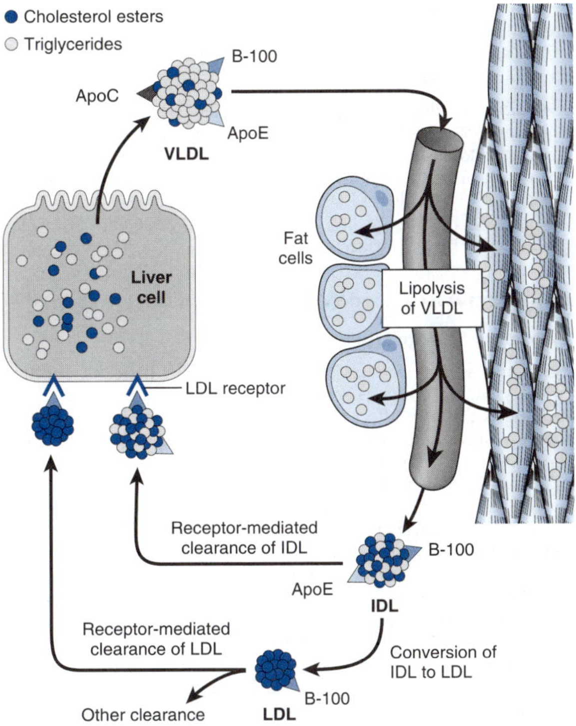

Figure 5-1 Schematic illustration of LDL metabolism and the role of the liver in its synthesis and clearance. Lipolysis of very low-density lipoprotein (VLDL) by lipoprotein lipase in the capillaries releases triglycerides that are then stored in fat cells and used as a source of energy in skeletal muscles. *ApoE,* Apoprotein E; *IDL,* intermediate-density lipoprotein.

through distinct *scavenger* receptors for chemically altered LDL (e.g., acetylated or oxidized).

- The transport and metabolism of LDL in the liver involve the following:
  - Binding to specific LDL plasma membrane receptors
  - Internalization and subsequent dissociation from its receptor in the early endosome, followed by transport to lysosomes
  - Lysosomal processing, leading to release of free cholesterol into cytoplasm through the action of NPC1 and 2 proteins (Niemann-Pick disease [NPC], type C)
- Free cholesterol affects three processes:
  - Suppresses cholesterol synthesis by inhibiting the rate-limiting enzyme hydroxymethylglutaryl coenzyme A reductase
  - Activates enzymes that esterify cholesterol
  - Suppresses LDL receptor synthesis, thereby limiting further cholesterol transport

Without intracellular cholesterol feedback inhibition of these processes, total circulating cholesterol levels increase. Heterozygotes occur at a frequency of approximately 1 in 500 in the general population and have two to threefold elevated cholesterol levels; homozygotes have five to sixfold cholesterol elevations, with early onset of severe atherosclerosis and the possibility of cardiovascular events (e.g., myocardial infarction) before age 20. Xanthomas of the skin are also more prominent.

The various LDL receptor mutations (more than 900 described to date) fall into five general classes:

- *Class I:* Inadequate LDL receptor protein synthesis (rare)
- *Class II:* Abnormal LDL receptor folding leading to retention in the endoplasmic reticulum (common)
- *Class III:* Reduced binding capacity of LDL receptor protein
- *Class IV:* Inability of LDL receptor to internalize
- *Class V:* Inability of LDL and receptor to dissociate, with recycling to the cell surface

Disorders Associated With Defects in Enzymes (p. 149)

Lysosomal Storage Diseases (p. 149)

Lysosomal storage diseases result from a genetic deficiency of functional lysosomal enzymes or other proteins essential for their activity; mutations can also affect the targeting of lysosomal enzymes after their synthesis in the endoplasmic reticulum (enzymes destined for the lysosome are tagged by appending a terminal mannose-6-phosphate residue during transit through the Golgi apparatus). In the absence of adequate lysosomal processing, catabolism of complex substrates is impaired, leading to accumulation of partially degraded metabolites within lysosomes. The lysosomes, enlarged with undigested macromolecules, can interfere with normal cell function; there is also deficient recycling of constituent nutrients. Because lysosomal function is critical for autophagy, such storage disorders lead to the accumulation of "autophagic substrates" (e.g., effete mitochondria and other organelles, as well as polyubiquinated proteins). Failure to clear dysfunctional mitochondria can lead to increased apoptosis and generate greater quantities of oxygen-derived free radicals.

Therapeutic approaches include the following:

- Enzyme replacement
- Substrate reduction
- Molecular "chaperones" to assist in the normal folding of mutant proteins

Lysosomal storage diseases are classified on the basis of the biochemical nature of the accumulated metabolite (Table 5-6). The tissues affected and the resultant clinical features depend on where the material to be degraded is normally located and in which sites it is typically catabolized. Because macrophages are particularly rich in lysosomes and are responsible for degradation of several substrates, organs with abundant macrophages (e.g., liver and spleen) are often affected.

Tay-Sachs Disease (p. 151)

Tay-Sachs disease results from mutations in the α-subunit of the hexosaminidase enzyme complex; it is the most common of the three G_{M2} gangliosidoses resulting from lysosomal G_{M2} ganglioside accumulation (all have similar clinical outcomes). It is most common in Jews of Eastern European (Ashkenazic) origin. Antenatal diagnosis and carrier detection are possible by DNA probe analysis and enzyme assays on cells obtained from amniocentesis.

Because neurons are rich in gangliosides, they are the cell type most severely affected; thus typical clinical features are motor and mental deterioration commencing at approximately 6 months of age, blindness, and death by age 2 to 3 years.

***Morphology** (p. 151).*

- Neuronal ballooning with lipid-filled cytoplasmic vacuoles
- Progressive neuronal destruction with microglial proliferation
- Accumulation of lipids in retinal ganglion cells, rendering them pale in color, thus accentuating the normal red color of the macular choroid *(cherry-red spot).*

Niemann-Pick Disease, Types A and B (p. 152)

NPC, types A and B are related disorders associated with sphingomyelinase deficiency (more than 100 mutations are described); sphingomyelin accumulation is most prominent in mononuclear phagocytes but can also affect neurons. Like Tay-Sachs, these disorders are common in Ashkenazic Jews. Acid sphingomyelinase is an *imprinted* gene (see later) that is preferentially expressed from the maternal chromosome due to paternal gene epigenetic silencing.

Type A is more common; it is a severe, infantile form of the disease clinically manifest at birth and with death occurring typically within 3 years. Affected cells are engorged with numerous small vacuoles that impart cytoplasmic foaminess:

- Diffuse neuronal involvement, leading eventually to cell death and central nervous system (CNS) atrophy; a retinal cherry-red spot similar to that seen in Tay-Sachs occurs in approximately half the patients.
- Extreme accumulation of lipids in mononuclear phagocytes, yielding massive hepatosplenomegaly and lymphadenopathy, with bone marrow infiltration.
- Visceral involvement mainly affecting the gastrointestinal tract and lungs.

Type B is associated with organomegaly but not CNS involvement, and patients typically survive into adulthood.

Niemann-Pick Disease, Type C (p. 153)

NPC, type C is distinct from types A and B and is more common than both combined. It is due to mutations in either *NPC1* (95% of cases) or *NPC2,* coding for proteins involved in cholesterol transport from lysosomes to the cytosol. Cholesterol and gangliosides are both accumulated and can present with hydrops fetalis, neonatal hepatitis, or (most commonly) progressive neurologic degeneration

TABLE 5-6 Lysosomal Storage Diseases

Glycogenosis		
Type 2—Pompe disease	α-1,4-Glucosidase (lysosomal glucosidase)	Glycogen
Sphingolipidoses		
G_{M1} gangliosidosis Type 1—infantile, generalized Type 2—juvenile	G_{M1} ganglioside β-galactosidase	G_{M1} ganglioside, galactose-containing oligosaccharides
G_{M2} gangliosidosis	Hexosaminidase-α subunit	G_{M2} ganglioside
Tay-Sachs disease	Hexosaminidase-β subunit	G_{M2} ganglioside
Sandhoff disease	Ganglioside activator protein	G_{M2} ganglioside
Sulfatidoses		
Metachromatic leukodystrophy	Arylsulfatase A	Sulfatide
Multiple sulfatase deficiency	Arylsulfatases A, B, C; steroid sulfatase; iduronate sulfatase; heparan N-sulfatase	Sulfatide, steroid sulfate, heparan sulfate, dermatan sulfate
Krabbe disease	Galactosylceramidase	Galactocerebroside
Fabry disease	α-Galactosidase A	Ceramide trihexoside
Gaucher disease	Glucocerebrosidase	Glucocerebroside
NPC: types A and B	Sphingomyelinase	Sphingomyelin
MPS		
MPS I-H (Hurler)	α-L-Iduronidase	Dermatan sulfate, heparan sulfate
MPS II (Hunter)	L-Iduronosulfate sulfatase	
Mucolipidoses (ML)		
I-cell disease (ML II) and pseudo-Hurler polydystrophy	Deficiency of phosphorylating enzymes essential for the formation of mannose-6-phosphate recognition marker; acid hydrolases lacking the recognition marker cannot be targeted to the lysosomes but are secreted extracellularly	Mucopolysaccharide, glycolipid
Other Diseases of Complex Carbohydrates		
Fucosidosis	α-Fucosidase	Fucose-containing sphingolipids and glycoprotein fragments
Mannosidosis	α-Mannosidase	Mannose-containing oligosaccharides
Aspartylglycosaminuria	Aspartylglycosamine amide hydrolase	Aspartyl-2-deoxy-2-acetamido-glycosylamine
Other Lysosomal Storage Diseases		
Wolman disease	Acid lipase	Cholesterol esters, triglycerides
Acid phosphate deficiency	Lysosomal acid phosphatase	Phosphate esters

beginning in childhood with ataxia, dystonia, and psychomotor regression.

Gaucher Disease (p. 153)

Gaucher disease refers to a cluster of autosomal recessive disorders involving mutations leading to diminished glucocerebrosidase activity; cleavage of ceramide (derived from cell membranes of senescent leukocytes and red blood cells as well as from turnover of brain gangliosides) is impaired. Glucocerebroside accumulation occurs in mononuclear phagocytes and (in some forms) the CNS. Disease manifestations are secondary to the burden of stored material, as well as macrophage activation and local cytokine production. Three variants are identified:

- *Type I* is most common form (99% of cases) and occurs in adults with a higher incidence in European Jews; there is reduced but detectable levels of enzyme activity. This chronic, *non-neuronopathic* form is associated with glucocerebroside storage in mononuclear phagocytes. Although there is no brain involvement, patients have massive splenomegaly and lymphadenopathy, and marrow involvement leads to bone erosions that can cause pathologic fractures; pancytopenia or thrombocytopenia results from hypersplenism; lifespan is not markedly affected.
- *Type II* is the *acute neuronopathic form,* affecting infants but without a Jewish predilection. It is associated with hepatosplenomegaly but progressive CNS deterioration predominates, with death at a young age.
- *Type III* is intermediate with systemic involvement of macrophages, as well as progressive neurologic disease beginning in adolescence.

Morphology *(p.153).* Affected cells (Gaucher cells) are distended with periodic acid-Schiff (PAS)-positive material with a fibrillary appearance resembling "crumpled tissue paper" (composed of elongated lysosomes containing stored lipid in bilayer stacks).

Clinical Features *(p.154).* Prenatal diagnosis is possible by enzyme assay of amniotic fluid or by DNA probe analysis, although there are more than 150 known mutations. Replacement therapy with recombinant enzymes is effective but expensive; bone marrow transplant and/or gene transfer into bone marrow cells, as well as substrate reduction therapy, is being evaluated.

Mucopolysaccharidoses (p. 154)

Mucopolysaccharidoses (MPS) are a group of disorders resulting from inherited deficiencies of enzymes that degrade glycosaminoglycans (abundant in the extracellular matrix of connective tissues). Accumulated substrates include heparan sulfate, dermatan sulfate, keratan sulfate, and chondroitin sulfate.

Several MPS clinical variants (numbered I to VII) are known, each resulting from the deficiency of one specific enzyme; all are autosomal recessive except MPS II *(Hunter syndrome),* which is X-linked recessive. Severity relates to the degree of enzyme deficiency; in general, all forms are progressive and are characterized by the following:

- Coarse facial features
- Hepatosplenomegaly
- Corneal clouding
- Valve and subendothelial arterial thickening
- Joint stiffness
- Mental retardation

Morphology *(p.154).* Affected cells are distended with clear cytoplasm (balloon cells) containing PAS-positive material. Accumulated mucopolysaccharides are found in many cell types, including mononuclear phagocytes, fibroblasts, endothelial cells, intimal smooth muscle cells, and neurons.

Clinical Features *(p. 155).* The two most well-characterized syndromes are as follows:

- *Hurler syndrome* (MPS 1-H), due to α-L-iduronidase deficiency; a severe form with onset at 6 to 24 months and death by age 6 to 10 years, usually due to cardiovascular complications.
- *Hunter syndrome* (MPS II), lacking corneal opacification and with a generally milder course.

Glycogen Storage Diseases (Glycogenoses) (p. 155)

Glycogen storage diseases result from hereditary deficiencies in the synthesis or catabolism of glycogen (Fig. 5-2); disorders may be restricted to specific tissues or can be systemic. On the basis of specific enzymatic deficiencies and resultant clinical pictures, the glycogenoses are divided into three major groups:

- *Hepatic form* due to deficiencies in enzymes that primarily influence liver glycogen catabolism; these are characterized by low blood glucose (hypoglycemia) and hepatic glycogen accumulation. The prototype is von Gierke disease (type I) due to glucose-6-phosphatase deficiency (converts glucose 6-phosphate to glucose); others include deficiencies in liver phosphorylase or debranching enzyme (Fig. 5-2).
- *Myopathic form* characterized by deficiencies of enzymes that fuel glycolysis in striated muscles. These characteristically present with muscle weakness and cramping after exercise without exercise-induced rises in blood lactate; skeletal muscles show glycogen accumulation. McArdle disease (type V) is due to deficient muscle phosphorylase.
- *Miscellaneous forms* associated with α-glucosidase deficiency (acid maltase) or lack of branching enzyme; these lead typically to glycogen overload in many organs and early death. Type II glycogenosis, or Pompe disease, results from deficiency of the lysosomal enzyme acid maltase (α-glucosidase). As in other lysosomal storage diseases, many organs are involved; however, cardiac involvement is most prominent in this disorder.

Disorders Associated With Defects in Proteins That Regulate Cell Growth (p. 157)

Normal cellular growth and differentiation is regulated by proteins deriving from proto-oncogenes and tumor suppressor genes. Mutations in these genes are important in tumor pathogenesis (see Chapter 7); nevertheless, only approximately 5% of all cancers are due to germline mutations (most are autosomal dominant), and the vast majority of cancer-associated mutations in these genes occur de novo in somatic cells.

Complex Multigenic Disorders (p. 158)

Such disorders result from the interplay of variant forms of genes and environmental factors. Genetic variants with at least two different alleles and an incidence in the population ≥1% are called *polymorphisms*. Complex genetic disorders occur when several polymorphisms—individually with modest effects and low

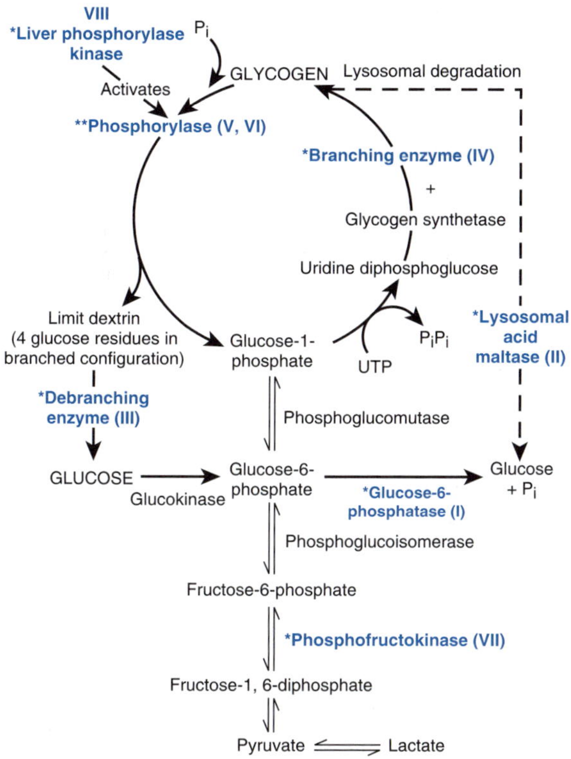

Figure 5-2 Glycogen metabolic pathways and the associated enzymatic deficiencies (marked with "*") leading to glycogenoses; roman numerals indicate the type of glycogen storage disease. Types V and VI result from muscle and liver phosphorylase deficiencies, respectively. *(Modified from Hers H et al.: Glycogen storage diseases. In Scriver CR, Beaudet AL, Charles R, Sly WS, Valle D [eds]:* The Metabolic Basis of Inherited Diseases, *6th ed. New York, NY: McGraw-Hill, 1989, p. 425.)*

penetrance—are inherited together. Not all polymorphisms are equally important; although 20 to 30 genes are implicated in type 1 diabetes mellitus, six to seven are most important, and certain HLA alleles make up >50% of the risk. Some polymorphisms are disease specific, whereas others crop up in multiple mechanistically related diseases (i.e., immune-mediated disorders). Moreover, environmental influences significantly modify the risk of expression.

Chromosomal Disorders (p. 158)

Cytogenetic disorders may be due to alterations in the *number* or in the *structure* of chromosomes. Karyotypes are given as total number of chromosomes, followed by the sex chromosome complement, and then abnormalities in ascending numerical order (e.g., a male with trisomy 21 is designated: 47,XY,+21). The short arm is designated *p* (for *petite*); the long arm is designated as *q* (next letter in the alphabet). Giemsa staining leads to characteristic light

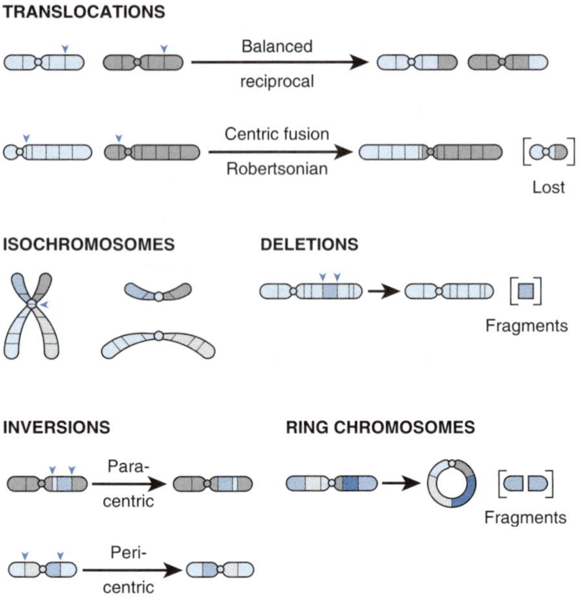

Figure 5-3 Types of chromosomal rearrangements.

and dark bands for each chromosome, so-called G banding. In a banded karyotype (400 to 800 bands per haploid set), the various regions are demarcated by prominent bands, numbered sequentially starting from the centromere going outward. Bands are further subsegmented; thus *Xp21.2* denotes a chromosome segment located on the short arm of the X chromosome in region 2, band 1, and sub-band 2.

Numerical Disorders

Numerical disorders are as follows:

- *Monosomy,* associated with one less normal chromosome
- *Trisomy,* associated with one extra chromosome
- *Mosaicism,* associated with one or more populations of cells, some with normal chromosomal complement, others with extra or missing chromosomes

Numerical disorders of chromosomes result from errors during cell division. Monosomy and trisomy usually result from chromosomal nondisjunction during gametogenesis (the first meiotic division), whereas mosaics are produced when mitotic errors occur in the zygote. Monosomy of autosomes usually results in early fetal death and spontaneous abortion, whereas trisomies can be better tolerated, and similar imbalances in sex chromosomes are usually compatible with life.

Structural Abnormalities of Chromosomes (p. 159) (Fig. 5-3)

- *Deletion:* Loss of a terminal or interstitial (midpiece) segment of a chromosome.

- *Translocation:* Involves transfer of a segment of one chromosome to another:
  - *Balanced reciprocal,* involving exchange of chromosomal material between two chromosomes with no net gain or loss of genetic material.
  - *Robertsonian (centric) fusion,* or reciprocal translocation between two acrocentric chromosomes involving the short arm of one and the long arm of the other; transfer of segments leads to formation of one abnormally large chromosome and one extremely small one. The latter is usually lost. This translocation predisposes to the formation of abnormal (unbalanced) gametes.
- *Isochromosome:* Formed when one arm (short or long) is lost and the remaining arm is duplicated, resulting in a chromosome of two short arms only or of two long arms. In live births the most common isochromosome involves the X chromosome, designated i(X)(q10), with resulting duplication (and thus trisomy) of genes on the long arm and deletion (with monosomy) for genes on the short arm.
- *Inversion:* Rearrangement associated with two breaks in a chromosome, followed by inversion and reincorporation of the broken segment.
- *Ring chromosome:* Deletion affecting both ends, followed by fusion of the damaged ends.

Cytogenetic Disorders Involving Autosomes (p. 161)

Trisomy 21 (Down Syndrome) *(p. 161)*

This is the most common chromosomal disorder (1 in 700 births) and a major cause of mental retardation:

- Approximately 95% have a complete extra chromosome 21 (e.g., 47,XY,+21). In 95% of these cases the extra chromosome is maternal in origin. The incidence is strongly influenced by maternal age: 1 in 1550 births in women younger than 20 years; 1 in 25 in women older than 45 years.
- Approximately 4% of all cases have extra chromosomal material derived from a parental chromosome bearing a translocation of the long arm of chromosome 21 to chromosome 22 or 14. Because the fertilized ovum already possesses two normal autosomes 21, the translocated chromosomal fragment provides the same triple-gene dosage as trisomy 21. Such cases are frequently (but not always) familial because the parent is a carrier of a robertsonian translocation. Maternal age has no impact.
- Mosaic variants make up approximately 1% of all cases; they have a mixture of cells with normal chromosome numbers and cells with an extra chromosome 21. Maternal age has no impact.
- Clinical features include the following (Fig. 5-4, *A*):
  - Flat faces with oblique palpebral fissures and epicanthic folds; simian hand creases.
  - Severe mental retardation.
  - Forty percent will have congenital heart disease, especially endocardial cushion defects, responsible for the majority of deaths in infancy and childhood.
  - Tenfold to twentyfold increased risk of acute leukemia.
  - Abnormal immune responses leading to recurrent infections and thyroid autoimmunity.
  - Premature Alzheimer disease.

Other Trisomies (p. 163)

Trisomy 18 (*Edwards syndrome;* Fig. 5-4, *B*) and trisomy 13 (*Patau syndrome;* Fig. 5-4, *C*) occur much less commonly than trisomy 21; both are associated with increased maternal age. Affected infants have severe malformations and usually die within the first year of life.

Chromosome 22q11.2 Deletion Syndrome (p. 163)

Chromosome 22q11.2 deletion syndrome is fairly common (1 in 4000 births) and is due to a small deletion of band 11.2 on the long arm of chromosome 22. The clinical features associated with this deletion (see later) constitute a spectrum that includes *DiGeorge syndrome* (see Chapter 6) and *velocardiofacial syndrome.* T-cell immunodeficiency and hypocalcemia are more prominent in some cases (DiGeorge syndrome), whereas facial dysmorphology and cardiac malformations are more prominent in others (velocardiofacial syndrome):

- Congenital heart defects
- Abnormalities of palate
- Facial dysmorphism
- Developmental delay
- Increased incidence of psychiatric disorders (schizophrenia, bipolar, attention deficit hyperactivity disorder)

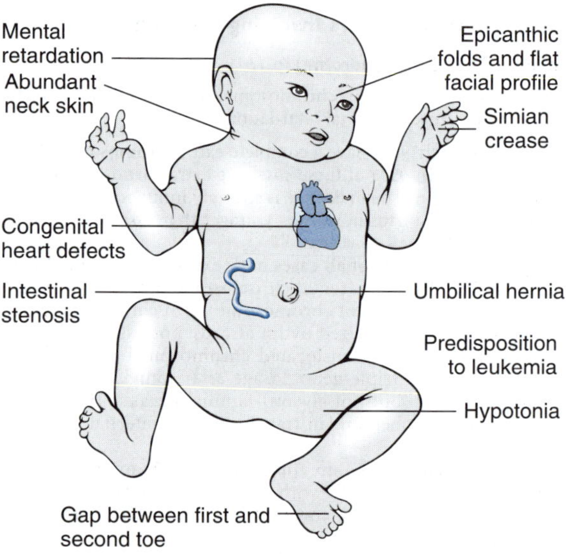

TRISOMY 21: DOWN SYNDROME

Incidence: 1 in 700 births

Karyotypes:

Trisomy 21 type:	47,XX, +21
Translocation type:	46,XX,der(14;21)(q10;q10),+21
Mosaic type:	46,XX/47,XX, +21

A

Figure 5-4 Clinical features and karyotypes of selected autosomal trisomies.

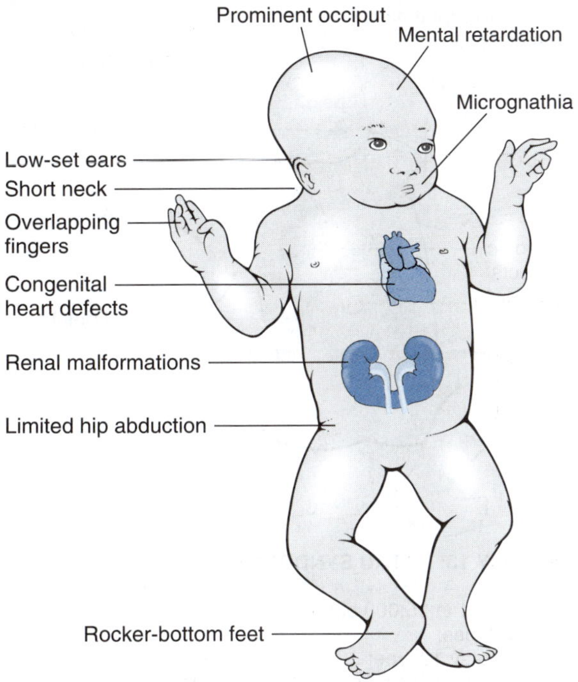

TRISOMY 18: EDWARDS SYNDROME

Incidence: 1 in 8000 births

Karyotypes:

Trisomy 18 type:	47,XX, +18
Mosaic type:	46,XX/47,XX, +18

B

Figure 5-4, cont'd

- Variable T-cell deficiency
- Hypoparathyroidism

Cytogenetic Disorders Involving Sex Chromosomes (p. 164)

Imbalances in sex chromosomes are more common than autosomal imbalances because they are typically better tolerated. For example, the milder nature of X chromosome-associated aberrations is related to the fact that there is normally random inactivation of one X chromosome (Lyon hypothesis):

- Random inactivation of either paternal or maternal X chromosome occurs early in embryogenesis and leads to the formation of a Barr body.
- Normal females are functional mosaics with two cell populations, one with an inactivated paternal X chromosome and the other with an inactivated maternal X chromosome.
- With extra X chromosomes, all but one X chromosome is inactivated.

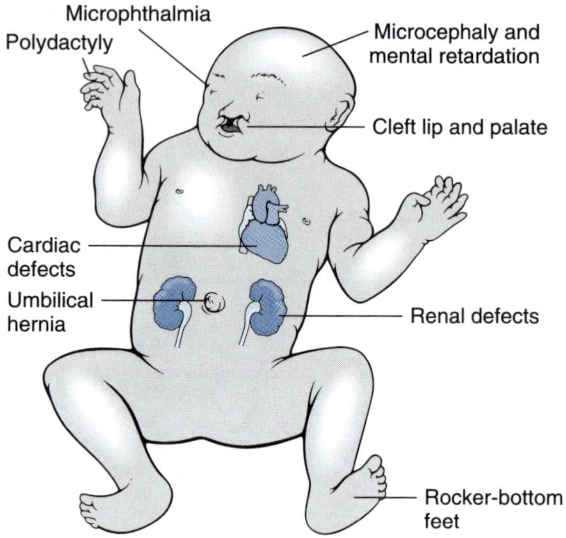

TRISOMY 13: PATAU SYNDROME

Incidence: 1 in 15,000 births

Karyotypes:

Trisomy 13 type:	47,XX, +13
Translocation type:	46,XX,+13,der(13;14)(q10;q10)
Mosaic type:	46,XX/47,XX, +13

C

Figure 5-4, cont'd

Because numerical aberrations of X chromosomes (extra or missing) are nevertheless associated with somatic and gonadal abnormalities, the Lyon hypothesis is modified as follows:

- Both X chromosomes are required for normal gametogenesis; the inactivated X is selectively reactivated in germ cells during gamete formation.
- X-inactivation spares certain regions of the chromosome necessary for normal growth and development; up to 20% of the genes on the short arm of any "inactivated" X chromosome escape inactivation.

The Y chromosome is both necessary and sufficient for male development. Regardless of the number of X chromosomes, the presence of a single Y drives development toward the male sex.

Klinefelter Syndrome *(p. 165)*

Klinefelter syndrome is male hypogonadism associated with two or more X chromosomes and at least one Y chromosome. It has an incidence of approximately 1 in 660 live male birth; 47,XXY is most common (90% of cases) with the remainder being mosaics (e.g., 46,XY/47,XXY). Clinical features include the following:

- Male infertility
- Eunuchoid body habitus

- Minimal or no mental retardation
- High incidence of type 2 diabetes mellitus (low testosterone causes relative insulin resistance)
- Failure of male secondary sexual characteristics
- Gynecomastia with twentyfold increased risk of breast cancer relative to normal males; female distribution of hair
- Atrophic testes
- Plasma follicle-stimulating hormone and estrogen levels elevated; testosterone levels low
- Osteoporosis and fractures due to sex hormone imbalance

The hypogonadism and other clinical features are explained by the pattern of X-inactivation. For example, the gene encoding the androgen receptor is on the X chromosome. It has highly polymorphous CAG trinucleotide repeats, with longer CAG repeats leading to less receptor activity; fortuitously (or not) the X chromosome with the shorter CAG repeats is preferentially inactivated.

Turner Syndrome (p. 166)

Turner syndrome is hypogonadism in phenotypic females resulting from complete or partial monosomy of X chromosome; 45,X occurs in approximately 57% of cases, with partial deletions of the X chromosome and mosaics (e.g., 45,X/46,XX) making up the rest. Sensitive techniques suggest 75% of Turner syndrome patients may actually be mosaics. Isochromosomes of the long arm with deletion of the short arm (46,X,i[Xq]) and ring chromosomes with deletions of both long and short arms also yield a Turner phenotype. The karyotypic variability explains the heterogeneity of the Turner phenotype (45,X is most severely affected). In 75% of cases the X chromosome is maternal in origin, suggesting that the primary defect may be in paternal gametogenesis. Clinical features include the following:

- Lymphedema of neck, hands, and feet
- Webbing of neck (due to early lymphatic dilation)
- Short stature
- Broad chest and widely spaced nipples
- Primary amenorrhea
- Failure of development of normal secondary sex characteristics
- Ovaries severely atrophic and fibrous (streak ovaries)
- Congenital heart disease, particularly aortic coarctation

Hypogonadism and the absence of secondary sexual maturation occur because both X chromosomes are necessary for normal oogenesis and ovarian development; affected patients thus have an accelerated loss of oocytes and essentially undergo menopause before they experience menarche. The short stature comes from the loss of both (expressed) copies of the short stature homeobox gene *(SHOX)* on the X chromosome which affects height. The mechanisms of the cardiac malformations are unknown.

Hermaphroditism and Pseudohermaphroditism (p. 167)

- *True hermaphrodites* are extremely rare (ovaries and testes are both present, either combined as an ovotestis or with one gonad on each side). Fifty percent have 46,XX karyotype; most others are 46,XX/46,XY mosaics, with very few being 46,XY. Testes in a 46,XX individual implies cryptic chimerism of the *SRY* gene (dictates testicular differentiation) or possibly a Y-to-autosome translocation.
- *Female pseudohermaphrodites* have a 46,XX karyotype with normal ovaries and internal genitalia but ambiguous or virilized

external genitalia. The most common cause is androgenic steroid exposure during gestation (e.g., due to congenital adrenal hyperplasia or androgen-secreting maternal tumors).

- *Male pseudohermaphrodites* have Y chromosomes; the gonads are therefore exclusively testes, but external genitalia are either ambiguous or completely female. The condition results from defective virilization of the male embryo because of reduced androgen synthesis or resistance to action of androgens. The most common form is *complete testicular feminization*, an X-linked disorder associated with mutations in the androgen receptor gene located on Xq11-Xq12.

Single-Gene Disorders With Nonclassic Inheritance (p. 168)

Diseases Caused by Trinucleotide Repeat Mutations

(p. 168) (Table 5-7)

Approximately 40 disorders, including Huntington disease, myotonic dystrophy, Friedrich ataxia, fragile X syndrome, and multiple types of spinocerebellar ataxia, are associated with the expansion of stretches of trinucleotides; neurodegenerative changes dominate the clinical picture:

- Most of these repeats contain guanine (G) and cytosine (C) nucleotides, and they can occur in noncoding regions (fragile X) or coding regions (Huntington disease).
- Expansions in coding regions (typically CAG trinucleotides) lead to the production of polyglutamine tracts in the proteins and subsequent aberrant folding with aggregation (with large intranuclear inclusions), mitochondrial dysfunction, an unfolded protein stress response, and apoptosis (Fig. 5-5).
- Expansions in noncoding regions suppress the synthesis of the affected protein (Fig. 5-5).
- The proclivity for trinucleotide expansion depends on the sex of the transmitting parent; in fragile X, expansions occur in oogenesis, whereas in Huntington disease, they occur during spermatogenesis.

Fragile X Syndrome and Fragile X Tremor/Ataxia (p. 169)

Fragile X syndrome is prototypical of these disorders; it is a common cause of familial mental retardation. It is characterized cytogenetically by a "fragile site" on Xq27.3 visualized as a discontinuity of chromosomal staining when cells are grown in folate-deficient medium.

- The site on Xq has multiple CGG nucleotide repeats in the 5′-untranslated region of the *familial mental retardation-1 (FMR1)* gene. In normal individuals the average number of repeats is 29 (range of 6 to 55), whereas affected individuals have 200 to 4000 repeats; patients with *premutations* (clinically silent) have 55 to 200 CGG repeats.
- In carrier females the premutations undergo amplification during oogenesis, resulting in full mutations that are then passed on to progeny. The worsening of clinical presentation with succeeding generations is called *anticipation.*
- Because the mutations are carried on the X chromosome, this is an X-linked recessive disorder. However, because premutations are amplified only during oogenesis, the transmission pattern

TABLE 5-7 Examples of Trinucleotide Repeat Disorders

Disease	Gene	Locus	Protein	Repeat	Number of Repeats	
					Normal	Disease
Expansions Affecting Noncoding Regions						
Fragile X syndrome	*FMRI (FRAXA)*	Xq27.3	FMRP	CGG	6-55	55-200 (pre); >230 (full)
Friedreich ataxia	*FXN*	9q21.1	Frataxin	GAA	7-34	34-80 (pre); >100 (full)
Myotonic dystrophy	*DMPK*	19q13.3	Myotonic dystrophy protein kinase (DMPK)	CTG	5-37	34-80 (pre); >100 (full)
Expansions Affecting Coding Regions						
Spinobulbar muscular atrophy (Kennedy disease)	*AR*	Xq12	Androgen receptor (AR)	CAG	9-36	38-62
Huntington disease	*HTT*	4p16.3	Huntingtin	CAG	6-35	36-121
Dentatorubral-pallidoluysian atrophy (Haw River syndrome)	*ATNL*	12p13.31	Atrophin-1	CAG	6-35	49-88
Spinocerebellar ataxia type 1	*ATXN1*	6p23	Ataxin-1	CAG	6-44	39-82
Spinocerebellar ataxia type 2	*ATXN2*	12q24.1	Ataxin-2	CAG	15-31	36-63
Spinocerebellar ataxia type 3 (Machado-Joseph disease)	*ATXN3*	14q21	Ataxin-3	CAG	12-40	55-84
Spinocerebellar ataxia type 6	*CACNA2A*	19p13.3	α1A-Voltage-dependent calcium channel subunit	CAG	4-18	21-33
Spinocerebellar ataxia type 7	*ATXN7*	3p14.1	Ataxin-7	CAG	4-35	37-306

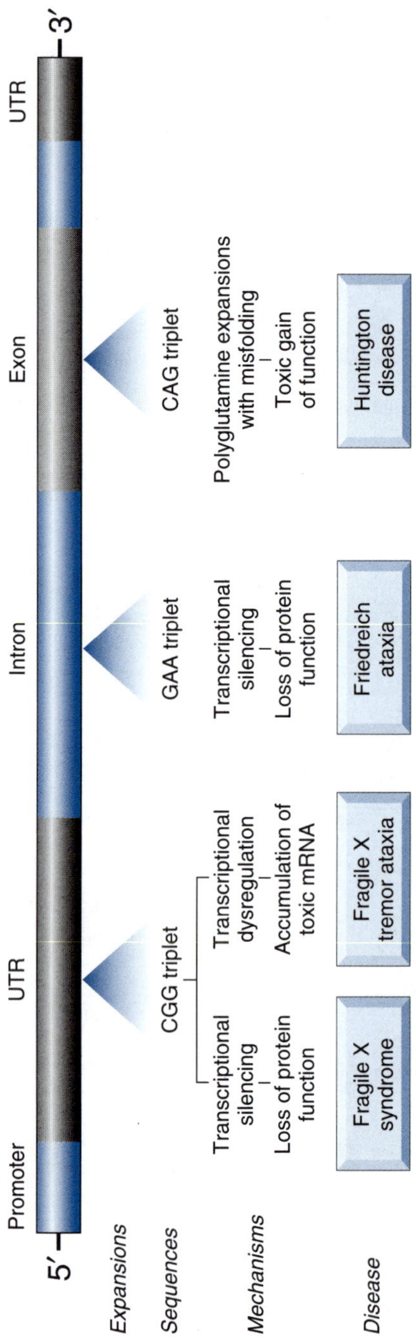

Figure 5-5 Sites of expansion and the affected sequence in selected diseases caused by nucleotide repeat mutations. *UTR,* Untranslated region.

differs from classic X-linked disorders. Consequently, carrier males with premutations do not typically have any symptoms and do not transmit the disease; conversely, almost all sons and approximately 50% of daughters of carrier females are affected. Carrier females are also affected (i.e., mentally retarded) at a 30% to 50% frequency, which is much higher than in typical X-linked disorders.

- Expansion of the trinucleotide repeats in *FMR1* beyond 230 copies leads to abnormal gene methylation and transcriptional suppression.
- The molecular basis of fragile X syndrome is related to loss of function of the FMR protein (FMRP), a cytoplasmic protein abundant in brain and testis. FMRP is an RNA-binding protein associated with polyribosomes; it suppresses the translation of certain transcripts at synaptic junctions. Loss of FMRP leads to increased protein translation, and the resulting imbalance adversely impacts neuronal function with permanent changes in synaptic activity.
- Affected males have severe mental retardation, and 80% have enlarged testes. Other physical features, such as an elongated face and large mandible, are inconsistent.
- Carriers of premutations also get premature ovarian failure (females) and progressive neurodegeneration (males).

Fragile X Tremor/Ataxia *(p. 171)*

CGG premutations in the *FMR1* gene in *carriers* can also cause the phenotypically distinct fragile X tremor/ataxia syndrome. Instead of being methylated and silenced, the *FMR1* gene in these cases continues to be transcribed, leading to a "toxic" overproduction of mRNA that sequesters RNA-binding proteins in the nucleus. As a result, there is premature (before age 40) ovarian failure in carrier females, and transmitting males have a progressive neurodegenerative disorder that begins in their 50s.

Mutations in Mitochondrial Genes—Leber Hereditary Optic Neuropathy (p. 171)

Ova contain multiple mitochondria, whereas spermatozoa contain few; hence the mitochondrial content of zygotes is derived almost entirely from the ovum (sperm mitochondria also tend to be selectively degraded after formation of the fertilized zygote). Thus mitochondrial DNA (mtDNA) is transmitted entirely by females, and diseases resulting from mutations in mitochondrial genes are *maternally inherited.*

- Affected females transmit the disease to all their offspring—male and female; daughters and not sons pass the disease further along to progeny.
- Expression of disorders resulting from mutations in mitochondrial genes is unpredictable. When a cell carrying normal and mutant mtDNA divides, the proportion of normal and mutant DNA in the daughter cells is random and quite variable (a situation called *heteroplasmy*). There is also a threshold effect related to a minimum number of mutant mtDNA required to see oxidative dysfunction.
- mtDNA encodes 22 tRNAs, 2 rRNAs, and 13 genes for proteins involved in oxidative phosphorylation. Consequently, mtDNA mutations predominantly affect organs heavily dependent on mitochondrial energy metabolism, such as the neuromuscular system, liver, heart, and kidney. Prototypical is Leber hereditary optic neuropathy resulting in progressive

blindness, neurologic dysfunction, and cardiac conduction defects.

Genomic Imprinting (p. 172)

This is an epigenetic process resulting in differential inactivation of either maternal or paternal alleles of certain genes. *Maternal imprinting* refers to transcriptional silencing of the maternal allele, whereas *paternal imprinting* refers to inactivation of the paternal allele. Imprinting occurs in the ovum or sperm before fertilization and then is stably transmitted to all somatic cells. The process involves differential DNA methylation or histone H4 deacetylation, leading to selective gene inactivation; 200 to 600 genes are estimated to be imprinted, and although some may occur in isolation, most are clustered in groups regulated by common *cis*-acting elements.

Prader-Willi Syndrome and Angelman Syndrome (p. 172)

Prader-Willi syndrome and Angelman syndrome are uncommon genetic disorders caused by deletion of neighboring regions on chromosome 15 (15q12). In this region there are both maternally and paternally imprinted genes. Prader-Willi syndrome occurs when the paternal 15q12 is deleted, leaving behind only the "silenced" maternal gene product; Angelman syndrome involves deletion of the maternal 15q12 region, leaving behind only the "silenced" paternal gene.

- *Prader-Willi syndrome* is characterized by mental retardation, short stature, hypotonia, obesity, and hypogonadism. In some cases an entire paternal chromosome 15 is absent, replaced instead by two maternally derived (and therefore silenced) chromosomes 15 (uniparental disomy).
- *Angelman syndrome* patients exhibit mental retardation, ataxia, seizures, and inappropriate laughter. These can also occur through uniparental disomy (receipt of only two paternal chromosomes 15).

In Angelman syndrome the affected paternally imprinted gene is *UBE3A,* coding for a ubiquitin protein-ligase with a role in directing proteasomal degradation of a variety of intracellular proteins in particular regions of the brain. The converse gene(s) in Prader-Willi syndrome are not known, although a gene encoding small nuclear riboprotein N—involved in gene splicing—has been implicated.

Gonadal Mosaicism (p. 174)

Gonadal mosaicism results from mutations that selectively affect cells embryologically destined to form gonads. Because germ cells are affected, one or more offspring can manifest disease even though somatic cells are uninvolved and the affected individual is phenotypically normal.

Molecular Genetic Diagnosis (p. 174)

The analysis of disease at the nucleic acid level permits exquisite specificity and sensitivity—enabled by the amplification and analysis of minute amounts of material, even from individual cells. The considerations for appropriate tissue sampling (e.g., peripheral blood, tumor tissue, sputum sample) include whether a disorder is constitutional (present in every cell type) or somatic (restricted to specific tissues); infectious pathogens may be localized to a specific site.

Diagnostic Methods and Indications for Testing (p. 174)

Indications for Analysis of Inherited Genetic Alterations (p. 174)

- Prenatal evaluation can be performed on specimens obtained from amniocentesis, chorionic villus sampling, umbilical cord blood, or free DNA in maternal blood (10% of which is fetal in origin); it is indicated in the following settings:
  - Advanced maternal age
  - Parent with a known balanced chromosomal rearrangement
  - Fetal abnormalities on ultrasound
  - Children at risk for specific genetic disorders based on family history
- Postnatal evaluation is commonly performed on peripheral blood lymphocytes and is based on clinical suspicion:
  - Multiple congenital anomalies
  - Suspected metabolic syndrome
  - Unexplained mental retardation or developmental delay
  - Suspected aneuploidy (e.g., Down syndrome)
  - Suspected monogenic disease
- Evaluation in older patients can be performed on peripheral blood or specific tissues for disorders manifesting at later stages:
  - Inherited cancer syndromes
  - Atypically mild monogenic disease (e.g., attenuated cystic fibrosis)
  - Neurodegenerative disorders (e.g., Huntington disease)

Indications for Analysis of Acquired Genetic Alterations (p. 175)

- Diagnosis and management of malignancy:
  - Specific mutations or cytogenetic alterations that are hallmarks of certain tumors (e.g., *BCR-ABL* in chronic myelogenous leukemia)
  - Determination of clonality as an indicator of malignancy
  - Identification of genetic alterations that can influence therapy (e.g., epidermal growth factor [EGF] receptor mutations in lung cancer)
  - Determination of treatment efficacy (presence of residual disease)
  - Detection of therapy-resistant secondary mutations
- Diagnosis and management of infectious disease:
  - Detection of specific microorganism (e.g., human immunodeficiency virus [HIV], mycobacteria)
  - Identification of specifically drug-resistant microbes
  - Determination of treatment efficacy (e.g., viral loads in hepatitis C)

Polymerase Chain Reaction and Detection of DNA Sequence Alterations (p. 175)

Polymerase chain reaction (PCR)-based techniques allow the amplification of small amounts of target DNA; these amplified fragments may then be analyzed by the following:

- *Sanger sequencing.* Amplified DNA is mixed with DNA polymerase, a primer sequence, unlabeled nucleotides (A, C, G, and T), and four "dead-end" (dideoxy terminator) nucleotides that are tagged with different fluorescent labels. The subsequent reaction generates DNA species of all possible lengths, each labeled by a single fluorescent tag that corresponds to the incorporation of the terminator base at its end. After capillary electrophoresis to separate the DNA fragments by molecular weight, the sequence can be "read" by simple inspection.

- *Pyrosequencing.* This approach takes advantage of the release of pyrophosphate when a nucleotide is incorporated into a growing DNA strand. Using a single sequence primer, individual nucleotides (A, C, G, or T) are added to the reaction mixture; if one or more of a particular nucleotide are incorporated this is reflected by a luciferase-linked reporter assay and quantitated by a photodetector. This technique is more sensitive to sequence variants than Sanger sequencing and can detect as little as 5% mutated alleles in a background of normal alleles (as for cancer cells in a largely nonmalignant host stroma).
- *Single-base primer extension.* This approach is used when identifying mutations at a specific nucleotide position and can detect frequencies as low as 1% to 2%. The primer sequence is designed to bind just one base upstream of the target nucleotide position. Differently tagged terminator fluorescent nucleotides are then added, and a single base polymerase extension is performed, with the subsequent determination of the relative amounts of wild-type and variant fluorescent signals.
- *Restriction fragment length analysis.* DNA from a sample is digested with restriction enzymes (endonucleases that cleave at only specific target sequences). If a mutation affects the restriction site, then wild-type and mutant PCR products will yield different length bands after electrophoresis.
- *Amplicon length analysis.* Mutations that affect DNA length (e.g., deletions or expansions) can be detected by using PCR primers that span the region of expansion or deletion. These can then be detected and quantified after electrophoresis.
- *Real-time PCR.* This variation on the basic PCR technique uses the incorporation of fluorophore-tagged nucleotides to quantify how much of a particular sequence is present. Larger quantities will lead to a brighter signal sooner; lower frequency sequences do not generate a signal until additional rounds of PCR amplification.

Molecular Analysis of Genomic Alterations (p. 176)

Large deletions, duplications, or complex rearrangements may not be amenable to PCR-based techniques. In those cases, hybridization approaches are used.

Fluorescence in Situ Hybridization (p. 177)

Fluorescence in situ hybridization (FISH) uses fluorescently labeled DNA probes that bind to specific chromosomal regions. FISH can be used on nondividing cells, from a variety of preparations (including fixed archival material). It is used to detect chromosomal abnormalities (aneuploidy and rearrangements), deletions, and gene amplifications.

Multiplex Ligation-Dependent Probe Amplification (p. 177)

Multiplex ligation-dependent probe amplification (MLPA) blends DNA hybridization, DNA ligation, and PCR amplification to detect deletions and duplications of any size. Pairs of primers are bound side by side to a single strand of target DNA and ligated; these can then serve as a template for PCR amplification. If the target DNA is in some way modified, one or the other probe will not bind and ligation (and subsequent amplification) will not occur.

Southern Blotting (p. 177)

Southern blotting uses hybridization of a sequence-specific probe to restriction enzyme-digested DNA that has been separated by gel electrophoresis. Bands of different size relative to normal indicate a genetic anomaly.

Cytogenomic Array Technology (p. 177)

Cytogenomic array technology includes *array-based comparative genomic hybridization (array CGH)* and *single nucleotide polymorphism (SNP) genotyping arrays:*

- In *array CGH,* test DNA and normal DNA are typically labeled with either green or red fluorescent probes; these are then allowed to competitively bind to an array spotted with DNA probes that span the genome at regularly spaced intervals. The relative fluorescence intensity of binding is compared at each spot; if binding is equivalent from both samples, the result is a yellow spot, if one or the other predominates (due to overexpression or a mutation that affects the ability to hybridize), red or green fluorescence will predominate.
- *SNP genotyping arrays* have a similar approach but use probes designed to detect SNPs, common DNA polymorphisms occurring approximately each thousand nucleotides through exons, introns, and regulatory sequences.

Polymorphic Markers and Molecular Diagnosis (p. 178)

Two DNA loci even 100,000 base pairs apart on the same chromosome are still highly likely to cosegregate during meiosis (i.e., are said to exhibit *linkage*). Thus if the exact nature of a disease-causing genetic alteration is not known, molecular analysis can still take advantage of the linkage phenomenon with other nearby known marker loci to establish a relative risk; a disease "haplotype" can be defined by a panel of marker loci that cosegregate with the putative disease allele(s). Marker loci in linkage studies are naturally occurring *polymorphisms* (i.e., normal variants in DNA sequences); these include the following:

- *SNPs* are physical landmarks in the genome and are stably transmitted through generations.
- *Repeat-length polymorphisms* are represented by *microsatellite repeats* (repeats of 2 to 6 base pairs, usually less than 1 kb in length) and *minisatellite repeats* (15- to 70-base pair repeat motifs, 1 to 3 kb long). The lengths of such repeats are variable in the population but are stably transmitted across generations, so they can be linked to putative disease alleles. These are also easy to analyze by gel electrophoresis with PCR primers that flank the repeat sequences.

Polymorphisms and Genome-Wide Analyses (p. 179)

Classical linkage analysis is limited when a disease allele has low penetrance or is only one of several genes that contribute to a multifactorial phenotype. This problem can be circumvented by GWAS that study the linkage of genetic variants (SNPs and repeat polymorphisms) among large cohorts in the general population with and without disease (rather than families). In GWAS, polymorphisms that are over-represented in a disease population are assumed to link to causal candidate genes.

Epigenetic Alterations (p. 180)

These are heritable chemical modifications of DNA or chromatin (e.g., methylation of DNA or acetylation of histones) that do not modify the primary DNA sequence but impact genetic expression. Examples include imprinting and X-inactivation. Analysis requires treating DNA with chemicals (e.g., sodium bisulfite) that convert unmethylated or methylated nucleotides to a species that can be uniquely detected or by using antibodies to precipitate modified histones and then sequence the associated DNA.

RNA Analysis (p. 180)

Although mRNA is overall less stable than DNA, sequencing mRNA expression patterns can be useful for the following:

- Quantification of RNA viruses (e.g., hepatitis C and HIV)
- Chromosomal translocations where the breakpoint is scattered over a large stretch of intronic sequence. After DNA splicing to make mRNA, rearrangements may be more readily detected.

Next-Generation Sequencing (p. 180)

Next-generation sequencing (NGS) describes a number of newer technologies that produce huge amounts of sequence data relatively inexpensively in a massively parallel fashion. As opposed to Sanger sequencing that requires a simple, homogeneous, intact DNA template, NGS technologies can sequence DNA with extreme heterogeneity. Individual bits of DNA are isolated and amplified using PCR; these amplified species are then simultaneously sequenced, typically yielding short "reads" of 500 bases or less.

Bioinformatics

The staggering amount of individual data from the NGS reads must then be stitched together to yield a complete sequence:

- *Alignment.* Using sophisticated computational techniques, the short sequencing reads are mapped onto a reference genome.
- *Variant calling.* The aligned sequence and the reference genome are compared; the more reads that cover a particular sequence, the greater the "depth" of the read, and the greater the likelihood that a variant will be detected. If there is sufficient evidence of a difference from the reference genome, a variant "call" is made.
- *Variant annotation and interpretation.* Called variants can be evaluated as to gene names, coding changes and predicted protein effects, and databases of previously described benign and pathogenic variations. This allows the assignment of likely significance.

Clinical Applications of Next-Generation Sequencing DNA Sequencing

For sequencing, genomic DNA is fragmented into smaller segments (<500 base pairs), and instrument-compatible oligonucleotide linker sequences are added to generate a *library.*

- *Targeted sequencing* means that only a subset of genes (e.g., using custom complementary probes) are initially selected for NGS preparation; this can range from a few dozen genes to almost a thousand.
- *Whole exome sequencing* is targeted sequencing that uses thousands of custom probes to extract the 1.5% of the genome that contains protein-coding exons.
- *Whole genome sequencing (WGS)* involves comprehensive sequencing of the entire genome; due to costs, WGS is usually performed at a lower sequencing depth and may lack the ability to detect low-frequency mutations in heterogeneous samples.

6 Diseases of the Immune System

The immune system evolved primarily to defend against microbial invasion; it accomplishes this by distinguishing self from nonself (exogenous or foreign) molecules and marshalling an impressive armamentarium of effector mechanisms to neutralize or destroy perceived invaders. The normal immune response (i.e., the pathways leading to the recognition and elimination of nonself) involves both *innate* (nonspecific) and *adaptive* (antigen-specific) components. The fundamentals of normal immunity are well reviewed in pages 186 to 200 of *Robbins and Cotran Pathologic Basis of Disease,* 9th ed. and summarized briefly here:

- The initial response to microbial infection is mediated through *innate immunity,* comprising epithelial barriers, monocyte or macrophages, neutrophils, dendritic cells, natural killer (NK) cells, mast cells, and soluble proteins, such as those involved in the complement cascade. Innate immunity typically manifests as inflammation; unlike adaptive immunity, it does not have fine antigen specificity or memory (p. 186).
- Innate immunity uses *pattern recognition receptors* (e.g., Toll-like receptors [TLRs]) to recognize molecules either expressed by microbes *(pathogen-associated molecular patterns)* or produced by injured or necrotic cells *(damage-associated molecular patterns)* (p. 187).
- *NK cells* (p. 192) can kill microbially infected cells or cells that are damaged beyond repair; their cytocidal activity is normally inhibited by surface receptors that recognize major histocompatibility complex (MHC) molecules (p. 194) that healthy cells express.
- The adaptive immune system is facilitated by lymphocytes—characterized by their expression of specific receptors for antigens. Although each lymphocyte can recognize only one distinct antigenic conformation, the cumulative population of lymphocytes in any individual can potentially recognize 10^9 different specificities. The defenses related to adaptive immunity develop more slowly than innate immunity (p. 189).
- *T (thymus-derived) lymphocytes* express antigen receptors called T-cell receptors (TCRs); these recognize peptide fragments of protein antigens bound to MHC molecules on the surface of antigen-presenting cells (APCs) (e.g., dendritic cells and macrophages) (p. 190).
- *B (bone marrow-derived) lymphocytes* recognize antigens via membrane-bound antibodies; after antigen binding, B cells are activated to become plasma cells that produce secreted antibodies (p. 191).
- *APCs* capture microbes and other antigens, transport them to lymphoid organs, and display them in association with MHC molecules for recognition by lymphocytes (p. 191); MHC molecules in humans are called human leukocyte antigens (HLAs). Such recognition leads to activation, with proliferation and

differentiation into effector and memory cells (p. 196). The most efficient APCs are dendritic cells.

- The cells of the immune system are organized into discrete tissues: the *generative lymphoid organs*—bone marrow and thymus—are the sites where mature lymphocytes are produced; the *peripheral lymphoid organs*—lymph nodes, spleen, and mucosal lymphoid tissues—are the sites where immune responses occur (p. 193).
- *Cellular immunity* (p. 197) is mediated through T lymphocytes, designed to combat cell-associated microbes (e.g., phagocytosed microbes and microbes in the cytoplasm of infected cells). *Humoral immunity* (p. 198) is mediated by antibodies and is effective against extracellular microbes (in the circulation and mucosal lumens).
- *CD4+ helper T cells* help B cells to make antibodies, activate macrophages to destroy ingested microbes, stimulate recruitment of leukocytes, and regulate all immune responses to protein antigens (p. 197). The functions of CD4+ T cells are mediated by secreted proteins called *cytokines* (p. 196). CD8+ cytotoxic T lymphocytes (CTLs) kill cells that express antigens in the cytoplasm that are seen as foreign (e.g., virus-infected and tumor cells) and can also produce cytokines (p. 196).
- Antibodies secreted by plasma cells neutralize microbes and block their infectivity and promote the phagocytosis and destruction of pathogens. Antibodies also confer passive immunity to neonates (p. 198).

Hypersensitivity: Immunologically Mediated Tissue Injury (p. 200)

Injurious immune responses are called *hypersensitivity reactions;* these represent excessive responses to an antigenic stimulus, attributable to imbalances between effector and regulatory mechanisms. Pathology related to the immune system can be a result of responses to exogenous environmental antigens or to endogenous self-antigens *(autoimmune disease).* Hypersensitivity responses are often associated with particular susceptibility genes (e.g., HLA).

Classification of Hypersensitivity Diseases (p. 200)

Hypersensitivity responses are divided into four general categories based on the underlying mechanisms of immune injury (Table 6-1).

Immediate (Type I) Hypersensitivity (p. 201)

Immediate (type I) hypersensitivity is also called "allergy"; it is mediated by immunoglobulin E (IgE) antibodies directed against specific antigens (allergens). These responses can be localized to a specific site or have systemic manifestations. Susceptibility to immediate hypersensitivity reactions *(atopy)* is genetically determined, with affected individuals having higher IgE titers and more interleukin-4 (IL-4)-producing T_H2 cells than the general population; there is linkage to the certain HLA alleles and to the chromosome 5q31 region that encodes the cytokines IL-4, IL-5, IL-9, IL-13, and granulocyte-monocyte colony stimulating factor (GM-CSF).

IgE synthesis requires T_H2 CD4+ helper T-cell responses; in particular, IL-4 and IL-13 induce and enhance B cell IgE synthesis. T_H2 cells also produce other cytokines that contribute to the type I hypersensitivity response; thus IL-4 promotes the development of additional T_H2 cells, and IL-5 is involved in the development and activation of *eosinophils*—important effector cells in type I hypersensitivity responses.

TABLE 6-1 Mechanisms of Immunologically Mediated Hypersensitivity Reactions

Type of Reaction	Prototypic Disorder	Immune Mechanisms	Pathologic Lesions
Immediate (type I) hypersensitivity	Anaphylaxis; allergies; bronchial asthma (atopic forms)	Production of IgE antibody → immediate release of vasoactive amines and other mediators from mast cells; later recruitment of inflammatory cells	Vascular dilation, edema, smooth muscle contraction, mucus production, tissue injury, inflammation
Antibody-mediated (type II) hypersensitivity	Autoimmune hemolytic anemia; Goodpasture syndrome	Production of IgG, IgM → binds to antigen on target cell or tissue → phagocytosis or lysis of target cell by activated complement or Fc receptors; recruitment of leukocytes	Phagocytosis and lysis of cells; inflammation; in some diseases, functional derangements without cell or tissue injury
Immune complex–mediated (type III) hypersensitivity	SLE; some forms of glomerulonephritis; serum sickness; Arthus reaction	Deposition of antigen-antibody complexes → complement activation → recruitment of leukocytes by complement products and Fc receptors → release of enzymes and other toxic molecules	Inflammation, necrotizing vasculitis (fibrinoid necrosis)
Cell-mediated (type IV) hypersensitivity	Contact dermatitis; multiple sclerosis; type 1 diabetes; rheumatoid arthritis; inflammatory bowel disease; tuberculosis	Activated T lymphocytes → (1) release of cytokines → inflammation and macrophage activation; (2) T cell–mediated cytotoxicity	Perivascular cellular infiltrates; edema; granuloma formation; cell destruction

Sensitization and Activation of Mast Cells (p. 202)

IgE antibodies synthesized in response to an allergen are bound to mast cells via specific high-affinity surface Fc receptors (FcεR1). On re-exposure, the allergen binds to and cross-links the IgE-FcεR1 and results in an immediate reaction (minutes), followed by late-phase reactions (hours) due to the following:

- Release *(degranulation)* of preformed vesicles containing *primary mediators*
- de novo synthesis and release of *secondary mediators*

Mast cells can also be activated by other stimuli (yielding responses similar to those elicited by allergens):

- Complement fragments C3a and C5a *(anaphylatoxins)* binding to surface receptors
- Chemokines (chemotactic peptides, e.g., IL-8) and adenosine
- Drugs, such as codeine and morphine

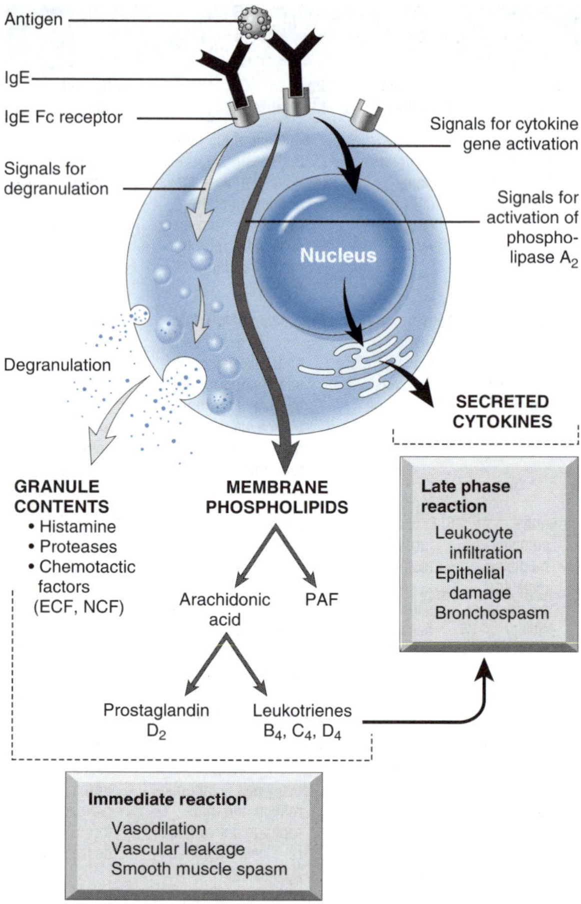

Figure 6-1 Activation of mast cells through the cross-linking of surface IgE receptors, with subsequent release of mediators responsible for immediate- and late-phase responses. *ECF,* Eosinophil chemotactic protein; *NCF,* neutrophil chemotactic protein.

- Melittin (in bee venom)
- Physical stimuli, such as sunlight, trauma, exercise, and heat or cold (20% to 30% of immediate hypersensitivity reactions are triggered by nonantigenic stimuli)

Mediators of Immediate Hypersensitivity *(p. 203)*

The consequences of mast cell activation are schematized in Figure 6-1:

- An *initial rapid response* (5 to 30 minutes) is characterized by vasodilation, increased vascular permeability, bronchial smooth muscle contraction, and glandular secretions. This is driven by *preformed mediators* stored in secretory vacuoles and typically resolves within 60 minutes:
    - *Biogenic amines* (e.g., histamine): Bronchial smooth muscle contraction, increased vascular permeability and dilation, and increased mucous secretion

- *Enzymes* contained in granule matrix (e.g., chymase, tryptase): Generate kinins and activated complement by cleaving precursor proteins
- *Proteoglycans* (e.g., heparin)

- A *second (delayed) phase,* with onset 2 to 24 hours after initial allergen exposure is characterized by inflammatory cell infiltrates and tissue damage (especially epithelium). It can persist for days and is driven by lipid mediators and cytokines produced by the activated mast cells:
  - *Lipid mediators* are produced from precursors released from mast cell membranes by phospholipase A_2
  - *Leukotriene B_4*: Highly chemotactic for neutrophils, monocytes, and eosinophils
  - *Leukotrienes C_4, D_4,* and *E_4*: Thousand-fold more potent than histamine for increasing vascular permeability and bronchial smooth muscle contraction
  - *Prostaglandin D_2*: Intense bronchospasm and mucous secretion
  - *Platelet-activating factor (PAF):* Platelet aggregation, histamine release, bronchoconstriction, vasodilation, and increased vascular permeability; chemotactic for neutrophils and eosinophils and can cause activation with degranulation
  - *Cytokine mediators* recruit and activate inflammatory cells; these include tumor necrosis factor (TNF), IL-1, and chemokines. IL-4 released from mast cells amplifies the T_H2 response.

Systemic Anaphylaxis (p. 204)

Typically follows parenteral or oral administration of foreign proteins, drugs (e.g., penicillin), food (e.g., peanuts), or insect toxins (e.g., bee venom). The severity reflects the level of sensitization; even minuscule doses can induce anaphylactic shock in a sensitized host. Pruritus, urticaria, and erythema occur minutes after exposure, followed by bronchoconstriction and laryngeal edema; this can escalate into laryngeal obstruction, hypotensive shock, and death within minutes to hours.

Local Immediate Hypersensitivity Reactions (p. 205)

Approximately 10% to 20% of the population suffers from localized allergic symptoms (e.g., urticaria, angioedema, rhinitis, and asthma) to common inhaled or ingested allergens (e.g., pollens, house dust, and animal dander).

Antibody-Mediated (Type II) Hypersensitivity *(p. 205)*

Antibody-mediated (type II) hypersensitivity is mediated by antibodies against extrinsic or endogenous antigens present on cell surfaces or in the extracellular matrix; complement activation also plays a significant role. The subsequent injury is a consequence of three mechanisms (Fig. 6-2); examples are listed in Table 6-2:

- *Opsonization and phagocytosis:* Cells can be directly lysed by the C5 to C9 complement membrane attack complex (MAC) or can be *opsonized* (enhanced phagocytosis) as a result of fixation of antibody or C3b fragments. Bound antibody can also cause cell lysis (without phagocytosis) by cells bearing Fc receptors (e.g., NK cells), so-called *antibody-dependent cell-mediated cytotoxicity (ADCC).*
- *Inflammation:* Antibodies (and subsequent complement activation) lead to recruitment and activation of antigen nonspecific inflammatory cells (neutrophils and macrophages). These release injurious proteases and reactive oxygen species that lead to tissue pathology.

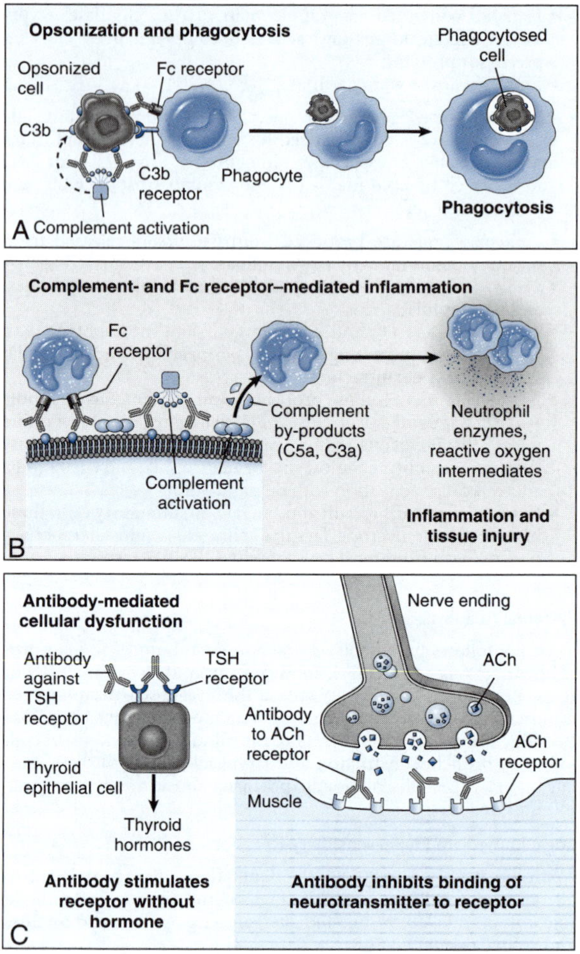

Figure 6-2 Mechanisms of antibody-mediated injury. A, Opsonization of cells by antibodies and complement components and ingestion by phagocytes. **B,** Inflammation induced by antibody binding to leukocyte Fc receptors and by activated complement fragments. **C,** Antireceptor antibodies disturb receptor function (e.g., anti-acetylcholine [ACh] receptor antibodies impair neuromuscular synaptic transmission in myasthenia gravis or anti-thyroid-stimulating hormone [TSH] receptor antibodies activate thyroid epithelial cells in Graves disease).

- *Cellular dysfunction:* Certain antibodies can inappropriately activate or block normal cellular or hormonal function, without causing tissue damage.

Immune Complex-Mediated (Type III) Hypersensitivity *(p. 207)*

Immune complex-mediated (type III) hypersensitivity is mediated by antigen-antibody complexes—immune complexes—forming either in the circulation or at sites of antigen deposition. Antigens can be exogenous (e.g., infectious agents) or endogenous; immune complex-mediated disease can be either systemic or local. Examples are given in Table 6-3.

TABLE 6-2 Examples of Antibody-Mediated Diseases (Type II Hypersensitivity)

Disease	Target Antigen	Mechanisms of Disease	Clinicopathologic Manifestations
Autoimmune hemolytic anemia	Erythrocyte membrane proteins (Rh blood group antigens, blood group antigen)	Opsonization and phagocytosis of erythrocytes	Hemolysis, anemia
Autoimmune thrombocytopenic purpura	Platelet membrane proteins (GpIIb:IIIa or GpIb/IX)	Opsonization and phagocytosis of platelets	Bleeding
Pemphigus vulgaris	Proteins in intercellular junctions of epidermal cells (cadherin)	Antibody-mediated activation of proteases, disruption of intercellular adhesions	Skin vesicles (bullae)
Vasculitis caused by ANCA	Neutrophil granule proteins, presumably released from activated neutrophils	Neutrophil degranulation and inflammation	Vasculitis
Goodpasture syndrome	Noncollagenous protein in basement membranes of kidney glomeruli and lung alveoli	Complement- and Fc receptor-mediated inflammation	Nephritis, lung hemorrhage
Acute rheumatic fever	Streptococcal cell wall antigen; antibody cross-reacts with myocardial antigen	Inflammation, macrophage activation	Myocarditis, arthritis
Myasthenia gravis	Acetylcholine receptor	Antibody inhibits acetylcholine binding, downmodulates receptors	Muscle weakness, paralysis
Graves disease (hyperthyroidism)	TSH receptor	Antibody-mediated stimulation of TSH receptors	Hyperthyroidism
Insulin-resistant diabetes	Insulin receptor	Antibody inhibits binding of insulin	Hyperglycemia, ketoacidosis
Pernicious anemia	Intrinsic factor of gastric parietal cells	Neutralization of intrinsic factor, decreased absorption of vitamin B_{12}	Abnormal erythropoiesis, anemia

ANCA, Antineutrophil cytoplasmic antibodies; *TSH,* thyroid-stimulating hormone.
From Abbas AK, Lichtman H: *Cellular and Molecular Immunology,* ed 5. Philadelphia, PA, 2003, Saunders.

TABLE 6-3 Examples of Immune Complex–Mediated Diseases

Disease	Antigen Involved	Clinicopathologic Manifestations
SLE	DNA, nucleoproteins, others	Nephritis, arthritis, vasculitis
Polyarteritis nodosa	Hepatitis B virus surface antigen (in some cases)	Vasculitis
Poststreptococcal glomerulonephritis	Streptococcal cell wall antigen(s); may be "planted" in glomerular basement membrane	Nephritis
Acute glomerulonephritis	Bacterial antigens *(Treponema);* parasite antigens (malaria, schistosomes); tumor antigens	Nephritis
Reactive arthritis	Bacterial antigens *(Yersinia)*	Acute arthritis
Arthus reaction	Various foreign proteins	Cutaneous vasculitis
Serum sickness	Various proteins (e.g., foreign serum [anti-thymocyte globulin])	Arthritis, vasculitis, nephritis

- *Systemic immune complex disease* (p. 207) results from the deposition of circulating immune complexes; it can occur as a response to inoculation of a large volume of exogenous antigen *(acute serum sickness)* or can result from antibody responses to endogenous antigens (e.g., *lupus erythematosus*) or infectious agents (e.g., *polyarteritis nodosa*). The process is divided into three phases:
  - *Formation of immune complexes.* Newly synthesized antibodies typically arise approximately a week after antigen inoculation; the antibodies then bind to the foreign molecules to form circulating immune complexes.
  - *Deposition of immune complexes.* Propensity for deposition depends on the physicochemical nature of the complexes (charge, size, etc.) and local vascular characteristics (e.g., fenestration, permeability). Deposition is greatest with medium-sized complexes (slight antigen excess) and in vascular beds that filter (e.g., glomerulus and synovium).
  - *Injury caused by immune complexes.* Immune complex deposition activates the complement cascade; subsequent tissue injury derives from complement-mediated inflammation and cells bearing Fc receptors.

Single large antigen exposures tend to induce acute, self-limited disease that resolves as the inciting antigen is eliminated (e.g., poststreptococcal glomerulonephritis); repeated or prolonged exposure leads to chronic, recurrent tissue injury (e.g., lupus).

Morphology (p. 208)

The classic lesion is *acute vasculitis* with vessel wall necrosis and intense neutrophil accumulation. Necrotic tissue and protein accumulations composed of immune complexes, complement, and exuded serum proteins contribute to a smudgy, eosinophilic deposition, so-called *fibrinoid necrosis.* Superimposed thrombosis and downstream tissue necrosis may also be present. Immune complexes and complement can be visualized by immunofluorescence or by electron microscopy (electron-dense deposits). In chronic lesions there is intimal thickening and vascular and/or parenchymal scarring.

Local Immune Complex Disease (Arthus Reaction) (p. 208)

Local immune complex disease is characterized by a localized vasculitis and tissue necrosis; it occurs when the formation or deposition of immune complexes is extremely localized (e.g., *intracutaneous* antigen injection in previously sensitized hosts carrying the appropriate circulating antibody).

T Cell–Mediated (Type IV) Hypersensitivity (p. 208)

T cell–mediated (type IV) hypersensitivity is mediated by antigen-specific T lymphocytes and includes delayed-type hypersensitivity (DTH) (CD4+ T cells) and T cell–mediated cytotoxicity (CD8+ T cells) (Fig. 6-3). T cell–associated hypersensitivity responses cause a number of chronic inflammatory and autoimmune diseases (Table 6-4).

CD4+ T Cell–Mediated Inflammation (p. 208)

CD4+ T cell–mediated inflammation can be of two major types; responses associated with T_H1 CD4+ T cells are predominated by macrophages, whereas those driven by T_H17 CD4+ T cells are characterized by neutrophil-dominated infiltration.

Activation of CD4+ T Cells

Recognition of processed peptide antigens on APCs leads to production of IL-2, an autocrine proliferation factor. Whether proliferating CD4+ T cells differentiate into T_H1 or T_H17 lineages depends on the cytokine environment at the time of initial T-cell activation. IL-12 production by APCs induces T_H1 cells, which in turn produce interferon-γ (IFN-γ) that promotes further T_H1 development and thus amplifies the reaction. Conversely, IL-1, IL-6, IL-23, and transforming growth factor-β (TGF-β) will stimulate differentiation to T_H17 cells.

Responses of Differentiated Effector T Cells

- The major effector cytokine of activated T_H1 cells is IFN-γ; it activates macrophages, increases class II histocompatibility molecule expression (improving antigen presentation capacity), induces TNF-α and IL-1 production (promoting inflammation), and increases IL-12 secretion (amplifying the T_H1 process). Activated macrophages then clear the offending agent; sustained activation (or the inability to clear the stimulus) can result in greater inflammation and tissue injury.
- Stimulated T_H17 cells secrete IL-17, IL-22, and other cytokines that recruit and activate neutrophils and monocytes—and IL-21 that amplifies the T_H17 response.

Clinical Examples of CD4+ T Cell–Mediated Inflammatory Reactions

- The classic DTH response is the *tuberculin reaction* to intracutaneous injection of purified protein derivative (PPD) derived from the tubercle bacillus. Prior tuberculosis infection results in circulating PPD-responsive memory CD4+ T cells; subsequent PPD injection into such an individual leads to the recruitment and activation of these cells beginning at 6 to 8 hours and peaking at 24 to 72 hours (the *delayed* in DTH). Histologically there is a perivascular mononuclear cell infiltrate (CD4+ T cells and macrophages) with evidence of endothelial activation.
- *Granulomatous inflammation* occurs when persistent or non-degradable antigens (e.g., foreign bodies) lead to chronic

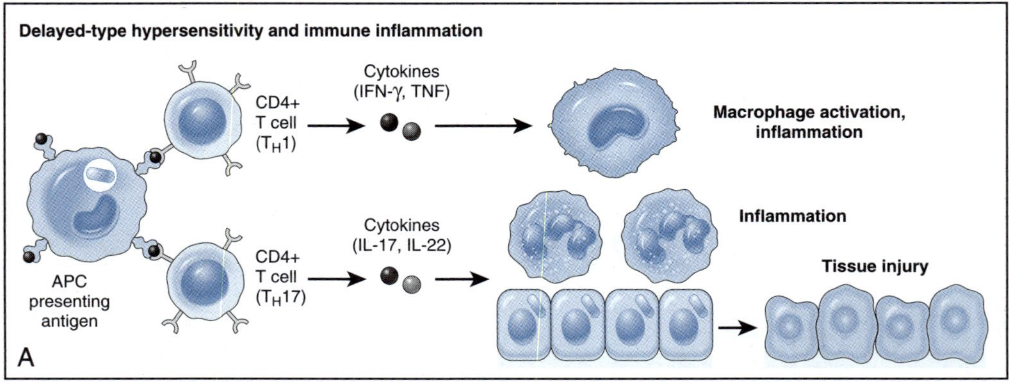

Figure 6-3 Mechanisms of T cell–mediated (type IV) hypersensitivity reactions. A, In DTH reactions, CD4+ T cells (and sometimes CD8+ T cells) respond to local antigens by secreting cytokines that recruit and activate inflammatory cells leading to tissue injury.

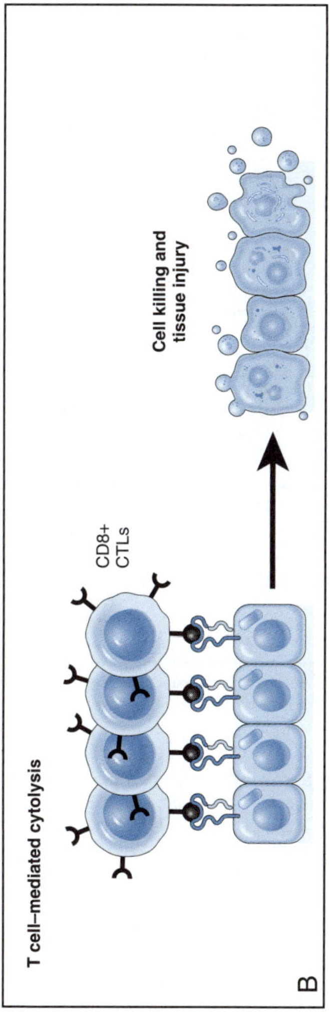

Figure 6-3, cont'd **B,** In some diseases, CD8+ CTLs directly kill tissue cells. *CD,* Cluster designation antigen.

TABLE 6-4 T Cell–Mediated Diseases

Disease	Specificity of Pathogenic T Cells	Principal Mechanisms of Tissue Injury	Clinicopathologic Manifestations
Rheumatoid arthritis	Collagen? Citrullinated self-proteins?	Inflammation mediated by T_H17 (and T_H1?) cytokines; role of antibodies and immune complexes?	Chronic arthritis with inflammation, destruction of articular cartilage
Multiple sclerosis	Protein antigens in myelin (e.g., myelin basic protein)	Inflammation mediated by T_H1 and T_H17 cytokines, myelin destruction by activated macrophages	Demyelination in CNS with perivascular inflammation; paralysis
Type 1 diabetes mellitus	Antigens of pancreatic islet β cells (insulin, glutamic acid decarboxylase, others)	T cell–mediated inflammation, destruction of islet cells by CTLs	Insulitis (chronic inflammation in islets), destruction of β cells; diabetes
Inflammatory bowel disease	Enteric bacteria; self-antigens?	Inflammation mediated by T_H1 and T_H17 cytokines	Chronic intestinal inflammation, obstruction
Psoriasis	Unknown	Inflammation mediated mainly by T_H17 cytokines	Destructive plaques in the skin
Contact sensitivity	Various environmental chemicals (e.g., urushiol from poison ivy or poison oak)	Inflammation mediated by T_H1 (and T_H17?) cytokines	Epidermal necrosis, dermal inflammation, causing skin rash and blisters

Examples of human T cell–mediated diseases are listed. In many cases, the specificity of the T cells and the mechanisms of tissue injury are inferred based on the similarity with experimental animal models of the diseases.

macrophage activation manifesting as large *epithelioid* cells; nodules of these activated cells are called *granulomas.*

- *Contact dermatitis* is another example of a DTH response, in this case to modified self; an example is poison ivy and exposure to its active constituent, urushiol, which binds to host proteins and alters their antigenicity.

Reactions of CD8+ T Cells: Cell-Mediated Cytotoxicity (p. 211)

Generation of CD8+ CTLs is the principal pattern of response to many viral infections and to tumor cells; CTLs also contribute to allograft rejection. CTL-induced injury is mediated by perforin-granzyme and Fas-Fas ligand (FasL) pathways that ultimately induce apoptosis.

Autoimmune Diseases (p. 211)

Immune reactions against self-antigens—autoimmunity—result from breakdown in *self-tolerance,* the normal state of nonresponsiveness to one's own antigens. Autoimmune diseases can be mediated by self-reactive antibodies and/or T cells (Table 6-5).

TABLE 6-5 Autoimmune Diseases	
Organ-Specific	**Systemic**
Diseases Mediated by Antibodies	
Autoimmune hemolytic anemia	SLE
Autoimmune thrombocytopenia	
Autoimmune atrophic gastritis of pernicious anemia	
Myasthenia gravis	
Graves disease	
Goodpasture syndrome	
Diseases Mediated by T Cells*	
Type 1 diabetes mellitus	Rheumatoid arthritis
Multiple sclerosis	Systemic sclerosis (scleroderma)†
Sjögren syndrome†	
Diseases Postulated to be Autoimmune	
Inflammatory bowel diseases (Crohn disease, ulcerative colitis)‡	
Primary biliary cirrhosis†	Polyarteritis nodosa†
Autoimmune (chronic active) hepatitis	Inflammatory myopathies†

*A role for T cells has been demonstrated in these disorders, but antibodies may also be involved in tissue injury.
†An autoimmune basis of these disorders is suspected but the supporting evidence is not strong.
‡These disorders may result from excessive immune responses to commensal enteric microbes, autoimmunity, or a combination of the two.

Immunologic Tolerance *(p. 212)*

The mechanisms of self-tolerance can be either central or peripheral:

Central Tolerance (p. 212)

Central tolerance refers to the process by which T and B cells that recognize self-antigens are either killed *(negative selection)* or rendered harmless. Many self-antigens are expressed in the thymus and presented by thymic APCs; when developing T cells with high-affinity TCRs for these self-antigens encounter thymic APC, they are deleted. A protein called *autoimmune regulator (AIRE)* is responsible for inducing the self-antigen expression, and interestingly, mutations in AIRE result in an autoimmune polyendocrinopathy (see Chapter 24). In additional, some autoreactive T cells are not deleted but rather develop into regulatory T cells.

When developing B cells strongly recognize self-antigens, they frequently reactivate the machinery for immunoglobulin rearrangement, generating new nonreactive B-cell receptors *(receptor editing)*. If receptor editing does not occur, self-reactive B cells also undergo apoptosis.

However, clonal deletion is not perfect, and numerous "normal" T and B cells can be found with receptors that recognize self-antigens. Unless muzzled by the elements of peripheral tolerance, they can cause autoimmune disease.

Peripheral Tolerance (p. 213)

Autoreactive cells that escape central regulatory mechanisms can be removed or inactivated in the periphery through one of the following pathways:

- *Anergy:* Irreversible functional inactivation may occur when T cells recognize self-antigen in the absence of necessary costimulatory signals (e.g., via B7-CD28 interactions).

Alternatively, APCs can inhibit T-cell activation by signals transmitted through T-cell CTLA-4 or PD-1 receptors. If self-reactive B cells encounter antigen in peripheral tissues in the absence of T-cell help, they lose the capacity for any subsequent antigenic stimulation.

- *Suppression by regulatory T cells:* Regulatory T cells—CD4+ cells expressing CD25 (the α-chain of the IL-2 receptor) and the Foxp3 transcription factor—may inhibit lymphocyte activation and effector functions by secreting cytokines, such as IL-10 and TGF-β. Mutations in *Foxp3* cause a severe autoimmune disease called IPEX (immune dysregulation, polyendocrinopathy, enteropathy, X-linked). Regulatory T cells are also likely important for maintaining maternal tolerance to the developing fetus (that expresses paternal antigens).
- *Deletion by apoptosis:* Self-antigens that are abundant in the peripheral tissue may cause persistent activation of self-reactive T cells, leading to either increased relative expression of proapoptotic molecules (e.g., Bim) or expression of FasL on these cells. Increased FasL expression will induce apoptosis of the T cells by engaging Fas coexpressed on these cells; self-reactive B cells expressing Fas can also be deleted by the FasL-positive T cells. Mutations in the *FAS* gene lead to *autoimmune lymphoproliferative syndrome (ALPS).*
- *Antigen sequestration:* Immune-privileged sites, such as testis, eye, and brain, may sequester tissue antigens across a relatively impermeant blood-tissue barrier. Release of such previously "privileged" antigens (e.g., due to physical injury) is the postulated mechanism for posttraumatic orchitis and uveitis.

Mechanisms of Autoimmunity: General Principles *(p. 214)*

Autoimmunity arises through some combination of susceptibility genes and environmental triggers (especially infections), such that the immune system experiences the following:

- Defective tolerance or regulation of immune responses
- Abnormal display of self-antigens (e.g., those arising from modifications due to stress or injury)
- Inflammation-driven lymphocyte activation

Role of Susceptibility Genes (p. 215)

Most autoimmune disorders are complex multigenic disorders. Although many are associated with specific histocompatibility molecule HLA alleles (potentially related to effects on negative selection or regulatory T-cell development), the expression of particular HLA molecules is not—by itself—the cause of autoimmunity. As described previously, defects in pathways that normally regulate either peripheral or central tolerance have also been demonstrated (e.g., *AIRE,* Fas-FasL, CTLA-4, IL-2 receptor, and *Foxp3*). Polymorphisms in other genes have also been implicated:

- *PTPN-22*—encoding a tyrosine phosphatase—is associated with multiple autoimmune disorders (e.g., type 1 diabetes mellitus and rheumatoid arthritis); a defective phosphatase would not adequately counter the activity of lymphocyte tyrosine kinases and could thus lead to excessive activation.
- *NOD-2*—part of the sensing mechanism for intracellular microbes—is associated with inflammatory bowel disease; defective NOD-2 could allow increased entry and subsequent inflammation to otherwise well-tolerated commensal gastrointestinal (GI) organisms.

- IL-2 and IL-7 receptors are associated with multiple sclerosis; polymorphisms may affect regulatory T-cell development and maintenance.

Role of Infections

Autoimmune disease onset is often temporally associated with infection. This may occur secondary to costimulator upregulation, which overwhelms peripheral tolerance mechanisms. Infection might also break tolerance by *molecular mimicry;* if a microbe shares epitopes with self-antigens, immune responses directed against the pathogen could cross-react with and damage normal tissues. Tissue injury occurring in the course of response to infection can also structurally alter self-antigens or release normal self-antigens; these molecules would then activate T cells that are not tolerant to the altered or previously cryptic antigens. The normal skin and gut microbiome may also influence the development of autoimmunity by impacting the relative proportions of effector and regulatory T cells.

General Features of Autoimmune Disease *(p. 217)*

Once induced, autoimmune diseases tend to be progressive (albeit with occasional relapses and remissions). This is in part due to intrinsic amplification loops that the immune system employs to allow initially small numbers of responsive cells to eventually overcome infection. In addition, immune responses are subject to the phenomenon of *epitope spreading;* many possible epitopes within self-antigens are not normally presented to developing T cells, and thus there is no opportunity to develop tolerance to such *cryptic* peptides. However, if such epitopes become recognizable in postnatal life as a result of molecular alteration of self-antigens, T cells reactive to them can cause persistent autoimmunity. The phenomenon is called *epitope spreading* because the immune response "spreads" to determinants that were not initially recognized.

The clinical and pathologic consequences of a specific autoimmune disease will be influenced by the nature of the response; thus T_H1 responses will have a macrophage-rich inflammation and substantial antibody-mediated elements, whereas neutrophil-mediated injury will predominate in T_H17 responses. Different autoimmune diseases also show substantial clinical and pathologic overlaps, so that precise classification may not be possible.

Systemic Lupus Erythematosus (p. 218)

Systemic lupus erythematosus (SLE) is the prototypical systemic autoimmune disorder, characterized by numerous autoantibodies, especially *antinuclear antibodies (ANAs).* Incidence approaches 1 in 2500 in some general populations; the female-male ratio is 9:1 with 1 in 700 women of childbearing age affected. The prevalence is twofold to threefold higher in blacks and Hispanics than in white populations.

Spectrum of Autoantibodies in Systemic Lupus Erythematosus *(p. 218)*

ANAs are typically detected by indirect immunofluorescence. The patterns of immunofluorescence (e.g., homogeneous, peripheral, speckled, nucleolar), although nonspecific, can suggest the type of circulating autoantibody. ANAs also occur in other autoimmune disorders (and in up to 10% of normal individuals) (Table 6-6), but *anti-double-stranded DNA (anti-dsDNA) and anti-Smith antigen antibodies strongly suggest SLE.*

In addition to ANAs, SLE patients produce other autoantibodies, some directed against blood elements (red blood cells, platelets,

TABLE 6-6 Autoantibodies in Systemic Autoimmune Diseases

Disease	Specificity of Autoantibody	% Positive	Association With Specific Disease Features
SLE	Double-stranded DNA	40-60	Nephritis; specific for SLE
	U1-RNP	30-40	
	Smith (Sm) antigen (core protein of small RNP particles)	20-30	Specific for SLE
	Ro (SS-A)/La (SS-B) nucleoproteins	30-50	Congenital heart block; neonatal lupus
	Phospholipid-protein complexes (anti-PL)	30-40	Antiphospholipid syndrome (in ~10% of SLE patients)
	Multiple nuclear antigens ("generic ANAs")	95-100	Found in other autoimmune diseases, not specific.
Systemic sclerosis	DNA topoisomerase 1	30-70	Diffuse skin disease, lung disease; specific for systemic sclerosis
	Centromeric proteins (CENPs) A, B, C	20-40	Limited skin disease, ischemic digital loss, pulmonary hypertension
	RNA polymerase III	15-20	Acute onset, scleroderma renal crisis, cancer
Sjögren syndrome	Ro/SS-A La/SS-B	70-95	
Autoimmune myositis	Histidyl aminoacyl-tRNA synthetase, Jo1	25	Interstitial lung disease, Raynaud phenomenon
	Mi-2 nuclear antigen	5-10	Dermatomyositis, skin rash
	MDA5 (cytoplasmic receptor for viral RNA)	20-35 (Japanese)	Vascular skin lesions, interstitial lung disease
	TIF1γ nuclear protein	15-20	Dermatomyositis, cancer
Rheumatoid arthritis	Cyclic citrullinated peptides (CCP); various citrullinated proteins	60-80	Specific for rheumatoid arthritis
	Rheumatoid factor (not specific)	60-70	

Listed autoantibodies are associated with high frequencies with particular diseases. "Generic" ANAs, which may react against many nuclear antigens, are positive in a large fraction of patients with SLE but are also positive in other autoimmune diseases. Percent positive refers to the approximate percentage of patients who test positive for each antibody.

The table was compiled with the help of Dr. Antony Rosen, Johns Hopkins University.

leukocytes). Moreover, 30% to 40% of SLE patients have antibodies to phospholipid-associated proteins *(antiphospholipid antibodies);* these are antibodies that recognize epitopes that are revealed when proteins complex with phospholipids. Some bind to cardiolipin antigen, giving rise to a false-positive result for syphilis. Others interfere with (prolong) in vitro coagulation assays; these so-called *lupus anticoagulants* actually exert a *pro*coagulant effect in vivo, causing a hypercoagulable state with vascular thrombosis, recurrent spontaneous miscarriages, or focal cerebral or ocular ischemia *(secondary antiphospholipid antibody syndrome).*

Etiology and Pathogenesis of Systemic Lupus Erythematosus (p. 219)

- *Genetic factors:* Monozygotic twin concordance (>20%) and familial and HLA clustering strongly implicate a genetic predisposition. Although the cause is unknown, the presence of a plethora of autoantibodies suggests a basic defect in the maintenance of B-cell tolerance. Congenital deficiencies in certain complement components (C2, C4, or C1q) may also impair immune complex clearance and favor tissue deposition.
- *Immunologic factors:* Defective elimination of self-reactive B cells and ineffective peripheral tolerance mechanisms are most important; inappropriate B-cell activation by nuclear RNA and DNA via TLRs or activation via abnormal elaboration of type I interferons or other cytokines may contribute. Finally, CD4+ T cells specific for nucleosomal antigens may escape tolerance.
- *Environmental factors:* Ultraviolet (UV) light exacerbates SLE by driving apoptosis, increasing IL-1 production by keratinocytes, and potentially by altering DNA to increase its immunogenicity. Estrogen is also implicated because of the gender and age predilection of the disease, and certain drugs (e.g., hydralazine and procainamide) can directly induce SLE-like responses.

A Model for the Pathogenesis of Systemic Lupus Erythematosus (p. 221)

Cell injury (e.g., UV and other environmental insults) leads to apoptosis and an increased burden of nuclear antigens. Defective B- and T-cell tolerance leads to autoantibodies directed against the nuclear antigens, with the resulting immune complexes being ingested by B cells and dendritic cells; subsequent TLR engagement causes further cellular activation, cytokine production, and augmented autoantibody synthesis, which causes more apoptosis in a self-amplifying loop.

Mechanisms of Tissue Injury (p. 221)

Tissue damage occurs primarily through formation of immune complexes (type III hypersensitivity) or by antibody-mediated injury to blood cells (type II hypersensitivity). Although ANAs cannot penetrate cells, these circulating autoantibodies may nevertheless form immune complexes with intracellular contents released from otherwise damaged cells. The secondary antiphospholipid antibody syndrome results in thrombotic complications, and the neuropsychiatric manifestations of lupus have been attributed to antibodies directed against neurons or neurotransmitter receptors.

***Morphology** (p. 222).* Although any organ can be involved, the most characteristic tissues affected are skin, blood vessels, kidneys, and connective tissue. *Classically there is a type III hypersensitivity response with acute necrotizing vasculitis and fibrinoid deposits, involving small arteries and arterioles.* Immunoglobulin, dsDNA, and C3 can be found in vessel walls, and a perivascular lymphocytic infiltrate is frequently present. In chronic cases, vessels show a fibrous thickening and luminal narrowing.

- *Kidney* is involved in virtually all cases of SLE; the principal mechanism of injury is immune complex deposition. Five patterns of *lupus nephritis* are recognized with increasing degrees of cellular infiltration, microvascular thrombosis, and vascular wall deposition; in turn, these are associated with increasing degrees of hematuria, proteinuria, hypertension, and renal insufficiency.
- *Skin: Malar erythema* is the classic lesion *(butterfly rash)*, along with variable cutaneous lesions ranging from erythema to bullae occurring elsewhere. Sunlight exacerbates the lesions. Microscopically there is basal layer degeneration with dermal-epidermal junction immunoglobulin and complement deposits. The dermis shows variable fibrosis, perivascular mononuclear cell infiltrates, and vascular fibrinoid change.
- *Joints:* There is a *nonspecific, nonerosive synovitis* with minimal joint deformity.
- *Central nervous system (CNS):* Neuropsychiatric manifestations are probably secondary to endothelial injury and occlusion (antiphospholipid antibodies) or impaired neuronal function as a result of autoantibodies to a synaptic membrane antigen.
- *Pericarditis and other serosal cavity involvement:* Serositis is initially fibrinous with focal vasculitis, fibrinoid necrosis, and edema; this progresses to adhesions, possibly obliterating serosal cavities (i.e., the pericardial sac).
- *Cardiovascular system:* Principal involvement is pericarditis; myocarditis is much less common, and—although a classic finding—*nonbacterial verrucous (Libman-Sacks) endocarditis* happens infrequently. The latter features numerous small, warty vegetations (1 to 3 mm) on the inflow or outflow surfaces (or both) of the mitral and tricuspid valves. There may also be diffuse leaflet thickening of the mitral or aortic valves with functional stenosis or insufficiency. There is an increasing incidence of accelerated coronary atherosclerosis, potentially attributable to exacerbation of traditional risk factors (e.g., hypertension, hypercholesterolemia) and immune complex– and antiphospholipid antibody–mediated vascular injury.
- *Spleen:* Splenomegaly with capsular thickening and follicular hyperplasia are common. Penicilliary artery perivascular fibrosis is characteristic, producing an *onion-skin* appearance.
- *Lungs:* Pleuritis and/or effusions occur in 50% of patients; there is also chronic interstitial fibrosis and secondary pulmonary hypertension.

Clinical Features *(p. 225).* The clinical manifestations of SLE are protean. It can present insidiously as a systemic, chronic, recurrent, febrile illness with symptoms referable to virtually any tissue but especially joints, skin, kidneys, and serosal membranes. Autoantibodies to hematologic components may induce thrombocytopenia, leukopenia, and anemia. The course of the disease is highly variable; rarely it is fulminant with death in weeks to months.

- Occasionally may cause minimal symptoms (hematuria, rash) and remit even without treatment.
- More often the disease is characterized by recurrent flares and remissions over many years and is held in check by immunosuppressive regimens.
- Five-year survival is 90%; ten-year survival is 80%; death is most commonly caused by renal failure or intercurrent infections.

Chronic Discoid Lupus Erythematosus (p. 225)

This disease is limited to cutaneous lesions that grossly and microscopically mimic SLE. Only 35% of patients have a positive ANA. As in SLE there is deposition of immunoglobulin and C3 at the dermal-epidermal junction. After many years, 5% to 10% of affected individuals develop systemic manifestations.

Drug-Induced Lupus Erythematosus (p. 226)

Hydralazine, procainamide, isoniazid, D-penicillamine, and other agents can induce a positive ANA (up to 80% of patients taking procainamide); anti-TNF therapy can also do so. Nevertheless, less than a third will have lupus symptomatology; although there is multiorgan involvement, renal and CNS disease is uncommon. Anti-dsDNA antibodies are rare, but antihistone antibodies are common. There may be HLA associations that are distinct for each drug (*HLA-DR4* for hydralazine and *HLA-DR6* for procainamide). Drug-related lupus erythematosus usually remits after removal of the offending agent.

Rheumatoid Arthritis (see Chapter 26)

Sjögren Syndrome (p. 226)

Sjögren syndrome is characterized by dry eyes *(keratoconjunctivitis sicca)* and dry mouth *(xerostomia)*, resulting from immune-mediated lacrimal and salivary gland destruction. Approximately 40% of cases occur in isolation (the primary form or *sicca syndrome*); the remainder are associated with other autoimmune diseases (e.g., rheumatoid arthritis [most common], SLE, or scleroderma); 90% of patients are women between ages 35 and 45.

- Most patients have rheumatoid factor (an IgM autoantibody that binds self IgG) without having rheumatoid arthritis; ANAs against ribonucleoproteins SS-A (Ro) and SS-B (La) are especially common (Table 6-4).
- Injury is probably a consequence of both cellular and humoral mechanisms; it is most likely initiated by CD4+ T cells reacting to an unknown self-antigen after an initiating infectious injury. Epstein-Barr virus (EBV) and hepatitis C have been implicated, and patients infected with human T-cell lymphotropic virus (HTLV) type 1 develop similar lesions.

Morphology (p. 227)

The lacrimal and salivary glands (other exocrine glands may also be involved) initially show a periductal lymphocytic infiltrate with ductal epithelial hyperplasia and luminal obstruction. This is followed by acinar atrophy, fibrosis, and eventual fatty replacement, with an expanding lymphocyte infiltrate that can develop lymphoid follicles and germinal centers. Changes secondary due to loss of glandular secretion include corneal inflammation, erosion, ulceration, and atrophy of oral mucosa with inflammatory fissuring and ulceration; patients frequently develop nasal drying and crusting, and rarely septal perforation. Laryngitis, bronchitis, or pneumonitis can result from respiratory involvement.

Clinical Features (p. 227)

Xerostomia makes swallowing foods difficult, and the keratoconjunctivitis can markedly affect vision. Extraglandular involvement occurs in a third of patients, with synovitis, pulmonary fibrosis, and peripheral neuropathy; although glomerular lesions are rare, renal tubular dysfunction (e.g., renal tubular acidosis and phosphaturia) occur commonly in association with tubulointerstitial nephritis. Adenopathy may occur with pleomorphic lymph node infiltrates, and there is a fortyfold increased risk of developing B-cell lymphoma. *Mikulicz syndrome* is a term for lacrimal and salivary gland enlargement from any cause; distinguishing Sjögren syndrome from other etiologies (e.g., sarcoidosis, leukemia, lymphoma) requires lip biopsy (to examine minor salivary glands).

Systemic Sclerosis (Scleroderma) (p. 228)

Scleroderma is a chronic autoimmune inflammatory disorder characterized by widespread vascular injury and progressive perivascular and interstitial fibrosis of multiple organs. Cutaneous involvement is greatest (where it may be confined for years), although the fibrosis frequently involves the GI tract, kidneys, heart, muscles, and lung. The female-male ratio is 3:1, with peak incidence in the 50- to 60-year age group. There are two major clinical categories:

- *Diffuse scleroderma* with widespread skin involvement and rapid progression, with early visceral involvement.
- *Limited scleroderma* with limited cutaneous involvement, late visceral involvement, and a relatively benign course. Patients with limited disease can also develop *c*alcinosis, *R*aynaud phenomenon, *e*sophageal dysmotility, *s*clerodactyly, and *t*elangiectasia, or *CREST syndrome.*

Etiology and Pathogenesis (p. 228)

- *Autoimmunity:* Current speculation is that CD4+ T cells respond to yet unidentified antigens and release cytokines (e.g., TGF-β and IL-13) that activate additional inflammatory cells and fibroblasts. Inappropriate humoral immunity is also triggered, producing a number of autoantibodies, including ANAs (Table 6-6); these are good markers of disease but may not necessarily cause injury:
  - *Anti-topoisomerase I* (anti-Scl-70) is highly specific and is associated with diffuse scleroderma and pulmonary fibrosis.
  - *Anti-centromere* antibody is found more commonly in patients with limited disease and CREST syndrome.
- *Vascular damage:* Microvascular injury is a hallmark feature of systemic sclerosis and indeed may be the primary inciting pathology. Although the cause of the injury is unknown, it is speculated to be a consequence of either direct autoimmune attack or a by-product of chronic perivascular inflammation. Regardless, repeated cycles of endothelial injury followed by platelet aggregation lead to the release of a number of growth factors and cytokines (e.g., platelet-derived growth factor [PDGF], TGF-β) that ultimately induce vascular smooth muscle and fibroblast proliferation, as well as matrix synthesis that narrows the vascular lumen.
- *Fibrosis:* This results not only from scarring in the setting of ischemic injury but also because of fibrogenic cytokine elaboration and hyper-responsiveness of fibroblasts to the various growth factors.

Morphology *(p. 229).* Vessels throughout the body exhibit perivascular lymphocytic infiltrates with focal vascular occlusion and edema; this is temporally followed by progressive perivascular fibrosis and vascular hyaline thickening. The manifestation of these vascular changes varies with the tissue type:

- *Skin* grossly exhibits diffuse sclerosis with atrophy. Affected areas are initially edematous with a doughy consistency. Eventually, fibrotic fingers become tapered and claw-like with diminished mobility, and the face becomes a drawn mask. Focal vascular obliteration causes ulceration, and fingertips may undergo autoamputation.
- *Alimentary tract* shows progressive atrophy and fibrosis of the muscularis, most prominently in the esophagus, where it assumes a rubber-hose consistency. Throughout the GI tract, there is mucosal thinning, ulceration, and scarring.

- *Musculoskeletal system:* Inflammatory synovitis progressing to fibrosis is common; joint destruction is uncommon. Muscle involvement begins proximally with edema and mononuclear perivascular infiltrates, progressing to interstitial fibrosis with myofiber degeneration.
- *Kidneys* are affected in two thirds of patients; *renal failure accounts for 50% of deaths in systemic sclerosis.* The most prominent changes are in vessel walls (especially interlobular arteries) with intimal proliferation and deposition of mucinous or collagenous material. Hypertension is present in 30% of cases, 10% of which have a malignant course. Hypertension further accentuates the vascular changes, often resulting in fibrinoid necrosis with thrombosis and necrosis.
- *Lungs:* Lungs show variable fibrosis of small pulmonary vessels with diffuse interstitial and alveolar fibrosis, progressing in some cases to honeycombing.
- *Heart:* Perivascular infiltrates with interstitial fibrosis occasionally evolve into a restrictive cardiomyopathy. There may also be conduction system involvement with resultant arrhythmias.

Clinical Features *(p. 229).* Although sharing features with SLE, rheumatoid arthritis and polymyositis, the striking feature of systemic sclerosis is the cutaneous fibrosis. Other associated clinical findings include the following:

- *Raynaud phenomenon* (episodic arteriolar constriction in the extremities) occurs in virtually all patients and precedes other symptoms in more than 70%.
- Dysphagia from esophageal fibrosis (50% of patients).
- GI involvement leading to malabsorption, intestinal pain, or obstruction.
- Pulmonary fibrosis, causing respiratory or right-sided heart failure.
- Direct cardiac involvement, which can induce arrhythmias or heart failure secondary to microvascular infarction.
- Development of malignant hypertension, potentially culminating in fatal renal failure.

Inflammatory Myopathies (see Chapter 27)

Mixed Connective Tissue Disease *(p. 231)*

This may not be a distinct entity but rather a heterogeneous subgroup of other autoimmune disorders (SLE, polymyositis, and systemic sclerosis) and can with time evolve into classic SLE or scleroderma. It is characterized by the following:

- High antibody titers to U1 ribonucleoprotein (Table 6-6)
- Modest initial renal involvement
- Good initial response to steroids
- Serious complications are pulmonary hypertension and progressive renal disease

Polyarteritis Nodosa and Other Vasculitides (see Chapter 11)

IgG_4-Related Disease *(p. 231)*

This is a collection of disorders—now described in virtually every tissue—characterized by fibrosis and obliterative phlebitis, with inflammatory infiltrates dominated by T cells and IgG_4 antibody–producing plasma cells; serum IgG_4 levels are also often elevated but may not contribute to the pathologic lesions. B-cell depletion affords some clinical benefit. This entity includes *Mikulicz syndrome* (involving salivary and lacrimal glands), *Riedel thyroiditis, idiopathic retroperitoneal fibrosis, autoimmune pancreatitis,* and *inflammatory pseudotumors* of the orbit, lungs, and kidneys.

Rejection of Transplant Tissues (p. 231)

Transplant rejection involves the mechanisms of immune-mediated damage discussed previously, including CTL and DTH responses, and antibody-mediated injury. Grafts between individuals of the same species are called *allografts;* grafts between different species are called *xenografts.*

Mechanisms of Recognition and Rejection of Allografts (p. 231)

The host immune system is triggered by the presence of foreign HLA histocompatibility molecules on the endothelium and parenchymal cells of the transplanted tissue (Fig. 6-4). HLA molecules occur in two forms, class I and class II, that drive distinct aspects of the specific immune response (see also pp. 194-196 of *Robbins and Cotran Pathologic Basis of Disease,* 9th ed.).

- *Class I molecules* are expressed on all nucleated cells; they are heterodimers composed of a polymorphic heavy-chain glycoprotein (coded on one of three closely linked loci: HLA-A, HLA-B, and HLA-C) and a nonpolymorphic β2-microglobulin. Class I molecules bind peptide fragments derived from *endogenous proteins* (e.g., viral products in a virally infected cell) and present these processed antigens to CD8+ CTL, resulting in their activation.
- *Class II molecules* are confined to APCs, including dendritic cells, macrophages, B cells, and activated T cells; they are heterodimers composed of noncovalently associated α and β chains coded in the HLA-D region (with three serologically defined subloci DP, DQ, and DR). Class II molecules bind peptide fragments derived from *exogenous proteins* and present these processed antigens to CD4+ helper T lymphocytes, resulting in their activation.

Host T cells recognize allograft HLA by two pathways:

- *Direct pathway:* Host T cells recognize donor HLA on APC derived from the donor; the most important cells in this process are donor dendritic cells. Host CD8+ T cells recognize donor class I HLA molecules and mature into CTL; host CD4+ T cells recognize donor class II HLA molecules; they proliferate and differentiate to form T_H1 (and possibly T_H17) effector cell populations.
- *Indirect pathway:* Host T cells recognize donor HLA after processing and presentation on host APCs (analogous to any other exogenous processed antigen). Therefore the principal response is a DTH mediated by CD4+ T lymphocytes.

The frequency of T cells that can recognize foreign antigens in a graft is much higher than the frequency of T cells specific for any particular microbe; thus allograft responses are much stronger than typical pathogen-specific responses.

Following lymphocyte activation, rejection is mediated by the following (Fig. 6-4):

- Direct CTL–mediated parenchymal and endothelial cytolysis.
- Macrophage-mediated damage.
- Cytokine-mediated vascular and parenchymal dysfunction.
- Microvascular injury will also cause downstream tissue ischemia.
- *Antibody-mediated responses* can also be important; these tend to induce injury to endothelial cells rather than parenchymal cells.

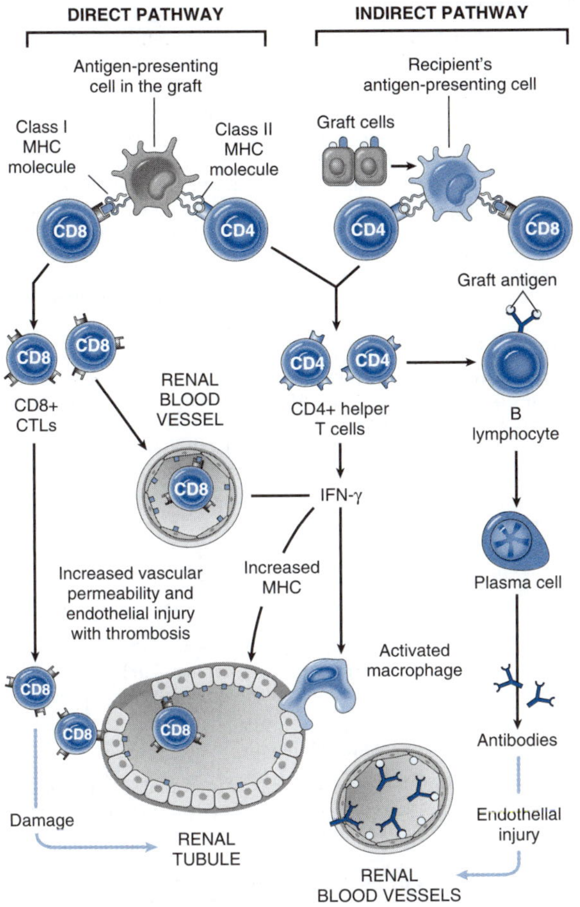

Figure 6-4 Recognition and rejection of histoincompatible grafts. In the direct pathway, class I and class II antigens on donor APCs are recognized by host CD8+ CTL and CD4+ helper T cells, respectively. CD4+ cells proliferate and produce cytokines that induce tissue damage by a local DTH response, stimulating B cells and CD8+ T cells. CD8+ T cells responding to graft antigens differentiate into CTL that directly kill graft cells. In the indirect pathway, graft antigens are displayed by host APC and primarily activate CD4+ T cells; these in turn damage the graft by DTH mechanisms, including the induction of autoantibodies. Although the example shown involves a renal transplant, the same principles apply to all solid organ allografts.

Hyperacute Rejection *(p. 233)*

Hyperacute rejection occurs when the recipient has been previously sensitized to graft antigens (e.g., by blood transfusion or pregnancy). Preformed circulating antibody binds to graft endothelial HLA with an immediate (minutes to days) complement- and ADCC-mediated injury. Grossly the organ is cyanotic, mottled, and flaccid. Microscopically the lesions resemble immune complex–mediated disease; immunoglobulin and complement are deposited in the vessel walls with endothelial injury, fibrin-platelet microthombi, neutrophil infiltrates, and arteriolar fibrinoid necrosis followed by distal parenchymal infarction.

Acute Rejection (p. 233)

Acute rejection typically occurs within days to months of transplantation or after cessation of immunosuppressive therapy. Both cellular and humoral mechanisms can contribute.

- *Acute cellular rejection* is characterized by an interstitial mononuclear cell infiltrate (macrophages and both CD4+ and CD8+ T cells).
- *Acute humoral rejection* is mediated by newly synthesized (not preformed) antidonor antibodies that cause a necrotizing vasculitis with consequent thrombosis. Complement activation contributes, and complement C4d deposition in vascular beds is used as a diagnostic feature of humoral rejection. A subacute vasculitis may also occur, with intimal thickening (by proliferating fibroblasts and macrophages); resultant vascular narrowing can cause infarction.

Chronic Rejection (p. 234)

Chronic rejection occurs over months to years and is characterized by progressive organ dysfunction. *Morphologically* arteries show dense obliterative intimal fibrosis, causing allograft ischemia.

Based on the mechanisms of allograft rejection, *methods of increasing graft survival* (p. 234) include the following:

- HLA matching between donor and recipient
- Inhibiting inflation (e.g., steroids)
- Immunosuppressive therapy blocking T-cell activation or costimulation, including inhibiting the following:
  - IL-2 production (e.g., calcineurin inhibitors, such as cyclosporine and tacrolimus)
  - IL-2 signaling (e.g., rapamycin)
  - T lymphocyte proliferation (e.g., mycophenolate)
  - B7-CD28 costimulatory molecule interactions
- T-cell destruction (anti-T-cell antibodies)
- Plasmapheresis or anti-B-cell therapy

Immunosuppression carries the risk of increased susceptibility to opportunistic infections (e.g., polyoma virus) and certain malignancies (e.g., EBV-induced lymphomas).

Transplantation of Hematopoietic Stem Cells (p. 236)

Hematopoietic stem cell (HSC) transplantation is facilitated by harvesting HSC from the umbilical cord of newborns (a rich source) or by mobilizing these precursor cells from the marrow into the peripheral blood by administering hematopoietic growth factors. Bone marrow transplantation—used for treating hematologic malignancies (e.g., leukemia), aplastic anemia, or immunodeficiency states—requires lethal levels of irradiation (and/or chemotherapy) to eradicate any malignant cells, create a satisfactory graft bed, and minimize host rejection of the grafted marrow. Besides the significant toxicity of the "conditioning regimen," complications include graft-versus-host disease (GVHD) and immunodeficiency.

Graft-Versus-Host Disease

Immunocompetent donor lymphocytes in an HLA-nonidentical recipient recognize host cells as foreign and induce CD8+ and CD4+ T cell–mediated injury. Any tissues can be affected but host immune cells (immunosuppression), biliary epithelium (jaundice), skin (desquamative rash), and GI mucosa (bloody diarrhea) bear the brunt of the attack. In *chronic GVHD,* ongoing cutaneous and GI injury can resemble that seen in systemic sclerosis. Reactivation of cytomegalovirus infection, particularly in the lung, can be fatal.

Immunodeficiency

Immunocompromise can result from the original myeloablative protocol, a delay in repopulation of the lymphoid tissues, and/or graft destruction of host immune cells. Patients are thus susceptible to a number of opportunistic infections, particularly cytomegalovirus.

GVHD and the infectious complications of bone marrow transplantation can be lethal; HLA matching and selective donor marrow T-cell depletion (and/or immunosuppression) can minimize the severity. Unfortunately, T cell–depleted marrow engrafts poorly, and in leukemic patients the malignancy relapse rate is increased when T cell–depleted marrow is used (donor T cells exert a potent *graft-versus-leukemia* effect).

Immunodeficiency Syndromes (p. 237)

- *Primary immunodeficiencies* are usually hereditary and manifest between 6 months and 2 years of life as maternal antibody protection is lost.
- *Secondary immunodeficiencies* result from altered immune function due to infections, malnutrition, aging, immunosuppression, irradiation, chemotherapy, or autoimmunity.

Defects in Innate Immunity (p. 237) (Table 6-7)

Defects in Leukocyte Function (p. 237)

- *Inherited defects in leukocyte adhesion* lead to recurrent bacterial infections due to defective leukocyte recruitment.
    - *Leukocyte adhesion deficiency type 1:* Defective synthesis of the β_2 chain shared by LFA-1 and Mac-1 integrins
    - *Leukocyte adhesion deficiency type 2:* Absence of the sialyl-Lewis X ligand for E- and P-selectins
- *Inherited defects in phagolysosome function* cause susceptibility to infections due to neutropenia, defective degranulation, and delayed microbial killing.
    - *Chediak-Higashi syndrome* is an autosomal recessive disorder caused by mutations in a cytosolic protein (LYST) involved in lysosomal trafficking.
- *Inherited defects in microbicidal activity* lead to recurrent bacterial infections; granulomatous inflammation occurs as a compensatory response when the initial neutrophil-mediated killing is inadequate to contain microbes.
    - *Chronic granulomatous disease* results from mutations in the phagocyte oxidase complex, culminating in deficient superoxide production.
- *Defects in TLR signaling* are rare and typically have restricted clinical phenotypes.
    - Mutations in TLR3 (a viral RNA receptor) lead to recurrent herpes simplex encephalitis.
    - Defects in MyD88 (a downstream adaptor protein for several TLRs) are associated with destructive bacterial pneumonias.

Defects Affecting the Complement System (p. 238)

- Deficiency of the C2 (most common) or C4 complement components is classically associated with increased viral and bacterial infections but can also manifest as an SLE-like autoimmune disease.

- Alternate pathway (properdin and factor D) deficits are rare; these lead to recurrent pyogenic infections. Defects in the mannose-binding lectin pathway of complement activation have similar manifestations.
- C3 deficiency leads to severe recurrent pyogenic infections, as well as increased susceptibility to immune complex–mediated glomerulonephritis (the latter presumably due to poor immune complex clearance in the absence of complement).
- Defects in C5 to C9 are associated with recurrent neisserial infections.
- C1 inhibitor (C1INH) deficiency leads to the autosomal dominant entity *hereditary angioedema.* C1INH normally inhibits proteases, such as C1r and C1s in the complement cascade, factor XIIa in coagulation, and kallikrein, and unregulated activity by those enzymes leads to increased complement, clotting, and bradykinin activation with recurrent episodes of cutaneous and mucosal edema.
- Hereditary or acquired mutations in membrane-bound, complement-regulatory proteins can cause *paroxysmal nocturnal hemoglobinuria* (see Chapter 14) and *hemolytic uremic syndrome* (see Chapter 20).

Defects in Lymphocyte Maturation (p. 238) (Fig. 6-5)

Severe Combined Immunodeficiency Disease (*p. 239*)

Severe combined immunodeficiency disease (SCID) is a heterogeneous group of X-linked and autosomal recessive disorders characterized by

TABLE 6-7 Defects in Innate Immunity

Disease	Defect
Defects in Leukocyte Function	
Leukocyte adhesion deficiency 1	Defective leukocyte adhesion because of mutations in β chain of CD11/CD18 integrins
Leukocyte adhesion deficiency 2	Defective leukocyte adhesion because of mutations in fucosyl transferase required for synthesis of sialylated oligosaccharide (receptor for selectins)
Chédiak-Higashi syndrome	Decreased leukocyte functions because of mutations affecting protein involved in lysosomal membrane traffic
Chronic granulomatous disease	Decreased oxidative burst
X-linked	Phagocyte oxidase (membrane component)
Autosomal recessive	Phagocyte oxidase (cytoplasmic components)
Myeloperoxidase deficiency	Decreased microbial killing because of defective MPO-H_2O_2 system
Defects in the Complement System	
C2, C4 deficiency	Defective classical pathway activation, results in reduced resistance to infection and reduced clearance of immune complexes
C3 deficiency	Defects in all complement functions
Deficiency of complement regulatory proteins	Excessive complement activation; clinical syndromes include angioedema, paroxysmal hemoglobinuria, others

The table lists some of the more common inherited immune deficiencies affecting phagocytic leukocytes and the complement system.

Modified in part from Gallin JI: Disorders of phagocytic cells. In Gallin JI, Goldstein IM, Snyderman R (eds): *Inflammation: Basic Principles and Clinical Correlates,* 2nd ed. New York, NY: Raven Press, 1992, pp 860, 861.

defects in both T- and B-cell function, impacting both cellular and humoral immunity. Lymphoid tissues are diffusely hypoplastic, and patients are susceptible to recurrent, severe infections from a wide range of bacterial, viral, and fungal organisms. Without bone marrow transplantation, SCID is usually fatal within 1 year; X-linked SCID was the first human disease to be successfully treated by replacing a defective gene in a stem cell.

- *X-linked SCID* (50% to 60% of SCID) results from mutations in the signal-transducing γ chain (γc) subunit common to several

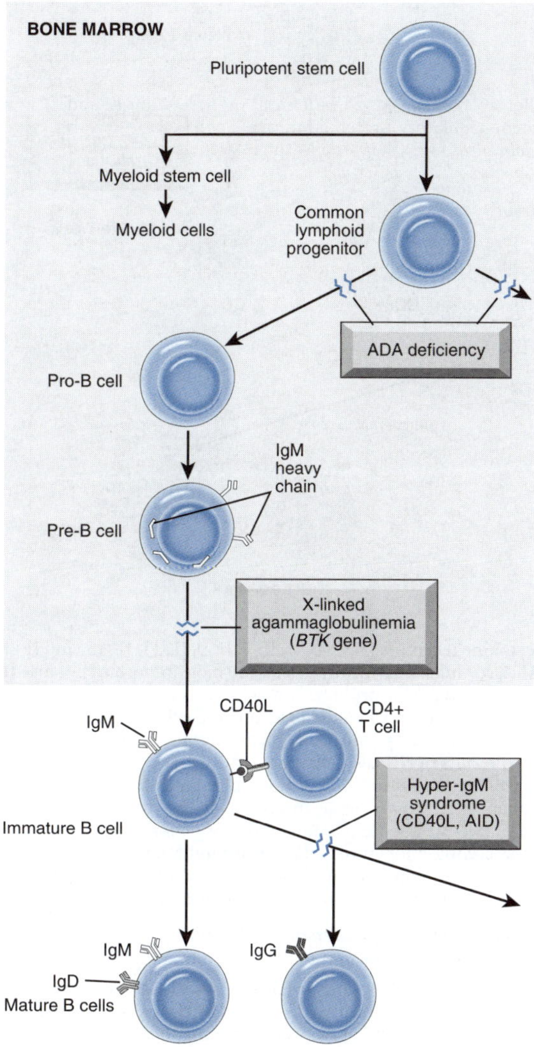

Figure 6-5 Schematic of lymphocyte development and sites of blockade for some of the primary immunodeficiency disorders; affected genes are indicated in parentheses. *BTK,* Bruton tyrosine kinase; *CD40L,* CD40 ligand; *SCID,* severe combined immune deficiency.

Continued

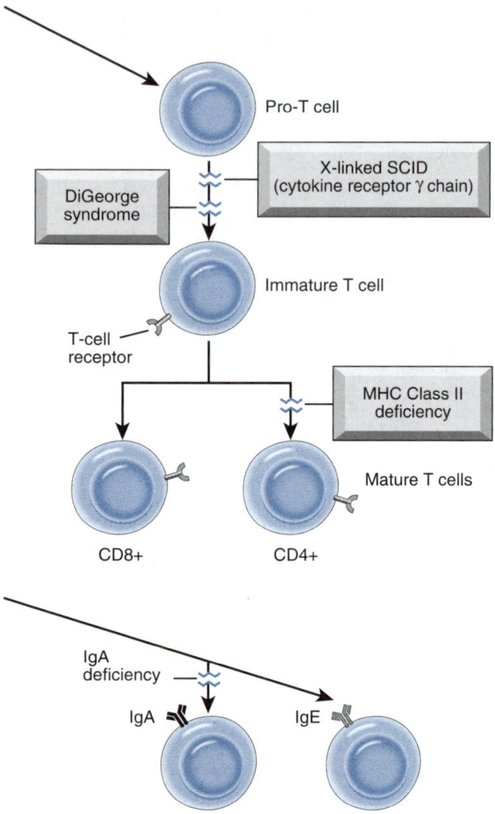

Figure 6-5, cont'd

cytokine receptors (IL-2, IL-4, IL-7, IL-9, IL-11, IL-15, and IL-21). IL-7 stimulatory pathway defects are most important because IL-7 is required for the proliferation of lymphoid progenitors, especially in the T-cell lineage, and inadequate T-cell help severely impacts B-cell antibody production. Ineffective IL-15 receptor signaling also results in NK cell deficiency.

- *Autosomal recessive SCID* is most commonly due to *adenosine deaminase* (ADA) *deficiency;* this results in the accumulation of lymphotoxic metabolites, including deoxyadenosine and deoxy-ATP. Less common forms of SCID involve mutations in the antigen receptor recombination machinery or signaling pathways, including Jak3 kinase (transduces the activation signal from the γc subunit).

X-Linked Agammaglobulinemia (Bruton Agammaglobulinemia) *(p. 240)*

X-linked agammaglobulinemia (Bruton agammaglobulinemia) is one of the more common primary immunodeficiency syndromes. It presents at about 6 months of age—after maternal-derived antibodies have been depleted—as *recurrent bacterial infections* (typically *Haemophilus influenzae, Streptococcus pneumoniae,* or *Staphylococcus aureus* that require antibody opsonization for clearance). Cell-mediated immune function is normal, but there is virtually no serum immunoglobulin.

Thus viral and fungal infections are usually not problematic; nevertheless, enterovirus, echovirus (causing a fatal encephalitis), and vaccine-associated poliovirus (causing paralysis) can still cause disease because they are normally neutralized by circulating antibodies. *Giardia lamblia,* an intestinal parasite neutralized by IgA, can also cause persistent infections.

- Affected individuals lack mature B cells due to mutations in the B-cell tyrosine kinase *(BTK)* gene; *BTK* is normally expressed in early B cells and is critical for transduction of signals from the antigen receptor complex that drive B-cell maturation. Pre-B cells are present in normal numbers in marrow, but lymph nodes and spleen lack germinal centers, and plasma cells are absent from all tissues.
- T-cell numbers and function are entirely normal.
- Increased incidence (up to 35%) of autoimmune connective tissue diseases; chronic infections and/or a breakdown in self-tolerance are implicated.
- Therapy involves immunoglobulin replacement therapy from normal donor serum.

DiGeorge Syndrome (Thymic Hypoplasia) *(p. 241)*

DiGeorge syndrome (thymic hypoplasia) is a multiorgan disorder resulting from congenital failure of development of the third and fourth pharyngeal pouches and absence of the organs that normally arise from them; 90% of cases are associated with deletion of a gene mapping to 22q11. Features include the following:

- Thymic hypoplasia or aplasia: T-cell deficiency with lack of cell-mediated responses (especially to fungi and viruses); immunoglobulin levels be normal or reduced depending on the severity of the T-cell deficiency.
- Parathyroid hypoplasia: Abnormal calcium regulation with hypocalcemic tetany.
- Congenital defects of heart and great vessels.
- Dysmorphic facies.

Defects in Lymphocyte Activation and Function (p. 241)

Hyper-IgM Syndrome *(p. 241)*

Hyper-IgM syndrome is characterized by the production of IgM without IgG, IgA, or IgE antibodies; it results from failure of T cells to support B-cell immunoglobulin *isotype switching.* Such switching depends on interaction of T-cell CD40 ligand (CD40L) with B-cell CD40. In 70% of patients the disease is X-linked due to mutation of the *CD40L* gene encoded on the X chromosome (Xq26). In the remainder there are mutations in CD40 or in *activation-induced deaminase (AID);* the latter is a DNA-editing enzyme required for isotype switching. Features include the following:

- Lack of opsonizing IgG leads to recurrent bacterial infections.
- Patients are also susceptible to *Pneumocystis jiroveci* because T-cell-macrophage interactions in cell-mediated immune responses also involve CD40-CD40L binding.
- Many of the IgM antibodies react with blood cells, resulting in autoimmune hemolytic anemia, thrombocytopenia, or neutropenia.

Common Variable Immunodeficiency *(p. 241)*

Common variable immunodeficiency is a heterogeneous group of disorders, congenital and acquired, sporadic and familial. The common feature is hypogammaglobulinemia in the absence of other well-defined causes; generally all immunoglobulin classes are affected, but occasionally only IgG. The pathogenesis may involve intrinsic B-cell defects in maturation or survival or, more commonly, defective B-cell development secondary to T-cell shortcomings. Clinical features include the following:

- Initial presentation similar to X-linked agammaglobulinemia (i.e., recurrent sinopulmonary infections, serious enterovirus infections, and persistent *G. lamblia* infections).
- Affecting both sexes equally with onset in late childhood or adolescence.
- Adenopathy with hyperplastic B-cell zones, reflecting intact B-cell proliferation but lack of IgG-mediated feedback inhibition.
- Increased incidence of autoimmune diseases (20%) and lymphoid malignancies.

Isolated Immunoglobulin A Deficiency (p. 242)

Isolated IgA deficiency is a common immunodeficiency (in the United States, 1 in 600 people of European descent) with *virtually absent serum and secretory IgA* (also occasionally IgG_2 and IgG_4 subclasses). It can be familial or acquired after toxoplasmosis, measles, or other viral infection. The basic defect is failure of IgA-positive B cells to mature; immature forms are present in normal numbers. Features include the following:

- Mucosal immunity is most affected. Although usually asymptomatic, patients can have recurrent sinopulmonary and GI infections.
- Increased incidence of respiratory tract allergies and autoimmune diseases (SLE, rheumatoid arthritis).
- Patients can have antibodies directed against IgA, and transfusion of IgA-containing blood products can induce anaphylaxis.

X-Linked Lymphoproliferative Syndrome (p. 242)

X-linked lymphoproliferative syndrome is characterized by the inability to clear EBV, leading to fulminant mononucleosis, as well as EBV-associated B-cell tumors. Eighty percent of cases are caused by mutations in an adaptor molecule (*SLAM-associated protein* [SAP]) that interacts with cell surface receptors that activate T, B, and NK cells. SAP defects lead to poor T- and NK-cell activation, as well as inadequate follicular helper T-cell activation; the latter results in meager germinal center formation and poor production of high-affinity antibodies.

Immunodeficiencies Associated With Systemic Diseases (p. 242)

Wiskott-Aldrich Syndrome (p. 242)

Wiskott-Aldrich syndrome is an X-linked disorder characterized by recurrent infections. It is caused by mutations in the gene for Wiskott-Aldrich syndrome protein (WASP) located at Xp11.23; WASP links cell surface receptors and intracellular cytoskeleton and may be important for cell migration and signal transduction. Features include the following:

- Relatively normal thymus, but peripheral lymphoid T-cell depletion with subsequent defective cellular immunity.
- No antibody production to polysaccharides and poor response to protein antigens.
- Increased incidence of non-Hodgkin B-cell lymphoma.

Ataxia Telangiectasia (p. 242)

Ataxia telangiectasia is an autosomal recessive disorder caused by mutations of the *ataxia telangiectasia mutated (ATM)* gene on chromosome 11; it is characterized by abnormal gait (ataxia), vascular malformations (telangiectasias), neurologic deficits, increased tumor incidence, and immunodeficiency that may affect both T and B cells. The T-cell defects are associated with thymic hypoplasia, whereas the B-cell deficits involve reduced production of isotype-switched antibodies. ATM is a protein kinase that can sense DNA double-strand breaks (DSBs) and activate *p53* to initiate cell cycle arrest and/or apoptosis; it also stabilizes DSB during immunoglobulin V(D)J recombination, and abnormal ATM may thus lead to defective antigen receptor generation.

Secondary Immunodeficiencies (p. 243)

As a group these are substantially more common than primary immune deficiencies and can result from various infections, malnutrition, aging, immunosuppression, irradiation, chemotherapy, or autoimmunity.

Acquired Immunodeficiency Syndrome (p. 243)

Acquired immunodeficiency syndrome (AIDS) is caused by the retrovirus human immunodeficiency virus (HIV); it is characterized by profound suppression of T cell–mediated immunity, leading to opportunistic infections, secondary neoplasms, and neurologic disorders.

Epidemiology (p. 236)

Transmission of HIV occurs through the following:

- *Sexual contact:* Seventy-five percent of all cases worldwide have this mode of transmission; virus is carried in semen and vaginal secretions (as free virus and within infected lymphocytes) and enters the host via mucosal abrasions (rectal, oral, vaginal) or direct mucosal cell contact. Transmission occurs by direct inoculation into the blood stream or infection of host mucosal dendritic cells or CD4+ T cells. Transmission is enhanced by concurrent sexually transmitted diseases, either by causing increased mucosal ulceration or by increasing the numbers of virus-containing inflammatory cells in genital fluids.
- *Parenteral inoculation:* Intravenous drug users constitute the dominant population, with recipients of blood product concentrates (e.g., hemophiliacs) or blood transfusions now being substantially less common (less than 1 in 2 million blood transfusions in the United States). Risk of transmission from accidental needlestick is less than 0.3%, and antiretroviral therapy postexposure reduces the risk an additional eightfold. Risk of transmission from insect bites is virtually impossible.
- *Vertical transmission from infected mothers to fetuses or newborns:* This may be transplacental in utero, during delivery through an infected birth canal, or through ingestion of breast milk. The majority of children with AIDS have had transplacental or perinatal transmission; the risk of transmission from infected mothers ranges from 7% to 49% but is virtually eliminated by maternal antiretroviral therapy. Risk is increased with high viral load and chorioamnionitis.

In the United States, five major risk groups are identified:

- *Homosexual and bisexual men:* Approximately half of the reported cases of AIDS. This mode of transmission appears to be in decline.
- *Intravenous drug users (without a history of homosexual contact):* Approximately 20% of all patients.
- *Hemophiliacs:* Approximately 0.5% of cases; mainly those receiving large amounts of pooled factor VIII or IX concentrates before 1985.

- *Blood or component recipients (excluding hemophiliacs):* Approximately 1% of all patients. Ten percent of pediatric AIDS patients presumably developed their infection through blood or blood products received before 1985.
- *Heterosexual contact:* Approximately 20% of patients acquire the disease through heterosexual contacts with other high-risk groups; approximately a third of new cases are attributable to this route. Outside the United States and Europe, male-to-female transmission (most through vaginal intercourse) is the most common mode of spread; female-to-male transmission is still uncommon in the United States (twentyfold less common than male-to-female heterosexual transmission).

In approximately 5% of cases, no risk factors can be identified. HIV is *not* transmitted by casual (nonsexual) contact.

Etiology: The Properties of Human Immunodeficiency Virus (p. 245)

HIV is a nontransforming retrovirus in the lentivirus family; it causes immunodeficiency by destruction of target T cells. There are two different but genetically related forms; HIV-1 is most commonly associated with AIDS in the United States, Europe, and Central Africa, whereas HIV-2 causes a similar disease in India and West Africa.

- The HIV-1 lipid envelope, derived from the infected host membrane during budding, is studded with two viral glycoproteins, gp120 and gp41; both are critical for HIV infection.
- There is substantial variability in the envelope proteins, making vaccine targeting against specific antigenic structures extremely difficult.
- The virus core contains the capsid protein p24, nucleocapsid protein p7/p9, two copies of genomic RNA, and three viral enzymes: protease, integrase, and reverse transcriptase.
- p24 is the most readily detectable viral antigen and is the target in most diagnostic antibody assays.
- The viral genome contains typical retroviral *gag, pol,* and *env* genes; the *gag* and *pol* gene products are synthesized as a larger precursor protein that must be proteolytically processed. Components of antiviral therapy are thus directed against the protease, as well as the retroviral polymerase.
- Besides the typical retroviral *gag, pol,* and *env* genes, HIV has several genes not present in other retroviruses important for viral synthesis and assembly. These genes include *tat, vpu, vif, nef,* and *rev;* for example, *tat* and *rev* regulate HIV transcription and may be therapeutic targets.

Pathogenesis of Human Immunodeficiency Virus Infection and Acquired Immunodeficiency Syndrome (p. 245)

Depletion of CD4+ helper T cells (and impaired functioning of any surviving helper T cells) causes profound immunosuppression and constitutes the central pathogenic pathway of AIDS; the CNS is another important target.

Life Cycle of Human Immunodeficiency Virus (p. 246)

- The CD4 antigen (also present at lower levels on monocytes, macrophages, and dendritic cells) is the high-affinity receptor for the HIV gp120 protein.
- HIV gp120 must also bind coreceptors on target cells to facilitate cell entry; the major coreceptors are chemokine receptors CCR5 and CXCR4. CCR5 is found mainly on monocyte or macrophage

lineages; consequently, HIVs using this coreceptor are denoted M-tropic. Conversely, CXCR4 is mostly found on T lymphocytes, and viruses using that coreceptor are denoted T-tropic. M-tropic viruses typically constitute the majority of HIV in the blood of acutely infected individuals; over the course of an infection the more virulent T-tropic viruses will accumulate. Individuals with mutations in the CCR5 coreceptor (approximately 1% of the Caucasian American population are homozygous) are resistant to infection by M-tropic HIV strains.

- After gp120 interacts with CD4 and one of the coreceptors, the noncovalently linked gp41 protein undergoes a conformational change that allows the virus to be internalized.
- The genome undergoes reverse transcription, generating double-stranded complementary (proviral) DNA. HIV causes productive infections only in memory and activated T cells; naïve T cells are "protected" by the activity of a cytidine deaminase that introduces cytosine-to-uracil mutations in the proviral DNA. This enzyme is inactivated by previous T-cell activation.
- In quiescent T cells, the proviral DNA remains in the cytoplasm as a linear episomal form. However, in proliferating T cells (e.g., after antigenic stimulation), the proviral DNA circularizes, enters the nucleus, and is integrated into the host genome.
- After integration, proviral DNA may be silent (latent) for months to years; alternatively, proviral DNA can be transcribed in activated cells to make viral particles. Cell activation results in nuclear translocation of the NF-κB transcription factor; it binds to the long-terminal-repeat sequences that flank the HIV genome and induces viral transcripts.

Mechanisms of T-Cell Depletion in Human Immunodeficiency Virus Infection (p. 248)

Most T-cell loss is attributable to the direct cytopathic effect of replicating virus; this may be due to interference with normal host cell protein synthesis or to increased membrane permeability associated with viral budding. Other mechanisms that contribute to T-cell loss include the following:

- Progressive destruction of the architecture and cellular composition of the lymphoid organs, including cells important for maintaining a cytokine environment conducive to CD4+ maturation.
- Chronic activation of uninfected cells (responding to HIV or opportunistic infections), leading eventually to *activation-induced cell death.*
- Fusion of infected and noninfected cells via gp120 (forming syncytia or giant cells) leading to cell death.
- Binding of soluble gp120 to noninfected CD4+ T cells leading to activation of apoptotic pathways or to CTL-mediated killing.
- In addition to cell death, HIV infection also causes qualitative defects in T-cell function including diminished T_H1 responses (relative to T_H2), defective intracellular signaling, and reduced antigen-induced T-cell proliferation.

Human Immunodeficiency Virus Infection of Non-T Cells (p. 249)

- Infected monocytes and macrophages bud relatively small amounts of virus and are refractory to HIV cytopathic effects; these infected monocytes or macrophages can thus act as HIV reservoirs (potentially transferring virus to T cells during antigen presentation), as well as vehicles for viral transport, especially to the CNS.
- Mucosal dendritic cells transport virus to regional lymph nodes. Nodal follicular dendritic cells are important HIV reservoirs; viral particles coated with anti-HIV antibodies attach to the dendritic

cell Fc receptors and can continually infect T cells as they come in close contact during passage through lymph nodes.
- Despite defects in T-cell help—and therefore the inability to mount antibody responses to newly encountered antigen—there is also paradoxical polyclonal B-cell activation. This can occur through reactivation or reinfection with cytomegalovirus and/or EBV, direct activation by gp41, or increased IL-6 production by infected macrophages.

Pathogenesis of Central Nervous System Involvement (p. 250)

CNS involvement occurs predominantly through infected monocytes that circulate to the brain and either directly release toxic cytokines (IL-1, TNF, etc.), induce neuronal NO production via gp41, or cause neuron damage via soluble gp120.

Natural History of Human Immunodeficiency Virus Infection (p. 250)

HIV infection can be divided into three phases (Fig. 6-6):

- *Primary infection, virus dissemination, and the acute retroviral syndrome* (p. 250) are characterized by transient viremia, widespread seeding of mucosal lymphoid tissue and infection of memory T cells (expressing CCR5), a temporary (but substantial) fall in CD4+ T cells, followed by antibody seroconversion and partial control of viral replication by generation of CD8+ antiviral T cells. Clinically a self-limited acute illness (the *acute retroviral syndrome*) will occur in 40% to 90% of infected individuals with sore throat, fatigue, myalgias, fever, rash, adenopathy, and/or weight loss. Mucosal infection often leads to epithelial damage and microbial invasion across the defective barrier. Mucosal infection allows epithelial dendritic cells to capture and subsequently deliver the virus to lymph nodes where CD4+ T cells become infected through direct cell-cell contact.
  Clinical improvement and a partial recovery in CD4+ T-cell counts occur within 6 to 12 weeks; the level of circulating CD4+ T cells is the most reliable short-term indicator of disease progression. The viral load at the end of the acute phase also reflects the balance between HIV production and host defenses. This viral set point is an important predictor of the rate of progression of HIV disease; high viral loads at the end of the acute phase portend rapid progression to AIDS.
- *Chronic infection* (p. 252) is characterized by clinical latency (absence of symptoms) despite ongoing vigorous viral replication; lymph nodes and spleen are the major sites of viral production. There is initially a brisk regeneration of T cells, but eventually recurrent viral infection and associated T-cell death lead to progressive depletion. Concomitant with T-cell loss is a decline in immune function and an increasing viral burden, with a shift to T-tropic viruses. Patients may develop minor opportunistic infections such as oral candidiasis. The period of clinical latency is typically 7 to 10 years in untreated patients, although *rapid progressors* may see this period truncated to 2 to 3 years, and 5% to 15% will be *long-term nonprogressors* who remain symptom-free, with stable CD4 counts and low viral loads, for 10 or more years; 1% are *elite controllers* with a vigorous anti-HIV response and undetectable plasma virus.
- *AIDS* (p. 252) is heralded by a rapid decline in host defenses manifested by low CD4+ counts and a dramatic increase in viral burden; patients frequently present with prolonged fever, weight loss, and diarrhea, followed by serious opportunistic infections, secondary neoplasms, or neurologic disease *(AIDS indicator diseases)*.

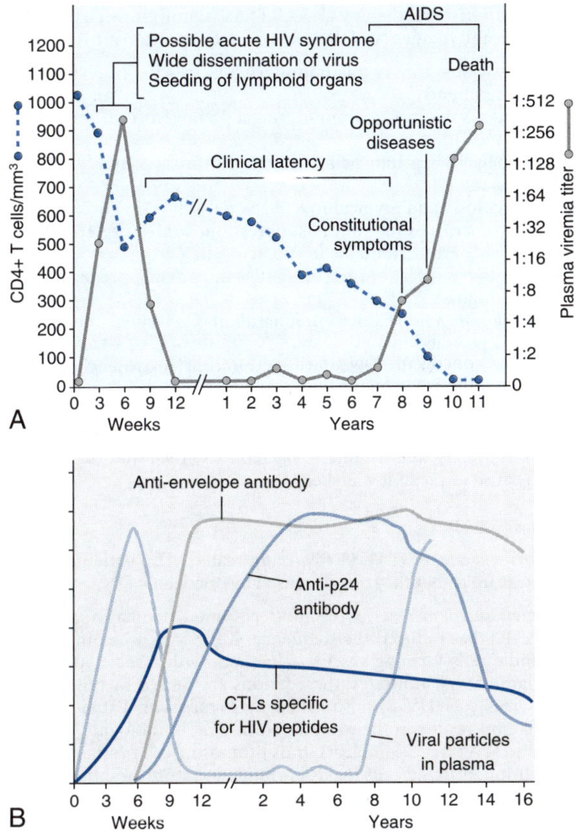

Figure 6-6 Clinical course of HIV infection. A, After initial infection, there is widespread viral dissemination and a sharp decrease in peripheral CD4+ T-cell counts. With the ensuing immune response to HIV the viral load is diminished followed by a prolonged period of clinical latency; during this period, viral replication continues. The CD4+ T-cell count gradually decreases during the following years, until it reaches a critical level below which constitutional symptoms and various opportunistic diseases supervene. **B,** Immune response to HIV infection. A CTL response to HIV is detectable 2 to 3 weeks after the initial infection, peaking at 9 to 12 weeks. Marked expansion of virus-specific CD8+ T-cell clones occurs during this time; the humoral immune response peaks at about 12 weeks. *(**A,** Redrawn from Fauci AS, Lane HC: Human immunodeficiency virus disease: AIDS and related conditions. In Fauci AS, Braunwald E, Isselbacher K, Wilson J, Martin J, Kasper D, Hauser S, Longo D (eds):* Harrison's Principles of Internal Medicine, *14th ed. New York, NY: McGraw-Hill, 1997, p 1791.)*

Clinical Features of Acquired Immunodeficiency Syndrome *(p. 252)*

These run the gamut from asymptomatic to the acute retroviral syndrome to life-threatening infection or malignancy. The clinical features of full-blown AIDS include the following that are discussed next.

Opportunistic Infections (p. 252)

Opportunistic infections account for the majority of deaths in untreated patients with AIDS; most cases represent reactivation of latent infections rather than de novo infections. The advent of highly active antiretroviral therapy (HAART) has significantly changed the spectrum and frequency of these secondary opportunistic infections.

- *Pneumocystis jiroveci* pneumonia occurs in 15% to 30% of untreated patients.
- *Candida* is the most common fungal pathogen (oral, vaginal, or esophageal).
- Cytomegalovirus may be systemic but more commonly involves the eye and GI tract.
- Tuberculosis and atypical mycobacterial infections occur late in the setting of severe immunosuppression; a third of AIDS deaths worldwide are attributable to tuberculosis.
- *Cryptococcus* infections occur in 10% of patients, predominantly as meningitis.
- *Toxoplasma gondii* causes encephalitis and is responsible for 50% of CNS mass lesions.
- JC papovavirus causes progressive multifocal leukoencephalopathy.
- Herpes simplex virus manifests as chronic mucocutaneous ulcerations.
- *Cryptosporidium, Isospora belli,* microsporidia, and atypical mycobacteria, as well as enteric bacteria (*Shigella* and *Salmonella*) can cause intractable diarrhea.

Tumors (p. 253)

Tumors will occur in 25% to 40% of untreated AIDS patients; a common feature is that they are all caused by oncogenic DNA viruses:

- *Kaposi sarcoma (KS)* is the most common neoplasm, although HAART has reduced the frequency. KS lesions are composed of spindle cells forming vascular channels, with associated chronic inflammatory infiltrates; these lesions are caused by human herpesvirus 8 (HHV-8), also called *KS herpesvirus.* Latent HHV-8 infection results in the production of viral homologues of cyclin D and several p53 inhibitors, thus promoting cell proliferation. In addition, infected cells make a proinflammatory viral homologue of IL-6 and a G protein–coupled receptor that induces the release of vascular endothelial growth factor. Besides infecting endothelial cells to produce KS, HHV-8-infected B cells may also be the source of *primary effusion lymphomas* in AIDS patients. AIDS-associated KS is quite distinct from the sporadic form of KS in non-HIV-infected individuals (see Chapter 11).
- *Lymphomas* may be systemic, CNS, or body cavity based; 10% of AIDS patients will eventually develop such tumors. Aggressive non-Hodgkin B-cell lymphomas, especially involving extranodal sites (such as the CNS), are characteristic. The etiology for many of these lymphomas is a sustained polyclonal B-cell proliferation driven by EBV infection, followed by the emergence of an oligoclonal or monoclonal population. Alternatively, the germinal center B-cell hyperplasia that occurs early in HIV infections may drive lymphomagenesis by increasing B-cell proliferation, thus allowing the coincidental acquisition of oncogene mutations (e.g., in *MYC* and *BCL6*).
- *Other tumors* include squamous cell carcinoma of the uterine cervix and anus, likely reflecting greater susceptibility to HPV infection.

Central Nervous System Disease (p. 255)

CNS disease occurs in 40% to 60% of patients. In addition to opportunistic infections and tumors, patients can present with acute aseptic meningitis, vacuolar myelopathy, and peripheral neuropathy. Most common is a progressive encephalopathy, designated *AIDS-dementia complex* (see Chapter 28).

Effect of Antiretroviral Therapy on the Clinical Course of Human Immunodeficiency Virus Infection (p. 255)

- HAART involves more than 25 compounds in six distinct drug categories; triple drug regimens in compliant patients are effective in reducing viral burden to nondetectable levels indefinitely, with gradual recovery of T-cell counts. Morbidity and mortality have dropped commensurately.
- Treated patients still carry viral DNA in their lymphoid tissues and can spread the infection or can develop active infection if treatment is stopped.
- Long-term HAART can also cause toxicities, including fat redistribution, insulin resistance, premature cardiovascular disease, and renal and hepatic dysfunction.
- *Immune reconstitution inflammatory syndrome* can occur as a consequence of a recovering immune system in the presence of a heavy burden of persistent microbes (e.g., atypical mycobacteria or *Pneumocystis*).

Morphology *(p. 256).* With the exception of the CNS, the tissue changes in AIDS are neither specific nor diagnostic; the pathologic features are those of the various opportunistic infections and neoplasms (discussed elsewhere in the organ-specific chapters).

- *Lymph nodes:* Adenopathy in early HIV infection reflects the initial polyclonal B-cell proliferation (and hypergammaglobulinemia), showing nonspecific, predominantly follicular hyperplasia with mantle zone attenuation and intense medullary plasmacytosis. HIV particles can be demonstrated in germinal centers by in situ hybridization, localized mainly on the surface of follicular dendritic cells. With progression to full-blown AIDS, the lymphoid follicles become involuted *(burned out)*, with general lymphocyte depletion and follicular disruption. Similar lymphoid depletion occurs in the spleen and thymus.
- *Inflammatory responses to infections* may be sparse or atypical, and infectious organisms may not be apparent without special stains.

Amyloidosis (p. 256)

Amyloid is a heterogeneous group of fibrillar proteins that *share the ability to aggregate into an insoluble, cross-beta-pleated sheet tertiary conformation;* amyloid fibrils accumulate extracellularly in tissues due either to excess synthesis or resistance to catabolism. As amyloid accumulates, it produces pressure atrophy of adjacent parenchyma. Depending on tissue distribution and degree of involvement, the clinical effects of amyloid can range from life threatening to an asymptomatic incidental finding at autopsy.

Properties of Amyloid Proteins (p. 257)

By electron microscopy, amyloid is composed predominantly (95%) of nonbranching fibrils 7.5 to 10 nm in diameter, associated with a minor (5%) amount of *P component* and other glycoproteins. Of more than 20 distinct forms thus identified, three are most common (Table 6-8):

- *Amyloid light chain* (AL): Immunoglobulin light chains (or amino-terminal fragments thereof) derived from plasma cells and associated with plasma cell tumors (e.g., multiple myeloma); lambda light chain amyloid occurs more often than kappa.

TABLE 6-8 Classification of Amyloidosis

Clinicopathologic Category	Associated Diseases	Major Fibril Protein	Chemically Related Precursor Protein
Systemic (Generalized) Amyloidosis			
Immunocyte dyscrasias with amyloidosis (primary amyloidosis)	Multiple myeloma and other monoclonal plasma cell proliferations	AL	Immunoglobulin light chains, chiefly λ type
Reactive systemic amyloidosis (secondary amyloidosis)	Chronic inflammatory conditions	AA	SAA
Hemodialysis-associated amyloidosis	Chronic renal failure	$A\beta_2m$	β_2-microglobulin
Hereditary Amyloidosis			
Familial Mediterranean fever		AA	SAA
Familial amyloidotic neuropathies (several types)		ATTR	TTR
Systemic senile amyloidosis		ATTR	TTR
Localized Amyloidosis			
Senile cerebral	Alzheimer disease	Aβ	APP
Isolated atrial amyloidosis	Congestive heart failure, mitral valve insufficiency	AANF	Atrial natriuretic factor
Endocrine			
Islets of Langerhans	Type 2 diabetes mellitus	AIAPP	Islet amyloid peptide
	Medullary carcinoma of thyroid	A Cal	Calcitonin

- *Amyloid-associated* (AA): An 8500-dalton nonimmunoglobulin protein derived from a larger serum precursor called *SAA* (serum amyloid-associated) protein synthesized by hepatocytes as part of the "acute phase response"; AA amyloid is associated with chronic inflammatory states.
- *β-Amyloid* (Aβ): A 4000-dalton peptide that forms the core of cerebral plaques and deposits within cerebral vessel walls in Alzheimer disease; it derives from a transmembrane amyloid precursor protein (see Chapter 28).

Other less common forms of amyloid include the following:

- *Transthyretin (TTR):* A normal serum protein that binds and transports thyroxine and retinol. Excess amounts of normal TTR can deposit in geriatric hearts (senile systemic amyloidosis), whereas mutant forms of the protein are deposited in a group of hereditary diseases called *familial amyloid polyneuropathy.*
- *β_2-microglobulin:* The smaller nonpolymorphic peptide component of class I HLA molecules and a normal serum protein; it is deposited in a form of amyloidosis that complicates long-term hemodialysis.

Pathogenesis and Classification of Amyloidosis (p. 258)

Proteins that form amyloid are either:

- Normal proteins that have a propensity to fold improperly and associate to form fibrils; overproduction (or defective catabolism) will thus lead to deposition.
- Mutant proteins that are prone to misfolding and aggregation; even "normal" levels of synthesis can cause deposition.

Amyloidosis is subdivided into systemic (generalized) and localized (tissue-specific) forms and is further classified on the basis of predisposing conditions (Table 6-8).

Systemic amyloidosis is associated with the following conditions:

- *Primary amyloidosis: Immunocyte dyscrasias with amyloidosis* is due to AL-type amyloid; it occurs in 5% to 15% of patients with multiple myeloma (see Chapter 13). Malignant plasma cells synthesize abnormal quantities of a single immunoglobulin (*M spike* on serum protein electrophoresis) or immunoglobulin light chain (*Bence Jones* protein). The vast majority of cases of AL-type systemic amyloidosis are *not* associated with *overt* B-cell neoplasms but nevertheless have elevated monoclonal immunoglobulins, light chains, or both.
- *Reactive secondary amyloidosis* is due to AA-type amyloid. Secondary amyloidosis is associated with chronic inflammatory states (infectious and noninfectious) (e.g., rheumatoid arthritis, scleroderma, dermatomyositis, bronchiectasis, chronic osteomyelitis), and nonimmunocyte tumors (e.g., Hodgkin lymphoma and renal cell carcinoma).
- *Heredofamilial amyloidosis* includes a number of rare entities, often confined to specific geographic locations. The most common and best characterized form is *familial Mediterranean fever,* a recurrent, febrile illness caused by overproduction of IL-1; this is caused by mutations in the *pyrin* protein involved in regulating cytokine production. The amyloid is of AA type, suggesting that chronic inflammation plays a pivotal role.
- *Hemodialysis-associated amyloidosis* is due to deposition (in joints, synovium, and tendon sheaths) of β_2-microglobulin not filtered by normal dialysis membranes; improved filters have reduced the incidence of this entity.

Localized amyloidosis is amyloid confined to a single organ or tissue:

- Localized forms of AL immunocyte-derived amyloid with associated plasma cell infiltrates; nodular deposits can occur in lung, larynx, skin, bladder, and tongue and periorbitally.
- *Endocrine amyloid* occurs in tumors associated with hormone synthesis (e.g., thyroid medullary carcinoma making procalcitonin that deposits as amyloid fibrils).
- *Amyloid of aging* occurs typically in the eighth and ninth decades and is most commonly due to deposition of nonmutant TTR. Although amyloid distribution is systemic, the dominant involvement is of the heart, presenting as a restrictive cardiomyopathy or arrhythmias. In addition to sporadic senile systemic amyloidosis, another form—more common in blacks—occurs due to mutant TTR.

Morphology (p. 260)

In general there is no consistent or distinctive pattern of organ involvement for the systemic amyloidoses, except perhaps hemodialysis-associated amyloid. Macroscopically, affected tissues are enlarged, waxy, and firm. Microscopically, routine stains reveal only amorphous, acellular, hyaline, eosinophilic extracellular material. With special stains (e.g., Congo red), amyloid is salmon-pink, and characteristic yellow-green birefringence may be seen using polarized light.

- *Kidneys:* Initial mesangial and subendothelial, progressing to complete glomerular hyalinization. Peritubular deposits begin in the tubular basement membrane and gradually extend into the interstitium. Hyaline thickening of arterial and arteriolar walls with narrowing lumen eventually causes ischemia with tubular atrophy and interstitial fibrosis.
- *Spleen* may be enlarged (up to 800 g). Amyloid deposits begin between cells. With time, one of two patterns emerges:
  - *Sago spleen:* Deposits are limited to the splenic follicles, giving rise to tapioca-like granules on gross inspection.
  - *Lardaceous spleen:* Amyloid largely spares the follicles and is deposited in the red pulp. Fusion of deposits forms large geographic areas of amyloid.
- *Liver* shows hepatomegaly. Microscopically amyloid first deposits in the space of Disse, gradually encroaching on parenchyma and sinusoids to produce pressure atrophy with massive hepatic replacement.
- *Heart:* Distinctive (although not always present) are minute, typically atrial, pink-gray subendocardial droplets representing focal amyloid accumulations. Vascular and subepicardial deposits may also occur. Microscopically there are interstitial and perimyocyte deposits, progressively leading to pressure atrophy.
- *Other organs:* Nodular deposits in the tongue can cause macroglossia *(tumor-forming amyloid of the tongue).* Deposits on the carpal ligament of the wrist (e.g., in hemodialysis-associated amyloid) can cause carpal tunnel syndrome.

Clinical Features *(p. 262)*

- Renal involvement can give rise to proteinuria and nephrotic syndrome (see Chapter 20). Cardiac amyloid can present as insidious congestive heart failure or arrhythmias, and GI amyloidosis can present with malabsorption. Vascular involvement can lead to vessel fragility with occasionally massive hemorrhage in the setting of relatively minimal trauma. AL amyloid can also bind and inactivate coagulation factor X, promoting a bleeding diathesis.
- Diagnosis is made on the basis of biopsy and characteristic Congo red stain. Favored biopsy sites are the kidney (when renal manifestations are present) and the rectum or gingiva (in systemic disease). Abdominal fat pad aspirates can also yield diagnostic tissue but has low sensitivity.
- In amyloidosis associated with B-cell dyscrasias, serum and urine electrophoresis and bone marrow biopsy (for plasmacytosis) are indicated.
- In systemic amyloidosis, the prognosis is poor. Median survival after diagnosis in the setting of B-cell dyscrasias is approximately 2 years, and myeloma-associated amyloid is worse. Reactive amyloidosis may have a slightly better outlook, depending on the ability to control the underlying condition.

7 Neoplasia

Nomenclature (p. 266)

The terms *neoplasm* (literally "new growth") and *tumor* are used interchangeably; these refer to abnormal masses of tissue, the growth of which are virtually autonomous and exceed that of normal tissues. In contrast to non-neoplastic proliferations, the growth of tumors persists after cessation of the initiating stimulus. A more modern definition includes the newer insight that tumor growth is driven by acquired mutations that confer a proliferative advantage and are passed to progeny in a clonal fashion from a single initial malignant cell.

Tumors are broadly classified based on clinical behaviors:

- *Benign*—with an "innocent" behavior characterized by a localized lesion without spread to other sites and amenable to surgical resection; the patient typically survives—although there are exceptions.
- *Malignant*—called *cancers,* with aggressive behavior including invasion and destruction of adjacent tissues, and capacity for spread to other sites *(metastasis).*

All tumors have two basic components:

- Clonal expansions of neoplastic cells constituting the tumor parenchyma
- Supporting stroma composed of non-neoplastic connective tissue and blood vessels; abundant collagenous stroma is called *desmoplasia,* and such tumors will be rock hard or *scirrhous.*

The type of neoplasm is based on the characteristics of its parenchyma. Tumor nomenclature is summarized in Table 7-1).

Benign tumors (p. 266) typically end with the suffix *-oma;* benign mesenchymal tumors include lipoma, fibroma, angioma, osteoma, and leiomyoma. The nomenclature for benign epithelial tumors also typically uses the *-oma* suffix but in addition incorporates elements of histogenesis, macroscopic appearance, and microscopic architecture:

- *Adenomas:* Epithelial tumors arising in glands or forming glandular patterns
- *Cystadenomas:* Adenomas producing large cystic masses, common in ovary
- *Papillomas:* Epithelial tumors forming gross or microscopic fingerlike projections
- *Polyp:* Tumor projecting macroscopically above the mucosa (e.g., a colon polyp)

It is worth emphasizing that some tumors do not follow the *-oma* rule; for example, melanoma, lymphoma, and mesothelioma are all malignant.

Malignant tumors (p. 266) are categorized as the following:

- *Carcinomas* derived from epithelial cells.
- *Sarcomas* of mesenchymal cell origin.

TABLE 7-1 Nomenclature of Tumors

Tissue of Origin	Benign	Malignant
Composed of One Parenchymal Cell Type		
Tumors of Mesenchymal Origin		
Connective tissue and derivatives	Fibroma Lipoma Chondroma Osteoma	Fibrosarcoma Liposarcoma Chondrosarcoma Osteogenic sarcoma
Vessels and Surface Coverings		
Blood vessels	Hemangioma	Angiosarcoma
Lymph vessels	Lymphangioma	Lymphangiosarcoma
Mesothelium	Benign fibrous tumor	Mesothelioma
Brain coverings	Meningioma	Invasive meningioma
Blood Cells and Related Cells		
Hematopoietic cells		Leukemias
Lymphoid tissue		Lymphomas
Muscle		
Smooth	Leiomyoma	Leiomyosarcoma
Striated	Rhabdomyoma	Rhabdomyosarcoma
Tumors of Epithelial Origin		
Stratified squamous	Squamous cell papilloma	Squamous cell carcinoma
Basal cells of skin or adnexa		Basal cell carcinoma
Epithelial lining of glands or ducts	Adenoma Papilloma Cystadenoma	Adenocarcinoma Papillary carcinomas Cystadenocarcinoma
Respiratory passages	Bronchial adenoma	Bronchogenic carcinoma
Renal epithelium	Renal tubular adenoma	Renal cell carcinoma
Liver cells	Hepatic adenoma	Hepatocellular carcinoma
Urinary tract epithelium (transitional)	Transitional cell papilloma	Transitional cell carcinoma
Placental epithelium	Hydatidiform mole	Choriocarcinoma
Testicular epithelium (germ cells)		Seminoma Embryonal carcinoma
Tumors of Melanocytes	Nevus	Malignant melanoma
More Than One Neoplastic Cell Type—Mixed Tumors, Usually Derived From One Germ Cell Layer		
Salivary glands	Pleomorphic adenoma (mixed tumor of salivary origin)	Malignant mixed tumor of salivary gland origin
Renal anlage		Wilms tumor
More Than One Neoplastic Cell Type Derived From More Than One Germ Cell Layer—Teratogenous		
Totipotential cells in gonads or in embryonic rests	Mature teratoma, dermoid cyst	Immature teratoma, teratocarcinoma

- Mesenchymal tumors of blood-forming cells are called *leukemias,* and tumors of lymphocytes or their precursors are called *lymphomas.*

The nomenclature for specific malignant tumors is based on their appearance and/or presumed cell of origin (Table 7-1). Malignant epithelial tumors resembling stratified squamous epithelium are denoted *squamous cell carcinoma,* whereas those with glandular growth patterns are called *adenocarcinomas.* Sarcomas are designated by the appropriate cell prefix (e.g., smooth muscle malignancies are *leiomyosarcomas*). Not infrequently, neoplasms composed of poorly differentiated unrecognizable cells can only be designated as undifferentiated malignant tumors.

Some tumors appear to have more than one parenchymal cell type:

- *Mixed tumors* derive from a neoplastic clone of a single germ cell layer that differentiates into more than one cell type (e.g., mixed salivary gland tumors containing epithelial cells and myxoid stroma).
- *Teratomas* are composed of various parenchymal cell types representative of more than one germ cell layer. They arise from totipotential cells capable of forming endodermal, ectodermal, and mesenchymal tissues and can have both benign and malignant forms. Such tumors typically occur in testis or ovary or rarely midline embryonic rests.

Two *non-neoplastic* lesions that should not be confused with malignancy:

- *Choristomas:* Ectopic rests of nontransformed tissues (e.g., pancreatic cells under the small bowel mucosa).
- *Hamartomas:* Masses of disorganized tissue indigenous to a particular site (i.e., lung hamartomas exhibit cartilage, bronchi, and blood vessels); many are clonal with characteristic acquired chromosomal abnormalities.

Characteristics of Benign and Malignant Neoplasms (p. 267)

Classification of a tumor as benign or malignant ultimately depends on its clinical behavior; however, morphologic evaluation (and increasingly molecular profiling) allows categorization based on degree of differentiation, local invasion, and metastasis. Although malignant tumors tend to grow faster than benign neoplasms, this is not a consistent finding; indeed some malignancies can be exceedingly slow growing and indolent.

The general features used to distinguish benign and malignant tumors are summarized in Table 7-2 and Figure 7-1. Again, remember these are only broad generalizations, and there are *always* exceptions.

Differentiation and Anaplasia (p. 268)

Differentiation refers to how closely tumor cells histologically (and functionally) resemble their normal cell counterparts; lack of differentiation is called *anaplasia.* In general, neoplastic cells in benign lesions are well differentiated; cells in malignant neoplasms can range from well differentiated to completely undifferentiated. Well-differentiated tumors, whether benign or malignant, tend to retain the functional characteristics of their normal counterparts

TABLE 7-2 Comparisons Between Benign and Malignant Tumors

Characteristics	Benign	Malignant
Differentiation or anaplasia	Well differentiated; structure sometimes typical of tissue of origin	Some lack of differentiation (anaplasia); structure often atypical
Rate of growth	Usually progressive and slow; may come to a standstill or regress; mitotic figures rare and normal	Erratic, may be slow to rapid; mitotic figures may be numerous and abnormal
Local invasion	Usually cohesive, expansile, well-demarcated masses that do not invade or infiltrate surrounding normal tissues	Locally invasive, infiltrating surrounding tissue; sometimes may be misleadingly cohesive and expansile
Metastasis	Absent	Frequent; more likely with large undifferentiated primary tumors

(e.g., hormone production by endocrine tumors or keratin production by squamous epithelial tumors). Malignant cells can revert to embryologic phenotypes or express proteins not elaborated by the original cell of origin.

Histologic changes in tumors include the following:

- *Pleomorphism:* Variation in the shape and size of cells and/or nuclei
- *Abnormal nuclear morphology:* Darkly stained *(hyperchromatic)* nuclei with irregularly clumped chromatin, prominent nucleoli, and increased nuclear-to-cytoplasmic ratios (approaching 1:1 versus normal ratios of 1:4 or 1:6)
- *Abundant and/or atypical mitoses* reflecting increased proliferative activity and abnormal cell division (e.g., tripolar mitoses, so-called *Mercedes-Benz* sign)
- *Loss of polarity:* Disturbed orientation and tendency for forming anarchic, disorganized masses
- *Tumor giant cells* with single polyploid nuclei or multiple nuclei
- *Ischemic necrosis* due to insufficient vascular supply

Metaplasia and Dysplasia (p. 270)

Metaplasia is defined as the replacement of one mature cell type with another mature cell type, often associated with tissue damage, repair, and regeneration (e.g., stratified squamous epithelium replacing respiratory epithelium in the bronchioles of smokers [see Chapter 2]).

Dysplasia is the term used to describe the constellation of histologic changes seen in a neoplasm. Dysplasia (literally "disordered growth") refers to loss of cellular uniformity and architectural organization and can range from mild to severe. Dysplasia can occur adjacent to frank malignancy and in many cases antedates the development of cancer. However, *dysplasia does not equate to malignancy,* and moreover, *dysplastic cells do not necessarily progress to cancer;* removal of the inciting stimulus from dysplastic epithelium (e.g., chronic irritation) can result in reversion to complete normalcy. When dysplastic changes are marked and *involve the entire thickness of an epithelium,* the lesion is considered a preinvasive neoplasm and is referred to as *carcinoma in situ.* This lesion can be forerunner to invasive carcinoma.

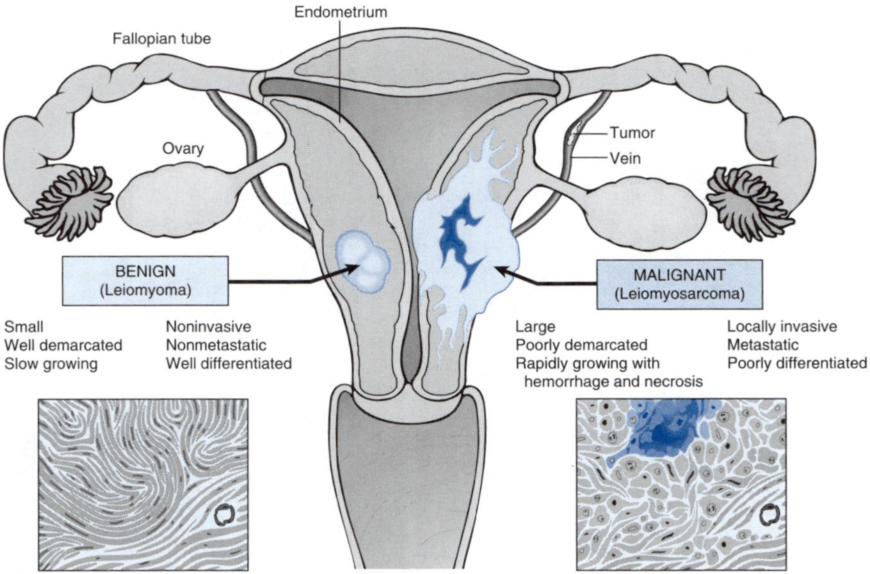

Figure 7-1 Comparison of the general features between benign and malignant neoplasms, using uterine myometrial tumors as examples. A benign tumor of myometrium is the leiomyoma, whereas the malignant tumor of the same origin is a leiomyosarcoma.

Local Invasion (p. 271)

Most benign tumors grow as cohesive, expansile masses that develop a surrounding rim of condensed connective tissue, or *capsule.* These tumors do not penetrate the capsule or the surrounding normal tissues, and the plane of cleavage between the capsule and the surrounding tissues facilitates surgical enucleation.

Malignant neoplasms are typically invasive and infiltrative, destroying surrounding normal tissues. They commonly lack a well-defined capsule and cleavage plane, making simple excision impossible. Consequently, surgery requires removal of a considerable margin of healthy and apparently uninvolved tissue.

Metastasis (p. 272)

Metastasis involves invasion of lymphatics, blood vessels, or body cavities by tumor, followed by transport and growth of secondary tumor cell masses discontinuous from the primary tumor. *This is the single most important feature distinguishing benign from malignant.* In general the likelihood of metastatic spread increases with lack of differentiation, local invasion, rapid growth, and large size. Almost all malignant tumors can metastasize; central nervous system (CNS) tumors and cutaneous basal cell carcinomas do so only rarely.

Pathways of Spread (p. 273)

Cancer dissemination occurs by three routes:

- *Seeding of body cavities and surfaces* (p. 273) occurs by dispersion into peritoneal, pleural, pericardial, subarachnoid, or joint spaces. Ovarian carcinoma typically spreads transperitoneally to the surface of abdominal viscera, often without deeper invasion. Mucus-secreting appendiceal carcinomas can fill the peritoneum with a gelatinous neoplastic mass called *pseudomyxoma peritonei.*
- *Lymphatic spread* (p. 273) transports tumor cells to regional nodes and ultimately throughout the body. Although tumors do not contain functional lymphatics, lymphatic vessels at tumor margins appear sufficient. Lymph nodes draining tumors are frequently enlarged; this can result from metastatic tumor cell proliferation or from reactive hyperplasia to tumor antigens. Biopsy of the proximal *sentinel lymph node* draining a tumor can allow accurate assessment of tumor metastasis.
- *Hematogenous spread* (p. 274) is typical of sarcomas but also is the favored route for certain carcinomas (e.g., renal). Because of their thinner walls, veins are more frequently invaded than arteries, and metastasis follows the pattern of venous flow; understandably, lung and liver are the most common sites of hematogenous metastases.

Epidemiology (p. 275)

Epidemiologic studies allow the identification of environmental, racial, gender, and cultural risk factors and also shed light on pathogenic mechanisms.

The Global Impact of Cancer (p. 275)

In the United States, prostate, lung, and colon or rectum malignancies are the most common cancers in men; breast, lung, and colon or rectum cancers are the most common in women (Fig. 7-2). The good news is that cancer death rates in developed countries have declined 18.4% in men and 10.4% in women since 1990.

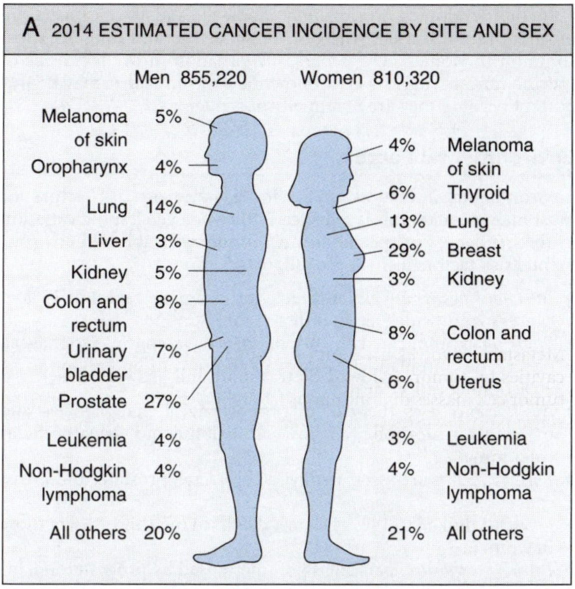

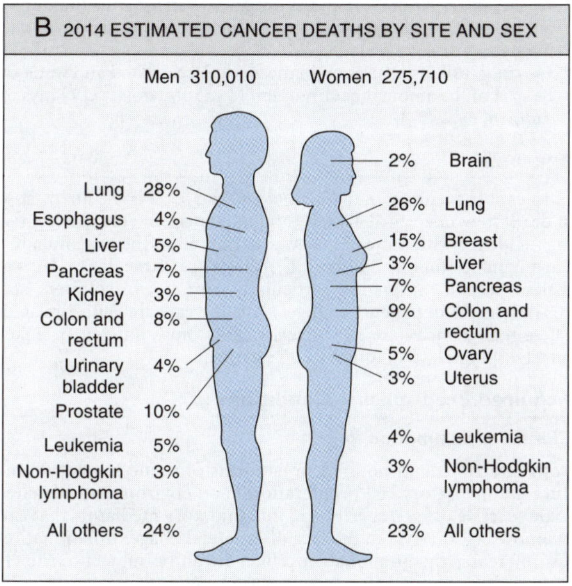

Figure 7-2 Cancer incidence **(A)** and mortality **(B)** by site and sex for the U.S. population. The data exclude basal cell and squamous cell skin cancers and in situ carcinomas, except urinary bladder. *(Adapted from American Cancer Society Cancer Statistics, 2011).*

In the developing world, lung, stomach, and liver cancers are most common in men, whereas breast, cervix, and lung are most common in women. The geographic variation in the incidence of specific cancers suggests environmental exposures that may be important because they are potentially preventable.

Environmental Factors (p. 276)

Environmental influences appear to be dominant risk factors for most malignancies; this is reflected in the wide geographic variation in the incidences of specific forms of cancer. Established environmental risk factors include the following:

- *Infectious agents* are either directly or indirectly causal in 15% of cancers worldwide (see later discussion).
- *Smoking* is implicated in oropharyngeal, laryngeal, esophageal, pancreatic, and bladder cancers, in addition to underlying some 90% of lung cancer deaths.
- *Alcohol* increases the risk of oropharyngeal malignancies and by causing alcoholic cirrhosis contributes to hepatocellular carcinoma.
- *Dietary factors* are associated with colorectal, prostate, and breast cancers.
- *Obesity* is linked to 14% of cancer deaths in men and 20% of those in women.
- *Estrogen exposure,* particularly if unopposed by progesterone, increases the risk of breast and endometrial cancer; thus the timing and number of pregnancies can influence lifelong cancer risk in women.
- *Carcinogens* may be present in the workplace or food and water or be part of the ambient environment (e.g., ultraviolet (UV) rays or radon) (Table 7-3).

Age (p. 278)

Most cancer occurs in individuals older than 55; it is the main cause of death in women aged 40 to 79 and in men aged 60 to 79. The rising incidence with increasing age is attributed to the accumulation of somatic mutations and decline in immune surveillance. Nevertheless, certain cancers are particularly common in children, and 10% of deaths in patients younger than 15 years are cancer related. These malignancies are not typically carcinomas but rather leukemia, lymphoma, CNS tumors, and sarcomas.

Acquired Predisposing Conditions (p.278)

Chronic Inflammation (p. 279)

Both infectious and noninfectious forms of tissue injury will induce compensatory cell proliferation in an environment of genotoxic reactive oxygen species and inflammatory mediators that can promote cell survival in the face of genetic damage. Inflammation also increases the pool of stem cells that can be subject to the effects of mutagens. When inflammation persists over years, cells with potentially oncogenic mutations can survive and expand (Table 7-4).

Precursor Lesions (p. 279)

Defined as local morphologic changes that are associated with increased risk of malignant transformation, these include metaplasia (e.g., *Barrett esophagus* or squamous metaplasia in bronchial epithelium), hyperplasia (e.g., endometrial hyperplasia in response to prolonged unopposed estrogens), and certain benign neoplasms

TABLE 7-3 Occupational Cancers

Agents or Groups of Agents	Human Cancers for Which Reasonable Evidence Is Available	Typical Use or Occurrence
Arsenic and arsenic compounds	Lung carcinoma, skin carcinoma	By-product of metal smelting; component of alloys, electrical and semiconductor devices, medications and herbicides, fungicides, and animal dips
Asbestos	Lung, esophageal, gastric, and colon carcinoma; mesothelioma	Formerly used for many applications because of fire, heat, and friction resistance; still found in existing construction as well as fire-resistant textiles, friction materials (i.e., brake linings), underlayment and roofing papers, and floor tiles
Benzene	Acute myeloid leukemia	Principal component of light oil; despite known risk, many applications exist in printing and lithography, paint, rubber, dry cleaning, adhesives and coatings, and detergents; formerly widely used as solvent and fumigant
Beryllium and beryllium compounds	Lung carcinoma	Missile fuel and space vehicles; hardener for lightweight metal alloys, particularly in aerospace applications and nuclear reactors
Cadmium and cadmium compounds	Prostate carcinoma	Uses include yellow pigments and phosphors; found in solders; used in batteries and as alloy and in metal platings and coatings
Chromium compounds	Lung carcinoma	Component of metal alloys, paints, pigments, and preservatives
Nickel compounds	Lung and oropharyngeal carcinoma	Nickel plating; component of ferrous alloys, ceramics, and batteries; by-product of stainless-steel arc welding
Radon and its decay products	Lung carcinoma	From decay of minerals containing uranium; potentially serious hazard in quarries and underground mines
Vinyl chloride	Hepatic angiosarcoma	Refrigerant; monomer for vinyl polymers; adhesive for plastics; formerly inert

Modified from Stellman JM, Stellman SD: Cancer and workplace. *CA Cancer J Clin* 1996;46:70.

(e.g., colonic *villous adenoma* which—left untreated—progresses to cancer in approximately half of cases). Although cancer can arise in previously benign tumors, this is uncommon, and most malignant tumors arise de novo.

Immunodeficiency States *(p. 279)*

Immune compromise—particularly related to deficits in T-cell immunity—increases the risk of malignancy, especially those caused by oncogenic viruses (e.g., lymphomas associated with Epstein-Barr virus [EBV]).

TABLE 7-4 Chronic Inflammatory States and Cancer

Pathologic Condition	Associated Neoplasm(s)	Etiologic Agent
Asbestosis, silicosis	Mesothelioma, lung carcinoma	Asbestos fibers, silica particles
Inflammatory bowel disease	Colorectal carcinoma	
Lichen sclerosis	Vulvar squamous cell carcinoma	
Pancreatitis	Pancreatic carcinoma	Alcoholism, germline mutations (e.g., in the trypsinogen gene)
Chronic cholecystitis	Gallbladder cancer	Bile acids, bacteria, gallbladder stones
Reflux esophagitis, Barrett esophagus	Esophageal carcinoma	Gastric acid
Sjögren syndrome, Hashimoto thyroiditis	MALT lymphoma	
Opisthorchis, cholangitis	Cholangiocarcinoma, colon carcinoma	Liver flukes *(Opisthorchis viverrini)*
Gastritis and ulcers	Gastric adenocarcinoma, MALT lymphoma	*Helicobacter pylori*
Hepatitis	Hepatocellular carcinoma	HBV and/or HCV
Osteomyelitis	Carcinoma in draining sinuses	Bacterial infection
Chronic cervicitis	Cervical carcinoma	HPV
Chronic cystitis	Bladder carcinoma	Schistosomiasis

Adapted from Tlsty TD, Coussens LM: Tumor stroma and regulation of cancer development. *Ann Rev Pathol Mech Dis* 2006;1:119.

Genetic Predisposition and Interactions Between Environmental and Inherited Factors (p. 279)

Approximately 95% of malignancies arise sporadically (i.e., do not have an apparent inherited familial basis). Nevertheless, germline mutations that increase cancer risk—often in tumor suppressor genes—do occur. Importantly, the presence of an inherited component does not necessarily doom the affected individual to cancer, nor does lack of a family history preclude a heritable mutation, particularly when tumor development depends on the interaction of multiple genes or requires additional environmental factors.

Molecular Basis of Cancer: Role of Genetic and Epigenetic Alterations (p. 280)

The molecular pathogenesis of cancer is schematized in Figure 7-3; the following are fundamental principles:

- *Nonlethal genetic damage underlies carcinogenesis;* genetic injury can be inherited in the germline or acquired in somatic cells through spontaneous mutation or environmental exposures.
- Tumors develop as clonal progeny of a single genetically damaged progenitor cell. Although tumors begin as monoclonal

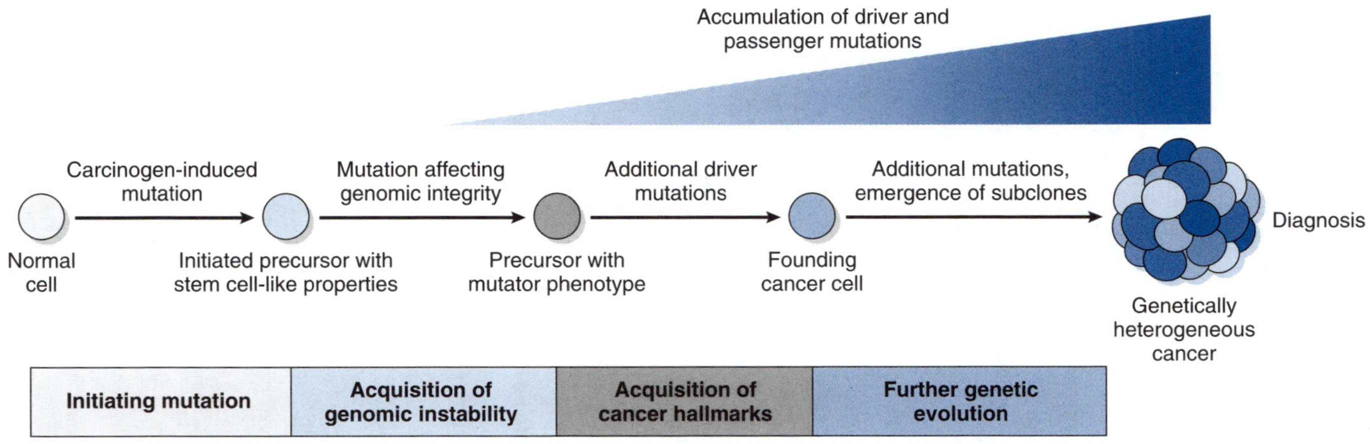

Figure 7-3 Development of a cancer through stepwise acquisition of complementary mutations. The order in which various driver mutations occur in initiated precursor cells is not known and may vary from tumor to tumor.

proliferations, by the time they are clinically evident (approximately 1 g or 10^9 cells), they are extremely heterogeneous.

- Four classes of normal regulatory genes are the targets of genetic damage:
  - Growth-promoting proto-oncogenes
  - Growth-inhibiting tumor-suppressor genes
  - Genes that regulate apoptosis
  - Genes that regulate DNA repair; defective DNA repair predisposes to genomic mutations *(mutator phenotype)*
- Carcinogenesis is a multistep process. The attributes of malignancy *(cancer hallmarks)*—for example, invasiveness, excessive growth, escape from the immune system—are acquired incrementally, a process called *tumor progression.* At the genetic level, progression results from accumulation of successive mutations. Tumors also genetically "evolve" in a Darwinian survival of the fittest because malignant cells compete for limiting metabolic resources, and defective cells die by apoptosis. Thus tumors progressively become more aggressive; chemotherapy and radiotherapy also select for resistant clones.
- *Driver mutations* contribute to the development of a malignant phenotype (as opposed to *passenger mutations* that occur due to genetic instability but which may have no phenotypic consequence). The first driver mutation that starts a cell toward malignancy is an *initiating mutation* and is typically maintained in all progeny cells. Because no single mutation is fully transforming, the development of cancer requires that the "initiated" cell acquire additional drivers—gradually over time. The relative permanence of such "initiated" cells supports the concept that cancers may arise from stemlike cells, with the capacity for long-term persistence and self-renewal.
- *Loss-of-function* mutations in genes responsible for maintaining genomic integrity are common early steps; these lead to genomic instability and increase the likelihood of developing additional driver mutations.
- In addition to DNA mutations, epigenetic changes (e.g., DNA methylation and histone modification) also contribute to malignancy by altering gene transcription (e.g., by silencing tumor suppressors).

Cellular and Molecular Hallmarks of Cancer (p. 282)

Certain fundamental changes in cell physiology contribute to development of the malignant phenotype:

- Self-sufficiency in growth signals (proliferation without external stimuli)
- Insensitivity to growth-inhibitory signals
- Altered cellular metabolism (switch to aerobic glycolysis, *Warburg effect*)
- Evasion of apoptosis
- Limitless replicative potential (related to telomere maintenance)
- Sustained angiogenesis to provide adequate nutrition and waste removal
- Ability to invade and metastasize
- Ability to escape immune recognition and regulation

Self-Sufficiency in Growth Signals: Oncogenes (p. 283)

Normal cell proliferation involves the following steps:

- Growth factor binding to cell surface receptor
- Transient and limited activation of the receptor and associated membrane or cytoplasmic signal-transduction proteins
- Nuclear transmission via second messengers

- Induction and activation of nuclear regulatory factors that initiate DNA transcription
- Entry into and progression through the cell cycle

Cancer is characterized by proliferation in the absence of growth-promoting signals. *Oncogenes* are genes that promote autonomous cell growth in cancer cells; their unmutated normal counterparts are *proto-oncogenes.* Proteins encoded by proto-oncogenes may function as growth factors or their receptors, transcription factors, or cell cycle components. *Oncoproteins* are the protein products of oncogenes; they resemble the normal products of proto-oncogenes except that they are devoid of normal regulatory elements, and their synthesis may be independent of normal growth stimuli.

Proto-Oncogenes, Oncogenes, and Oncoproteins *(p. 284)*

Mutations convert proto-oncogenes into constitutively active oncogenes that endow the cell with growth self-sufficiency. These can fall in the following categories (Table 7-5) that are discussed next.

TABLE 7-5 Selected Oncogenes, Their Mode of Activation, and Associated Human Tumors

Category	Proto-Oncogene	Mode of Activation in Tumor	Associated Human Tumor
Growth Factors			
PDGF-β chain	*PDGFB*	Overexpression	Astrocytoma
Fibroblast growth factors	*HST1* *FGF3*	Overexpression Amplification	Osteosarcoma Stomach cancer Bladder cancer Breast cancer Melanoma
TGF-α	*TGFA*	Overexpression	Astrocytomas
HGF	*HGF*	Overexpression	Hepatocellular carcinomas Thyroid cancer
Growth Factor Receptors			
EGF-receptor family	*ERBB1 (EGFR)* ERBB2 (HER)	Mutation Amplification	Adenocarcinoma of lung Breast carcinoma
FMS-like tyrosine kinase 3	*FLT3*	Point mutation	Leukemia
Receptor for neurotrophic factors	*RET*	Point mutation	Multiple endocrine neoplasia 2A and B, familial medullary thyroid carcinomas
PDGF receptor	*PDGFRB*	Overexpression, translocation	Gliomas, leukemias
Receptor for KIT ligand	*KIT*	Point mutation	GI stromal tumors, seminomas, leukemias
ALK receptor	*ALK*	Translocation, fusion gene formation Point mutation	Adenocarcinoma of lung, certain lymphomas Neuroblastoma

Continued

TABLE 7-5 Selected Oncogenes, Their Mode of Activation, and Associated Human Tumors—cont'd

Category	Proto-Oncogene	Mode of Activation in Tumor	Associated Human Tumor
Proteins Involved in Signal Transduction			
GTP-binding (G) proteins	*KRAS*	Point mutation	Colon, lung, and pancreatic tumors
	HRAS	Point mutation	Bladder and kidney tumors
	NRAS	Point mutation	Melanomas, hematologic malignancies
	GNAQ	Point mutation	Uveal melanoma
	GNAS	Point mutation	Pituitary adenoma, other endocrine tumors
Nonreceptor tyrosine kinase	*ABL*	Translocation	Chronic myelogenous leukemia
		Point mutation	Acute lymphoblastic leukemia
BRAF	Point mutation, translocation	*BRAF*	Point mutation, translocation
Notch signal transduction	*NOTCH1*	Point mutation, translocation Gene rearrangement	Leukemias, lymphomas, breast carcinoma
JAK-STAT signal transduction	*JAK2*	Translocation	Myeloproliferative disorders Acute lymphoblastic leukemia
Nuclear Regulatory Proteins			
Transcriptional activators	*MYC*	Translocation	Burkitt lymphoma
	N-MYC	Amplification	Neuroblastoma
Cell Cycle Regulators			
Cyclins	*CCND1* (Cyclin D1)	Translocation	Mantle cell lymphoma, multiple myeloma
		Amplification	Breast and esophageal cancers
CDK	*CDK4*	Amplification or point mutation	Glioblastoma, melanoma, sarcoma

Growth Factors (p. 285)

Tumors can acquire the ability to produce growth factors to which they are also responsive—leading to an autocrine stimulation loop; in most cases the growth factor gene is not mutated. Growth factor-driven division is not in itself sufficient for neoplastic transformation but rather increases the risk of acquiring mutations during increased proliferation.

Growth Factor Receptors (p. 285)

Several oncogenes encode growth factor receptors; mutations in these can drive malignant transformation by resulting in constitutive activation:

- Activation in the absence of ligand binding (e.g., point mutations in *ERBB1* [encoding the epidermal growth factor receptor] occur in a subset of lung adenocarcinomas)

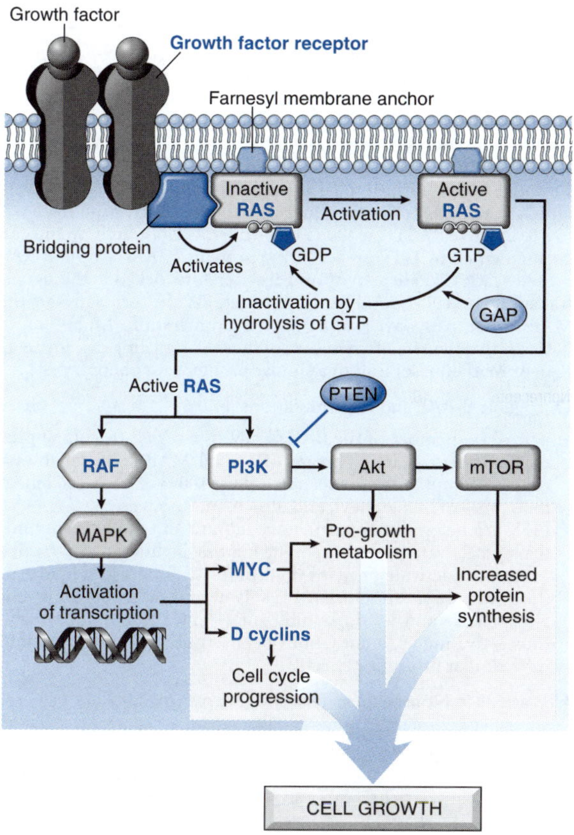

Figure 7-4 Growth factor signaling pathways in cancer. Growth factor receptors, as well as RAS, PI3K, MYC, and D cyclins, are all proto-oncogenes that can be affected by mutations in various malignancies. GAPs increase GTP hydrolysis and thus inactivate RAS; PTEN serves the same function for PI3K. *mTOR,* Mammalian target of rapamycin.

- Overexpression that renders cells more sensitive to smaller quantities of growth factor (e.g., *ERBB2,* encoding HER2 tyrosine kinase receptors in breast cancers).
- Gene rearrangements that activate receptor tyrosine kinases (e.g., echinoderm microtubule-associated protein-like 4 [EML4] fusion with anaplastic lymphoma kinase [ALK] in a subset of lung adenocarcinomas)

Antibody blockade of overexpressed receptors or small molecule inhibition of constitutively active receptors allow *targeted therapy* of tumors.

Downstream Components of the Receptor Tyrosine Kinase Signaling Pathway (p. 286)

Receptor tyrosine kinase activation stimulates RAS, which in turn drives the mitogen-activated protein (MAP) kinase cascade, and the phosphatidylinositol kinase (PI3K)-AKT pathways. Gain-of-function mutations in these downstream proteins can mediate cell growth independent of receptor kinase-ligand interactions (Fig. 7-4).

RAS Mutations (p. 286)

RAS is a family of guanine triphosphate (GTP)-binding proteins *(G proteins);* mutated RAS proteins are present in 15% to 20% of all human tumors, although the frequency can be much higher (e.g., 90% of pancreatic and cholangiocarcinomas and 50% of colon, endometrial, and thyroid cancers); most differ from their normal counterparts by point mutations. Normal RAS proteins alternate between activated (GTP-bound) signal-transmitting and inactive (guanosine diphosphate [GDP]-bound) quiescent forms. Conversion from active to inactive RAS is mediated by intrinsic GTPase activity and can be augmented by GTPase-activating proteins (GAPs). Mutant RAS proteins lack GTPase activity and are therefore locked in the signal-transmitting GTP-bound form; activated RAS in turn activates the MAP kinase pathway, leading to cell proliferation. Mutations in GAPs or in downstream members of the RAS signaling cascade (e.g., RAF or MAP kinase) lead to a similar proliferative phenotype.

Oncogenic B-RAF and PI3K Mutations (p. 286)

- B-RAF (a member of the RAF family) is a serine-threonine protein kinase that sits upstream of several MAP kinase pathways (Fig. 7-4); mutations are seen in almost 100% of hairy cell leukemias, 80% of benign nevi, and 60% of melanomas.
- PI3K is a heterodimer (regulatory subunit and catalytic subunit) that can activate serine-threonine kinases, including AKT (which in turn can activate proteins that stimulate protein and lipid synthesis or inhibit apoptosis). PI3K is negatively regulated by the phosphatase and tensin homologue (PTEN) tumor suppressor; thus activating PI3K mutations or inactivating PTEN mutations have similar protumor effects.

Alterations in Nonreceptor Tyrosine Kinases (p. 287)

The activity of these tyrosine kinases influences cell proliferation. Thus c-*ABL* codes for a tyrosine kinase whose activity is normally tightly regulated; however, in chronic myeloid leukemia (CML), translocation of c-*ABL* with fusion to the *BCR* gene produces a hybrid protein that self-associates through the BCR moiety and exhibits potent, unregulated tyrosine kinase activity. Inhibitors of the BCR-ABL kinase thus have high therapeutic efficacy in treating CML. Other examples include activating point mutations in the JAK2 tyrosine kinase; these mutant forms constitutively activate STAT transcription factors and are associated with polycythemia vera and primary myelofibrosis.

Transcription Factors (p. 288)

Growth autonomy can also occur through mutations in nuclear transcription factors (e.g., *MYC, JUN, FOS, REL,* and *MYB* oncogenes) that regulate the expression of growth-related genes.

***MYC Oncogene** (p.288).* The MYC oncogene is most commonly involved in human tumors; the proto-oncogene is rapidly induced when quiescent cells are signaled to divide and likely functions by activating genes involved in proliferation. These include the D cyclins, genes that drive ribosomal synthesis, proteins involved in metabolic switching, and telomerase expression. MYC overexpression (e.g., due to gene amplification, gene translocations, or altered posttranslational regulation) leads to malignancy.

Cyclins and Cyclin-Dependent Kinases (p. 288)

Loss of cell cycle control is central to malignant transformation. Autonomous growth can be driven by overexpression or mutation (with increased activity) of cyclins or cyclin-dependent kinases (CDKs), or by mutation (with loss of activity) of CDK inhibitors; indeed, dysregulation of cyclin D, CDK 4, Rb, or the CDK inhibitor p16/INK4a is seen in the vast majority of human cancers (see also Chapter 1 regarding cell cycle regulation). The G_1/S transition (where DNA damage must be identified and repaired before replication) and the G_2/M transition (where fidelity of DNA synthesis must be verified before mitosis) are critical cell cycle checkpoints; mutations in the damage sensors or repair mechanisms are a major source of genetic instability in cancer cells.

Insensitivity to Growth Inhibition: Tumor Suppressor Genes (p. 290)

Tumor suppressors form a network of checkpoints that prevent uncontrolled growth; tumor suppressor proteins may also be involved in cellular differentiation. Many of these tumor suppressors (e.g., Rb and p53) detect genotoxic stress and shut down cell proliferation before a new mutation can be permanently embedded in the genome; loss of function can therefore lead to unregulated cell growth and genetic instability. The protein products of tumor suppressors can be transcription factors, cell cycle inhibitors, signal transduction molecules, receptors, or involved in DNA damage repair (Table 7-6).

In general, both alleles of a tumor suppressor gene must be mutated for carcinogenesis to occur; because heterozygous cells have adequate tumor suppressor activity, the mutation of the second

TABLE 7-6 Cell Cycle Components and Inhibitors That Are Frequently Mutated in Cancer

Cell Cycle Component	Main Function
Cyclins and Cyclin-Dependent Kinases	
CDK4; D cyclins	Form a complex that phosphorylates Rb, allowing the cell to progress through the G_1 restriction point
Cell Cycle Inhibitors	
CIP-KIP family: p21, p27 (CDKN1A-D)	Block the cell cycle by binding to cyclin-CDK complexes p21 is induced by the tumor suppressor p53 p27 responds to growth suppressors such as TGF-β
INK4-ARF family (CDKN2A-C)	p16/INK4a binds to cyclin D-CDK4 and promotes the inhibitory effects of Rb p14/ARF increases p53 levels by inhibiting MDM2 activity
Cell Cycle Checkpoint Components	
Rb	Tumor suppressive "pocket" protein that binds E2F transcription factors in its hypophosphorylated state, preventing G_1/S transition; also interacts with several transcription factors that regulate differentiation
p53	Tumor suppressor altered in the majority of cancers; causes cell cycle arrest and apoptosis. Acts mainly through p21 to cause cell cycle arrest. Causes apoptosis by inducing the transcription of pro-apoptotic genes such as *BAX*. Levels of p53 are negatively regulated by MDM2 through a feedback loop. p53 is required for the G_1/S checkpoint and is a main component of the G_2/M checkpoint

normal tumor suppressor (leading to carcinogenesis) is also referred to as *loss of heterozygosity (LOH)*. In some cases there is a germline mutation (e.g., in familial retinoblastoma due to *Rb* mutations); subsequent mutation of the normal *Rb* gene leads to increased cellular proliferation at a fairly high frequency (10,000-fold greater than the general population). In comparison, sporadic retinoblastoma is extremely uncommon since this requires concurrent mutation of both *Rb* genes in the same cell.

Rb: Governor of Proliferation (p. 292)

The *Rb* gene is the prototypic tumor-suppressor gene. Among other activities, its gene product regulates the advancement of cells through the G_1/S checkpoint. By sequestering E2F less efficiently, *Rb* mutations lead to increased E2F transcription factor activity, and cells can thus cycle in the absence of a growth stimulus. Several oncogenic DNA viruses (e.g., human papillomavirus [HPV]) synthesize proteins that bind to Rb and displace the E2F transcription factors, thereby contributing to persistent cell cycling.

TP53: Guardian of the Genome (p. 293)

The p53 protein prevents the propagation of genetically defective cells (p63 and p73 are related family members with similar activities). Loss-of-function mutations in *TP53* are found in more than 50% of cancers; patients with germline *TP53* mutations (e.g., *Li-Fraumeni syndrome*) have a twenty-fivefold greater risk of malignancy (e.g., leukemias, sarcomas, breast cancer, and brain tumors) due to inactivation of the normal allele in somatic cells. Similar to the Rb protein, p53 can also be functionally inactivated by products of DNA oncogenic viruses.

- When cells are "stressed" (e.g., by damage to DNA), p53 undergoes posttranslational phosphorylation, releasing it from an associated MDM2 protein that normally targets it for degradation. The sensing of DNA damage is accomplished through two protein kinases, *ataxia-telangiectasia mutated (ATM)* and *ataxia-telangiectasia and Rad3-related (ATR)*.
- The unshackled p53 then acts as a transcription factor for additional genes (including miRNAs) that arrest the cell cycle and promote DNA repair; for example, G_1 cell cycle arrest is mediated largely through p53-dependent transcription of the CDK inhibitor p21.
- If DNA can be repaired during the cell cycle arrest, MDM2 transcription increases and p53 is subsequently degraded, allowing the cell to progress into S phase.
- If DNA damage cannot be repaired, p53 induces cellular senescence by altering E2F signaling pathways or can induce apoptosis by increasing transcription of proapoptotic genes.

The p53 status of a tumor has important therapeutic implications because chemotherapy and radiotherapy mediate their effects by inducing DNA damage and provoking p53-driven apoptosis. By losing its ability to direct DNA repair or cell death, defective p53 renders cells relatively resistant to therapies and promotes a "mutator phenotype" prone to rapid accumulation of additional mutations.

Adenomatous Polyposis Coli: Gatekeeper of Colonic Neoplasia (p. 296)

Adenomatous polyposis coli (APC) genes are a class of tumor suppressors that downregulate growth-promoting signals in the WNT signaling pathway. APC protein is a negative regulator of β-catenin activity; it binds and regulates the degradation of cytoplasmic β-catenin. During normal embryonic development, WNT binding to its surface receptor causes APC dissociation from β-catenin, allowing β-catenin to enter the nucleus and drive proliferation. In the absence of normal APC, cells respond as if under continuous WNT signaling; cytoplasmic β-catenin levels increase, resulting in increased nuclear translocation and ultimately increased transcription of c-*MYC, cyclin D1,* and other genes. Those born with one mutant *APC* allele develop thousands of adenomatous polyps in the colon, of which one or more develop into colonic cancers (see Chapter 17). Approximately 70% to 80% of sporadic colon cancers also exhibit *APC* LOH; β-catenin mutations are also seen in over 50% of hepatoblastomas, and over 20% of hepatocellular carcinomas. E-cadherins that facilitate cell-cell interactions also interact with β-catenin; loss of intercellular adhesion (due to injury or mutation) results in increased cytoplasmic β-catenin that can also drive cellular proliferation.

CDKN2A *(p. 297)*

This locus encodes two proteins; p16/INK4a is a CDK inhibitor that blocks Rb phosphorylation and thus maintains the Rb checkpoint, whereas p14/ARF inhibits MDM2 and thereby prevents p53 destruction. Mutations occur in bladder, head and neck tumors, and certain leukemias, and gene activity can also be silenced by epigenetic hypermethylation in cervical cancers.

TGF-β Pathway *(p. 298)*

Transforming growth factor-β (TGF-β) receptor ligation causes intracellular signaling (via e.g., SMAD 2 and SMAD 4) that upregulates the expression of growth inhibitory genes, including CDK inhibitors. Mutations affecting the TGF-β receptor are common in colon, gastric, and endometrial malignancies; mutations inactivating SMAD4 are common in pancreatic cancers.

PTEN *(p. 298)*

PTEN is a *p*hosphatase and *ten*sin homologue; it is a membrane-associated phosphatase that acts as a tumor suppressor brake on the prosurvival-progrowth PI3K-AKT pathway. Germline mutations in *PTEN* underlie the Cowden syndrome, characterized by frequent benign skin appendage tumors and increased risk of epithelial malignancies, such as breast, endometrial, and thyroid cancers.

NF1 *(p. 298)*

NF1 is a tumor-suppressor gene coding for *neurofibromin;* the protein has a GTPase activity that regulates signal transduction through RAS. *NF1* LOH impairs the conversion of active (GTP-bound) RAS to inactive (GDP-bound) RAS; cells are thus continuously stimulated to divide. Germline inheritance of one mutant allele of *NF-1* predisposes to the development of numerous benign neurofibromas when the second NF-1 gene is lost or mutated (neurofibromatosis type I); some progress to malignancy.

NF2 *(p. 298)*

NF2 codes for *neurobromin 2* or *merlin, a protein* related to erythrocyte protein 4.1 and the ezrin, radixin, and moesin family of membrane-cytoskeletal related proteins. Cells lacking merlin fail to establish stable cell-cell junctions and are insensitive to normal cell-cell contact growth arrest signals. Germline mutations are associated with benign bilateral schwannomas of the acoustic nerve, and somatic mutations are associated with sporadic ependymomas and meningiomas.

WT1 (p. 298)

Mutational inactivation of *WT1* (either germline or somatic) is associated with the development of Wilms tumors. The WT1 protein is a transcriptional activator of genes involved in renal and gonadal differentiation; the tumorigenic function of WT1 deficiency relates to its role in genitourinary differentiation.

PATCHED (p. 298)

PTCH1 is a tumor suppressor gene encoding the cell membrane protein PATCHED1, a negative regulator of the Hedgehog signaling pathway. In the absence of PATCHED proteins, there is unopposed Hedgehog activation of the normal PATCH receptor, leading to increased expression of *N-myc* and D cyclins. Germline mutations in *PTCH1* cause Gorlin syndrome (nevoid basal cell carcinoma syndrome) with increased risk of cutaneous basal cell carcinomas and medulloblastoma; *PTCH1* mutations are also present in sporadic cases of basal cell carcinomas and medulloblastomas.

von Hippel-Lindau (p. 299)

Germline loss-of-function mutations of the von Hippel-Lindau (VHL) gene are associated with hereditary renal cell cancer, pheochromocytomas, hemangioblastomas of the CNS, and retinal angiomas. The VHL protein is part of a ubiquitin ligase complex involved in the degradation of hypoxia-inducible transcription factor 1α (HIF1α); mutations in VHL lead to increased cytoplasmic HIF1α and subsequent increased nuclear translocation that drives cell growth and angiogenic factor production.

Serine-Threonine Kinase 11 (p. 299)

The serine-threonine kinase 11 (STK11) protein is involved in regulating cellular metabolism; loss-of-function mutations cause *Peutz-Jeghers syndrome,* an autosomal dominant disorder associated with benign gastrointestinal (GI) polyps and an increased risk of GI and pancreatic carcinomas.

Growth-Promoting Metabolic Alterations: The Warburg Effect (p. 300)

Even with ample oxygen, malignant cells (and indeed all rapidly dividing cells) often switch their metabolism to ferment glucose to lactose (by glycolysis) rather than metabolize it—with greater adenosine triphosphate (ATP) production—through oxidative phosphorylation. Called *aerobic glycolysis* or the *Warburg effect,* this phenomenon also forms the basis by which tumors can be imaged via positron emission tomography after the avid uptake of ^{18}F-fluorodeoxyglucose (a nonmetabolizable derivative of glucose). The reason for the paradoxical shift to a less energy-efficient metabolism is that the aerobic glycolysis shunts more metabolites into intermediates that can be used to support cellular synthetic pathways; at the same time, mitochondria become less important for generating ATP and more important for generating metabolic precursors (Fig. 7-5).

The PI3K-AKT pathway is an important regulatory node for the metabolic changes that occur, increasing the transport and glycolysis of glucose and stimulating lipid and protein synthesis. Another mechanism involves the activation of receptor tyrosine kinases that can phosphorylate the M2 isoform of pyruvate kinase; this dampens the conversion of phosphoenolpyruvate to pyruvate at the end of glycolysis, creating a bottleneck that allows the accumulation of upstream glycolytic intermediates for DNA, RNA, and protein synthesis. Finally, MYC upregulates several glycolytic enzymes, as well as glutaminase, the latter critical for mitochondrial utilization

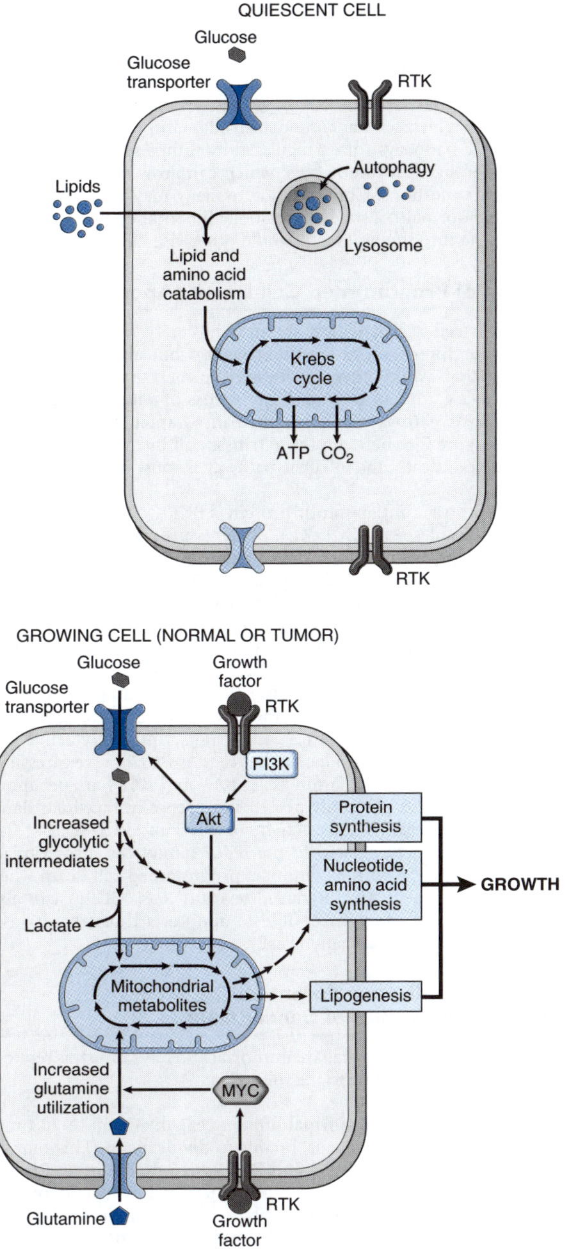

Figure 7-5 Metabolism and cell growth. Quiescent cells rely mainly on the tricarboxylic acid (TCA or Krebs) cycle for ATP production; in the setting of starvation, autophagy can provide metabolic substrates. Proliferating cells upregulate glucose and glutamine transport, providing the carbon sources for nucleotides, proteins, and lipids. In cancers, oncogenic mutations (e.g., growth factor receptor pathways or MYC) deregulate the pathways leading to aerobic glycolysis (Warburg effect).

of glutamine. Interestingly many tumor suppressors have activities that oppose the Warburg effect.

Autophagy (p.301)

Cells that are nutrient starved can sustain themselves by cannibalizing their own intracellular contents, an adaptation called *autophagy*. Autophagic pathways (often regulated by tumor suppressor genes) may be deranged in tumor cells, which can grow despite marginal metabolic conditions. Conversely, autophagy may help tumor cells to become dormant, a state of metabolic hibernation that can make them resistant to therapies that would otherwise kill dividing cells.

Evasion of Programmed Cell Death (Apoptosis) (p. 301)

Neoplastic cell accumulation requires not only oncogene activation and/or tumor suppressor inactivation but also mutations in pathways that would otherwise induce the aberrant cell to undergo apoptosis (e.g., due to DNA damage or loss of adhesion). The major apoptosis pathways are described in Chapter 2, and summarized in Figure 7-6; between the extrinsic and intrinsic pathways of apoptotic cell death, the intrinsic pathway is most often disabled in malignancy.

The prototypic antiapoptotic protein is BCL-2, which, along with related molecules (e.g., BCL-XL), prevents programmed cell death by limiting the exit of cytochrome c from mitochondria (recall that cytochrome c and apoptotic peptidase activating factor-1 [APAF-1] complexes activate the proteolytic enzyme caspase 9 pathway). Overexpression of *BCL2* extends cell survival; if such cells are already genetically unstable, they will continue to accrue additional oncogene and tumor suppressor gene mutations. *BCL2* overexpression in follicular B-cell lymphomas is the classic example of this antiapoptotic mechanism; 85% of these lymphomas have a t(14;18) translocation juxtaposing *BCL2* with a transcriptionally active immunoglobulin heavy chain locus; the result is *BCL2* overexpression. Other genes of the *BCL2* family (e.g., *BAX and BAK*) are proapoptotic, and so-called BH3-only proteins can sense intracellular damage signals and neutralize the activity of BCL2 and BCL-XL.

Genes not directly related to the *BCL2* family can also regulate apoptosis; thus *p53* normally induces programmed cell death when DNA repair is ineffective. Reduced levels of Fas (CD95) can also render tumor cells less susceptible to apoptosis through extrinsic pathways involving Fas ligand (FasL).

Limitless Replicative Potential: The Stem Cell-Like Properties of Cancer Cells (p. 303)

All cancers contain cells that are immortal and have limitless replicative potential. This is due to the following:

- *Evasion of senescence.* Normal human cells divide 60 to 70 times and then become senescent, unable to divide again. This may be due to upregulation of p53 and INK4a/p16 maintaining Rb in a hypophosphorylated state. In malignancy the Rb-dependent G_1/S cell cycle checkpoint is disrupted by acquired genetic and epigenetic changes allowing additional rounds of replication.
- *Evasion of mitotic crisis.* Increased replicative capacity alone is insufficient to confer immortality. Telomerase (normally expressed only in germ cells and stem cells) is not active in most somatic cells; as a consequence, chromosomal telomeres progressively shorten with each division until DNA replication can no longer proceed. Indeed shortened telomeres are interpreted by DNA

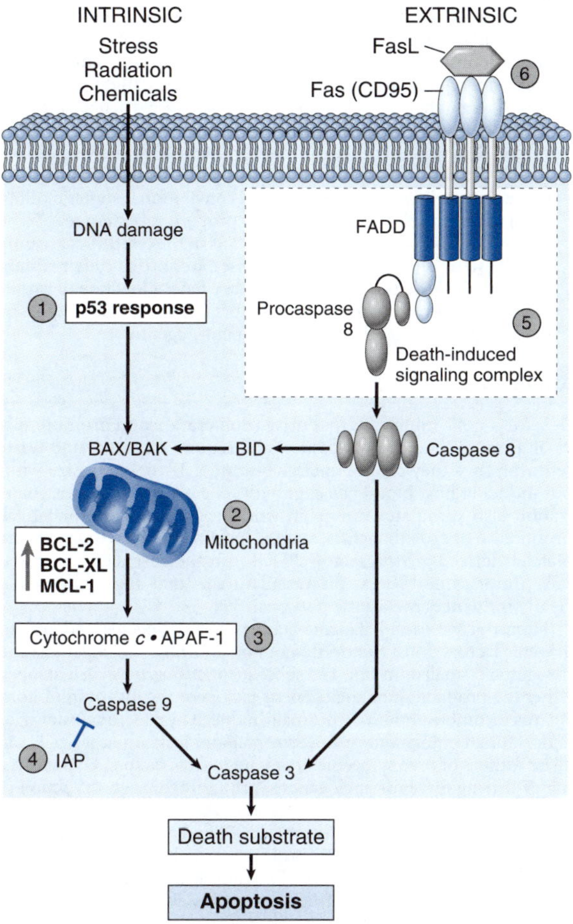

Figure 7-6 Intrinsic and extrinsic pathways of apoptosis, and strategies used by tumor cells to evade cell death. (1) Loss of p53 leads to reduced function of proapoptotic factors, such as BAX. (2) Increased BCL-2, BCL-XL, and/or MCL-1 leading to reduction in the egress of cytochrome from mitochondria. (3) Reduction in APAF-1. (4) Upregulation of inhibitors of apoptosis (IAP) (5) Reduced Fas expression. (6) Inactivation of death-induced signaling complex. *FADD,* Fas-associated protein with death domain.

repair machinery as double-strand breaks, leading to *mitotic crisis* with cell cycle arrest via p53 and Rb. If p53 and Rb mutations disable these checkpoints, nonhomologous end-joining pathways swing into action, leading to the fusion of the shortened ends of two chromosomes. Such inappropriate repair system activation leads to dicentric chromosomes that are then torn asunder at anaphase, resulting in a new round of double-strand breaks. The resulting genetic instability of multiple cycles of bridge-fusion-breakage leads to cell death. Cancer cells overcome these limitations by reactivating telomerase or occasionally through DNA recombination that also elongates telomeres; more than 90% of human tumors show increased telomerase activity.

- *Self-renewal.* In addition to expressing telomerase and avoiding the genetic and epigenetic alterations that trigger senescence, *stem cells* are immortal because they are also capable of self-renewal (i.e., they undergo *asymmetric division* to generate a daughter stem cell as well as a daughter cell that proceeds along a particular differentiation pathway). Because cancers are likewise immortal, the logical conclusion is that they must also contain self-renewing cells—so-called *cancer stem cells.* This may happen by transformation of a tissue stem cell or by conversion of a conventional somatic cell to a transformed cell with the acquired property of "stemness." The concept of cancer stem cells is important in the context of treating cancer; stem cells (cancer or otherwise) are intrinsically resistant to most cytotoxic therapies because they have a low rate of proliferation and because they express factors (e.g., multiple drug resistance-1) that counteract chemotherapeutic agents.

Angiogenesis (p. 305)

Despite genetic mutations that drive proliferation and promote survival, tumors (like normal tissues) still require nutrients and waste removal; thus they cannot enlarge beyond a 1- to 2-mm size without inducing host blood vessel growth *(angiogenesis).* Neovascularization also stimulates tumor growth through the endothelial cell production of growth factors, such as insulin-like growth factor and platelet-derived growth factor (PDGF). In the absence of new vessels, tumor cannot access the vasculature so that angiogenesis also clearly influences metastatic potential.

Tumor growth is a balancing act between angiogenic and antiangiogenic factors. Most tumors do not initially induce angiogenesis and thus remain small or in situ. The subsequent *angiogenic switch* involves either the production of angiogenesis factors or the loss of inhibitors, such as thrombospondin-1 (normally induced by p53), angiostatin, or endostatin. Tumors and/or host stromal and inflammatory cells can all be sources of proangiogenic or antiangiogenic factors. Hypoxia is a major driving force for angiogenesis, primarily through the action of the HIF1α transcription factor. Endothelial growth proteins include *vascular endothelium growth factor (VEGF)* and *basic fibroblast growth factor (bFGF)* (see Chapter 2); proteases can also release preformed angiogenic mediators (e.g., bFGF) from the extracellular matrix (ECM). It is noteworthy that new tumor vessels differ from normal vasculature by being dilated and leaky with slow and abnormal flow.

Angiogenesis inhibitors (e.g., the monoclonal antibody bevacizumab that neutralizes VEGF activity) have not been as effective as anticipated in the treatment of cancer—potentially related to other strategies to drive angiogenesis or to access vessels.

Invasion and Metastasis (p. 306)

The steps involved in invasion and metastasis are depicted in Figure 7-7. Cells within a primary tumor are heterogeneous with respect to the various requisite metastatic attributes; consequently, only a distinct minority can complete all the steps and form distant tumors.

Invasion of Extracellular Matrix *(p. 306)*

To metastasize, tumor cells must dissociate from adjacent cells, and then degrade, adhere, and migrate through ECM.

- *Detachment:* In normal epithelial cells, loss of integrin attachment to the ECM typically induces programmed cell death; clearly tumor cells become resistant to such apoptotic pathways. Epithelial cells also bind each other through adhesion molecules, including

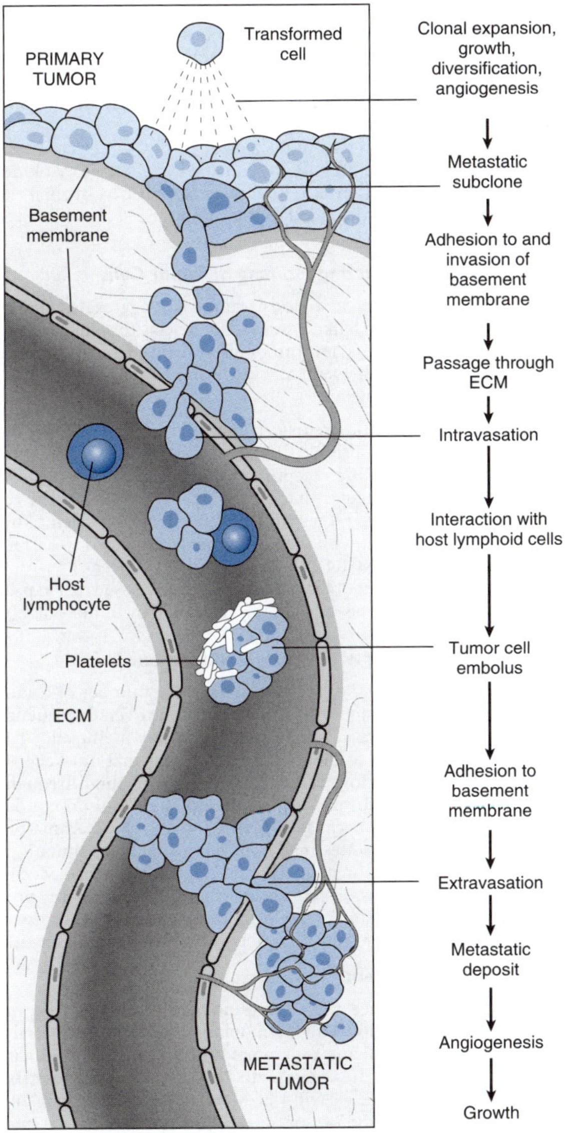

Figure 7-7 The metastatic cascade: sequential steps involved in the hematogenous spread of a tumor.

a family of glycoproteins called *cadherins*. In several carcinomas, there is downregulation of epithelial (E)-cadherins (or their intracellular linkers called *catenins*), thereby reducing cellular cohesion.

- *ECM degradation:* Tumors elaborate proteases or can induce stromal cell to produce them. Although tumor cells can rapidly squeeze between ECM fibers, matrix degradation creates ready passage for migration; in addition, ECM degradation releases a host of growth factors. Thus matrix metalloproteinase 9 (MMP9) degrades epithelial and vascular basement membrane type IV collagen, in addition to releasing ECM-sequestered pools of VEGF.

- *ECM attachment:* Invading cells must express adhesion molecules that allow interaction with the ECM. Conversely, catabolism of the ECM (e.g., via MMP9) can create novel binding sites that promote tumor cell migration.
- *Migration:* In addition to diminished adhesivity, tumor cells have increased locomotion, in part attributable to autocrine cytokines and motility factors; they also migrate in response to stromal cell chemotactic factors, degraded ECM components, and liberated stromal growth factors.

Vascular Dissemination and Homing of Tumor Cells (p. 308)

Tumor cells embolize in the bloodstream as self-aggregates and by adhering to circulating leukocytes and platelets; this may confer some protection from host antitumor effector mechanisms. Exactly where tumor cell emboli eventually lodge and begin growing is influenced by the following:

- Vascular and lymphatic drainage from the site of the primary tumor (discussed previously).
- Interaction with specific receptors. Certain tumor cells express CD44 adhesion molecules that avidly bind high endothelial venules in lymph nodes. Other tumors exhibit specific chemokine receptors that interact with ligands uniquely expressed in certain vascular beds (e.g. CXCR4 and CCR7 in breast cancer).
- The microenvironment of the organ or site (e.g., a tissue rich in protease inhibitors might be resistant to penetration by tumor cells).

Molecular Genetics of Metastasis Development (p. 309)

Relative to the number of cells in a tumor or the number of tumor cells present in the circulation at a given time, the overall frequency of metastases is remarkably small. This metastatic inefficiency has been classically ascribed to the multiple mutations that must accrue in any individual cell. However, some tumors show high frequencies of cells with the requisite "metastatic signature" but do not develop secondary spread because of host stromal and inflammatory countermeasures. Metastases may also require that any mutations occur specifically in tumor stem cells and not just the progeny cells. Finally, specific "metastases suppressor genes" or "metastases promoter genes" (e.g., miRNA) have been described that also impact the capacity of primary lesions to develop secondary tumor spread.

Role of Stromal Elements in Metastasis (p. 309)

Tumors clearly influence their surrounding stroma (e.g., by inducing neovascularization and desmoplastic matrix). Conversely, host stromal cells, ECM, and inflammatory cells can also modulate (inhibit *and* augment) tumor growth (e.g., by secreting matrix-degrading proteases and cleaving ECM to release angiogenic and growth factors). Successful tumors co-opt these pathways; however, because these are products of normal nontransformed cells, they are also tantalizing targets of therapy.

Evasion of Host Defense (p. 310)

There is substantial evidence that the immune system is normally capable of recognizing and eliminating malignant cells *(immune surveillance):*

- Lymphocytes infiltrate tumors, and there is reactive hyperplasia of lymph nodes that drain cancers.

- Experimental systems demonstrate that tumors can be eliminated by host immunity.
- There is increased incidence of certain tumors in immunodeficient patients.
- Direct demonstration of tumor-specific T cells and antibodies in patients.
- Response of malignancies to immune modulation.

The fact that tumors *do* arise in immunocompetent hosts implies that surveillance is imperfect and that malignancies can somehow suppress or otherwise become "invisible" to host immune cells.

Tumor Antigens *(p. 310)*

The main classes of tumor antigens that can elicit a host immune response include the following:

- *Products of mutated genes*—essentially variant proteins that the immune system has not previously "seen." These can be proteolytically processed and complexed with class I major histocompatibility complex (MHC) molecules and are recognized by CD8+ cytotoxic T lymphocytes. Antigen processing cells can also phagocytize necrotic tumor cells and present variant peptides complexed with class II MHC molecules to stimulate CD4+ helper T cells.
- *Overexpressed or aberrantly expressed cellular proteins.* These are normal cellular proteins, but because of local overproduction (e.g., tyrosinase in melanoma) or production in new locations that are not immune-privileged (e.g., cancer-testis antigens), they can break tolerance or otherwise induce immune responses.
- *Tumor antigens produced by oncogenic viruses.* Viruses (particularly DNA viruses, such as human papilloma and EBVs) produce a number of virus-specific proteins that can induce potent immune responses.
- *Oncofetal antigens.* These proteins are normally expressed at high levels during fetal development but usually only at very low levels (if at all) in normal adult tissues. Because these antigens have not previously been seen by a "mature" immune system, expression by tumors can be perceived as foreign. Although many oncofetal antigens can thus potentially induce immune responses, these proteins can also be upregulated at sites of inflammation and injury. Consequently, oncofetal antigens are probably *not* important targets of antitumor immunity inflammatory states, although they can be used as biomarkers to aid in diagnosis or management (e.g., carcinoembryonic antigen [CEA] and α-fetoprotein (AFP]).
- *Altered cell surface glycolipids and glycoproteins.* Abnormal forms or higher than normal levels of surface glycoproteins and glycolipids can be used as both therapeutic targets and diagnostic markers.
- *Cell type-specific differentiation antigens.* Proteins that are normally present on the cell of origin of a particular tumor (e.g., CD20 on B cells) do not induce immune responses. However, they can be used to identify the origin of a malignancy or as targets for immunotherapy (e.g., monoclonal antibody).

Antitumor Effector Mechanisms *(p. 312)*

Cell-mediated immunity—CD8+ cytotoxic T cells, natural killer (NK) cells, and activated macrophages—is the dominant antitumor mechanism. In general, antitumor antibodies play a much lesser role.

Immune Surveillance and Escape *(p. 312)*

The heterogeneity of tumors and the selection pressures imposed by immune surveillance allows the development of malignant cell variants that can evade immune recognition or killing. Mechanisms of immune escape include the following:

- *Outgrowth of antigen-negative variants.*
- *Loss of MHC expression.* Although this may diminish cytotoxic T-cell killing, NK cell killing may be augmented in the setting of reduced MHC expression.
- *Activation of immunoregulatory pathways.* This includes downregulation of costimulators or upregulation of surface proteins that induce lymphocyte cell death (PD-L1 or PD-L2). Tumors can also induce the production of regulatory T cells.
- *Secretion of immunosuppressive factors,* such as TGF-β, interleukin 10, and prostaglandin E_2.

Genomic Instability (p. 314)

DNA repair pathways do not directly influence cell proliferation; rather, they act indirectly by correcting DNA errors that occur spontaneously during cell division or subsequent to mutagenic chemicals or irradiation. Thus *DNA repair genes are not directly oncogenic;* however, defective proteins permit mutations to occur in other genes. Inherited mutations in DNA repair proteins greatly increase the risk of carcinogenesis *(genomic instability syndromes),* and defects in DNA repair pathways also occur in sporadic malignancies. Defects can occur in three types of DNA repair systems:

- Mismatch repair
- Nucleotide excision repair
- Recombination repair

Hereditary Nonpolyposis Colon Cancer Syndrome (p. 314)

Patients inherit one defective copy of DNA repair genes involved in *mismatch repair* (e.g., *MSH2* and *MLH1*), with a second hit occurring in a colonic epithelial cell. Loss of the normal "spell checker" function of the mismatch repair enzymes leads to gradual accumulation of errors in multiple genes including proto-oncogenes and tumor suppressor genes. Mismatch repair mutations are heralded by *microsatellite instability.* Microsatellites are tandem repeats of 1 to 6 nucleotides scattered throughout the genome; in normal tissues the length of these remains constant. Variation of microsatellite length is a hallmark of mismatch repair defects.

Xeroderma Pigmentosum (p. 314)

Nucleotide excision repair genes are specifically required for correcting UV light-induced pyrimidine dimer formation. Patients with defects in these genes develop skin cancers due to UV mutagenic effects.

Diseases With Defects in DNA Repair by Homologous Recombination (p. 314)

These autosomal recessive disorders (e.g., Bloom syndrome, Fanconi anemia, and ataxia-telangiectasia) are characterized by hypersensitivity to DNA-damaging agents (e.g., ionizing radiation or chemical cross-linking agents). In ataxia-telangiectasia, *ATM* gene mutations yield a protein kinase unable to sense DNA double-strand breaks; whereas normal ATM protein phosphorylates p53, leading to cell cycle arrest or apoptosis, defective ATM allows DNA-damaged cells to proliferate and accumulate additional mutations. In Bloom syndrome the mutated protein is a helicase normally involved in DNA repair by homologous recombination.

Mutations in *BRCA-1* or *BRCA-2* account for 25% of cases of familial breast cancer; patients who inherit defective copies of

BRCA-1 also have an increased risk of developing ovarian or prostate cancers, whereas patients with defective germline *BRCA-2* have increased risk for cancers of ovary, prostate, pancreas, stomach, bile ducts, and melanocytes. Both genes are involved in the repair of double-strand DNA breaks by homologous recombination. Interestingly these genes are rarely inactivated in sporadic breast cancers.

Cancers Resulting From Mutations Induced by Regulated Genomic Instability: Lymphoid Neoplasms *(p. 315)*

Normal adaptive immunity requires that B and T cells diversify their antigen receptor repertoire through recombinase gene products (RAG1 and RAG2) and antigen-induced cytosine deaminase (AID). Errors that occur during these normal gene rearrangements are ironically responsible for driving many of the mutations that cause lymphoid neoplasms (see Chapter 13).

Cancer-Enabling Inflammation (p. 315)

Infiltrating cancers provoke chronic inflammatory responses that not only cause systemic signs and symptoms (anemia, fatigue, and cachexia) but can also beneficially impact the tumor:

- Release of growth factors that promote proliferation or proteases that liberate factors from the ECM
- Removal of growth suppressors (e.g., the degradation of adhesion molecules)
- Enhanced resistance to cell death (e.g., through cell and stromal interactions that promote survival in the setting of stresses, such as DNA damage)
- Induction of angiogenesis
- Facilitating invasion and metastasis (e.g., by degrading ECM or by inducing tumor cell mobility)
- Contributing to immune evasion (e.g., by driving the activation of M2 macrophages [see Chapter 3])

Dysregulation of Cancer-Associated Genes (p. 316)

In addition to oncogene activation or tumor suppressor inactivation, large chromosomal changes (visible by karyotyping) and epigenetic changes (e.g., DNA methylation) can induce malignancy.

Chromosomal Changes *(p. 316)*

Translocations (p. 316; common in hematopoietic malignancies) and inversions can activate proto-oncogenes by the following:

- Shifting proto-oncogenes away from normal regulatory elements, resulting in overexpression. In the case of the t(8:14)(q24:q32) translocation in Burkitt lymphoma, the tightly regulated c-*myc* gene moves to the immunoglobulin heavy chain gene locus resulting in its overexpression.
- Forming new hybrid genes that fortuitously encode growth-promoting chimeric molecules. In the reciprocal t(9:22) translocation *(Philadelphia chromosome)* a truncated portion of the c-*abl* proto-oncogene is joined with the *BCR* (breakpoint cluster region) gene to form a fusion protein that has constitutive kinase activity.
- Transcription factors (activators or repressors) can also be important partners in neoplastic gene fusions. An example is a reciprocal translocation between chromosomes 15 and 17, generating a PML-RARα (promyelocytic-retinoic acid receptorα) chimeric protein. The resulting oncoprotein recruits transcriptional repressors that interferes with the expression of genes required for myeloid differ-

entiation, thus causing acute promyelocytic leukemia. Fortunately this functional blockade can be overcome by treatment with all-*trans* retinoic acid, causing a conformational change that displaces the repressor complexes, and for normal differentiation.

Deletions (p. 317)

Deletions are more common in nonhematopoietic solid tumors and are typically attributable to loss of a critical tumor suppressor gene (e.g., 13q14 deletions containing the *Rb* gene, or deletion of the *VHL* tumor suppressor gene on chromosome 3p in renal cell carcinomas).

Gene Amplification (p. 318)

Reduplication and amplification of DNA sequences may underlie the proto-oncogene activation associated with overexpression. Examples include *N-myc* overexpression in 25% to 30% of neuroblastomas and *ERB-B2* overexpression in 20% of breast cancers.

Chromothrypsis (p. 318)

Literally "chromosome shattering," chromothrypsis represents dramatic chromosomal rearrangements that can only be appreciated with whole chromosome sequencing. Such chromosomal catastrophes are observed in 1% to 2% of cancers but occur in a high frequency of osteosarcomas and gliomas. In such tumors, DNA repair mechanisms appear to haphazardly stitch DNA sequences together, leading to random oncogene activation and tumor suppressor inactivation.

Epigenetic Changes (p. 319)

Posttranslational modification of histones (e.g., acetylation) and DNA methylation—without changes in the primary DNA sequence—can influence gene expression including silencing tumor suppressor genes (e.g., *p14ARF* in GI cancers and *p16INK4a* in various malignancies). Therapeutic strategies to demethylate selected DNA sequences may be efficacious in these cases.

Noncoding RNAs and Cancer (p. 320)

MicroRNAs (miRNAs) are small noncoding single-stranded RNAs that are incorporated into silencing complexes and can mediate post-transcriptional gene silencing (see Chapter 1). Deletions of miRNA sequences can drive oncogene expression, whereas overactivity can inhibit tumor suppressor gene function. Thus miRNA-200 is important for invasion and metastasis, whereas miRNA-155 upregulates genes that promote proliferation, including *MYC.* Conversely, deletions of miRNA-15 and miRNA-16 lead to the upregulation of antiapoptotic BCL-2 in chronic lymphocytic leukemias.

Long intervening noncoding RNAs (lincRNAs) can regulate the activity of chromatin "writers" that modify histones and thereby control gene expression; other noncoding RNA species also have roles in post-transcriptional gene silencing or affect the maturation of ribosomes.

Molecular Basis of Multistep Carcinogenesis (p. 320)

No single genetic alteration is sufficient to induce cancers in vivo. A variety of controls influenced by multiple categories of genes—oncogenes, tumor suppressor genes, apoptosis-regulating genes, senescence-modulating genes—must be lost for the emergence of cancer cells. This situation is exemplified by the colon adenoma-to-carcinoma sequence (Fig. 7-8); the evolution of benign adenomas to carcinomas is marked by increasing and additive effects of

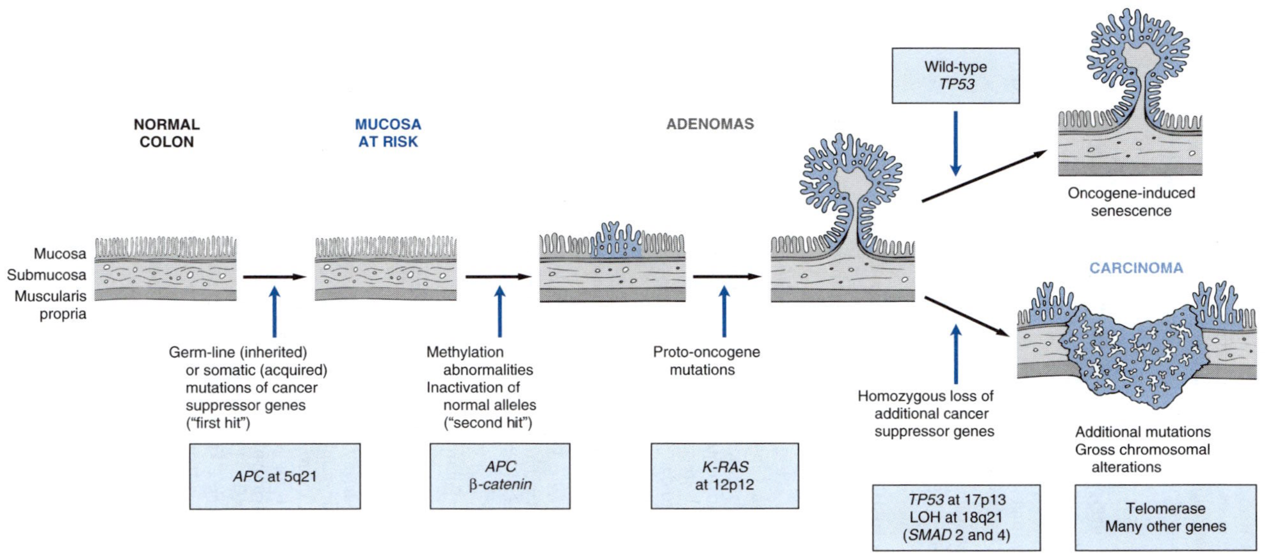

Figure 7-8 Molecular model for the evolution of colorectal cancers in the adenoma-carcinoma sequence. Although *APC* mutation is an early event and loss of *p53* occurs late in tumorigenesis, the timing for other changes can be quite variable. Note also that individual tumors may not have all the changes listed or may have other "passenger mutations" that occur as a result of genomic instability but are not necessarily causally related to oncogenesis. *Top right,* Cells that gain oncogene signaling without loss of *TP53* eventually enter oncogene-induced senescence.

mutations. The accumulation of mutations with increasing genetic instability can be promoted by loss of *p53,* DNA repair genes, or both. Over time, tumors acquire additional changes that result in greater malignant potential (e.g., accelerated growth, invasiveness, angiogenesis, and the ability to form distant metastases). Despite the fact that tumors are initially *monoclonal in origin, by the time they become clinically evident, they are extremely heterogeneous.*

Carcinogenic Agents and Their Cellular Interactions (p. 321)

Environmental agents that cause genetic damage and induce neoplastic transformation include the following:

- Chemical carcinogens
- Radiant energy
- Oncogenic viruses and other microbes

Steps Involved in Chemical Carcinogenesis (p. 322)

Neoplastic transformation brought about by chemicals is broadly divided into two stages:

- *Initiation* refers to the induction of certain irreversible changes (mutations) in the genome. All initiating chemical carcinogens are highly reactive electrophiles that target nucleophilic DNA, RNA, and proteins, inflicting nonlethal damage that cannot be adequately repaired. Mutated cells can then pass on the DNA changes to daughter cells. Initiated cells are not transformed cells; they do not have growth autonomy or unique phenotypic characteristics. However, in contrast to normal cells, they give rise to tumors when appropriately stimulated by promoting agents.
- *Promotion* refers to the process of tumor induction in *previously initiated cells.* This occurs by enhancing the proliferation of initiated cells. The effect of promoters is relatively short-lived and reversible; promoters do not affect DNA and are nontumorigenic by themselves.

Initiators fall in two categories:

- ***Direct-acting agents*** (p. 322) require no metabolic conversion to become carcinogenic (e.g., many alkylating agents used for chemotherapy)
- ***Indirect-acting agents*** (p. 323) require metabolic conversion, most commonly through cytochrome P-450 mixed function oxidases; examples of such indirect-acting agents are polycyclic hydrocarbons and benzo[*a*]pyrene. The mixed-function oxidases have polymorphisms within the population that can influence their activity. Thus smokers with a highly inducible form of the P-450 gene *CYP1A1* have a sevenfold higher risk of developing lung cancer than smokers with a different genotype.

Metabolic pathways can also inactivate carcinogens and the carcinogenic potential of any given molecule is therefore a balance of activation and inactivation.

Molecular Targets of Chemical Carcinogens (p. 323)

Interaction of carcinogens with DNA induces mutations by altering the primary sequence; although any gene can be mutated, oncogenes and tumor suppressors are especially important targets (e.g., *RAS* and *p53*). Because specific sequences can be targeted by certain chemicals, an analysis of the mutations found in human tumors can sometimes identify a culprit carcinogen.

Promotion of Chemical Carcinogenesis (p. 324)

Unrepaired DNA alterations are essential first steps in *initiating* tumors; however, the damaged DNA template must also be replicated to make the changes permanent. Thus for initiation to occur, carcinogen-altered cells must undergo at least one cycle of replication to "fix" the change in the DNA. Quiescent cells may never be affected by chemical carcinogens unless a mitotic stimulus is also provided.

Thus the initial mutagenic event in most instances requires subsequent exposure to *promoters* to induce cellular proliferation. These can include various drugs, phenols, and phorbol esters. Other examples of promoters include unopposed estrogenic stimulation of endometrium and breast, and chronic inflammatory processes associated with ongoing tissue repair (e.g., chronic hepatitis and inflammatory bowel disease).

Radiation Carcinogenesis (p. 324)

Radiant energy, in the form of UV rays or ionizing radiation, is carcinogenic.

Ultraviolet Rays (p. 324)

Sun-derived UV radiation, especially UVB (280 to 320 nm), can cause skin cancer. At greatest risk are fair-skinned people who live in sunny climes or have less ozone protection; carcinomas and melanomas of exposed skin are particularly common in Australia and New Zealand. Risk of nonmelanoma skin cancers is associated with cumulative exposure; melanoma risk is associated with intense intermittent exposures (e.g., sunbathing). Damage to DNA occurs through the formation of pyrimidine dimers; repair of these dimers requires nucleotide excision mechanisms that can be mutated in *xeroderma pigmentosum* or can be overwhelmed, leading to nontemplated DNA-repair mechanisms that are error-prone.

Ionizing Radiation (p. 325)

Radiation from electromagnetic (e.g., x-rays) and particulate (e.g., α and β particles or neutrons) sources are all carcinogenic. The ability of ionizing radiation to cause cancer lies in its ability to induce DNA mutations; these can occur directly or indirectly by the generation of free radicals from water or oxygen.

In humans there is a hierarchy of cellular vulnerability to radiation-induced neoplasms:

- Most common are myeloid leukemias, followed by thyroid cancer in children.
- Cancers of the breast and lung are less commonly radiation induced.
- Skin, bone, and gut are the least susceptible to radiation carcinogenesis.

Microbial Carcinogenesis (p. 325)

Although a variety of DNA and RNA viruses cause cancer in animals, relatively few are yet implicated in human cancers.

Oncogenic RNA Viruses (p. 325)

Human T-lymphotropic virus 1 (HTLV-1) is a retrovirus causing a T-cell leukemia and/or lymphoma that is endemic in Japan and the Caribbean but occurs sporadically elsewhere. HTLV-1 has a CD4+ T-cell tropism, and infection requires transmission of infected cells (sexual intercourse, blood products, or breastfeeding). Leukemia develops in 3% to 5% of infected individuals, after a 40- to 60-year latency. The transforming activity resides in a viral-encoded Tax protein that inactivates p16/INK4a and enhances cyclin D activation, thus leading to increased cell replication. Tax also interferes with DNA repair mechanisms, leading to genomic instability, and activates NF-κB, a transcription factor that regulates several proapoptotic and antiapoptotic genes. The resulting T-cell proliferation and genomic instability eventually result in the emergence of a monoclonal neoplastic population.

Oncogenic DNA Viruses *(p. 326)*

Oncogenic DNA viruses integrate into the host cell genome forming a stable association. The virus cannot complete its replicative cycle because essential viral genes are interrupted during viral DNA integration; consequently the virus may remain latent for years. Viral genes that are transcribed early in the viral life cycle are typically important for cellular transformation.

Human Papillomavirus (p. 326)

Approximately 70 genetically distinct types of HPV have been identified. Some types (e.g., 1, 2, 4, and 7) cause benign squamous papillomas (warts) in humans; the viral genome is typically not integrated, remaining as an episome. Integration appears to be a requisite step in oncogenesis:

- Genital warts with low malignant potential are caused by distinct HPV types (*low-risk* types [e.g., HPV-6 and HPV-11]).
- Cervical squamous cell cancers contain HPV types 16 or 18 in more than 90% of cases.
- In HPV-associated cervical carcinomas, random integration of the viral genome into host DNA interrupts the viral DNA within the E1/E2 open reading frame; this leads to loss of the E2 viral repressor and subsequent overexpression of the E6 and E7 viral proteins. These proteins transform cells by binding to and increasing the degradation of p53 and Rb tumor suppressor proteins, respectively; E7 also inactivates the CDK inhibitors p21 and p27.
- HPV infection alone is typically not sufficient for carcinogenesis; cigarette smoking, coinfections, dietary deficiencies, and hormones are also implicated in cervical carcinoma pathogenesis. Immune suppression (e.g., due to HIV) also increases the risk of cervical malignancy.

Epstein-Barr Virus (p. 327)

This is a herpesvirus that infects B cells and oropharyngeal epithelium. B cells are latently infected becoming immortalized, acquiring the ability for indefinite propagation. The immortalization is largely mediated through the action of the EBV latent membrane protein-1 (LMP-1) that constitutively activates NF-κB and JAK-STAT pathways to promote B-cell proliferation and survival. A second gene, *EBNA-2,* encodes a nuclear protein that also constitutively activates a variety of host proteins such as cyclin D and *src* proto-oncogenes. In immunocompetent hosts, EBV-driven B-cell proliferation is readily checked; immune system inactivation is key to EBV-related oncogenesis. EBV is associated with multiple human cancers:

- *Burkitt lymphoma* is a B-cell tumor associated with a t(8;14) translocation or other translocations that inactivate *c-MYC;* it need not be associated with EBV, and indeed in nonendemic areas of the world, 80% of the tumors do not contain the EBV genome. However, in central Africa and New Guinea, where Burkitt lymphoma is the major childhood malignancy, 90% of tumors contain the

EBV genome. Thus EBV alone does not cause Burkitt lymphoma. However, in patients with subtle or overt immune dysregulation (e.g., due to chronic malaria) unchecked B-cell proliferation may lead to additional mutations (including the t(8;14) translocation) that allow autonomous replication.

- *B-cell lymphomas in immunosuppressed patients* (AIDS, transplant recipients) have polyclonal B-cell proliferations that transform into monoclonal lymphomas. In transplant recipients, withdrawal of immunosuppressive drugs can cause regression of such EBV-induced proliferations.
- A subset of *Hodgkin lymphomas* is associated with EBV (see Chapter 13), as are rare forms of T-cell lymphoma and NK cell lymphoma.
- *Nasopharyngeal carcinoma* is endemic in southern China and some other locales; the EBV genome is found in all such tumors, and LMP-1 is implicated in driving cell proliferation. As in Burkitt lymphoma, EBV probably acts in concert with other factors to induce malignant transformation.

Hepatitis B and C Viruses (p. 328)

Approximately 70% to 85% of hepatocellular carcinomas worldwide are due to hepatitis B virus (HBV) or hepatitis C virus (HCV) infections. The mechanism is multifactorial but the dominant effect is immunologically mediated chronic inflammation:

- By causing hepatocellular injury and resulting regenerative hyperplasia, the pool of mitotically active cells subject to damage by carcinogenic agents is increased.
- Activated immune cells also produce a plethora of mediators (e.g., reactive oxygen species) that are mutagenic.
- HBV encodes a regulatory element called *HBx* that can inactivate p53, as well as cause transcriptional activation of several proto-oncogenes.

Helicobacter Pylori (p. 329)

Helicobacter pylori causes no clinical consequences in the great majority of infected individuals; however, in 3% of cases infection can lead to gastric carcinoma through pathways involving prolonged chronic inflammation. Strains associated with adenocarcinoma also express a cytotoxin-associated A *(CagA)* gene that induces unregulated proliferation.

H. pylori is also associated with gastric lymphomas. Prolonged infection induces *H. pylori*-reactive T cells that secrete cytokines that promote polyclonal B-cell proliferation. These proliferating cells eventually become monoclonal and T-cell independent by accumulating mutations (e.g., t[11:18] translocations). The resultant tumor is called *marginal zone lymphoma* or *MALToma* (for *m*ucosa-*a*ssociated *l*ymphoid *t*issue lymphoma; see Chapter 13).

Clinical Aspects of Neoplasia (p. 329)

Although malignant tumors are more threatening than benign, any tumor can cause morbidity and mortality.

Local and Hormonal Effects (p. 330)

- *Location:* Intracranial tumors (e.g., pituitary adenoma) can expand and destroy the remaining pituitary gland, giving rise to an endocrine disorder; tumors of the GI tract may cause obstruction of the bowel or may ulcerate and cause bleeding.

- *Hormone production:* These may cause paraneoplastic syndromes, such as hypoglycemia (insulin production) or hypercalcemia (parathyroid hormone [PTH]-producing tumors).

Cancer Cachexia (p. 330)

Loss of body fat, lean body mass, and profound weakness are referred to as *cancer cachexia.* Its cause is multifactorial but is largely driven by TNF and other cytokines elaborated by inflammatory cells in response to tumors:

- Loss of appetite
- Metabolic changes causing reduced synthesis and storage of fat and increased mobilization of fatty acids from adipocytes
- Increase catabolism of muscle and adipose tissue by ubiquitin-proteasome pathways

Paraneoplastic Syndromes (p. 330)

These are tumor-associated syndromes in which the symptoms are not directly related to the spread of the tumor or to the elaboration of hormones indigenous to the tumor tissue; they occur in approximately 10% of patients with cancer. Paraneoplastic syndromes may be the earliest clinical manifestations of a neoplasm and can mimic distant spread (Table 7-7). The most common syndromes include the following:

- *Endocrinopathies:* Some nonendocrine cancers produce hormones or hormonelike factors (ectopic hormone production). Thus small cell lung cancer causes *Cushing syndrome* by elaborating adrenocorticotropic hormone (ACTH); 50% of patients with this endocrinopathy have lung carcinoma.
- *Hypercalcemia* is the most common paraneoplastic syndrome. It is caused by bone resorption resulting from the elaboration of PTH-like peptides. Cancer-associated hypercalcemia due to osteolysis induced by bony metastases is *not* considered a paraneoplastic syndrome.
- *Neuropathic paraneoplastic syndromes* include peripheral neuropathies, cortical cerebellar degeneration, and myasthenic syndromes. In most cases the mechanisms are thought to involve autoantibodies against tumor antigens that cross-react with normal host tissues.
- *Thrombotic diatheses* result from production of thromboplastic substances by tumor cells and manifest as disseminated intravascular coagulation, migratory thrombophlebitis *(Trousseau syndrome),* or valvular vegetations *(nonbacterial thrombotic endocarditis).*

Grading and Staging of Tumors (p. 332)

This assessment provides a semiquantitative estimate of the clinical gravity of a tumor. Both histologic grading and clinical staging are valuable for prognostication and for planning therapy, although staging has proved to be of greater clinical value.

- *Grading* is based primarily on the degree of differentiation (how well the tumor resembles its normal counterpart), and occasionally, architectural features or number of mitoses. In general, higher-grade tumors (more poorly differentiated) are more aggressive than lower-grade tumors.
- *Staging* is based on the size of the primary tumor and the extent of local and distant spread. The major system currently used is the American Joint Committee on Cancer (AJCC) staging; the classification involves a TNM designation—T for tumor (size and

TABLE 7-7 Paraneoplastic Syndromes

Clinical Syndromes	Major Forms of Underlying Cancer	Causal Mechanism
Endocrinopathies		
Cushing syndrome	Small-cell carcinoma of lung Pancreatic carcinoma Neural tumors	ACTH or ACTH-like substance
Syndrome of inappropriate antidiuretic hormone secretion	Small-cell carcinoma of lung Intracranial neoplasms	Antidiuretic hormone or atrial natriuretic hormones
Hypercalcemia	Squamous cell carcinoma of lung Breast carcinoma Renal carcinoma Adult T-cell leukemia and/or lymphoma	Parathyroid hormone-related protein (PTHRP), TGF-α, TNF, IL-1
Hypoglycemia	Ovarian carcinoma Fibrosarcoma Other mesenchymal sarcomas	Insulin or insulin-like substance
Polycythemia	Renal carcinoma Cerebellar hemangioma Hepatocellular carcinoma	Erythropoietin
Nerve and Muscle Syndromes		
Myasthenia	Bronchogenic carcinoma Thymic neoplasms	Immunologic
Disorders of the central and peripheral nervous system		Breast carcinoma
Dermatologic Disorders		
Acanthosis nigricans	Gastric carcinoma	Immunologic; secretion of epidermal growth factor
	Lung carcinoma Uterine carcinoma	
Dermatomyositis	Bronchogenic carcinoma Breast carcinoma	Immunologic
Osseous, Articular, and Soft Tissue Changes		
Hypertrophic osteoarthropathy and clubbing of the fingers	Bronchogenic carcinoma Thymic neoplasms	Unknown
Vascular and Hematologic Changes		
Venous thrombosis (Trousseau phenomenon)	Pancreatic carcinoma	Tumor products (mucins that activate clotting)
	Bronchogenic carcinoma Other cancers	
Disseminated intravascular coagulation	Acute promyelocytic leukemia Prostatic carcinoma	Tumor products that activate clotting
Nonbacterial thrombotic endocarditis	Advanced cancers	Hypercoagulability
Red cell aplasia	Thymic neoplasms	Unknown
Others		
Nephrotic syndrome	Various cancers	Tumor antigens, immune complexes

IL, Interleukin; *TNF*, tumor necrosis factor.

local invasion), N for regional lymph node involvement, and M for distant metastases.

Laboratory Diagnosis of Cancer (p. 332)

Histologic and Cytologic Methods (p. 332)

Histologic examination is the most important method of diagnosis. In addition to traditional formalin-fixed and paraffin-embedded sections, quick-frozen sections provide rapid diagnoses during procedures. Proper histologic diagnosis requires complete clinical data (age, gender, site, previous therapy, etc.), good tissue preservation, and adequate specimen sampling.

Cytologic interpretation is based chiefly on changes in the appearance of individual cells. In the hands of experts, false-positive results are uncommon, but false-negative results do occur because of sampling errors. When possible, cytologic diagnosis must be confirmed by biopsy before therapeutic intervention.

- *Fine-needle aspiration* involves aspiration of cells and fluids from tumors or masses; improved imaging techniques allow the sampling of deep as well as more readily palpated lesions
- *Cytologic (Pap) smears* involve examination of shed cells; exfoliative cytologic examination is used most commonly in the diagnosis of cancer of the uterine cervix and tumors of the stomach, bronchus, endometrium, and urinary bladder.

Immunohistochemistry (p. 334)

Immunohistochemistry detects cell products or surface markers using specific antibodies. Antibody binding is visualized by fluorescent labels or chemical reactions that generate a colored product. Immunohistochemistry is useful in the following settings:

- Diagnosis of undifferentiated tumors by the detection of tissue-specific intermediate filaments or other markers
- Determination of the site of origin of metastases by using reagents that identify specific cell types (e.g., prostate-specific antigen for prostate cancer)
- Detection of molecules that have prognostic or therapeutic significance (e.g., immunochemical detection of hormone receptors in breast cancer) or products of proto-oncogenes (e.g., *ERB-B2* on breast cancers)

Flow Cytometry (p. 334)

Flow cytometry can be used to rapidly and quantitatively measure the presence of membrane antigens or DNA content of tumor cells. It is routinely used in the diagnosis and classification of leukemias and lymphomas.

Circulating Tumor Cells (p. 334)

Circulating tumor cells can be captured and isolated using three-dimensional flow cells coated with antibodies specific for the tumor cells of interest. Although currently only a research tool, these devices have the potential to permit early diagnosis, assess risk of metastasis, and analyze response to therapy.

Molecular and Cytogenetic Diagnostics (p. 334)

- *Diagnosis of malignancy:* In lymphocytic lesions, polymerase chain reaction (PCR) can distinguish monoclonal (neoplastic) and polyclonal (reactive) proliferations. Fluorescence in situ hybridization (FISH)- or PCR-based detection of characteristic translocations can also diagnose specific malignancies, and unique translocations detected by PCR can distinguish similar-appearing tumors (e.g., small, round blue cell tumors in children). *Spectral karyotyping* can analyze all chromosomes from a single cell using a pallet of fluorochromes; it can detect even small translocations or insertions and determine the origin of chromosome fragments.

- *Prognosis of malignancy:* Certain genetic alterations are associated with poor prognosis; identification of these can stratify treatment. Thus N-myc amplifications bode ill for neuroblastomas, and HER-2-NEU overexpression in breast cancer is an indication for monoclonal antibody therapy against the ERBB2 receptor.
- *Detection of residual disease:* The ability to detect extremely small numbers of malignant cells can be useful for evaluating therapy efficacy or for assessing tumor recurrence. Thus the PCR-based detection of the *BCR-ABL* fusion gene product aids in determining whether tumor kill has been effective or if the tumor has recurred.
- *Diagnosis of hereditary predisposition to cancers* (e.g., breast cancer and endocrine neoplasms) can be detected by mutational analysis of *BRCA-1, BRCA-2,* and *RET* genes, allowing family screening and risk stratification.

Molecular Profiles of Tumors: The Future of Cancer Diagnostics (p. 335)

Technologic innovation now allows entire genome sequencing, genome-wide assessment of epigenetic modifications *(epigenome),* evaluation of all RNA transcripts *(transcriptome),* analysis of multiple proteins *(proteome),* or characterization of cellular metabolites *(metabolome).* Because RNA is prone to degradation, its sequencing is less applicable to the variety of clinical specimens. Consequently, massively parallel DNA sequencing (NextGen sequencing) is the mainstay for cataloguing the genomic alterations in human cancers. Although whole genome sequencing is possible, most clinical efforts now focus on the sequencing of therapeutically "actionable" genetic lesions. Thus most diagnostic labs have developed strategies to simultaneously sequence several hundred exons of key genes. DNA arrays are also used to identify changes in copy number (amplifications and deletions).

Tumor Markers (p. 337)

Tumor markers are tumor-derived or -associated molecules that are detected in blood or other body fluids. These are not primary methods of diagnosis but rather diagnostic adjuncts that can be used for screening large populations. They are also useful in determining therapeutic responses or tumor recurrence. In most cases tumor markers are not specific for malignancy so that elevated levels must be interpreted in the context of other possible pathologies (Table 7-8).

Examples include the following:

- *Prostate-specific antigen (PSA)* elaborated by prostate epithelium; elevated levels can reflect malignancy or can also be seen with benign prostatic hypertrophy or prostatic inflammation.
- *CEA* is normally produced by fetal gut, liver, and pancreas and can be elaborated by cancers of the colon, pancreas, stomach, and breast, as well as in non-neoplastic conditions (e.g., alcoholic cirrhosis, hepatitis, and ulcerative colitis).
- *AFP* is normally produced by fetal yolk sac and liver; elevated levels occur in liver and testicular germ cell tumors but also occur in non-neoplastic conditions, such as cirrhosis and hepatitis.

TABLE 7-8 Selected Tumor Markers

Tumor Markers	Tumor Types
Hormones	
Human chorionic gonadotropin	Trophoblastic tumors, nonseminomatous testicular tumors
Calcitonin	Medullary carcinoma of thyroid
Catecholamine and metabolites	Pheochromocytoma and related tumors
Ectopic hormones	Adrenocorticotropic hormone (ACTH) in small-cell cancer of lung
Oncofetal Antigens	
AFP	Liver cell cancer, nonseminomatous germ cell tumors of testis
CEA	Carcinomas of the colon, pancreas, lung, stomach, and heart
Isoenzymes	
Prostatic acid phosphatase	Prostate cancer
Neuron-specific enolase	Small-cell cancer of lung, neuroblastoma
Specific Proteins	
Immunoglobulins	Multiple myeloma and other gammopathies
Prostate-specific antigen and prostate-specific membrane antigen	Prostate cancer
Mucins and Other Glycoproteins	
CA-125	Ovarian cancer
CA-19-9	Colon cancer, pancreatic cancer
CA-15-3	Breast cancer
Cell-Free DNA Markers	
TP53, APC, RAS mutants in stool and serum	Colon cancer
TP53, RAS mutants in stool and serum	Pancreatic cancer
TP53, RAS mutants in sputum and serum	Lung cancer
TP53 mutants in urine	Bladder cancer

8

Infectious Diseases

General Principles of Microbial Pathogenesis (p. 341)

Despite vaccines and antibiotics, infectious diseases significantly contribute to the mortality in elderly individuals and those who are immunosuppressed or have chronic diseases. In developing countries, infectious diseases—abetted by malnutrition and unsanitary living conditions—constitute six of the top 10 causes of mortality, with the majority occurring in children from respiratory or diarrheal illness.

How Microorganisms Cause Disease (p. 342)

Humans harbor a complex ecosystem of microbial flora (the *microbiome*) with 10 times more microbes than human cells. Most of these microorganisms are commensals that occupy niches that might otherwise be filled by pathogens. However, when normal host defenses are attenuated, even "healthy" microbial flora can cause pathologic infections. Most infectious diseases are caused by noncommensal organisms with a wide range of virulence. Highly infectious microbes produce disease in healthy individuals, whereas other microbes are minimally pathogenic, requiring large exposures and/or significant failures of host defenses.

Routes of Entry of Microbes (p. 342)

Barriers that prevent microbes from entering the body include intact skin and mucosal surfaces, their secretory products (lysozyme in tears, acid in stomach), and cells and proteins of host immunity. In the skin and gastrointestinal (GI) tract, a substantial population of normal flora also prevents new microbes from gaining admission by eliminating unfilled niches. Successful microorganisms either take advantage of barrier failure or have virulence factors that enable them to circumvent these barricades.

- *Skin* (p. 342) includes a keratinized outer layer, fatty acids, and low pH.
    - These barriers can be breached directly (e.g., schistosomiasis) or by skin damage that allows access of otherwise less virulent microbes (e.g., macerated skin, cuts, burns, intravenous lines, or insect bites).
- *GI tract* (p. 342) includes gastric acid, pancreatic bile, lytic enzymes, a mucous layer, defensins, and secreted immunoglobulin A (IgA).
    - These barriers are lost in the setting of low gastric acidity, antibiotics that alter the normal flora, loss of pancreatic function, or diminished bowel motility.

- *Respiratory tract* (p. 343) includes bronchial epithelium ciliary activity, a mucous layer, defensins, secreted IgA, and alveolar macrophages.
  - Compromises to these barriers include when the mucociliary clearance mechanism is disrupted (e.g., by smoking) and when host macrophage clearance is ineffective (e.g., in tuberculosis).
- *Urogenital tract* (p. 343) includes frequent bladder flushing with urine; in the vagina, catabolism of glycogen by normal commensal lactobacilli lowers the pH and reduces fungal growth.
  - These barriers are lost with bladder atonia, flow obstruction, or reflux; antibiotics will kill the lactobacilli and render the vagina susceptible to candidal infection.
- *Vertical transmission* (p. 344) reflects infection from mother to fetus or newborn child.
  - Placental-fetal transmission during pregnancy. Effects on fetal development will depend on when during gestation the infection occurs; rubella infection during the first trimester can be devastating, whereas the same infection in the third trimester has little effect.
  - Transmission during birth (e.g., gonococcus and chlamydia).
  - Postnatal transmission in maternal milk (e.g., cytomegalovirus [CMV], human immunodeficiency virus [HIV], and hepatitis B virus [HBV]).

Spread and Dissemination of Microbes Within the Body *(p. 344)*

Some microbes proliferate locally; others penetrate the epithelial barrier and spread distally via lymphatics, blood, or nerves, so that disease manifestations occur at sites distant from organism entry. After gaining access to a new host, most organisms have a predilection for a specific site(s), so-called tissue *tropism.* The consequences of the spread of pathogens depend on microbial virulence, magnitude and pattern of seeding, and the host immune response. Thus sporadic dispersal in the bloodstream of low-virulence microbes (such as occurs with tooth brushing) is generally well tolerated; however, disseminated bacteremia can have substantial morbidity and even mortality, owing to the potential for a systemic inflammatory response syndrome (see Chapter 4).

Release From the Body and Transmission of Microbes *(p. 345)*

For purposes of microbial propagation, exit strategies are as important as how an organism initially infects its host. Microbes can be transmitted person to person via respiratory, fecal-oral, sexual, or transplacental routes. Animal-to-human transmission can occur through direct contact or ingestion *(zoonotic infections);* alternatively, insect or arthropod vectors may passively spread infection or serve as required hosts for pathogen replication and development. Some microbes are hardy and can survive extended periods in dust, food, or water; others may need quick transmission and require direct person-to-person contact.

Host-Pathogen Interactions (p. 345)

Host Defenses Against Infection *(p. 345)*

In addition to host barrier function, the innate and adaptive immune systems are critical to preventing infection or in ultimately eradicating it (see Chapter 6). In some cases a stalemate between host and microorganism results in a state of microbial latency without much pathology. However, subsequent diminution of host immunity can result in aggressive reactivation and disease (e.g., latent Epstein-Barr virus [EBV] or tuberculosis infections).

Immune Evasion by Microbes (p. 345)

Immune evasion is an important determinant of microbial virulence. Mechanisms include the following (Fig. 8-1):

- *Antigenic variation:* This is important for escaping antibody-mediated host defenses that can block microbial adhesion or facilitate phagocytosis and complement activation. Mechanisms of antigenic variation include wholesale genetic switching, recombination events, and mutation (Table 8-1).
- *Resistance to antimicrobial peptides (e.g., defensins and cathelicidins):* Accomplished by altering membrane surface charge and

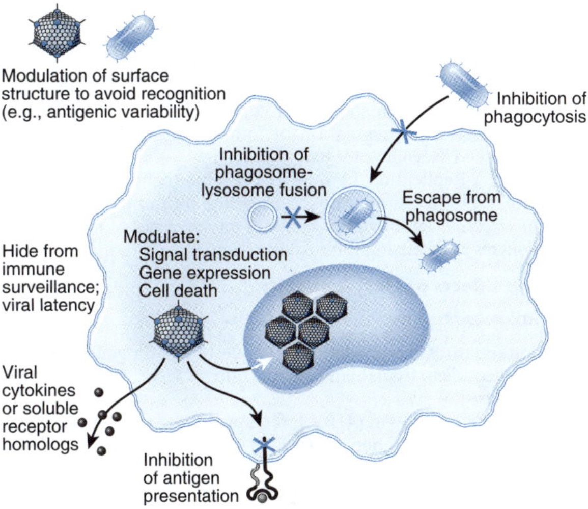

Figure 8-1 An overview of mechanisms used by viral and bacterial pathogens to evade innate and adaptive immunity. *(Modified with permission from Finlay B, Mcfadden G: Anti-immunology: evasion of the host immune system by bacterial and viral pathogens.* Cell *2006;124:767-782.)*

TABLE 8-1 Mechanisms of Antigenic Variation

Type	Example	Disease
High mutation rate	HIV Influenza virus	AIDS Influenza
Genetic reassortment	Influenza virus Rotavirus	Influenza Diarrhea
Genetic rearrangement (e.g., gene recombination, gene conversion, site-specific inversion)	*B. burgdorferi* *N. gonorrhoeae* *Trypanosoma* sp. *Plasmodium* sp.	Lyme disease Gonorrhea African sleeping sickness Malaria
Large diversity of serotypes	Rhinoviruses *S. pneumoniae*	Colds Pneumonia Meningitis

hydrophobicity to inhibit peptide binding or by producing proteases to degrade peptides or pumps to export them.
- *Resistance to phagocyte killing:* Components of some microbial capsules can prevent phagocytosis or complement-mediated lysis. Microbes can also resist intracellular cytotoxicity or produce proteins that kill phagocytes, prevent their migration, or diminish their oxidative burst.
- *Evasion of apoptosis and manipulation of host cell metabolism:* Proteins that modulate host cell apoptosis or autophagy pathways can allow viruses or other intracellular pathogens sufficient time to replicate, enter latency, or even transform the cell.
- *Resistance to cytokine-, chemokine-, and complement-mediated host defense:* Microbial proteins can degrade or inhibit host cell protein mediators of immunity; viruses can produce cytokine homologues that function as antagonists.
- *Evasion of recognition by CD4+ helper T cells and CD8+ cytotoxic T cells:* This can occur by downregulating major histocompatibility complex (MHC) molecules required for presenting antigen fragments to T cells.
- *Exploit immunoregulatory mechanisms to downregulate T-cell responses:* "T-cell exhaustion" is a consequence of chronic infections, driven by upregulation of immune inhibitory pathways, such as PD-1 (see Chapter 6).
- *Lying low:* Replication in sites inaccessible to host immune response, rapid invasion of host cells before immune responses become effective, latent viral infections, parasitic cysts, and infecting leukocytes and causing their dysfunction.

Injurious Effects of Host Immunity *(p. 347)*

Host immune responses to microbes cause pathology:

- Granulomatous responses can sequester pathogens but can cause secondary tissue damage and fibrosis (e.g., *Mycobacterium tuberculosis*).
- Liver damage following HBV infection is due to the immune destruction of infected hepatocytes.
- Antibodies directed against bacterial antigens may cross-react with host molecules (e.g., rheumatic heart disease) or may form immune complexes that lodge in vascular beds (e.g., poststreptococcal glomerulonephritis).
- Chronic inflammation and epithelial injury may lead to malignancy (e.g., *Helicobacter pylori* and gastric cancer).

Infections in People With Immunodeficiencies *(p. 347)*

The nature of the infections depends on which effector mechanisms are impaired.

- Genetic immunodeficiencies
  - *Antibody deficiencies:* X-linked agammaglobulinemia is associated with *Streptococcus pneumoniae, Haemophilus influenzae, Staphylococcus aureus,* rotavirus, and enterovirus infections.
  - *Complement proteins:* Associated with infections due to encapsulated bacteria (e.g., *S. pneumoniae* for early complement components and *Neisseria meningitidis* for late [C5 to C9] elements).
  - *Neutrophil function:* Infections from *S. aureus,* gram-negative bacteria, and fungi.
  - *T-cell deficiencies:* Infections due to intracellular pathogens (e.g., viruses and some parasites); defects in T_H1 generation increase the risk of infections by atypical mycobacteria, and defects in T_H17 generation are associated with chronic mucocutaneous candidiasis.

- Acquired immunodeficiencies: HIV annihilation of T-helper cells is associated with a variety of infections; many were well-recognized pathogens before acquired immunodeficiency syndrome (AIDS), while others (Kaposi sarcoma herpesvirus [KSHV], cryptococcus, and *Pneumocystis*) were uncommon. Malnutrition also broadly impairs immune defenses.
- Immunosuppression in organ transplantation or during bone marrow engraftment renders patients susceptible to virtually all organisms, including common environmental microbes (*Aspergillus* and *Pseudomonas*).
- Diseases of organs other than the immune system also render patients susceptible to specific organisms. Lack of splenic function in sickle cell disease increases risk of infection by encapsulated bacteria *(S. pneumoniae),* and patients with cystic fibrosis commonly get *Pseudomonas* infections.

Host Damage (p. 348)

Infectious disease results from the interaction of microbial virulence characteristics and host immune responses. Infectious agents cause damage by the following:

- Entering cells and directly causing cell death
- Releasing toxins that kill cells at a distance
- Releasing enzymes that degrade tissue components
- Damage blood vessels, causing ischemic necrosis
- Inducing host inflammatory cell responses that directly or indirectly injure tissues

Mechanisms of Viral Injury *(p. 348) (Fig. 8-2)*

Viruses have tissue *tropisms* that will dictate which tissue(s) will be injured. Determinants of viral tropisms include the following:

- Binding to specific cell surface proteins (HIV binds to CD4 and the CXCR4 chemokine receptor on T cells).
- Cell type-specific proteases may be necessary to enable binding (host protease activation of influenza virus hemagglutinin).
- Cell type-specific transcription factors (JC virus can proliferate only in oligodendroglia).
- Physical barriers, local temperature, and pH (enteroviruses resist gut acid and enzymes).

Once inside cells, viruses cause injury by the following:

- Direct cytopathic effects
  - Inhibiting host DNA, RNA, or protein synthesis
  - Producing degradative enzymes or toxic proteins
  - Inducing apoptosis
  - Damaging the plasma membrane (HIV)
  - Lysing cells (rhinoviruses and influenza viruses)
- Inducing an antiviral host immune response
  - Cytotoxic T cells or natural killer (NK) cells
- Transformation of infected cells (see Chapter 7)

Mechanisms of Bacterial Injury *(p. 349)*

Bacterial Virulence (p. 349)

Microbial damage depends on the ability of infecting bacteria to adhere to host cells, invade cells and tissues, or deliver toxins.

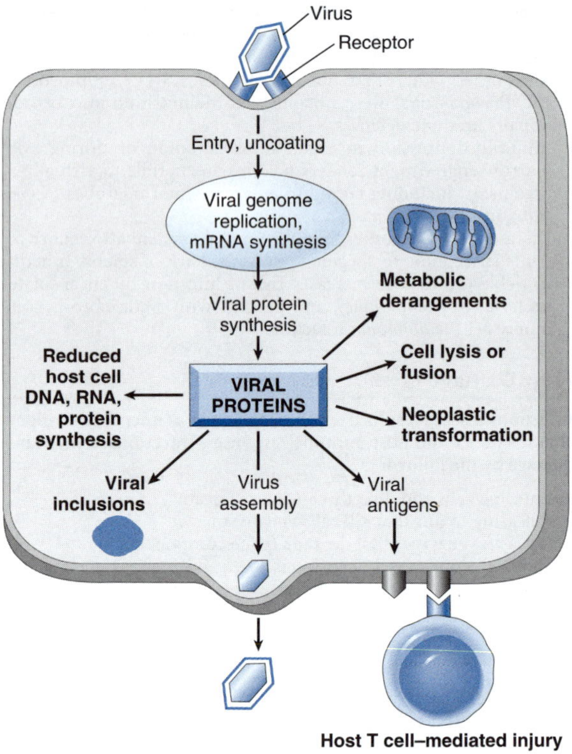

Figure 8-2 Mechanisms by which viruses can cause cellular injury.

- Virulence genes are frequently clustered together in the microbe genome as *pathogenicity islands.*
- Plasmids and bacteriophages are mobile genetic elements that can encode and transfer virulence factors between different bacteria (e.g., toxins or antibiotic resistance).
- In large microbial populations, virulence factor expression may be coordinated by the secretion of peptides that turn on specific genes in the population, a process called *quorum sensing.*
- Communities of bacteria—particularly in association with artificial surfaces (e.g., catheters and artificial joints)—can form *biofilms,* where the organisms live within a viscous polysaccharide "slime" that facilitates adhesion and also frustrates attempts at immune cell clearance or antibiotic permeation.

Bacterial Adherence to Host Cells (p. 349)

Bacterial *adhesins* are surface molecules that bind to specific host cells or matrix; besides being the first step in infection, adhesin specificities can also influence tissue tropisms.

Pili are filamentous bacterial surface proteins that can also mediate adhesion. In addition, these can be targeted by immune responses; pilus variation is a mechanism used by *Neisseria gonorrhoeae* to escape immune clearance.

Virulence of Intracellular Bacteria (p. 350)

Intracellular bacteria can kill host cells by rapid replication and lysis (*Shigella* and *Escherichia coli*). Alternatively, they may permit continued host cell viability while evading intracellular defenses and proliferating within endosomes *(M. tuberculosis)* or cytoplasm *(Listeria monocytogenes)*.

Bacterial Toxins (p. 350)

Bacterial toxins may be either endotoxins (intrinsic components of the cell wall) or exotoxins (secreted by the bacteria).

- *Endotoxin* (lipopolysaccharide [LPS]) is a cell wall component of gram-negative bacteria composed of a common long-chain fatty acid (lipid A) and a variable carbohydrate chain (O antigen). Low doses of the lipid A component elicit protective inflammatory cell recruitment and cytokine production. However, higher doses contribute to septic shock, disseminated intravascular coagulation, and adult respiratory distress syndrome.
- *Exotoxins* damage host tissues by several mechanisms:
  - Enzymes destroy tissue integrity by digesting structural proteins
  - Exotoxins alter intracellular signaling; a number of exotoxins have a binding (B) subunit that delivers a toxic active (A) component into the cell cytoplasm, where it modifies signaling pathways to cause cell dysfunction or death (e.g., in diptheria, anthrax, or cholera).
  - Neurotoxins that block neurotransmitter release, causing paralysis (e.g., in botulism and tetanus).
  - Superantigens stimulate large numbers of T cells by linking T-cell receptors with class II MHC molecules on antigen-presenting cells; the result is massive T-cell proliferation and cytokine release (e.g., toxic shock syndrome due to *S. aureus*).

Sexually Transmitted Infections (p. 351, and see Chapters 21 and 22) (Table 8-2)

- Groups at greater risk for sexually transmitted infections (STIs) include adolescents, men who have sex with men, and intravenous drug users. STIs in children, unless acquired during birth, suggest sexual abuse.
- STI transmission requires direct person-to-person contact because the pathogens do not survive in the environment; transmission often occurs from asymptomatic persons.
- Infection with one STI-associated organism increases the risk for additional STIs; this is because the risk factors are the same, and mucosal injury facilitates coinfection by multiple agents.
- STI in pregnancy can be spread to the fetus either in utero or at delivery, resulting in severe damage.

Spectrum of Inflammatory Responses to Infection (p. 351)

Although microbes have impressive molecular diversity, tissue responses to them follow five basic histologic patterns (see later; Table 8-3). Important caveats are as follows:

- Similar patterns can occur secondary to physical or chemical injury or in primary inflammatory disorders.
- Different types of host reactions often occur at the same time due to overlapping infections or processes.
- The same microbe can cause different patterns in different patients due to host idiosyncratic responses (e.g., granulomas in patients exhibiting *tuberculoid leprosy* and tissue necrosis in patients exhibiting *lepromatous leprosy*).

Suppurative (Purulent) Inflammation *(p. 352)*

Suppurative (purulent) inflammation is usually caused by pyogenic bacteria, mostly extracellular gram-positive cocci and gram-negative rods.

TABLE 8-2 Classification of Important Sexually Transmitted Diseases

Pathogens	Disease or Syndrome and Population Principally Affected		
	Males	*Females*	*Both*
Viruses			
HSV			Primary and recurrent herpes, neonatal herpes
HBV			Hepatitis
Human papillomavirus	Cancer of penis (some cases)	Cervical dysplasia and cancer, vulvar cancer	Condyloma acuminatum
HIV	AIDS		
Chlamydiae			
C. trachomatis	Urethritis, epididymitis, proctitis	Urethral syndrome, cervicitis, bartholinitis, salpingitis and sequelae	Lymphogranuloma venereum
Mycoplasmas			
Ureaplasma urealyticum	Urethritis		
Bacteria			
N. gonorrhoeae	Epididymitis, prostatitis, urethral stricture	Cervicitis, endometritis, bartholinitis, salpingitis, and sequelae (infertility, ectopic pregnancy, recurrent salpingitis)	Urethritis, proctitis, pharyngitis, disseminated gonococcal infection
T. pallidum			Syphilis
H. ducreyi			Chancroid
K. granulomatis			Granuloma inguinale (donovanosis)
Protozoa			
Trichomonas vaginalis	Urethritis, balanitis	Vaginitis	

- Increased vascular permeability and neutrophil recruitment by bacterial chemoattractants.
- Lesions vary from tiny microabscesses to entire lung lobes; these may resolve without sequelae (pneumococcal pneumonia) or may scar *(Klebsiella)*.

Mononuclear and Granulomatous Inflammation (p. 352)

Mononuclear and granulomatous inflammations are patterns typical for viruses, intracellular bacteria, spirochetes, intracellular parasites, and helminths.

- The cell type that predominates depends on the host response to a particular pathogen: plasma cells in chancres of primary syphilis, lymphocytes in viral infections of the brain, or macrophages in *Myobacterium avium-intracellulare* infections of AIDS patients.
- Granulomatous inflammation, characterized by accumulation of activated macrophages, occurs with resistant organisms that evoke a strong T-cell response *(M. tuberculosis)*.

TABLE 8-3 Spectrum of Inflammatory Responses to Infection

Type of Response	Pathogenesis	Examples
Suppurative (Purulent) Infection	Increased vascular permeability Leukocyte infiltration (neutrophils) Chemoattractants from bacteria Formation of "pus"	Staphylococcal pneumonia Tissue abscesses
Mononuclear and granulomatous inflammation	Mononuclear cell infiltrates (monocytes, macrophages, plasma cells, lymphocytes) Cell-mediated immune response to pathogens ("persistent antigen") Formation of granulomata	Syphilis Tuberculosis
Cytopathic-cytoproliferative reactions	Viral transformation of cells Necrosis or proliferation (including multinucleation) Linked to neoplasia	Human papillomavirus herpesvirus
Tissue necrosis	Toxin- or lysis-mediated destruction Lack of inflammatory cells Rapidly progressive processes	*C. perfringens* Hepatitis B
Chronic inflammation or scarring	Repetitive injury leads to fibrosis Loss of normal parenchyma	Chronic hepatitis (cirrhosis)
No reaction	Severe immune compromise	*M. avium* in untreated AIDS (T-cell deficiency) Mucormycosis in bone marrow transplant patients (neutropenia)

Cytopathic-Cytoproliferative Reaction (p. 353)

Cytopathic-cytoproliferative reaction usually occurs in viral infections; there is cell proliferation and necrosis with sparse inflammation.

- Other features include inclusion bodies (herpesevirus), fused cells (measles viruses), blisters (herpesviruses), or warty excrescences (papillomaviruses).

Tissue Necrosis (p. 353)

Tissue necrosis is caused by rampant viral infections (fulminant HBV infection), secreted bacterial toxins *(Clostridium perfringens)*, or direct protozoan cytolysis of host cells *(Entamoeba histolytica);* there is severe tissue necrosis in the absence of inflammation.

Chronic Inflammation and Scarring (p. 353)

Outcomes range from complete healing to scarring; excessive scarring can cause dysfunction. Inflammation can be severe despite a paucity of organisms *(M. tuberculosis)*.

Special Techniques for Diagnosing Infectious Agents (p. 353)

Some infectious agents can be directly observed in routine hematoxylin and eosin-stained sections (e.g., CMV inclusion bodies,

Candida and *Mucor*, most protozoans, and all helminths). However, most microbes are best visualized after special stains that take advantage of particular cell wall characteristics. Cultures of fluids or lesional tissues may be performed to speciate organisms and to determine drug sensitivity. Antibody titers to specific pathogens can also be used to diagnose infection; IgM antibodies suggest an acute infection, whereas IgG antibodies suggest something more remote. Nucleic acid amplification tests are used to diagnose *M. tuberculosis*, *Neisseria gonnorrhoeae*, and *Chlamydia trachomatis* and to quantify HIV, HBV, and HCV to monitor response to treatment.

Viral Infections (p. 354; Table 8-4)

Viral infections can be transient, chronic latent, or chronic productive or can promote cellular transformation and malignancy.

TABLE 8-4 Selected Human Viruses and Viral Diseases

Organ System	Species	Disease
Respiratory	Adenovirus	Upper and lower respiratory tract infections, conjunctivitis, diarrhea
	Rhinovirus	Upper respiratory tract infection
	Influenza viruses A, B	Influenza
	Respiratory syncytial virus	Bronchiolitis, pneumonia
Digestive	Mumps virus	Mumps, pancreatitis, orchitis
	Rotavirus	Childhood gastroenteritis
	Norovirus	Gastroenteritis
	Hepatitis A virus	Acute viral hepatitis
	Hepatitis B virus	Acute or chronic hepatitis
	Hepatitis D virus	With HBV, acute or chronic hepatitis
	Hepatitis C virus	Acute or chronic hepatitis
	Hepatitis E virus	Enterically transmitted hepatitis
Systemic with skin eruptions	Measles virus	Measles (rubeola)
	Rubella virus	German measles (rubella)
	VZV	Chickenpox, shingles
	HSV-1	Oral herpes ("cold sore")
	HSV-2	Genital herpes
Systemic with hematopoietic disorders	CMV	CID
	EBV	Infectious mononucleosis
	HIV-1 and HIV-2	AIDS
Arboviral and hemorrhagic fevers	Dengue virus 1-4	Dengue hemorrhagic fever
	Yellow fever virus	Yellow fever
Skin or genital warts	Papillomavirus	Condyloma; cervical carcinoma
CNS	Poliovirus	Poliomyelitis
	JC virus	Progressive multifocal leukoencephalopathy (opportunistic)

Acute (Transient) Infections (p. 354)

Viruses that cause transient infections are structurally heterogeneous, but each elicits an immune response that effectively eliminates the virus.

Measles (p. 355)

Measles is an RNA paramyxovirus transmitted by respiratory droplets; it is a leading cause of vaccine-preventable morbidity and mortality worldwide.

- Initial replication is within upper respiratory epithelial cells, with subsequent spread to local lymphoid tissue and then systemically.
- Ulcerated oral mucosal lesions near Stensen ducts form pathognomonic *Koplik spots.* There is marked lymphoid follicular and germinal center hyperplasia, with pathognomonic multinucleated giant cells with eosinophilic inclusion bodies, called *Warthin-Finkeldey cells* (also seen in lungs and sputum).
- Infection can cause croup, pneumonia, diarrhea, keratitis (with scarring and blindness), and encephalitis.
- T cell–mediated responses control the initial infection; the characteristic measles rash is due to hypersensitivity to measles-infected cutaneous cells. Antibody-mediated immunity protects against reinfection.
- Subacute sclerosing panencephalitis and inclusion body encephalitis (in immunocompromised individuals) are rare late complications.

Mumps (p. 355)

Mumps is a paramyxovirus spread by respiratory droplets.

- Initial replication is in lymph nodes draining the upper respiratory tract, followed by hematogenous spread to salivary glands and other sites.
- Infection of salivary gland ductal epithelium leads to desquamation, edema, and inflammation and thus the classic salivary gland swelling and pain.
- Spread can also occur to testes, ovary, pancreas, and central nervous system (CNS); aseptic meningitis is the most common extrasalivary gland complication (10% of infections).
- In mumps orchitis, swelling contained within the tunica albuginea can compromise the vascular supply and cause infarction.

Poliovirus Infection (p. 356)

Poliovirus infection is a spherical, unencapsulated RNA enterovirus transmitted by the fecal-oral route; other enteroviruses cause diarrhea and rashes (coxsackievirus A), conjunctivitis (enterovirus 70), meningitis (coxsackievirus and echovirus), and myopericarditis (coxsackievirus B).

- The virus infects via CD155, a surface molecule not present in other species; there are no nonhuman reservoirs.
- Multiplication in intestinal mucosa and lymph nodes is followed by a transient viremia and fever; nervous system involvement may occur by systemic viremia or retrograde transport via motor neurons. Antiviral antibodies control the disease.
- Although usually asymptomatic, poliovirus invades the CNS in 1 of 100 infected persons, replicating in motor neurons of the spinal cord (causing muscular paralysis) or brain stem *(bulbar poliomyelitis).*

West Nile Virus (p. 356)

West Nile virus is an arthropod-borne flavivirus *(arbovirus);* the group also includes the pathogens causing dengue and yellow fever. It is transmitted by mosquitos (birds being the major viral reservoir) but has also been transmitted by transfusion, organ transplant, and breast milk and transplacentally.

- Initial replication occurs in skin dendritic cells, which carry virus to lymph nodes for further expansion; subsequent hematogenous spread can lead to CNS neuronal infection. Rare complications include hepatitis, myocarditis, or pancreatitis. Immunosuppressed and elderly individuals are at greatest risk.
- CNS complications (meningitis, encephalitis, meningoencephalitis) develop in approximately 1 of 150 clinically apparent infections. Meningoencephalitis carries a 10% mortality rate; survivors can have long-term cognitive and neurologic impairment.

Viral Hemorrhagic Fever (p. 357)

Viral hemorrhagic fever (e.g., Ebola, Marburg, and Lassa) is a systemic infection caused by enveloped RNA viruses from four different families (arenaviruses, filoviruses, bunyaviruses, and flaviviruses).

- Transmission occurs through contact with infected insects or animals. Consequently, the viruses are normally geographically restricted to their hosts' habitat; humans are not the natural reservoir but can often transmit infection to other humans.
- Manifestations range from mild, acute disease (fever, headache, rash, myalgia, neutropenia, and thrombocytopenia) to severe, life-threatening hemodynamic deterioration and shock.
- Most of these viruses infect endothelial cells and thus hemorrhagic manifestations can be secondary to endothelial or platelet dysfunction. However, macrophage and dendritic cell infection can also result in profound cytokine release.

Latent Infections (Herpesvirus Infections) (p. 357)

Latency is defined as the persistence of viral genomes that do not produce infectious virus. Subsequent dissemination and/or tissue injury stem from reactivation of the latent virus. There are eight types of human herpesvirus (HHV), which are large, encapsulated double-stranded DNA viruses; three subgroups are defined by the most common infected cell and the site of latency.

- α-Group infects epithelium and produces latent infections of neurons (herpes simplex virus [HSV]-1, HSV-2, and varicella-zoster virus [VZV]).
- β-Group infects lymphocytes and can be latent in a variety of cell types (CMV, HHV-6 and -7).
- γ-Group causes latency in lymphoid cells (EBV and KSHV/HHV-8).

Herpes Simplex Viruses (p. 357)

HSV replicate in skin and mucous membranes at the site of initial inoculation (usually oropharynx or genitals), causing vesicular lesions.

- After epithelial infection, viruses spread to associated sensory neurons and then by retrograde axonal transport to the sensory neuron ganglia to establish latent infections. During reactivation, virus spreads from regional ganglia back to skin or mucous membranes.
- HSV lesions range from self-limited cold sores and gingivostomatitis (HSV-1) to genital sores (mainly HSV-2) to life-threatening

disseminated visceral infections (hepatitis and bronchopneumonitis) and encephalitis.

- HSV-1 is also the major infectious cause of corneal blindness in the United States. *Herpes epithelial keratitis* reflects virus-induced cytolysis of the superficial corneal epithelium. *Herpes stromal keratitis* results in mononuclear cell infiltrates around keratinocytes and endothelial cells; subsequent neovascularization, scarring, and corneal opacification leads to blindness.
- Classic HSV lesions include large, pink-purple, virion-containing intranuclear inclusions *(Cowdry type A inclusions)*, as well as inclusion-bearing multinucleated syncytia.

Varicella-Zoster Virus *(p. 358)*

VZV is transmitted by aerosols, disseminates hematogenously, and causes widespread vesicular skin lesions. Acute VZV infection causes *chickenpox;* reactivation of latent VZV causes *shingles* (or *herpes zoster*).

- Like HSV, VZV infects mucous membranes, skin, and neurons, establishing a latent infection in sensory ganglia.
- Shingles occurs when latent VZV in dorsal root ganglia reactivates, infecting sensory nerves that carry viruses to the skin and causing painful vesicular lesions, typically in a dermatomal distribution.
- VZV can also cause interstitial pneumonia, encephalitis, transverse myelitis, and necrotizing visceral lesions, particularly in immunocompromised hosts.
- Skin lesions evolve rapidly from macules to vesicles, classically resembling "a dew drop on a rose petal." Histologically vesicles contain epithelial cell blisters and intranuclear inclusions similar to HSV.

Cytomegalovirus *(p. 359)*

CMV is carried in breast milk, respiratory droplets, blood, and saliva and can have transplacental ("congenital"), venereal, fecal-oral, transfusion, or organ transplantation modes of transmission.

- Infections are usually asymptomatic in immunocompetent hosts but can manifest as a *mononucleosis-like syndrome* (fever, atypical lymphocytosis, lymphadenopathy, and hepatosplenomegaly). CMV can infect dendritic cells and cause transient but severe immunosuppression; viruses remain latent in leukocytes.
- In immunosuppressed patients, CMV can cause life-threatening colitis or pneumonitis; hepatitis, chorioretinitis, and meningoencephalitis are also significant morbidities. CMV is the most common opportunistic viral pathogen in AIDS.
- Although 95% of congenitally infected infants are asymptomatic, CMV can produce *cytomegalic inclusion disease (CID);* manifestations are similar to erythroblastosis fetalis and include intrauterine growth retardation, hemolytic anemia, jaundice, and encephalitis. Infants who survive usually have permanent deficits including deafness and mental retardation.
- CMV infection causes marked cellular enlargement, with characteristic large intranuclear inclusions surrounded by a clear halo, and smaller basophilic cytoplasmic inclusions.

Chronic Productive Infections (p. 360)

In some infections the immune system cannot eliminate the virus, resulting in persistent viremia. High mutation rates (e.g., in HIV and HBV) may be a mechanism to evade the immune system. HIV is covered in Chapter 6; HBV is discussed in Chapter 18.

Transforming Viral Infections (p. 360)

These are viruses implicated in causing human cancer (see also Chapter 7).

Epstein-Barr Virus *(p. 360)*

EBV infections occur through close contact, including saliva, blood, or venereal transmission.

- EBV infection begins in nasopharyngeal and oropharyngeal epithelial cells, followed by infection of B cells in underlying lymphoid tissues; virus binds to CD21, the complement C3d receptor.
- In a minority of infected B cells, EBV has a productive lytic infection, releasing more virions. In most cells, EBV establishes a latent infection via genes that can induce B-cell proliferation as well as production of nonspecific antibodies *(heterophile antibodies);* these antibodies can agglutinate sheep or horse erythrocytes in the laboratory (allowing a presumptive EBV diagnosis) but do not react with EBV.
- EBV causes *infectious mononucleosis,* a benign, self-limited disease characterized by fever, fatigue, sore throat, lymphocytosis, generalized lymphadenopathy, and splenomegaly; hepatitis and rash can also occur. Symptoms are secondary to the host immune response:
  - CD8+ cytotoxic T cells (the *atypical lymphocytes* seen in the blood) recognize and lyse EBV-infected B cells.
  - Reactive proliferation of these T cells leads to lymphadenopathy and splenomegaly.
- Persistence of EBV in a small population of latently infected cells can result in late reactivation and B-cell proliferation. In immunocompromised individuals, EBV is associated with B-cell lymphoma (see Chapter 13); EBV also contributes to some cases of *Burkitt lymphoma.*

Bacterial Infections (p. 362; Table 8-5)

Gram-Positive Bacterial Infections (p. 362)

Staphylococcal Infections *(p. 362)*

Staphylococcal infections are distinctive for local destructiveness; the organisms are pyogenic (pus-forming) cocci that grow in clusters.

- *S. aureus* cause a variety of skin infections *(boils, carbuncles, impetigo),* osteomyelitis, pneumonia, endocarditis, food poisoning, and toxic shock syndrome.
- Less virulent staphylococci cause opportunistic infections in intravenous drug abusers, and in patients with catheters or prosthetic heart valves *(Staphylococcus epidermidis); Staphylococcus saprophyticus* is a common cause of urinary tract infections.
- Virulence factors include the following:
  - Surface proteins that allow host cell adherence
  - Enzymes that degrade host proteins, promoting invasion and tissue destruction
  - Toxins that damage host cell membranes *(hemolysins)* or induce skin sloughing (exfoliative toxins), vomiting (enterotoxins), or shock (superantigens)

TABLE 8-5 Selected Human Bacterial Pathogens and Associated Diseases

Organ System	Species	Frequent Disease Presentations
Respiratory	*S. pyogenes*	Pharyngitis
	Corynebacterium diphtheriae	Diphtheria
	B. pertussis	Pertussis
	S. pneumoniae	Lobar pneumonia
	M. tuberculosis	Tuberculosis
	Legionella pneumophila	Legionnaire disease
GI	*H. pylori*	Peptic ulcers
	Vibrio cholerae, enterotoxigenic *E. coli*	Noninflammatory gastroenteritis
	Shigella species, *Salmonella* species, *Campylobacter jejuni*, enterohemorrhagic *E. coli*	Inflammatory gastroenteritis
	Salmonella typhi	Enteric (typhoid) fever
	C. difficile	Pseudomembranous colitis
Nervous system	*N. meningitidis, S. pneumoniae, H. influenza, L. monocytogenes*	Acute meningitis
	C. tetani, C. botulinum	Paralytic intoxications, tetanus and botulism
Urogenital	*E. coli, P. aeruginosa, Enterococcus* species	Urinary tract infections
	N. gonorrhoeae	Gonorrhea
	C. trachomatis	Chlamydia
	T. pallidum	Syphilis
Skin and adjacent soft tissue	*S. aureus*	Abscess, cellulitis
	S. pyogenes	Impetigo, erysipelas, necrotizing fasciitis
	C. perfringens	Gas gangrene
	B. anthracis	Cutaneous anthrax
	P. aeruginosa	Burn infections
	M. leprae	Leprosy
Disseminated infections	*Y. pestis*	Plague
	B. burgdorferi	Lyme disease
	Brucella species	Brucellosis (undulant fever)
Disseminated neonatal infection	*S. agalactiae, L. monocytogenes*	Neonatal bacteremia, meningitis
	T. pallidum	Congenital syphilis

- Antibiotic resistance is a growing problem with *S. aureus* infections; methicillin-resistant *S. aureus* (MRSA) can now be a virulent community-acquired infection.

Streptococcal and Enterococcal Infections (p. 364)

Streptococcal and enterococcal infections are cocci that grow in pairs or chains. The streptococci are classified by their pattern of hemolysis on blood agar: β (complete or clear hemolysis), α (partial or green hemolysis), and γ (no hemolysis, rarely pathogenic).

- β-Hemolytic streptococci are grouped by their carbohydrate (Lancefield) antigens:
  - Group A *(Streptococcus pyogenes)* causes pharyngitis, scarlet fever, erysipelas, impetigo, rheumatic fever, toxic shock syndrome, necrotizing fasciitis, and glomerulonephritis.

- Group B *(Streptococcus agalactiae)* colonizes the female genital tract and causes chorioamnionitis in pregnancy, as well as neonatal sepsis and meningitis.

- α-Hemolytic streptococci include *S. pneumoniae,* a common cause of adult community-acquired pneumonia and meningitis.
- Viridans-group includes both α- and γ-hemolytic streptococci that are normal oral flora but are common causes of endocarditis; *Streptococcus mutans* is the major cause of dental caries (metabolizes sucrose to lactic acid which demineralizes tooth enamel).
- *Enterococci* cause endocarditis and urinary tract infections; many are antibiotic resistant.
- Streptococcal virulence factors include the following:
    - Capsules that resist phagocytosis (*S. pyogenes* and *S. pneumoniae*).
    - *M proteins* that inhibit complement activation *(S. pyogenes).*
    - Exotoxins that cause fever and rash *(S. pyogenes)* in scarlet fever.
    - *Pneumolysin* destroys host-cell membranes and damages tissue *(S. pneumoniae).*
- Enterococci have an antiphagocytic capsule and produce enzymes that degrade host tissues.
- Streptococcal infections are characterized by diffuse interstitial neutrophilic infiltrates with minimal host tissue destruction (except for some virulent strains of *S. pyogenes* that cause a rapidly progressive fasciitis and have been dubbed "flesh-eating bacteria").

Diphtheria *(p. 365)*

Diphtheria is caused by *Corynebacterium diptheriae,* a slender gram-positive rod with clubbed ends; it is passed as an aerosol or through skin exudates.

- Diphtheria is a life-threatening disease characterized by an oropharyngeal fibrinosuppurative exudate; *C. diphtheriae* growth in this membrane elaborates an exotoxin that injures heart, nerves, and other organs.
- Diphtheria toxin is a phage-encoded two-part (A-B) toxin that blocks host protein synthesis. The B fragment binds to the cell surface and facilitates entry of the A subunit; the A subunit blocks protein synthesis by adenosine diphosphate (ADP) ribosylation (and inactivation) of elongation factor-2.

Listeriosis *(p. 366)*

L. monocytogenes is a gram-positive, facultative intracellular bacillus causing severe foodborne infections.

- *Listeria* causes sepsis and meningitis in elderly and immunosuppressed people and placental infections in pregnant women with consequent neonatal infections.
- *L. monocytogenes* express leucine-rich proteins called *internalins* that bind epithelial E-cadherin and promote internalization; the bacillus then uses listeriolysin O and two phospholipases to degrade the phagolysosome membrane and escape into the cytoplasm.
- In the cytoplasm a bacterial protein (ActA) induces actin polymerization to propel the bacteria into adjacent cells.
- Resting macrophages internalize but do not kill *Listeria;* macrophages activated by interferon-γ effectively phagocytize and kill the bacterium.
- *L. monocytogenes* evokes exudative inflammation with numerous neutrophils.

Anthrax (p. 366)

Bacillus anthracis is a spore-forming, gram-positive bacillus prevalent in animals having contact with spore-contaminated soil.

- Humans contract anthrax through exposure to contaminated animal products or powdered spores (a biologic weapon).
- Three major anthrax syndromes are known; in all cases, lesions are characterized by necrosis with neutrophil and macrophage exudates:
  - *Cutaneous:* Painless, pruritic papules that become edematous vesicles followed by a black eschar
  - *Inhalation:* Rapidly leads to sepsis, shock, and frequently death
  - *GI:* Contracted by eating contaminated meat; causes severe, bloody diarrhea and often death
- Anthrax toxin is composed of a B subunit involved in toxin endocytosis and A subunits of two different types:
  - *Edema factor* converts adenosine triphosphate (ATP) to cyclic adenosine monophosphate (cAMP), which causes cellular water efflux.
  - *Lethal factor* is a protease that causes cell death by destroying mitogen-activated protein kinase kinases.

Nocardia (p. 367)

Nocardia are aerobic, gram-positive bacteria growing in branched chains; they also stain with modified acid-fast protocols (Fite-Faraco stain).

- *Nocardia* are found in soil and cause opportunistic infections in immunocompromised hosts.
- *Nocardia asteroides* causes indolent respiratory infections often with CNS dissemination; *Nocardia brasiliensis* infects the skin.
- *Nocardia* elicit suppurative responses, surrounded by granulation tissue and fibrosis.

Gram-Negative Bacterial Infections (p. 367)

Neisserial Infections (p. 368)

Neisserial infections are caused by aerobic, gram-negative diplococci; they usually have stringent in vitro growth requirements (e.g., sheep blood-enriched ["chocolate"] agar).

- *N. meningitidis* is an important cause of bacterial meningitis, particularly in children younger than age 2; there are 13 different serotypes.
  - Bacteria colonize the oropharynx (10% of the population is colonized at any one time) and are spread by respiratory droplets.
  - Meningitis occurs when people encounter serotypes to which they are not previously immune (e.g., in military barracks or college dormitories).
- *Neisseria gonorrhoeae* is the second most common sexually transmitted bacterial infection in the United States (after *Chlamydia*).
  - In males it causes symptomatic urethritis; in women it is often asymptomatic and can lead to pelvic inflammatory disease, infertility, and ectopic pregnancy.
  - Disseminated adult infections cause septic arthritis and hemorrhagic rash.
  - Neonatal infections cause blindness and, rarely, sepsis.

- Virulence factors include a capsule that inhibits opsonization and antigenic variation to escape the immune response:
  - Adhesive pili undergo genetic recombination.
  - Outer membrane adhesive OPA proteins (so-called because they make colonies opaque) undergo 5-nucleotide frameshifts.
  - Host defects in complement lead to more severe infections.

Pertussis *(p. 368)*

Pertussis is caused by *Bordetella pertussis,* a gram-negative coccobacillus; it is a highly communicable illness characterized by paroxysms of violent coughing (whooping cough). The incidence has increased in recent years with epidemics in 2005, 2010, and 2012, potentially due to a less-effective acellular vaccine.

- Coordinated expression of virulence factors is regulated by the *Bordetella* virulence gene *(bvg)* locus:
  - Hemagglutinin binds to respiratory epithelium carbohydrates and macrophage Mac-1 integrins.
  - Pertussis toxin ADP ribosylates and inactivates guanine nucleotide-binding proteins; G proteins cannot transduce signals, and bronchial epithelium cilia are paralyzed.
- Infection causes laryngotracheobronchitis with mucosal erosion, and mucopurulent exudates associated with striking peripheral lymphocytosis.

Pseudomonas Infection *(p. 369)*

Pseudomonas infection is due to *Pseudomonas aeruginosa,* an opportunistic aerobic, gram-negative bacillus.

- This pathogen is frequently seen in patients with cystic fibrosis, burns, or neutropenia and is a common hospital-acquired infection. It also causes corneal keratitis in contact wearers and external otitis (swimmer's ear) in normal hosts.
- Virulence factors include the following:
  - Pili and adherence proteins that bind to epithelial cells and lung mucin.
  - Endotoxin that cause gram-negative sepsis and disseminated intravascular coagulation.
  - Exotoxin A that inhibits protein synthesis by the same mechanism as diphtheria toxin.
  - Phospholipase C that lyses red cells and degrades surfactant, and an elastase that degrades IgG and extracellular matrix (ECM).
  - Iron-containing compounds that are toxic to endothelium.
  - In patients with cystic fibrosis the organism secretes an exopolysaccharide (alginate) that forms a slimy biofilm that protects bacteria from antibodies, complement, phagocytes, and antibiotics.
- *Pseudomonas* pneumonia can cause extensive tissue necrosis by vascular invasion with subsequent thrombosis. Skin infections give rise to well-demarcated necrotic and hemorrhagic skin lesions, *ecthyma gangrenosum.*

Plague *(p. 370)*

Yersinia is a gram-negative, facultative intracellular bacterium with three clinically important species:

- *Yersinia pestis* causes plague; it is transmitted from rodents to humans by aerosols or fleabites.

- *Yersinia enterocolitica* and *Yersinia pseudotuberculosis* cause fecal-oral transmitted ileitis and mesenteric lymphadenitis.
- *Yersinia* proliferate in lymphoid tissues; virulence factors include the following:
    - *Yersinia* toxins (called *Yops*) that are injected into host phagocytes by a syringelike mechanism; the toxins block phagocytosis and cytokine production.
    - A biofilm that obstructs the flea GI tract, forcing it to regurgitate before feeding and thus ensuring infection.
- Plague causes massive lymph node enlargement *(buboes)*, pneumonia, and sepsis, with massive bacterial proliferation, tissue necrosis, and neutrophilic infiltrates.

Chancroid (Soft Chancre) *(p. 370)*

Chancroid (soft chancre) is an acute, venereal, ulcerative genital infection caused by *Haemophilus ducreyi,* most common in Africa and Southeast Asia; the ulcerations probably serve as important cofactors in HIV transmission.

Granuloma Inguinale *(p. 370)*

Granuloma inguinale is a sexually transmitted disease caused by *Klebsiella granulomatis,* a minute, encapsulated coccobacillus.

- Infection begins as a papule on the genitalia or extragenital sites (oral mucosa or pharynx) that ulcerates and granulates to form a soft, painless mass, with prominent epithelial hyperplasia at the borders.
- Left untreated, the lesion may scar and cause urethral, vulvar, or anal strictures; it is also associated with lymphatic scarring and lymphedema of the external genitalia.

Mycobacteria (p. 371)

Mycobacteria are aerobic bacilli that grow in chains and have a waxy cell wall composed of mycolic acid; the cell wall retains certain dyes after acid treatment (hence the name *acid-fast bacilli*).

Tuberculosis *(p. 371)*

Tuberculosis is caused by *M. tuberculosis;* it affects over one billion people worldwide and kills 1.4 million people annually. There are approximately 10,000 new cases of tuberculosis in the United States annually, mostly in immigrant, homeless, jailed, or HIV-infected individuals. It is transmitted person to person as an aerosol and increasingly is multidrug resistant.

- *Infection* represents only the presence of organisms and in most cases does not cause clinical *disease.*
- *M. tuberculosis* secretes no toxins, and its virulence is based on the properties of its cell wall.
- Host recognition of tuberculosis organisms involves multiple innate pathogen-associated molecular patterns (lipoproetins and glycolipids) triggering Toll-like receptors (TLR)-2 and -9.
- Outcomes of infection depend on host immunity (Fig. 8-3); responses can both control infections and contribute to the pathologic manifestations of disease:
    - Infection leads to the induction of a T_H1-mediated delayed hypersensitivity response (see Chapter 6) that activates macrophages (via interferon-γ) to the following:
        - Promote endocytosis and killing via nitric oxide (NO) and/or autophagy

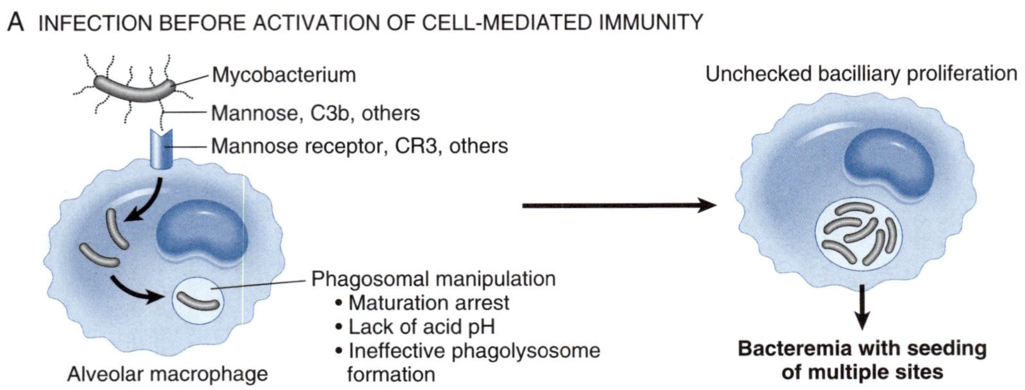

Figure 8-3 The sequence of events following inhalation of *M. tuberculosis* and the development of cell-mediated immunity. A, Events occurring during early infection, before activation of T cell–mediated immunity.

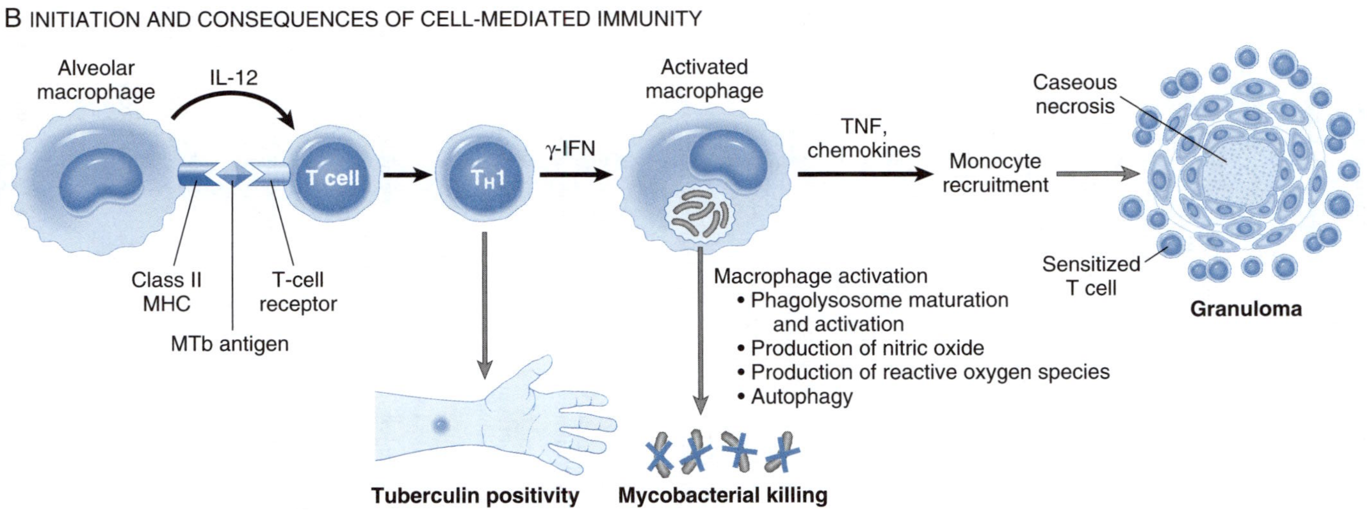

Figure 8-3, cont'd **B,** The generation and consequences of T cell–mediated immunity. Resistance to the organism corresponds to the appearance of a positive tuberculin test. *γ-IFN,* Interferon-γ; *MTB, M. tuberculosis.*

        - Promote cytocidal activity through tumor necrosis factor and defensin production
        - Surround microbes with granulomatous inflammation

    - *Caseating granulomas* are characteristic; central necrosis is surrounded by lymphocytes and activated macrophages.
    - T-cell immunity to mycobacteria can be detected by a tuberculin skin test (purified protein derivative [PPD]); the test signifies only prior T-cell sensitization to mycobacterial antigens and does not discriminate infection and disease.

- In most individuals (95%), primary infection is asymptomatic.
    - Granulomas formed in response to infection typically involve the lung apex and draining lymph node: these are called a *Ghon complex.*
    - Eventual control of the infection leaves behind only a small residua—a tiny fibrocalcific nodule at the site where viable organisms may remain within granulomas, dormant for decades.
- Five percent of primary infections are symptomatic, with lobar consolidation, hilar adenopathy, and pleural effusions.
    - Rarely, hematogenous spread leads to tuberculous meningitis and systemic *miliary tuberculosis.*
    - More than 50% of patients with severe immune deficiency will have extrapulmonary involvement.
- Secondary tuberculosis occurs in a previously exposed host, classically involving the lung apices.
    - If immunity wanes, the infection can reactivate to produce communicable disease with substantial morbidity and mortality.
    - Classically, because of prior T-cell sensitization, there is more tissue damage with apical pulmonary cavitation, and increased systemic manifestations with low-grade fever, night sweats, and weight loss.
- HIV is associated with an increased risk of tuberculosis, due to diminished T-cell immunity.
- Diagnosis of tuberculosis can be made by the following:
    - Identifying acid-fast bacilli in sputum or tissue
    - Culture from sputum or tissue (allows drug sensitivity testing)
    - Polymerase chain reaction (highly sensitive)

Mycobacterium Avium Complex *(p. 376)*

These common environmental bacteria cause widely disseminated infections in immunocompromised hosts characterized by abundant acid-fast organisms within macrophages.

Leprosy *(p. 377)*

Leprosy, also known as Hansen disease, is a slowly progressive infection caused by *Mycobacterium leprae;* it affects skin and peripheral nerves with resultant deformities.

- Inhaled *M. leprae* are phagocytized by pulmonary macrophages and disseminated hematogenously; however, they replicate only in cooler tissues of the periphery.
- *M. leprae* secretes no toxins, and its virulence is based on the properties of its cell wall.
- Leprosy has two patterns of disease (depending on the host immune response):
    - *Tuberculoid leprosy:* Associated with a T_H1 response (IFN-γ), with extensive granulomatous inflammation with few bacilli.

Clinically there are insidious, dry, scaly skin lesions lacking sensation, with asymmetric peripheral nerve involvement. Local anesthesia with skin and muscle atrophy increases the risk of trauma with chronic ulcers, and autoamputation of digits.
- *Lepromatous (anergic) leprosy:* Associated with a relatively ineffective T_H2 response, with large collections of lipid-laden macrophages overstuffed with bacilli. Clinically there are disfiguring cutaneous thickening and nodules, with nervous system damage due to mycobacterial invasion into perineural macrophages and Schwann cells. The testes are usually extensively involved leading to sterility.

Spirochetes (p. 378)

Spirochetes are gram-negative, corkscrew-shaped bacteria with flagella; an outer sheath membrane can mask bacterial antigens from host immune responses.

Syphilis (p. 378)

Syphilis is caused by *Treponema pallidum,* transmitted venereally or transplacentally (congenital syphilis). A T_H1 delayed-type hypersensitivity response with macrophage activation appears important in reining in the infection, but can also be the cause of disease manifestations (e.g., aortitis).

- *Primary syphilis* occurs about 3 weeks after contact:
  - A firm, nontender, raised, red lesion *(chancre)* forms on the penis, cervix, vaginal wall, or anus; this will heal even without therapy.
  - Treponemes are plentiful (visualizable with silver or immunofluorescent stains) at the chancre surface; there is an exudate composed of plasma cells, macrophages, and lymphocytes, with a proliferative endarteritis.
  - Treponemes spread lymphohematogenously throughout the body even before the chancre appears.
- *Secondary syphilis* occurs 2 to 10 weeks later in 75% of untreated patients, due to spread and proliferation of spirochetes in skin (including palms and soles) and mucocutaneous tissues (especially mouth).
  - Superficial lesions with erosions are painless and contain infectious spirochetes. Mucocutaneous lesions show plasma cell infiltrates and obliterative endarteritis.
  - Lymphadenopathy, mild fever, malaise, and weight loss are common.
- *Tertiary syphilis* occurs in one third of untreated patients, after a long latent period (>5 years).
  - Cardiovascular syphilis (>80% of tertiary syphilis) results in aortitis (due to endarteritis of the aortic vasa vasorum) with aortic root and arch aneurysms and aortic valve insufficiency.
  - Neurosyphilis can be symptomatic (meningovascular disease, *tabes dorsalis,* or diffuse brain parenchymal disease, so-called *general paresis*) or asymptomatic (cerebrospinal fluid [CSF] abnormalities only, with pleocytosis, increased protein, and decreased glucose).
  - "Benign" tertiary syphilis is associated with necrotic, rubbery masses (*gummas* due to delayed-type hypersensitivity to the organisms), which form in various sites (bone, skin, oral mucosa).
- *Congenital syphilis* usually occurs when the mother has primary or secondary syphilis.

- Intrauterine or perinatal death will occur in 50% of untreated cases.
- Early *(infantile)* congenital syphilis includes nasal discharge, a bullous rash with skin sloughing, hepatomegaly, and skeletal abnormalities (nose and lower legs are most distinctive). Diffuse lung or liver fibrosis can also occur.
- Late *(tardive)* manifestations include notched central incisors, deafness, and interstitial keratitis with blindness *(Hutchinson triad).*

- Serologic tests for syphilis:
  - Treponemal antibody tests measure antibodies reactive with *T. pallidum.*
  - Nontreponemal tests (venereal disease research laboratory [VDRL], rapid plasma reagin [RPR]) measure antibody to cardiolipin, a phospholipid in treponemes and normal tissues.
  - Both tests become positive approximately 6 weeks after infection but are only moderately sensitive (70% to 85%) for primary syphilis; they are >95% sensitive for secondary syphilis. Nontreponemal test may become negative with time or treatment, but treponemal antibody tests remain positive and are very sensitive for tertiary and latent syphilis.

Lyme Disease *(p. 381)*

Lyme disease is caused by *Borrelia burgdorferi* transmitted from rodents by *Ixodes* ticks; it is divided into three stages.

- *Stage 1 (weeks):* Spirochetes multiply at the site of the tick bite, causing an expanding erythema, often with a pale center *(erythema chronicum migrans),* fever, and lymphadenopathy.
- *Stage 2 (weeks to months):* Spirochetes spread hematogenously, causing secondary skin lesions, lymphadenopathy, migratory joint and muscle pain, cardiac arrhythmias, and meningitis.
- *Stage 3 (years):* Chronic and occasionally destructive arthritis; less commonly there is encephalitis and polyneuropathy.

B. burgdorferi evades antibody-mediated immunity through antigenic variation.

The bacterium does not make toxins; rather the pathology associated with infection is due to host immune responses. A distinctive feature of Lyme arthritis is an arteritis resembling that seen in lupus erythematosus.

Anaerobic Bacteria (p. 382)

These organisms normally reside in niches with low oxygen tension (intestine, vagina, oral recesses); they cause disease when they disproportionately expand (e.g., *Clostridium difficile* colitis following antibiotic treatment) or when introduced into sterile sites. Environmental anaerobes also cause disease (e.g., tetanus, botulism).

Abscesses Caused by Anaerobes *(p. 382)*

Abscesses caused by anaerobes usually contain two to three different species of mixed bacteria flora; for each aerobic or facultative bacterial species present, there are one to two anaerobic species. The usual culprits are commensal bacteria from adjacent sites (e.g., oropharynx, intestines, or female genital tract), so that "normal flora" are typically cultured from abscesses.

- In head and neck abscesses, *Prevotella* and *Porphyromonas* are the usual anaerobes, whereas *S. aureus* and *S. pyogenes* are typical facultative aerobes.

- In abdominal abscesses, *Bacteroides fragilis, Peptostreptococcus,* and *Clostridium* species are the common anaerobes, typically admixed with facultative *E. coli.*
- In genital tract abscesses in women, the anaerobes include *Prevotella* species, often mixed with facultative *E. coli* or *S. agalactiae.*
- Anaerobic abscesses are typically foul smelling and poorly circumscribed but otherwise pathologically resemble other pyogenic infections.

Clostridial Infections (p. 382)

Clostridial infections are due to gram-positive bacillus anaerobes that produce spores in the soil.

- *C. perfringens* and *Clostridium septicum* cause cellulitis and muscle necrosis in wounds *(gas gangrene),* food poisoning, and small bowel infection in ischemic or neutropenic patients.
  - *C. perfringens* secretes 14 toxins, the most important being α-toxin; this has multiple activities, including *phospholipase C* that degrades erythrocyte, muscle, and platelet cell membranes, and sphingomyelinase that causes nerve sheath damage.
  - *C. perfringens* enterotoxin lyses GI epithelial cells and disrupts tight junctions, causing diarrhea.
  - Gas gangrene exhibits marked edema and enzymatic necrosis of involved tissues; fermentation gas bubbles, hemolysis, and thrombosis with minimal inflammation are also characteristic.
- *Clostridium tetani* in wounds (or the umbilical stump of newborns) releases a neurotoxin (tetanospasmin) that causes *tetanus*—convulsive contractions of skeletal muscles—by blocking release of γ-aminobutyric acid, a neurotransmitter that inhibits motor neuron activity.
- *Clostridium botulinum* grows in canned foods; it releases a neurotoxin that causes flaccid paralysis of respiratory and skeletal muscles *(botulism)* by blocking acetylcholine release. Botulism toxin (Botox) is used in cosmetic surgery for its ability to paralyze strategically selected facial muscles.
- *C. difficile* overgrows other intestinal flora in antibiotic-treated patients and releases two glucosyl transferase toxins, causing *pseudomembranous colitis.*
  - Toxin A stimulates chemokine production to recruit leukocytes.
  - Toxin B (used for diagnosing *C. difficile* infections) causes cytopathic effects in cultured cells.

Obligate Intracellular Bacteria (p. 383)

Although some of these bacteria can survive in the extracellular environment, they can only proliferate within cells. They are well adapted to the intracellular environment with membrane transporters to capture amino acids and ATP.

Chlamydial Infections (p. 383)

Chlamydial infections are caused by small gram-negative bacteria; *C. trachomatis* exists in two forms:

- A metabolically inactive but infectious sporelike *elementary body* (EB). The EB is internalized by receptor-mediated endocytosis.
- Inside host cell endosomes the EB differentiates into the metabolically active *reticulate body* (RB); the RB replicates to form new EB for release.

Specific *C. trachomatis* diseases are caused by particular serotypes:

- *Trachoma,* an ocular infection of children (serotypes A, B, and C).

- Urogenital infections and conjunctivitis are caused by serotypes D through K. Chlamydia is the most common bacterial sexually transmitted infection in the world. Although frequently asymptomatic, urogenital infections can cause epididymitis, prostatitis, pelvic inflammatory disease, pharyngitis, conjunctivitis, perihepatic inflammation, and proctitis.
  - Infections exhibit a mucopurulent discharge containing neutrophils but no visible organisms by Gram stain.
  - The Centers for Disease Control and Prevention (CDC) recommends treating both *C. trachomatis* and *N. gonorrhoeae* when either is diagnosed, due to frequent coinfections.
- Lymphogranuloma venereum (serotypes L1, L2, and L3) is a sporadic genital infection in the United States and Western Europe; it is endemic in parts of Asia, Africa, the Caribbean, and South America.
  - Two to six weeks after infection, organism growth and host immune response in draining lymph nodes lead to painful adenopathy.
  - Lesions contain a mixed granulomatous and neutrophilic response with irregular foci of necrosis *(stellate abscesses);* chlamydial inclusions can be seen in epithelial or inflammatory cells.

Rickettsial Infections *(p. 384)*

Rickettsial infections are caused by gram-negative bacilli transmitted by arthropod vectors. They primarily infect endothelial cells, causing endothelial swelling, thrombosis, and vessel wall necrosis. Vascular thrombosis and increased permeability cause hypovolemic shock, pulmonary edema, and CNS manifestations. NK cell and cytotoxic T-cell responses are necessary to contain and eradicate infections.

- *Epidemic typhus (Rickettsia prowazekii)* is transmitted by body lice.
  - Lesions range from a rash with small hemorrhages to skin necrosis and gangrene with internal organ hemorrhages.
  - CNS typhus nodules show microglial proliferations with T-cell and macrophage infiltration.
- *Rocky Mountain spotted fever (Rickettsia rickettsii)* is transmitted by dog ticks.
  - A hemorrhagic rash extends over the entire body, including the palms of the hands and soles of the feet.
  - Vascular lesions in the CNS may involve larger vessels and produce microinfarcts.
  - Noncardiogenic pulmonary edema is the major cause of death.
- *Ehrlichiosis* is transmitted by ticks.
  - The bacteria predominantly infects neutrophils (*Anaplasma phagocytophilum* and *Ehrlichia ewingii*) or macrophages *(Ehrlichia chaffeensis)* with characteristic intracytoplasmic inclusions *(morulae).*
  - Infection is characterized by fever, headache, and malaise, progressing to respiratory insufficiency, renal failure, and shock.

Fungal Infections (p. 385)

Fungi are eukaryotes with cell walls. They grow as single cells or chains that typically propagate by budding *(yeasts)* or as multicelluar filaments that grow and divide at their tips *(molds); dimorphic fungi* assume a yeast form at body temperature and a mold form at room temperature.

Mycoses (fungal infections) include the following:

- *Superficial and cutaneous mycoses:* Common, limited to superficial keratinized layers of skin, hair, and nails
- *Subcutaneous mycoses:* Involve skin, subcutaneous tissues, and lymphatics and rarely disseminate
- *Endemic mycoses:* Caused by dimorphic fungi, capable of causing serious systemic illness in healthy individuals
- *Opportunistic mycoses:* Can cause life-threatening infections in immunocompromised hosts or in patients with vascular catheters or prosthetic devices

Yeast (p. 386)

Candidiasis (p. 386)

Candida species are part of the normal flora of the skin, mouth, and GI tract; they occur as yeast and pseudohyphal forms. *Candida* causes superficial infections in healthy individuals; disseminated visceral infections in neutropenic patients occur when skin or mucosal barriers are breached.

- *Candida* virulence factors include the following:
  - Adhesins that mediate binding to host cells
  - Enzymes that contribute to invasiveness
  - Catalases that aid intracellular survival by resisting phagocyte oxidative killing
  - Adenosine that blocks neutrophil degranulation and oxygen radical production
  - Ability to grow as biofilms on devices, thereby frustrating immune responses and antifungal agents
- Innate and T-cell responses are important for protection:
  - Neutrophil and macrophage phagocytosis and oxidative killing are the first-line defense; these are induced as a T_H17 response after *Candida* β-1,3-glucan engages Dectin-1 on dendritic cells and promotes interleukin (IL)-6 and IL-23 production.
  - Yeast forms induce a protective T_H1 response; filamentous forms tend to induce a nonprotective T_H2 response.
- *Candida* grows best on warm, moist surfaces; in healthy individuals it can cause vaginitis and diaper rash.
- Superficial infections of the mouth and vagina are most common, producing superficial curdy white patches; these are easily detached to reveal a reddened, irritated mucosa.
- Chronic mucocutaneous candidiasis occurs in persons with AIDS, with defective T-cell immunity, or with polyendocrine deficiencies (hypoparathyroidism, hypoadrenalism, and hypothyroidism).
- Severe, invasive candidiasis occurs via bloodborne dissemination in neutropenic persons; typically, microabscesses (with fungi in the center) are surrounded by areas of tissue necrosis.

Cryptococcosis (p. 387)

Cryptococcus neoformans is an encapsulated yeast; in tissues the capsule stains bright red with mucicarmine, and in CSF it is negatively stained with India ink.

- Virulence factors include the following:
  - A capsular polysaccharide (glucuronoxylomannan) inhibits phagocytosis, leukocyte migration, and inflammatory cell recruitment.

  - Regular alteration in the size and structure of the capsule polysaccharide allows immune evasion.
  - Laccase, an enzyme that induces formation of a melaninlike pigment with antioxidant properties.
  - Enzymes that degrade fibronectin and basement membrane proteins and aids in tissue invasion.

- In healthy individuals *C. neoformans* can form solitary pulmonary granulomata (with reactivation if immunity wanes) and rarely causes meningoencephalitis.
- It presents as an opportunistic infection in patients with AIDS, leukemia or lymphoid malignancies, lupus, sarcoidosis, or organ transplants, or those receiving high-dose corticosteroids. In such patients the major lesions involve the CNS, occurring as gray matter cysts ("soap bubble lesions"), occasionally with no inflammatory response.

Molds (p. 388)

Aspergillosis *(p. 388)*

Aspergillus (*fumigatus* is the most common species) is a ubiquitous mold transmitted by airborne conidia; it grows as septated hyphae branching at acute angles occasionally with spore-producing fruiting bodies. It causes allergy (allergic bronchopulmonary aspergillosis) in healthy individuals and severe sinusitis, pneumonia, and invasive disease in immunocompromised hosts.

- Neutrophils and macrophages are the major host defenses, killing by phagocytosis and reactive oxygen species. Macrophages recognize *Aspergillus* through TLR2 and Dectin-1. Neutropenia is a major risk factor.
- Virulence factors include the following:
  - Adhesion to albumin, surfactant, and a variety of ECM proteins
  - Antioxidant defenses, including melanin pigment, mannitol, catalases, and superoxide dismutase
  - Phospholipases, proteases, and toxins, including *aflatoxin* (synthesized by fungus growing on peanuts), a cause of liver cancer in Africa
- Preexisting pulmonary lesions caused by tuberculosis, bronchiectasis, old infarcts, or abscesses can develop secondary *Aspergillus* colonization *(aspergillomas)* without tissue invasion.
- Invasive aspergillosis in immunosuppressed hosts usually presents as necrotizing pneumonia (forming "target lesions") but often develops widespread hematogenous dissemination.
- *Aspergillus* tends to invade blood vessels with resulting thrombosis; consequently, areas of hemorrhage and infarction are superimposed on necrotizing inflammation.

Zygomycosis (Mucormycosis) *(p. 389)*

Zygomycosis (mucormycosis) is an opportunistic infection in neutropenic patients and diabetics caused by *Zygomycetes* molds (*Mucor, Absidia, Rhizopus,* and *Cunninghamella*). Zygomycetes are nonseptated with right-angle branching.

- The primary site of infection (nasal sinuses, lungs, or GI tract) depends on whether the spores are inhaled or ingested.
- Macrophages recognize *Mucor* via TLR2, yielding a proinflammatory cascade of IL-6 and tumor necrosis factor (TNF); neutrophils can kill hyphae after germination.

- Increased free iron increases *Mucor* growth; diabetes increases the probability of infection by increasing the availability of free iron through ketoacidosis.
- In diabetics, fungus may spread from nasal sinuses to the orbit or brain.
- These fungi commonly invade arterial walls and cause necrosis.

Dimorphic Fungi (p. 390)

Dimorphic fungi include *Blastomyces, Histoplasma,* and *Coccidiomyces;* discussed in Chapter 15.

Parasitic Infections (p. 390; Table 8-6)

Protozoa (p. 390)

These are unicellular, eukaryotic organisms; parasitic protozoa are transmitted by insects or by the fecal-oral route. In humans they mainly occupy the intestine or blood (extracellular or intracellular).

Malaria (p. 390)

Malaria is an intracellular parasite affecting 160 million people worldwide and killing more than 500,000 annually (90% of these deaths occur in sub-Saharan Africa). *Plasmodium falciparum* causes severe malaria; *vivax, ovale,* and *malariae* species cause less severe disease. All species are transmitted by female *Anopheles* mosquitoes; mass spraying to eliminate the mosquito vector was previously effective, but environmental concerns and insecticide-resistant mosquitoes have frustrated this approach.

- The *Plasmodium* life cycle is schematized in Figure 8-4:
  - From the mosquito salivary gland, *sporozoites* in the bloodstream invade via the hepatocyte receptor for thrombospondin and properdin.

TABLE 8-6 Selected Human Protozoal Diseases

Location	Species	Disease
Luminal or epithelial	*E. histolytica*	Amebic dysentery; liver abscess
	Balantidium coli	Colitis
	Giardia lamblia	Diarrheal disease, malabsorption
	Isospora belli, Cryptosporidium sp.	Chronic enterocolitis or malabsorption or both
	T. vaginalis	Urethritis, vaginitis
CNS	*Naegleria fowleri*	Meningoencephalitis
	Acanthamoeba sp.	Meningoencephalitis or ophthalmitis
Bloodstream	*Plasmodium* sp.	Malaria
	Babesia microti, B. bovis	Babesiosis
	Trypanosoma sp.	African sleeping sickness
Intracellular	*T. cruzi*	Chagas disease
	Leishmania donovani	Kala-azar
	Leishmania sp.	Cutaneous and mucocutaneous leishmaniasis
	Toxoplasma gondii	Toxoplasmosis

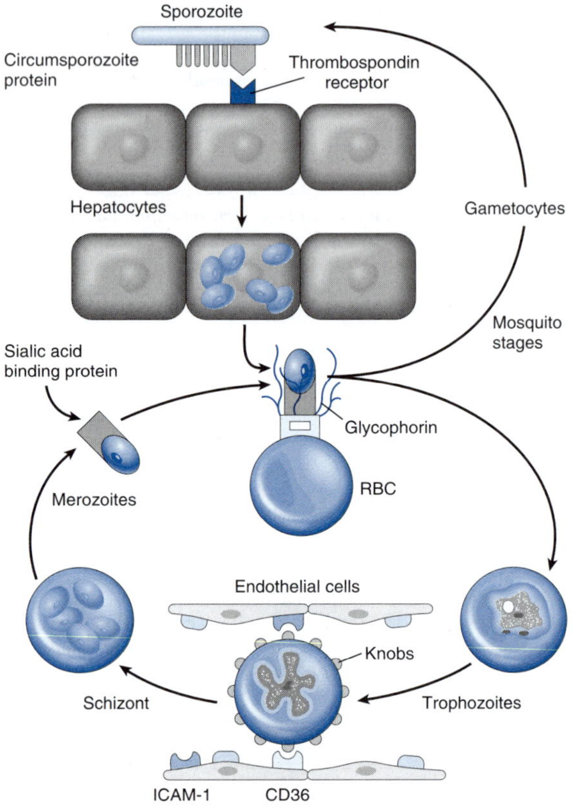

Figure 8-4 Life cycle of *P. falciparum*. Both exoerythocytic and erythrocytic stages are depicted. *ICAM-1,* Intercellular adhesion molecule 1; *RBC,* red blood cell. *(Based on a drawing courtesy of Dr. Jeffrey Joseph, Beth Israel-Deaconess Hospital, Boston, MA.)*

- Parasites multiply rapidly causing hepatocyte rupture and release of *merozoites* (asexual, haploid).
- Merozoites bind to sialic acid residues on erythrocyte glycophorin and are internalized.
- In erythrocytes, parasites hydrolyze red blood cell hemoglobin to generate characteristic *hemozoin* pigment and undergo development.
- *Trophozoites* (single chromatin mass) divide to form *schizonts* (multiple chromatin masses) that form new merozoites.
- Merozoites released by red cell lysis cause another round of erythrocyte infection.
- A small fraction of the parasites within red blood cells develop into sexual forms *(gametocytes)* that infect mosquitoes when they feed.

- The greater pathogenicity of *P. falciparum* stems from its ability to trigger the following:
  - Infect erythrocytes of any age; other species infect only new or old cells.
  - Cause infected erythrocytes to clump together or adhere to small vessel endothelium (via "knobs" on erythrocyte surfaces

that bind to endothelial cells), causing vascular occlusion. Ischemia due to such occlusions causes the manifestations of cerebral malaria.
  - Induce high levels of cytokines, such as TNF and interferon-γ that suppress red cell production, cause fever, and stimulate nitric oxide production. This occurs through release of glycosylphosphatidylinositol (GPI)-linked proteins (including merozoite surface antigens) from infected erythrocytes.
  - Use antigenic variation to continuously modify surface proteins.
- Resistance to *Plasmodium* occurs through the following:
  - Heritable erythrocyte traits (common in areas of the world where malaria is endemic):
    - Sickle cell trait (HbS), hemoglobin C (HbC), loss of globin genes (α- or β-thalassemia) and erythrocyte glucose-6-phosphatase deficiency all lessen malaria severity by reducing parasite proliferation and increasing erythrocyte clearance by macrophages.
    - Absence of Duffy blood group antigen prevents *Plasmodium vivax* binding to erythrocytes.
  - Antibody and T cell–mediated repertoires that develop after chronic infection.

Babesiosis *(p. 392)*

Babesiosis is caused by malaria-like protozoans transmitted from white-footed mice to humans by *Ixodes* ticks or rarely, contracted through blood transfusion.

- *Babesia* cause fever and, through erythrocyte parasitization, hemolytic anemia.
- *Babesia* resemble malaria schizonts but lack hemozoin pigment, are more pleomorphic, and form characteristic tetrads.

Leishmaniasis *(p. 392)*

Leishmaniasis is a chronic inflammatory disease of skin, mucous membranes, and viscera caused by *Leishmania* species, obligate intracellular parasites transmitted by sandfly bites. The life cycle involves two forms:

- Promastigotes develop and live extracellularly in the sandfly vector.
- Amastigotes multiply intracellularly in the macrophages of mammalian hosts.
  - When sandflies bite infected hosts, infected macrophages are ingested; amastigotes differentiate into promastigotes in the insect digestive tract and migrate to the salivary gland.
  - Subsequent bite of a second host delivers the promastigotes; these are phagocytized by macrophages and undergo transformation in phagolysosomes into amastigotes that then proliferate.
- Disease manifestations vary with the species and host responses. Thus whether a patient develops cutaneous disease, mucocutaneous disease, or visceral disease depends on which organism is in play; there are also different agents in the Old World versus the New World.
- Virulence factors include the following:
  - *Lipophosphoglycan* on promastigotes activates complement (leading to C3b deposition on the parasite surface and

increasing phagocytosis) but also inhibits complement action (by preventing membrane attack complex assembly).
- *gp63* on promastigotes binds fibronectin to promote promastigote adhesion to macrophages; it also cleaves complement and lysosomal antimicrobial enzymes to frustrate killing.
- A proton pump in amastigotes reduces macrophage phagolysosome acidity.

- Activation of macrophages by IFN-γ is necessary for adequate host defense; activated macrophages kill parasites through reactive oxygen species and NO.

African Trypanosomiasis (p. 394)

African trypanosomiasis is caused by extracellular parasites transmitted by tsetse flies.

- *Trypanosoma brucei rhodesiense* (East Africa) is acute and virulent, and *Trypanosoma brucei gambiense* (West Africa) is chronic.
- Trypanosomiasis is a disease of intermittent fevers, lymphadenopathy, progressive brain dysfunction (sleeping sickness), cachexia, and death.
    - In the fly, parasites multiply in the stomach and then in salivary glands before becoming nondividing but infective trypomastigotes.
    - A chancre forms at the insect bite site; large numbers of parasites are surrounded by a dense, largely mononuclear, inflammatory infiltrate.
    - Lymph nodes and spleen enlarge as a result of hyperplasia and infiltration by lymphocytes, plasma cells, and parasite-laden macrophages.
    - When parasites breach the blood-brain barrier, they induce a leptomeningitis and a demyelinating panencephalitis.
- Virulence factors include antigenic variation of a surface glycoprotein (VSG) specified by several different genes; as antibody responses clear one population of organisms expressing a particular VSG (causing a fever spike), a small number undergo genetic rearrangement and produce a new VSG.

Chagas Disease (p. 394)

Chagas disease is caused by *Trypanosoma cruzi,* an intracellular protozoan transmitted between animals (cats, dogs, rodents) and humans by "kissing bugs" (triatomids or reduviids) that pass parasites in their feces as they bite. Disease can also be transmitted by ingestion of food products contaminated by reduviid bugs or their feces.

- *T. cruzi* requires brief acid exposure in phagolysosomes to stimulate *amastigote* development; the organism then proliferates in the cytoplasm before developing flagella and rupturing the cell, traversing the blood to infect smooth, skeletal, and cardiac muscle.
- Acute Chagas disease has the following:
    - Is generally mild with cardiac damage secondary to direct invasion and associated inflammation.
    - Is rarely severe with high parasitemia, fever, and progressive cardiac dilation and failure.
- Chronic Chagas disease occurs in 20% of patients, with late manifestations up to 5 to 15 years later:
    - Myocardial inflammation causing cardiomyopathy and arrhythmias.
    - Damage to the myenteric plexus causing colon and esophageal dilation.

Metazoa (p. 395)

Metazoa are multicellular, eukaryotic organisms, typically contracted by eating undercooked meat, through insect bites, or by direct host invasion through the skin. Depending on the organism, they may ultimately dwell in the host intestine, skin, lung, liver, muscle, blood vessels, or lymphatics.

Strongyloidiasis (p. 395)

Strongyloides stercoralis larvae live in the soil.

- Larvae directly penetrate the skin of humans, traveling in the circulation to the lungs. From there they migrate up the trachea and are swallowed. Adult female worms produce eggs asexually in the mucosa of the small intestine; passed larvae contaminate soil to complete the cycle.
- In immunocompetent hosts there may be diarrhea and malabsorption; larvae are present in the duodenal crypts with an underlying eosinophil-rich infiltrate.
- In immunocompromised hosts larvae hatched in the gut can invade colonic mucosa and reinitiate infection. Such uncontrolled autoinfection results in massive larval burdens with widespread invasion—occasionally complicated by sepsis caused by bacteria carried into the bloodstream by parasites.

Tapeworms (Cestodes): Cysticercosis and Hydatid Disease (p. 395)

Disease is caused by larval development after the ingestion of eggs; *Taenia solium* causes *cysticercosis* and *Echinococcus granulosus* causes *hydatid disease.*

- Tapeworms have complex life cycles requiring two hosts—a definitive host, where the worm reaches sexual maturity, and an intermediate host.
- *T. solium* are transmitted to humans in two ways with distinct outcomes:
  - Larval cysts (cysticerci) ingested in pork attach to the intestinal wall where they mature and produce egg-laden proglottids (segments) that are passed in stool.
  - If intermediate hosts (pigs or humans) ingest eggs in feces-contaminated food or water, hatching larvae penetrate the gut wall, and disseminate to encyst in many organs, including the brain (causing severe neurologic manifestations).
- Humans are accidental hosts for *E. granulosus* and *E. multilocularis;* these are normally passed only between the definitive (dog or fox) and intermediate (sheep and rodents) hosts.
  - Hydatid disease is caused by ingestion of echinoccal eggs in food contaminated with dog or fox feces.
  - Eggs hatch in the duodenum and invade the liver, lungs, or bones, where they form cysts.
- *T. saginata* (beef) and *Diphyllobothrium latum* (fish) are acquired by eating undercooked meat; in humans these parasites live only in the gut and do not form cysticerci.

Trichinosis (p. 396)

Trichinella spiralis is typically acquired by ingestion of larvae in undercooked pork; pigs are infected by eating contaminated meat.

- In the gut, larvae develop into adults that mate and produce new larvae; these disseminate hematogenously and penetrate muscle cells causing fever, myalgias, eosinophilia, and periorbital edema.

- Intracellular organisms increase dramatically in size and encapsulate; they may persist for years subverting the cell to become a "nurse cell-parasite complex" surrounded by an eosinophil-rich infiltrate and a new host vascular plexus.
- *T. spiralis* stimulates T_H2 cells that activate eosinophils and mast cells (typical antinematodal inflammatory response; see Chapter 6) and increase gut contractility to expel worms. Organisms usually die after a number of years, leaving behind characteristic calcified scars.

Schistosomiasis *(p. 397)*

Schistosomiasis is caused by *Schistosoma mansoni* (Latin America, Africa, and the Middle East), *Schistosoma haematobium* (Africa), and *Schistosoma japonicum* or *Schistosoma mekongi* (East Asia); these are transmitted from freshwater snails.

- Larvae penetrate human skin, migrate through the vasculature, and settle in the pelvic *(S. haematobium)* or portal (all others) venous systems.
- Females produce eggs that may disseminate and are shed in urine or stool. Proteases produced by eggs and the host inflammatory response are necessary for eggs to penetrate mucosa (bladder or intestine) and be shed.
- Much of the pathology associated with schistosomiasis is caused by host inflammatory responses. The immune response is directed against eggs; early responses are T_H1-dominated, whereas in chronic infections, T_H2 responses predominate. Hepatic fibrosis is a serious manifestation of chronic schistosomiasis, in which T_H2 cells and alternatively activated macrophages may play a key role.
- Both T-cell populations contribute to granuloma formation (often eosinophil-rich) and fibrosis; urinary schistosmiasis is also associated with urinary bladder squamous cell carcinoma.

Lymphatic Filariasis *(p. 398)*

Lymphatic filariasis is caused by two nematodes, *Wuchereria bancrofti* (90% of cases) and *Brugia malayi;* larvae are contracted from infected mosquitoes.

- Larvae develop into adults in lymphatic channels; those mate and release microfilariae that enter the bloodstream and can then infect secondary mosquitoes.
- Damage to lymphatics is mediated by T_H1-mediated inflammation, although T_H2 inflammation can also occur; differences in host immune responses likely account for the different manifestations of filariasis:
    - Asymptomatic microfilaremia
    - Recurrent lymphadenitis
    - Chronic lymphadenitis with swelling of the dependent limb or scrotum *(elephantiasis)*
    - Tropical pulmonary eosinophilia
- Virulence factors include the following:
    - Antioxidant glycoproteins protect from oxygen radical injury.
    - Homologues of cystatins, cysteine protease inhibitors, impair antigen presentation.
    - Serpins (serine protease inhibitors) inhibit neutrophil proteases.
    - Homologues of TGF-β bind to host TGF-β receptors, and downregulate inflammatory responses.

- Rickettsia-like *Wolbachia* bacteria infect filaria and are needed for nematode development and reproduction; these may also release LPS and stimulate inflammation.

Onchocerciasis (p. 399)

Onchocerca volvulus is a filarial nematode transmitted by black flies; it causes "river blindness," the second-most common cause of blindness in sub-Saharan Africa. The pathologic consequences of infection are mostly attributable to host inflammatory responses.

- Nematodes mate in the host dermis, surrounded by host inflammatory cells that produce a subcutaneous nodule *(onchocercoma)*.
- Female worms release large numbers of microfilariae, which accumulate in the skin and eye chambers, causing pruritic dermatitis and blindness.
- Treatment includes doxycycline to kill the symbiotic *Wolbachia* bacteria that live inside *O. volvulus* and are required for worm fertility.

Emerging Infectious Diseases (p. 400)

The list of disease-causing microorganisms is constantly expanding (Table 8-7).

- Some are recent discoveries due to difficulty in culturing (e.g., *Helicobacter* gastritis, hepatitis B and C, and legionnaire pneumonia).

TABLE 8-7 Some Recently Recognized Infectious Agents and Manifestations

Date Recognized	Infectious Agent	Manifestations
1977	Ebola virus	Epidemic Ebola hemorrhagic fever
	Hantaan virus	Hemorrhagic fever with renal syndrome
	L. pneumophila	Legionnaire disease
	C. jejuni	Enteritis
1980	HTLV-I	T-cell lymphoma or leukemia, HTLV-associated myelopathy
1981	*S. aureus*	Toxic shock syndrome
1982	*E. coli* 0157:H7	Hemorrhagic colitis, hemolytic-uremic syndrome
	B. burgdorferi	Lyme disease
1983	HIV	AIDS
	H. pylori	Gastric ulcers
1988	Hepatitis E	Enterically transmitted hepatitis
1989	Hepatitis C	Hepatitis C
1992	*V. cholerae* 0139	New epidemic cholera strain
	Bartonella henselae	Cat-scratch disease
1995	KSHV (HHV-8)	Kaposi sarcoma in AIDS
1999	West Nile virus	West Nile fever, neuroinvasive disease
2003	SARS coronavirus	SARS

HTLV, Human T-cell lymphotropic virus.

- Some are genuinely new to humans (e.g., HIV [causing AIDS], *B. burgdorferi* [causing Lyme disease], and the coronavirus causing severe acute respiratory syndrome [SARS]).
- Some have become more common as a result of therapeutic or AIDS-induced immunosuppression (e.g., CMV, KSHV, *M. avium-intracellulare, Pneumocystis jiroveci,* and *Cryptosporidium parvum*).
- Some have been previously well recognized in one region but are only recently entering a new population or geographic locale (e.g., West Nile virus).
- Human demographics and behaviors are important variables in the emergence of new infectious diseases; thus reforestation of the eastern United States led to the expansion of the populations of animal vectors (mice and deer) for Lyme disease. Antibiotic resistance led to the emergence of increasingly virulent microorganisms (e.g., methicillin-resistant staphylococcus). Dense populations of domesticated animals (chickens and pigs) led to the acquisition of unique traits in common pathogens (e.g., H1N1 influenza) or the emergence of unique pathogens that cross species barriers (e.g., the coronavirus that causes SARS).

Agents of Bioterrorism (p. 401)

These pathogens are those that pose the greatest danger due to efficient disease transmission, significant morbidity and mortality, relative ease of production and distribution, difficulty in defending against, or the ability to provoke alarm and fear in the general public.

- Category A agents pose the greatest risk; they are readily disseminated and/or transmitted from person to person, can cause high mortality, and are likely to be societally disruptive. Smallpox falls in this category.
- Category B agents are relatively easy to disseminate (often they are foodborne or waterborne) but have lower morbidity and mortality. Examples include *Brucella, Vibrio cholerae,* and ricin toxins.
- Category C agents include emerging pathogens that have the potential for being engineered for mass dissemination, with high morbidity and mortality; examples include Hantavirus and Nipah virus.

9 Environmental and Nutritional Diseases

Environmental diseases refer to conditions caused by exposure to chemical or physical agents in the ambient, workplace, or personal environment (e.g., diet, drugs, alcohol, and tobacco), including diseases of nutritional origin (overnutrition or undernutrition). Exposures may be acute or represent chronic contact with low-level contaminants. Worldwide, two million people die annually due to occupation-related injury or illness; malnutrition affects one in seven people worldwide, disproportionately affecting children and accounting for more than 50% of global childhood mortality.

Environmental Effects on Global Disease Burden (p. 404)

Global health data are reported using a disability-adjusted life year (DALY) metric that combines years lost to premature mortality and years lived with illness and disability within a population. By this measure the burden of disease imposed by environmental causes (including infectious and nutritional diseases) shows several trends over the period between 1990 and 2010:

- Mortality due to human immunodeficiency virus (HIV) or acquired immunodeficiency syndrome (AIDS) and associated infections peaked in 2006.
- Since 1990 there has been an almost 40% increase in noncommunicable diseases (e.g., cancer, diabetes, and cardiovascular disease) and an almost 10% increase in deaths from injuries, both attributable in part to the aging of the world's population (from a mean age of 26.1 to a mean age of 29.5 years).
- Global life expectancy *free of disability* rose from 54.4 to 58.3 years for men and from 57.8 years to 61.8 years for women.
- Undernutrition is the single leading global cause of health loss; one third of the disease burden in developing countries is nutrition related.
- Coronary and cerebrovascular diseases are the leading causes of death in developed countries; major risk factors include obesity, smoking, and high cholesterol.
- Infections constitute a significant global health burden; 5 of the top 10 causes of death in developing countries are infectious diseases. In the postnatal period 50% of all deaths before the age of 5 are attributable to pneumonia, diarrheal illnesses, and malaria.
    - Malnutrition increases the risk of infection.
    - Drug-resistant strains (due to clinical and agricultural antibiotic use) are the most important group of pathogens.
    - Vector-borne diseases constitute almost a third of newly emerging infections and in many cases can be linked to environmental changes, including global warming.

Health Effects of Climate Change (p. 405)

The dominant greenhouse gases—water vapor, carbon dioxide, methane, and ozone—trap energy from the earth that would otherwise radiate into space and have led to an ever-accelerating rate of temperature rise in the past half-century. The major culprit in this global warming is carbon dioxide; its level in 2012 (391 ppm) was higher than any time in 650,000 years. The rise is attributable to the burning of fossil fuels, as well as the loss of carbon fixation through deforestation. Depending on the model, global temperatures are predicted to rise 2 to 5° C by 2100. Although the outcome will depend on the tempo and extent of change, and the ability of humankind to mitigate such changes, global warming will inevitably impact human disease:

- Cardiovascular and respiratory diseases will be amplified by heat waves and air pollution.
- Gastroenteritis and infection epidemics will be impacted by water and food contamination following flooding and other environmental disruptions.
- Vector-borne infectious diseases are expected to increase as vector numbers and geographic distributions are altered.
- Malnutrition will increase as crop productivity wanes.
- Melting of polar ice will raise sea levels by as much as 16.5 feet, displacing the 10% of the world population that lives in low-lying areas, and likely fomenting war, poverty, and political unrest—a recipe for malnutrition, infectious diseases, and death.

Toxicity of Chemical and Physical Agents (p. 406)

Toxicology studies the distribution, effects, and mechanisms of action of toxic agents. Xenobiotics are exogenous agents in the environment that may be inhaled, ingested, or directly absorbed. Four billion pounds of toxic chemicals, including 72 million pounds of known carcinogens are released annually in the United States. Moreover, of the approximately 100,000 chemicals in commercial use in the United States, very few have been formally tested for adverse health effects.

- Toxicity depends on the structural properties of a compound and the administered dose. Low doses of a given agent may be well tolerated *or even therapeutic,* whereas greater amounts are toxic.
- Toxic compounds may act locally at the site of entry into the body or in other tissues after bloodstream transport.
- A lipophilic (fat-soluble) compound will have increased blood transport by associating with lipoproteins and will cross plasma membranes more readily.
- Compounds may be excreted in urine, feces, or expired air or may accumulate in bone, fat, brain, or other tissues.
- Some agents act directly and may be rendered less toxic (or more readily excreted) by metabolic activity; other compounds may become toxic only after being metabolized.
- Drug-metabolizing enzymes are divided into two general groups:
  - Phase I:
    - Hydrolysis, oxidation, or reduction.
    - The most important catalyst is the cytochrome P-450 (CYP-450) enzyme system, comprising a large family of heme-containing endoplasmic reticulum enzymes.

- Variation in CYP enzymatic activity can be due to genetic polymorphisms or to compounds that augment or reduce CYP expression; tobacco and alcohol can enhance expression, whereas malnutrition can diminish it.
- Enzymatic activity releases oxygen-derived free radicals.

- Phase II:
  - Glucuronidation, sulfation, methylation, and conjugation.
  - Generally increase water solubility and hence excretion.

Environmental Pollution (p. 407)

Air Pollution (p. 407)

Air pollution is a significant cause of global morbidity and mortality, particularly for individuals with preexisting pulmonary or cardiac disease.

Outdoor Air Pollution (p. 407)

Lung is the major organ impacted, although other tissues can be affected by air pollutants, such as carbon monoxide (CO) and lead. In the lung, inflammation, increased airway reactivity, diminished mucociliary clearance, and increased infections all commonly occur.

- *Ozone* forms from the interaction of oxygen and ultraviolet (UV) radiation. Stratospheric ozone is critical in absorbing solar UV radiation; loss due to chlorofluorocarbon use increases skin cancer risk. However, ozone in the lower atmosphere is a major component of smog, which also contains nitrogen oxides and volatile organic compounds from industrial emissions and motor vehicle exhaust.
  Ozone toxicity occurs through the subsequent generation of free radicals; these injure alveolar epithelium and induce release of inflammatory mediators. The outcome is cough (upper airway hyper-reactivity), chest discomfort, and pulmonary inflammation; the consequences are more severe in patients with asthma or emphysema.
- *Sulfur dioxide* is produced by the combustion of coal and oil, copper smelting, and paper manufacture. It is converted into sulfuric acid and sulfur trioxide that cause burning, dyspnea, and airway hyper-reactivity.
- *Particulate matter* (soot) is emitted by coal, oil, and diesel combustion; deposition and clearance of inhaled particulates depend on their size and shape with particles <10 μm being most deleterious (larger particles are usually trapped in nasal mucus or by the upper respiratory mucociliary clearance mechanisms). Toxic effects are attributed to macrophage and neutrophil uptake, with subsequent inflammatory mediator production.
- *CO* is a colorless, odorless, tasteless, nonirritating gas produced by incomplete oxidation of carbonaceous materials (internal combustion engines, wood burning, cigarette smoking, etc.). Ambient low-level exposure may contribute to impaired respiratory function; chronic poisoning in confined spaces (tunnels, toll takers, underground garages) can cause serious injury. Acute lethality occurs through central nervous system (CNS) depression and systemic hypoxia (CO has 200-fold greater affinity for hemoglobin than oxygen). Acute poisoning is characterized by a cherry-red coloring of the victim due to high levels of carboxyhemoglobin.

Indoor Air Pollution (*p. 409*)

Levels of indoor air pollutants have increased, owing to improved insulation and fewer air leaks in homes, coupled with increasing reliance on air conditioning rather than open-window ventilation. Tobacco smoke, CO, nitrogen dioxide, and carcinogenic polycyclic aromatic hydrocarbons (from cooking) are all complicit. The following are some of the major indoor air pollutants:

- *Wood smoke* is a complex mixture of particulates and other toxic components (e.g., polycyclic hydrocarbons); these are directly irritating, can increase the incidence of respiratory infections, and are potentially carcinogenic.
- *Bioaerosols* include the bacterial aerosols responsible for *Legionella* pneumonia, and allergens from pet danders, dust mites, and molds.
- *Radon* is a radioactive gas formed as a decay product of uranium found naturally in the soil. Low-level radon in some homes may increase cancer risk in smokers.
- *Formaldehyde* is a soluble, volatile chemical used in the manufacture of many consumer products; it can cause acute irritation of the eyes and upper respiratory tract and is classified as a carcinogen.

Metals as Environmental Pollutants (p. 410)

Lead (*p. 410*)

Lead is present in many forms in the environment:

- Air associated with spray painting, foundries, and gasoline combustion
- Soil and house dusts contaminated with leaded paint
- Water supplied through lead plumbing

Inhalation is the most important route of occupational exposure, but lead toxicity can also occur with oral intake. Infants and children are particularly vulnerable due to greater gastrointestinal (GI) absorption and a more permeable blood-brain barrier. Lead binds to protein sulfhydryl groups and competes with calcium ions in a variety of metabolic pathways; 80% to 85% of absorbed lead accumulates in bones and teeth. The toxic effects of lead are attributable to the following:

- Neurotoxicity due to altered calcium homeostasis that disrupts neurotransmitter release. In children this typically presents as psychomotor impairment; in adults a peripheral demyelinating neuropathy is more common.
- Inhibition of enzymes involved in heme synthesis (δ-aminolevulinic acid dehydratase) and iron incorporation (ferrochelatase), leading to microcytic, hypochromic anemia (erythrocytes exhibit a characteristic punctate basophilic stippling).
- Altered cartilage remodeling in epiphyses (this leads to characteristic radiodense "lead lines") and inhibition of bone healing.
- GI changes include abdominal pain and anorexia (lead "colic").

Mercury (*p. 412*)

Mercury exposure occurs primarily through the following:

- Methyl mercury-contaminated fish that concentrate environmental mercury over a millionfold
- Mercury vapors released by metallic mercury in dental amalgams
- Mercury used in gold mining that contaminates water run-off

Mercury toxicity is related to its binding affinity for cellular sulfhydryl groups. Renal tubular epithelium is especially susceptible, and the high lipid solubility of methyl mercury facilitates accumulation in the CNS, particularly in developing brains; in utero exposure can cause cerebral palsy, deafness, blindness, and mental retardation.

Arsenic (p. 412)

Arsenic is found naturally in soil and water and is used in herbicides and as a wood preservative. The trivalent forms are most toxic (e.g., arsenic trioxide and sodium arsenite). Ingestion leads to GI, cardiovascular, and neurologic sequelae by inhibiting mitochondrial oxidative phosphorylation. Chronic low-level exposure increases the risk of skin and lung cancer.

Cadmium (p. 413)

Cadmium is an environmental pollutant generated by mining, electroplating, and the production and improper disposal of nickel-cadmium batteries. Ingestion of contaminated food (after uptake by plants grown in contaminated soil) is the most common route of human exposure. Toxicity follows cellular import via ZIP8 zinc transporters; alveolar epithelial damage leads to obstructive lung disease, and renal tubular damage causes end-stage kidney disease; skeletal abnormalities may be related to calcium loss. An increased risk of lung cancer is attributed to DNA damage induced by reactive oxygen species.

Occupational Health Risks: Industrial and Agricultural Exposures (p. 413)

More than 10 million injuries and 65,000 deaths annually in the United States are due to work-related illness or accident. Occupational exposures contribute to diseases that range from mild respiratory irritation to lung cancer and leukemia; all organ systems can be affected (Table 9-1).

- *Organic solvents,* such as chloroform and carbon tetrachloride, are widely used as industrial solvents and cleaning agents. These compounds are readily absorbed through the lungs, skin, and GI tract. In addition to acute CNS depression, they can cause liver and kidney toxicity. *Aromatic hydrocarbons,* such as benzene, are metabolized by CYP2E1 to toxic metabolites that disrupt marrow hematopoiesis, leading to dose-dependent aplasia and an increased risk of acute myeloid leukemia.
- *Polycyclic hydrocarbons* are produced during fossil fuel combustion and by steel foundries. These are potent carcinogens, and occupational exposure is associated with an increased risk of lung and bladder cancers.
- *Organochlorines* are synthetic lipophilic compounds that resist degradation; these include pesticides, such as dichlorodiphenyltrichloroethane *(DDT)* and nonpesticides, such as polychlorinated biphenyl (PCB) and dioxin. Most are endocrine disrupters with antiestrogen and antiandrogenic effects.
    - *Dioxins and PCBs* can also cause a foliculitis or dermatosis called chloracne, as well as hepatic and CNS abnormalities; they activate CYP and thus can alter drug metabolism.
- *Mineral dust inhalation* (coal, silica, asbestos, beryllium) can cause chronic, non-neoplastic but diffusely fibrosing *pneumoconioses* (see Chapter 15).

TABLE 9-1 Human Diseases Associated With Occupational Exposures

Organ	Effect	Toxicant
Cardiovascular system	Heart disease	CO, lead, solvents, cobalt, cadmium
Respiratory system	Nasal cancer	Isopropyl alcohol, wood dust
	Lung cancer	Radon, asbestos, silica, bis(chloromethyl)ether, nickel, arsenic, chromium, mustard gas
	Chronic obstructive lung disease	Grain dust, coal dust, cadmium
	Hypersensitivity	Beryllium, isocyanates
	Irritation	Ammonia, sulfur oxides, formaldehyde
	Fibrosis	Silica, asbestos, cobalt
Nervous system	Peripheral neuropathies	Solvents, acrylamide, methyl chloride, mercury, lead, arsenic, DDT
	Ataxic gait	Chlordane, toluene, acrylamide, mercury
	CNS depression	Alcohols, ketones, aldehydes, solvents
	Cataracts	UV radiation
Urinary system	Toxicity	Mercury, lead, glycol ethers, solvents
	Bladder cancer	Naphthylamines, 4-aminobiphenyl, benzidine, rubber products
Reproductive system	Male infertility	Lead, phthalate plasticizers
	Female infertility	Cadmium, lead
	Teratogenesis	Mercury, PCBs
Hematopoietic system	Leukemia	Benzene, radon, uranium
Skin	Folliculitis and acneiform dermatosis	PCBs, dioxins, herbicides
	Cancer	UV radiation
GI tract	Liver angiosarcoma	Vinyl chloride

Data from Leigh JP, Markowitz SB, Fahs M, Shin C, Landrigan PJ: Occupational injury and illness in the United States. Estimates of costs, morbidity, and mortality. *Arch Intern Med* 157:1557, 1997; Mitchell FL: Hazardous waste. In Rom WN (ed): *Environmental and Occupational Medicine,* ed 2, Boston, MA: Little, Brown, 1992, p 1275; Levi PE: Classes of toxic chemicals. In Hodgson E, Levi PE (eds): *A Textbook of Modern Toxicology,* Stamford, CT: Appleton & Lange, 1997, p 229.

- *Vinyl chloride* monomers used to produce polyvinyl chloride resins is associated with angiosarcoma of the liver.
- *Bisphenol A* (BPA) is widely used in the synthesis of polycarbonate food and water containers; exposure leads to endocrine disruption.

Effects of Tobacco (p. 414)

Cigarette smoking is responsible for over 400,000 deaths annually in the United States and 4 million deaths worldwide; lung cancer (one third of the total) and cardiovascular and chronic pulmonary disease account for the vast majority of the mortality. Indeed, tobacco use is the most common exogenous cause of human malignancy, responsible for 90% of lung cancers. Within 5 years of smoking cessation, overall mortality and—more specifically—risk of death from cardiovascular disease are markedly reduced. Lung cancer risk decreases by 21% within 5 years, but the excess risk persists for 30 years.

- Cigarette smoke contains 2000 to 4000 constituents; more than 60 are known carcinogens.
- Nicotine is an addictive alkaloid found naturally in tobacco leaves; binding to CNS receptors releases catecholamines that increase heart rate, blood pressure, and cardiac contractility.

Smoking and Lung Cancer (p. 415)

Polycyclic hydrocarbons, benzopyrene, and nitrosamines in cigarette smoke are potent carcinogens, especially after CYP modification. Cancer risk is dose-related (smoking more cigarettes increases risk), and smoking synergizes with other carcinogenic influences in causing lung carcinoma (e.g., asbestos or radiation exposures). In addition to lung cancer, tobacco contributes to cancer development in the oral cavity, esophagus, pancreas, and bladder; smoke and smokeless tobacco both interact with alcohol in driving laryngeal cancer.

Smoking and Other Diseases (p. 416)

Formaldehyde, phenol, and nitrogen oxides in cigarette smoke are directly irritating, inducing tracheobronchial inflammation and increased mucus output *(bronchitis);* leukocyte recruitment leads to increased elastase production and subsequent *emphysema.*

- Cigarette smoking is strongly linked to development of atherosclerosis and myocardial infarction; increased platelet aggregation, endothelial dysfunction, and myocardial hypoxia are all implicated.
- Maternal smoking causes fetal hypoxia with intrauterine growth retardation and increases the risk of spontaneous abortions and preterm births.
- *Second-hand* smoke *(environmental smoke)* also increases the risk of lung cancer, ischemic heart disease, and acute myocardial infarction; relative risk of lung cancer in nonsmokers exposed to second-hand smoke is 1.3 times greater than individuals not exposed to environmental smoke. Passive smoke inhalation in nonsmokers is estimated by measuring serum *cotinine,* a metabolite of nicotine.

Effects of Alcohol (p. 417)

- There are 10 million alcoholics in the United States. Approximately 100,000 deaths are attributable to alcohol abuse each year, with the majority due to drunken driving or alcohol-related homicides and suicides; 15% of alcohol-related deaths are due to cirrhosis. Worldwide, alcohol accounts for 3.2% of all death annually.
- A blood alcohol concentration of 80 mg/dL is the legal definition for drunk driving in most states; drowsiness typically occurs at 200 mg/dL, stupor at 300 mg/dL, and coma (with possible respiratory arrest) at higher concentrations. Alcohol effects vary depending on age, gender, and body fat; for the *average individual,* 80 mg/dL occurs after 36 oz of beer, 15 oz of wine, or 4 to 5 oz of 80-proof distilled spirits. Chronic alcoholics can tolerate greater volumes due to hepatic CYP induction.

- After consumption, alcohol is absorbed unaltered in the stomach and small bowel; less than 10% is excreted unchanged in the urine, sweat, and breath.
- Ethanol is metabolized to acetaldehyde in hepatocytes mainly by cytosolic alcohol dehydrogenase (ADH); at high blood alcohol levels, the micro-osomal ethanol-oxidizing system (MEOS) also participates, whereas liver catalase metabolizes less than 5%. Hepatic acetaldehyde dehydrogenase (ALDH) then converts acetaldehyde to acetate that can be used by normal mitochondrial metabolic pathways (Fig. 9-1).
- Induction of CYP (especially CYP2E1) by alcohol accelerates the metabolism of other drugs by the MEOS. However, when alcohol is present in high concentrations, it competes for the enzyme complex and the metabolism of other compounds can be delayed.
- The metabolism of ethanol is directly responsible for most of its toxic and chronic effects:
    - Acetaldehyde is responsible for many of the acute toxicities of alcohol and the development of oral cancers. ADH and ALDH isoforms influence the relative rates of metabolite generation. Thus approximately half of Asians have low ALDH activity due to one copy of an inactive ALDH enzyme; homozygotes cannot oxidize acetaldehyde at all, and alcohol consumption is associated with nausea, flushing, tachycardia, and hyperventilation.
    - ADH oxidation of alcohol reduces nicotinamide adenine dinucleotide (NAD) to NADH; because NAD is required for fatty acid oxidation and for converting lactic acid to pyruvate, alcohol consumption leads to liver fat accumulation.
    - CYPE21 oxidation of alcohol leads to the formation of reactive oxygen species that can cause liver injury by membrane peroxidation; alcohol in the GI tract also induces release of endotoxins from gut flora with subsequent inflammatory cytokine production.

Adverse alcohol effects are due to the following:

- *Acute alcohol injury* including hepatic steatosis (fatty change), gastritis and ulceration, and the depression of CNS activity.
- *Chronic alcoholism,* affecting virtually all organs, with substantial morbidity and mortality:
    - *Liver* is the main site of injury; in addition to fatty change, alcoholic hepatitis and cirrhosis can result (see Chapter 18). Cirrhosis is associated with portal hypertension and increased risk of hepatocellular carcinoma.
    - *GI tract:* Massive bleeding may result from acute gastritis and ulceration or as a consequence of esophageal varices due to portal hypertension.
    - *Nervous system:* Thiamine deficiency (due to poor nutrition) is common in chronic alcoholics; it causes peripheral neuropathies and the Wernicke-Korsakoff syndrome (see Chapter 28), as well as cerebral atrophy, cerebellar degeneration, and optic neuropathy.
    - *Cardiovascular system:* Chronic alcoholism can cause a dilated cardiomyopathy and is associated with an increased incidence of hypertension. Liver injury due to alcohol excess will reduce high-density lipoprotein (HDL) production and increase cardiovascular risk.
    - *Pancreas:* Alcohol use increases the risk of acute and chronic pancreatitis (see Chapter 19).
    - *Fetal alcohol syndrome:* This is characterized by growth and developmental defects, including microcephaly, facial dysmorphology, and malformations of the brain, cardiovascular

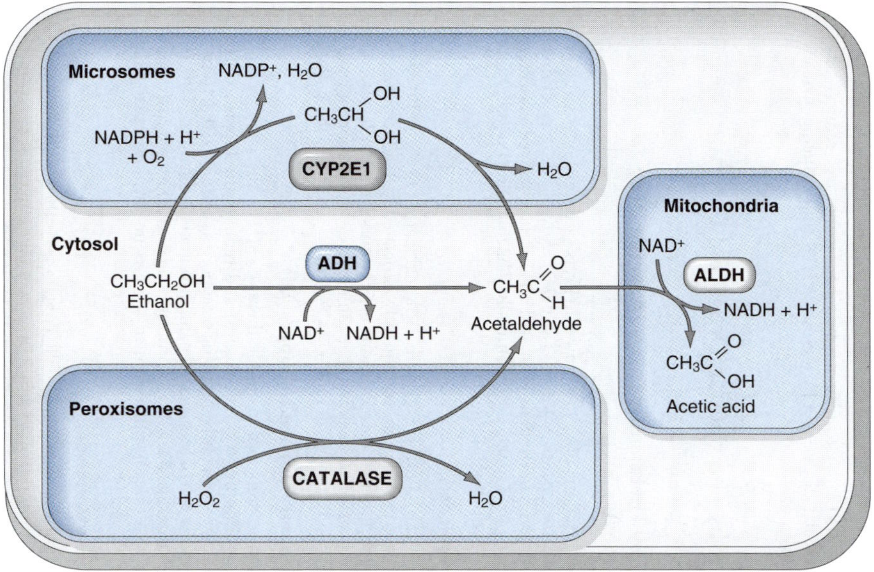

Figure 9-1 **Metabolism of ethanol: oxidation of ethanol to acetaldehyde by three different routes and the generation of acetic acid.** Note that oxidation by ADH takes place in the cytosol; the cytochrome P-450 system and its CYP2E1 isoform are located in the endoplasmic reticulum (microsomes), and catalase is located in peroxisomes. Oxidation of acetaldehyde by ALDH occurs in mitochondria. ADH oxidation is the most important route; catalase is involved in only 5% of ethanol metabolism. Oxidation through CYPs may also generate reactive oxygen species (not shown). *(From Parkinson A: Biotransformation of xenobiotics. In Klassen CD [ed]:* Casarett and Doull's Toxicology: The Basic Science of Poisons, *6th ed. New York, NY: McGraw-Hill, 2001, p 133.)*

system, and genitourinary system. Consumption during the first trimester is most harmful, although the minimal absolute amount consumed is difficult to establish; frequent or binge drinking occurs in 6% of pregnant women, and fetal alcohol syndrome affects 0.1% to 0.5% of children born in the United States.

- *Ethanol and cancer:* Alcohol use is associated with increased cancer rates in the oral cavity, pharynx, esophagus, liver, and possibly breast. The acetaldehyde metabolite may act as a tumor promoter.

Potential beneficial effects of alcohol:

- *Cardiovascular system:* In moderation, alcohol can reduce cardiovascular disease risk by increasing HDL and reducing platelet aggregation.

Injury by Therapeutic Drugs and Drugs of Abuse (p. 419)

Injury by Therapeutic Drugs (Adverse Drug Reactions) (p. 419)

Adverse reactions refer to untoward effects of drugs given in conventional therapeutic settings (Table 9-2). Adverse drug reactions are common, affecting an estimated 10% of hospitalized patients, accounting for 140,000 deaths annually. The following therapies are common culprits.

Anticoagulants (p. 420)

Warfarin (a vitamin K antagonist) and dabigatran (a thrombin inhibitor) are the drugs most frequently associated with adverse reactions; the principal complications are thrombosis when levels are subtherapeutic and bleeding that can occur even with appropriate dosing.

Menopausal Hormone Therapy (p. 421)

Although menopausal hormone therapy (MHT) alleviates menopausal symptoms (e.g., hot flashes) and reduces the incidence of fractures (presumably by reducing osteoporosis), prolonged therapy increases the risk of breast cancer and thromboembolism. In women younger than age 60, MHT is protective against atherosclerosis and coronary disease; in older women there is no cardiovascular risk benefit.

Oral Contraceptives (p. 421)

Oral contraceptives (OCs) usually contain a synthetic estradiol and variable amounts of a progestin or can contain progestins alone that prevent ovulation and/or implantation. Lower estrogen content is associated with fewer side effects; these are dependent on dosage and delivery modality, and most current OC formulations have the following risk profiles:

- *Cancer:* OCs do not increase the risk of breast cancer and are protective for ovarian and endometrial cancers. Cervical cancer risk may be increased for women infected with human papillomavirus.
- *Thromboembolism:* OC use results in a threefold to sixfold increased risk of venous thrombosis and pulmonary thromboembolism, due to increased hepatic synthesis of coagulation factors.

TABLE 9-2 Some Common Adverse Drug Reactions and Their Agents

Reaction	Major Offenders
Bone Marrow and Blood Cells*	
Granulocytopenia, aplastic anemia, pancytopenia	Antineoplastic agents, immunosuppressives, and chloramphenicol
Hemolytic anemia, thrombocytopenia	Penicillin, methyldopa, quinidine, heparin
Cutaneous	
Urticaria, macules, papules, vesicles, petechiae, exfoliative dermatitis, fixed drug eruptions, abnormal pigmentation	Antineoplastic agents, sulfonamides, hydantoins, some antibiotics, and many other agents
Cardiac	
Arrhythmias	Theophylline, hydantoins, digoxin
Cardiomyopathy	Doxorubicin, daunorubicin
Renal	
Glomerulonephritis	Penicillamine
Acute tubular necrosis	Aminoglycoside antibiotics, cyclosporin, amphotericin B
Tubulointerstitial disease with papillary necrosis	Phenacetin, salicylates
Pulmonary	
Asthma	Salicylates
Acute pneumonitis	Nitrofurantoin
Interstitial fibrosis	Busulfan, nitrofurantoin, bleomycin
Hepatic	
Fatty change	Tetracycline
Diffuse hepatocellular damage	Halothane, isoniazid, acetaminophen
Cholestasis	Chlorpromazine, estrogens, contraceptive agents
Systemic	
Anaphylaxis	Penicillin
Lupus erythematosus syndrome (drug-induced lupus)	Hydralazine, procainamide
CNS	
Tinnitus and dizziness	Salicylates
Acute dystonic reactions and parkinsonian syndrome	Phenothiazine antipsychotics
Respiratory depression	Sedatives

*Affected in almost half of all drug-related deaths.

Risk is further increased in carriers of mutations in factor V or prothrombin. It is important to remember that the risk of thromboembolism associated with OCs is twofold to sixfold *lower* than the risk of thromboembolism associated with pregnancy.

- *Cardiovascular disease:* OCs do not increase the risk of myocardial infarction in nonsmokers; however, risk approximately doubles in smokers older than age 35.
- *Hepatic adenoma:* There is a well-defined association between OC and this benign tumor.

Anabolic Steroids (p. 422)

Anabolic steroids are synthetic versions of testosterone; these are used at 10 to 100 times therapeutic doses to achieve enhanced athletic performance. In males, high doses inhibit luteinizing hormone/follicle stimulating hormone (LH/FSH) production and lead to testicular atrophy; catabolism of the anabolic steroids leads to increased estrogens and causes gynecomastia. In adolescents, use can lead to stunted growth; women will experience virilization and menstrual dysfunction. Additional effects include psychiatric changes, premature myocardial infarctions, and hepatic cholestasis.

Acetaminophen (p. 422)

Acetaminophen is the most commonly used analgesic in the United States; it is also responsible for more than 50% of acute liver failure in the United States, with a 30% mortality. At therapeutic doses, >95% is metabolized by phase II hepatic enzymes with urinary excretion as sulfate or glucuronate conjugates. The remainder is primarily metabolized by hepatic CYP2E to a highly reactive metabolite (*N*-acetyl-*p*-benzoquinoneimine [NAPQ1]) that is conjugated by glutathione before it can cause any harm. In overdoses, glutathione stores are depleted making the liver susceptible to reactive free radical injury; moreover, excess NAPQ1 complexes with hepatocyte membrane proteins and mitochondria, causing their dysfunction or degradation. In overdoses, therapy involves the administration of N-acetylcysteine to help to maintain glutathione store.

Aspirin (Acetylsalicylic Acid) (p. 422)

Overdose initially causes respiratory alkalosis, followed by potentially fatal metabolic acidosis. *Chronic aspirin toxicity (salicylism)* can develop in persons taking ≥3 g daily; it is manifested by headache, dizziness, ringing in the ears (tinnitus), difficulty in hearing, mental confusion, drowsiness, nausea, vomiting, and diarrhea. The most common adverse effects of aspirin are acute erosive gastritis and ulcers; bleeding may be exacerbated by aspirin inhibition of platelet cyclooxygenase and the inability to make thromboxane A_2 to drive platelet aggregation. Long-term ingestion (years) of analgesic mixtures of aspirin and phenacetin is associated with renal papillary necrosis (*analgesic nephropathy;* see Chapter 20).

Injury by Nontherapeutic Agents (Drug Abuse) (p. 423)

Common drugs of abuse, and their molecular targets, are listed in Table 9-3.

Cocaine (p. 423)

Cocaine is extracted from coca leaves and snorted or injected as the water-soluble cocaine hydrochloride; it is often diluted with powder look-alikes (e.g., talcum). Crack cocaine is the crystallized form of the pure alkaloid; its effects are the same, but its weight-for-weight potency is substantially greater. Cocaine induces euphoria and stimulation; there is no physical dependence, although psychologic withdrawal can be profound.

- *Cardiovascular effects* are due to excess dopaminergic and adrenergic stimulation (cocaine blocks neurotransmitter reuptake and increases synaptic release of norepinephrine). The consequences are tachycardia, hypertension, and vascular spasm; in the coronary artery circulation, vasoconstriction can cause myocardial infarction. Cocaine causes arrhythmias through the enhanced sympathetic activity, as well as by disrupting normal myocardial K^+, Na^+, and Ca^{2+} channel transport.
- *CNS effects* include hyperpyrexia (due to disrupted dopaminergic signaling) and seizures.

TABLE 9-3 Common Drugs of Abuse

Class	Molecular Target	Example
Opioid narcotics	Mu opioid receptor (agonist)	Heroin, hydromorphone (Dilaudid) Oxycodone (Percodan, Percocet, Oxycontin) Methadone (Dolophine) Meperidine (Demerol)
Sedative-hypnotics	$GABA_A$ receptor (agonist)	Barbiturates Ethanol Methaqualone (Quaalude) Glutethimide (Doriden) Ethchlorvynol (Placidyl)
Psychomotor stimulants	Dopamine transporter (antagonist) Serotonin receptors (toxicity)	Cocaine Amphetamines MDMA (ecstasy)
Phencyclidine-like drugs	NMDA glutamate receptor channel (antagonist)	Phencyclidine (PCP, angel dust) Ketamine
Cannabinoids	CBI cannabinoid receptors (agonist)	Marijuana Hashish
Hallucinogens	Serotonin 5-HT_2 receptors (agonist)	Lysergic acid diethylamide (LSD) Mescaline Psilocybin

5-HT_2, 5-Hydroxytryptamine; *GABA*, γ-aminobutyric acid; *NMDA*, *N*-methyl D-aspartate.
Data from Hyman SE: A 28-year-old man addicted to cocaine. *JAMA* 286:2586, 2001.

- In *pregnancy*, cocaine may reduce placental blood flow leading to fetal hypoxia and neurologic deficits or spontaneous abortions.
- *Other effects* of chronic use include dilated cardiomyopathy and nasal septum perforation.

Opiates (p. 424)

Heroin is an alkaloid of the poppy plant, injected subcutaneously or intravenously along with any adulterants. *Oxycodone*, an oral synthetic opiate, now exceeds heroin as a cause of opiate-related deaths in the United States. Opiates induce euphoria, hallucinations, somnolence, and sedation and are physically addictive. Adverse effects include the following:

- *Sudden death*, most commonly due to overdose leading to respiratory depression, pulmonary edema, and/or arrhythmia
- *Pulmonary* edema

For individuals who use an intravenous route of administration, there are additional risks:

- *Pulmonary* foreign body granulomas to particulate matter.
- *Infection* due to contaminated needles or dirty skin at sites of injection. Tricuspid valve endocarditis is a frequent sequelae, most often caused by normal skin flora. Sharing of needles is also a route for viral hepatitis and HIV transmission.
- *Skin* pathology, such as cellulitis, abscesses, and ulcerations, as well as thrombosed vessels.
- *Renal* pathology, such as amyloidosis (secondary to chronic skin infections) and focal, segmental glomerulosclerosis; both result in proteinuria and nephrotic syndrome.

Amphetamines and Related Drugs *(p. 424)*

Methamphetamine (p. 424) (also known as "speed") is an addictive drug that induces CNS dopamine release and thereby slows glutamate release; administration induces euphoria. Long-term use can lead to violent behavior, confusion, paranoia, and hallucinations.

3,4-Methylenedioxymethamphetamine (MDMA; p. 425) (also known as "ecstasy") induces euphoria and hallucinogen-like feelings via enhanced CNS serotonin release.

Marijuana *(p. 425)*

Marijuana is isolated from the hemp plant *Cannabis sativa;* the major psychoactive substance is Δ^9-tetrahydrocannibinol (THC). THC binds to endogenous cannabinoid receptors (the normal ligands are *endocannabinoids*) that modulate the hypothalamic-pituitary-adrenal axis and regulate appetite, food intake, energy balance, fertility, and sexual behavior. Acute THC use distorts sensory perception and impairs motor coordination; it can also increase heart rate and blood pressure. Smoking marijuana is associated with the characteristic effects of inhaling gases from burning plant fibers (e.g., bronchitis, pharyngitis, and chronic obstructive pulmonary diseases). Notably, the typical behaviors associated with marijuana smoking (deeper inhalation and breath holding) also lead to a threefold increased deposition of tars and particulates compared to standard cigarette smoking. THC has therapeutic benefit in treated chemotherapy-induced nausea and chronic pain syndromes.

Other Drugs *(p. 425)*

Inhalation of organic fumes (e.g., paint thinner, glues) causes acute behavioral changes (aggression, suicidal ideation, etc.) and chronically can lead to cognitive abnormalities and mild-to-severe dementia.

So-called "bath salts" are a new set of methylenedioxypyrovalerone-containing compounds with amphetamine-like effects. Snorting or ingestion can result in agitation, psychosis, myocardial infarction, or suicide.

Injury by Physical Agents (p. 426)

Mechanical Trauma (p. 426)

Mechanical forces can injure soft tissues, bones, or head; outcomes depend on the shape of the colliding object, force imparted, and tissues that bear the brunt of impact. Bone and head injuries with unique features are described in Chapters 26 and 28.

Thermal Injury (p. 426)

Thermal Burns *(p. 426)*

Burn injury and smoke inhalation cause approximately 3500 deaths annually in the United States; shock, sepsis, and respiratory insufficiency are the greatest threats to life. The clinical significance of burns depends on the following:

- Depth of the burn
  - Superficial (confined to epidermis; formerly first degree)
  - Partial thickness (involving the dermis; formerly second degree)
  - Full-thickness (extending to subcutaneous tissue; formerly third or fourth degree)

- Percentage of body surface involved
  - Burns involving more than 20% of surface area lead to rapid fluid mobilizations and potentially hypovolemic shock.
  - Burns induce a hypermetabolic state; thus injury involving 40% of surface area causes a doubling of metabolic demand.
  - The greater the surface area involved, the greater the risk of infection; in addition to loss of barrier function and vast swaths of necrotic debris, burn injury causes depressed systemic innate and adaptive responses and compromises local blood flow that reduces local inflammatory recruitment. Opportunistic organisms, such as *Pseudomonas,* and antibiotic-resistant strains of hospital-acquired microbes, such as *Staphylococcus aureus* and *Candida,* are common.
- Internal injuries from inhalation of hot and toxic fumes
  - Airway and lung parenchymal injury typically develops within 1 to 2 days of exposure and can involve direct thermal injury or chemical toxicity.
  - Water-soluble gases (chlorine, sulfur oxides, and ammonia) react with water to form acids and alkalis that cause substantial upper airway edema and inflammation.
  - Lipid-soluble gases (nitrous oxide, burning plastic) reach deeper airways and cause pneumonitis.
- Promptness and efficacy of postburn therapy
  - Fluid and electrolyte management
  - Prevention or control of wound infection

Hyperthermia *(p. 427)*

Prolonged exposure to elevated ambient temperatures can result in the following:

- *Heat cramps* (cramping of voluntary muscles) occur from loss of electrolytes through sweating; core body temperature is maintained.
- *Heat exhaustion* is the most common heat syndrome. It results from a failure of the cardiovascular system to compensate for hypovolemia, secondary to water depletion. Its onset is sudden with prostration and collapse.
- *Heat stroke* is associated with high ambient temperatures, high humidity, and exertion. Thermoregulatory mechanisms fail, sweating ceases, and core body temperature markedly elevates (e.g., to 40° C). The body responds with generalized peripheral vasodilation with peripheral pooling of blood and a decreased effective circulating blood volume. Necrosis of muscles and myocardium can occur associated with systemic effects, such as arrhythmias and disseminated intravascular coagulation.

Mutations in the ryanodine receptor type I—responsible for regulating skeletal muscle sarcoplasmic reticulum calcium release—can cause *malignant hyperthermia,* a rare situation in which common anesthetics cause profound muscle contraction and elevated core body temperature.

Hypothermia *(p. 427)*

Hypothermia occurs with prolonged exposure to low ambient temperature. At a core temperature of 90° F, individuals lose consciousness; with further cooling, bradycardia and atrial fibrillation occur.

- Freezing of cells and tissues causes direct injury through the crystallization of intracellular and extracellular water.

- Indirect injury occurs due to circulatory changes. Slowly falling temperatures may induce vasoconstriction and increased vascular permeability, leading to edematous changes (e.g., *trench foot*). Persistent low temperatures may cause ischemic injury.

Electrical Injury (p. 427)

The passage of an electric current through the body may be without effect; may cause sudden death by disruption of neural regulatory impulses or cardiac conduction pathways; or may cause thermal injury. Variables include the following:

- Current strength, duration, and path; alternating current induces tetanic muscle spasm and prolongs the duration of exposure by causing involuntary clutching.
- Tissue resistance varies inversely with water content; dry skin is resistant, but wet skin has greatly decreased resistance. The greater the tissue resistance, the greater the heat generated.

Injury Produced by Ionizing Radiation (p. 428)

Radiation is energy traveling in the form of waves or high-speed particles; it has a wide range of energies spanning the electromagnetic spectrum:

- *Nonionizing radiation* includes UV and infrared light, radiowaves, microwaves, and soundwaves; these sources are characterized by relatively longer wavelengths and lower frequencies and can produce vibration and rotation of atoms but have insufficient energy to displace bound electrons.
- *Ionizing radiation* includes x-rays and gamma rays, high-energy neutrons, alpha particles (composed of two neutrons and two protons), and beta particles (essentially electrons); these are typically of short wavelengths and high frequency and have sufficient energy to remove electrons from biologic molecules.

Radiation Units (p. 428)

Radiation doses are measured in three different ways—the amount of radiation emitted by a source, the radiation dose absorbed by a tissue, and the biologic effect of radiation:

- *Curie (Ci)* reflects the amount of radiation emitted from a source; it represents the disintegrations per second of a radioisotope such that 1 Ci = 3.7×10^{10} disintegrations per second.
- *Gray (Gy)* reflects the energy absorbed by a target tissue per unit mass; 1 Gy corresponds to 10^4 ergs/g of tissue. This was previously expressed as "radiation absorbed dose" or "Rad" where 1 Rad = 10^{-4} Gy.
- *Sievert (Sv)* reflects the biologic effect of a particular radiation dose (this was previously expressed by the term "rem"); some forms of radiation cause more injury than others, and some tissues are more susceptible. The *equivalent* dose—expressed in Sv—is the absorbed dose (expressed in Gy) multiplied by the relative biologic effectiveness of the type of radiation. For x-rays, 1 mSv = 1 mGy.

Main Determinants of the Biologic Effects of Ionizing Radiation (p. 428)

- *Rate of delivery:* A single dose can cause greater injury than divided or fractionated doses of the same cumulative amount. This is exploited in tumor therapy; normal tissues have intact repair pathways, and divided doses allow time for cellular repair, whereas tumor cells putatively have poorer repair mechanisms and will not recover between doses.

- *Field size:* A single low dose of external radiation administered to the whole body is potentially more lethal than higher doses administered regionally with shielding.
- *Cell proliferation:* Because DNA is the main target of radiation injury, rapidly dividing cells are more susceptible than quiescent cells. Except at very high doses that impair DNA transcription, DNA damage is compatible with survival in nondividing cells. Rapidly dividing normal cells (e.g., bone marrow, gonads, GI epithelium) may be exquisitely sensitive to radiation injury because DNA damage can induce growth arrest and apoptosis.
- *Oxygen effects and hypoxia:* The generation of reactive oxygen species from water ionization is the major pathway by which DNA damage is initiated by radiation. Poorly vascularized tissues with relative hypoxia will therefore be less sensitive to radiation injury.
- *Vascular damage:* Endothelial cells are moderately sensitive to radiation injury; their damage leads to the production of proinflammatory cytokines and vascular wall healing with luminal narrowing that will cause progressive tissue ischemia.

The acute effects of ionizing radiation range from overt necrosis at high doses (>10 Gy), killing of proliferating cells at intermediate doses (1 to 2 Gy), to no histopathologic effect at ≤0.5 Gy. If cells undergo extensive DNA damage or if they are unable to repair this damage, they may undergo apoptosis. Surviving cells may show delayed effects of radiation injury: mutations, chromosomal aberrations, and genetic instability. These genetically damaged cells may become malignant and cause cancers.

Total Body Irradiation *(p. 430)*

Whole-body exposures of <1 Sv produce little or no effect. However, greater exposures cause *acute radiation syndromes,* which at progressively higher doses involve the hematopoietic, GI, and CNS (Table 9-4).

Acute Effects on Hematopoietic and Lymphoid Systems *(p. 430)*

With high doses and large fields, peripheral lymphopenia with spleen and lymph node atrophy can develop within hours; at sublethal doses, repopulation occurs over weeks to months. Hematopoietic precursors are similarly sensitive, resulting in a marrow aplasia; very high doses kill stem cells and will cause a permanent aplastic anemia. Reflecting their relative peripheral longevity, granulocyte numbers are first affected (approximately 12- to 24-hour lifespan), followed by platelets (10-day lifespan), and finally erythrocytes (120-day lifespan); full recovery may require months.

Fibrosis *(p. 430)*

Fibrosis can occur in the radiation field weeks to months after exposure. This occurs primarily as a consequence of replacing dead tissue with scar but is also due to vascular injury (described previously), destruction of tissue stem cells, and the release of inflammatory cytokines that promote fibroblast activation and matrix synthesis.

DNA Damage and Carcinogenesis *(p. 430)*

DNA damage from radiation includes single-base damage, single- and double-strand breaks (DSBs), and DNA-protein cross-links. In surviving cells, damage is repaired by a variety of mechanisms; DSBs are most serious, and repair requires either homologous recombination or nonhomologous end-joining (see Chapter 7). The latter is most common and also leads to mutations, including deletions,

TABLE 9-4 Effects of Total Body Ionizing Radiation

	0-1 Sv	1-2 Sv	2-10 Sv	10-20 Sv	>50 Sv
Main site of injury	None	Lymphocytes	Bone marrow	Small bowel	Brain
Main signs and symptoms	None	Moderate granulocytopenia Lymphopenia	Leukopenia, hemorrhage, hair loss, vomiting	Diarrhea, fever, electrolyte imbalance, vomiting	Ataxia, coma, convulsions, vomiting
Time of development	—	1 day to 1 wk	2-6 wk	5-14 days	1-4 h
Lethality	None	None	Variable (0%-80%)	100%	100%

duplications, inversions, or translocations. In the absence of cell cycle checkpoint controls, such mutations may initiate carcinogenesis.

Cancer Risks From Exposures to Radiation *(p. 431)*

Although the level of radiation that increases cancer risk is difficult to unambiguously identify, any mutation has the potential to drive carcinogenesis. Doses >100 mSv clearly increase risk, but risk for doses in the range of 5 to 100 mSv is more difficult to quantify. To put this in context, a single chest x-ray delivers 0.01 mSv and computed chest tomography delivers 10 mSv.

Nutritional Diseases (p. 432)

Dietary Insufficiency (p. 432)

An appropriate diet provides adequate caloric intake to satisfy energy needs, amino acids and fats for protein and lipid synthesis, and necessary vitamins and minerals. In primary malnutrition, one or more components are missing; in secondary malnutrition, the nutrient supply is sufficient, but inadequate intake (e.g., due to anorexia), malabsorption, impaired use or storage, excess loss, or increased demand supervene. Poverty is a major determinant for primary malnutrition, although ignorance or failure of dietary supplement can contribute (e.g., iron deficiency in infants exclusively receiving formula diets). Illness (e.g., cancers and infection) can dramatically increase metabolic demand, and alcoholism often leads to vitamin deficiencies due to diminished intake, abnormal use, or increased loss.

Protein-Energy Malnutrition (p. 433)

Protein-energy malnutrition (PEM) is characterized by inadequate dietary intake of protein and calories (or malabsorption) with resultant muscle, fat, and weight loss, lethargy, and generalized weakness. A body mass index (BMI) <16 kg/m^2 is considered malnutrition; BMI is defined as weight (kg)/height^2 (m^2), where $nl = 18.5 - 25$ kg/m^2. More practically a child whose weight falls to less than 80% of normal is considered to be malnourished. Other helpful measures are fat stores, muscle mass, and circulating levels of serum proteins (e.g., albumin and transferrin). In elderly nursing home patients >5% weight loss associated with PEM increases mortality risk fivefold.

Marasmus and Kwashiorkor *(p. 433)*

Marasmus and kwashiorkor are two ends of the PEM spectrum but also have substantial overlap:

- Marasmus:
    - Weight loss of ≥60% compared to normal for sex and age.
    - Growth retardation and loss of muscle mass.
    - Protein and fat are mobilized from the *somatic compartment* of the body (largely skeletal muscle and subcutaneous fat); this provides energy from amino acids and triglycerides.
    - Serum protein levels are largely maintained.
    - Diminished leptin synthesis may drive increased pituitary-adrenal axis production of glucocorticoids that induce lipolysis.
    - Anemia and immune deficiency are common, with recurrent infections.
- Kwashiorkor:
    - Occurs when protein deprivation is relatively greater than overall calorie reduction.

- Associated with protein loss from the *visceral compartment* of the body (largely liver); there is relative sparing of muscle and adipose tissue.
- Resulting hypoalbuminemia causes generalized edema that may mask weight loss.
- An enlarged fatty liver is due to inadequate lipoprotein synthesis and thus hepatic accumulation of peripherally mobilized triglycerides.
- Apathy, listlessness, and anorexia occur.
- Small bowel mucosal atrophy (reversible) can lead to malabsorption.
- Immune deficiency is common, with secondary infections.

Protein-Energy Malnutrition in the Developed World *(p. 434)*

PEM in the developed world occurs in chronically ill, geriatric, and bedridden individuals; half of older nursing home residents are estimated to be malnourished. A 5% weight loss associated with PEM correlates with a fivefold increased mortality risk, related to infections, sepsis, and impaired wound healing.

Cachexia *(p. 435)*

Cachexia is a term used to describe PEM that occurs in chronically ill patients (e.g., with cancer or AIDS). Cachexia occurs in approximately 50% of cancer patients and is the cause of death in a third (often due to atrophy of muscles of respiration). Tumors cause cachexia via proteolysis-inducing factor (PIF) and lipid-mobilizing factor, the latter likely by driving the production of proinflammatory cytokines, such as tumor necrosis factor and interleukin (IL)-6. PIF and the inflammatory cytokines cause skeletal muscle catabolism through NF-κB-induced activation of ubiquitin-proteasome pathways.

Anorexia Nervosa and Bulimia (p. 435)

These disorders occur as a result of obsession with body image; altered serotonin metabolism is implicated:

- Anorexia nervosa is self-induced starvation.
  - Highest death rate of any psychiatric disorder.
  - Clinical findings are similar to those in severe PEM.
  - Amenorrhea is common due to suppression of the hypothalamus-pituitary axis.
  - Decreased thyroid hormone production causes cold intolerance, bradycardia, constipation, dry scaly skin, and hair thinning.
  - Decreased bone density is associated with low estrogen levels.
  - Sudden death due to arrhythmias in the setting of hypokalemia.
- Bulimia is characterized by food binging followed by self-induced vomiting; diuretic or laxative abuse may also occur.
  - More common than anorexia, afflicting 1% to 2% of women and 0.1% of men.
  - Better overall prognosis.
  - Amenorrhea is less common due to relatively normal weights and hormonal levels.
  - Medical complications are related to persistent vomiting and include electrolyte abnormalities (hypokalemia) that can cause arrhythmias, aspiration of gastric contents, and esophageal or gastric laceration.

Vitamin Deficiencies (p. 435)

Thirteen vitamins are necessary for health. Nine are water soluble and are primarily renally excreted. Four—vitamins A, D, E, and K—are fat soluble and thus readily stored but also may be poorly taken up in malabsorption syndromes. Vitamins D and K, biotin, and niacin can be synthesized endogenously, but dietary intake is also generally necessary. Table 9-5 is a summary of the essential vitamins and their deficiency syndromes. Table 9-6 is the equivalent table for selected trace elements.

TABLE 9-5 Vitamins: Major Functions and Deficiency Syndromes

Vitamin	Functions	Deficiency Syndrome
Fat-Soluble		
Vitamin A	A component of visual pigment Maintenance of specialized epithelia Maintenance of resistance to infection	Night blindness, xerophthalmia, blindness Squamous metaplasia Vulnerability to infection, particularly measles
Vitamin D	Facilitates intestinal absorption of calcium and phosphorus and mineralization of bone	Rickets in children Osteomalacia in adults
Vitamin E	Major antioxidant; scavenges free radicals	Spinocerebellar degeneration
Vitamin K	Cofactor in hepatic carboxylation of procoagulants—factors II (prothrombin), VII, IX, and X; and protein C and protein S	Bleeding diathesis
Water-Soluble		
Vitamin B_1 (thiamine)	As pyrophosphate, is coenzyme in decarboxylation reactions	Dry and wet beriberi, Wernicke syndrome, Korsakoff syndrome
Vitamin B_2 (riboflavin)	Converted to coenzymes flavin mononucleotide and flavin adenine dinucleotide, cofactors for many enzymes in intermediary metabolism	Ariboflavinosis, cheilosis, stomatitis, glossitis, dermatitis, corneal vascularization
Niacin	Incorporated into NAD and NAD phosphate, involved in a variety of redox reactions	Pellagra—three "Ds": dementia, dermatitis, diarrhea
Vitamin B_6 (pyridoxine)	Derivatives serve as coenzymes in many intermediary reactions	Cheilosis, glossitis, dermatitis, peripheral neuropathy
Vitamin B_{12}	Required for normal folate metabolism and DNA synthesis Maintenance of myelinization of spinal cord tracts	Combined system disease (megaloblastic pernicious anemia and degeneration of posterolateral spinal cord tracts)
Vitamin C	Serves in many oxidation-reduction (redox) reactions and hydroxylation of collagen	Scurvy
Folate	Essential for transfer and use of 1-carbon units in DNA synthesis	Megaloblastic anemia, neural tube defects
Pantothenic acid	Incorporated in coenzyme A	No nonexperimental syndrome recognized
Biotin	Cofactor in carboxylation reactions	No clearly defined clinical syndrome

TABLE 9-6 Functions of Trace Metals and Deficiency Syndromes

Nutrient	Functions	Deficiency Syndromes
Iron	Essential component of hemoglobin as well as a number of iron-containing metalloenzymes	Hypochromic microcytic anemia
Zinc	Component of enzymes, principally oxidases	Acrodermatitis enteropathica, growth retardation, infertility
Iodine	Component of thyroid hormone	Goiter and hypothyroidism
Selenium	Component of glutathione peroxidase	Myopathy, rarely cardiomyopathy
Copper	Component of cytochrome *c* oxidase, dopamine β-hydroxylase, tyrosinase, lysyl oxidase, and unknown enzymes involved in cross-linking keratin	Muscle weakness, neurologic defects, hypopigmentation, abnormal collagen cross-linking
Manganese	Component of metalloenzymes, including oxidoreductases, hydrolases, and lipases	No well-defined deficiency syndrome
Fluoride	Mechanism unknown	Dental caries

Vitamin deficiency may be primary (dietary in origin) or secondary to abnormalities of absorption, transport, storage, loss, or metabolic conversion. Isolated single-vitamin deficiencies are relatively uncommon.

Vitamin A (p. 436)

Vitamin A is a group of related compounds with similar activities. *Retinol* is the transport and storage form of vitamin A; *retinal* is the aldehyde, and *retinoic acid* the acid form. Dietary intake includes preformed vitamin A (found in meat, eggs, milk) and carotenoids (primarily β-carotene, found in yellow and leafy green vegetables); carotenoids are efficiently metabolized to active vitamin A and constitute approximately a third of dietary intake. Ninety percent of vitamin A is stored in the perisinusoidal stellate (Ito) cells in the liver and in healthy adults constitutes a 6-month reserve. Retinol is transported bound to retinol-binding protein, synthesized in the liver.

Function (p. 436)

- Maintenance of normal vision: Rhodopsin (rods) and iodopsins (cones) are synthesized from retinal and membrane protein opsins. Photons convert bound 11-*cis* retinal to all *trans*-retinal triggering opsin conformational changes that are ultimately converted into nerve impulses that enable vision. Most all-*trans* retinal is reduced to retinol and is lost to the retina, thus requiring constant replenishing.
- Cell growth and differentiation: Interaction of retinoic acid with intracellular receptors (RARs) releases repressor molecules and permits heterodimer formation with retinoic X receptors (RXRs); these then activate a variety of genes by binding to specific promoter elements. Vitamin A deficiency leads to squamous metaplasia of epithelium.

- Metabolic effects of retinoids: Interaction of retinoic acid with RXR leads to heterodimer formation with other nuclear receptors involved in regulating metabolism and vitamin D activity. Peroxisome proliferator-activated receptors (PPARs) interact with RXR and are key regulators of lipid metabolism and adipogenesis.
- Enhancing immunity to infections, in part by maintaining epithelial integrity.
- Host resistance to infections.

Vitamin A Deficiency (p. 437)

Vitamin A deficiency affects vision (especially in reduced light [night blindness]), immunity, and the normal differentiation of various epithelia.

- *Xerophthalmia* (dry eye) occurs when conjunctival and lacrimal epithelium become keratinized; this causes conjunctival dryness (xerosis), formation of small opaque spots on the cornea due to keratin debris (Bitot spots), and eventual destruction of the cornea (keratomalacia) with blindness.
- Keratinizing metaplasia of epithelial surfaces results in respiratory tract infections due to airway squamous metaplasia and causes renal and urinary bladder calculi due to desquamation of keratinized epithelium.

Vitamin A Toxicity (p. 438)

- Acute manifestations include headache, vomiting, stupor, and papilledema.
- Chronic toxicity is associated with weight loss, nausea and vomiting, lip dryness, and bone and joint pain. Retinoic acid activates osteoclasts, leading to increased bone resorption and risk of fracture.
- Synthetic retinoids can be teratogenic and should be avoided in pregnancy.

Vitamin D (p. 438)

Vitamin D is critical for maintenance of normal plasma levels of calcium and phosphorus and is therefore involved in maintaining normal bone mineralization and neuromuscular transmission.

Metabolism of Vitamin D (p. 438)

Metabolism of vitamin D is outlined in Figure 9-2, *A:*

- Vitamin D_3 (cholecalciferol, hereinafter vitamin D) is absorbed in the gut (10% of requirement) or synthesized by UV-induced conversion from a 7-dehydrolcholesterol precursor in the skin; limited sun exposure or melanin in dark skin may result in less conversion.
- Vitamin D is transported to liver bound to a plasma α_1-globulin (D-binding protein) where it is converted to 25-hydroxyvitamin D (25[OH]D) by a 25-hydroxylase CYP.
- In the kidney, α_1-hydroxylase converts 25(OH)D to 1,25$(OH)_2$D, the most biologically active form; the enzyme activity is regulated:
  - 1,25$(OH)_2$D feedback inhibits α_1-hydroxylase activity.
  - Parathyroid hormone (PTH) (induced by low calcium) activates α_1-hydroxylase.
  - Hypophosphatemia activates α_1-hydroxylase.

Function (p. 438)

Vitamin D is essentially a steroid hormone that binds to high-affinity intracellular receptors and induces their association with RXR. The heterodimer binds to promoters of vitamin D target genes in small

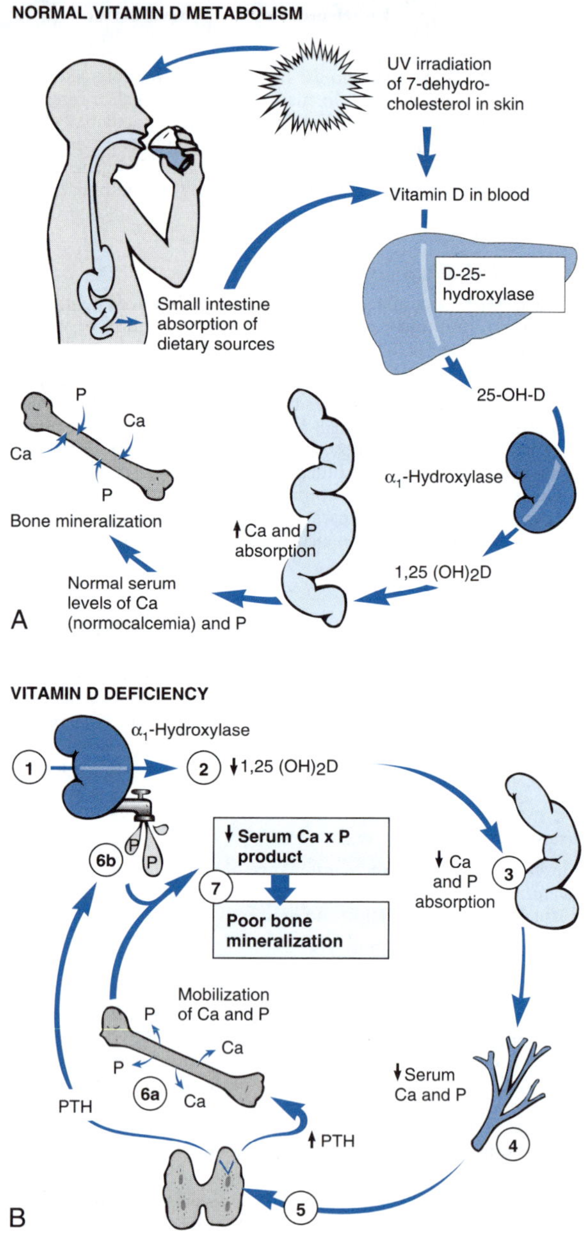

Figure 9-2 **A,** Vitamin D metabolism. Vitamin D is produced from 7-dehydrocholesterol in the skin or is ingested in the diet. It is converted by liver to 25(OH)D and by kidney to 1,25(OH)$_2$D (1,25-dihydroxyvitamin D), the active form of the vitamin. 1,25(OH)$_2$D stimulates the expression of RANKL, an important regulator of osteoclast maturation and function, on osteoblasts and enhances the intestinal absorption of calcium and phosphorus in the intestine. **B,** Vitamin D deficiency. Inadequate substrate for the renal α_1-hydroxylase (1), results in a deficiency of 1,25(OH)$_2$D (2), and insufficient calcium and phosphorus absorption from the gut (3), with consequently depressed serum levels of both (4). Hypocalcemia activates the parathyroid glands (5), with PTH release causing mobilization of calcium and phosphorus from bone (6a). PTH also induces renal calcium retention and phosphate wasting (6b); this maintains serum calcium near normal levels, but with low serum phosphate, mineralization is impaired (7).

bowel, bone, and kidney to regulate plasma calcium and phosphorus (see later); it also has immunomodulatory and antiproliferative effects. Vitamin D can also bind to membrane receptors that directly activate protein kinase C and open calcium channels.

Effects of Vitamin D on Calcium and Phosphorus Homeostasis (p. 439)

- *Intestinal calcium absorption* is augmented by vitamin D-induced increases in TRPV6, a calcium transport channel.
- *Renal tubular epithelial resorption of calcium* is augmented by vitamin D-induced increases of TRPV5, another calcium transport channel.
- *Osteoclast maturation and activity* is induced by vitamin D-driven increases of RANKL expression on osteoblasts (see Chapter 26).
- *Bone mineralization* is increased by vitamin D-induced stimulation of osteoblasts to synthesize osteocalcin, a protein involved in calcium deposition.

Deficiency States (p. 440)

Deficiency states are schematized in Figure 9-2, *B*.

- Vitamin D deficiency primarily results from inadequate intake, inadequate sun exposure, or altered vitamin D absorption or metabolism (e.g., renal disease).
- Deficiency causes deficient absorption of calcium and phosphorus from the gut with consequent depressed serum levels of both.
- Hypocalcemia activates the parathyroid glands, causing PTH-induced mobilization of calcium and phosphorus from bone; PTH also induces calcium retention in the urine with phosphate wasting. Although serum levels of calcium may thereby be maintained, the phosphate level is low, impairing bone mineralization.
- Vitamin D deficiency causes *rickets* in growing children and *osteomalacia* in adults; both forms of skeletal disease arise from an excess of unmineralized matrix.
- In *rickets,* inadequate provisional calcification of epiphyseal cartilage deranges endochondral bone growth, resulting in skeletal deformation, including frontal bossing, deformation of the chest plate, lumbar lordosis, and bowing legs.
- In osteomalacia, newly formed osteoid is inadequately mineralized leading to weakening of the bone and increased susceptibility to fracture.

Nonskeletal Effects of Vitamin D (p. 441)

1,25$(OH)_2$D can be synthesized by macrophages and a variety of epithelia; vitamin D receptors are also present in numerous tissues that do not regulate calcium and phosphorus homeostasis. Vitamin D activity in these cells may be related to innate immunity; moreover, of the 200+ genes whose expression is regulated by vitamin D, several influence cell proliferation, differentiation, apoptosis, and angiogenesis. Chronic vitamin D insufficiency is associated with 30% to 50% increased incidence of colon, prostate, and breast cancers.

Vitamin D Toxicity (p. 442)

Vitamin D toxicity due to overingestion can cause hypercalcemia and cause metastatic calcification in soft tissues.

Vitamin C (Ascorbic Acid) *(p. 442)*

Vitamin C (ascorbic acid) is present in many foods and is abundant in fruits and vegetables, so that all but the most restricted diets provide adequate amounts.

Function (p. 443)

- Activating prolyl and lysyl hydroxylases, providing for hydroxylation of procollagen and thereby facilitating collagen cross-linking.
- Scavenging free radicals and regenerating the antioxidant form of vitamin E.

Deficiency States (p. 443)

Insufficient vitamin C leads to *scurvy,* characterized in children by inadequate osteoid (and therefore bone formation) and by hemorrhage and poor healing in all ages due to poor collagen cross-linking.

Vitamin C Excess (p. 443)

Supraphysiologic doses of vitamin C do not protect against the common cold but do have a mild antihistamine effect; likewise there is no efficacy in cancer prevention. Bioavailability of vitamin C is limited by intrinsic instability, modest intestinal absorption, and rapid urinary excretion. Toxicities of overdosing include possible iron overload (vitamin C increases elemental iron uptake), hemolytic anemia in the setting of glucose-6-phosphate dehydrogenase deficiency, and calcium oxalate kidney stones.

Obesity (p. 444)

Obesity is a massive problem (pun not intended). Individuals with BMI ≥30 kg/m^2 are considered obese; those with BMI between 25 and 30 kg/m^2 are overweight. By these standards, 66% of adults in the United States are overweight or obese, and 16% of children are overweight. Excess adiposity is associated with increased incidence of type 2 diabetes mellitus, dyslipidemias, cardiovascular disease, hypertension, and cancer. The World Health Organization estimates that by 2015, 700 million adults globally will be obese.

Obesity is a simple consequence of caloric imbalance with intake greater than expenditure; however, the regulation of the neural and humoral mechanisms controlling appetite, satiety, and energy balance is complex (Fig. 9-3):

- Peripheral sites generate signals to indicate adequacy of metabolites or stores; *leptin* and *adiponectin* in fat cells, *ghrelin* in the stomach, *peptide YY (PYY)* from ileum and colon, and *insulin* from the pancreas.
- The arcuate nucleus in the hypothalamus integrates the peripheral input and outputs efferent signals through pro-opiomelanocortin (POMC) and cocaine and amphetamine-regulated transcript (CART) neurons, as well as neurons containing neuropeptide Y (NPY) and agouti-related peptide (agRP).
- The efferent output to second-order hypothalamic neurons controls food intake and energy expenditure.
  - POMC/CART neurons enhance energy expenditure and weight loss by production of anorexigenic α-melanocyte-stimulating hormone that binds to melanocortin receptors.
  - NPY/AgRP neurons promote food intake and weight gain.

Leptin (p. 444)

Leptin is a peptide hormone secreted by adipose tissue when fat stores are abundant. Leptin stimulates hypothalamic POMC/CART neurons and inhibits NPY/AgRP neurons; food intake is accordingly diminished. If adipose stores are low, leptin secretion is diminished and food intake is increased. Through other circuits, an abundance

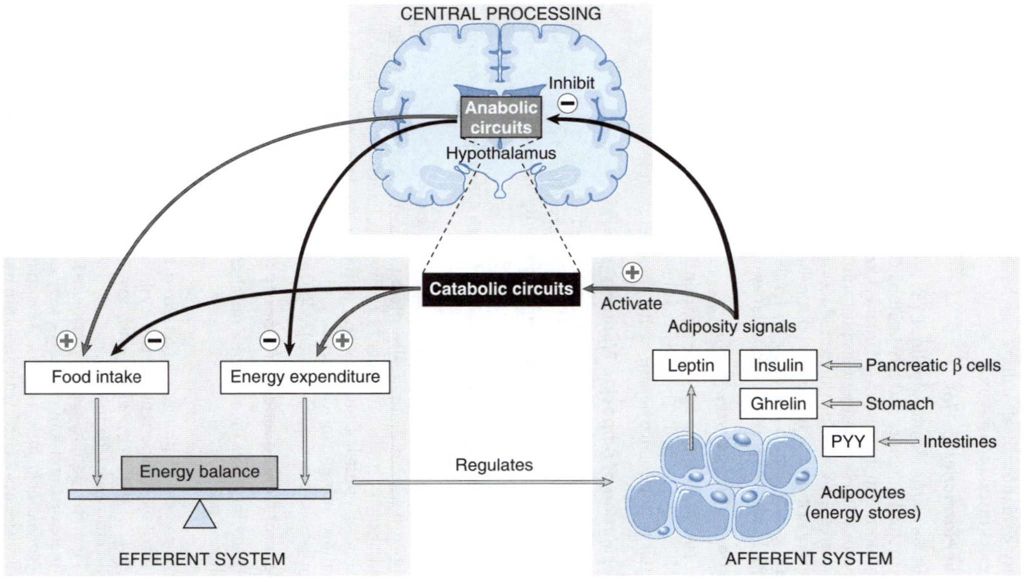

Figure 9-3 Regulation of energy balance. Adipose tissues generate signals that influence hypothalamic activity, which centrally regulates appetite and satiety. Adipose tissue signals cecrease food intake by inhibiting anabolic circuits, and enhance energy expenditure by activating catabolic circuits.

of leptin also stimulates physical activity, heat production, and energy expenditure. Loss of function in the leptin signaling pathway is a rare cause of massive obesity; melanocortin receptor mutations account for perhaps 5% of severe obesity.

Adiponectin *(p. 446)*

Adiponectin is a polypeptide hormone produced by adipocytes; it diminishes liver influx of triglycerides and stimulates skeletal muscle fatty oxidation. It also decreases hepatic gluconeogenesis and increases insulin sensitivity.

Gut Hormones *(p. 446)*

Gut hormones include ghrelin, PYY, and insulin; these act as short-term meal initiators and terminators. Ghrelin is the only known gut hormone that increases food intake, likely acting through NPT/AgRP neurons; in obese individuals postprandial ghrelin suppression is attenuated. PYY administration reduces food intake; PYY levels are low during fasting and increase after meals, and PYY levels are increased after gastric bypass surgery. PYY levels are generally low in patients with Prader-Willi syndrome and may contribute to their obesity.

Actions of Adipocytes *(p. 446)*

Adipose tissue is also a source of proinflammatory cytokines, such as TNF, IL-6, and IL-1. These lead to chronic subclinical inflammatory states that influence hepatic acute-phase reactant levels.

Regulation of Adipocyte Numbers *(p. 447)*

Absolute adipocyte number is established during childhood and adolescence and does not significantly vary after that time. Thus weight loss is due to reduced volume of adipocytes but no change in their quantity.

Other Emerging Factors Associated With Obesity: Role of the Gut Microbiome *(p. 447)*

Diet can influence the bacterial makeup of the colon, and gut microbial flora can dramatically affect the host's ability to catabolize and absorb certain nutrients (e.g., fiber). Changes in gut flora can also alter epithelial integrity and influence the levels of GI inflammation. Subsequent changes in gut PYY expression (among other hormones) can modulate the feedback regulation of appetite.

General Consequences of Obesity *(p. 447)*

Obesity increases the risk for a number of conditions, including the following:

- *Metabolic syndrome,* characterized by visceral adiposity, insulin resistance, hypertension, and dyslipidemia.
- *Type 2 diabetes mellitus,* with insulin resistance and hyperinsulinemia (see Chapter 24).
- Hypertension, hypertriglyceridemia, and low HDL cholesterol all increase the risk of *coronary artery disease.*
- *Nonalcoholic fatty liver disease* is marked by fatty change that can also be associated with inflammation and focal liver cell injury and can progress to cirrhosis (see Chapter 18).
- *Cholelithiasis* (gallstones) is 6 times more common in obese than in lean individuals.
- *Hypoventilation syndrome* is a group of respiratory abnormalities in obese individuals associated with hypersomnolence, polycythemia, and right-sided heart failure (cor pulmonale).
- *Osteoarthritis* is attributable to the cumulative effects of added wear and tear on the joints.

Obesity and Cancer (p. 448)

Between 4% and 7% of cancers are associated with obesity. High BMI is strongly correlated with esophageal adenocarcinoma and cancers of pancreas, thyroid, colon, breast, endometrium, kidney, and gallbladder.

Increased risk is attributed to peripheral insulin resistance and the associated hyperinsulinemia. High insulin levels activate a variety of kinases (e.g., phosphatidylinositol-3-kinase and Ras) that influence proliferation; hyperinsulinemia also induces insulin-like growth factor-1 production, a peptide that is mitogenic and antiapoptotic. The proinflammatory state associated with obesity may promote carcinogenesis (see Chapter 7). Finally, obesity influences the production of steroid hormones that regulate growth and differentiation of breast, uterus, and other tissues; greater adiposity increases adrenal and ovarian synthesis of androgens, and fat cell aromatases increase estrogen production from androgen precursors.

Diet, Cancer, and Atherosclerosis (p. 448)

Diet and Cancer (p. 448)

Epidemiologic studies demonstrate impressive geographic and population variation in cancer incidence, some of which can be associated with diet.

- *Exogenous carcinogens:* Examples include aflatoxin in the development of hepatocellular carcinoma and the possible carcinogenicity of selected food additives, artificial sweeteners, and pesticide contaminants.
- *Endogenous synthesis of carcinogens from dietary components:* Examples include nitrosamines and nitrosamides derived from amides in digested proteins, derived from nitrites in food preservatives, or produced by gut flora reduction of vegetable nitrates. Increased fat intake also increases bile acid production that modifies GI flora; subsequent bile acid catabolism produces carcinogenic metabolites. Conversely, increased dietary fiber can bind and remove potential carcinogens, while also decreasing bowel transit time, thus effectively lessening mucosal exposure to noxious metabolites. Although attractive hypotheses, the data are conflicting.
- *Lack of protective factors:* Selenium, β-carotene, and vitamins C and E are presumed to be anticarcinogenic by virtue of their antioxidant properties; the data again are incomplete.

Diet and Atherosclerosis (p. 449)

Reduced consumption of cholesterol and saturated animal fats and increased levels of unsaturated fatty acids can potentially lower serum cholesterol levels and may lessen atherosclerotic complications. However, consumption of omega-3 fatty acids has not been shown to be protective against cardiovascular complications. Caloric restriction, related to effects on sirtuin activation and insulin lowering, lowers the risk of atherosclerosis and also extends lifespan.

10 Diseases of Infancy and Childhood

The major causes of death in infancy and childhood are listed in Table 10-1; the greatest mortality is in the first year and declines progressively until accidents and suicide supervene beginning in the middle teens. The relative incidences of the various causes of mortality also depend on age, with congenital anomalies, prematurity, and sudden infant death syndrome (SIDS) topping the list in the first year of life; overall, congenital anomalies and malignancies are the most important causes across all pediatric age groups.

Congenital Anomalies (p. 452)

Congenital anomalies are morphologic defects present at birth; occasionally these become apparent only later in life. Approximately 3% of newborns in the United States have a congenital anomaly; clearly such abnormalities are still compatible with life. However, it is estimated that >20% of all fertilized ova are so anomalous that they never develop into a viable conceptus.

DEFINITIONS (p. 452)

Malformation: *Intrinsic* disturbance in morphogenesis; these are typically multifactorial and not caused by a single genetic defect.

Disruption: *Extrinsic* disturbance in morphogenesis causing a secondary destruction of a previously developmentally normal tissue; disruptions are not heritable. The classic example is an *amniotic band,* resulting from an amniotic rupture that causes a fibrous band that encircles, compresses, or attaches to a developing body part.

Deformations: These are common, affecting 2% of neonates, and—like disruptions—result from an *external* disturbance in morphogenesis. Deformations are caused by localized or generalized compression by abnormal mechanical forces and manifest as abnormalities in shape, form, or position (e.g., clubfeet). Most have a low risk of recurrence. The most common underlying factor is *uterine constraint:*

- Maternal factors include first pregnancies, a small uterus, or leiomyomas.
- Fetal and placental factors include oligohydramnios, multiple fetuses, or abnormal fetal presentations.

Sequence: Constellation of anomalies resulting from one initiating aberration that leads to multiple secondary effects. A classic example is the *oligohydramnios (Potter) sequence.* Thus oligohydramnios (decreased amniotic fluid) can occur through a variety of mechanisms: renal agenesis (fetal urine is a major component of amniotic fluid), placental insufficiency due to maternal hypertension, or an amniotic leak. Regardless of the cause, oligohydramnios leads in sequence to fetal compression with characteristic findings, including facial flattening, hand and foot malpositioning, hip dislocation, and chest compression with lung hypoplasia (Fig. 10-1).

Syndrome: Combination of anomalies that cannot be explained on the basis of one initiating aberration and a subsequent cascade. Most syndromes are caused by a single pathology that simultaneously affects several tissues (e.g., viral infection or chromosomal abnormality).

Organ-specific terms include the following:

- *Agenesis:* Complete absence of an organ and its associated primordium
- *Aplasia:* Absence of an organ due to growth failure of the primordium
- *Atresia:* Absence of an opening, usually of a hollow visceral organ (e.g., intestine)
- *Hypoplasia:* Underdevelopment of an organ, with decreased numbers of cells
- *Hyperplasia:* Enlargement of an organ associated with increased numbers of cells
- *Hypertrophy:* Increased organ size due to increased cell size
- *Hypotrophy:* Decreased organ size due to decreased cell size
- *Dysplasia:* In the context of malformations, refers to abnormal cellular organization

Causes of Anomalies (p. 454)

The causes of congenital anomalies are known in only 25% to 50% of cases; these are grouped into three major categories (Table 10-2):

Genetic Causes (p. 454)

- *Chromosomal abnormalities* are present in 10% to 15% of live-born infants with congenital anomalies, although it is important to note that 80% to 90% of fetuses with chromosomal abnormalities die in utero. Most cytogenetic aberrations arise as defects in gametogenesis and are therefore not familial. The most common chromosomal abnormalities in live-born infants are (in order) as follows:
  - Trisomy 21 (Down syndrome)
  - Klinefelter syndrome (47,XXY)
  - Turner syndrome (45,XO)
  - Trisomies 13 (Patau) and 18 (Edwards) (see Chapter 5)
- *Single-gene mutations* are relatively uncommon but follow mendelian patterns of inheritance; many involve loss of function in genes that drive organogenesis or development (e.g., Hedgehog signaling pathway and holoprosencephaly developmental defects of the forebrain and midface).

Environmental Influences (p. 454)

- *Viruses* (p. 454): The effect is related to gestational age at time of infection. Fortunately vaccination has reduced the incidence of such in utero infections.
- *Drugs and other chemicals* (p. 454): These cause <1% of congenital anomalies. Teratogens include thalidomide, folate antagonists, androgenic hormones, anticonvulsants, and 13-*cis*-retinoic acid.
- *Alcohol:* Alcohol is the most widely used teratogen; it is responsible for several structural anomalies, as well as cognitive and behavioral deficits, collectively termed *fetal alcohol spectrum disorders.* The most severely affected infants have a classic teratogenic phenotype called *fetal alcohol syndrome:* growth retardation, microcephaly, atrial septal defects, short palpebral fissures, and maxillary hypoplasia.

TABLE 10-1 Cause of Death Related With Age

Causes*	Rate†
Younger Than 1 yr	**660.6**
Congenital malformations, deformations, and chromosomal anomalies	
Disorders related to short gestation and low birth weight	
SIDS	
Newborn affected by maternal complications of pregnancy	
Accidents (unintentional injuries)	
Newborn affected by complications of placenta, cord, and membranes	
Bacterial sepsis of newborn	
Respiratory distress of newborn	
Diseases of the circulatory system	
Neonatal hemorrhage	
1-4 yr	**28.3**
Accidents (unintentional injuries)	
Congenital malformations, deformations, and chromosomal abnormalities	
Assault (homicide)	
Malignant neoplasms	
Diseases of the heart‡	
5-9 yr	**12.5**
Accidents (unintentional injuries)	
Malignant neoplasms	
Congenital malformations, deformations, and chromosomal abnormalities	
Assault (homicide)	
Influenza and pneumonia	
10-14 yr	**15.7**
Accidents (unintentional injuries)	
Malignant neoplasms	
Intentional self-harm (suicide)	
Assault (homicide)	
Congenital malformations, deformations, and chromosomal anomalies	

*Causes are listed in decreasing order of frequency. All causes and rates are based on 2008 (final) and 2009 (preliminary) data.
†Rates are expressed per 100,000 population from all causes within each age group.
‡Excludes congenital heart disease.
Data source: Centers for Disease Control and Prevention/NCHS, National Vital Statistics System: mortality, 2009 and 2008 (www.cdc.gov/nchs/nvss/mortality_tables.htm).

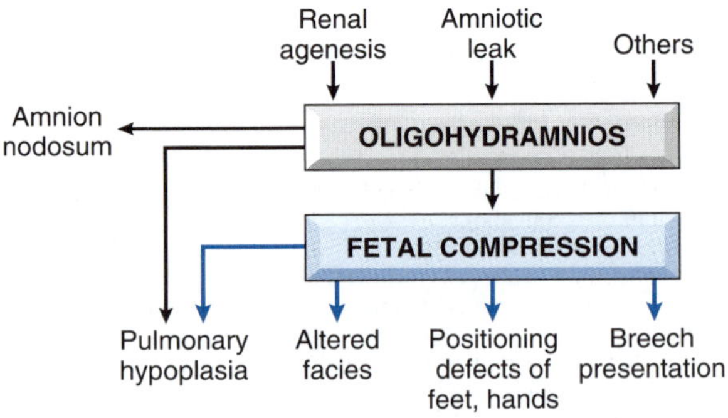

Figure 10-1 Schematic diagram of the oligohydramnios sequence.

TABLE 10-2 Causes of Congenital Anomalies in Humans

Cause	Frequency (%)
Genetic	
Chromosomal aberrations	10-15
Mendelian inheritance	2-10
Environmental	
Maternal/placental infections	2-3
Rubella	
Toxoplasmosis	
Syphilis	
Cytomegalovirus	
HIV	
Maternal disease states	6-8
Diabetes	
PKU	
Endocrinopathies	
Drugs and chemicals	1
Alcohol	
Folic acid antagonists	
Androgens	
Phenytoin	
Thalidomide	
Warfarin	
13-*cis*-retinoic acid	
Others	
Irradiations	1
Multifactorial (Multiple Genes and Environmental Influences)	**20-25**
Unknown	**40-60**

Data from Stevenson RE, Hall JG, Goodman RM (eds): *Human Malformations and Related Anomalies,* New York, NY: Oxford University Press, 1993, p 115.

- *Maternal smoking:* Maternal smoking during pregnancy is associated with higher incidences of spontaneous abortions, premature labor, placental abnormalities, low birth weight, and SIDS.
- *Maternal diabetes (p. 455):* The incidence of major malformations in diabetic mothers is 6% to 10%. Maternal hyperglycemia-induced fetal hyperinsulinemia causes increased body fat, muscle mass and organomegaly *(fetal macrosomia),* cardiac anomalies, neural tube defects, and other central nervous system (CNS) malformations.

Multifactorial Inheritance (p. 455)

Anomalies may involve the interaction of environmental factors with mutated genes; independently these may have no or minimal effect. For example, neural tube defects require a genetic predisposition *and* low maternal folate.

Pathogenesis (p. 455)

- The timing of any teratogenic insult influences the nature and incidence of the anomaly produced—a given agent can have significantly different outcomes depending on when it is encountered (Fig. 10-2).
  - In the early *embryonic period* (first 3 weeks after fertilization), injury either kills so many cells that death and spontaneous abortion results or such a limited number of cells that the fetus can recover without much consequence.

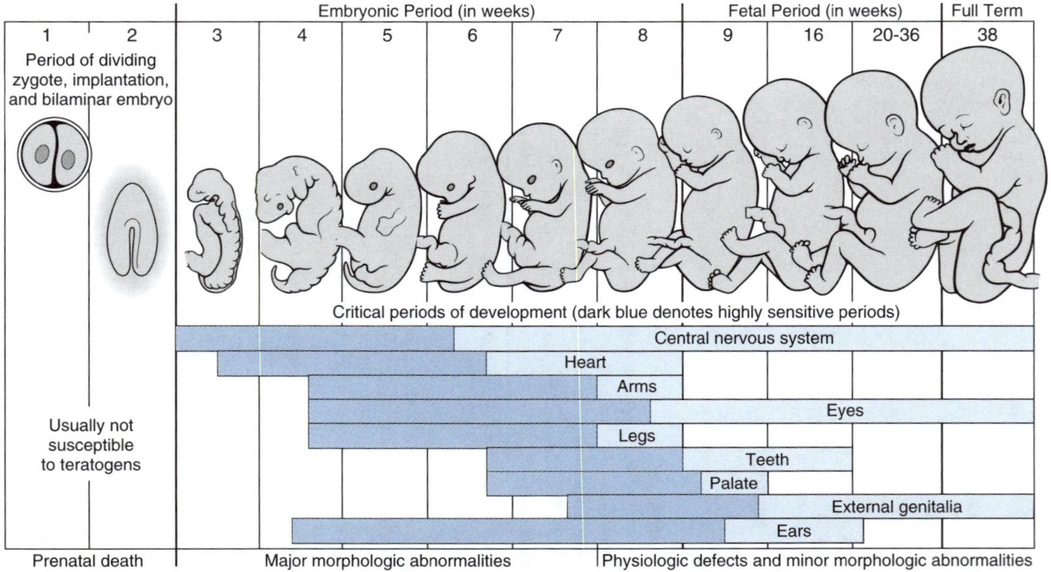

Figure 10-2 Critical periods of development for various organ systems and the resultant malformations. *(Modified and redrawn from Moore KL, Persaud TVN (eds):* The Developing Human, *5th ed. Philadelphia, PA: Saunders, 1993, p 156.)*

- Between the third and ninth week of the *embryonic period,* organs are developing from germ layers and the embryo is exquisitely sensitive to teratogenesis.
- The *fetal period* following organogenesis is marked chiefly by further maturation and growth, with greatly reduced sensitivity to teratogenic agents. However, the fetus is susceptible to growth retardation.

- Teratogens and genetic defects can act on the same developmental pathways and result in similar anomalies.
  - Valproic acid (an antiseizure medication) is teratogenic through disruption of the expression of several homeobox *(HOX)* transcription factors; moreover, *HOX* gene mutations give rise to congenital anomalies that mimic the valproate embryopathy.
  - Vitamin A (retinol) as all *trans*-retinoic acid is essential for normal development and differentiation; its absence during embryogenesis affects eyes, diaphragm, lungs, and genitourinary and cardiovascular systems. Conversely, excessive exposure is teratogenic, with characteristic CNS, cardiac, and craniofacial (e.g., cleft palate) abnormalities. The consequences are attributed to retinoic acid-mediated deregulation of transforming growth factor-β (TGF-β) signaling; notably, mutations of TGF-β pathway components can recapitulate retinoic acid embryopathy.

Prematurity and Fetal Growth Restriction (p. 456)

Morbidity and mortality rates are greater for infants born before the normal gestation period is completed; prematurity is the second most common cause of neonatal mortality after congenital anomalies. Babies born before the thirty-seventh week of gestation are considered *preterm* (12% of births in the United States); those born after the forty-second week are denoted *postterm.* Infants who fail to grow normally during gestation are also at increased risk, but a small full-term neonate will generally have fewer adverse consequences than a premature infant of the same weight. To take into account both developmental age *and* weight, infants are classified as the following:

- Appropriate for gestational age (10th to 90th percentiles)
- Small for gestational age (below 10th percentile)
- Large for gestational age (above 90th percentile)

Fetal Growth Restriction (p. 456)

Major risk factors for prematurity are as follows:

- *Preterm* (before 37 weeks) *premature rupture of membranes (PPROM)* complicates 3% of pregnancies and is the most common cause of prematurity (33%). PPROM is associated with maternal smoking or malnutrition, preterm labor, and gestational vaginal bleeding. The pathophysiology involves placental inflammation and matrix metalloproteinase activation.
- *Intrauterine infection* (25% of preterm births), with inflammation of the placental membrane (chorioamnionitis) and/or umbilical cord (funisitis). Organisms include *Ureaplasma urealyticum, Mycoplasma hominis, Gardnerella vaginalis, Trichomonas, gonorrhea,* and *Chlamydia.* Toll-like receptor (TLR) activation may deregulate prostaglandin production, leading to uterine smooth muscle contraction.
- *Uterine, cervical, and placental structural abnormalities* (e.g., uterine fibroids or "cervical incompetence").
- *Multiple gestation* (twin pregnancy).

Infants with fetal growth restriction (FGR; also called intrauterine growth retardation) are small for gestational age. Three main factors contribute to FGR:

- *Fetal abnormalities* (p. 457): Despite adequate maternal nutritional supply, there is compromised fetal growth potential; typically there is symmetric growth restriction—all organ systems are proportionately affected. Causes include the following:
  - Chromosomal abnormalities (e.g., triploidy and trisomy 18, 13, and 21)
  - Congenital anomalies
  - Congenital infections, most commonly the TORCH group (*to*xoplasmosis, *r*ubella, *c*ytomegalovirus, *h*erpesvirus)
- *Placental abnormalities* (p. 457): Vigorous fetal growth in the third trimester demands adequate placental growth and development; defects in placental supply typically cause asymmetric growth retardation, with relative sparing of the brain. Causes include the following:
  - Umbilical-placental vascular anomalies (single umbilical artery, abnormal insertion, etc.)
  - Placental abruption
  - Placenta previa (low-lying placenta)
  - Placental thrombosis and infarctions
  - Placental infections
  - Multiple gestations
- *Maternal abnormalities* (p. 457): The causes of FGR are the most common; essentially all these result in decreased placental blood supply. These impose significant risks for CNS dysfunction, learning disability, hearing or visual impairment. Causes include the following:
  - Preeclampsia
  - Hypertension
  - Inherited thrombophilias (e.g., factor V Leiden mutations)
  - Acquired thrombophilias (e.g., antiphospholipid antibody syndrome)
  - Malnutrition
  - Narcotic or alcohol intake
  - Cigarette smoking
  - Certain drugs (e.g., teratogens)

Neonatal Respiratory Distress Syndrome (p. 457)

Among many causes of neonatal respiratory distress (e.g., maternal sedation, blood or amniotic fluid aspiration, fetal head injury, or umbilical cord around the neck), the most common is respiratory distress syndrome (RDS), also known as *hyaline membrane disease.*

Pathogenesis (p. 457) (Fig. 10-3)

Lung immaturity is the most important substrate; the incidence of RDS is 60% in infants born before 28 weeks of gestation and <5% in infants born after 37 weeks. Inadequate pulmonary surfactant is the key feature; surfactant synthesis by type II pneumocytes (see Chapter 15) is accelerated beginning at 35 weeks of gestation, with production of phospholipids and glycoproteins that impact innate immunity and alveolar surface tension:

- Decreased surfactant results in increased alveolar surface tension, progressive alveolar atelectasis, and increasing inspiratory pressures required to expand alveoli.
- Hypoxemia results in acidosis, pulmonary vasoconstriction, pulmonary hypoperfusion, capillary endothelial and alveolar epithelial damage, and plasma leakage into alveoli.

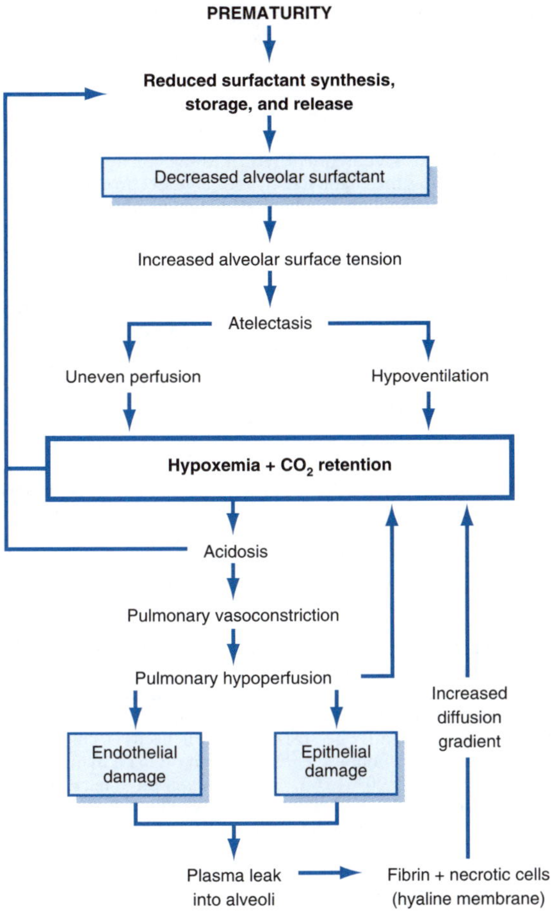

Figure 10-3 Schematic outline of the pathophysiology of respiratory distress syndrome (see text).

- Plasma proteins combine with fibrin and necrotic alveolar pneumocytes to form *hyaline membranes* that further impede gas exchange.
- *Corticosteroids* reduce RDS by inducing surfactant lipid and apoprotein production. Increased fetal insulin levels (due to maternal diabetes) suppress surfactant production.

Morphology (p. 458)

Grossly, lungs are solid, airless, and reddish purple. Microscopically alveoli are poorly developed and frequently collapsed; proteinaceous "membranes" line respiratory bronchioles, alveolar ducts, and alveoli.

Clinical Features (p. 458)

The typical infant with RDS is preterm but appropriate for gestational age. Lung maturity (reflecting surfactant synthesis) is assessed by measuring the amniotic fluid lecithin-sphingomyelin ratio. Antenatal corticosteroid therapy can induce surfactant production. If delivery cannot be delayed until there is adequate surfactant synthesis, therapy involves surfactant replacement and oxygen therapy.

In uncomplicated cases, recovery begins in 3 to 4 days; however, because of high-concentration oxygen therapy, infants are at risk for developing *retinopathy of prematurity* and *bronchopulmonary dysplasia* (BPD).

- Retinopathy occurs when hyperoxic therapy reduces vascular endothelial growth factor (VEGF) expression, resulting in endothelial cell apoptosis; subsequent return to the "relative" hypoxia of room air causes the characteristic retinal vessel proliferation.
- BPD is attributed to impaired alveolar septation in the setting of hyperoxia, hyperventilation, and inflammatory cytokines; BPD is manifested by decreased alveolar number *(alveolar hypoplasia)* and a dysmorphic capillary configuration.

Infants recovering from RDS may also have other complications of prematurity, including patent ductus arteriosus, intraventricular hemorrhage, and necrotizing enterocolitis (NEC).

Necrotizing Enterocolitis (p. 459)

NEC occurs most commonly in premature infants; the incidence is inversely proportional to gestational age (10% of very low birth weight infants ≤1500 g). Predisposing conditions include bacterial colonization of the gut and enteral feeding that induce inflammatory mediators; in particular, platelet activating factor production is implicated in promoting enterocyte apoptosis and increased intercellular permeability. This augments transmural bacterial migration with a vicious cycle of associated inflammation and mucosal necrosis.

NEC typically involves the terminal ileum, cecum, and right colon. Affected infants present with bloody stools, abdominal distention, and progressive circulatory collapse; gas within the intestinal wall *(pneumatosis intestinalis)* can occur. Microscopically there is mucosal to transmural coagulative necrosis, ulceration, bacterial colonization, and submucosal gas bubbles. Early NEC can often be managed conservatively, although 20% to 60% require resection of necrotic bowel segments, and perinatal mortality is high; survivors may have post-NEC bowel strictures due to healing-associated fibrosis.

Perinatal Infections (p. 459)

Infections are typically either transcervical (ascending) or transplacental (hematologic); occasionally, ascending microbes infect the endometrium and then the fetus via the chorionic villi.

Transcervical (Ascending) Infections (p. 459)

Most bacterial and a few viral infections occur via the cervicovaginal route. Infection may be acquired in utero by inhaling infected amniotic fluid into the lungs or at parturition by passing through an infected birth canal. Preterm birth is a common outcome, due either to inflammation-mediated damage to the amniotic sac or to neutrophil release of prostaglandins that precipitate the induction of labor. In the fetus, pneumonia, sepsis, and meningitis are the most common sequelae.

Transplacental (Hematologic) Infections (p. 460)

Most parasitic (e.g., toxoplasma, malaria) and viral infections, as well as a few bacterial infections (*Listeria,* syphilis), enter the fetal bloodstream via chorionic villi. Infection may occur at any time during gestation or occasionally at parturition (hepatitis B and human immunodeficiency virus [HIV]). Sequelae are highly variable, depending on the gestational timing and microorganism; adverse outcomes include spontaneous abortion, stillbirth, hydrops fetalis (see later), and congenital anemia (parvovirus B19).

TORCH infections all have similar manifestations, including fever, encephalitis, chorioretinitis, hepatosplenomegaly, pneumonitis, myocarditis, hemolytic anemia, and vesicular or hemorrhagic skin lesions; long-term sequelae include growth and mental retardation, cataracts, congenital cardiac anomalies, and bone defects.

Sepsis (p. 460)

Early-onset (first 7 days of life) sepsis is most commonly due to group B streptococcus, acquired at or shortly before birth; in addition to sepsis, infants present with pneumonia and occasionally meningitis. Late onset (up to 3 months) is often due to *Listeria* or *Candida.*

Fetal Hydrops (p. 461)

Fetal hydrops refers to fetal edema fluid collection during intrauterine growth; Table 10-3 lists the possible causes. Accumulation can be variable, ranging from severe and generalized (*hydrops fetalis,* usually lethal) to more localized, nonlethal forms (e.g., isolated pleural and peritoneal effusions or postnuchal fluid accumulations [cystic hygroma]).

TABLE 10-3 Selected Causes of Nonimmune Fetal Hydrops
Cardiovascular
Malformations
Tachyarrhythmia
High-output failure
Chromosomal
Turner syndrome
Trisomy 21, trisomy 18
Thoracic Causes
Cystic adenomatoid malformation
Diaphragmatic hernia
Fetal Anemia
Homozygous α-thalassemia
Parvovirus B19
Immune hydrops (Rh and ABO)
Twin Gestation
Twin-to-twin transfusion
Infection (Excluding Parvovirus)
Cytomegalovirus
Syphilis
Toxoplasmosis
Genitourinary Tract Malformations
Tumors
Genetic/Metabolic Disorders

Note: The cause of fetal hydrops may be undetermined ("idiopathic") in up to 20% of cases.
Data from Machin GA: Hydrops, cystic hygroma, hydrothorax, pericardial effusions, and fetal ascites. In Gilbert-Barness E, Kapur RP, Oligny LL, Siebert JR (eds): *Potter's Pathology of the Fetus, Infant, and Child,* St Louis, MO: Mosby, 2007, p 33.

Immune Hydrops (p. 461)

Immune hydrops is a hemolytic disorder caused by blood group incompatibility between mother and fetus. If fetal erythrocytes express paternal antigens that are foreign to the mother, those will elicit antibody responses that can cause red cell hemolysis. The most important molecules are the Rh D antigen and ABO blood group antigens.

Etiology and Pathogenesis (*p. 461; Fig. 10-4*)

The underlying basis of disease is the immunization of the mother by antigens present on fetal erythrocytes, followed by free passage of maternal antibodies across the placenta and into the fetus. These antibodies bind to erythrocytes and mediate complement-dependent lysis and/or phagocytosis by Fc receptor-bearing cells.

- Fetal erythrocytes can reach the maternal circulation during childbirth or during the last trimester of pregnancy (due to loss of the cytotrophoblast barrier).
- The first exposure to the antigenic stimulus elicits immunoglobulin M (IgM) antibodies that do not cross the placenta; however, subsequent pregnancies can elicit brisk maternal IgG responses that do cross the placenta.

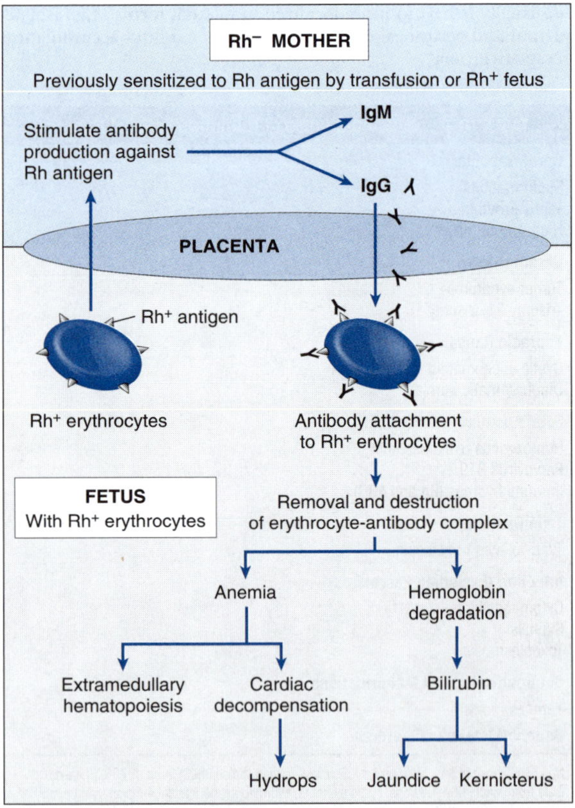

Figure 10-4 Pathogenesis of immune hydrops (see text).

- In Rh-negative mothers, prophylaxis with anti-D immunoglobulin at the time of initial delivery usually prevents sensitization and subsequent hemolytic disease.
- Although ABO incompatibility is more common than Rh incompatibility, hemolytic disease is rare in such mismatches because of the following:
    - Most ABO antibodies are IgM and do not cross the placenta.
    - Neonatal erythrocytes express A and B antigens poorly.
    - Many cells in addition to red blood cells express A/B antigens and therefore adsorb the majority of any antibody that enters the fetal bloodstream.
- Concurrent ABO incompatibility tends to reduce Rh immunization because any leaked red blood cells are promptly coated by maternal antibodies to A/B and cleared.

Anemia is a major sequela. If mild, fetal extramedullary hematopoiesis can keep pace. If severe, there is progressive heart and liver ischemia; liver injury leads to diminished protein synthesis, whereas cardiac hypoxia causes decompensation and failure. The combination of reduced oncotic pressure and increased venous hydrostatic pressure (heart failure) results in generalized edema.

Jaundice develops because hemolysis produces unconjugated bilirubin; this passes across the poorly developed fetal blood-brain barrier and causes CNS injury *(kernicterus).*

Nonimmune Hydrops (p. 462)

Major causes include the following:

- *Cardiovascular defects;* congenital defects or arrhythmias can all lead to congestive failure.
- *Chromosomal anomalies* (Turner syndrome, trisomies 21 and 18), often due to cardiac structural abnormalities. In Turner syndrome, aberrant lymphatic drainage in the neck can lead to local fluid accumulations *(cystic hygromas).*
- *Fetal anemia unrelated to immune hemolysis* (e.g., homozygous α-thalassemia or parvovirus B19; in the latter, virus replicates within erythroid precursors [normoblasts], leading to apoptosis and aplastic anemia).
- Monozygous twin pregnancies and twin-twin transfusions via anastomoses between the two circulations (10% of nonimmune hydrops).

Morphology (p. 462)

Anatomic findings vary with hydrops severity and the underlying cause. With fetal anemia, both fetus and placenta are pale; there is hepatosplenomegaly from cardiac failure and congestion. Except in parvovirus infections, the bone marrow exhibits compensatory erythroid hyperplasia, and multiple organs exhibit extramedullary hematopoiesis; increased hematopoiesis deposits large numbers of immature red blood cells in the peripheral blood (hence the name *erythroblastosis fetalis*).

Inborn Errors of Metabolism and Other Genetic Disorders (p. 464)

Phenylketonuria (p. 464)

Phenylketonuria (PKU) is an autosomal recessive disease, affecting 1 in 10,000 Caucasian infants. It is most commonly associated with biallelic mutations of the gene encoding *phenylalanine hydroxylase*

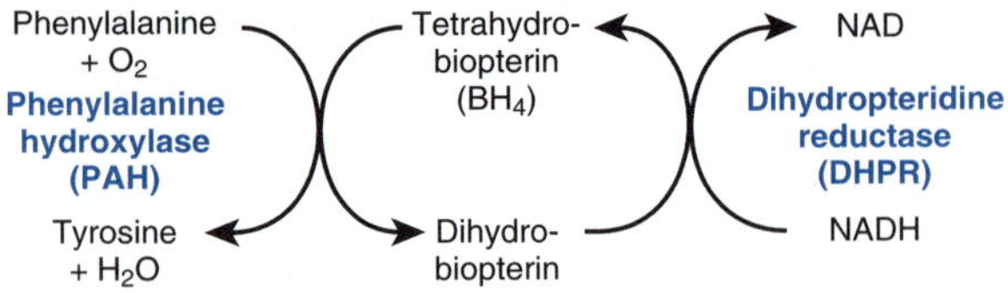

Figure 10-5 The PAH system. Deficiency of PAH or dihydropteridine reductase (DHPR) can give rise to PKU.

(PAH) responsible for the conversion of phenylalanine to tyrosine; approximately 2% of PKU cases are caused by defects in regenerating tetrahydrobiopterin (BH_4), a necessary cofactor for PAH activity (Fig. 10-5). There are more than 500 PAH disease-associated alleles, with disease severity correlating with the level of enzyme activity and the related increase in phenylalanine. Some PAH mutations result in only modestly elevated phenylalanine levels without neurologic sequelae, so-called *benign hyperphenylalaninemia.*

Although normal at birth, affected infants exhibit rising plasma phenylalanine within the first few weeks of life, followed by impaired brain development and mental retardation. Affected individuals also present with seizures, decreased pigmentation (due to reduced tyrosine and thus reduced melanin synthesis), and eczema. Screening for elevated phenylalanine metabolite in the urine allows early diagnosis, and subsequent phenylalanine dietary restriction prevents most clinical sequelae. Phenylalanine and its metabolites are teratogenic—infants born to PKU mothers with high phenylalanine levels are microcephalic and mentally retarded.

Galactosemia (p. 465)

Intestinal mucosal lactase converts lactose into glucose and galactose; galactose is then metabolized to glucose by three additional enzymes (Fig. 10-6). Enzymatic defects lead to accumulation of toxic metabolites *(galactosemia).* The most common and clinically significant form is an autosomal recessive mutation in *galactose-1-phosphate uridyl transferase (GALT);* affected patients accumulate galactose-1-phosphate, as well as elevated levels of galactitol (a polyol of galactose) and galactonate (an oxidized galactose metabolite).

The clinical picture is variable, depending on the GALT mutations. Classically infants present with failure to thrive and vomiting and diarrhea after milk ingestion. Important pathologic sequelae include hepatomegaly due to hepatic fat accumulation, cirrhosis, cataracts, and nonspecific CNS alterations (including mental retardation).

Urinary screening reveals the presence of an abnormal reducing sugar. Removal of dietary galactose for at least the first 2 years of life prevents most of the consequences. Nevertheless, older patients may exhibit speech disorders, ataxia, and gonadal failure.

Cystic Fibrosis (Mucoviscidosis) (p. 466)

Cystic fibrosis (CF) is an autosomal recessive disorder that affects epithelial cell ion transport and causes abnormal fluid secretion in exocrine glands, as well as in respiratory, gastrointestinal, and reproductive mucosa. It occurs in 1 of 2500 live births in the United States (1 in 20 carrier frequency among Caucasians but lower in other groups) and is the most common lethal genetic disease affecting Caucasian populations. Heterozygote carriers also have a higher

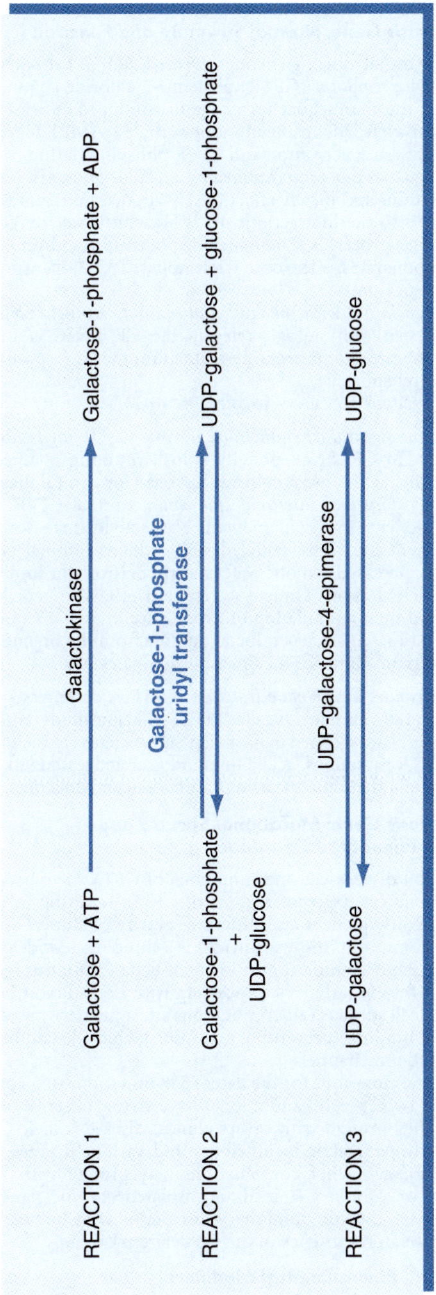

Figure 10-6 Pathway of galactose metabolism. *ADP,* Adenosine diphosphate; *UDP,* uridine diphosphate.

incidence of respiratory and pancreatic pathology relative to the general population.

Cystic Fibrosis Gene: Normal Structure and Function *(p. 466)*

- The gene mutated in CF encodes the *cystic fibrosis transmembrane conductance regulator* (CFTR) protein—a chloride channel; activation of the channel occurs via agonist-induced increases in intracellular cyclic adenosine monophosphate (cAMP), followed by protein kinase A activation and CFTR phosphorylation.
- *CFTR regulates other ion channels and cellular processes.* Although CF mutations specifically affect the CFTR, disease manifestations are related to the interactions of CFTR with other ion channels and cellular processes. These include potassium, sodium and gap junction channels, adenosine triphosphate (ATP) transport, and mucus secretion.
- *CFTR association with the epithelial sodium channel (ENaC)* has the most pathophysiologic relevance to CF. ENaC is an apical membrane protein in exocrine epithelium that is responsible for sodium transport.
- *CFTR functions are tissue-specific* (Fig. 10-7).
    - In *eccrine sweat duct epithelium,* normal CFTR *augments* ENaC activity. In CF, ENaC activity is lost, resulting in hypertonic sweat (hence the sweat chloride test used for clinical diagnosis).
    - In *respiratory and intestinal epithelium,* normal CFTR *inhibits* ENaC activity. In CF, augmented ENaC activity increases sodium movement into cells; coupled with reduced luminal chloride, there is increased osmotic water resorption from the lumen leading to dehydration of mucus secretions. Defective mucociliary action and the accumulation of hyperconcentrated, viscous secretions ultimately obstruct ductal outflow from the organs (hence the alternate name for the disease—*mucoviscidosis*).
- *CFTR mediates bicarbonate transport.* CFTR is coexpressed with a family of anion exchangers called SLC26. Alkaline fluids (containing bicarbonate) are secreted in normal tissues, whereas in the setting of some CFTR mutations, acidic fluids are secreted leading to an acid environment that causes mucin precipitation and duct obstruction.

Cystic Fibrosis Gene: Mutational Spectra and Genotype-Phenotype Correlation *(p. 467)*

At least 1800 disease-causing mutations of *CFTR* have been identified; these affect different regions of CFTR, resulting in distinct functional consequences and differing severity of clinical sequelae. The most common (70% worldwide) is a three-nucleotide deletion coding for phenylalanine at position 508 (delta F508); this results in defective intracellular CFTR processing with degradation before it reaches the cell surface. Other mutations affect primary protein synthesis, ATP binding (preventing activation), chloride conductance, or associated ion channels.

Patients homozygous for the delta F508 mutation (or a combination of any two "severe" mutations) have virtual absence of CFTR function; they present with severe clinical disease (*classic* CF), including early pancreatic insufficiency and various degrees of pulmonary damage. Other combinations may present with features of *atypical* or *variant CF,* including isolated chronic pancreatitis and late-onset chronic pulmonary disease, or with infertility only (caused by bilateral absence of the vas deferens).

Genetic and Environmental Modifiers *(p. 469)*

Genetic and environmental modifiers impact CF severity. Thus reduced expression of mannose-binding lectin 2 (involved in microbial

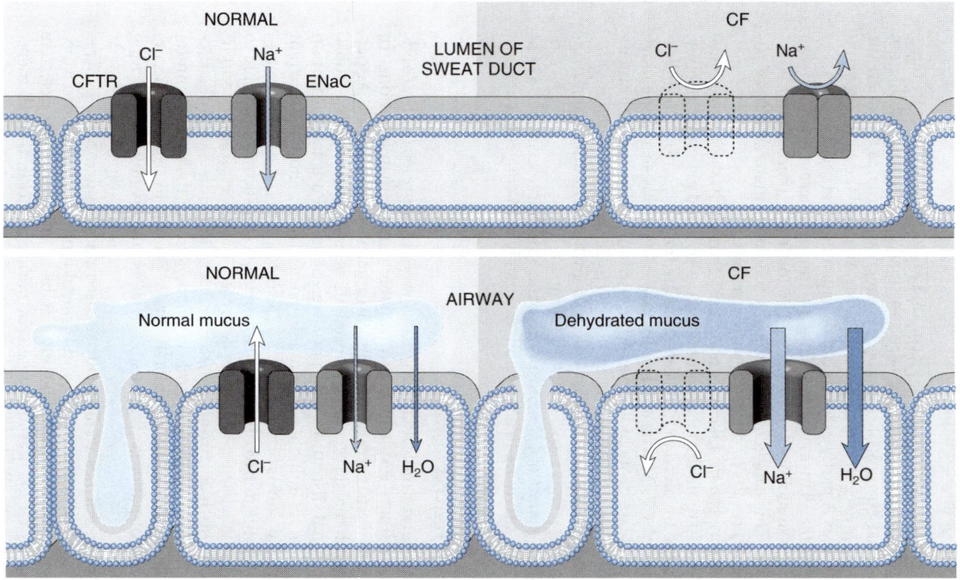

Figure 10-7 Chloride channel defect in the sweat duct *(top)* causes increased chloride and sodium concentration in sweat. In the airway *(bottom)*, patients with CF have decreased chloride secretion and increased sodium and water reabsorption, leading to dehydration of the mucus layer coating epithelial cells, defective mucociliary action, and mucus plugging of airways.

opsonization) confers a threefold increased risk of end-stage lung disease; polymorphisms that influence TGF-β expression (a direct inhibitor of CFTR function) also exacerbate the pulmonary phenotype.

The nature of secondary pulmonary infections (e.g., *Pseudomonas*—with more or less mucoid polysaccharide biofilm production) will also impact subsequent inflammation and lung destruction.

Morphology (p. 469)

Features are variable depending on the affected epithelium and the severity of involvement:

- *Pancreas:* Abnormalities occur in 85% to 90% of patients, ranging from mucus accumulation in small ducts with mild dilation to total atrophy of the exocrine pancreas. Absence of pancreatic exocrine secretions impairs fat absorption and the resulting avitaminosis A partly explains ductal squamous metaplasia.
- *Intestine:* Thick viscous plugs of mucus *(meconium ileus)* can cause small bowel obstruction (5% to 10% of affected infants).
- *Liver:* Bile canalicular plugging by mucinous material (5% of patients) results in diffuse hepatic cirrhosis.
- *Salivary glands:* Like pancreas, these commonly show progressive duct dilation, ductal squamous metaplasia, and glandular atrophy.
- *Lungs:* Involved in most cases and are the most serious complication of CF. Mucus cell hyperplasia and viscous secretions block and dilate bronchioles. Superimposed infections and pulmonary abscesses are common. *Staphylococcus aureus, Haemophilus influenzae,* and *Pseudomonas aeruginosa* are most common; *Burkholderia cepacia* is associated with fulminant illness.
- *Male genital tract:* Azoospermia and infertility occur in 95% of males surviving to adulthood, frequently with congenital absence of the vas deferens.

Clinical Features (p. 470)

The different molecular variants as well as the presence of secondary modifiers result in highly variable clinical manifestations. In classic CF, pancreatic exocrine insufficiency is universal, associated with malabsorption that presents as large, foul-smelling stools, abdominal distention, and poor weight gain. Poor fat absorption results in fat-soluble vitamin deficiencies (A, D, and K). Recurrent sinonasal polyps occur in 10% to 25% of patients, and 95% of males are infertile due to obstructive azospermia (most commonly due to congenital absence of the vas deferens). Cardiorespiratory complications, such as chronic cough, persistent lung infections, obstructive pulmonary disease, and *cor pulmonale,* are the most common causes of death (approximately 80%); chronic liver disease occurs in 15% of patients. The mean life expectancy is now approaching 40 years.

Treatment has traditionally focused on antimicrobials, pancreatic enzyme replacement, and bilateral lung transplantation. More recently, "potentiator" therapy has been introduced for defective forms of CFTR that are present at normal levels in the cell membrane; the orally bioavailable agents partially restore normal ion transport function.

Sudden Infant Death Syndrome (p. 471)

SIDS is officially defined by the National Institute of Clinical Health and Human Development as: "sudden death of an infant less than 1 year of age, that remains unexplained after a thorough case investigation, including performance of a complete autopsy, examination

TABLE 10-4 Risk Factors and Postmortem Findings Associated With Sudden Infant Death Syndrome*

Parental

Young maternal age (age younger than 20 years)
Maternal smoking during pregnancy
Drug abuse in *either* parent, specifically paternal marijuana and maternal opiate, cocaine use
Short intergestational intervals
Late or no prenatal care
Low socioeconomic group
African-American and American Indian ethnicity (? socioeconomic factors)

Infant

Brain stem abnormalities, associated with delayed development of arousal and cardiorespiratory control
Prematurity and/or low birth weight
Male sex
Product of a multiple birth
SIDS in a prior sibling
Antecedent respiratory infections
Germline polymorphisms in autonomic nervous system genes

Environment

Prone or side sleep position
Sleeping on a soft surface
Hyperthermia
Co-sleeping in first 3 months of life

*SIDS is not the only cause of SUIDs, but rather is a *diagnosis of exclusion.* Therefore, performance of an autopsy may often reveal findings that would explain the cause of an SUID. These cases should *not,* strictly speaking, be labeled as "SIDS."

of the death scene, and review of the clinical history." Thus by definition SIDS is a diagnosis of exclusion and a disease of unknown cause; nevertheless there are several known risk factors (Table 10-4). Infants usually die while asleep, mostly in the prone or side position. Most SIDS deaths occur between 2 and 4 months of life, and 90% within 6 months of birth; in the United States it is the leading cause of death in children between 1 month and 1 year of age and the third leading cause of infant death overall.

In comparison, sudden death in infancy with an anatomical or biochemical basis uncovered at autopsy should not be labeled as SIDS but rather as "sudden unexpected infant death" (SUID) (Table 10-5).

Morphology (p. 472)

Autopsy findings are usually subtle and of uncertain significance. Multiple petechiae (thymus, visceral and parietal pleura, epicardium) and histologic evidence of recent infection in the upper respiratory tract are common. The CNS demonstrates astrogliosis of the brain stem and cerebellum; arcuate nucleus hypoplasia may be present.

Pathogenesis (p. 472)

Pathogenesis is poorly understood; SIDS is most likely a heterogeneous, multifactorial disorder. The most compelling hypothesis is that SIDS reflects developmental immaturity of critical brain stem regions (e.g., arcuate nucleus) involved in arousal and cardiorespiratory control and that environmental influences (e.g., infection) further fatally impair these regulatory mechanisms.

TABLE 10-5 Postmortem Abnormalities Detected in Cases of Sudden Unexpected Infant Death*

Infections
- Viral myocarditis
- Bronchopneumonia

Unsuspected congenital anomaly
- Congenital aortic stenosis
- Anomalous origin of the left coronary artery from the pulmonary artery

Traumatic child abuse
- Intentional suffocation (filicide)

Genetic and metabolic defects
- Long QT syndrome (*SCN5A* and *KCNQ1* mutations)
- Fatty acid oxidation disorders (*MCAD, LCHAD, SCHAD* mutations)
- Histiocytoid cardiomyopathy (*MTCYB* mutations)
- Abnormal inflammatory responsiveness (partial deletions in *C4a* and *C4b*)

*SIDS is not the only cause of sudden unexpected death in infancy but rather is a *diagnosis of exclusion.* Therefore an autopsy may often reveal findings that would explain the cause of sudden unexpected death. These cases should *not,* strictly speaking, be labeled "SIDS."

C4, Complement component 4; *KCNQ1,* potassium voltage-gated channel, KQT-like subfamily, member 1; *LCHAD,* long-chain 3-hydroxyacyl coenzyme A dehydrogenase; *MCAD,* medium-chain acyl coenzyme A dehydrogenase; *MTCYB,* mitochondrial cytochrome *b; SCHAD,* short-chain 3-hydroxyacyl coenzyme A dehydrogenase; *SCN5A,* sodium channel, voltage-gated, type V, alpha polypeptide.

Tumors and Tumorlike Lesions of Infancy and Childhood (p. 473)

Benign tumors are much more common than malignant tumors; however, 2% of all cancers occur in infancy and childhood, and these are the leading cause of death (after accidents) in U.S. children aged 4 to 14 years.

Because displaced tissue masses can be present from birth, distinguishing true tumors from "tumorlike" lesions can be difficult; the latter are frequently histologically normal and grow at approximately the same rate as the infant.

- *Heterotopia* (also called *choristomas*) represents microscopically normal cells or tissues present in abnormal locations (e.g., a rest of pancreatic tissue in the wall of the stomach); these cells are usually of little significance but can be the origin of true neoplasms (e.g., adrenal carcinoma in an ovary).
- *Hamartomas* are excessive (but focal) overgrowth of mature cells or tissues native to the organ or site in which they occur that do not recapitulate normal architecture (e.g., a hamartoma of cartilaginous tissue in the lung parenchyma). These are histologically benign but can be clinically significant.

Benign Tumors and Tumorlike Lesions (p. 473)

The most common neoplasms of childhood are often "soft-tissue tumors" of mesenchymal origin; in comparison, the most common tumors of adults—benign or malignant—are of epithelial derivation.

Hemangiomas (p. 474) are the most common tumors of infancy; most are cutaneous, with a predilection for face and scalp. They may enlarge along with the growth of the child but commonly spontaneously regress; they rarely become malignant. Hemangiomas may represent one facet of hereditary disorders, such as *von Hippel-Lindau disease* (see Chapter 28).

Lymphatic tumors (p. 474) may occur on the skin but also within deeper regions of the neck, axilla, mediastinum, and retroperitoneal tissue. They tend to increase in size and depending on location become clinically significant if they encroach on vital structures. Histologically lymphangiomas are composed of cystic and cavernous lymphatic spaces, with variable numbers of associated lymphocytes.

Fibrous tumors (p. 474) range from sparsely cellular proliferations *(fibromatosis)* to richly cellular lesions indistinguishable from adult fibrosarcomas. The histology does not predict the biology of the infantile tumors. Thus as compared to their malignant adult counterparts, congenital-infantile fibrosarcomas have an excellent prognosis; in these tumors a characteristic chromosomal translocation produces an *ETV6-NTRK3* fusion gene that codes for a constitutively active tyrosine kinase.

Teratoma (p. 474) incidence has two peaks: at age 2 and again in late adolescence. Those occurring in infancy and childhood are congenital lesions, with 40% arising in the sacrococcygeal region.

- Approximately 10% of sacrococcygeal teratomas are associated with congenital anomalies, primarily defects of the hindgut and cloacal region, and other midline defects.
- Approximately 75% are benign mature teratomas, whereas 12% are unequivocally malignant and lethal; the remainder—designated immature teratomas—contain mature and immature tissue, with malignant potential correlating with the percentage of immature tissues.

Malignant Tumors (p. 475)

Childhood malignancies differ biologically and histologically from their adult counterparts by the following:

- Incidence and type of tumor
- A close relationship between abnormal development (teratogenesis) and tumor induction (oncogenesis)
- A greater prevalence of underlying familial or genetic germline aberrations
- A tendency to spontaneously regress or cytodifferentiate
- Better survival and cure rates, with attention being increasingly focused on preventing subsequent therapy-induced malignancies

Incidence and Types (p. 475)

The most frequent childhood cancers involve the following:

- Hematopoietic system (leukemia, some lymphomas)
- CNS (astrocytoma, medulloblastoma, ependymoma)
- Adrenal medulla (neuroblastoma)
- Retina (retinoblastoma)
- Soft tissue (rhabdomyosarcoma)
- Bone (Ewing sarcoma, osteogenic sarcoma)
- Kidney (Wilms tumor)

Leukemia accounts for more deaths in children younger than 15 years of age than all other tumors combined.

Many pediatric cancers tend to have a more primitive, *embryonal* rather than a frankly anaplastic histology, with features of organogenesis consistent with the site of origin (hence the suffix "-blastoma"). Such tumors are often collectively labeled as "small, round blue cell tumors"; included in this designation are lymphoma, Wilms tumor, rhabdomyosarcoma, Ewing sarcoma/peripheral neuroectodermal tumor [PNET]), neuroblastoma, medulloblastoma, and retinoblastoma.

Neuroblastic Tumors *(p. 475)*

Neuroblastic tumors arise in the adrenal medulla or sympathetic ganglia. Characteristic features include spontaneous regression, spontaneous or therapy-induced differentiation into mature elements, and a wide range of biologic behaviors; neuroblastoma is the most important entity in this group. Most neuroblastic tumors occur sporadically, but 1% to 2% are familial, associated with *anaplastic lymphoma kinases (ALK)* mutations. In high-risk subsets of neuroblastic tumors, the 5-year survival is only 40%.

Morphology (p. 476)

Neuroblastoma is the most common histologic subtype; 40% occur in the adrenal. These tumors are characterized by sheets of small, round blue neuroblasts within a neurofibrillary background (neuropil) and characteristic *Homer Wright pseudorosettes.* Some tumors display variable differentiation toward ganglion cells, accompanied by the appearance of a so-called "schwannian stroma" (organized fascicles of neuritic processes, Schwann cells, and fibroblasts). Depending on the degree of differentiation, these latter tumors are called *ganglioneuroblastomas* or *ganglioneuromas.*

Clinical Course and Prognostic Features (p. 477)

Prognosis is based on staging (size and spread), patient age (<18 months is favorable), histologic features (schwannian stroma is favorable), and specific genetic changes (near-normal ploidy and *N-MYC* amplification are unfavorable). In addition to local infiltration and lymph node spread, hematogenous spread commonly involves the liver, lungs, bones, and marrow. Approximately 90% of neuroblastomas produce catecholamines; elevated blood or urine catecholamine metabolites can aid in diagnosis. Newer therapeutic approaches involve retinoids to direct differentiation of neuroblastomas into mature tissues, and tyrosine kinase inhibitors.

Wilms Tumor *(p. 479)*

Wilms tumor of the kidney occurs in approximately 1 in 10,000 children; it is usually diagnosed between ages 2 and 5 years. Although malignant, the overall survival rate is >90%.

Pathogenesis and Genetics (p. 479)

Most (90%) of tumors are sporadic; bilateral tumors occur in 5% to 10% of patients and are presumed related to germline mutations; the tumors in this group are associated with malformation syndromes, all involving chromosome 11p:

- *W*ilms tumor, *a*niridia, *g*enital anomalies, mental *r*etardation *(WAGR) syndrome* are associated with a deletion on chromosome 11p band 13; patients have a 33% chance of developing Wilms tumor. The deleted chromosomal segment contains the Wilms tumor 1 *(WT1)* and aniridia *(PAX6)* genes. *WT1* encodes a DNA-binding transcription factor critical for normal renal and gonadal development; patients heterozygous for the deletion ("first hit") can develop a Wilms tumor when the second *WT1* allele acquires a frameshift or nonsense mutation ("second hit").
- *Denys-Drash syndrome* patients have gonadal dysgenesis and nephropathy (diffuse mesangial sclerosis) leading to renal failure; 90% develop Wilms tumors. The genetic abnormality is a dominant negative mutation in the *WT1* gene that affects DNA binding; Wilms tumors arise when the wild-type *WT1* allele is also inactivated. Denys-Drash patients are also at increased risk for gonadoblastomas.

- *Beckwith-Wiedemann syndrome* patients have enlarged body organs, hemihypertrophy, adrenal cytomegaly, and a predisposition to developing Wilms and other primitive tumors; the genetic abnormality is localized to chromosome 11p band 15.5 distal to the *WT1* locus. Several candidate genes map to this locus, including insulin-like growth factor 2 *(IGF2); IGF2* is normally imprinted (transcribed from only one parental allele) but demonstrates loss of imprinting (biallelic expression) in many of the tumors.
- Less than 10% of sporadic Wilms tumors are associated with *WT1* mutations, indicating that there are other tumorigenic pathways. In 10% of sporadic tumors, gain-of-function mutations in β-catenin are implicated.

Morphology (p. 480)

Wilms tumors are soft, large, well-circumscribed renal masses characterized by triphasic histologic features: (1) blastema, (2) immature stroma, and (3) tubules—an attempt to recapitulate nephrogenesis. Histologic anaplasia (approximately 5% of tumors) is associated with a worse prognosis. *Nephrogenic rests* are putative precursor lesions of Wilms tumors and are seen in renal parenchyma adjacent to 40% of unilateral tumors. This frequency rises to nearly 100% in bilateral Wilms tumors, so that identifying rests on a unilateral Wilms tumor resection mandates watchful waiting for a malignancy on the contralateral side.

Clinical Features (p. 481)

Patients typically present with large abdominal masses; hematuria, pain, hypertension, or bowel obstruction are common. Resection and some combination of radiotherapy and chemotherapy will be curative in 85% of patients, although second malignancies related to earlier treatment can occur.

Systemic Pathology: Diseases of Organ Systems

11

Blood Vessels

Vascular Structure and Function (p. 483)

- All vessels except capillaries share a three-layered architecture consisting of an endothelium-lined intima, a surrounding smooth muscle media, and supportive adventitia, admixed with extracellular matrix (ECM).
- The smooth muscle cell (SMC) and matrix content of arteries, veins, and capillaries vary according to hemodynamic demands (e.g., pressure, pulsatility) and functional requirements.
- Many disorders affect only particular types of vessels and therefore have characteristic anatomic distributions.
    - Atherosclerosis affects elastic and muscular arteries.
    - Hypertension is a consequence of increased tone in small muscular arteries and arterioles.
    - Different vasculitides characteristically affect only vessels of a certain caliber.
    - Inflammatory cell exudation and increased permeability occur primarily at postcapillary venules.
    - The relatively thinner walls of veins permits greater compliance of those vessels but also allows veins to be more easily extrinsically compressed and/or infiltrated by tumors and inflammation.

Vascular Anomalies (p. 485)

- *Variants of the usual anatomic pattern* of vascular supply are important during surgery and vascular interventions.
- *Berry aneurysms* are outpouchings in cerebral vessels due to congenital wall weakness; rupture can cause fatal intracerebral hemorrhage (see Chapter 28).
- *Arteriovenous fistulas* are abnormal communications between arteries and veins. They can be congenital or secondary to trauma, surgery, inflammation, or a healed ruptured aneurysm. Fistula rupture can cause extensive hemorrhage, and large fistulas can create significant left-to-right vascular shunting, with increased venous return that leads to high-output heart failure.
- *Fibromuscular dysplasia* is focal, irregular thickening and attenuation of the arterial wall due to intimal and medial hyperplasia and fibrosis. In the renal artery the associated luminal stenosis causes renovascular hypertension (see later); areas of medial thinning can also lead to aneurysm formation with possible vascular rupture.

Vascular Wall Response to Injury (p. 485)

Endothelial Cells (p. 485)

Normal endothelial function maintains vessel wall homeostasis and circulatory function through the following:

- Maintenance of a permeability barrier
- Elaboration of prothrombotic, antithrombotic, and fibrinolytic mediators
- ECM production
- Modulation of blood flow and vasomotor tone
- Regulation of inflammation
- Regulation of cell growth

Endothelial cells (ECs) in different portions of the vascular tree have distinct expression profiles, behaviors, and even morphologic appearance (e.g., fenestrated in liver sinusoids and glomerular capillaries versus contributing to the blood-brain barrier in the central nervous system).

Endothelial Dysfunction (p. 486)

Endothelial dysfunction is defined as an altered phenotype that affects vasoreactivity, induces a thrombogenic surface, or is abnormally adhesive for inflammatory cells (Fig. 11-1).

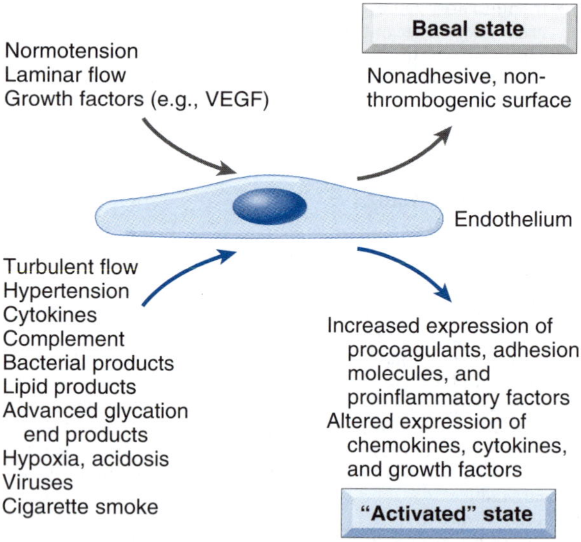

Figure 11-1 Basal and activated EC states. Normal blood pressure, laminar flow, and low growth factor levels promote a basal EC state that maintains a nonthrombotic, nonadhesive surface with appropriate vascular wall smooth muscle tone. Injury or exposure to certain mediators results in endothelial activation, a state where ECs develop a procoagulant surface that can be adhesive for inflammatory cells and also express factors that cause smooth muscle contraction and/or proliferation and matrix synthesis.

Vascular Smooth Muscle Cells (p. 486)

Vascular SMCs are the dominant cell type of the vessel media and can do the following:

- Migrate and proliferate in response to various mediators (e.g., platelet-derived growth factor, endothelin, thrombin, and fibroblast growth factor)
- Elaborate cytokines and growth factors
- Synthesize and remodel ECM
- Constrict or dilate in response to physiologic or pharmacologic stimuli

Intimal Thickening: A Stereotyped Response to Vascular Injury *(p. 486)*

Regardless of the nature of injury (traumatic, inflammatory, toxic, infectious, etc.), injured endothelium and underlying vessel wall "heal" by stimulating SMC ingrowth and ECM production, leading to intimal thickening, a so-called *neointima.* The neointimal cells have a proliferative and synthetic phenotype distinct from the underlying media, and the cells may derive from vessel wall or circulating precursors. In small-to-medium–sized vessels (e.g., coronary artery) such intimal thickening can cause luminal stenosis and downstream tissue ischemia.

Hypertensive Vascular Disease (p. 487)

Blood pressure needs to be maintained within certain parameters to prevent untoward consequences. *Hypotension* (low pressure) leads to inadequate organ perfusion—causing dysfunction or tissue death, whereas *hypertension* (high pressure) can cause significant vessel and end-organ damage. Indeed hypertension is a major risk factor for coronary heart disease, cerebrovascular accidents, heart failure, renal failure, and aortic dissection.

Blood pressure is a continuously distributed variable, and detrimental effects increase continuously as the pressure rises; thus no rigidly defined level distinguishes safety from risk, and other concomitant risk factors (e.g., diabetes) can lower the threshold for what is deleterious. Nevertheless, clinically significant hypertension is defined as sustained diastolic pressures >89 mm Hg or systolic pressures >139 mm Hg; by these criteria 29% of the U.S. population is hypertensive.

Less than 5% of hypertensive patients will have a rapidly rising blood pressure that can cause death within 1 to 2 years if untreated. Such *malignant hypertension* is characterized by systolic blood pressure >200 mm Hg, diastolic pressure >120 mm Hg, renal failure, and retinal hemorrhages.

Blood Pressure Regulation (p. 488)

Blood pressure is the product of cardiac output and peripheral vascular resistance, which are in turn influenced by genetic and environmental factors (Fig. 11-2).

- Cardiac output is determined by myocardial contractility, heart rate, and blood volume. Blood volume is affected by the following:
  - Sodium load
  - Mineralocorticoids (aldosterone)
  - Natriuretic peptides induce sodium excretion; these are produced by atrial and ventricular myocardium in response to volume expansion.

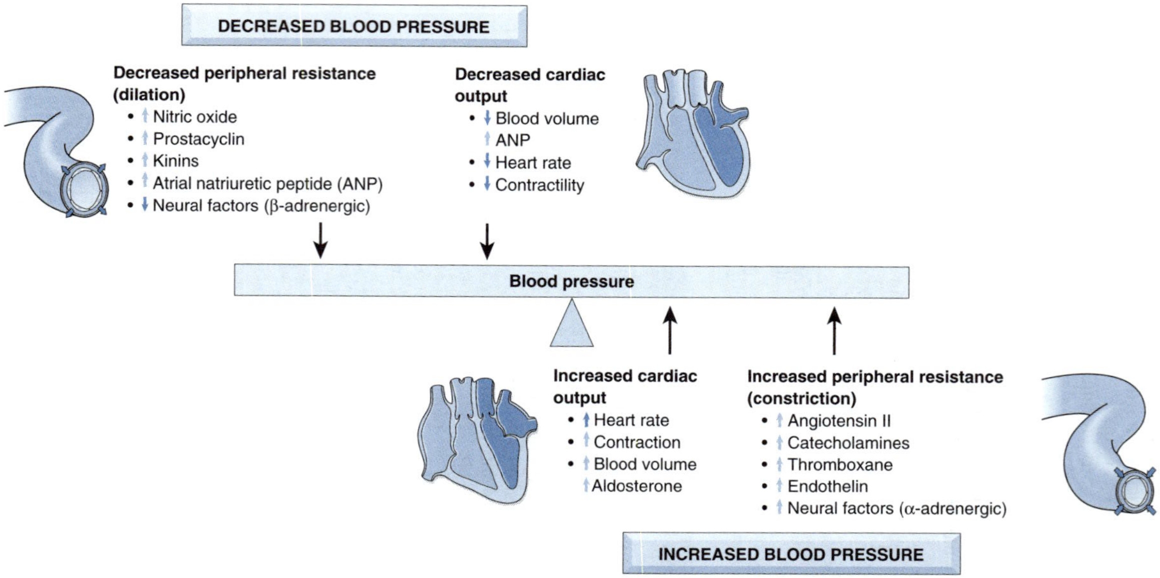

Figure 11-2 Blood pressure regulation. Diverse influences on cardiac output (e.g., blood volume and myocardial contractility) and peripheral resistance (neural, humoral, and local effectors) impact the output blood pressure. *Dark blue arrows* designate dominant effects.

- Peripheral resistance is determined primarily at the level of the arterioles.
  - Vasoconstrictors: Angiotensin II, catecholamines, thromboxane, leukotrienes, and endothelin
  - Vasodilators: Kinins, prostaglandins, nitric oxide, and adenosine
- Regional autoregulation occurs when increased blood flow leads to local vasoconstriction; local hypoxia or acidosis can also cause vasodilation.
- Kidneys have a major influence on blood pressure by producing renin in the setting of hypotension:
  - Renin converts angiotensinogen to angiotensin I, which is subsequently converted to angiotensin II.
  - Angiotensin II causes vasoconstriction.
  - Angiotensin II also increases blood volume by inducing aldosterone production that increases renal sodium resorption.

Pathogenesis of Hypertension (p. 490)

Mechanisms of Essential Hypertension *(p. 490)*

In 90% to 95% of cases, hypertension is idiopathic *(essential hypertension)* (Table 11-1). This does not mean that there is no cause but rather that cumulative effects of nongenetic environmental factors (e.g., stress, salt intake) and multiple (individually minor) genetic

TABLE 11-1 Types and Causes of Hypertension
Essential Hypertension
Secondary Hypertension
Renal
Acute glomerulonephritis
Chronic renal disease
Polycystic disease
Renal artery stenosis
Renal artery fibromuscular dysplasia
Renal vasculitis
Renin-producing tumors
Endocrine
Adrenocortical hyperfunction (Cushing syndrome, primary aldosteronism, congenital adrenal hyperplasia, licorice ingestion)
Exogenous hormones (glucocorticoids, estrogen [including pregnancy induced and oral contraceptives], sympathomimetics, tyramine-containing foods, and monoamine oxidase inhibitors)
Pheochromocytoma
Acromegaly
Hypothyroidism (myxedema)
Hyperthyroidism (thyrotoxicosis)
Pregnancy induced
Cardiovascular
Coarctation of aorta
PAN (or other vasculitides)
Increased intravascular volume
Increased cardiac output
Rigidity of the aorta
Neurologic
Psychogenic
Increased intracranial pressure
Sleep apnea
Acute stress, including surgery

polymorphisms in vasomotor tone or blood volume regulation conspire to cause high blood pressure.

Sodium homeostasis is a key element of blood volume control and is primarily regulated at the level of renal sodium resorption in the distal tubule; this in turn is largely influenced by the renin-angiotensin system that regulates aldosterone production. Although *single gene disorders* in these pathways (Table 11-1) are rare causes of hypertension, it is apparent that subtle variations in their activity might influence blood pressure in the broader population:

- Mutations in enzymes that influence aldosterone synthesis (11β-hydroxylase, 17α-hydroxylase) lead to increased aldosterone production.
- Mutations in the renal epithelial Na^+ channel protein lead to increased sodium resorption *(Liddle syndrome).*

Pathogenesis of Secondary Hypertension (p. 490)

In the remainder of cases *(secondary hypertension),* causes include intrinsic renal disease, renal artery stenosis (renovascular hypertension), endocrine abnormalities, vascular malformations, or neurologic disorders (Table 11-1).

Vascular Pathology in Hypertension (p. 490)

Hypertension accelerates the development of atherosclerosis and also causes arteriolar structural changes that potentiate both aortic dissection and cerebrovascular hemorrhage. Hypertension is also associated with the following two forms of small arteriolar disease:

- *Hyaline arteriolosclerosis* is due to EC injury, with subsequent plasma leakage into arteriolar walls and increased SMC matrix synthesis. The same lesions occur in diabetic angiopathy due to EC hyperglycemic injury. Microscopically there is diffuse, pink, hyaline arteriolar wall thickening, with associated luminal stenosis.
- *Hyperplastic arteriolosclerosis* occurs in malignant hypertension; there is concentric laminated *(onion-skin)* arteriolar thickening with reduplicated basement membrane and SMC proliferation, frequently associated with fibrin deposition and wall necrosis, so-called *necrotizing arteriolitis.*

Arteriosclerosis (p. 491)

Arteriosclerosis is a term denoting arterial wall thickening and loss of elasticity; the following three patterns are recognized:

- *Arteriolosclerosis,* primarily affecting small- and medium-sized arteries and arterioles and associated with downstream ischemia (see previous discussion).
- *Mönckeberg medial sclerosis,* characterized by medial calcification in muscular arteries, typically occurring after age 50. The calcific deposits are nonobstructive and not usually clinically significant.
- *Atherosclerosis,* the most frequent and clinically important (see the following).

Atherosclerosis (p. 491)

Atherosclerosis is a slowly progressive disease of large- to medium-sized muscular and elastic arteries. The lesions are characterized by elevated intimal-based plaques composed of lipids, proliferating

SMC, inflammatory cells, and increased ECM. They cause pathology by the following:

- Mechanically obstructing flow, especially in smaller-bore vessels
- Plaque rupture leading to vessel thrombosis
- Weakening the underlying vessel wall, leading to aneurysm formation

Epidemiology (p. 491)

The prevalence and severity of atherosclerosis and its complications are related to a number of risk factors, some constitutional and some modifiable. The major classic risk factors emerging from the Framingham Heart Study are family history, hypercholesterolemia, hypertension, smoking, and diabetes; the number of risk factors increases disease incidence in an approximately multiplicative way.

Constitutional Risk Factors *(p. 492)*

- *Genetics:* Family history is the most significant independent risk factor for atherosclerosis. Monogenic disorders, such as familial hypercholesterolemia, account for only a minor percentage, and numerous genetic polymorphisms (including predilection for hypertension and diabetes) are contributory.
- ***Age:*** Atherosclerotic burden progressively increases with age, typically reaching a critical mass with clinical manifestations beginning between ages 40 and 60.
- ***Gender:*** Relative to age-matched males, premenopausal women are relatively protected against atherosclerosis and its complications. In postmenopausal women, the risk rapidly increases and can exceed that for men. In addition to affecting the progression of atherosclerosis, female gender also influences hemostasis, infarct healing, and myocardial remodeling.

Modifiable Major Risk Factors *(p. 492)*

- *Hyperlipidemia and hypercholesterolemia:* Increased risk is associated with increased low-density lipoprotein (LDL) and decreased high-density lipoprotein (HDL, clears cholesterol from vessel wall lesions). Levels can be favorably modified by diet, exercise, moderate alcohol intake, and statins (inhibitors of hydroxymethylglutaryl-CoA reductase, the rate-limiting enzyme in cholesterol biosynthesis).
- *Hypertension:* Both diastolic and systolic hypertension are important, and independent of other risk factors; high blood pressure increases the risk of atherosclerotic ischemic heart disease by 60%.
- *Smoking:* Smoking of one pack of cigarettes daily over several years doubles the death rate from ischemic heart disease.
- *Diabetes mellitus:* Directly and indirectly (by inducing hypercholesterolemia), diabetes accelerates atherosclerosis, and doubles the risk of myocardial infarction, as well as markedly increasing the risk of stroke or extremity gangrene.

Additional Risk Factors *(p. 493)*

Up to 20% of all cardiovascular events occur in the absence of the major identified risk factors, suggesting other contributions:

- *Inflammation:* Present at all stages of atherosclerosis development, inflammation plays a significant causal role. A number of circulating markers of inflammation correlate with risk of ischemic heart disease; C-reactive protein (CRP, a liver-synthesized acute phase reactant involved in bacterial recognition and complement activation) has emerged as one of the simplest and most sensitive to measure. It strongly and independently predicts risk of cardiovascular events, even in apparently healthy individuals.

- *Hyperhomocysteinemia:* Elevated levels of homocysteine are associated with increased atherosclerotic vascular disease. Levels are increased in the setting of low folate or vitamin B_{12} or with hereditary homocystinuria.
- *Metabolic syndrome:* A constellation of findings, including central obesity, hypertension, glucose intolerance, dyslipidemia, and a systemic proinflammatory state. Adipose tissue proinflammatory cytokines have been implicated.
- *Lipoprotein(a):* This is an altered form of LDL; elevated levels confer increased risk independent of LDL or total cholesterol levels.
- *Factors affecting hemostasis:* Systemic markers of hemostasis or fibrinolysis are predictors of risk for atherosclerotic events.
- *Other factors:* These include difficult-to-quantitate risks, such as type A personality and obesity (the latter is confounded by commonly accompanying hypertension, diabetes, hyperlipidemia, etc.)

Pathogenesis of Atherosclerosis (p. 494)

Atherosclerosis is a chronic inflammatory and healing response of the arterial wall to EC injury. In turn, EC injury causes increased endothelial permeability, white blood cell and platelet adhesion, and coagulation activation. These events induce chemical mediator (e.g., growth factors and inflammatory mediators) release and activation, followed by recruitment and subsequent proliferation of SMCs in the intima to produce the characteristic intimal lesion (Fig. 11-3).

Endothelial Injury *(p. 494)*

Even without the loss of EC, *EC dysfunction* will result in increased adhesivity and procoagulant activity; injury mechanisms include hypercholesterolemia, hemodynamic disturbances (e.g., disturbed flow), smoking, hypertension, toxins, and infectious agents. Regardless of the inciting stimulus, the vessel responds with a fairly stereotyped intimal thickening; in the presence of circulating lipids, typical atheromas ensue.

Hemodynamic Disturbances *(p. 495)*

Despite presumably uniformly distributed injurious agents (hypercholesterolemia, cigarette toxins, hyperglycemia, etc.), atherosclerotic plaques are not randomly distributed and in fact characteristically develop at vascular branch points and other areas of disturbed flow. Indeed, nonturbulent laminar flow activates EC genes whose products are *protective* against atherosclerosis.

Lipids *(p. 495)*

Defects in lipid uptake, metabolism, or binding to circulating apoproteins can lead to elevated lipids. Increased circulating levels accumulate in the vessel wall and cause EC dysfunction by increasing local oxygen free radical formation. Accumulated lipoproteins also become oxidized; oxidized LDL in particular are directly toxic to ECs and SMCs, causing dysfunction. Moreover, oxidized LDL are ingested by macrophages through scavenger receptors, causing the formation of *foam cells* and leading to proinflammatory macrophage activation.

Inflammation *(p. 496)*

Dysfunctional ECs express increased levels of adhesion molecules (e.g., vascular cell adhesion molecule-1 [VCAM-1]), promoting increased inflammatory cell recruitment. Subsequent T-cell and macrophage accumulation and activation lead to local increased

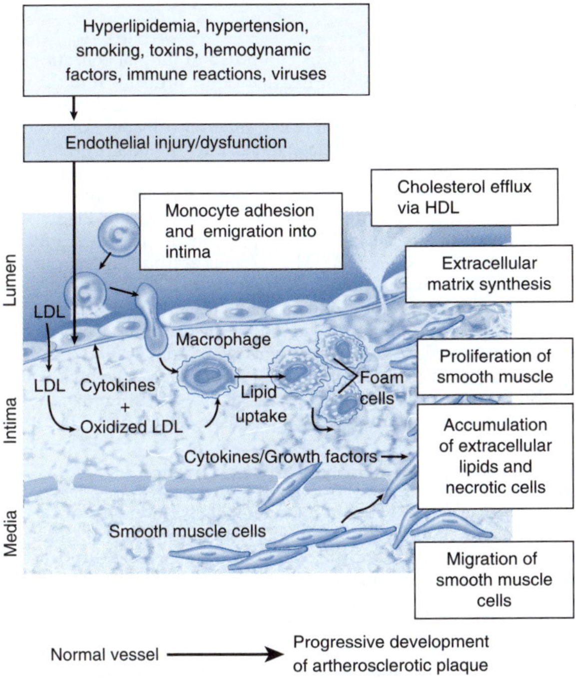

Figure 11-3 Sequence of cellular interactions in atherosclerosis. A host of noxious insults (e.g., hyperlipidemia, hyperglycemia, hypertension, smoking) cause endothelial injury or dysfunction. This results in monocyte and platelet adhesion, with subsequent cytokine and growth factor release. In response to the elaborated cytokines and chemokines, SMCs migrate to the intima, proliferate, and produce ECM, including collagen and proteoglycans. Foam cells in atheromatous plaques derive from macrophages and SMCs that have accumulated modified lipids (e.g., oxidized and aggregated LDL) via scavenger and LDL-receptor-related proteins. Extracellular lipid is derived from insudation from the vessel lumen, particularly in the presence of hypercholesterolemia, as well as from degenerating foam cells. Cholesterol accumulation in the plaque reflects an imbalance between influx and efflux; HDL likely helps to clear cholesterol from these accumulations.

cytokine production that drives SMC proliferation and matrix synthesis.

Infection (p. 496)

Herpesvirus, cytomegalovirus, and *Chlamydia pneumoniae* have all been detected in atherosclerotic plaques. It is not clear whether this is coincidence (these are common organisms) or causal (e.g., by driving inflammatory responses).

Smooth Muscle Proliferation and Matrix Synthesis (p. 496)

SMC precursors recruited from the circulation or the vessel wall are induced to proliferate and synthesize ECM through the activities of platelet-derived growth factor (released by adherent platelets and inflammatory cells), fibroblast growth factor, and transforming growth factor (TGF)-α.

Activated inflammatory cells can also cause medial SMC apoptosis and increase ECM degradation, leading to unstable plaques (see later).

Morphology (p. 496)

- *Fatty streaks* are early lesions composed of intimal collections of foamy macrophages and SMCs that gently protrude into the vascular lumen. These can occur at virtually any age and even in infants and occur at sites that often will eventually develop atherosclerotic plaques. Nevertheless, not all fatty streaks are destined to become atheromatous plaques.
- The characteristic atheromatous plaque (*atheroma* or *fibrofatty plaque*) is a raised, white-yellow, intimal-based lesion. Plaques are composed of superficial fibrous caps containing SMCs, inflammatory cells, and dense ECM overlying necrotic cores, containing dead cells, lipid, cholesterol (manifesting as empty "clefts" on most routine processing), foam cells, and plasma proteins; small blood vessels proliferate at the intimal-medial interface.
- Plaques are denoted as *complicated* when they exhibit calcification, hemorrhage, fissuring, or ulceration; such changes are often also associated with local thrombosis, medial thinning, cholesterol microemboli, and aneurysmal dilation.

Consequences of Atherosclerotic Disease (p. 499)

Atherosclerosis is a dynamic process with periods of growth and remodeling beginning in childhood (Fig. 11-4). Most plaques are typically asymptomatic for decades until manifesting through one of the following mechanisms:

Atherosclerotic Stenosis (p. 500)

Atherosclerotic stenosis restricts blood flow to downstream tissues; restricted flow can cause tissue atrophy or infarction, depending on the degree of stenosis, tempo of narrowing, and metabolic demands of the affected tissues.

- Slow insidious narrowing of vascular lumens occurs by gradual accumulation of plaque matrix.
- At early stages of stenosis, outward remodeling of the vessel media (leading to overall vessel dilation) can preserve the luminal diameter.
- At approximately 70% stenosis *(critical stenosis)*, the vascular supply typically becomes inadequate to meet demand, and ischemia supervenes.

Acute Plaque Change (p. 500)

Acute plaque change means that there is plaque erosion, frank rupture, or hemorrhage into the plaque (which expands the plaque volume and can increase luminal stenosis). When plaques are disrupted, the blood can be exposed to highly thrombogenic plaque contents or subendothelial basement membrane, leading to partial or complete vascular thrombosis.

- In most cases of myocardial infarction, plaque disruption and associated precipitous thrombosis occur at areas of subcritical stenoses (i.e., <70%).
- Intrinsic factors that influence disruption include plaque structure and composition (Fig. 11-5).
    - *Vulnerable plaques* have large deformable atheromatous cores, thin fibrous caps, and/or increased inflammatory cell content (leading to the elaboration of matrix metalloproteinases [MMPs] that degrade ECM).
    - *Stable plaques* have minimal atheromatous cores and thicker well-collagenized fibrous caps, with relatively less inflammation.

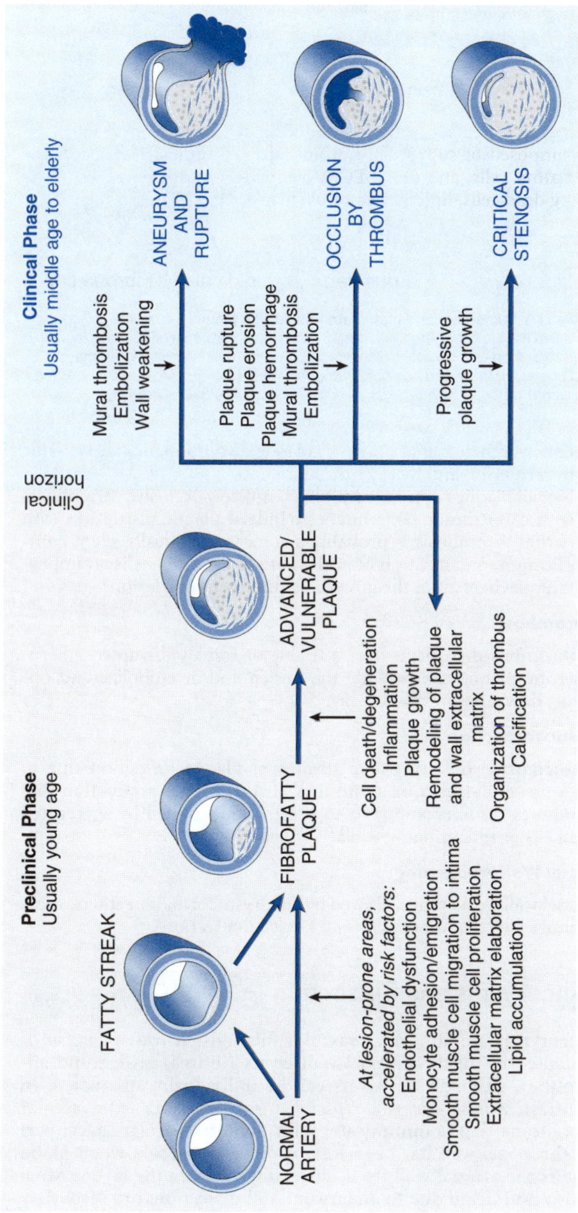

Figure 11-4 The natural history, morphologic features, main pathogenic events, and clinical complications of atherosclerosis.

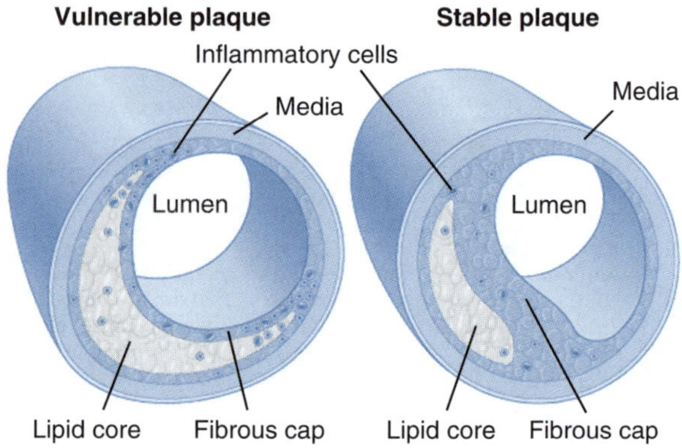

Figure 11-5 Vulnerable and stable atherosclerotic plaque. *Vulnerable plaques* have thin fibrous caps, large lipid cores, and greater inflammation. Stable plaques have thickened and densely collagenous fibrous caps with minimal inflammation and underlying atheromatous core. *(Adapted from Libby P: Molecular bases of the acute coronary syndromes.* Circulation *91:2844-2850, 1995.)*

- Extrinsic factors that influence plaque disruption include systemic hypertension and focal vasoconstriction.
- Not all plaque ruptures result in completely occlusive thromboses with catastrophic consequences. Indeed plaque disruption with partial thrombosis is probably a common, clinically silent complication; organization of such subtotal thromboses is an important mechanism in the growth of atherosclerotic lesions.

Thrombosis (p. 501)

A thrombus that forms over a friable or frankly disrupted atherosclerotic plaque can occlude the lumen and/or embolize and obstruct downstream vessels.

Vasoconstriction (p. 501)

Vasoconstriction can occur at sites of plaque formation due to endothelial dysfunction (with loss of nitric oxide production that promotes vasorelaxation) or to products elaborated by aggregated platelets or inflammatory cells.

Vessel Wall Weakening

Vessel wall weakening followed by aneurysm formation and possible rupture (see the Aneurysms and Dissection section).

Aneurysms and Dissection (p. 501)

Aneurysms are abnormal vascular dilations. A *true aneurysm* is bounded by all three vessel wall layers (intima, media, and adventitia), although the layers can be individually attenuated. In contrast, a *false aneurysm (pseudoaneurysm)* is an extravascular hematoma that communicates with the intravascular space; part of the vessel wall has been lost. A *dissection* occurs when blood enters the arterial wall itself, dissecting between the layers. Morbidity and death due to aneurysms and dissections are secondary to the following:

- Rupture
- Impingement on adjacent structures

- Occlusion of proximal vessels by extrinsic pressure or superimposed thrombosis
- Embolism from a mural thrombus

Pathogenesis of Aneurysms (p. 501)

Arteries are dynamically remodeling, and the various constituents are constantly turning over. Aneurysms occur due to the following:

- *Poor intrinsic quality of the vessel matrix:* In *Marfan syndrome,* inadequate fibrillin synthesis leads to aberrant TGF-β activation and progressive loss of elastic tissue matrix; in *Loeys-Dietz syndrome,* TGF-β receptor mutations likewise cause elastic tissue loss. In both cases, aneurysms result from progressive remodeling of the inelastic media. Defective collagen III synthesis in *Ehlers-Danlos syndrome* or defective collagen cross-linking in vitamin C deficiency *(scurvy)* also leads to aneurysm formation.
- *Imbalance of matrix synthesis and degradation:* Increased MMP activity by inflammatory cells (e.g., in atherosclerotic plaque or in vasculitis) can cause a net loss of medial ECM.
- *Loss of medial SMCs or change in SMC synthesis:* Ischemia of the innermost aspect of the aortic media occurs when thick atherosclerotic plaque impedes adequate oxygen and nutritional diffusion from the lumen. Similarly mid-medial ischemia of the aorta can occur when vessels of the vasa vasorum are stenosed due to inflammation or hypertension. Such ischemia is reflected in SMC loss and/or "degenerative changes," with loss of normal ECM synthesis and increased production of amorphous ground substance (glycosaminoglycan). These changes are collectively denoted as *cystic medial degeneration* and can be seen in a variety of settings, including Marfan syndrome or scurvy.

The most common causes of aortic aneurysms are *atherosclerosis* (particularly in the abdominal aorta) and *hypertension* (particularly in the ascending thoracic aorta). Other causes include syphilis, trauma, vasculitis, and congenital defects (e.g., berry aneurysms). Aneurysms due to infections *(mycotic aneurysms)* can originate from septic embolization (e.g., from bacterial endocarditis), an adjacent suppurative process, or systemic bacteremia. The intense acute inflammation in mycotic aneurysms accelerates vascular wall destruction and potentiates rapid aneurysmal dilation.

Abdominal Aortic Aneurysm (p. 502)

Abdominal aortic aneurysms (AAAs) are true aneurysms; they classically occur in male smokers over age 50 and are located below the renal arteries and above the iliac bifurcation. Pathogenesis involves medial SMC loss and increased matrix degradation by MMP; histology reveals severe complex atherosclerosis with markedly attenuated media. Due to the aneurysmal dilation and abnormal vascular flow, the lumen typically contains a laminated, poorly organized mural thrombus.

Complications include occlusion of a branch vessel, atheroembolism, compression of adjacent structures, or rupture. Risk of rupture increases with the maximal diameter of the AAA: it is low if an aneurysm is smaller than 5 cm but 11% annually when it is 5 to 6 cm and 25% per year when it is >6 cm. The operative mortality rate is 5% for unruptured aneurysms but more than 50% after rupture. Because aortic atherosclerosis is usually accompanied by severe coronary atherosclerosis, patients with AAA also have a high incidence of ischemic heart disease.

Inflammatory AAAs constitute 5% to 10% of AAAs; these characteristically occur in younger patients and are characterized by an exuberant transmural lymphoplasmacytic infiltrate and dense periaortic fibrosis. A subset of inflammatory AAAs may actually be a vascular manifestation of a recently recognized entity called *immunoglobulin G4 (IgG4)-related disease.* This is a steroid-sensitive disorder associated with high plasma levels of IgG4; fibrosis and infiltrating IgG4-expressing plasma cells can also affect the pancreas, biliary system, and salivary gland.

Thoracic Aortic Aneurysm (p. 503)

The most common etiology is hypertension, although Marfan and Loeys-Dietz syndromes are increasingly recognized; syphilis is a rare cause in the United States. Signs and symptoms are referable to aortic root dilation (aortic valve insufficiency), rupture, or encroachment on mediastinal structures, including airways (dyspnea), esophagus (dysphagia), recurrent laryngeal nerves (cough), or vertebral bodies (bony pain).

Aortic Dissection (p. 504)

Dissection of blood within the aortic media often leads to rupture, causing sudden death through massive hemorrhage or cardiac tamponade. Aortic dissection is not usually associated with marked preexisting aortic dilation and occurs principally in the following two groups:

- Hypertensive males 40 to 60 years old; the aortas typically exhibit variable degrees of cystic medial degeneration.
- Younger individuals with connective tissue defects that affect the aorta (e.g., Marfan syndrome).

Other causes of aortic dissection include trauma, complications from therapeutic or diagnostic arterial cannulation, and hormonal and physiologic changes associated with pregnancy. Dissection is uncommon in atherosclerosis or in other conditions with medial scarring, presumably because the fibrosis limits dissection propagation.

Pathogenesis *(p. 504)*

Medial degeneration (described previously) is the important underlying substrate; the trigger for the intimal tear that begins the dissection is often unknown. Nevertheless, once the tear is initiated, blood flow under systemic pressures advances the dissection plane. In some cases, rupture of the penetrating vessels of the vasa vasorum can give rise to an intramural hematoma without an intimal tear.

Morphology *(p. 504)*

The most common preexisting histologic change is cystic medial degeneration, most often without accompanying inflammation. The vast majority of dissections begin as a tear within the first 10 cm above the aortic valve annulus. The dissection plane can extend retrograde to the heart (causing coronary compression or hemopericardium with tamponade) and/or anterograde, extending into the great arteries or other major branches. Rupture through the wall of the aorta will cause massive hemorrhage; occasionally reentry into the lumen will give rise to a double-barreled aorta *(chronic dissection).*

Clinical Features (p. 505)

The complications of dissection depend on the portion of the aorta affected; dissections are classified into the following:

- The more common (and dangerous) *proximal* lesions, involving the ascending aorta (called *type A*)
- *Distal lesions not involving the ascending part* and usually beginning distal to the subclavian artery *(type B)*

The classic presentation involves sudden onset of excruciating pain, usually beginning in the anterior chest, radiating to the back, and moving downward as the dissection progresses. Death is usually the result of rupture into the pericardium, thorax, or abdomen; early recognition, institution of antihypertensive therapy, and surgical plication allow 65% to 75% survival.

Vasculitis (p. 505)

Vasculitis is vessel wall inflammation; symptoms are typically referable to the ischemia that occurs in the downstream tissues (due to vessel injury and thrombosis), as well as constitutional manifestations, such as fever, myalgias, arthralgias, and malaise. Any vessel can be involved, but many of the vasculitides have a predilection for specific vascular sizes or beds. Vasculitides are classified according to vessel size and site, lesion histology, clinical manifestations, and pathogenesis (Fig. 11-6). The two most common pathogenic mechanisms are immune-mediated inflammation and infections; physical and chemical injury (irradiation, trauma, toxins, etc.) can also be causal.

Noninfectious Vasculitis (p. 506)

Immune Complex–Associated Vasculitis (p. 506)

Immune complex–associated vasculitis is caused by vascular deposition of circulating antigen-antibody complexes (e.g., DNA/anti-DNA complexes in systemic lupus erythematosus [SLE]). Vascular injury arises from complement activation or the recruitment of Fc receptor-bearing cells (see Chapter 6). Although the nature of the initiating antigen is not always known, immune complex deposition typically underlies the vasculitis associated with drug hypersensitivities (antibodies against the agent itself or directed against modified self-proteins); in vasculitis secondary to viral infections, antibodies can be directed against viral proteins (e.g., hepatitis B surface antigen in 30% of patients with polyarteritis nodosa [PAN]).

Antineutrophil Cytoplasmic Antibodies (p. 507)

Antineutrophil cytoplasmic antibodies (ANCAs) are a heterogeneous group of autoantibodies directed against the constituents of neutrophil primary granules, monocyte lysosomes, or EC:

- *Antiproteinase 3 (PR3-ANCA),* directed against a neutrophil azurophilic granule constituent; also called *cytoplasmic ANCA (c-ANCA).* This is characteristically associated with *granulomatosis with polyangiitis* (GPA, previously called *Wegener granulomatosis;* see later).
- *Antimyeloperoxidase (MPO-ANCA),* directed against the lysosomal constituent involved in generating oxygen free radicals; also called *perinuclear ANCA (p-ANCA).* This antibody is characteristically seen in *microscopic polyangiitis* or *Churg-Strauss syndrome.*

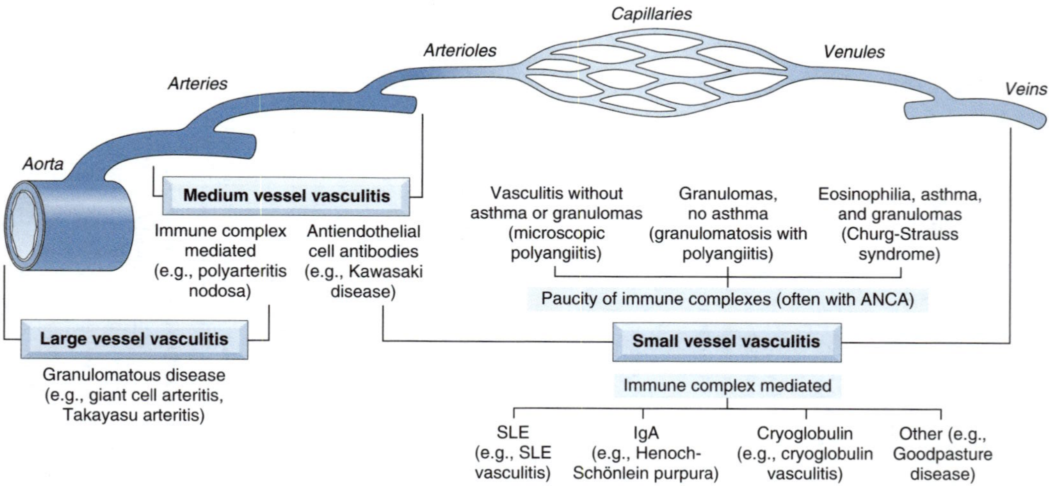

Figure 11-6 Vascular sites typically involved with the more common forms of vasculitis, as well as their presumptive etiologies. Note that there is a substantial overlap in distributions.

ANCAs are useful diagnostic markers for ANCA-associated vasculitides, and titers often mirror inflammation levels, suggesting a pathogenic association. These autoantibodies may be induced via cross-reactive microbial antigens; once formed, they can directly activate neutrophils and thereby cause release of proteolytic enzymes and reactive oxygen species that damage endothelium.

Antiendothelial Cell Antibodies *(p. 507)*

Antiendothelial cell antibodies may underlie certain vasculitides, such as *Kawasaki disease* (see later).

Giant Cell (Temporal) Arteritis (p. 507)

The most common form of vasculitis in the U.S. elderly population; it is characterized by focal granulomatous inflammation of medium- and small-sized arteries, chiefly cranial vessels (most commonly the temporal arteries). It can also involve the aorta *(giant cell aortitis)*. The primary etiology is likely a T cell–mediated immune response to vessel wall antigen(s).

Morphology *(p. 508)*

- Granulomatous vasculitis with elastic tissue fragmentation; multinucleated giant cells are seen in up to 75% of cases.
- Intimal and adventitial fibrosis with medial scarring and luminal narrowing.

Clinical Features *(p. 508)*

Temporal arteritis typically presents with headache and facial pain; most patients also have systemic symptoms, including a flulike syndrome with fever, fatigue, and weight loss. Ophthalmic artery involvement with ocular symptoms appears abruptly in approximately 50% of patients and can cause permanent blindness. The disease responds well to steroids or antitumor necrosis factor (TNF) therapies.

Takayasu Arteritis (p. 508)

This is a granulomatous vasculitis of medium-to-large arteries characterized by transmural fibrous thickening of the aortic arch and virtual obliteration of the great vessel branches. An immune etiology is likely causal.

Morphology *(p. 509)*

- *Grossly* there is irregular aortic thickening with intimal hyperplasia.
- *Microscopically,* early stages show adventitial perivascular (vasa vasorum) mononuclear cell infiltrates, followed in later stages by medial fibrosis, with granulomas and acellular intimal thickening; the changes are indistinguishable from giant cell arteritis.

Clinical Features *(p. 509)*

Initial symptoms are usually nonspecific (fatigue, fever, weight loss). Ocular and neurologic disturbances and marked weakening of upper extremity perfusion pressures (hence the name *pulseless disease*) are common. The pulmonary artery is involved in half of cases, and coronaries and renal arteries can also be affected; hypertension occurs secondary to the renal artery disease. Takayasu arteritis is diagnosed when the affected patient is less than 50 years old; the same gross and histologic features in older individuals are designated as giant cell aortitis.

Polyarteritis Nodosa (p. 509)

PAN is a systemic disease characterized by necrotizing vasculitis involving small-to-medium arteries; kidney, heart, liver, and gastrointestinal (GI) tract are involved in descending order, and the pulmonary circulation is spared. Immune complex deposition is causal in the third of cases associated with chronic hepatitis, but the etiology of the classic idiopathic and cutaneous forms of PAN is unknown. ANCAs are not involved.

Morphology (p. 509)

PAN lesions are sharply demarcated and often induce thrombosis, causing distal ischemic injury. Lesions at different histologic stages may be present concurrently.

- *Acute* lesions are characterized by sharply circumscribed arterial *fibrinoid necrosis* (hyaline proteinaceous depositions in a degenerating vessel wall), with associated neutrophilic infiltrates that may extend into the adventitia.
- *Healed* lesions show only marked fibrotic thickening of the artery, with associated elastic lamina fragmentation and occasionally aneurysmal dilation.

Clinical Features (p. 510)

PAN is largely a disease of young adults, with nonspecific systemic symptoms (fever, malaise, weight loss) and clinical presentations related to the tissues involved (e.g., hematuria, albuminuria, and hypertension [kidneys]). Untreated, the disease is generally fatal, but a 90% remission rate is achieved with immunosuppressive therapy.

Kawasaki Disease (p. 510)

An acute febrile, usually self-limited illness of infants and children associated with a medium-large vessel arteritis. The etiology is a T-cell hypersensitivity to yet unidentified antigens.

Morphology (p. 510)

Lesions resemble those of PAN.

Clinical Features (p. 510)

Also known as mucocutaneous lymph node syndrome, the disease is typically heralded by fever, lymphadenopathy, skin rash, and oral or conjunctival erythema. Its clinical significance stems largely from its propensity to cause coronary arteritis (20% of untreated patients), forming aneurysms that rupture or thrombose and leading to myocardial infarction. Aspirin and intravenous gamma globulin reduce the arteritis incidence approximately fivefold.

Microscopic Polyangiitis (p. 510)

A necrotizing vasculitis of vessels (arterioles, capillaries, and venules) smaller than those involved in PAN, with lesions typically all at the same histologic stage. In some cases an antibody response to drugs, microbes, or tumor proteins (typically lymphoproliferative disorders) has been implicated with immune complex deposition. However, most lesions are "pauci-immune," and MPO-ANCAs are increasingly implicated.

Morphology (p. 510)

There is typically fibrinoid necrosis, although affected vessels may show only fragmented neutrophilic nuclei within and around vessel walls *(leukocytoclastic vasculitis)*. Necrotizing glomerulonephritis (90% of patients) and pulmonary capillaritis are particularly common. Little or no immunoglobulin deposition is seen in most lesions.

Clinical Features *(p. 511)*

The clinical features depend on the vascular bed involved and can include hemoptysis, hematuria and proteinuria, purpura, or bowel pain and bleeding. Cyclosporine and steroids induce remission and improve long-term survival.

Churg-Strauss Syndrome (p. 511)

Also called *allergic granulomatosis and angiitis,* this is a small-vessel necrotizing vasculitis associated with asthma, allergic rhinitis, peripheral eosinophilia, and extravascular necrotizing granulomas. ANCAs are identified in <50% of cases. Vascular lesions resemble PAN but are also characteristically accompanied by eosinophils and granulomas. Eosinophilic infiltrates are causally implicated in the cardiomyopathy that develops in 60% of patients; the cardiac involvement is the cause of mortality in approximately half the patients.

Behçet Disease (p. 511)

Behçet disease is a small- to medium-vessel neutrophilic vasculitis, typically presenting as a triad of the following:

- Recurrent oral aphthous ulcers
- Genital ulcers
- Uveitis

Other vessel beds can also be involved, and disease mortality is related to severe neurologic involvement or rupture of vascular aneurysms. Steroids or TNF-antagonist therapies are generally effective.

Granulomatosis With Polyangiitis (Previously Called Wegener Granulomatosis) (p. 511)

GPA *(previously called Wegener granulomatosis)* is a necrotizing vasculitis associated with a triad of the following:

- Necrotizing or granulomatous vasculitis of small-to-medium vessels mostly in the lung and upper airway
- Necrotizing granulomas of the upper and lower respiratory tract
- Glomerulonephritis

A T-cell hypersensitivity to an inhaled agent or microbe is likely causal, although PR3-ANCAs are present in 95% of cases.

Morphology *(p. 512)*

- Granulomas with geographic necrosis and accompanying vasculitis.
- Granulomas may coalesce to produce nodules that cavitate.
- Renal lesions vary from focal and segmental necrosis and scarring to proliferative (crescentic) glomerulonephritis.

Clinical Features *(p. 512)*

Males over age 40 are the most commonly affected group. Without treatment, there is 80% 1-year mortality; treatment with cyclophosphamide, steroids, and TNF antagonists is largely effective.

Thromboangiitis Obliterans (Buerger Disease) (p. 512)

Typically encountered in heavy cigarette smokers <35 years old, this is a segmental, thrombosing, acute, and chronic inflammation of intermediate and small arteries and veins in the extremities. A T-cell hypersensitivity response to smoke-modified self-antigens is implicated.

Morphology (p. 512)

- Acute lesions include neutrophilic infiltrates with mural thrombi containing microabscesses, often with giant cell formation and secondary involvement of the adjacent vein and nerve.
- Late lesions show thrombus organization and recanalization.

Clinical Features (p. 512)

The clinical features include nodular phlebitis, Raynaudlike cold sensitivity (see later), and leg claudication. The vascular insufficiency can lead to excruciating pain (even at rest, suggesting neural involvement), skin ulcers, and ultimately gangrene.

Vasculitis Associated With Other Noninfectious Disorders (p. 512)

Vasculitis that clinically and histologically resembles PAN or hypersensitivity angiitis may be attributable to other disorders, such as rheumatoid arthritis, malignancy, or antiphospholipid antibody syndrome. Identifying the underlying etiology has important therapeutic implications (e.g., immunosuppression versus anticoagulation).

Infectious Vasculitis (p. 513)

Arteritis can be caused by direct invasion from an adjacent source (especially *Aspergillus* and *Mucor*) or originate from septic embolization (e.g., from bacterial endocarditis). Vascular infections can result in mycotic aneurysms or cause thrombosis and downstream infarction.

Disorders of Blood Vessel Hyper-Reactivity (p. 513)

Raynaud Phenomenon (p. 513)

Raynaud phenomenon results from exaggerated vasoconstriction of digital (and sometimes facial) arteries and arterioles, producing pain, pallor, and even cyanosis; prolonged vasospasm can result in tissue necrosis. Raynaud phenomenon can be the initial manifestation in up to 10% of patients with immune-mediated vasculitides.

- *Primary Raynaud phenomenon* occurs in 3% to 5% of the general population and most commonly affects young women; it reflects exaggerated vasomotor responses to cold or emotion. The clinical course is usually benign.
- *Secondary Raynaud phenomenon* is vascular insufficiency due to arterial narrowing induced by other conditions (e.g., atherosclerosis, SLE, systemic sclerosis [scleroderma], or Buerger disease).

Myocardial Vessel Vasospasm (p. 514)

Vasoactive mediators can precipitate prolonged myocardial vessel contraction; such constriction can result in ischemia and infarction. Causal agents can be endogenous (e.g., epinephrine released by pheochromocytomas) or exogenous (e.g., cocaine). Elevated thyroid hormone causes a similar effect by increasing the sensitivity of vessels to circulating catecholamines; autoantibodies and T cells in scleroderma (see Chapter 6) can cause vascular instability and vasospasm. Extreme psychological stress (with catecholamine release) can also lead to pathologic vasospasm. Elevated levels of catechols also increase heart rate and myocardial contractility, exacerbating ischemia caused by the vasospasm. The outcome may be sudden cardiac death (likely caused by a fatal arrhythmia) or an ischemic dilated cardiomyopathy, so-called *Takotsubo cardiomyopathy.* Histologically, acute cases can exhibit microscopic areas of *contraction band necrosis;* microscopic foci of granulation tissue and/or scar can be seen in subacute and chronic cases.

Veins and Lymphatics (p. 514)

Vein disorders are extremely common; 90% involve *varicose veins* or *thrombophlebitis* and/or *phlebothrombosis.*

Varicose Veins (p. 514)

These are typically superficial lower extremity veins that are dilated and tortuous due to chronically elevated intraluminal pressure. They occur in 10% to 30% of adults; obesity and pregnancy increase the risk. Other causes include hereditary venous defects and prolonged dependent leg position.

Vein dilation renders the valves incompetent, with vascular stasis, persistent edema, and trophic skin changes, ultimately resulting in stasis dermatitis; affected tissues may have impaired circulation and poor healing with *varicose ulcers.* Although thrombosis is common, superficial varicosities are rarely sources of clinically significant emboli.

Varicosities in two other sites are clinically important:

- *Esophageal varices* are typically due to portal vein hypertension (secondary to cirrhosis or hepatic or portal vein thrombosis); portal hypertension opens portosystemic shunts with increased flow into veins at the gastroesophageal junction (esophageal varices), rectum (hemorrhoids), and periumbilical veins *(caput medusa).* Esophageal varices are most important because their rupture can lead to exsanguination.
- *Hemorrhoids* can also result from primary dilation of the anorectal venous plexus (e.g., secondary to pregnancy or chronic constipation). They can ulcerate and bleed or thrombose and become painfully inflamed.

Thrombophlebitis and Phlebothrombosis (p. 514)

These are largely interchangeable terms for venous thrombosis and inflammation. Predisposing factors for *deep vein thrombosis (DVT)* include congestive heart failure, prolonged immobilization, local infection, or systemic hypercoagulability (e.g., neoplasia, pregnancy, or the postoperative state). Although 90% of thromboses occur in deep leg veins, the periprostatic plexus in men and ovarian and pelvic veins in women are other important sites. *In contrast to superficial vein thromboses, DVT are common sources of pulmonary emboli.*

Migratory thrombophlebitis (Trousseau syndrome) is a malignancy-associated hypercoagulability due to procoagulant elaboration (see Chapter 7); it is characterized by sporadic thrombosis at various sites.

Superior and Inferior Vena Cava Syndromes (p. 515)

- Superior vena cava (SVC) syndrome is usually caused by neoplasms compressing or invading the SVC (e.g., primary bronchogenic carcinoma). The resulting vascular obstruction produces a distinctive dusky cyanosis and marked dilation of head, neck, and arm veins.

- Inferior vena cava (IVC) syndrome is caused by extrinsic IVC compression. In addition, certain neoplasms, particularly hepatocellular and renal cell carcinomas, tend to grow within veins and ultimately obstruct the IVC. IVC obstruction induces marked leg edema, distention of the lower abdominal superficial collateral veins, and—when renal veins are involved—massive proteinuria.

Lymphangitis and Lymphedema (p. 515)

Lymphangitis denotes the inflammation occurring when infections spread into lymphatics; β-hemolytic streptococci are a common cause. Lymphangitis presents as painful subcutaneous red streaks, often with tender regional lymphadenopathy *(lymphadenitis)*. Dilated lymphatics are filled with neutrophils and macrophages; inflammation can extend into adjacent tissues with cellulitis or abscess formation.

Lymphedema is due to lymphatic obstruction and dilation, with associated increases in interstitial fluid. Primary hereditary causes include *Milroy disease* (primary lymphatic agenesis). Common secondary causes of lymphedema are as follows:

- Malignancy
- Surgical resection of regional lymph nodes
- Postradiation fibrosis
- Filariasis
- Postinflammatory thrombosis with lymphatic scarring

Prolonged lymphedema causes interstitial fibrosis, and in cutaneous tissues causes a *peau d'orange* (orange peel) appearance, with associated ulcers and *brawny induration.* Rupture of obstructed lymphatics in a body cavity leads to milky *chylous* accumulations.

Vascular Tumors (p. 515)

Primary tumors of blood vessels and lymphatics run the gamut from common, benign *hemangiomas* to intermediate, locally aggressive lesions to rare, highly malignant *angiosarcomas.* Congenital or developmental malformations and non-neoplastic reactive vascular proliferations (e.g., *bacillary angiomatosis*) can also present as tumorlike lesions.

Vascular neoplasms can be EC-derived or arise from cells that support or surround blood vessels. In general, benign vascular neoplasms are composed of well-formed vascular channels lined by EC; at the other end of the spectrum, malignant tumors show few or poorly developed vascular channels with solid, cellular, anaplastic endothelial proliferation.

Benign Tumors and Tumorlike Conditions (p. 516)

Vascular Ectasias (p. 516)

Vascular ectasias are common lesions characterized by local dilations of preexisting vessels; they are *not* true neoplasms.

- *Nevus flammeus* (p. 516) is the classic "birthmark." It is a macular cutaneous lesion that histologically shows only dermal vessel dilation; most eventually regress. *Port-wine stains* are an important variant that tend to persist and grow along with the child, thickening the involved skin. *Sturge-Weber syndrome* is characterized by port-wine stains in association with leptomeningeal angiomatous masses, mental retardation, seizures, hemiplegia, and skull radiopacities.

- *Spider telangiectasias* (p. 516) are minute subcutaneous arterioles, often pulsatile, arranged in radial fashion around a central core. They typically occur above the waist and are associated with hyperestrogenic states (e.g., pregnancy or cirrhosis).
- *Hereditary hemorrhagic telangiectasia (Osler-Weber-Rendu disease)* (p. 516) is a rare, autosomal dominant disorder caused by mutations in genes encoding components of the TGF-β signaling pathway; the disease is characterized by multiple small (<5 mm) aneurysmal telangiectasias on skin and mucous membranes. Patients present with epistaxis, hemoptysis, or GI or genitourinary bleeding.

Hemangiomas *(p. 516)*

Hemangiomas are very common lesions, accounting for 7% of all benign pediatric tumors.

- *Capillary hemangiomas* (p. 516) are the most common type of vascular tumor, occurring primarily in skin or mucous membranes. These are unencapsulated lesions 1 mm to several centimeters in size, composed of closely packed aggregates of capillary-sized, thin-walled vessels. They may be partially or completely thrombosed. The *juvenile (strawberry) hemangioma* variant is present at birth in 1 of 200 children, grows rapidly for a few months, and begins regressing at 1 to 3 years; most disappear by age 7.
- *Cavernous hemangiomas* (p. 516) are unencapsulated lesions usually 1 to 2 cm in diameter (with rare giant forms), exhibiting large, thin-walled vascular spaces. In addition to the skin, the liver is a common site, and lesions can also occur in the central nervous system or other viscera. These can be locally destructive and generally do not regress; thrombosis and dystrophic calcification are common. Cavernous hemangiomas in the cerebellum, brain stem, or eye grounds are associated with angiomatous or cystic neoplasms in pancreas and liver in *von Hippel-Lindau disease* (see Chapter 28).
- *Pyogenic granulomas* (p. 516) are an ulcerated polypoid variant of capillary hemangiomas, often following trauma. Composed of proliferating capillaries with interspersed edema and inflammatory infiltrates, they resemble exuberant granulation tissue. Pregnancy tumor *(granuloma gravidarum)* is essentially the same lesion, occurring in gingiva of 1% of pregnant women and regressing postpartum.

Lymphangiomas *(p. 516)*

Lymphangiomas are the benign lymphatic analog of hemangiomas.

- *Simple (capillary) lymphangiomas* (p. 516) are 1 to 2 cm, exudate-filled, blisterlike blebs composed of small lymphatic channels lined by EC; they have a predilection for head, neck, and axillary subcutaneous tissue.
- *Cavernous lymphangiomas (cystic hygromas)* (p. 517) are the analog to cavernous hemangioma, occurring in children in the neck or axilla (and rarely retroperitoneally). They can occasionally be large (up to 15 cm) and produce gross deformities; they are not well encapsulated, and complete surgical resection can be difficult.

Glomus Tumor (Glomangioma) *(p. 517)*

Glomus tumor (glomangioma) is a benign, exquisitely painful tumor of modified SMCs arising from the glomus body, a specialized arteriovenous structure involved in thermoregulation. Tumors occur most commonly in the distal phalanges, especially beneath nail beds. Excision is curative.

Tumors are <1 cm and may be pinpoint; they consist of aggregates, nests, and masses of specialized glomus cells associated with branching vascular channels.

Bacillary Angiomatosis *(p. 517)*

Bacillary angiomatosis is a vascular proliferation resulting from opportunistic infection in an immunocompromised host; lesions can involve skin, bone, brain, and other organs. It is caused by a gram-negative bacillus of the *Bartonella* family. The vascular proliferation results from hypoxia-inducing factor 1α (HIF-1α) induction, which in turn drives vascular endothelial growth factor (VEGF) production. Treatment with erythromycin is curative.

Intermediate-Grade (Borderline) Tumors (p. 518)

Kaposi Sarcoma *(p. 518)*

Kaposi sarcoma (KS) is a vascular neoplasm caused by human herpesvirus 8 (HHV-8), also called Kaposi sarcoma-associated herpesvirus (KSHV). Epidemiologically KS is categorized into the following four varieties:

- *Chronic or classic or European KS* occurs typically in elderly men of Eastern European (especially Ashkenazi Jew) or Mediterranean descent; it is not associated with human immunodeficiency virus (HIV). Lesions are red-purple cutaneous plaques and nodules on the lower extremities, rarely with visceral involvement.
- *Lymphadenopathic or African or endemic KS* has the same general geographic distribution as Burkitt lymphoma; it typically occurs in individuals younger than age 40 and is not associated with HIV. Cutaneous lesions are sparse, and KS occurs largely in lymph node but with occasional visceral involvement (often in prepubertal children) can be quite aggressive (3-year mortality of 100%).
- *Transplant-associated KS* occurs in patients receiving chronic immunosuppression. Nodal, mucosal, and visceral involvement can be aggressive (and fatal); lesions may regress when immunosuppression is discontinued.
- *Acquired immunodeficiency syndrome (AIDS)–associated (epidemic) KS* may occur anywhere in the skin and mucous membranes, lymph nodes, GI tract, or viscera. Wide visceral dissemination can occur early. With current antiretroviral therapies, the incidence in the United States AIDS population is now just 2% to 3%; most patients die of opportunistic infections and not KS. In combination with the endemic form of the disease (see previous text), KS constitutes the most common tumor in central Africa.

Pathogenesis (p. 518)

HHV-8 is both necessary and sufficient for KS development, although a local proliferative milieu (potentially related to inflammatory cell cytokine production) is an important cofactor in disease pathogenesis and clinical expression.

Morphology (p. 518)

Three stages of lesions are recognized as the following:

- *Patches* are pink-purple macules, usually confined to the distal lower extremities. Microscopically these contain dilated, irregular EC-lined spaces, with interspersed lymphocytes, plasma cells, and macrophages (sometimes containing hemosiderin).
- *Raised plaques* have dilated, jagged vascular channels lined by plump spindle cells accompanied by perivascular aggregates of similar spindled cells.

- *Nodular lesions* are more distinctly neoplastic and often herald lymph node and visceral involvement, particularly in the African and AIDS-associated diseases. Microscopically lesions consist of sheets of plump, spindle-shaped cells creating slitlike vascular spaces filled with erythrocytes; there are intermingled small vessels, with marked hemorrhage and mononuclear inflammatory cell infiltration.

Clinical Features (p. 519)

The course varies widely, depending on the clinical setting; most primary KSHV infections are asymptomatic. Classic KS is generally restricted to the skin, and surgical resection is usually adequate for an excellent prognosis. Radiation and/or chemotherapy is generally effective for the lymphadenopathic form, and withdrawal of immunosuppression can ameliorate the transplantation-associated form. For AIDS-associated KS, antiretroviral therapy is helpful; interferon-α, angiogenesis inhibitors, and blockade of intracellular kinase pathways are also used.

Hemangioendotheliomas *(p. 519)*

Hemangioendotheliomas are neoplasms with clinical behaviors straddling benign and malignant. *Epithelioid hemangioepithelioma* is an example; most lesions are cured by excision, although 40% may recur and 20% eventually metastasize, and 15% of patients may die from their tumor.

Malignant Tumors (p. 519)

Angiosarcomas *(p. 519)*

Angiosarcomas are malignant endothelial neoplasms on a spectrum from well-differentiated *(hemangiosarcoma)* to anaplastic; they can occur anywhere but tend to arise in skin, soft tissue, breast, and liver. Angiosarcomas are aggressive tumors and metastasize readily; 5-year survival rates are approximately 30%.

Hepatic angiosarcomas are associated with exposure to arsenic (some pesticides), polyvinylchloride (some plastics), and Thorotrast (a radiocontrast agent no longer used).

Angiosarcomas can also develop in long-term chronic lymphedema—classically in the ipsilateral arm years after radical mastectomy for breast cancer; the tumor putatively arises from dilated lymphatic vessels *(lymphangiosarcoma)*. Angiosarcomas may also be induced by radiation and are rarely associated with foreign bodies.

Morphology (p. 519)

Cutaneous lesions begin as small, well-demarcated red nodules evolving into large, fleshy, gray-white, soft tissue masses. *Microscopically* all degrees of differentiation are found, from plump anaplastic EC to undifferentiated lesions with marked cellular atypia (including giant cells) and lacking vascular lumens.

Hemangiopericytomas *(p. 520)*

Hemangiopericytomas are pericyte tumors, commonly arising on the lower extremities or in the retroperitoneum; 50% metastasize. Presenting as slowly enlarging, painless masses, they consist of branching capillary channels encased by nests and masses of spindle-shaped to round cells extrinsic to the EC basement membrane.

Pathology of Vascular Intervention (p. 520)

In the same way that various forms of vascular wall injury result in healing that leads to intimal hyperplasia (e.g., in atherosclerosis), the trauma consequent to vascular intervention tends to induce a concentric intimal thickening composed of recruited SMC and associated ECM.

Endovascular Stenting (p. 520)

Angioplasty dilates arterial stenoses (typically coronary arteries) using a balloon catheter. Balloon dilation of an atherosclerotic vessel causes plaque fracture and medial dissection; complications include abrupt reclosure (uncommon) and proliferative restenosis in 30% to 50% of patients within the 4 to 6 months. Angioplasty is rarely now performed without concurrent stent placement.

Vascular stents are expandable tubes of metallic mesh that preserve luminal patency at angioplasty sites. Stents can ameliorate the untoward effects of angioplasty by providing a larger and more regular lumen, acting as a scaffold to support the intimal flaps and dissections that occur during angioplasty, limiting elastic recoil and preventing vascular spasm, and increasing blood flow. Nevertheless, both early thrombosis and late intimal thickening can occur and lead to vascular occlusion. Use of anticoagulation and incorporation of antiproliferative drugs in the stents *(drug eluting stents)* are current therapeutic approaches to ameliorate such *in-stent restenosis.*

Vascular Replacement (p. 521)

Large-diameter (>10 cm) synthetic grafts in high-flow locations, such as the aorta, perform well. In contrast, small-diameter vascular conduits (≤6 to 8 mm)—either synthetic or derived from autologous saphenous vein—perform less durably. Graft failure is related to thrombotic occlusion (early) or intimal fibrous hyperplasia (months to years), either generalized (vein grafts) or specifically at anastomotic sites (synthetic grafts).

The patency of saphenous veins used as coronary artery bypass grafts is 50% at 10 years. In comparison, internal mammary arteries used as coronary bypass grafts have more than 90% patency at 10 years.

12 The Heart

Cardiac Structure and Specializations (p. 523)

Volume and/or pressure overloads lead to dilated chamber size and/or to increased atrial or ventricular wall thickness; increased myocardial mass occurs through myocyte *hypertrophy*, and heart enlargement is termed *cardiomegaly*.

Myocardium (p. 524)

The heart contracts (during *systole*) and relaxes (during *diastole*). The amount of force generated during systole is determined by the distance each sarcomere contracts through the coordinated ratcheting of myosin over actin myofilaments. Moderate ventricular dilation during diastole creates a greater distance over which the sarcomere can subsequently shorten and augment the force of systolic contraction—thus accommodating variations in volume and pressure demands. However, with excessive dilation the overlap of the actin and myosin filaments is reduced and the force of contraction decreases sharply, leading to heart failure.

Some atrial cells have distinctive cytoplasmic electron-dense storage granules that contain *atrial natriuretic peptide*, a peptide hormone that promotes arterial vasodilation and stimulates renal salt and water elimination (*natriuresis* and *diuresis*).

The coordinated beating of cardiac myocytes depends on the cell-to-cell movement of calcium through *gap junctions* at the lateral borders of adjacent myocytes and at intercalated discs. Abnormalities in the spatial distribution of gap junctions can cause electromechanical dysfunction *(arrhythmia)* and/or heart failure.

Valves (p. 524)

Valve function depends on the mobility, pliability, and structural integrity of the *leaflets* of the *atrioventricular* (AV) valves (tricuspid and mitral) or *cusps* of the *semilunar valves* (aortic and pulmonary). Semilunar valve function depends on the integrity and coordinated movements of the cuspal attachments; aortic root dilation can hinder coaptation of the valve cusps and lead to valvular regurgitation. AV valve function depends on the leaflets as well as tendinous cords and the attached papillary muscles of the ventricular wall. Left ventricular dilation, a ruptured tendinous cord, or papillary muscle dysfunction can all cause valvular insufficiency.

Pathologic changes include damage to collagen that weakens the leaflets (e.g., mitral valve prolapse [MVP]), nodular calcification (calcific aortic stenosis), and fibrotic thickening (e.g., rheumatic heart disease [RHD]).

Conduction System (p. 524)

Heart rate and rhythm are coordinated through specialized excitatory and conducting myocytes within the cardiac conduction system. The cells of the cardiac conduction system depolarize spontaneously, enabling them to function as cardiac pacemakers. The frequency of electrical impulses is sensitive to autonomic neural inputs (e.g., vagal stimulation), extrinsic adrenergic agents (e.g., adrenaline), hypoxia, and potassium concentration (i.e., hyperkalemia can block signal transmission altogether). Because the normal rate of spontaneous depolarization in the sinoatrial (SA) node (60 to 100 beats/minute) is faster than the other components, it normally sets the pace. The AV node has a gatekeeper function; by delaying the transmission of signals from the atria to the ventricles, it ensures that atrial contraction precedes ventricular systole.

Blood Supply (p. 525)

Cardiac myocytes rely almost exclusively on oxidative phosphorylation for their energy needs. Besides a high density of mitochondria (20% to 30% of myocyte volume), myocardial energy generation also requires a constant supply of oxygenated blood—rendering myocardium extremely vulnerable to ischemia. The right and left coronary arteries function as end arteries, although anatomically most hearts have numerous intercoronary anastomoses (connections called collateral circulation). Blood flow to the myocardium occurs during ventricular diastole, following closure of the aortic valve, and when the microcirculation is not compressed by cardiac contraction. At rest, diastole comprises approximately two thirds of the cardiac cycle; with tachycardia (increased heart rate), the relative duration of diastole also shortens, thus potentially compromising cardiac perfusion.

Cardiac Stem Cells (p. 525)

There are bone marrow-derived precursors—as well as a small population of stem cells within the myocardium—that are capable of repopulating the mammalian heart; the intramyocardial stem cells constitute 5% to 10% of normal atrial cellularity, but only 1 in 100,000 cells in a normal ventricle. Cardiac stem cells have a very slow rate of proliferation that progressively decreases with age. Although stem cell numbers and progeny do increase to a limited extent after myocardial injury or hypertrophy, hearts that suffer myocardial cell loss (e.g., due to infarction) do not recover any significant function in the necrotic zone.

Effects of Aging on the Heart (p. 525)

- Reduced ventricular cavity size (base-to-apex) leads to bulging of the basal ventricular septum and partial functional outflow tract obstruction *(sigmoid septum)*.
- Valve sclerosis and calcification lead to stenosis (aortic valve).
- Valve degenerative changes lead to insufficiency (mitral valve).
- Reduced myocyte number and increased interstitial fibrosis cause reduced contractility and compliance.
- The aorta becomes progressively stiffer due to loss of elastic tissue and increased collagen deposition; this causes higher systemic pressures and cardiac hypertrophy.
- Accumulated atherosclerosis leads to coronary stenosis and ischemia or to vulnerable plaques that can abruptly rupture and thrombose.

Overview of Cardiac Pathophysiology (p. 526)

Cardiac disease occurs as a consequence of one (or more) of the following general mechanisms:

- *Pump failure,* due either to poor contractile function or inability to relax to allow filling.
- *Flow obstruction* (e.g., due to atherosclerosis, thrombosis, hypertension, or valvular stenosis).
- *Regurgitant flow* (e.g., due to valvular insufficiency), output from each contraction is directed backward causing volume overload and diminished forward flow.
- *Shunted flow* that allows abnormal blood flow either right to left (bypassing the lungs) or left to right (causing volume overload).
- *Abnormal cardiac conduction* leading to uncoordinated myocardial contractions.
- *Rupture of the heart or major vessels.*

Heart Failure (p. 526)

Congestive heart failure (CHF) is the common end point of many forms of heart disease and affects 2% of the U.S. population; it is the cause of death in approximately 300,000 patients annually. CHF occurs when impaired function renders the heart unable to maintain output sufficient for the metabolic requirements of the body or can only do so at elevated filling pressures. CHF is characterized by diminished cardiac output (forward failure), accumulation of blood in the venous system (backward failure), or both.

When cardiac function is impaired or the workload increases, the following compensatory mechanisms attempt to maintain arterial pressure and organ perfusion:

- *Frank-Starling mechanism:* Increased filling pressures dilate the heart and thereby increase functional cross-bridges in the sarcomeres, enhancing contractility.
- *Myocardial hypertrophy* with increased expression of contractile apparatus.
- *Activation of neurohumoral systems.*
  - Autonomic nervous system adrenergic stimulation, increasing heart rate, contractility, and vascular resistance
  - Modulating blood volume and pressures by activation of the renin-angiotensin-aldosterone axis and release of atrial natriuretic peptide

Although initially adaptive, these compensatory changes impose further demands on cardiac function. Moreover, when superimposed on further pathologic insults, such as myocyte apoptosis, cytoskeletal changes, and increased extracellular matrix, CHF may supervene.

- Most frequently heart failure occurs due to progressive deterioration of myocardial contractile function *(systolic dysfunction);* causes include ischemia, pressure or volume overload due to valvular disease, or primary myocardial failure.
- Occasionally CHF results from the inability of the heart chamber to relax and fill during diastole *(diastolic dysfunction);* causes include hypertrophy (most common), fibrosis, amyloid deposition, or constrictive pericarditis. This occurs more commonly over age 65 and more so in women than men.

Cardiac Hypertrophy: Pathophysiology and Progression to Heart Failure (p. 527)

Because adult myocytes cannot classically proliferate, the heart responds to pressure or volume overload by increasing myocyte size *(myocyte hypertrophy);* similar hypertrophy is stimulated by chronic trophic signals (e.g., β-adrenergic signaling). The result is a larger and heavier heart. Notably, similar compensatory changes can occur in residual viable myocardium after nonlethal myocardial infarction (MI).

In *pressure-overload hypertrophy* (e.g., due to hypertension or aortic stenosis), new sarcomeres are assembled in parallel to the long axes of cells, expanding the cross-sectional area of myocytes in ventricles and causing a concentric increase in wall thickness. In *volume-overload hypertrophy* (e.g., due to valvular insufficiency), new sarcomeres are assembled in series, causing ventricular dilation. Heart *weight,* rather than wall thickness, is the best measure of hypertrophy in dilated hearts.

Individual myocytes exhibit increased DNA ploidy, increased numbers of mitochondria, and increased numbers of sarcomeres. The genetic expression pattern also shifts to a more embryonic phenotype, including fetal isoforms of β-myosin heavy chain, natriuretic peptides, and collagen.

Although hypertrophy is initially adaptive, it can make myocytes vulnerable to injury. The capillary density does not increase in proportion to the cell size increase or metabolic demands. Hypertrophy is also accompanied by interstitial matrix deposition that can diminish cardiac compliance.

Heart failure with volume or pressure overload may eventually result from a combination of (1) aberrant myocyte metabolism, (2) alterations in intracellular calcium flux, (3) apoptosis, and (4) genetic reprogramming. Increased heart mass is also an independent risk factor for sudden (presumably arrhythmic) cardiac death (Fig. 12-1).

Physiologic hypertrophy (with aerobic exercise) is a volume-load hypertrophy that tends also to induce beneficial effects, including increased capillary density and decreased resting heart rate and blood pressure.

Left-Sided Heart Failure (p. 529)

Major causes include ischemic heart disease (IHD), hypertension, aortic and mitral valve disease, and intrinsic myocardial disease. Left-sided failure can be due to either systolic failure (inadequate contractile function) or diastolic dysfunction leading to poor filling; left-sided heart failure is manifested by the following:

- *Pulmonary congestion and edema* due to regurgitant flow or impaired pulmonary outflow
- *Left atrial dilation with atrial fibrillation*
- *Reduced renal perfusion:*
  - Salt and water retention
  - Ischemic acute kidney injury (AKI)
  - Impaired waste excretion, causing prerenal azotemia
- *Hypoxic encephalopathy* due to reduced central nervous system perfusion

Right-Sided Heart Failure (p. 530)

Right-sided heart failure is most commonly caused by left-sided failure; thus in most cases patients present with biventricular CHF.

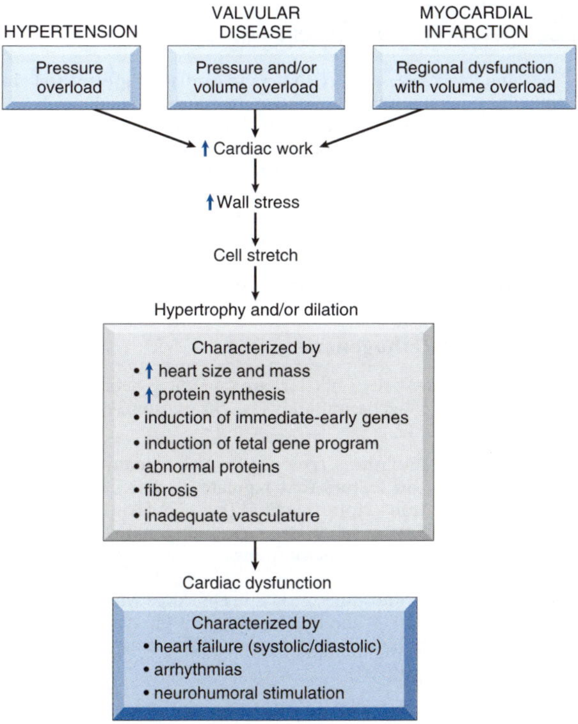

Figure 12-1 Schematic representation of the causes and consequences of cardiac hypertrophy.

Isolated right-sided heart failure is caused by tricuspid or pulmonic valvular disease or by intrinsic pulmonary or pulmonary vasculature disease, causing functional right ventricular outflow obstruction (cor pulmonale). Right-sided failure is manifested by the following:

- Right atrial and ventricular dilation and hypertrophy.
- *Edema,* typically in dependent peripheral locations (e.g., feet, ankles, sacrum) with *serous effusions* in pericardial, pleural, or peritoneal spaces.
- *Hepatomegaly with centrilobular congestion and atrophy,* producing a *nutmeg* appearance *(chronic passive congestion).* With severe hypoxia, there is *centrilobular necrosis,* and elevated right-sided pressures cause central hemorrhage. Subsequent central fibrosis creates *cardiac sclerosis.*
- *Congestive splenomegaly* with sinusoidal dilation, focal hemorrhages, hemosiderin deposits, and fibrosis.
- *Renal congestion,* hypoxic injury, and AKI (more marked in right- versus left-sided CHF).

Therapies for CHF are primarily pharmacologic; they include diuretics to relieve fluid overload, angiotensin-converting enzyme inhibitors to block the renin-angiotensin-aldosterone axis, and β-1 blockers to lower adrenergic tone. Newer approaches include mechanical assist devices and resynchronization of electrical impulses to maximize cardiac efficiency.

Congenital Heart Disease (p. 531)

Congenital heart disease (CHD) refers to cardiac or great vessel abnormalities present at birth; most are attributable to faulty embryogenesis during gestational weeks 3 to 8, when major cardiovascular structures develop. Severe anomalies are incompatible with intrauterine survival; thus defects that permit development to birth generally involve only specific chambers or regions, with the remainder of the heart being normal. Congenital disorders constitute the most common cardiac disease among children, with an incidence of 1% of live births; the incidence is higher in premature infants and stillborns. The most frequent disorders (constituting 85% of cases) are listed in Table 12-1.

Etiology and Pathogenesis (p. 532)

- The main known causes of CHD are sporadic genetic abnormalities, either single-gene mutations or chromosomal deletions or additions Table 12-2.
    - Single-gene mutations typically involve signaling pathways or transcription factors that regulate cardiac development; some of the transcription factors (e.g., GATA-4) are mutated in rare forms of adult-onset cardiomyopathy, suggesting an additional role in maintaining normal postnatal cardiac function.
    - Deletion of chromosome 22q11.2 in DiGeorge syndrome affects the development of the third and fourth pharyngeal pouches with thymic, parathyroid, and cardiac defects.

TABLE 12-1 Frequencies of Congenital Cardiac Malformations*

Malformation	Incidence per Million Live Births	%
VSD	4482	42
ASD	1043	10
Pulmonary stenosis	836	8
PDA	781	7
TOF	577	5
Coarctation of aorta	492	5
AV septal defect	396	4
Aortic stenosis	388	4
TGA	388	4
Truncus arteriosus	136	1
Total anomalous pulmonary venous connection	120	1
Tricuspid atresia	118	1
Total	9757	

*Presented as upper quartile of 44 published studies. Percentages do not add to 100% owing to rounding.

From Hoffman JIE, Kaplan S: The incidence of congenital heart disease. *J Am Coll Cardiol* 39:1890, 2002.

- The *most common genetic cause of CHD is trisomy 21* (Down syndrome); 40% of Down syndrome patients will have one or more cardiac defects.

- Beyond known associations, genetics likely also contributes to many lesions; first-degree relatives of affected patients are at increased risk of CHD relative to the general population.
- Environmental (e.g., congenital rubella infection or teratogens) and maternal factors (e.g., gestational diabetes) also contribute to the incidence of CHD.

Clinical Features *(p. 533)*

Children with CHD have direct hemodynamic sequelae, as well as retarded development and failure to thrive. They are at increased risk for chronic illness and infective endocarditis (IE) (due to abnormal valves or endocardial injury from jet lesions).

CHD lesions are either *obstructions* or *shunts.*

- *Obstructions* include abnormal narrowing of chambers, valves, or vessels; a complete obstruction is called an *atresia.*
- *Shunts* denote abnormal communications between heart chambers, between vessels, or between chambers and vessels. Depending on pressure relationships, blood is shunted from right-to-left or from left-to-right (more common).
    - ***Right-to-left shunts*** bypass the lungs, leading to hypoxia and tissue *cyanosis.* Right-to-left shunts also allow venous emboli to enter the systemic circulation *(paradoxical emboli).* Secondary findings in long-standing cyanotic heart disease include finger and toe *clubbing* (also called hypertrophic osteoarthropathy), and polycythemia.

TABLE 12-2 Selected Examples of Gene Defects Associated With CHD*

Disorder	Gene(s)	Gene Product Function
Nonsyndromic		
ASD or conduction defects	*NKX2.5*	Transcription factor
ASD or VSD	*GATA4*	Transcription factor
TOF	*ZFPM2* or *NKX2.5*	Transcription factors
Syndromic†		
Alagille syndrome—pulmonary artery stenosis or TOF	*JAG1* or *NOTCH2*	Signaling proteins or receptors
Char syndrome—PDA	*TFAP2B*	Transcription factor
CHARGE syndrome—ASD, VSD, PDA, or hypoplastic right side of the heart	*CHD7*	Helicase-binding protein
DiGeorge syndrome—ASD, VSD, or outflow tract obstruction	*TBX1*	Transcription factor
Holt-Oram syndrome—ASD, VSD, or conduction defect	*TBX5*	Transcription factor
Noonan syndrome—pulmonary valve stenosis, VSD, or HCM	*PTPN11, KRAS, SOS1*	Signaling proteins

*Different mutations can cause the same phenotype, and mutations in some genes can cause multiple phenotypes (e.g., *NKX2.5*). Many of these congenital lesions also can occur sporadically, without specific genetic mutation.

†Only the cardiac manifestations of the syndrome are listed; the other skeletal, facial, neurologic, and visceral changes are not.

ASD, Atrial septal defect; *CHARGE,* posterior *c*oloboma, *h*eart defect, choanal *a*tresia, *r*etardation, *g*enital and *e*ar anomalies; *PDA,* patent ductus arteriosus; *VSD,* ventricular septal defect.

- ***Left-to-right shunts*** cause pulmonary volume overload. If prolonged, the vasculature responds with medial hypertrophy and increased vascular resistance to maintain normal pulmonary capillary and venous pressures. As pulmonary resistance approaches systemic levels, a right-to-left shunt occurs *(Eisenmenger syndrome).* Once there is significant pulmonary hypertension, the underlying structural defects are no longer candidates for surgical correction.

- Altered hemodynamics usually cause chamber dilation and/or hypertrophy. However, defects occasionally lead to diminished chamber volume and muscle mass. This is called *hypoplasia* if it occurs during development or *atrophy* if it occurs postnatally.

Left-to-Right Shunts (p. 533)

The major congenital left-to-right shunts are as follows (Fig. 12-2):

- Atrial septal defect (ASD)
- Ventricular septal defect (VSD)
- Patent ductus arteriosus (PDA)

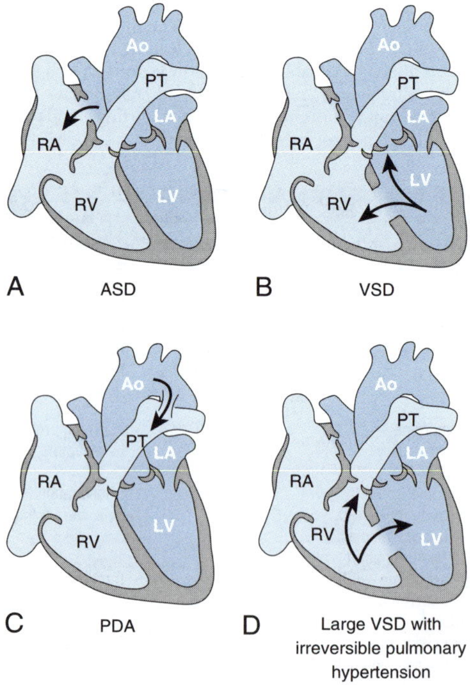

Figure 12-2 Schematics of the most important congenital left-to-right shunts (*arrows* indicate the direction of blood flow). A, ASD. **B,** VSD. With VSD the shunt is left-to-right, with equilibration of pressures in both ventricles. Pressure hypertrophy of the right ventricle and volume hypertrophy of the left ventricle are generally present. **C,** PDA. **D,** Large VSD with irreversible pulmonary hypertension. Long-standing pressure-volume overload in the pulmonary circulation leads to increased resistance, eventually with sufficient right ventricular hypertrophy to generate pressures in excess of the left ventricle; at that point, flow reversal occurs with a right-to-left shunt, so-called *Eisenmenger syndrome. Ao,* Aorta; *LA,* left atrium; *LV,* left ventricle; *PT,* pulmonary trunk; *RA,* right atrium; *RV,* right ventricle.

Atrial Septal Defects *(p. 534; Fig. 12-2, A)*

ASDs are the most common congenital cardiac anomalies seen in adults. Even large ASDs are usually asymptomatic until adulthood, when either right-sided heart failure can occur or right-sided hypertrophy and pulmonary hypertension can induce right-to-left shunting with cyanosis.

- *Primum type:* 5% of ASD; these occur adjacent to the mitral and tricuspid valves.
- *Secundum type:* 90% of ASD; results from deficient or fenestrated fossa ovalis in the central atrial septum and is usually not associated with other anomalies.
- *Sinus venosus type:* 5% of ASD; occurs near the superior vena cava entrance and can be associated with anomalous right pulmonary vein drainage.

Patent Foramen Ovale *(p. 534)*

Patent foramen ovale occurs when there is defective postnatal sealing of the fossa ovalis flap; these occur in 20% of individuals and can be a conduit for paradoxical emboli in the setting of elevated right-sided pressures.

Ventricular Septal Defect *(p. 535; Fig. 12-2, B)*

VSDs are the most common congenital cardiac anomaly overall. Depending on VSD size, the clinical outcome ranges from fulminant CHF to late cyanosis to spontaneous closure (50% of those <0.5 cm diameter). Surgical correction is desirable before right-sided overload and pulmonary hypertension develop.

- VSDs are frequently associated with other anomalies, particularly *tetralogy of Fallot (TOF),* but 20% to 30% are isolated.
- Ninety percent involve the membranous septum *(membranous VSD)* near the aortic valve, whereas the remainder are muscular.

Patent Ductus Arteriosus *(p. 535; Fig. 12-2, C)*

The ductus arteriosus (just distal to the left subclavian artery) allows blood flow between the aorta and pulmonary artery during fetal development, thus bypassing the lungs. The ductus normally closes within 1 to 2 days of life, as a consequence of increasing arterial oxygenation, reduced pulmonary vascular resistance, and declining prostaglandin E_2 levels. Closure is delayed when there is hypoxia (e.g., respiratory distress) or with defects, such as VSD, that increase pulmonary vascular pressures.

- Ninety percent of PDA are isolated defects; the remainder are associated with VSD, aortic coarctation, or valvular stenosis.
- Most are initially asymptomatic but produce a harsh continuous *machinery-like* heart murmur. Large PDA will cause right-sided volume and pressure overload.
- Early closure—surgically or with prostaglandin synthesis inhibitors—is advocated, unless other concurrent CHDs (e.g., aortic valve atresia) are present; in the latter case the PDA may be the only means to provide systemic perfusion.

With persistent left-to-right shunting of any cause, chronic pressure-volume overload in the pulmonary circulation eventually induces increased pulmonary vascular tone *(pulmonary hypertension).* As pulmonary vascular pressures rise, they eventually exceed the left-sided heart pressures, and a right-to-left shunt supervenes—so-called *Eisenmenger syndrome* (Fig. 12-2, *D*).

Right-to-Left Shunts (p. 535)

The major congenital right-to-left shunts are as follows (Fig. 12-3):

- TOF
- Transposition of the great arteries (TGA)

Tetralogy of Fallot (*p. 535; Fig. 12-3, A*)

The cardinal findings are as follows:

- VSD
- Pulmonary stenosis with right ventricle outflow obstruction
- Overriding aorta
- Right ventricular hypertrophy

Symptom severity is directly related to the extent of right ventricle outflow obstruction. With a large VSD and mild pulmonary stenosis, there is minimal left-to-right shunt and no cyanosis. More severe pulmonary stenosis produces a cyanotic right-to-left shunt.

With complete pulmonary obstruction, survival can occur only by flow through a PDA or dilated bronchial arteries. Surgical correction can be delayed provided that the child can tolerate the level of oxygenation. Pulmonary outflow stenosis protects the lung from volume and pressure overload, and right ventricular failure is rare.

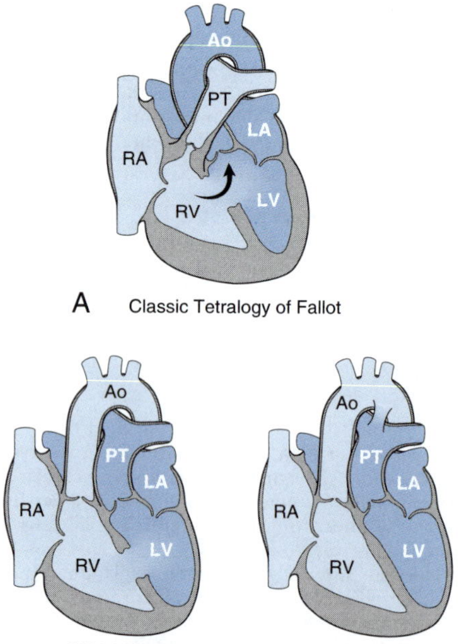

A Classic Tetralogy of Fallot

With VSD Without VSD

B Complete Transposition

Figure 12-3 Schematics of the most important congenital right-to-left shunts (*cyanotic CHD*). A, TOF. The direction of shunting across the VSD depends on the degree of the subpulmonic stenosis; if the pulmonary stenosis is severe, a right-to-left shunt results *(arrow)*. **B,** TGA, with and without VSD. *Ao,* Aorta; *LA,* left atrium; *LV,* left ventricle; *PT,* pulmonary trunk; *RA,* right atrium; *RV,* right ventricle.

Transposition of the Great Arteries *(p. 536; Fig. 12-3, B)*

Systemic and pulmonary venous return—to the right and left atria, respectively—are normal; however, the aorta arises from the right ventricle and the pulmonary artery from the left ventricle, so that the pulmonary and systemic circulations are functionally separated.

- Normal fetal development occurs because venous and systemic blood mix through the ductus arteriosus and a patent foramen ovale.
- Postnatal life critically depends on ongoing blood mixing (e.g., through a PDA, VSD, ASD, or patent foramen ovale).
- Prognosis depends on the severity of tissue hypoxia and the ability of the right ventricle to maintain systemic aortic pressures. Untreated, most infants die within months.

Obstructive Lesions (p. 537)

Although these will cause ventricular hypertrophy, none cause cyanosis unless there is an additional shunt present.

Coarctation of the Aorta *(p. 537) (Fig. 12-4)*

Coarctation of the aorta is a constriction of the aorta; 50% occur as isolated defects, the remainder with other anomalies, most commonly a bicuspid aortic valve (BAV). Males are affected twice as often as females, although coarcts are common in Turner syndrome. There is typically prominent left ventricular hypertrophy; additional clinical manifestations depend on the location and severity of the constriction and the ductus arteriosus patency.

- *Preductal* coarctation manifests early in life ("infantile form") and can be rapidly fatal. Survival depends on the ability of a PDA to provide adequate systemic blood flow.
- *Postductal* coarctation ("adult form") can be asymptomatic unless severe; effects are also dependent on ductus arteriosus patency:
  - Postductal coarctation without an associated PDA may be asymptomatic but classically manifests as upper extremity hypertension and lower extremity hypotension with arterial insufficiency

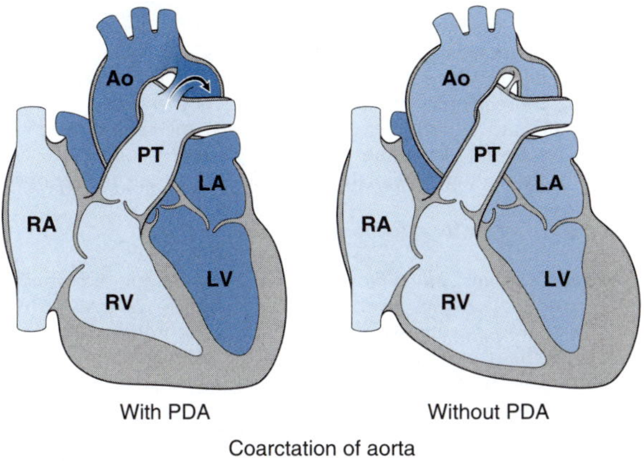

Figure 12-4 Schematic of aortic coarctation with and without PDA. *Ao,* Aorta; *LA,* left atrium; *LV,* left ventricle; *PDA,* patent ductus arteriosus; *PT,* pulmonary trunk; *RA,* right atrium; *RV,* right ventricle.

(claudication, cold sensitivity). Flow around the coarctation generally develops via internal mammary and axillary artery collaterals; such vascular dilation causes intercostal rib notching notable on x-rays.

- An associated PDA leads to right-to-left shunting with lower body cyanosis; long-term survival requires surgical intervention.
- Surgical resection and end-to-end anastomoses or conduit insertion yield an excellent outcome.

Pulmonary Stenosis and Atresia *(p. 537)*

Pulmonary stenosis and atresia can be isolated or occur with other anomalies (e.g., transposition or TOF).

- Valvular stenoses are associated with right ventricular hypertrophy and poststenotic pulmonary artery dilation.
- In subvalvular stenoses, the right ventricular pressures are not transmitted to the pulmonary circulation; the pulmonary trunk is not dilated and may be hypoplastic.
- In complete pulmonary atresia, blood flows to the lungs via an ASD and PDA, and the right ventricle is hypoplastic.

Aortic Stenosis and Atresia *(p. 537)*

- *Valvular aortic stenosis* can be caused by a small hypoplastic valve, thickened dysplastic cusps, or abnormal numbers of cusps (bicuspid or unicuspid); congenital aortic stenosis is an isolated lesion in 80% of cases.
- Infants with severe aortic stenosis or atresia can survive only via PDA flow to the aorta and coronaries; there is left ventricular underdevelopment (i.e., *hypoplastic left heart syndrome*).
- *Subaortic stenosis* due to a discrete ring or diffuse collar of endocardial fibrosis is associated with IE, left ventricle hypertrophy, poststenotic aortic dilation, and sudden death.
- *Supravalvular aortic stenosis* is a heritable form of aortic dysplasia with a thickened wall; it may be due to elastin gene mutations or part of a multiorgan developmental disorder due to partial chromosome 7 deletion (Williams-Beuren syndrome).

Ischemic Heart Disease (p. 538)

IHD comprises multiple pathophysiologically related syndromes related to myocardial ischemia (i.e., mismatch between metabolic demand and vascular supply of oxygenated blood to the heart muscle). The consequences are oxygen insufficiency *(hypoxia, anoxia)*, inadequate nutrient supply, and diminished metabolite removal. IHD is responsible for more than 400,000 deaths annually in the United States and approximately 7 million each year in developed countries.

Ischemia results from the following:

- *Reduced coronary blood flow;* >90% of cases are due to coronary atherosclerosis, vasospasm, and/or thrombosis. Atherosclerosis causes chronic progressive narrowing of the coronary lumens, a process that can be punctuated by acute plaque disruption and thrombosis (see Chapter 11). Uncommon causes of compromised flow include arteritis, emboli, and hypotension (e.g., shock).
- *Increased myocardial demand* (e.g., tachycardia, hypertrophy).
- *Hypoxia due to diminished oxygen transport* (nutrient supply and metabolite removal are not affected); causes include anemia, lung disease, cyanotic CHD, carbon monoxide poisoning, or cigarette smoking.

There are four overlapping ischemic syndromes, differing in severity and tempo:

- Angina pectoris ("chest pain")
- MI
- Chronic IHD
- Sudden cardiac death (SCD)

Unstable angina (see later), acute MI, and SCD constitute the *acute coronary syndromes*—typically precipitated by unpredictable and abrupt rupture or erosion of an atherosclerotic plaque with superimposed thrombosis and or vasospasm.

Angina Pectoris (p. 539)

This is paroxysmal substernal pain occurring when cardiac demand exceeds vascular supply; ischemia duration and severity are not sufficient to cause infarction. The pain itself is attributed to ischemia-induced release of adenosine, bradykinin, and other molecules that stimulate sympathetic and vagal afferent nerves. Importantly, not all ischemic episodes are perceived as pain; so-called *silent ischemia* is common in diabetic neuropathy and in geriatric patients.

Three patterns of angina are recognized:

- *Stable angina* reliably occurs with the same level of exertion and diminishes with rest; this is typically associated with ≥70% chronic stable stenosis (i.e., a fixed supply that becomes limiting with increased demand).
- *Prinzmetal angina* is due to vasospasm; symptoms are unrelated to exertion and respond promptly to vasodilators.
- *Unstable (crescendo) angina* is a pattern of pain occurring with successively lesser amounts of exertion or even at rest; it is often prolonged (>20 minutes) and is caused by atherosclerotic plaque disruption, typically without complete thrombotic obstruction to the vessel. Approximately half of such patients actually have myocardial necrosis; in the remainder, such unstable angina is a worrisome harbinger of impending MI.

Myocardial Infarction (p. 540)

MI is myocardial cell death caused by vascular occlusion. In the United States, 1.5 million MIs occur annually with risk increasing progressively with age; 10% occur in individuals ≤40 years old and 45% in people ≤65 years of age.

Pathogenesis *(p. 540)*

Coronary Arterial Occlusion (p. 540)

MIs are most commonly due to intraplaque hemorrhage or to plaque erosion or rupture with superimposed thrombosis. In 10% of cases, vascular occlusion is a consequence of vasospasm or embolization in the coronary circulation or due to smaller vessel obstruction (e.g., vasculitis, amyloidosis, sickle cell disease).

Myocardial Response (p. 540)

Coronary occlusion causes myocardial ischemia, dysfunction, and potentially myocyte death; the outcome depends on the severity and duration of flow deprivation (Fig. 12-5 and Table 12-3).

- Severe ischemia leads to adenosine triphosphate (ATP) depletion and loss of contractile function (but not cell death) within 60 seconds; this may precipitate myocardial failure long before there is cell death.

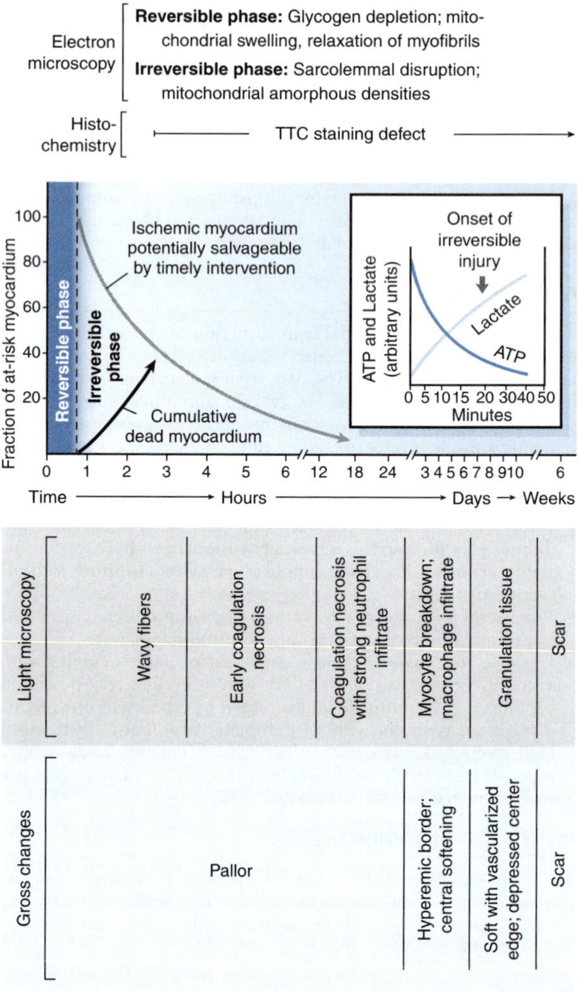

Figure 12-5 Temporal sequence of early biochemical findings and progression of necrosis after onset of severe myocardial ischemia. For approximately 30 minutes after the onset of even the most severe ischemia, myocardial injury is potentially reversible. Thereafter, progressive loss of viability occurs that is complete by 6 to 12 hours. The benefits of reperfusion are greatest when it is achieved early and are progressively lost when reperfusion is delayed. *ATP,* Adenosine triphosphate; *TTC,* triphenyl tetrazolium chloride (a substrate for lactate dehydrogenase enzyme that is lost from necrotic myocardium). *(Data from Schoen FJ: Pathologic considerations of the surgery of adult heart disease. In Edmunds LH (ed):* Cardiac Surgery in the Adult. *New York, NY: McGraw-Hill, 1997, p 85.)*

- Complete deprivation of blood flow for 20 to 30 minutes leads to irreversible myocardial injury.
- Severe compromise (but not complete blockage) of flow for prolonged periods (2 to 4 hours) will also cause irreversible injury; this delay before cell death underlies relatively later interventions to salvage "at risk" myocardium during an MI.

TABLE 12-3 Approximate Time of Onset of Key Events in Ischemic Cardiac Myocytes

Feature	Time
Onset of ATP depletion	**Seconds**
Loss of contractility	<2 min
ATP reduced	
to 50% of normal	10 min
to 10% of normal	40 min
Irreversible cell injury	20-40 min
Microvascular injury	>1 h

- Necrosis is usually complete within 6 hours of severe ischemia; however, with extensive coronary collateral circulation, necrosis can occur over a more protracted course (>12 hours).

Patterns of Infarction (p. 543)

The distribution of myocardial necrosis depends on the vessel involved (e.g., left anterior descending versus right coronary artery) and collateral perfusion, as well as the location of the occlusion within the vessel and the cause of diminished perfusion (Fig. 12-6).

- Many MIs occur within the distribution of a single coronary artery and are *transmural* (the full thickness of the ventricular wall); these are due to atherosclerosis and acute plaque change with thrombosis. These characteristically show electrocardiographic (ECG) ST elevations ("ST elevation MI").
- *Subendocardial* MIs are limited to the inner 30% to 50% of the ventricle and may involve more territory than is perfused by a single coronary. These result in "non-ST elevation MI." Causes include the following:
  - Lysis of a thrombotic occlusion before full-thickness infarction
  - Chronic atherosclerotic disease in the setting of increased myocardial demand (e.g., tachycardia) or systemically diminished supply (e.g., hypotension, anemia, lung disease)
- *Multifocal microinfarction* occurs with small vessel microembolization, vasculitis, or vascular spasm (e.g., due to endogenous epinephrine or drugs like cocaine). Catechols also increase myocardial contractility and heart rate, exacerbating ischemia caused by the vasospasm. Infarcts associated with microvascular infarcts can cause SCD (usually caused by a fatal arrhythmia) or an ischemic dilated cardiomyopathy (DCM). Indeed, vasospasm occurring in the setting of psychologic duress can lead to *takotsubo cardiomyopathy* (also called "broken heart syndrome"). Depending on the extent and location of the vascular involvement, microinfarctions show nonspecific changes or can even be electrocardiographically silent.

Morphology (p. 543)

After infarction, myocardium undergoes the following characteristic gross and microscopic changes (Fig. 12-3):

- *Gross changes*
  - **4 to 12 hours:** MIs are usually grossly inapparent but can be highlighted by histochemical stains; triphenyltetrazolium chloride (TTC) is a lactate dehydrogenase substrate; viable myocardium turns the substrate red-brown while nonviable areas are pale.

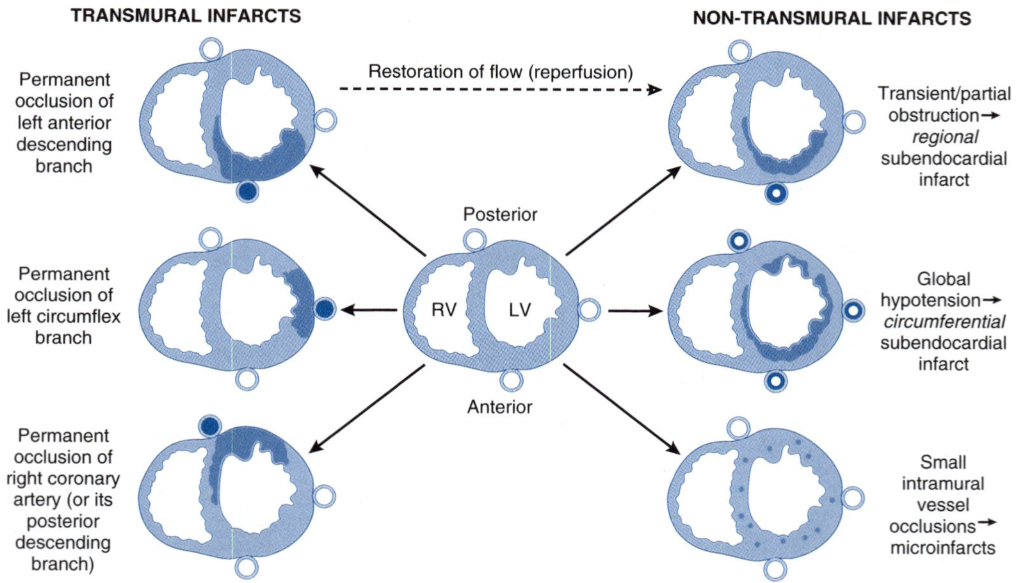

Figure 12-6 Distribution of myocardial ischemic necrosis correlates with the location and nature of decreased perfusion. *Left,* The positions of transmural acute infarcts resulting from occlusions of the major coronary arteries; *top to bottom,* left anterior descending, left circumflex, and right coronary arteries. *Right,* The types of infarcts that result from a partial or transient occlusion, global hypotension, or intramural small vessel occlusions.

  - **12 to 24 hours:** Infarcted tissue becomes apparent as pale-to-cyanotic areas.
  - **1 to 3 days:** Lesions become progressively more defined, yellow, and softened.
  - **3 to 7 days:** Hyperemic granulation tissue appears at the infarct edges.
  - **7 to 14 days:** Maximally yellow-tan and depressed infarct with red-gray infarct borders.
  - **1 to 2 months:** Gray-white fibrous scar progressively fills in the defect.
  - **>2 months:** Scarring is complete but can remodel with time.
- *Microscopic changes*
  - **<1 hr:** Intercellular edema and wavy myocytes at the infarct margin; coagulative necrosis is not yet evident.
  - **12 to 72 hr:** Dead myocytes become hypereosinophilic with loss of nuclei *(coagulative necrosis);* neutrophils also progressively infiltrate necrotic tissue.
  - **3 to 7 days:** Dead myocytes are digested by invading macrophages.
  - **7 to 10 days:** Granulation tissue progressively replaces necrotic tissue.
  - **>2 weeks:** Granulation tissue is progressively replaced by fibrous scar.

Infarct Modification by Reperfusion (p. 545)

Reflow to (*reperfusion* of) precariously injured cells (e.g., by intervention with thrombolytics) may restore viability but leave the cells poorly contractile *(stunned)* for 1 to 2 days. Reperfused myocardium is usually somewhat hemorrhagic due to ischemic vascular injury; irreversibly injured myocytes that are reperfused also show *contraction band necrosis* due to calcium overload and hypertetanic contraction. Finally, reperfusion can potentially cause additional injury by heightened recruitment of inflammatory cells, and perfusion-induced microvascular injury with capillary occlusion.

Clinical Features (p. 547)

MI diagnosis is based on symptoms (chest pain, nausea, diaphoresis, dyspnea), ECG changes, and serum elevation of cardiomyocyte-specific proteins released from dead cells (e.g., creatine kinase MB isoform [CK-MB] or various cardiac troponins [cTnT or cTnI]); CK-MB, cTnT, and cTnI are detectable in circulating blood by 3 to 12 hours after infarction, and CK-MB and cTnI levels peak at 24 hours; CK-MB returns to normal in 48 to 72 hours, cTnI in 5 to 10 days, and cTnT in 5 to 14 days. In up to 25% of patients (especially diabetic or geriatric), symptoms are absent ("silent MI"), although ECG changes are usually present, and biomarkers will be elevated.

- Nearly all transmural MIs affect the left ventricle; 15% also involve the right ventricle, particularly in posterior-inferior left ventricle infarcts. Isolated right ventricle infarction occurs in 1% to 3% of cases.
- Half of MI-associated deaths occur within the first hour, most before reaching a hospital. Overall mortality is 30% in the first year after an MI, with 3% to 4% mortality per annum thereafter.
- Therapies in the acute setting include anticoagulation, oxygen, nitrates, β-adrenergic blockade, angiotensin-converting enzyme inhibitors, and fibrinolytics; coronary angioplasting, stenting, or surgical bypass can also be performed.

Consequences and Complications of Myocardial Infarction (p. 547)

Consequences and complications depend on the size and location of injury, as well as functional myocardial reserves. Half of MI deaths occur in the first hour after onset, characteristically due to arrhythmia; most never reach the hospital. There is an approximately 5% in-hospital death rate associated with MIs; female gender, diabetes, and previous MI confer a poorer prognosis.

Therapies include the following:

- Morphine for pain and dyspnea
- Reperfusion to salvage myocardium
- Antiplatelet agents
- Anticoagulant therapy
- Nitrates to induce vasodilation
- β-blockers to reduce myocardial oxygen demand and reduce arrhythmia risk
- Antiarrhythmics
- Angiotensin-converting enzyme inhibitors to limit vascular dilation
- Oxygen supplementation

Complications include the following:

- Contractile dysfunction, approximately in proportion to the extent of infarction; effects include systemic hypotension and pulmonary edema (e.g., CHF). Severe pump failure ("cardiogenic shock") occurs in 10% to 15% of patients, typically with loss of ≥40% left ventricular mass. Cardiogenic shock has a 70% mortality rate.
- Arrhythmias.
- Ventricular rupture (1% to 2% of transmural MIs), typically within the first 10 days (median, 4 to 5 days). Rupture of the free wall causes pericardial tamponade; septal rupture causes a left-to-right shunt with right-sided volume overload.
- Papillary muscle infarction (+/− rupture) and/or dysfunction causes mitral regurgitation.
- Fibrinous pericarditis (Dressler syndrome) is common 2 to 3 days after an MI.
- Mural thrombosis adjacent to a noncontractile area can cause peripheral embolization.
- Stretching of a large area of transmural infarction *(expansion)* may heal into a *ventricular aneurysm;* both are prone to mural thrombosis.
- Infarction adjacent to existing MI *(extension).*

After an MI, noninfarcted myocardium undergoes hypertrophy and dilation *(ventricular remodeling).* Although initially this is hemodynamically beneficial, such changes can become substrate for aneurysms or for areas of secondary ischemia and arrhythmia. Long-term prognosis depends most importantly on residual left ventricular function and the extent of any vascular obstructions in vessels that perfuse the remaining viable myocardium. Overall mortality within the first year can be as high as 30%; each passing year is associated with an additional 3% to 4% mortality.

Chronic Ischemic Heart Disease (p. 550)

IHD represents progressive heart failure due to ischemic myocardial damage; it may result from postinfarction cardiac decompensation or slow ischemic myocyte degeneration.

- Invariably there is some degree of obstructive coronary atherosclerosis, often with evidence of prior healed infarcts. *Microscopically* there is myocyte hypertrophy, diffuse subendocardial myocyte vacuolization, and interstitial and replacement fibrosis.
- Patients need not have a prior diagnosed MI; diagnosis depends on excluding other causes of CHF.

Arrhythmias (p. 550)

Abnormal conduction can be sustained or sporadic *(paroxysmal)* and can initiate anywhere in the conduction system; atrial arrhythmias are designated as *supraventricular* to distinguish those with a ventricular origin. *Tachycardia* is an abnormally fast heart rate, and *bradycardia* is an abnormally slow heart rate; arrhythmias include irregular rhythm with normal ventricular contraction, chaotic depolarization without functional ventricular contraction *(ventricular fibrillation)*, or no electrical activity at all *(asystole)*. *Ischemic injury is the most common cause of rhythm disorders.*

- SA node damage (e.g., *sick sinus syndrome*) results in other fibers or even the AV node assuming pacemaker function, typically at a much slower intrinsic rate (causing bradycardia).
- Sporadically depolarizing atrial myocytes (*atrial fibrillation*, commonly associated with atrial dilation) lead to variable transmission through the AV node and an "irregularly irregular" heart rate.
- Dysfunctional AV nodes lead to *heart block* varying from P-R interval prolongation on the ECG *(first-degree heart block)* to intermittent transmission of the signal *(second-degree heart block)* to complete failure *(third-degree heart block)*.

Arrhythmias can be caused by the following:

- Abnormal gap junction structure or spatial distribution (occurring, e.g., in IHD and DCMs).
- Ischemia, myocyte hypertrophy, and inflammation (e.g., myocarditis or sarcoidosis).
- Deposition of nonconducting material (e.g., amyloid) or small areas of scarring.
- Heritable conditions. Some are associated with gross anatomic abnormalities (e.g., congenital anomalies, hypertrophic cardiomyopathy [HCM], MVP). Others are typically diagnosed by genetic testing. These so-called primary electrical abnormalities (Table 12-4) include several (usually autosomal dominant) *channelopathies*—mutations in genes that encode components of Na^+, K^+, or Ca^{2+} channels.

Sudden Cardiac Death (p. 551)

SCD is most commonly defined as *unexpected cardiac death within 1 hour of symptom onset.* More than 300,000 to 400,000 cases occur annually in the United States. Most are due to lethal arrhythmia, with IHD being the dominant cause. Although 80% to 90% of patients have significant atherosclerotic stenoses, only 10% to 20% have acute plaque disruption, and only 10% to 20% actually develop an MI (presuming they are successfully resuscitated from their "sudden death"), indicating that fatal arrhythmia (e.g., asystole or ventricular fibrillation) is the underlying cause of death. Arrhythmias are presumably triggered by conduction system scarring, acute ischemic injury, or electrical instability resulting from an ischemic focus. SCD can also be a consequence of myocardial hypertrophy (e.g., due to aortic valvular stenosis or HCM), hereditary or acquired conduction system abnormalities, electrolyte derangements, MVP, myocardial depositions, or myocarditis.

TABLE 12-4 Selected Examples of Causal Genes in Inherited Arrhythmogenic Diseases*

Disorder	Gene	Function
Long QT syndrome†	*KCNQ1*	K^+ channel (LOF)
	KCNH2	K^+ channel (LOF)
	SCN5A	Na^+ channel (GOF)
	CAV3	Caveolin, Na^+ current (GOF)
Short QT syndrome†	*KCNQ1*	K^+ channel (GOF)
	KCNH2	K^+ channel (GOF)
Brugada syndrome†	*SCN5A*	Na^+ channel (LOF)
	CACNB2b	Ca^{2+} channel (LOF)
	SCN1b	Na^+ channel (LOF)*
CPVT syndrome†	*RYR2*	Diastolic Ca^{2+} release (GOF)
	CASQ2	Diastolic Ca^{2+} release (LOF)

*Different mutations can cause the same general syndrome, and mutations in some genes can cause multiple different phenotypes; thus loss-of-function (LOF) mutations may cause long QT intervals, whereas gain-of-function (GOF) mutations result in short repolarization intervals.

†**Long QT syndrome** manifests as arrhythmias associated with excessive prolongation of the cardiac repolarization; patients often present with stress-induced syncope or SCD, and some forms are associated with swimming. **Short QT syndrome** patients have arrhythmias associated with abbreviated repolarization intervals; they can present with palpitations, syncope, and SCD. **Brugada syndrome** manifests as ECG abnormalities (ST segment elevations and right bundle branch block) in the absence of structural heart disease; patients classically present with syncope or SCD during rest or sleep or after large meals. CPVT does not have characteristic ECG changes; patients often present in childhood with life-threatening arrhythmias due to adrenergic stimulation (stress-related).

LOF, Loss-of-function mutations; *GOF,* gain-of-function mutations; *CPVT,* catecholaminergic polymorphic ventricular tachycardia.

Modified from Cerrone M, Priori SG: Genetics of sudden death: focus on inherited channelopathies. *Eur Heart J* 32:2109-2118, 2011.

Hypertensive Heart Disease (p. 552)

Systemic (Left-Sided) Hypertensive Heart Disease (p. 552)

Hypertrophy of the heart is an adaptive response to chronically elevated pressures; with continued overload, the result can be dysfunction, dilation, CHF, or SCD. The minimal criteria for diagnosing systemic hypertensive heart disease are a history or pathologic evidence of hypertension, and left ventricular hypertrophy (typically concentric) in the absence of other lesions that induce cardiac hypertrophy (e.g., aortic valve stenosis, aortic coarctation).

- Myocyte hypertrophy increases the content of contractile proteins. However, thickened myocardium reduces left ventricle compliance, impairing diastolic filling while increasing oxygen demand. Hypertrophy is also usually accompanied by interstitial fibrosis that also reduces compliance.
- Depending on the severity and duration of underlying hypertension (and adequacy of therapy) patients can have normal longevity, develop IHD as a consequence of the potentiating effects of hypertension and atherosclerosis, suffer the renal or cerebrovascular complications of hypertension, or experience progressive CHF or even SCD.

Pulmonary (Right-Sided) Hypertensive Heart Disease (*Cor Pulmonale*) (p. 553)

Cor pulmonale is the right-sided counterpart to systemic hypertensive heart disease; disorders that affect lung structure or function (e.g., emphysema or primary pulmonary hypertension) can cause pulmonary vascular hypertension, resulting in right ventricular hypertrophy, dilation, and/or failure. Recall that the most common cause of pulmonary venous hypertension is left-sided heart disease.

- *Acute cor pulmonale* with right ventricular dilation occurs after massive pulmonary embolization.
- *Chronic cor pulmonale* results from chronic right ventricular pressure overload (e.g., CHD or primary lung disease).

Valvular Heart Disease (p. 554)

Causes of *acquired* valvular heart disease (as opposed to congenital valvular disease, discussed previously) are as follows:

- Degeneration (e.g., calcific aortic stenosis, mitral annular calcification, MVP)
- Inflammatory processes (e.g., RHD)
- Infection (e.g., IE)
- Changes secondary to myocardial disease (e.g., IHD causing *ischemic mitral regurgitation*)

The clinical consequences depend on the valve involved, the degree of impairment, whether the lesion is stenotic (pressure overload) or regurgitant (volume overload), the tempo of onset, compensatory changes, and any comorbid disease.

Calcific Valvular Degeneration (p. 554)

Calcific Aortic Stenosis (p. 554)

Calcific aortic stenosis is a common (1% to 2% of the population) degenerative age-related lesion that typically manifests in individuals >70 years old. Although "wear and tear" has been cited as an etiology, newer data implicate chronic injury due to hypertension, hyperlipidemia, and inflammation.

Congenitally BAVs (p. 555) occur in approximately 1% of the population but are responsible for approximately half of adult aortic valve stenosis; the etiology for BAVs is unknown, although loss-of-function mutations in *NOTCH1* are described in some families. Symptomatic stenosis occurs at an earlier age (50 to 60 years) in patients with BAVs. Structural abnormalities of the aortic wall leading to dilation or dissection commonly accompany BAV, even if the valve is hemodynamically normal.

Morphology (p. 555)

- *Sclerosis* (valve fibrosis) is an early, hemodynamically inconsequential stage.
- Nodular, rigid calcific subendothelial masses on the valve outflow surface impede mobility and aortic outflow.
- In valves with three cusps there is no commissural fusion, and the thickening spares the cuspal free edges; in bicuspid valves there are two cusps, usually of unequal size with the larger cusp exhibiting a midline *raphe*, resulting from incomplete commissural separation; the pattern of sclerosis and calcification is comparable to valves with three cusps.
- Concentric left ventricular hypertrophy is common due to chronic pressure overload.

Clinical Features (p. 555)

Valvular stenosis leads to compensatory myocardial hypertrophy; subsequent decompensation is heralded by angina (reduced perfusion in hypertrophied myocardium), syncope (with increased risk of SCD), or CHF; if untreated, there is a 50% mortality within 2 to 5 years. Surgical valve replacement improves survival.

Mitral Annular Calcification (p. 556)

Mitral annular calcification is due to degenerative, noninflammatory calcific deposits, most commonly in women over age 60 or in individuals with MVP (see later). Although usually inconsequential, annular calcification can cause the following:

- Regurgitation due to poor systolic contraction of the mitral valve ring
- Stenosis due to poor leaflet excursion over bulky deposits
- Impingement on conduction pathways, causing arrhythmias
- Rarely, a focus for IE

Mitral Valve Prolapse (Myxomatous Degeneration of the Mitral Valve) (p. 556)

One or both mitral valve leaflets are enlarged, redundant, myxomatous, and floppy; they balloon back (prolapse) into the left atrium during systole. MVP affects 3% of the U.S. population, most commonly young women (7:1 female to male ratio). The etiology is uncertain; a high frequency in Marfan syndrome suggests abnormal extracellular matrix synthesis potentially related to dysregulated transforming growth factor (TGF)-β signaling.

Morphology (p. 556)

- *Grossly* redundancy and ballooning are seen with elongated, attenuated, or occasionally ruptured chordae tendineae.
- *Microscopically* the *fibrosa* layer (on which the strength of the leaflet depends) shows thinning and degeneration with myxomatous expansion of the *spongiosa.*
- Secondary changes include fibrous thickening of valve leaflets at points of contact, and thickened ventricular endocardium at sites of contact with prolapsing leaflets, with atrial thrombosis behind the ballooning cusps.

Clinical Features (p. 556)

Some patients also have aortic, tricuspid, or pulmonary valve myxomatous degeneration. *MVP is generally asymptomatic* and discovered only as a mid-systolic click on auscultation; more severe cases may also have mitral regurgitation. Importantly, 3% of patients will develop complications secondary to the following:

- IE
- Mitral insufficiency resulting in CHF
- Arrhythmias and/or SCD
- Embolization of atrial or leaflet thrombi

Rheumatic Fever and Rheumatic Heart Disease (p. 557)

Rheumatic fever (RF) is an acute inflammatory disease classically occurring in children after group A streptococcal infection (usually pharyngitis). It is attributed to host antistreptococcal antibodies and/or T cells that cross-react with cardiac antigens. The cell and antibody responses in turn cause progressive valve damage with fibrosis (RHD). Solitary mitral involvement occurs in 65% to 70% of cases, with combined aortic and mitral involvement in 20% to 25%; tricuspid and pulmonary valves are less frequently affected. RHD is virtually the only cause of acquired mitral valve stenosis.

Morphology (p. 558; Fig. 12-7)

- *Acute phase:*
  - *Aschoff bodies* are pathognomonic for RF; these are myocardial, pericardial, or endocardial foci of fibrinoid necrosis surrounded by mononuclear inflammatory cells. Activated macrophages in these lesions (so-called *Anitschkow cells*) have characteristic wavy chromatin aggregation, so-called "caterpillar cells."
  - Inflammatory valvulitis is characterized by beady fibrinous vegetations *(verrucae)* along the lines of valve closure.
  - Inflammatory foci are eventually replaced by scar.
- *Chronic (or healed) phase:*
  - Diffuse fibrous thickening of valve leaflets, with fibrous commissural fusion generating "fishmouth" or "buttonhole" stenoses.
  - Thickened, fused, and shortened chordae.
  - Subendocardial fibrosis, often in the left atrium (perhaps due to regurgitant valvular jets) constitute *MacCallum plaques.*

Clinical Features (p. 559)

Diagnosis of RF is based on clinical history and a constellation of findings (so-called *Jones criteria*) that include *erythema marginatum* (a skin rash), *Sydenham chorea* (a neurologic disorder with rapid, involuntary, purposeless movements), *carditis* (involving myocardium, endocardium, or pericardium), *subcutaneous nodules,* and/or *migratory large joint polyarthritis.* Death (most frequently secondary to *myocarditis*) occurs rarely in acute RF. Typically myocarditis and arthritis are transient and resolve without complications; however, valvular involvement can deform and scar the valve causing permanent dysfunction (RHD) and subsequent CHF. RHD is most likely when the first attack is in early childhood, is particularly severe, or if there are recurrent attacks. Changes secondary to mitral stenosis are as follows:

- Left atrial hypertrophy and enlargement, occasionally with mural thrombi
- Atrial fibrillation secondary to atrial dilation
- CHF with chronic pulmonary congestive changes
- Increased risk of IE

Infective Endocarditis (p. 559)

IE reflects microbial infection of valves, leading to friable vegetations composed of thrombotic debris and organisms, often with

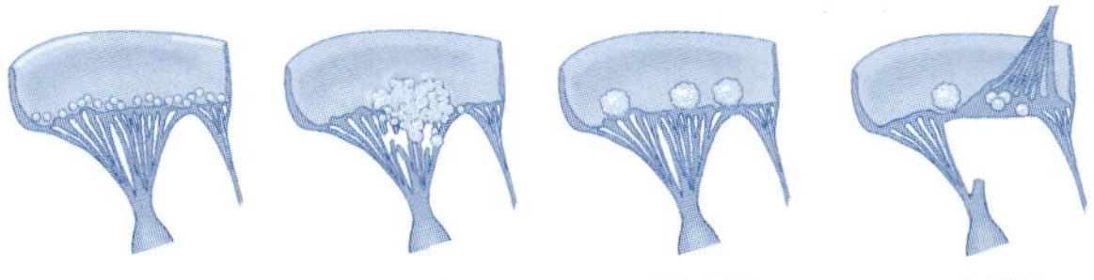

Figure 12-7 Comparison of the four major forms of vegetative endocarditis. The RF phase of RHD is marked by small, warty vegetations along the lines of closure of the valve leaflets. IE is characterized by large, irregular masses on the valve cusps that can extend onto the chordae. NBTE typically exhibits one or multiple small, bland vegetations, usually attached at the line of closure. Libman-Sacks endocarditis (LSE) has small or medium-sized vegetations on either or both sides of the valve leaflets.

valve damage. Traditionally these are classified as *acute* or *subacute* forms:

- *Acute IE* is caused by highly virulent organisms (e.g., *Staphylococcus aureus*), typically seeding a previously normal valve to produce necrotizing, ulcerative, and invasive infections. Clinically there is rapidly developing fever with rigors, malaise, and weakness. Larger vegetations can cause embolic complications.
- *Subacute IE* is typically caused by moderate-to-low virulence organisms (e.g., *Streptococcus viridans*) seeding an abnormal or previously injured valve; there is less valvular destruction than acute IE. This pattern occurs insidiously with nonspecific malaise, low-grade fever, weight loss, and a flulike syndrome. Vegetations tend to be small, such that embolic complications occur less frequently. The disease tends to have a protracted course even without treatment and has a lower mortality rate than acute IE.

Pathogenesis *(p. 559)*

IE is caused by bloodborne organisms, usually bacteria, which derive from infections elsewhere in the body, intravenous drug abuse, dental or surgical procedures, or otherwise trivial injury to gut, urinary tract, oropharynx, or skin. Contributory conditions include neutropenia and immunosuppression.

- Although endocarditis can occur on normal valves, infection is more likely to occur in the setting of previous valve pathology (e.g., CHD [particularly tight shunts or stenoses with jet streams], RHD, MVP, degenerative calcific stenoses, BAVs, or prosthetic valves).
- IE in intravenous drug abusers is most commonly caused by *S. aureus* infecting a normal valve; right-sided valves are involved more commonly than left.
- In addition to *S. viridans* (50% to 60% of cases), low-virulence organisms include enterococci and the so-called HASEK group of oral commensals (*Haemophilus, Actinobacillus, Cardiobacterium, Eikenella,* and *Kingella*).
- IE on prosthetic valves is caused most commonly by *Staphylococcus epidermidis;* sewing ring abscesses are a common feature.
- In 10% of IE, no organisms are identified ("culture-negative").

Morphology *(p. 560; Fig. 12-7)*

- Acute IE is typically characterized by bulky vegetations associated with underlying valve destruction; invasion into adjacent myocardium or aorta can cause abscesses. Distal embolization with septic infarcts or mycotic aneurysms can occur.
- Subacute IE has smaller vegetations with less valvular destruction.

Clinical Features *(p. 560)*

- Valvular and myocardial damage as described previously.
- Embolic complications as described previously.
- Renal injury, including embolic infarction or infection and antigen-antibody complex-mediated glomerulonephritis (with nephrotic syndrome, renal failure, or both).
- Diagnosis is confirmed by the Duke criteria (Table 12-5); blood cultures are critically important for directing therapy.

Noninfected Vegetations (p. 561)

Nonbacterial Thrombotic Endocarditis *(p. 561; Fig. 12-7)*

Nonbacterial thrombotic endocarditis (NBTE), also called *marantic endocarditis,* characteristically occurs in settings of cancer (particularly

TABLE 12-5 Diagnostic Criteria for Infective Endocarditis*

Pathologic Criteria

Microorganisms, demonstrated by culture or histologic examination, in a vegetation, embolus from a vegetation, or intracardiac abscess

Histologic confirmation of active endocarditis in vegetation or intracardiac abscess

Clinical Criteria

Major

Blood culture(s) positive for a characteristic organism or persistently positive for an unusual organism

Echocardiographic identification of a valve-related or implant-related mass or abscess, or partial separation of artificial valve

New valvular regurgitation

Minor

Predisposing heart lesion or intravenous drug use

Fever

Vascular lesions, including arterial petechiae, subungual or splinter hemorrhages, emboli, septic infarcts, mycotic aneurysm, intracranial hemorrhage, Janeway lesions†

Immunologic phenomena, including glomerulonephritis, Osler nodes,‡ Roth spots,§ rheumatoid factor

Microbiologic evidence, including a single culture positive for an unusual organism

Echocardiographic findings consistent with but not diagnostic of endocarditis, including worsening or changing of a preexistent murmur

*Diagnosis by these guidelines, often called the Duke Criteria, requires either pathologic or clinical criteria; if clinical criteria are used, 2 major, 1 major + 3 minor, or 5 minor criteria are required for diagnosis.

†Janeway lesions are small erythematous or hemorrhagic, macular, nontender lesions on the palms and soles and are the consequence of septic embolic events.

‡Osler nodes are small, tender subcutaneous nodules that develop in the pulp of the digits or occasionally more proximally in the fingers and persist for hours to several days.

§Roth spots are oval retinal hemorrhages with pale centers.

Modified from Durack DT, Lukes AS, Bright DK: New criteria for diagnosis of infective endocarditis: utilization of specific echocardiographic findings. *Am J Med* 96:200, 1994 and Karchmer AW: Infective endocarditis. In Braunwald E, Zipes DP, Libby P (eds): *Heart Disease. A Textbook of Cardiovascular Medicine,* 6th ed. Philadelphia, PA: Saunders, 2001, p 1723.

adenocarcinomas) or prolonged debilitating illness (e.g., renal failure, chronic sepsis) with disseminated intravascular coagulation or other hypercoagulable states.

- Small (1 to 5 mm), sterile, bland fibrin and platelet thrombi are loosely adherent to valve leaflets along closure lines, without significant inflammation or valve damage.
- Vegetations can embolize systemically.

Endocarditis of Systemic Lupus Erythematosus (Libman-Sacks Disease) (p. 562; Fig. 12-7)

Endocarditis of systemic lupus erythematosus (Libman-Sacks disease) occurs in systemic lupus erythematosus and in antiphospholipid syndrome, presumably due to immune complex deposition. Findings include small, fibrinous, sterile vegetations on *either* side of valve leaflets, with associated fibrinoid necrosis and inflammation. Valve scarring and deformation can result that resembles RHD and may require surgery.

Carcinoid Heart Disease (p. 562)

Carcinoid tumors (see Chapter 17) elaborate bioactive products (e.g., serotonin, kallikrein, bradykinins, histamine, prostaglandins, and tachykinins P and K). *Carcinoid syndrome* is a systemic disorder marked by flushing, diarrhea, dermatitis, and bronchoconstriction caused by the released mediators; *carcinoid heart disease* refers to the cardiac manifestations that occur in approximately half of carcinoid syndrome patients. The precise agent responsible is uncertain, although it is presumably rapidly metabolized in lung and liver because cardiac lesions do not occur unless there is extensive hepatic metastatic spread, and even then, right-sided heart lesions (valvular and endocardial) predominate.

Morphology (p. 562)

- Lesions are characterized by plaquelike intimal thickening (composed of smooth muscle cells and associated extracellular matrix) of the tricuspid and pulmonary valves and right ventricular outflow tract; left-sided lesions are uncommon except in primary pulmonary carcinoids.
- Tricuspid insufficiency and pulmonic stenosis are the typical valvular consequences.
- Similar lesions occur with drugs that have serotonergic effects (e.g., methylsergide, ergotamine, some antiparkinsonian medications, and fenfluramine [part of the fen-phen appetite suppressant combination with phentermine]).

Complications of Prosthetic Valves (p. 563)

Prosthetic valves are either mechanical (rigid, synthetic) or bioprosthetic (cryopreserved human valves or chemically fixed animal tissues). Approximately 60% of valve recipients will develop a significant valve-related complication within 10 years of surgical implantation:

- *Thromboembolic complications,* either local obstruction by thrombus or distal embolization are the major complications of mechanical valves; this complication necessitates long-term anticoagulation in such valve recipients, with the attendant risks of hemorrhagic stroke or other bleeding complication.
- *IE;* infection at the valve sewing ring often leads to ring abscesses and paravalvular regurgitation.
- *Structural deterioration* is uncommon with mechanical valves, but valvular calcification or degenerative tears often cause bioprosthetic valve failure.
- *Occlusion* due to tissue overgrowth, intravascular *hemolysis* due to high shear forces, or *paravalvular leak* due to poor healing.

Cardiomyopathies (p. 564)

Although myocardial dysfunction can occur secondary to ischemic, valvular, hypertensive, or other heart diseases, the term *cardiomyopathy* implies *principal* cardiac dysfunction. Causes of such myocardial disease can be *primary* (predominantly affecting heart) or *secondary* (part of a larger systemic disorder); they can be genetic or acquired, and increasingly a genetic basis is identified for cardiomyopathies previously classified as idiopathic:

- Infections (e.g., viral, bacterial, fungal, protozoal)
- Toxic exposures (e.g., alcohol, cobalt, chemotherapeutic agents)
- Metabolic disorders (e.g., hyperthyroidism, nutritional deficiency)
- Genetic abnormalities in cardiomyocytes (e.g., storage disorders, muscular dystrophies)

- Infiltrative lesions (e.g., sarcoid, carcinoma, radiation-induced fibrosis)
- Immunologic (e.g., autoimmune myocarditis, rejection)

Cardiomyopathy is divided into three main functional and pathophysiologic patterns: *dilated, hypertrophic,* and *restrictive* (Fig. 12-8 and Table 12-6). DCM is most common (90% of cases), and restrictive cardiomyopathy is least frequent; each pattern has a spectrum of severity, and clinical features can overlap.

Dilated Cardiomyopathy (p. 565)

DCM is characterized by gradual four-chamber hypertrophy and dilation; there is systolic dysfunction with hypocontraction. It typically presents as indolent, progressive CHF, with an end-stage annual mortality of 10% to 50%. Although the cause is frequently unknown *(idiopathic DCM)*, certain pathologic mechanisms can contribute (Fig. 12-9):

- *Genetic influences:* 20% to 50% of DCM is familial; autosomal dominant inheritance is most common. Known genetic abnormalities commonly involve cytoskeletal proteins (e.g., dystrophin in X-linked cardiomyopathy [Duchenne and Becker muscular dystrophies]). Others involve mutations of enzymes involved in

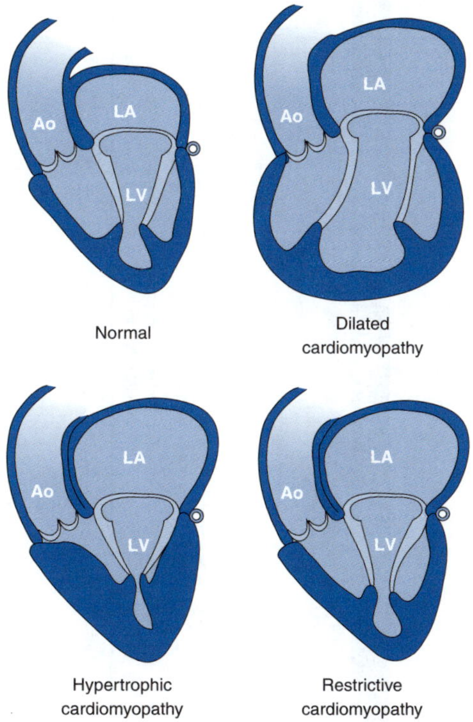

Figure 12-8 The three major morphologic patterns of cardiomyopathy. DCM leads primarily to systolic dysfunction, whereas restrictive and hypertrophic cardiomyopathies result in diastolic dysfunction. Note the changes in atrial and/or ventricular luminal dimensions and/or wall thickness. *Ao,* Aorta; *LA,* left atrium; *LV,* left ventricle.

TABLE 12-6 Cardiomyopathy and Indirect Myocardial Dysfunction: Functional Patterns and Causes

Functional Pattern	Left Ventricular Ejection Fraction*	Mechanisms of Heart Failure	Causes	Indirect Myocardial Dysfunction (Not Cardiomyopathy)
Dilated	<40%	Impairment of contractility (systolic dysfunction)	Idiopathic; alcohol; peripartum; genetic; myocarditis; hemochromatosis; chronic anemia; doxorubicin (Adriamycin); sarcoidosis	IHD; valvular heart disease; hypertensive heart disease; CHD
Hypertrophic	50%-80%	Impairment of compliance (diastolic dysfunction)	Genetic; Friedreich ataxia; storage diseases; infants of diabetic mothers	Hypertensive heart disease; aortic stenosis
Restrictive	45%-90%	Impairment of compliance (diastolic dysfunction)	Idiopathic; amyloidosis; radiation-induced fibrosis	Pericardial constriction

*Normal, approximately 50%-65%.

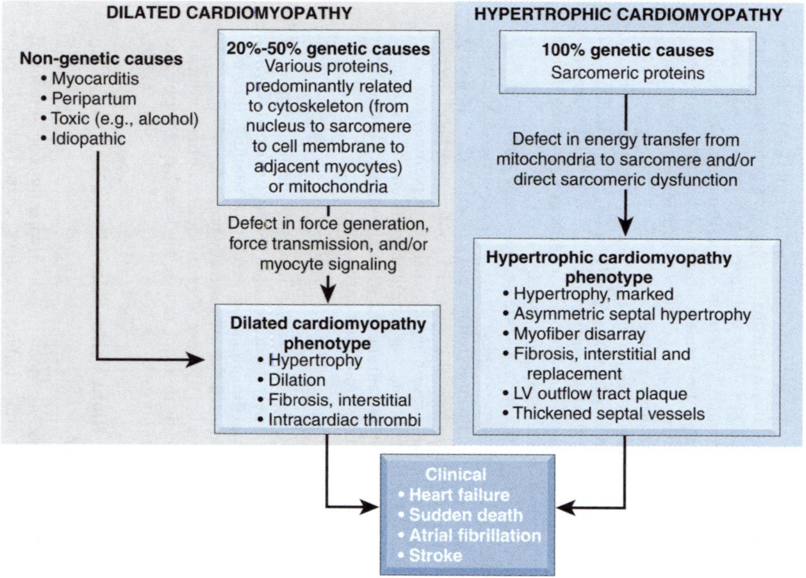

Figure 12-9 Causes and consequences of DCM and HCM. Some DCMs and virtually all HCMs are genetic in origin. The genetic causes of DCM involve mutations in any of a wide range of genes. They encode proteins predominantly of the cytoskeleton but also the sarcomere, mitochondria, and nuclear envelope. In contrast, all of the mutated genes that cause HCM encode proteins of the sarcomere. Although these two forms of cardiomyopathy differ greatly in subcellular basis and morphologic phenotypes, they share a common set of clinical complications. *LV,* Left ventricle.

fatty acid β-oxidation or mitochondrial gene deletions, causing abnormal oxidative phosphorylation.
- *Myocarditis* (see later discussion): Even after resolution of the infection, injury related to myocarditis can progress to DCM.
- *Alcohol and other toxins:* DCM can be caused by direct alcohol toxicity or to a metabolite (especially acetaldehyde). No morphologic features distinguish alcohol-induced cardiac damage from an alcohol-associated nutritional deficiency (e.g., inadequate thiamine) or from idiopathic DCM. Doxorubicin and tyrosine kinase inhibitors used for chemotherapy can also cause DCM, as can cobalt and—idiosyncratically—drugs such as lithium, phenothiazines, and chloroquine.
- *Peripartum cardiomyopathy* is a DCM presenting within the months before or after delivery. Although the mechanism is uncertain, the association with pregnancy suggests a potential role for chronic hypertension, volume overload, nutritional deficiencies, metabolic derangement, or immunologic response. Peripartum cardiomyopathy may also result from a microvascular angiogenic imbalance caused by placental-derived antiangiogenic proteins and leading to functional ischemia.
- *Iron overload* can cause DCM; the excess iron can occur secondary to hereditary hemochromatosis (see Chapter 18) or from multiple transfusions; the myocardial injury is attributed to interference with metal-dependent enzyme systems or to iron-mediated production of reactive oxygen species.
- *Supraphysiologic* stress (e.g., due to persistent tachycardia or hyperthyroidism) can progress to DCM. Excess catecholamines (e.g., due to pheochromocytomas) can cause DCM by inducing vasospasm with multifocal myocardial contraction band necrosis; cocaine or vasopressor agents, such as dopamine, can have similar consequences. Such a "catecholamine effect" also occurs in the setting of intense autonomic stimulation (e.g., secondary to intracranial lesions or emotional duress).

Morphology *(p. 567)*

- *Grossly* the heart is flabby with cardiomegaly (up to 900 g); wall thickness may not reflect the degree of hypertrophy due to dilation.
- Poor contractile function and stasis predispose to mural thrombi.
- Valves and coronary arteries are generally normal.
- *Microscopic changes* in DCM are often subtle and entirely nonspecific; most commonly there are diffuse myocyte hypertrophy and variable interstitial fibrosis.

Arrhythmogenic Right Ventricular Cardiomyopathy (p. 568)

Arrhythmogenic right ventricular cardiomyopathy is an autosomal dominant disorder (with variable penetrance) characterized by predominantly right-sided failure and arrhythmia. The defect is most commonly caused by defective adhesive molecules in desmosomes. Morphologically the right ventricular wall is severely thinned with myocyte loss and profound fatty infiltration. Death occurs secondary to progressive CHF or fatal arrhythmias.

Hypertrophic Cardiomyopathy (p. 568)

HCM is a common (1 in 500 individuals in the general population), clinically heterogeneous, genetic heart disease characterized by heavy, muscular, *hypercontractile*, poorly compliant hearts with poor diastolic relaxation; in a third of cases there is also ventricular outflow obstruction.

Pathogenesis *(p. 569)*

- HCM is caused by mutations of sarcomeric proteins (β-myosin heavy chain mutations being most common); most are autosomal dominant mutations with variable penetrance.
- Prognosis varies widely depending on the specific mutations.
- The pathogenic sequence leading from specific mutations to disease manifestations is not understood (Fig. 12-9). Different mutations in the same gene can even give rise to DCM or HCM.

Morphology *(p. 569)*

- Classically there is disproportionate thickening of the interventricular septum (asymmetric septal hypertrophy), although 10% have concentric hypertrophy.
- The left ventricular cavity is compressed into a *banana-like configuration* by the asymmetric bulging of the septum.
- Septal thickening at the level of the mitral valve compromises left ventricular systolic outflow by contact of the anterior mitral leaflet with the septum *(systolic anterior motion)*; this causes *hypertrophic obstructive cardiomyopathy,* reflected by a fibrous plaque on the septum.
- *Microscopically* there is marked myofiber hypertrophy, classically with helter-skelter *myocyte disarray,* accompanied by myofilament disorganization within muscle cells, most prominent in the interventricular septum. There is also patchy interstitial and replacement fibrosis.

Clinical Features *(p. 570)*

The major feature is reduced stroke volume due to a combination of impaired diastolic filling and left ventricular outflow tract obstruction.

- Due to increased ventricular pressures, massive myocyte hypertrophy, diminished stroke volume, and frequently abnormal intramyocardial arterioles, focal myocardial ischemia is common.
- HCM can be entirely asymptomatic. Symptomatic disease presents usually in young adults with dyspnea, angina, and/or near-syncope.
- The clinical course can be highly variable; major complications include atrial fibrillation with mural thrombus and embolization, IE, CHF, and SCD. Indeed HCM is one of the most common causes of sudden unexplained death in young athletes.

Restrictive Cardiomyopathy (p. 570)

Relatively rare and with multiple etiologies, this entity is marked by a restriction of ventricular filling leading to reduced cardiac output. Contractile function is usually normal. Ventricle size is normal, although there is typically biatrial dilation. Nonspecific interstitial myocardial fibrosis is usually present, but biopsy can frequently reveal a specific etiology. Causes include the following:

- *Endomyocardial fibrosis* is a disease mainly of African children and young adults; the cause is unknown. It is characterized by dense ventricular subendocardial fibrosis extending from the apex upward, often with superimposed organizing mural thrombus. Restrictive physiology results with reduced ventricular chamber volume and the endocardial fibrosis.
- *Loeffler endomyocarditis* is morphologically similar to endomyocardial fibrosis but is classically associated with peripheral eosinophilia and eosinophilic infiltration of multiple organs (especially the heart). The cardiac changes are probably due to toxic products of eosinophils, and the course can be rapidly fatal. A subset

of these patients have a myeloproliferative disorder with eosinophilia, associated chromosomal rearrangements of PDGF receptor genes; kinase inhibitors are effective in inducing hematologic remission.

- *Endocardial fibroelastosis* is an uncommon disorder of obscure etiology (and possibly the end point of different injuries), characterized by focal to diffuse, *fibroelastic* thickening of the endocardium, left ventricle greater than right. It occurs at all ages but is most common in patients ≤2 years. CHD are present in a third of cases.

Myocarditis (p. 570)

Infectious etiologies or primary autoimmune responses underlie myocarditis.

- The clinical spectrum is broad, from entirely asymptomatic to abrupt onset of arrhythmia, CHF, or SCD; most patients recover quickly and without sequelae, although DCM can occur (see earlier discussion).
- Most U.S. cases are viral in origin (e.g., coxsackievirus A and B, echovirus). Cardiac involvement occurs days to weeks after a primary viral infection; cardiac involvement can be due to a direct infection or secondary to immunologic cross-reactivity between pathogen and myocardium.
- *Trypanosoma cruzi* (causal organism in *Chagas disease*) causes myocarditis in the majority of infected individuals, with 10% dying acutely and others progressing to cardiac failure over 10 to 20 years.
- Toxin released by *Corynebacterium diptheriae* is responsible for the myocardial injury in diptheria.
- Myocarditis occurs in 5% of patients with Lyme disease *(Borrelia burgdorferi)*. Lyme myocarditis is usually mild and reversible but occasionally requires a temporary pacemaker for AV block.
- Myocarditis in acquired immunodeficiency syndrome (AIDS) patients is due either to inflammation and damage without a clear etiologic agent or directly to human immunodeficiency virus (HIV) or some other opportunistic pathogen.
- Noninfectious myocarditis may be immune mediated (e.g., associated with RF, systemic lupus erythematosus, or drug allergies).
- In some cases the cause is unknown (e.g., sarcoidosis, giant cell myocarditis) or the microbe is unidentifiable.

Morphology (p. 571)

Gross manifestations include a flabby heart often with four-chamber dilation and patchy hemorrhagic mottling.

- Mural thrombi can form in dilated chambers.
- Endocardium and valves are typically unaffected.
- Long-term remodeling can lead to dilation or hypertrophy.

Microscopically there is a myocardial inflammatory infiltrate with associated myocyte necrosis or degeneration. Lesions are often focal (and may be missed by routine endomyocardial biopsy). Inflammatory lesions typically resolve over days to weeks, leaving either no residua or variable interstitial and replacement fibrosis.

- In *Chagas disease,* trypanosomes parasitize myocytes and produce acute and chronic inflammation, including eosinophils.
- *Hypersensitivity myocarditis* is characterized by perivascular mononuclear and eosinophilic infiltrates; this variant is often induced by therapeutic drugs.

- In *giant cell myocarditis,* there is focal to occasionally extensive myocyte necrosis associated with multinucleated giant cells. This variant of myocarditis has a poor prognosis.

Other Causes of Myocardial Disease (p. 571)

Amyloidosis occurs as patchy nodular and perivascular/interstitial hyaline protein deposits; the amyloid nature of the protein is confirmed by Congo red staining, yielding a characteristic apple-green birefringence under polarized light. Cardiac amyloid can be secondary to systemic amyloidosis (see Chapter 6) or may be isolated (e.g., *senile cardiac amyloidosis* due to transthyretin deposition [transthyretin is a normal serum protein involved in *trans*porting *thy*roxine and *retin*ol]). Mutant forms of transthyretin (more common in African-Americans) can accelerate cardiac and systemic amyloidosis. Isolated atrial amyloid (of uncertain clinical significance) is due to atrial natriuretic peptide deposition. Amyloid accumulation typically causes a restrictive physiology, although DCM, arrhythmias, or CHF symptoms mimicking IHD can occur.

Pericardial Disease (p. 573)

Pericardial disease is typically secondary to diseases of adjacent structures or part of a systemic disorder; isolated disease is unusual.

Pericardial Effusion and Hemopericardium (p. 573)

The normal pericardial sac contains 30 to 50 mL of serous, *noninflammatory* fluid. Slow fluid accumulation (e.g., serous effusions) can be well tolerated, resulting in chronic collections greater than 500 mL; rapidly accumulating fluids (e.g., due to hemorrhage) can cause fatal *tamponade* with as little as 200 mL.

Pericarditis (p. 573)

Pericarditis is usually secondary to disorders involving the heart or mediastinal structures (e.g., after MI, surgery, trauma, radiation, tumors, infections); it can also be due to systemic abnormalities (e.g., uremia, autoimmune diseases). Acute primary pericarditis is chiefly viral in origin. Chronic pericarditis also occurs secondary to tuberculosis and fungal infections.

Acute Pericarditis *(p. 573)*

- *Serous pericarditis:* Although the etiology is frequently unknown, it is characteristically nonbacterial (e.g., RF, systemic lupus erythematosus, tumors, uremia, and primary viral infections). Microscopically there is scant pericardial acute and chronic inflammatory infiltration (mostly lymphocytes).
- *Fibrinous and serofibrinous pericarditis:* These are the most common forms of pericarditis, occurring as serous fluid mixed with a fibrinous exudate; patients classically present with a loud friction rub, pain, and fever. Causes include acute MI, postinfarction *(Dressler)* syndrome, cardiac surgery, uremia, irradiation, RF, SLE, and trauma. Exudates can be completely resolved or can organize, leaving fibrous adhesions.
- *Purulent (suppurative) pericarditis* usually signifies bacterial, fungal, or parasitic infection reaching the pericardium by direct extension, by hematogenous or lymphatic spread, or during cardiotomy. Purulent pericarditis is typically composed of 400 to 500 mL of a thin-to-creamy pus with marked inflammation and erythematous,

granular serosal surfaces. It presents with high fevers, rigors, and a friction rub and can organize to produce *mediastinopericarditis* or *constrictive pericarditis* (see following discussion).

- *Hemorrhagic pericarditis* denotes an exudate of blood admixed with fibrinous-to-suppurative effusion. Most commonly it follows cardiac surgery or is associated with tuberculosis or malignancy.
- *Caseous pericarditis* is due to tuberculosis (typically by direct extension from neighboring lymph nodes) or less commonly mycotic infection. This pattern is the most frequent antecedent to fibrocalcific constrictive pericarditis.

Chronic or Healed Pericarditis (p. 575)

Healing of acute lesions can lead to resolution or to pericardial fibrosis ranging from a thick, pearly, nonadherent, epicardial plaque ("soldier's plaque") to thin, delicate adhesions to massive fibrosis.

- *Adhesive mediastinopericarditis* obliterates the pericardial sac, and the parietal layer is tethered to mediastinal tissue. The heart thus contracts against all the surrounding attached structures, with subsequent hypertrophy and dilation.
- *Constrictive pericarditis* is marked by thick (up to 1 cm), dense, fibrous obliteration, often with calcification of the pericardial sac encasing the heart, limiting diastolic expansion and restricting cardiac output.

Heart Disease Associated With Rheumatologic Disorders (p. 575)

Rheumatoid arthritis involves the heart in 20% to 40% of severe chronic cases. Most common is fibrinous pericarditis; this can organize to form dense, fibrous, and potentially restrictive adhesions. Less frequently, granulomatous rheumatoid nodules involve the myocardium, endocardium, aortic root, or valves, where they are particularly damaging. Rheumatoid valvulitis can produce changes similar to those seen in RHD.

Tumors of the Heart (p. 575)

Cardiac metastases occur *much* more frequently than primary heart tumors; metastases can involve the pericardium (with or without effusions) or penetrate into the myocardium.

Primary Cardiac Tumors (p. 575)

- *Myxomas are the most common primary cardiac tumor in adults.* Usually isolated, 90% arise in the left atria in the region of the fossa ovale. Approximately 10% of patients with myxomas have an autosomal dominant *Carney syndrome,* with cardiac and extracardiac myxomas, pigmented skin lesions, and endocrine hyperactivity.
  - *Grossly,* myxomas range from 1 cm to >10 cm and are sessile-to-pedunculated masses varying from globular and hard to papillary and myxoid. They may cause symptoms by physical obstruction, trauma to the AV valves, or peripheral embolization.
  - *Microscopically* they are composed of stellate multipotential mesenchymal myxoma cells, embedded in an acid mucopolysaccharide matrix, with vessellike and glandlike structures.

- *Lipomas* are well-circumscribed benign accumulations of adipose tissue, more commonly in the left ventricle, right atrium, or septum. Symptoms depend on location and on encroachment on valve function or conduction pathways.
- *Papillary fibroelastomas* are sea-anemone-like lesions with centimeter-long filaments radiating out from a central core; they are characteristically found on valves and can cause emboli but are usually incidental findings at autopsy. Microscopically the filaments have a core of myxoid connective tissue with concentric elastic fibers, all covered by endothelium.
- *Rhabdomyomas* are the most common primary heart tumor in children; they can cause valvular or outflow tract obstruction. Approximately half of cases are associated with tuberous sclerosis (the remainder are spontaneous mutations), caused by defects in the *TSC1* and *TSC2* tumor suppressor genes. Microscopically, they are composed of large, rounded-to-polygonal cells rich in glycogen and containing myofibrils. Fixation and histologic processing leave characteristic artifactual cytoplasmic stranding radiating from the central nucleus to plasma membrane, forming so-called *spider cells.*
- *Angiosarcomas* and *rhabdomyosarcomas* are malignant neoplasms resembling their counterparts in other locations.

Cardiac Effects of Noncardiac Neoplasms (p. 576)

The heart can also be *indirectly* affected by tumors at other sites:

- Metastases or direct extension; 5% of patients dying from malignancy have heart involvement.
- Hypercoagulable states leading to NBTE.
- Carcinoid heart disease.
- Myeloma-associated amyloidosis.
- Pheochromocytoma-associated (catecholamine) heart disease.
- Effects of tumor therapy (e.g., radiation or cardiotoxic agents).

Cardiac Transplantation (p. 577)

Cardiac transplantation (approximately 3000 cases annually worldwide) is performed most commonly for DCM and IHD. The 1-year survival is 90%, with 5-year survival rates ≥60%. Cellular allograft rejection is characterized by interstitial lymphocytic inflammation with associated myocyte damage resembling myocarditis; severe rejection is accompanied by interstitial edema, and vascular injury leading to myocyte necrosis. Antibody-mediated rejection results from the production of donor-specific antibodies directed against major histocompatibility complex proteins that lead to complement activation and the recruitment of Fc-receptor-bearing cells. The major current long-term limitation to cardiac transplantation is progressive, diffuse, intimal proliferation of the coronary arteries *(graft arteriosclerosis)* causing downstream myocardial ischemia; 50% of patients will have significant disease by 5 years after transplantation. Other complications in immunosuppressed transplant recipients include opportunistic infections and malignancies, particularly B-cell lymphomas (due to Epstein-Barr virus).

13 Diseases of White Blood Cells, Lymph Nodes, Spleen, and Thymus

Development and Maintenance of Hematopoietic Tissues (p. 579)

- The hematopoietic system is traditionally (but somewhat artificially) divided into the *myeloid tissues,* which include the bone marrow and the cells derived from it: red cells, platelets, granulocytes, and monocytes; and the *lymphoid tissues,* consisting of the thymus, lymph nodes, and spleen.
- The formed blood elements have a common origin from hematopoietic stem cells (HSCs); the characteristic features of HSCs are their *pluripotency* (ability for one cell to produce all lineages) and *capacity for self-renewal.*
- HSCs give rise to several kinds of early progenitor cells with a restricted differentiation potential—ultimately producing mainly either myeloid cells or lymphoid cells. These early progenitors in turn give "birth" to progenitors that are further constrained to differentiation along particular lineages. Some of these cells are referred to as *colony-forming units* (CFUs) (Fig. 13-1).
- The self-renewing divisions of HSCs occur in specialized marrow niches where stromal cells and secreted factors maintain the appropriate milieu. Under stress conditions, other tissues (e.g., liver and spleen) can provide the requisite niche environment, leading to *extramedullary hematopoiesis.*
- Marrow responses to physiologic needs are regulated by lineage-specific hematopoietic growth factors acting on committed progenitor cells. Some growth factors (e.g., stem cell factor) may act on very early committed multipotent progenitors, whereas others (e.g., erythropoietin, granulocyte-macrophage colony–stimulating factor [GM-CSF]) act on committed progenitors with more restricted potential. Feedback loops mediated through growth factor production maintain the numbers of formed blood elements within appropriate ranges (Table 13-1).
- Tumors of hematopoietic origin are typically associated with mutations that either block progenitor cell maturation or abrogate their dependence on growth factors.

Disorders of White Cells (p. 582)

White blood cell disorders are broadly classified as either deficiency *(leukopenia),* or proliferation *(leukocytosis);* the latter can be reactive or neoplastic.

Leukopenia (p. 582)

Leukopenia can reflect decreased numbers of any of the specific leukocyte types; this most commonly involves neutrophils

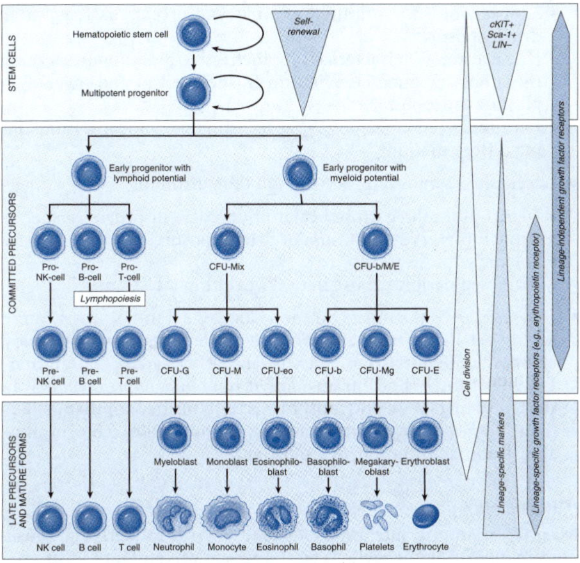

Figure 13-1 Differentiation of blood cells. *LIN*–, Negative for lineage-specific markers.

TABLE 13-1 Adult Reference Ranges for Blood Cells*

Cell Type	
White cells (×10³/µL)	4.8-10.8
Granulocytes (%)	40-70
Neutrophils (×10³/µL)	1.4-6.5
Lymphocytes (×10³/µL)	1.2-3.4
Monocytes (×10³/µL)	0.1-0.6
Eosinophils (×10³/µL)	0-0.5
Basophils (×10³/µL)	0-0.2
Red cells (×10⁶/µL)	4.3-5.0, men; 3.5-5.0, women
Platelets (×10³/µL)	150-450

*Reference ranges vary among laboratories. The reference ranges for the laboratory providing the result should always be used.

(*neutropenia,* granulocytopenia). *Lymphopenia* is less common; in addition to congenital immunodeficiency diseases, it can occur with human immunodeficiency virus (HIV) or other viral infections, glucocorticoid or cytotoxic drug therapy, autoimmune disorders, or malnutrition.

Neutropenia and Agranulocytosis (p. 582)

Pathogenesis (p. 582)

- Inadequate or ineffective granulopoiesis
  - HSC suppression, as in aplastic anemia (see Chapter 14)
  - Infiltrative marrow disorders (tumors, granulomatous disease)

- Suppression of committed granulocytic precursors (e.g., after drug exposure)
- Disease states characterized by ineffective granulopoiesis (e.g., megaloblastic anemias [vitamin B_{12} deficiency] and myelodysplastic syndromes [MDSs])
- Rare inherited conditions (e.g., Kostmann syndrome) impairing differentiation

- Accelerated removal or destruction of neutrophils
  - Neutrophil injury caused by immunologic disorders (e.g., systemic lupus erythematosus) or drug exposures
  - Splenic sequestration
  - Increased peripheral use in overwhelming infections

- *Drug toxicity* is the most common cause of agranulocytosis. Some agents act in a predictable dose-dependent fashion (i.e., many chemotherapeutic drugs, such as alkylating agents and antimetabolites). Others act in an *idiosyncratic and unpredictable* way related to metabolic polymorphisms or to the development of autoantibodies (e.g., chloramphenicol, sulfonamides, chlorpromazine, thiouracil, and phenylbutazone).

Morphology *(p. 583)*

Marrow anatomic alterations depend on the underlying cause. *Hypocellularity* occurs with agents that suppress granulocyte progenitor cell growth and survival; these may be granulocyte-specific or can potentially affect erythroid and megakaryocytic progenitors, leading to pancytopenia and aplastic anemia (empty marrow). *Hypercellularity* occurs in conditions with ineffective granulopoiesis (MDSs) or when there is increased peripheral destruction of neutrophils.

Clinical Features *(p. 583)*

Symptoms and signs relate to intercurrent infections and include malaise, chills, and fever, often with marked weakness and fatigability. Serious infections are most likely when the neutrophil count is $\leq$500 cells/mm^3. Ulcerating necrotizing lesions of the gingiva, buccal mucosa, or pharynx are characteristic. Severe, life-threatening, invasive bacterial or fungal infections can occur in the lungs, kidney, or urinary tract; neutropenic patients are at high risk for deep *Candida* or *Aspergillus* infections.

Infections are often fulminant; neutropenic patients are therefore treated with broad-spectrum antibiotics at the first sign of infection. Granulocyte colony–stimulating factor therapy decreases the duration and severity of the neutrophil nadir caused by chemotherapeutic drugs.

Reactive Proliferations of White Cells and Lymph Nodes (p. 583)

Leukocytosis (p. 583)

Leukocytosis occurs commonly in a variety of inflammatory states (Table 13-2). The peripheral leukocyte count is a function of the following: (1) the size of precursor pools in the marrow, circulation, and peripheral tissues; (2) rate of precursor release; (3) the proportion of cells adherent to the cell wall; and (4) the rate of extravasation into tissues. Infection is the major driving force for leukocytosis; inflammatory cytokines not only increase marrow egress but also increase proliferation and differentiation of committed precursors.

TABLE 13-2 Causes of Leukocytosis

Type of Leukocytosis	Causes
Neutrophilic leukocytosis	Acute bacterial infections, especially those caused by pyogenic organisms; sterile inflammation caused by, e.g., tissue necrosis (myocardial infarction, burns)
Eosinophilic leukocytosis (eosinophilia)	Allergic disorders, such as asthma, hay fever, parasitic infestations; drug reactions; certain malignancies (e.g., HL and some NHLs); autoimmune disorders (e.g., pemphigus, dermatitis herpetiformis) and some vasculitides; atheroembolic disease (transient)
Basophilic leukocytosis (basophilia)	Rare, often indicative of a myeloproliferative disease (e.g., CML)
Monocytosis	Chronic infections (e.g., tuberculosis), bacterial endocarditis, rickettsiosis, and malaria; autoimmune disorders (e.g., systemic lupus erythematosus); inflammatory bowel diseases (e.g., ulcerative colitis)
Lymphocytosis	Accompanies monocytosis in many disorders associated with chronic immunologic stimulation (e.g., tuberculosis, brucellosis); viral infections (e.g., hepatitis A, cytomegalovirus, EBV); *B. pertussis* infection

Growth factors can preferentially stimulate select lineages or more broadly induce several different leukocyte lines:

- *Polymorphonuclear leukocytosis* accompanies acute inflammation associated with infection or tissue necrosis. Sepsis or severe inflammatory disorders cause neutrophils to develop *toxic granulations* (coarse, dark cytoplasmic granules) and/or *Döhle bodies* (sky-blue, dilated endoplasmic reticulum).
- *Eosinophilic leukocytosis* (eosinophilia) can occur with allergic disorders, parasitic infestations, drug reactions, lymphomas, and some vasculitides.
- *Basophilic leukocytosis* (basophilia) is rare; it suggests an underlying myeloproliferative disease (e.g., chronic myelogenous leukemia [CML]).
- *Monocytosis* occurs with chronic infections (e.g., tuberculosis, bacterial endocarditis, and malaria), collagen vascular diseases (e.g., systemic lupus erythematosus), and inflammatory bowel diseases (e.g., ulcerative colitis).
- *Lymphocytosis* accompanies monocytosis in many disorders associated with chronic immunologic stimulation (e.g., tuberculosis, brucellosis), viral infections (e.g., hepatitis A, cytomegalovirus, Epstein-Barr virus [EBV]), and *Bordetella pertussis* infections.
- In childhood acute viral infections, atypical lymphocytes can appear in blood or bone marrow and simulate a lymphoid neoplasm. At other times, particularly with severe infections, copious immature granulocytes can appear in the blood and simulate myelogenous leukemia (so-called *leukemoid reaction*).

Lymphadenitis (p. 584)

Activation of resident immune cells in lymph nodes and spleen leads to morphologic changes in the lymphoid architecture. Following antigenic stimulation, the primary follicles enlarge and are transformed into *germinal centers,* highly dynamic structures in which B cells develop the capacity for making high-affinity antibodies; paracortical T cells may also be hyperplastic.

Acute Nonspecific Lymphadenitis *(p. 584)*

Acute nonspecific lymphadenitis can be localized or systemic.

- The *localized* form is commonly caused by direct microbiologic drainage, most frequently in the cervical area associated with dental or tonsillar infections.
- The *systemic* form is associated with bacteremia and viral infections, particularly in children.

Affected nodes are enlarged, tender, and (with extensive abscess formation) fluctuant. Histologically there are large germinal centers with numerous mitotic figures. With pyogenic organisms, a neutrophilic infiltrate occurs and the follicular centers can undergo necrosis. Overlying skin is frequently red; penetration of the infection to the skin surface produces draining sinuses. With control of the infection, lymph nodes can revert to their normal appearance, but scarring is common after suppurative reactions.

Chronic Nonspecific Lymphadenitis *(p. 585)*

Chronic nonspecific lymphadenitis is common in axillary and inguinal nodes and is characteristically nontender (due to slow enlargement).

Morphology *(p. 585)*

- *Follicular hyperplasia* is caused by inflammatory processes that activate B cells; these include rheumatoid arthritis, toxoplasmosis, and early stages of HIV infection. Follicular hyperplasia is distinguished by prominent large germinal centers (secondary follicles) surrounded by a rim of resting naïve B cells (the *mantle zone*):
  - Dark zones in the germinal centers contain proliferating blast-like B cells *(centroblasts).*
  - Light zones in the germinal center are composed of B cells with irregular or cleaved nuclear contours *(centrocytes).*
  - Interspersed are dendritic cells and *tingible-body macrophages* containing the nuclear debris of apoptotic B cells that failed to generate sufficiently high antibody affinities.
- Although follicular hyperplasia can be confused morphologically with follicular lymphomas, features favoring a reactive process include the following:
  - Preservation of the lymph node architecture
  - Marked variation in follicular shape and size
  - Frequent mitotic figures, phagocytic macrophages, and recognizable light and dark zones
- *Paracortical hyperplasia* is caused by stimuli that trigger T cell–mediated responses, such as acute viral infections (e.g., infectious mononucleosis). Paracortical hyperplasia is characterized by reactive changes within the T-cell regions of the lymph node:
  - Activated parafollicular T-cell immunoblasts (3 to 4 times larger than resting lymphocytes) proliferate and partially efface B-cell follicles.

Sinus histiocytosis (reticular hyperplasia) is nonspecific but is often observed in lymph nodes draining tissues involved by epithelial cancers. Sinus histiocytosis is characterized by prominent, distended lymphatic sinusoids caused by marked hypertrophy of lining endothelial cells and infiltration with macrophages (histiocytes).

Hemophagocytic Lymphohistiocytosis (p. 585)

Hemophagocytic lymphohistiocytosis (HLH) is a reactive condition marked by cytopenias and systemic inflammation related to macrophage (and cytotoxic CD8+ T cell) activation; it is also called *macrophage activation syndrome.* HLH can be familial or sporadic.

Pathogenesis (p. 585)

Activated macrophages in HLH phagocytose blood cell progenitors and formed elements. At the same time, macrophages and lymphocytes release mediators (interferon-γ, tumor necrosis factor [TNF-α], interleukin [IL]-6, and IL-12, as well as soluble IL-2 receptor) that suppress hematopoiesis and produce systemic inflammatory symptoms, leading to cytopenias and a shocklike picture.

Familial HLH—and some sporadic cases—are associated with mutations that affect the formation or release of cytotoxic granules from CD8+ T cells and natural killer (NK) cells. The most common trigger for HLH is infection, particularly with EBV.

Clinical Features (p. 586)

Most are febrile with hepatosplenomegaly. Hemophagocytosis can be visualized on bone marrow examination but is neither required nor sufficient for diagnosis. Anemia and thrombocytopenia are characteristic, with high plasma ferritin and soluble IL-2 receptor, consistent with severe inflammation. Elevated liver enzymes and triglyceride levels reflect an associated hepatitis, and there may be evidence of disseminated intravascular coagulation. Untreated patients can progress rapidly to multiorgan failure, shock, and death; familial HLH may survive less than 2 months. Treatment includes immunosuppression and chemotherapy. Familial and/or persistent or resistant disease may require HSC transplantation.

Neoplastic Proliferations of White Cells (p. 586)

White cell malignancies fall into three broad categories:

- *Lymphoid neoplasms,* encompassing tumors of B-cell, T-cell, or NK cell origin
- *Myeloid neoplasms,* originating from early hematopoietic progenitors
  - *Acute myeloid leukemias (AMLs):* Immature progenitor accumulation in the marrow
  - *MDSs:* Ineffective hematopoiesis
  - *Chronic myeloproliferative disorders (MPDs):* Increased production of one or more terminally differentiated myeloid elements
- *Histiocytoses,* representing proliferative lesions of macrophages ("histiocytes") and dendritic cells

Etiologic and Pathogenetic Factors in White Cell Neoplasia: Overview (p. 586)

Chromosomal translocations and other acquired mutations (p. 586). Nonrandom karyotypic abnormalities, most commonly *translocations,* are present in most white blood cell neoplasms. They can cause inappropriate expression of normal proteins or synthesis of novel fusion oncoproteins.

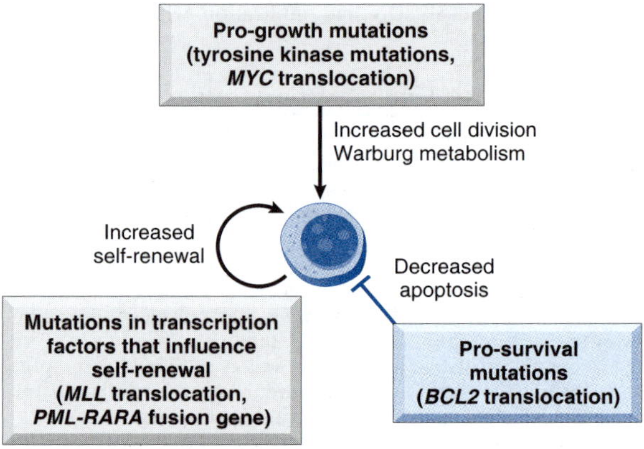

Figure 13-2 Pathogenesis of white cell malignancies. Various tumors harbor mutations that principally effect maturation or enhance self-renewal, drive growth, or prevent apoptosis. Exemplary examples of each type of mutation are listed; details are provided under specific tumor types.

- Altered genes often play crucial roles in the development, growth, or survival of the normal counterpart of the malignant cell; these may be dominant negative loss-of-function mutations or increased activity gain-of-function changes.
- Oncoproteins generated by genomic aberrations often block normal maturation, turn on progrowth signaling pathways, or protect cells against apoptosis (Fig. 13-2).
- Proto-oncogenes are often activated by errors that occur during antigen receptor rearrangement and diversification. Among lymphoid cells, oncogenic mutations occur most frequently in germinal center B cells during attempted antibody diversification. Thus after antigen stimulation, germinal center B cells upregulate activation-induced cytosine deaminase (AID), a DNA-modifying enzyme that allows immunoglobulin (Ig) class switching (e.g., IgM to IgG) and somatic hypermutation to increase antibody affinities. Remarkably the same AID enzyme can also induce *c-MYC/Ig* translocations that can put *c-MYC* oncogene expression under control of an Ig promoter and can also activate other proto-oncogenes, such as *BCL6,* a transcription factor important in many B-cell malignancies. Genomic instability can also be generated by the activities of the V(D) J recombinase responsible for antigen receptor variation.

Inherited Genetic Factors (p. 587)

Genetic diseases that promote genomic instability (e.g., Bloom syndrome, Fanconi anemia, and ataxia telangiectasia) increase the risk of leukemia. Down syndrome (trisomy 21) and neurofibromatosis type I are also associated with an increased incidence.

Viruses (p. 587)

Three viruses, human T-cell leukemia/lymphotropic virus type I (HTLV-1), EBV, and human herpesvirus (HHV-8), are implicated (see Chapter 7 for mechanisms). EBV is found in a subset of Burkitt lymphoma (BL), 30% to 40% of Hodgkin lymphoma (HL), many B-cell lymphomas occurring in the setting of T-cell immunodeficiency, and NK-cell lymphomas. HTLV-1 is associated with adult T-cell leukemia, and HHV-8 is found in unusual large B-cell lymphomas presenting as lymphomatous effusions.

Chronic Inflammation *(p. 587)*

Environmental agents that cause chronic immune stimulation can predispose to lymphoid neoplasia. The most clear-cut associations are *Helicobacter pylori* infection with gastric B-cell lymphoma and gluten-sensitive enteropathy with intestinal T-cell lymphoma. HIV-induced T-cell dysregulation also leads to early germinal center B-cell hyperplasia that can eventually lead to increased risk of B-cell lymphoma, arising in virtually any organ.

Iatrogenic Factors and Smoking *(p. 587)*

Radiotherapy and many cancer chemotherapies increase the risk of myeloid and lymphoid neoplasms, stemming from the mutagenic effects of such treatments on progenitor cells. The incidence of AML is increased from 1.3- to 2-fold in smokers, presumably due to carcinogens, such as benzene, in tobacco smoke.

Lymphoid Neoplasms (p. 588)

Definitions and Classifications *(p. 588)*

- *Leukemia:* Neoplasms with widespread involvement of bone marrow and often (but not always) the peripheral blood.
- *Lymphoma:* Proliferations that arise as discrete tissue masses (e.g., within lymph nodes, spleen, or extranodal tissues). Among the *lymphomas,* two broad categories are recognized:
  - *HL,* with important clinical and histologic distinctions
  - *Non-Hodgkin lymphoma* (NHL), comprising all forms besides HL
- *Plasma cell neoplasms* are another important group of lymphoid tumors; these typically arise in marrow (infrequently involving lymph nodes) and are composed of terminally differentiated B cells.

Whether a particular neoplasm is designated a "leukemia" or "lymphoma" is based on the *usual* tissue distribution. Thus entities formally classified as "lymphomas" can have leukemic presentations or may evolve to leukemias; similarly, tumors categorized as leukemias can occasionally arise as soft-tissue masses without marrow involvement.

As a corollary to this classification, lymphomas characteristically present as enlarged nontender lymph nodes, whereas the leukemias come to attention because of signs and symptoms related to the suppression of normal hematopoiesis (e.g., infection, bleeding, and/or anemia). The most common plasma cell neoplasm *(multiple myeloma)* causes bone destruction and often presents with pain and/or pathologic fractures.

The *World Health Organization (WHO)* classification scheme sorts the various lymphoid neoplasms into five broad categories based on clinical features, morphology, immunophenotype, and genotype:

- Precursor B (pre-B)-cell neoplasms (immature B cells)
- Peripheral B-cell neoplasms (mature B cells)
- Precursor T (pre-T)-cell neoplasms (immature T cells)
- Peripheral T-cell and NK-cell neoplasms (mature T cells and NK cells)
- HL (neoplasms of Reed-Sternberg [RS] cells)

Important principles regarding lymphoid neoplasms are as follows:

- Diagnosis requires histologic examination of lymph nodes or other involved tissues.

- In most lymphoid neoplasms, antigen receptor gene rearrangement precedes transformation; hence all daughter cells share the same antigen receptor sequence and synthesize identical proteins (either immunoglobulins or T-cell receptors). In contrast, normal immune responses are polyclonal. Thus clonality analyses of lymphoid populations can distinguish neoplastic versus reactive proliferations. Moreover, a unique antigen receptor rearrangement can be used as a highly specific clonal marker to detect small numbers of malignant cells.
- Most lymphoid neoplasms (85% to 90%) are of B-cell origin, with most of the remainder being T-cell tumors; only rare tumors are of NK-cell or histiocytic origin. Most lymphoid neoplasms resemble some recognizable stage of B- or T-cell development, a feature used in their classification (Fig. 13-3).
- Lymphoid neoplasms tend to disrupt normal immune regulatory mechanisms, leading frequently to immunologic dysfunction.
- Neoplastic B and T cells circulate widely but tend to home to and grow in areas where their normal counterparts reside.
- Although NHLs spread widely and somewhat unpredictably early in their course, HL spreads in an orderly fashion; hence staging in HL is of substantial utility in guiding therapy.
- The salient features (including genetic alterations) of the major types of lymphoid leukemias, NHLs, and plasma cell tumors are summarized in Table 13-3.

Precursor B- and T-Cell Neoplasms *(p. 590)*

Acute Lymphoblastic Leukemia or Lymphoma (p. 590)

Acute lymphoblastic leukemia or lymphomas (ALLs) are neoplasms of immature, pre-B or pre-T lymphocytes *(lymphoblasts).* These constitute the most common childhood cancers.

- Most (approximately 85%) are pre-B tumors manifesting as childhood acute leukemias with extensive marrow and peripheral blood involvement.
- Pre-T ALLs tend to present in adolescent boys as thymic "lymphomas" (50% to 70% of cases).

Pathogenesis *(p. 590).* Approximately 90% of ALLs have chromosomal changes. Many of the chromosomal aberrations dysregulate the expression or function of transcription factors that control normal B- and T-cell development and lead to maturation arrest. Pre-B and pre-T ALL (B-ALL and T-ALL, respectively) have different genetic aberrations, indicating that different molecular mechanisms underlie their pathogenesis. Characteristic changes include the following:

- *Hyperdiploidy* (>50 chromosomes) is most common, although hypodiploidy and balanced translocations also occur. Hyperdiploidy and hypodiploidy occur only in B-ALL.
- Seventy percent of T-ALLs have gain-of-function mutations in *NOTCH1,* a gene essential for T-cell development.
- Many B-ALLs have loss-of-function mutations in *PAX5, E2A,* or *EBF*—genes involved in B-cell development; they may also have balanced t(12;21) translocations involving genes that are important in early hematopoietic precursors.
- Importantly, *single mutations are not sufficient to cause ALL;* rather, additional, complementary mutations—that typically increase proliferation or survival—are necessary to convert a preleukemic clone into full-blown malignancy.

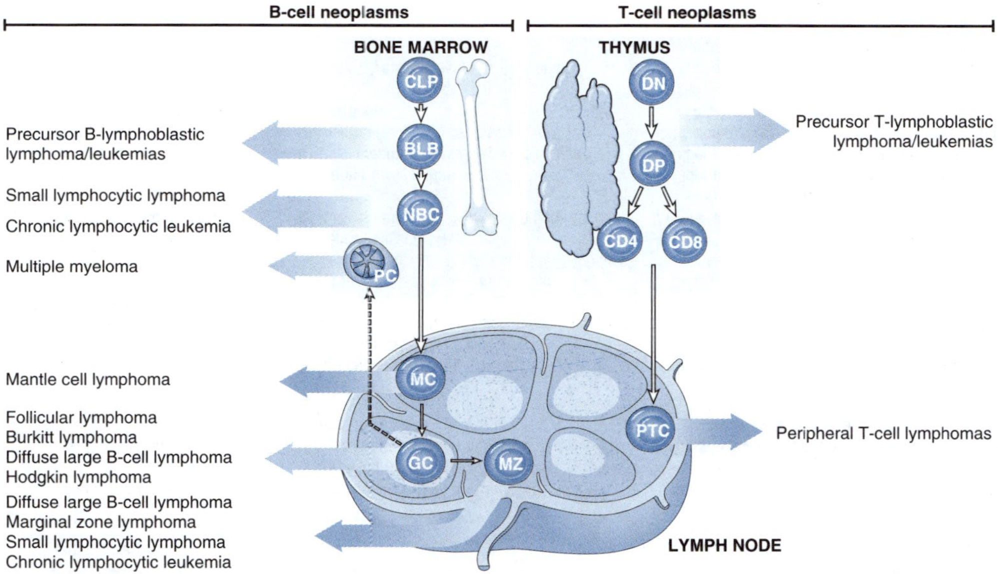

Figure 13-3 Origin of lymphoid neoplasms. Stages of B- and T-cell differentiation from which specific lymphoid tumors emerge are shown. *CLP,* Common lymphoid precursor; *BLB,* pre-B lymphoblast; *DN,* CD4/CD8 double-negative pro-T cell; *DP,* CD4/CD8 double-positive pre-T cell; *GC,* germinal-center B cell; *MC,* mantle B cell; *MZ,* marginal zone B cell; *NBC,* naive B cell; *PTC,* peripheral T cell.

TABLE 13-3 Summary of Major Types of Lymphoid Leukemias and NHLs

Diagnosis	Cell of Origin	Genotype	Salient Clinical Features
Neoplasms of Immature B and T Cells			
B-cell ALL*	Bone marrow pre-B cell	Diverse chromosomal translocations; t(12;21) involving *RUNX1* and *ETV6* present in 25%	Predominantly children; symptoms relating to marrow replacement and pancytopenia; aggressive
T-cell ALL	Pre-T cell (often of thymic origin)	Diverse chromosomal translocations, *NOTCH1* mutations (50%-70%)	Predominantly adolescent males; thymic masses and variable bone marrow involvement; aggressive
Neoplasms of Mature B Cells			
BL*	Germinal-center B cell	Translocations involving *MYC* and Ig loci, usually t(8;14); subset EBV associated	Adolescents or young adults with extranodal masses; uncommonly presents as "leukemia"; aggressive
DLBCL†	Germinal-center or postgerminal center B cell	Diverse chromosomal rearrangements, most often of *BCL6* (30%), *BCL2* (10%), or *MYC* (5%)	All ages, but most common in older adults; often appears as a rapidly growing mass; 30% extranodal; aggressive
Extranodal marginal zone lymphoma	Memory B cell	t(11;18), t(1;14), and t(14;18) creating *MALT1-IAP2, BCL10-IgH,* and *MALT1-IgH* fusion genes, respectively	Arises at extranodal sites in adults with chronic inflammatory diseases; may remain localized; indolent
Follicular lymphoma†	Germinal-center B cell	t(14;18) creating *BCL2-IgH* fusion gene	Older adults with generalized lymphadenopathy and marrow involvement; indolent
Hairy cell leukemia	Memory B cell	Activating *BRAF* mutations	Older males with pancytopenia and splenomegaly; indolent
Mantle cell lymphoma	NBC	t(11;14) creating *CyclinD1-IgH* fusion gene	Older males with disseminated disease; moderately aggressive
Multiple myeloma/solitary plasmacytoma†	Postgerminal-center bone marrow homing plasma cell	Diverse rearrangements involving *IgH;* 13q deletions	Myeloma: older adults with lytic bone lesions, pathologic fractures, hypercalcemia, and renal failure; moderately aggressive Plasmacytoma: isolated plasma cell masses in bone or soft tissue; indolent
SLL/CLL	NBC or memory B cell	Trisomy 12, deletions of 11q, 13q, and 17p	Older adults with bone marrow, lymph node, spleen, and liver disease; autoimmune hemolysis and thrombocytopenia in a minority; indolent

Neoplasms of Mature T Cells or NK Cells			
Adult T-cell leukemia/lymphoma	Helper T cell	HTLV-1 provirus present in tumor cells	Adults with cutaneous lesions, marrow involvement, and hypercalcemia; occurs mainly in Japan, West Africa, and the Caribbean; aggressive
Peripheral T-cell lymphoma, unspecified	Helper or cytotoxic T cell	No specific chromosomal abnormality	Mainly older adults; usually presents with lymphadenopathy; aggressive
Anaplastic large-cell lymphoma	Cytotoxic T cell	Rearrangements of *ALK* (anaplastic large cell lymphoma kinase) in a subset	Children and young adults, usually with lymph node and soft-tissue disease; aggressive
Extranodal NK/T-cell lymphoma	NK-cell (common) or cytotoxic T cell (rare)	EBV-associated; no specific chromosomal abnormality	Adults with destructive extranodal masses, most commonly sinonasal; aggressive
Mycosis fungoides/Sézary syndrome	Helper T cell	No specific chromosomal abnormality	Adult patients with cutaneous patches, plaques, nodules, or generalized erythema; indolent
Large granular lymphocytic leukemia	Two types: cytotoxic T cell and NK cell	Point mutations in *STAT3*	Adult patients with splenomegaly, neutropenia, and anemia, sometimes, accompanied by autoimmune disease

*Most common tumors in children

†Most common tumors in adults.

Morphology *(p. 591)*. In leukemic presentations the marrow is hypercellular and packed with lymphoblasts showing a high mitotic activity; tumor cells have scant basophilic cytoplasm with nuclei slightly larger than small lymphocytes exhibiting finely stippled chromatin and inconspicuous nucleoli; the nuclear membrane typically exhibits a convoluted appearance. Pre-B and pre-T lymphoblasts are morphologically identical.

Immunophenotype *(p. 592)*. Terminal deoxytransferase (TdT), a DNA polymerase expressed only by pre-B and pre-T lymphoblasts, is present in >95% of cases.

- Pre-B ALL cells are arrested at stages preceding surface Ig expression; most lymphoblasts express the pan B-cell antigen CD19 and the transcription factor PAX5, as well as CD10.
- Pre-T ALL cells are arrested at early intrathymic stages of maturation; the lymphoblasts often express CD1, CD2, CD5, and CD7.

Clinical Features *(p. 592)*. Approximately 2500 new cases of ALL are diagnosed each year in the United States. The peak incidence for B-ALL is 3 years of age, and the peak for T-ALL is adolescence; both B- and T-ALL occur less frequently in adults. The clinical features of ALL stem from accumulation of neoplastic blast cells in the marrow:

- *Abrupt stormy onset* within days to weeks of symptom onset.
- *Symptoms related to depressed marrow function* (e.g., fatigue due to anemia, fever due to infections in the setting of neutropenia, and bleeding due to thrombocytopenia).
- *Bone pain and tenderness,* due to marrow expansion and infiltration of the subperiosteum by blasts.
- *Generalized lymphadenopathy, splenomegaly, hepatomegaly,* and *testicular enlargement* due to neoplastic infiltration. Pre-T ALL with thymic involvement can cause compression of mediastinal vessels and airways and is also common in ALL.
- *Central nervous system manifestations* (e.g., headache, vomiting, and nerve palsies) due to meningeal spread.

Prognosis *(p. 592)*. With aggressive chemotherapy 95% of children with ALL achieve complete remission, and 75% to 85% are cured; however, ALL is the leading cause of cancer deaths in children. Approximately 35% to 40% of adults are cured.

- Features with worse prognosis are as follows:
  - Age <2 years (largely due to translocations involving the *MLL* gene)
  - Age >10 years
  - Peripheral blast counts >100,000/μL
  - Presence of t(9;22) (Philadelphia chromosome; see discussion later)
- Features with better prognosis include hyperploidy, trisomy of chromosomes 4, 7, and 10, and a t(12;21) translocation.

Peripheral B-Cell Neoplasms *(p. 593)*

Chronic Lymphocytic Leukemia and Small Lymphocytic Lymphoma (p. 593)

Chronic lymphocytic leukemia (CLL) and small lymphocytic lymphoma (SLL) are morphologically, phenotypically, and genotypically indistinguishable, differing only in the degree of peripheral blood lymphocytosis.

Pathogenesis *(p. 593).* Chromosomal translocations are rare in CLL and SLL. The most common findings are trisomy 12q and deletions of 13q12-14 (related to the loss of two microRNAs), 11q, or 17p; gain-of-function mutations in NOTCH1 receptor occur in 10% to 18% of CLL. Ig genes of several CLL/SLL are somatically hypermutated, suggesting that the cell of origin in those cases may be post-germinal center memory B cell; other CLL and SLL without such Ig hypermutation may derive from naïve B cells and tend to have a more aggressive behavior. Tumor growth is largely confined to the proliferation centers where tumor cells receive critical cues from the surrounding microenvironment (e.g., through ligation of the B-cell antigen receptor [membrane-bound Ig]); factors that induce NF-κB transcription factor production also promote neoplastic cell growth and survival. Signaling through the B-cell receptor is transduced by intracellular kinases, including Bruton tyrosine kinase (BTK); BTK inhibitors show clinical promise in this disease.

Morphology *(p. 593).* Lymph node architecture is diffusely effaced by small lymphocytes with round, slightly irregular nuclei; these are admixed with variable numbers of larger dividing cells *(prolymphocytes).* The mitotically active cells often cluster in loose aggregates *(proliferation centers)* that are pathognomonic for CLL and SLL. In CLL, peripheral smears contain increased numbers of small lymphocytes, some of which are disrupted, producing so-called *smudge cells.* Involvement of marrow, spleen, and liver is common.

Immunophenotype *(p. 594).* CLL and SLL cells express pan-B-cell markers (CD19 and CD20) as well as CD5, a marker found on a small subset of normal B cells. Low-level surface Ig expression (usually IgM) is typical.

Clinical Features *(p. 594).* CLL (defined as absolute lymphocyte count > 4000 cells/μL) is the most common adult leukemia in the Western world; 15,000 new cases arise each year in the United States, with a median age of 60 years and a 2:1 male predominance. A minority of cases do not have lymphocytosis and are classified as SLL (constituting 4% of NHL). Characteristic features include the following:

- Nonspecific symptoms (easy fatigability, weight loss, and anorexia)
- Generalized lymphadenopathy and hepatosplenomegaly (50% to 60%)
- Lymphocytosis in CLL, up to 200,000/μL
- Immune abnormalities, including hypogammaglobulinemia (common, leading to increased susceptibility to bacterial infections) and autoantibodies against erythrocytes or platelets (10% to 15%)

The prognosis is extremely variable, depending primarily on the clinical stage. Median survival is 4 to 6 years, but patients with minimal tumor burden often survive >10 years. Worse outcomes are associated with the following:

- Deletions of 11q or 17p
- Lack of somatic hypermutation
- Expression of ZAP-70, a protein that augments Ig receptor signaling activity

Transformation of CLL or SLL to a more aggressive histologic type is a common, ominous event; most patients survive less than 1 year. The following two forms are seen:

- *Prolymphocytic transformation* (15% to 30%) is heralded by worsening cytopenias, increasing splenomegaly, and large numbers of *prolymphocytes* in the circulation.

- *Transformation to diffuse large B-cell lymphoma (DLBCL) (Richter syndrome)* occurs in 5% to 10% of patients and presents as a rapidly enlarging mass within a lymph node or spleen.

Follicular Lymphoma (p. 594)

Follicular lymphoma is the most common form of NHL in the United States (15,000 to 20,000 cases per year). It arises from germinal center cells and is strongly associated with translocations involving *BCL2.*

Pathogenesis *(p. 594).* A characteristic t(14;18) translocation juxtaposes the *IgH* locus on chromosome 14 and the *BCL2* locus on chromosome 18, leading to BCL2 protein overexpression; BCL2 prevents apoptosis and promotes tumor cell survival. Mutations in the *MLL2* gene (encodes a histone methyltransferase that regulates gene expression) are also present in approximately 90% of cases.

Morphology *(p. 595).* In lymph nodes, follicular (nodular) and diffuse proliferations are composed of two principal cell types: *centrocytes*—small cells with cleaved nuclear contours and scant cytoplasm; and *centroblasts*—larger cells with open nuclear chromatin, several nucleoli, and modest amounts of cytoplasm. Centrocytes predominate in most tumors. Involvement of spleen, liver, and marrow is common; peripheral blood involvement occurs in 10% of patients.

Immunophenotype *(p. 595).* Neoplastic cells resemble normal follicular center B cells (CD19+, CD20+, CD10+, BCL6+, surface Ig+). More than 90% of tumor cells also express BCL2 protein (normal follicular center B cells are BCL2 negative).

Clinical Features *(p. 595).* Follicular lymphoma characteristically presents as painless, generalized lymphadenopathy in middle-aged adults. It is not curable but typically follows an indolent waxing-waning course with a median survival of 7 to 9 years. Histologic transformation to DLBCL occurs in 30% to 50% of cases; after transformation, median survival is <1 year.

Diffuse Large B-Cell Lymphoma (p. 595)

DLBCL is the most common form of NHL, with 25,000 new cases annually in the United States.

Pathogenesis *(p. 596).* DLBCL is a heterogeneous group of lymphomas. Nevertheless, two chromosomal rearrangements are relatively common:

- Thirty percent have *translocations involving the BCL6 locus,* suggested to be an inadvertent consequence of somatic hypermutation. *BLC6* encodes a zinc-finger transcription factor that regulates the development and growth of germinal center B cells; overexpression holds cells in a relatively undifferentiated and proliferative state. Somatic mutations in the *BCL6* promoter can also lead to aberrant BCL6 expression.
- Ten to twenty percent have a t(14;18) translocation, leading to overexpression of the antiapoptotic *BCL2* gene and may arise from transformation of previously unrecognized follicular lymphomas. Tumors with *BCL2* rearrangements also typically lack *BCL6* rearrangements, suggesting that these constitute distinct molecular classes of DLBCL.
- Mutations in histone acetyltransferases (that alter gene expression by modifying chromatin structure) are common in DLBCL,

and approximately 5% of these tumors are associated with *MYC* translocations (often following a more aggressive course).

Morphology *(p. 596).* Common features are a relatively large cell size (4 to 5 times the diameter of small lymphocytes) and a diffuse growth pattern obliterating the underlying architecture. The nuclear shape is variable and vesicular in appearance, with two to three nucleoli; the cytoplasm is moderately abundant and can be pale or basophilic.

Immunophenotype *(p. 596).* These mature B-cell tumors express pan-B-cell markers CD19 and CD20, with variable expression of germinal center B-cell markers, such as CD10 and BCL6; most have surface Ig.

Special subtypes associated with oncogenic herpesviruses (p. 596) are as follows:

- *Immunodeficiency-associated large B-cell lymphomas* occur in the setting of severe T-cell immunodeficiency (e.g., HIV and bone marrow transplantation). The neoplastic cells are often latently infected with EBV, which plays a critical pathogenic role. Restoration of T-cell immunity can lead to regression of the proliferations.
- *Primary effusion lymphomas* arise as malignant pleural or ascitic effusions, mostly in advanced HIV infection or the elderly. Tumor cells are anaplastic and lack T- or B-cell markers but have clonal Ig heavy (H) chain gene rearrangements. Tumor cells are infected with human KSHV/HHV-8, which play a causal role.

Clinical Features *(p. 596).* DLBCL occurs most frequently in older adults (median age of 60) as a rapidly enlarging, symptomatic mass at a single nodal or extranodal site (e.g., gastrointestinal tract, skin, bone, or brain). Involvement of liver, spleen, and marrow can occur but usually later in the course.

DLBCLs are aggressive, rapidly fatal tumors if left untreated. With intensive chemotherapy, complete remission is achieved in 60% to 80% of patients, and 40% to 50% are cured; anti-CD20 immunotherapy improves initial responses and overall outcomes. Patients with limited disease fare better than patients with widespread disease or a large bulky tumor mass.

Burkitt Lymphoma (p. 597)

BL occurs in three different settings; although they are histologically identical, they have distinct clinical, genotypic, and virologic features:

- African (endemic) BL
- Sporadic (nonendemic) BL
- A subset of aggressive lymphomas occurring in patients infected with HIV

Pathogenesis *(p. 597).* BL is associated with *c-MYC* gene (chromosome 8) translocations; the partner is usually the IgH locus (t[8;14]) but can be the Ig κ (t[2;8]) or λ (t[8;22]) light (L) chain loci. The outcome is *c-MYC* positioned adjacent to strong Ig enhancer and promoter elements that increase *c-MYC* expression. Inactivating p53 mutations are also common.

Virtually all African (endemic) tumors are latently infected with EBV; EBV is also present in 25% of HIV-associated tumors and 15% to 20% of sporadic cases. Molecular analysis shows that the viral

DNA configuration is identical in all tumor cells within a given case, indicating that infection precedes cellular transformation.

Morphology *(p. 597).* Involved tissues are diffusely effaced by intermediate-sized tumor cells with round-oval nuclei, coarse chromatin, several nucleoli, and moderate cytoplasm. A high mitotic index and numerous apoptotic cells are typical; apoptotic cells ingested by scattered macrophages with abundant, clear cytoplasm produce a characteristic "starry sky" appearance.

Immunophenotype *(p. 597).* Tumors comprise relatively mature B cells expressing surface IgM, CD19, CD20, CD10, and BCL6, consistent with a germinal center B-cell origin; BCL2 is rarely expressed.

Clinical Features *(p. 597).* Both endemic and sporadic BL occur largely in children or young adults; in the United States, BL accounts for 30% of childhood NHLs. Most tumors arise at extranodal sites as rapidly growing masses; endemic BL often presents in the mandible (with a predilection for kidneys, ovaries, and adrenals), whereas sporadic BL most often occurs as an ileocecal or peritoneal mass. Marrow and peripheral blood involvement is uncommon.

BL is aggressive but responds well to intensive chemotherapy; most children and young adults can be cured, whereas the outcome in older adults is more guarded.

Plasma Cell Neoplasms and Related Disorders (p. 598)

Plasma cell neoplasms and related disorders are neoplasms of terminally differentiated B cells. They represent the expansion of a single clone of Ig-secreting plasma cells, with resulting serum elevations in a single homogeneous Ig or its fragments. These tumors cause 15% of deaths due to lymphoid neoplasms; 15,000 cases of multiple myeloma (the most common and lethal form) occur annually in the United States.

A monoclonal Ig identified in the blood is called an *M component.* In many cases, neoplastic cells secrete excess free L or H chains; occasionally only L or H chains are produced. Because of their small size, free L chains are excreted in the urine (so-called *Bence Jones proteins*). Terms to describe abnormal Ig include monoclonal gammopathy, dysproteinemia, and paraproteinemia.

There are several different clinicopathologic entities associated with monoclonal gammopathies:

- ***Multiple myeloma*** is the most important plasma cell neoplasm, usually presenting as multifocal skeletal masses; variants include *solitary myeloma* and *smoldering myeloma.*
- *Waldenström macroglobulinemia* is a syndrome in which high levels of IgM lead to blood hyperviscosity.
- *H chain disease* (characterized by secretion of free H chain fragments) is a rare monoclonal gammopathy seen in association with, for example, lymphoplasmacytic lymphoma or small bowel marginal zone lymphomas in malnourished populations (so-called *Mediterranean lymphoma*).
- *Immunocyte-associated amyloidosis* results from monoclonal plasma cell proliferations that secrete L chains. Some patients have multiple myeloma, whereas others have only a minor clonal plasma cell population.
- *Monoclonal gammopathy of undetermined significance* (MGUS) is the designation for asymptomatic patients with M spikes on protein electrophoresis.

Multiple Myeloma (p. 599)

Multiple myeloma is a plasma cell neoplasm with a peak incidence at ages 65 to 70 years; it is characterized by multifocal destructive bony lesions.

Pathogenesis *(p. 599).*

- Ig genes show somatic hypermutation, indicating that the cell of origin is a postgerminal center B cell that has migrated to the marrow and differentiated into a plasma cell.
- Proliferation and survival are dependent on tumor cell and stromal cell cytokines, particularly IL-6.
- Factors produced by the tumor cells (e.g., MIP1α that drives stromal cell production of RANKL [receptor activator of NF-κB ligand]) lead to osteoclast activation and osteoblast inactivation; the net result is bone resorption with hypercalcemia and pathologic fractures.
- Translocations of the Ig H chain gene are common; translocation partners include *FGFR3* receptor gene and cell cycle regulatory genes cyclin D1 and cyclin D3. Deletions of chromosome 17p (involving *TP53*) and rearrangements involving *MYC* are associated with a poorer, more aggressive course.

Morphology *(p. 599)*

- Bone involvement by destructive plasma cell tumors (plasmacytomas) is most common in the vertebral column, ribs, skull, pelvis, and femur. Skull lesions have a sharply defined, punched-out radiologic appearance; generalized osteoporosis can also be seen.
- Away from overt masses, bone marrow shows increased numbers of plasma cells (>30% of total cells) often with abnormal features. The cells can diffusely infiltrate or occur as sheetlike masses that completely replace normal elements.
- High levels of M proteins cause erythrocytes in peripheral smears to stick together in linear arrays, so-called *rouleaux formation.*
- Bence Jones proteinuria leads to *myeloma kidney* (see Chapter 20).

Immunophenotype *(p. 599).* Plasma cell tumors are positive for the adhesion molecule CD138 (syndecan-1) and often express CD56.

Clinical Features *(p. 599).* Clinical features stem from organ infiltration (particularly bones) by neoplastic plasma cells, excess Ig production (often having abnormal physicochemical properties), and suppression of normal humoral immunity.

- *Bone infiltration, bone pain, and pathologic fractures due to bone resorption.* Secondary hypercalcemia contributes to renal disease and polyuria and can cause neurologic manifestations, including confusion, weakness, lethargy, and constipation.
- *Recurrent bacterial infections* result from decreased production of normal immunoglobulins.
- *Hyperviscosity syndrome* (see discussion later)
- *Renal insufficiency* (up to 50% of patients) is multifactorial; notably, L chains are toxic to tubular epithelial cells.
- Certain L chains are prone to causing *amyloidosis* of the amyloid light chain (AL) type (see Chapter 6)

In 99% of patients, electrophoresis reveals increased blood monoclonal Ig (M protein) and/or Bence Jones proteinuria. IgG (55%) and IgA (25%) are the most common M proteins. In 20% of patients, Bence Jones proteinuria is an isolated finding, and 1% of myelomas are nonsecretory.

Prognosis is variable but generally poor with median survivals of 4 to 6 years. If untreated, patients with multiple bony lesions survive only 6 to 12 months. Cyclin D1 translocations are associated with better outcomes; 13q or 17q deletions or t(4;14) portend a more aggressive course. Chemotherapy induces remission in 50% to 70%, and proteasome inhibitors are showing efficacy against myeloma cells; thalidomide has efficacy by blocking tumor-stromal interactions and by inhibiting angiogenesis. Infection and renal failure are the two most common causes of death.

- ***Solitary myelomas (plasmacytomas)*** (p. 601) represent 3% to 5% of plasma cell neoplasms. Modest elevations of serum or urinary M proteins occur in a minority. Solitary bony lesions almost inevitably progress to multiple myeloma but can take 10 to 20 years to do so. Extraosseous lesions often localize to lung, nasal sinuses, or oronasopharynx; these rarely disseminate and can be cured by local resection.
- ***Smoldering myeloma*** (p. 601) represents a middle ground between multiple myeloma and MGUS; plasma cells comprise 10% to 30% of marrow cellularity, and serum M protein is >3 g/dL, but patients are asymptomatic. Almost 75% will progress to myeloma within 15 years.

Monoclonal Gammopathy of Uncertain Significance (p. 601)

MGUS is the most common plasma cell dyscrasia. By definition, patients are asymptomatic; nevertheless, serum M proteins (<3 g/dL) are detected in 3% of people >50 years and 5% of people >70 years of age. Most patients follow a completely benign clinical course; however, 1% annually progress to a symptomatic monoclonal gammopathy, typically multiple myeloma.

Lymphoplasmacytic Lymphoma (p. 601)

Lymphoplasmacytic lymphoma is a B-cell neoplasm of older adults (sixth to seventh decade) that typically secretes monoclonal IgM, often in amounts sufficient to cause the *hyperviscosity syndrome* called *Waldenström macroglobulinemia.* Unlike multiple myeloma, H- and L-chain synthesis is balanced so that complications of excess L chains (e.g., amyloidosis or renal failure) are rare. Bony destruction is also not observed.

Pathogenesis *(p. 601).* Virtually all cases are associated with mutations in *MYD88,* encoding an adapter protein involved in signaling through the NF-κB and B-cell receptor pathways.

Morphology *(p. 601).* Diffuse marrow infiltrates of neoplastic lymphocytes, plasma cells, and plasmacytoid lymphocytes, mixed with reactive mast cells, are seen. With disseminated disease, similar polymorphous infiltrates can occur in lymph nodes, spleen, or liver.

Immunophenotype *(p. 601).* The lymphoid cells express CD20 and membrane Ig; the plasma cells secrete the same Ig as seen on the lymphoid cells.

Clinical Features *(p. 601).* Patients present with weakness, fatigue, and weight loss; half will have lymphadenopathy, hepatomegaly, and splenomegaly.

- Marrow infiltration causes anemia; this can be exacerbated by autoimmune hemolysis due to cold agglutinins of the IgM type (10% of patients).

- IgM secretion frequently results in a *hyperviscosity syndrome:*
  - *Visual impairment* due to venous congestion; there is striking *tortuosity* and distention of retinal veins, often with hemorrhages and exudates.
  - *Neurologic problems:* Headaches, dizziness, deafness, and stupor are attributable to sluggish blood flow and sludging.
  - *Bleeding* is related to the formation of complexes containing macroglobulins and clotting factors, as well as interference with platelet function.
  - *Cryoglobulinemia* resulting from precipitation of macroglobulins at low temperatures; symptoms include Raynaud phenomenon and cold urticaria.

Lymphoplasmacytic lymphoma is an incurable, progressive disease with a median survival time of 4 years. Symptoms related to IgM (such as hyperviscosity and hemolysis) can be treated with plasmapheresis.

Mantle Cell Lymphoma (p. 602)

Mantle cell lymphoma accounts for approximately 2.5% of NHLs in the United States and 7% to 9% of NHLs in Europe.

***Pathogenesis** (p. 602).* A distinctive t(11;14) translocation, detected in more than 70% of cases, results in the juxtaposition of the cyclin D1 and IgH loci and leads to cyclin D1 overexpression that promotes G1- to S-phase cell cycle progression.

***Morphology** (p. 602).* Tumor cells closely resemble the normal mantle zone B cells that surround germinal centers; they are small lymphocytes with irregular or clefted nuclei, condensed nuclear chromatin, inconspicuous nucleoli, and scant cytoplasm. Expansion of these cells in nodes can produce a nodular appearance or efface the normal architecture.

***Immunophenotype** (p. 603).* Tumor cells characteristically *overexpress cyclin D1;* most also express CD19, CD20, CD5, and moderate surface Ig. The IgH genes lack somatic hypermutation, consistent with a naïve B-cell origin.

***Clinical Features** (p. 603).* Males are affected more than females, and the typical age of onset is the fifth to sixth decades. Patients have generalized lymphadenopathy, and peripheral blood involvement occurs in 20% to 40% of patients. Extranodal disease is relatively common; marrow and splenic involvement (50% of patients) are not unusual, and there is frequently multifocal mucosal involvement of the small bowel and colon *(lymphomatoid polyposis).* The prognosis is poor with median survivals of 3 to 4 years; patients succumb to complications of organ dysfunction due to tumor infiltration.

Marginal Zone Lymphomas (p. 603)

Marginal zone lymphomas are a heterogeneous group of B-cell tumors arising in lymph nodes, spleen, or extranodal tissues. Because mucosa is a typical extranodal site, these are also called *m*ucosa-*a*ssociated *l*ymphoid *t*umors (or MALTomas). Although cells have different stages of B-lymphoid differentiation, *the predominant population resembles a normal marginal zone B cell;* there is evidence of Ig somatic hypermutation, suggesting an origin from memory B cells.

Notable characteristics of the extranodal marginal zone lymphomas are as follows:

- Tendency to occur at sites of *chronic immune or inflammatory reactions* (e.g., salivary glands in Sjögren disease, thyroid in Hashimoto thyroiditis, stomach in *H. pylori* infection).

- Lymphomas remain localized at sites of origin for long periods, spreading systemically only late in their course.
- Tumors can regress if the inciting stimulus (e.g., *Helicobacter*) is eradicated.

These features suggest that marginal zone lymphomas lie on a continuum between reactive hyperplasia and full-blown lymphoma. Following a reactive, polyclonal immune response, a monoclonal B-cell neoplasm emerges, probably due to acquired genetic changes; however, cell growth is still dependent on local factors (e.g., factors produced by reactive T-helper cells) for growth and survival. With additional genetic aberrations the neoplasm becomes factor-independent; (11;18), (1;14), or (11;14) translocations are relatively specific and lead to upregulation of BCL10 or MALT1—proteins that activate the NF-κB pathway and promote B-cell growth and survival. With further clonal evolution, distant spread and transformation to DLBCL can occur.

Hairy Cell Leukemia (p. 603)

Hairy cell leukemia constitutes approximately 2% of all leukemias; it predominantly affects middle-aged white men (male:female ratio of 5:1).

Pathogenesis (p. 603). More than 90% of cases are associated with activating point mutations in the serine/threonine kinase BRAF.

***Morphology** (p. 604).* The name derives from fine, hairlike projections on the tumor cells; routine blood smears reveal variably shaped nuclei and modest amounts of pale blue cytoplasm with threadlike or bleblike extensions. Because tumor cells are trapped in ECM, they frequently cannot be recovered from aspirates (so-called "dry tap") and can only be visualized on marrow biopsies. Splenic red pulp is usually heavily infiltrated, leading to white pulp obliteration and a beefy red gross appearance.

***Immunophenotype** (p. 604).* Cells typically express pan-B-cell markers (CD19 and CD20), surface Ig, CD11c, CD25, and CD103. Most tumors have hypermutated Ig genes, suggesting an origin from postgerminal center memory B cells.

***Clinical Features** (p. 604).* Clinical features result from marrow, liver, or splenic infiltration. *Splenomegaly,* often massive, is the most common and sometimes only abnormal physical finding. *Hepatomegaly* is less common and not as marked; lymphadenopathy is rare. *Pancytopenia,* resulting from marrow infiltration and splenic sequestration, occurs in more than 50% of cases. *Infections* are the presenting feature in one third of cases. Monocytopenia may contribute to the high incidence of atypical mycobacterial infections. This is an indolent disorder with good prognosis. It is exquisitely sensitive to certain chemotherapies, typically producing long-lasting remissions; BRAF inhibitors are efficacious for tumors that fail conventional therapies.

Peripheral T-Cell and NK-Cell Neoplasms *(p. 604)*

Peripheral T-cell and NK-cell neoplasms are a heterogeneous group united by phenotypes that resemble normal mature T or NK cells. Peripheral T-cell tumors account for 5% to 10% of NHLs in the United States and Europe, whereas NK-cell tumors are rare. Both types are more common in Asia.

Peripheral T-Cell Lymphomas, Unspecified (p. 604)

Peripheral T-cell lymphomas, unspecified is largely a "wastebasket" category for tumors that do not fit any other WHO criteria. No morphologic feature is pathognomonic, but certain findings are characteristic:

- Tumor cells diffusely efface lymph nodes and are commonly composed of a pleomorphic mixture of variably sized malignant T cells.
- Infiltrates of reactive cells (e.g., eosinophils and macrophages) are common, as is brisk angiogenesis.
- By definition, these all have a mature T-cell phenotype; they express pan-T-cell markers (e.g., CD2, CD3, CD5) and have clonal T-cell receptor rearrangements.

Most patients have generalized lymphadenopathy, sometimes with eosinophilia, pruritus, fever, and weight loss. Although cures are reported, the prognosis is worse than for comparably aggressive mature B-cell neoplasms (e.g., DLBCL).

Anaplastic Large-Cell Lymphoma (ALK Positive) (p. 604)

Anaplastic large-cell lymphoma is an entity defined by chromosomal rearrangements involving the *ALK* gene on chromosome 2p23. These rearrangements create *ALK* fusion genes that encode constitutively active forms of ALK—a tyrosine kinase upstream of JAK/STAT signaling pathways.

Tumor cells are large with reniform, embryoid, or horseshoe-shaped nuclei and voluminous cytoplasm.

These tumors occur most commonly in children and young adults, frequently involve soft tissues, and carry a very good prognosis; cure rates approach 80%. Most tumors express CD30, a member of the TNF receptor family; antibodies to CD30 show clinical promise. Morphologically similar tumors lacking *ALK* rearrangements usually arise in older adults and have a poor prognosis, similar to peripheral T-cell lymphoma, unspecified.

Adult T-Cell Leukemia or Lymphoma (p. 605)

Adult T-cell leukemia or lymphoma occurs in patients infected by *human T-cell leukemia retrovirus type 1 (HTLV-1);* it is most common where HTLV-1 is endemic (southern Japan, West Africa, and Caribbean basin). Tumor cells contain clonal HTLV-1 provirus, suggesting a pathogenic role; notably, HTLV-1 encodes a Tax protein that activates NF-κB and thereby enhances lymphocyte growth and survival. Tumor cells with multilobular (cloverleaf) nuclei are characteristic. Clinical findings include skin involvement, generalized lymphadenopathy and hepatosplenomegaly, peripheral blood lymphocytosis, and hypercalcemia. This is a rapidly fatal disease, often with mortality within a year, despite aggressive chemotherapy.

Mycosis Fungoides and Sézary Syndrome (p. 605)

Mycosis fungoides and Sézary syndrome are different manifestations of a tumor of CD4+ helper T cells that home to skin. Tumor cells characteristically express the CLA adhesion molecule, as well as CC4 and CCR10 chemokine receptors; all these surface molecules contribute to the cutaneous localization of tumor cells.

- *Mycosis fungoides* progresses from an inflammatory *premycotic phase* through a *plaque phase* to a *tumor phase.* Histologically the epidermis and upper dermis are infiltrated by neoplastic T cells with *cerebriform* nuclei (marked infolding of the nuclear membrane). Disease progression involves extracutaneous spread, most commonly to lymph nodes and marrow.
- *Sézary syndrome* is a variant in which skin involvement is manifested as a generalized exfoliative erythroderma with an associated leukemia of *Sézary* cells (also with cerebriform nuclei).

These tumors are usually indolent with median survivals of 8 to 9 years; transformation to aggressive T-cell lymphoma can be a terminal event.

Large Granular Lymphocytic Leukemia (p. 606)

Large granular lymphocytic leukemia is a rare neoplasm occurring mainly in adults. Between 30% and 40% have acquired mutations in the STAT3 transcription factor, which normally functions downstream of cytokine receptors; the result is cytokine-independent STAT3 activation.

- Tumor cells are large lymphocytes with abundant blue cytoplasm containing scattered coarse azurophilic granules. Marrow involvement is usually sparse; hepatic and splenic infiltrates are usually present.
- Two variants are recognized: CD3+ T-cell tumors and CD56+ NK-cell tumors.
- Despite the paucity of marrow involvement, *neutropenia* (with maturation arrest of myeloid elements in the marrow) and *anemia* dominate the clinical picture; *pure red blood cell aplasia* can rarely occur.
- There is also an increased incidence of *rheumatologic disorders;* some patients present with Felty syndrome, characterized by the triad of rheumatoid arthritis, splenomegaly, and neutropenia.
- The course is variable, being largely dependent on the severity of the cytopenias.

Extranodal NK or T-Cell Lymphoma (p. 606)

Extranodal NK or T-cell lymphoma is rare in the United States and Europe but constitutes 3% of Asian NHLs.

- It presents most commonly as a destructive nasopharyngeal mass; less common sites include skin or testis. Tumor cells infiltrate small vessels leading to extensive ischemic necrosis.
- Histologic appearance is variable; tumor cells can contain large *azurophilic granules* resembling those in normal NK cells.
- This lymphoma is highly associated with EBV; tumor cells in any given patient contain identical EBV episomes, indicating an origin from a single EBV-infected cell. Most tumors express NK-cell markers and lack T-cell receptor rearrangements, supporting an NK-cell origin.
- These are highly aggressive neoplasms that respond well to radiotherapy but are resistant to chemotherapy.

Hodgkin Lymphoma *(p. 606)*

HL accounts for 0.7% of all new cancers in the United States; the average age at diagnosis is 32 years. *As opposed to* NHL, which often occurs in extranodal sites and spreads in an unpredictable fashion, HL typifies the following:

- It arises in a single node or chain and spreads in a predictable way to anatomically contiguous lymphoid tissue.
- It is characterized by the presence of distinctive neoplastic giant cells called *RS* cells, derived primarily from germinal center or postgerminal center B cells. These cells release factors that induce the accumulation of the reactive lymphocytes, macrophages, and granulocytes that constitute >90% of tumor cellularity.

Classification *(p. 607)*

Pathogenesis (p. 607). In the vast majority of cases the Ig genes of RS cells have undergone both V(D)J recombination and somatic hypermutation, establishing an origin from germinal center or post-germinal center cells. Nevertheless, for unclear reasons, RS cells of classic HL fail to express most B cell–specific genes (including Ig).

- NF-κB transcription factor activation is a common event in classical HL, either through EBV infection or other mechanisms. This promotes lymphocyte survival and proliferation.
- The different kinds of tissue reaction observed in various HL subtypes are partly due to cytokines and chemokines secreted by the RS cells and reactive background cells. In turn, cytokines produced by the reactive cells may support the growth and survival of tumor cells (Fig. 13-4).
- RS cells are aneuploidy with diverse clonal chromosomal aberrations. In particular, copy number gains in the *c-REL* proto-oncogene on chromosome 2p are common and may contribute to increased NF-κB activity.

Morphology *(p. 607)*. *RS* cells and their variants are the neoplastic element; their identification is essential for histologic diagnosis:

- *Classic, diagnostic RS cells* are large (≥45 μm) with either a multi-lobed nucleus or multiple nuclei, each with a large, inclusion-like nucleolus approximately the size of a small lymphocyte (5-7 μm diameter); cytoplasm is abundant.
- *Mononuclear variants* contain only a single round or oblong nucleus with a large inclusion-like nucleolus.
- *Lacunar cells* have more delicate folded or multilobate nuclei surrounded by abundant pale cytoplasm that retracts during tissue processing, leaving the nucleus in an empty hole (the lacune).
- *Lymphohistiocytic variants (L&H cells)* have polypoid nuclei resembling popcorn kernels, inconspicuous nucleoli, and moderately abundant cytoplasm.

"Classic" RS cells express PAX5 (a B-cell transcription factor), CD15, and CD30 but are negative for other B- and T-cell markers

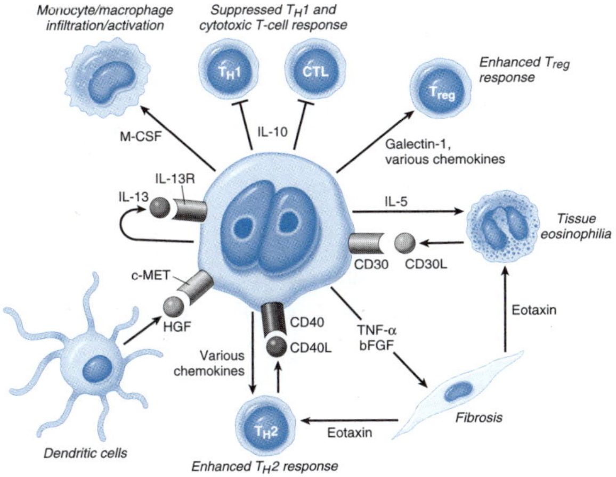

Figure 13-4 Signals mediating "cross-talk" between RS cells and surrounding normal cells in classical forms of HL. *CD30L,* CD30 ligand; *bFGF,* basic fibroblast growth factor; *M-CSF,* macrophage colony–stimulating factor; *HGF,* hepatocyte growth factor (binds to the c-MET receptor); *CTL,* CD8+ cytotoxic T cell; *T_H1* and *T_H2,* CD4+ T helper cell subsets; *Treg,* regulatory T cell.

and CD45. L&H variants express B-cell markers typical of germinal-center B cells (e.g., CD20 and BCL6) and are negative for CD15 and CD30.

Cells similar or identical in appearance to RS cells occur in other conditions (e.g., infectious mononucleosis, solid tissue cancers, and NHL). Thus RS cells must be present in an appropriate background of reactive, non-neoplastic inflammation to make the diagnosis.

There are five subtypes of HL in the standard WHO classification scheme, each with somewhat unique diagnostic and/or clinical features (Table 13-4):

1. **Nodular sclerosis type** is the most common form of HL, constituting 65% to 75% of cases; it tends to involve the lower cervical, supraclavicular, and mediastinal lymph nodes. This type is characterized by the presence of *lacunar variant* RS cells and *collagen bands* that divide the lymphoid tissue into circumscribed nodules. It is uncommonly associated with EBV. The prognosis is excellent.
2. **Mixed cellularity type** constitutes 20% to 25% of cases. It is more likely to be associated with older age, so-called B symptoms (fever and weight loss), and advanced tumor stage. Classic RS cells and

TABLE 13-4 Subtypes of Hodgkin Lymphoma

Subtype	Morphology and Immunophenotype	Typical Clinical Features
Nodular sclerosis	Frequent lacunar cells and occasional diagnostic RS cells; background infiltrate composed of T lymphocytes, eosinophils, macrophages, and plasma cells; fibrous bands dividing cellular areas into nodules. RS cells CD15+, CD30+; usually EBV–	Most common subtype; usually stage I or II disease; frequent mediastinal involvement; equal occurrence in males and females, most patients young adults
Mixed cellularity	Frequent mononuclear and diagnostic RS cells; background infiltrate rich in T lymphocytes, eosinophils, macrophages, plasma cells; RS cells CD15+, CD30+; 70% EBV+	More than 50% present with stage III or IV disease; M greater than F; biphasic incidence, peaking in young adults and again in adults older than 55 years
Lymphocyte rich	Frequent mononuclear and diagnostic RS cells; background infiltrate rich in T lymphocytes; RS cells CD15+, CD30+; 40% EBV+	Uncommon; M greater than F; tends to be seen in older adults
Lymphocyte depletion	Reticular variant: Frequent diagnostic RS cells and variants and a paucity of background reactive cells; RS cells CD15+, CD30+; most EBV+	Uncommon; more common in older men and HIV-infected individuals and in developing countries; often present with advanced disease
Lymphocyte predominance	Frequent L&H (popcorn cell) variants in a background of follicular dendritic cells and reactive B cells; RS cells CD20+, CD15–, C30–; EBV–	Uncommon; young males with cervical or axillary lymphadenopathy; mediastinal

mononuclear variants are usually plentiful and are infected by EBV in 70% of cases. The overall prognosis is good.
3. **Lymphocyte-rich type** is an uncommon variant. Reactive lymphocytes make up the vast majority of the non-neoplastic portion of the infiltrate, whereas mononuclear variants and diagnostic RS cells with a classical immunophenotype are reasonably common. This form is associated with EBV in approximately 40% of cases. Prognosis is very good to excellent.
4. **Lymphocyte-depletion type** is the least common form of HL (≤5%) and has a somewhat worse prognosis than other subtypes. RS cells and variants are frequent, and reactive cells are relatively sparse; RS cells are infected with EBV in more than 90% of cases. Advanced stage and systemic symptoms are common, and the overall prognosis is somewhat worse than the other varieties.
5. **Lymphocyte predominance type** accounts for approximately 5% of all cases, and typically presents with axillary or cervical lymphadenopathy. It is characterized by nodal effacement due to nodular infiltrates of small lymphocytes admixed with variable numbers of benign macrophages and *L&H RS cell variants* (classic RS cells are extremely difficult to find). There is no EBV association. The overall prognosis is excellent.

Clinical Features *(p. 610)*. HL typically presents with painless lymphadenopathy. Younger patients with more favorable histologic types tend to present in clinical stage I or II without systemic manifestations. Patients with disseminated disease (stages III and IV) and mixed cellularity or lymphocyte depletion types are more likely to present with B symptoms. Cutaneous anergy due to depressed cell-mediated immunity (attributed to factors released from RS cells that suppress T_H1 responses) is common.

Because HL spreads predictably from its site of origin to contiguous lymphoid groups and then on to spleen, liver, and marrow, staging is not only prognostically important but also guides therapy; patients with limited disease can be cured with local radiotherapy. Staging involves careful physical examination and several investigative procedures, including computed tomography of the abdomen and pelvis, chest radiography, and marrow biopsy.

Tumor burden (i.e., stage) rather than histologic type is the most important prognostic variable. The 5-year survival rate for stage I or IIA disease approaches 90%, and many are likely cured. Even with advanced disease (stage IVA or IVB), a 60% to 70% 5-year, disease-free survival rate is common.

Long-term HL survivors treated with alkylating chemotherapy and radiotherapy have an increased risk of developing second hematologic cancers (MDSs, acute myelogenous leukemia, NHL) or solid cancers of the lung, breast, stomach, skin, or soft tissues. Non-neoplastic complications of radiotherapy include pulmonary fibrosis and accelerated atherosclerosis.

Myeloid Neoplasms *(p. 611)*

The common feature of these neoplasms is an origin from hematopoietic progenitor cells. Myeloid neoplasms primarily involve the marrow with lesser involvement of the secondary hematopoietic organs (spleen, liver, and lymph nodes); clinical presentations are related to altered hematopoiesis. There are three broad categories:

- *AMLs* characterized by marrow accumulation of immature myeloid cells (blasts) that suppress normal hematopoiesis
- MDSs in which ineffective hematopoiesis leads to cytopenias
- MPDs characterized by increased production of one or more blood cell types

Acute Myeloid Leukemia (p. 611)

AML is a tumor of hematopoietic progenitors caused by acquired oncogenic mutations that impede differentiation, leading to the accumulation of immature myeloid blasts.

Classification *(p. 611)*. AML is quite heterogeneous, reflecting the complexities of myeloid cell differentiation. A new WHO system takes into account the molecular lesions that cause AML and is gaining favor largely because it predicts clinical outcome more reliably. In this classification (Table 13-5) AML is divided into four categories based on the presence or absence of characteristic cytogenetic abnormalities, the presence of dysplasia, prior exposure to drugs known to induce AML, and the type and degree of differentiation.

Pathogenesis *(p. 612)*. Most genetic aberrations in AML interfere with transcription factors required for normal myeloid cell differentiation. The most common chromosomal rearrangements, t(8;21) and inv(16), disrupt *RUNX1* and *CBFB* genes, respectively—encoding polypeptides that bind together to form a transcription factor complex required for normal hematopoiesis. In acute promyelocytic leukemia (APML), a t(15;17) translocation results in the fusion of the retinoic acid receptor-α gene *(RARα)* on chromosome 17 to the *PML* (for *promyelocytic leukemia*) gene on chromosome 15. The fusion product encodes an abnormal retinoic acid receptor that interacts with transcriptional repressors and thus blocks myeloid cell differentiation.

Some of the most commonly mutated genes in AML encode proteins that influence DNA methylation or histone modifications. Another 15% of tumors have mutations involving genes encoding

TABLE 13-5 Major Subtypes of AML in the WHO Classification

Class	Prognosis	FAB Subtype
I. AML With Genetic Aberrations		
AML with t(8;21)(q22;q22); *CBFα/ETO* fusion gene	Favorable	M2
AML with inv(16)(p13;q22); *CBFβ/MYH11* fusion gene	Favorable	M4eo
AML with t(15;17)(q22;11-12); *RARα/PML* fusion gene	Intermediate	M3, M3v
AML with t(11q23;v); diverse *MLL* fusion genes	Poor	M4, M5
AML with normal cytogenetics and mutated *NPM*	Favorable	Variable
II. AML With MDS-like Features		
With prior MDS	Poor	Variable
AML with multilineage dysplasia	Poor	Variable
AML with MDS-like cytogenetic aberrations	Poor	Variable
III. AML, Therapy Related	Very poor	Variable
IV. AML, Not Otherwise Specified		
AML, minimally differentiated	Intermediate	M0
AML without maturation	Intermediate	M1
AML with myelocytic maturation	Intermediate	M2
AML with myelomonocytic maturation	Intermediate	M4
AML with monocytic maturation	Intermediate	M5a, M5b
AML with erythroid maturation	Intermediate	M6a, M6b
AML with megakaryocytic maturation	Intermediate	M7

FAB, French-American-British; *MDS*, myelodysplasia; *NPM*, nucleophosmin.

components of the cohesin complex, proteins that regulate the three-dimensional structure of chromatin.

Mutations in genes that promote proliferation and survival (e.g., in tyrosine kinases) also likely synergize with transcription factor mutations to cause full-blown AML. Thus AML with the t(15;17) translocation frequently also has activating mutations in FLT3, a receptor tyrosine kinase that promotes cell growth and inhibits apoptosis.

The t(15;17) not only has pathogenic significance but also guides therapy. Thus tumors with this translocation respond to high doses of all-*trans* retinoic acid (ATRA); ATRA binds to the PML-RARα fusion protein and antagonizes its inhibitory effects on gene transcription.

Morphology *(p. 613).* The number of leukemic cells in the circulation is highly variable: >100,000 cells/μL in some but <10,000 cells/μL in 50% of patients. Occasionally the peripheral smear does not contain any blasts (aleukemic leukemia), and marrow biopsy is required for diagnosis. Myeloid versus lymphoid blasts are distinguished by immunohistochemistry specific for unique surface markers.

AML diagnosis is based on >20% myeloid blasts in the marrow; these will have different morphologic features, depending on the AML type.

- *Myeloblasts* have delicate nuclear chromatin, two to four nucleoli, and voluminous cytoplasm containing fine, azurophilic, peroxidase-positive granules or distinctive red-staining, peroxidase-positive, needlelike structures called *Auer rods.*
- *Monoblasts* have folded or lobulated nuclei, lack Auer rods, and usually do not express peroxidase but can be identified by staining for nonspecific esterase.

Immunophenotype *(p. 614).* AML is confirmed with markers of myeloid lineage, most often immature cells, such as CD33.

Cytogenetics *(p. 614).* A combination of standard cytogenetic techniques and high-resolution banding modalities reveal chromosomal abnormalities in 90% of cases. Several associations have emerged:

- AML arising de novo in patients with no risk factors is often associated with balanced chromosomal translocations (e.g., t(8;21), inv(16), and t(15;17)).
- AMLs that follow an MDS or occur after exposure to DNA-damaging agents (e.g., chemotherapy or radiation therapy) usually lack chromosomal translocations; instead they are commonly associated with deletions or monosomies involving chromosomes 5 and 7.
- AMLs occurring after treatment with drugs that inhibit the enzyme topoisomerase II are often associated with translocations involving the *MLL* gene on chromosome 11 at band q23.

Clinical Features *(p. 614).* Although AML constitutes 20% of childhood leukemias, it primarily affects adults, with incidence rising throughout life and peaking after age 60.

- Most patients present with findings related to *anemia, neutropenia,* and *thrombocytopenia,* most notably fatigue, fever, and spontaneous mucosal and cutaneous bleeding.
- The *bleeding diathesis* caused by thrombocytopenia is often the most striking clinical feature; cutaneous petechiae and ecchymoses, as well as hemorrhages into serosal linings, gingiva, and gastrointestinal and urinary tracts.

- *Procoagulants* released by leukemic cells, especially in APML, can produce *disseminated intravascular coagulation.*
- *Neutropenia leads to infections (frequently opportunistic [e.g., fungi]),* particularly in the oral cavity, skin, lungs, kidneys, urinary bladder, and colon.
- In AML with monocytic differentiation, gingival and skin infiltration *(leukemia cutis)* can occur.
- Central nervous system spread is less common than in ALL.
- Rarely, patients present with localized masses composed of myeloblasts (called *myeloblastomas* or *chloromas*). Without systemic treatment, these typically progress to typical AML.

Prognosis *(p. 614).* Prognosis is variable, depending on the underlying molecular pathogenesis. Overall, 60% achieve complete remission with chemotherapy, but only 15% to 30% remain disease-free for 5 years. AML with t(15;17) is curable in 80% of patients using ATRA and arsenic salts. AML arising out of an MDS (see following section) or after previous chemotherapy has a dismal prognosis, because *normal* HSCs in such patients have likely been damaged.

Myelodysplastic Syndromes (p. 614)

MDSs are a group of clonal stem cell disorders characterized by maturation defects associated with ineffective hematopoiesis and a high risk of transformation to AML. The marrow is partly or wholly replaced by the clonal progeny of a mutant multipotent stem cell that retains the capacity to differentiate but in a manner that is both ineffective and disordered. The marrow is usually hypercellular or normocellular, but the peripheral blood shows pancytopenia; myeloblasts are <10% of peripheral leukocytes.

MDS can be *idiopathic or primary*—developing insidiously in patients over age 50—or can be secondary to previous myelosuppressive chemotherapy or radiotherapy (usually appearing 2 to 8 years after treatment). All forms of MDS can transform to AML; transformation occurs most rapidly and with highest frequency in patients with therapy-related MDS.

Pathogenesis *(p. 614).* Although the pathogenesis is largely unknown, MDS is associated with a number of recurrently mutated genes:

- *Epigenetic factors* (similar to AML) that regulate DNA methylation and histone modifications.
- *RNA splicing factors.*
- *Transcription factors* required for normal myelopoiesis.
- *Loss-of-function mutations in the tumor suppressor gene* TP53 occur in 10% of MDS cases and correlate to poor clinical outcomes.

Progenitors undergo apoptosis at increased rates, a hallmark of ineffective hematopoiesis. Cytogenetic analysis can help to confirm an MDS diagnosis because certain chromosomal aberrations are characteristic. Thus both primary and therapy-related MDS are associated with monosomy 5 and monosomy 7, deletions of 5q and 7q, trisomy 8, and deletions of 20q.

Morphology *(p. 615).* The most characteristic finding is disordered (dysplastic) differentiation affecting all three lineages (erythroid, myeloid, and megakaryocytic).

- Erythroid lineage effects are as follows:
  - Ringed sideroblasts, erythroblasts with iron-laden mitochondria visible as perinuclear granules on Prussian blue stain.

  - Megaloblastoid maturation, resembling that seen in vitamin B_{12} or folate deficiency.
  - Nuclear budding abnormalities, producing misshapen nuclei, often with polypoid outlines.
- Granulocytic lineage effects are as follows:
  - Neutrophils with decreased numbers of secondary granules, toxic granulations, or Döhle bodies.
  - Pseudo-Pelger-Huët cells (neutrophils with only two nuclear lobes).
  - Myeloblasts may be increased but comprise <20% of overall marrow cellularity.
- *Megakaryocytic lineage effects:* Megakaryocytes with single nuclear lobes or multiple separate nuclei ("pawn ball" megakaryocytes).

***Clinical Features** (p. 615).* Mean age of onset is 70 years; half of patients are asymptomatic, and MDS is discovered only incidentally on routine blood testing. Symptoms that arise stem from pancytopenia. Median survival varies from 9 to 29 months (4 to 8 months for therapy-related MDS), but individuals in good prognostic groups can live ≥5 years. Death is related to infections and bleeding complications. Progression to AML occurs in 10% to 40% of individuals, accompanied by the appearance of additional clonal cytogenetic changes. In older patients, therapy is largely supportive (antibiotics and transfusions); in younger patients, HSC transplantation offers the best hope of long-term survival.

Myeloproliferative Disorders (p. 616)

The common pathogenic feature of these disorders is the presence of mutated, constitutively active tyrosine kinases. These tyrosine kinases circumvent normal proliferative control pathways that regulate hematopoiesis and lead to growth factor-independent proliferation and survival of marrow progenitors. These disorders are classified based on clinical, laboratory, and molecular criteria. Common clinical features include the following:

- Increased proliferative drive in the marrow
- Homing of HSCs to nonmarrow sites, causing extramedullary hematopoiesis
- Variable transformation to a spent phase characterized by marrow fibrosis and peripheral cytopenia
- Variable transformation to acute leukemia

Chronic Myelogenous Leukemia (p. 616)

CML is a neoplasm of pluripotent HSCs leading to preferential proliferation of granulocytic progenitors. It is distinguished from other MPDs by the presence of a *chimeric, constitutively active BCR-ABL tyrosine kinase.*

***Pathogenesis** (p. 617).* In >90% of CML the *BCR-ABL* fusion gene is generated by the reciprocal t(9;22) translocation designated as the Philadelphia chromosome. In the remaining cases the fusion gene is created by cytogenetically complex rearrangements.

- t(9;22) leads to fusion of portions of the *BCR* gene (chromosome 22) and the *ABL* gene (chromosome 9).
- The resultant *BCR-ABL* fusion gene directs the synthesis of a 210-kilodalton fusion protein with constitutive tyrosine kinase activity. The BCR portion provides a dimerization domain, leading to the activation of ABL kinase; ABL phosphorylates downstream targets to drive proliferation and survival.

Morphology *(p. 617)*. CML marrow specimens are markedly hypercellular, with most of the increased cellularity comprising maturing granulocytic precursors. Peripheral blood shows leukocytosis, often more than 100,000 cells/μL. A mixture of neutrophils, metamyelocytes, and myelocytes, with fewer than 10% myeloblasts, is typical. Peripheral blood eosinophilia, basophilia, and thrombocytosis are also common. Extramedullary hematopoiesis within the splenic red pulp produces marked splenomegaly, often complicated by focal infarction.

Clinical Features *(p. 617)*. CML primarily occurs in adults with a peak incidence from 50 to 60 years of age. Onset is insidious; initial symptoms (fatigability, weakness, weight loss, and anorexia) are due to anemia and hypermetabolism, owing to increased cell turnover. Other presentations are related to splenomegaly or splenic infarction.

- After a variable *stable phase* period averaging 3 years, 50% of patients enter an *accelerated phase* marked by worsening anemia and thrombocytopenia, increased basophilia, and refractoriness to treatment. Additional clonal cytogenetic abnormalities (e.g., trisomy 8, isochromosome 17q, or duplication of the Philadelphia chromosome) may appear.
- Within 6 to 12 months, the accelerated phase terminates in acute leukemia *(blast crisis)*.
- In the remaining 50%, blast crises occur abruptly without an intermediate accelerated phase.
- In 70% of patients, blasts have the morphologic and cytochemical features of myeloblasts; in approximately 30%, blasts are of pre-B-cell origin (lymphoid blast crisis).

CML is curable in 75% of patients by allogeneic bone marrow transplantation during the stable phase. Imatinib, a BCR-ABL kinase inhibitor, markedly decreases (but does not eliminate) the number of BCR-ABL-positive cells, and yields sustained hematologic remissions in 90% of patients. It also substantially decreases the risk of transformation to the accelerated phase and blast crisis; once in accelerated phase or blast crisis, CML is largely resistant to kinase inhibitor therapy.

Polycythemia Vera (PCV) (p. 618)

PCV is characterized by increased marrow production of erythrocytes, granulocytes, and platelets. However, the absolute increase in red blood cell mass is responsible for most of the clinical symptoms. PCV is strongly associated with activating point mutations in the JAK2 tyrosine kinase that participates in JAK-STAT signaling pathways.

Pathogenesis *(p. 618)*. Due to constitutive JAK2 signaling, progenitor cells in PCV have diminished requirements for erythropoietin and other hematopoietic growth factors, leading to substantial ongoing proliferation.

Morphology *(p. 618)*. There is hypercellular marrow involving all three lineages; 10% of patients have increased marrow reticulin fibers. Peripheral blood exhibits basophilia and abnormally large platelets. Late in the disease 15% to 20% of PCV patients progress to a spent phase with substantial marrow fibrosis that displaces hematopoietic cells. This in turn leads to *extramedullary hematopoiesis* in the spleen and liver, producing prominent organomegaly. Transformation to AML occurs in just 1% of patients.

Clinical Features *(p. 619).* PCV appears insidiously, usually in late middle age:

- *Erythrocytosis* causes patients to be plethoric and cyanotic due to vascular stagnation and deoxygenation. Headache, dizziness, and hypertension are common findings.
- *Basophilia* with histamine release may underlie gastrointestinal symptoms, increased tendency to peptic ulceration, and intense pruritus.
- *High cell turnover* causes hyperuricemia and symptomatic gout in 5% to 10% of cases.
- *Platelet dysfunction* coupled with abnormal blood flow leads to increased risk of both major bleeding and thrombotic events. Approximately 25% of patients first come to clinical attention with thrombosis; life-threatening hemorrhages occur in 5% to 10% of cases.

With no treatment, death from bleeding or thrombosis occurs within months. Simple phlebotomy to normalize the hematocrit results in median survival of approximately 10 years. JAK2 inhibitors are in clinical trials.

Essential Thrombocytosis (ET) (p. 619)

ET is an MPD arising in multipotent stem cells, but the increased proliferation and production is largely confined to the megakaryocytic elements. *ET is associated with activating point mutations in JAK2 (50% of cases) or MPL (5% to 10% of cases), a tyrosine kinase that is normally activated by thrombopoietin.* These mutations render megakaryocytic lineage progenitors thrombopoietin-independent and lead to hyperproliferation. Why some patients with *JAK2* mutations develop PCV and others ET is not understood.

Marrow cellularity is usually only mildly increased, but megakaryocytes are often markedly increased and include abnormally large forms. Peripheral smears reveal thrombocytosis and abnormally large platelets, accompanied by mild leukocytosis. Neoplastic extramedullary hematopoiesis can produce mild organomegaly (50% of cases). Uncommonly, ET can evolve to a spent phase of marrow fibrosis or transform to AML.

Qualitative and quantitative abnormalities in platelets underlie the major clinical manifestations of thrombosis and hemorrhage. *Erythromelalgia,* the throbbing and burning of hands and feet caused by occlusion of small arterioles by platelet aggregates, is a characteristic symptom.

ET has an indolent course; long asymptomatic periods are punctuated by thrombotic or hemorrhagic crises. Median survival time is 12 to 15 years.

Primary Myelofibrosis (p. 620)

Primary myelofibrosis is characterized by the development of obliterative marrow fibrosis, which—in turn—leads to diminished hematopoiesis, cytopenias, and extensive extramedullary hematopoiesis (spleens can be >4000 g).

Activating JAK2 mutations are present in 50% to 60% of cases and activating MPL mutations in 1% to 5%. The resulting marrow fibrosis and obliteration may be secondary to release of fibrogenic factors from neoplastic megakaryocytes; platelet-derived growth factor and TGF-β are both implicated. With displacement of hematopoietic elements to extramedullary sites (e.g., spleen, liver, and sometimes lymph nodes), the resulting blood cell production is often disordered.

Morphology *(p. 620)*

- Early, the marrow is often hypercellular and contains large, dysplastic, and abnormally clustered megakaryocytes. With progression, diffuse fibrosis displaces hematopoietic elements. Late in the course, the fibrotic marrow space can be largely converted to bone (osteosclerosis).
- Nucleated erythroid progenitors and early granulocytes are inappropriately released from the fibrotic marrow and sites of extramedullary hematopoiesis; their appearance in the circulation is termed *leukoerythroblastosis.* Other frequent peripheral blood findings include teardrop erythrocytes, increased basophils, and abnormally large platelets.
- Moderate-to-severe normochromic, normocytic anemia is common. The white blood cell count is usually normal or reduced but can be markedly elevated (80,000 to 100,000 cells/μL) during the early cellular marrow phase. Thrombocytopenia, often severe, appears with disease progression.

Clinical Features *(p. 621).* Primary myelofibrosis typically occurs in patients >60 years of age; it is less common than PCV or ET. It often presents with anemia or marked splenic enlargement. Nonspecific symptoms (e.g., fatigue, weight loss, and night sweats) result from increased metabolism associated with the expanded mass of hematopoietic cells. Owing to high cell turnover, hyperuricemia and secondary gout can complicate the picture. Prognosis is variable, with median survival periods of 3 to 5 years. Causes of death include infections, thrombotic episodes or bleeding related to platelet abnormalities, and transformation to AML (5% to 20% of cases). JAK2 inhibition is a therapeutic approach that reduces constitutional symptoms (e.g., fever and fatigue) even in patients without JAK2 mutations—suggesting that such symptoms may result from cytokine signaling via JAK-STAT in nontransformed cells.

Langerhans Cell Histiocytosis (p. 621)

There are three types of *histiocytoses* (an archaic term for proliferations of dendritic cells and macrophages):

- True histiocytic lymphomas (rare).
- Benign, reactive histiocytoses.
- Langerhans cell histiocytoses; these represent monoclonal neoplastic proliferations of an immature dendritic cell population; the most common mutation is an activating valine-to-glutamate substitution at residue 600 in BRAF, present in 55% to 60% of cases.

In this latter group the proliferating Langerhans cells have abundant, often vacuolated cytoplasm, with vesicular oval-to-indented nuclei; expression of HLA-DR, S100, and CD1a is characteristic. Electron microscopy also reveals cytoplasmic structures called *Birbeck granules;* these are pentalaminar tubules resembling tennis racquets and containing the protein *langerin.* Homing of the neoplastic Langerhans cells is dependent on their expression of CCR6 and CCR7.

Langerhans histiocytoses present as several different clinicopathologic entities:

- ***Multifocal multisystem Langerhans cell histiocytosis (Letterer-Siwe disease)*** is an aggressive, systemic disorder in which Langerhans cells infiltrate and proliferate within skin (there resembling a seborrheic eruption), spleen, liver, lung, and bone marrow;

anemia and destructive bony lesions are also seen. Usually occurring before age 2, Letterer-Siwe disease is rapidly fatal if untreated. Intensive chemotherapy yields 5-year survival rates of approximately 50%.

- ***Unifocal and multifocal unisystem Langerhans cell histiocytosis (eosinophilic granuloma)*** usually affects the skeleton as an erosive, expanding accumulation of Langerhans cells (commonly admixed with lymphocytes, plasma cells, neutrophils, and especially eosinophils) within calvarium, ribs, or femur; it can also occur in skin, lungs, or stomach. Lesions can be asymptomatic or painful; pathologic fractures may occur, and lesions can sometime expand into adjacent soft tissues. Involvement of the posterior hypothalamus causes diabetes insipidus in 50% of patients; indeed the triad of calvarial bone defects, diabetes insipidus, and exophthalmos is called *Hand-Schüller-Christian syndrome.* Lesions can remit spontaneously or may be cured by local excision or irradiation.
- ***Pulmonary Langerhans cell histiocytosis*** typically occurs in adult smokers and may represent a reactive hyperplasia rather than a true neoplasm; it can spontaneously regress with smoking cessation.

Spleen (p. 623)

The spleen has four functions that impact disease states:

1. Phagocytosis of blood cells and particulate matter
2. Antibody production
3. Hematopoiesis
4. Sequestration of formed blood elements

Splenomegaly (p. 624)

Splenomegaly is a common feature of hematolymphoid disorders, but spleens can be enlarged in a wide variety of non-neoplastic conditions (Table 13-6). *Hypersplenism* is a syndrome that can occur with splenic enlargement; it is characterized by reduction of one or more cellular elements of the blood (due to increased sequestration and splenic macrophage lysis). The cytopenias typically resolve after splenectomy.

Nonspecific Acute Splenitis (p. 624)

Splenic enlargement can occur with any bloodborne infection, largely due to the microbes themselves, as well as cytokine-induced proliferation. Grossly the spleen is red and extremely soft. Microscopically there is red pulp congestion with lymphoid follicle effacement, occasionally with white pulp follicular necrosis.

Congestive Splenomegaly (p. 624)

Passive chronic venous congestion and enlargement can result from the following:

- Systemic congestion, encountered in right-sided cardiac failure
- Intrahepatic derangement of portal venous drainage (e.g., due to cirrhosis)
- Extrahepatic portal vein obstruction (e.g., spontaneous portal vein thrombosis); inflammatory involvement of the portal vein *(pylephlebitis),* with intraperitoneal infections; and thrombosis of the splenic vein

There is moderate-to-marked splenic enlargement (1000 to 5000 g), with a thickened, fibrous capsule. Microscopically the red pulp is acutely congested but becomes increasingly fibrous and

TABLE 13-6 Disorders Associated With Splenomegaly

I. Infections
Nonspecific splenitis of various bloodborne infections (particularly infective endocarditis)
Infectious mononucleosis
Tuberculosis
Typhoid fever
Brucellosis
Cytomegalovirus
Syphilis
Malaria
Histoplasmosis
Toxoplasmosis
Kala-azar
Trypanosomiasis
Schistosomiasis
Leishmaniasis
Echinococcosis
II. Congestive States Related to Portal Hypertension
Cirrhosis of the liver
Portal or splenic vein thrombosis
Cardiac failure
III. Lymphohematogenous Disorders
HL
NHLs and lymphocytic leukemias
Multiple myeloma
MPDs
Hemolytic anemias
Thromobocytopenic purpura
IV. Immunologic Inflammatory Conditions
Rheumatoid arthritis
Systemic lupus erythematosus
V. Storage Diseases
Gaucher disease
Niemann-Pick disease
Mucopolysaccharidoses
VI. Miscellaneous
Amyloidosis
Primary neoplasms and cysts
Secondary neoplasms

cellular with time, leading to the vascular stasis and increased macrophage clearance.

Splenic Infarcts (p. 625)

Embolic infarcts occur in endocarditis and in severe atherosclerosis. Infarction due to enlargement and compromise of intrasplenic blood flow can occur in virtually any condition that causes significant splenomegaly (Table 13-5). Grossly infarcts are wedge-shaped and subcapsular. Fresh infarcts are hemorrhagic and red; older infarcts are yellow-gray and fibrotic.

Neoplasms (p. 625)

Neoplastic involvement of the spleen is rare except in cases of myeloid and lymphoid tumors. Benign splenic tumors include fibromas, osteomas, chondromas, lymphangiomas, and hemangiomas.

Congenital Anomalies (p. 625)

Complete absence of the spleen is rare and is usually associated with other congenital anomalies, such as *situs inversus;* hypoplasia is considerably more common. *Accessory spleens* are fairly common (up to a third of individuals) and can be found anywhere in the abdominal cavity.

Rupture (p. 625)

Splenic rupture is typically a sequela of blunt force trauma; so-called "spontaneous ruptures" without antecedent injury usually result from some minor physical insult to a spleen already rendered fragile due to an underlying disorder (e.g., infectious mononucleosis, other infections, or splenic neoplasms). Rupture leads to significant intraperitoneal hemorrhage and must be treated with prompt splenectomy to prevent exsanguination. Interestingly, chronically enlarged spleens often have reactive capsular fibrosis that resists rupture.

Thymus (p. 625)

Developmental Disorders (p. 626)

- *Thymic hypoplasia or aplasia* is accompanied by parathyroid aplasia and variable defects involving the heart and great vessels; these changes occur in *DiGeorge syndrome* (see Chapter 5).
- *Thymic cysts* are uncommon lesions lined by stratified or columnar epithelium; they are mostly developmental in origin and of little clinical significance. Occasionally, thymic cysts herald an adjacent thymic neoplasm, especially lymphoma or thymoma.

Thymic Hyperplasia (p. 626)

Thymic hyperplasia refers to the appearance of reactive B-cell lymphoid follicles within the thymus. It is seen in chronic inflammatory and immunologic states, particularly myasthenia gravis (65% to 75% of cases).

Thymomas (p. 626)

Thymomas are neoplasms derived from *thymic epithelial cells.* These may be: (1) cytologically benign and noninvasive; (2) cytologically benign but invasive or metastatic; or (3) cytologically malignant *(thymic carcinoma).*

Morphology (p. 627)

- *Grossly:* Thymomas are usually lobulated, firm, gray-white masses up to 15 to 20 cm; they can exhibit focal cystic necrosis and calcification. Most are encapsulated, but in 20% to 25% adjacent structures are invaded; benign tumors are typically well encapsulated.
- *Microscopically:*
  - *Noninvasive thymomas* are composed of medullary (spindled) and/or cortical (plump with rounded vesicular nuclei) epithelial cells, often with a sparse thymocyte infiltrate.
  - *Invasive thymomas* more commonly exhibit cortical-type epithelial cells and more numerous thymocytes. Occasionally,

neoplastic cells exhibit atypia, presaging a more aggressive phenotype. Invasive thymomas—by definition—penetrate through the capsule into surrounding structures.

- *Thymic carcinoma* represents 5% of thymomas; they are fleshy, invasive masses that are most commonly *squamous cell carcinomas.* The second most common variant is *lymphoepithelioma-like carcinoma,* microscopically resembling nasopharyngeal carcinomas, and in 50% of cases containing monoclonal EBV genomes.

Clinical Features *(p. 627)*

These are tumors primarily of adults >40 years of age; approximately 40% present with symptoms referable to compression of mediastinal structures and an additional 30% to 45% present with *myasthenia gravis.* Thymomas are associated with other paraneoplastic syndromes (e.g., acquired hypogammaglobulinemia, pure red blood cell aplasia, Graves disease, pernicious anemia, dermatomyositis and polymyositis, and Cushing syndrome). For minimally invasive lesions, complete excision results in >90% 5-year survivals; more extensive invasion is associated with 5-year survivals <50%.

Red Blood Cell and Bleeding Disorders

14

Anemias (p. 629)

Anemia is a reduction in the total circulating red blood cell (RBC) mass below normal limits; the consequences are reduced oxygen-carrying capacity and tissue hypoxia. Patients are pale, weak, and easily fatigued. Anemia is formally diagnosed based on a reduction in the hematocrit and/or hemoglobin concentration (Table 14-1). The classification of anemias is usually mechanistically based, as outlined in Table 14-2; the specifics of RBC morphology (size, shape, and hemoglobinization—as reflected in erythrocyte color) can often provide etiologic clues. Thus microcytic, hypochromic anemias suggest disorders of hemoglobin synthesis (most often iron deficiency), whereas macrocytic anemias suggest abnormalities in bone marrow erythroid precursor maturation; normochromic, normocytic anemias have diverse etiologies.

Anemias of Blood Loss (p. 631)

Clinical features depend on the rate of hemorrhage and whether it is external or internal; interstitial bleeding allows recapture of red cell iron, but bleeding into the gut or externally can lead to iron deficiency and hamper restoration of normal RBC counts.

- *Acute blood loss* (p. 631): Any clinical effects are due mainly to the loss of intravascular volume; shock and/or death can result. If the patient survives, fluid shifts from the interstitium rapidly restore the blood volume. However, there will be hemodilution and lowering of the hematocrit; the resulting reduction

TABLE 14-1 Adult Reference Ranges for Red Blood Cells*

Measurement (Units)	Men	Women
Hemoglobin (g/dL)	13.6-17.2	12.0-15.0
Hematocrit (%)	39-49	33-43
RBC count ($10^6/\mu L$)	4.3-5.9	3.5-5.0
Reticulocyte count (%)	0.5-1.5	
Mean cell volume (fL)	82-96	
Mean corpuscular hemoglobin (pg)	27-33	
Mean corpuscular hemoglobin concentration (g/dL)	33-37	
RBC distribution width (expressing the degree of anisocytosis)	11.5-14.5	

*Reference ranges vary among laboratories. The reference ranges for the laboratory providing the result should always be used in interpreting the test result.

TABLE 14-2 Classification of Anemia According to Underlying Mechanism

Mechanism	Specific Examples
Blood Loss	
Acute blood loss	Trauma
Chronic blood loss	GI tract lesions, gynecologic disturbances*
Increased Red Cell Destruction (Hemolysis)	
Inherited genetic defects	
Red cell membrane disorders	HS, hereditary elliptocytosis
Enzyme deficiencies	
Hexose monophosphate shunt enzyme deficiencies	G6PD deficiency, glutathione synthetase deficiency
Glycolytic enzyme deficiencies	Pyruvate kinase deficiency, hexokinase deficiency
Hemoglobin abnormalities	
Deficient globin synthesis	Thalassemia syndromes
Structurally abnormal globins (hemoglobinopathies)	Sickle cell disease, unstable hemoglobins
Acquired genetic defects	
Deficiency of phosphatidylinositol-linked glycoproteins	PNH
Antibody-mediated destruction	Hemolytic disease of the newborn (Rh disease), transfusion reactions, drug-induced, autoimmune disorders
Mechanical trauma	
Microangiopathic hemolytic anemias	Hemolytic uremic syndrome, DIC, thrombotic thrombocytopenia purpura
Cardiac traumatic hemolysis	Defective cardiac valves
Repetitive physical trauma	Bongo drumming, marathon running, karate chopping
Infections of red cells	Malaria, babesiosis
Toxic or chemical injury	Clostridial sepsis, snake venom, lead poisoning
Membrane lipid abnormalities	Abetalipoproteinemia, severe hepatocellular liver disease
Sequestration	Hypersplenism
Decreased Red Cell Production	
Inherited genetic defects	
Defects leading to stem cell depletion	Fanconi anemia, telomerase defects
Defects affecting erythroblast maturation	Thalassemia syndromes
Nutritional deficiencies	
Deficiencies affecting DNA synthesis	Vitamin B_{12} and folate deficiencies
Deficiencies affecting hemoglobin synthesis	Iron deficiency anemia
Erythropoietin deficiency	Renal failure, anemia of chronic disease
Immune-mediated injury of progenitors	Aplastic anemia, pure red cell aplasia
Inflammation-mediated iron sequestration	Anemia of chronic disease
Primary hematopoietic neoplasms	Acute leukemia, myelodysplasia, myeloproliferative disorders (see Chapter 13)

TABLE 14-2 Classification of Anemia According to Underlying Mechanism—cont'd

Mechanism	Specific Examples
Decreased Red Cell Production—cont'd	
Space-occupying marrow lesions	Metastatic neoplasms, granulomatous disease
Infections of red cell progenitors	Parvovirus B19 infection
Unknown mechanisms	Endocrine disorders, hepatocellular liver disease

*Most often cause of anemia is iron deficiency, not bleeding per se.

in oxygen-carrying capacity triggers renal erythropoietin production, with increased proliferation of committed erythroid progenitors. Release of new RBCs begins at day 5; it is heralded by increased numbers of reticulocytes (large, immature RBCs) peaking at 10% to 15% of the peripheral RBC count by day 7. Significant bleeding (with hypotension) also triggers an adrenergic response that mobilizes granulocytes from the intravascular marginated pool (causing leukocytosis); thrombocytosis also occurs due to increased platelet production.

- *Chronic blood loss* (p. 631): Anemia will occur only if the rate of loss exceeds the marrow regenerative capacity or when iron reserves are depleted.

Hemolytic Anemias (p. 631)

Hemolytic anemias feature premature RBC destruction (less than the normal 120-day lifespan), elevated erythropoietin with increased erythropoiesis, and increased hemoglobin catabolites (e.g., bilirubin). The excess serum bilirubin is unconjugated; the ultimate levels of hyperbilirubinemia depend on liver functional capacity and the rate of hemolysis; with normal livers, jaundice is rarely severe.

Hemolysis can occur in either extravascular or intravascular locations:

- *Extravascular hemolysis* occurs in macrophages of the spleen (and other organs). Predisposing factors include RBC membrane injury, reduced deformability, or opsonization. The principal clinical features are anemia, splenomegaly, and jaundice; modest reductions in haptoglobin (a serum protein that binds hemoglobin) also occur.
- *Intravascular hemolysis:* RBCs can be ruptured by mechanical injury (e.g., mechanical cardiac valves), complement fixation (e.g., mismatched blood transfusion), intracellular parasites (e.g., malaria), or extracellular toxins (e.g., clostridial enzymes). Patients exhibit anemia, hemoglobinemia, hemoglobinuria, hemosiderinuria, and jaundice; there is markedly reduced serum haptoglobin. Free hemoglobin can be oxidized to methemoglobin. Both forms of the protein are excreted in the urine (imparting a brown color) or are resorbed by renal proximal tubules; iron released from hemoglobin can accumulate in tubular cells (renal hemosiderosis).

Hereditary Spherocytosis (p. 632)

Hereditary spherocytosis (HS) is due to cytoskeletal or membrane protein defects that render RBCs spheroidal and less deformable and thus vulnerable to splenic sequestration and destruction; it is autosomal dominant in 75% of patients.

Pathogenesis (p. 632)

Insufficiency in several different proteins (spectrin, ankyrin, band 3, or band 4.2) can cause HS; all lead to reduced density of membrane skeletal components, which in turn causes reduced stability of the lipid bilayer and loss of membrane fragments as RBCs age. Compound heterozygosity for two defective alleles typically causes a more severe phenotype. Reduction in surface area causes RBCs to assume a spheroidal shape with diminished deformability and a propensity for being trapped and destroyed by splenic macrophages.

Morphology (p. 633)

Spherocytic RBCs are small and lack central pallor; there is reticulocytosis and marrow erythroid hyperplasia. Marked splenic congestion is seen with prominent erythrophagocytosis in the cords of Billroth.

Clinical Features (p. 633)

Diagnosis depends on family history, hematologic findings, and increased RBC osmotic fragility; the mean RBC hemoglobin concentration is increased due to cellular dehydration. Anemia, moderate splenomegaly, and jaundice are characteristic. Although the clinical course is typically stable due to compensatory increases in erythropoiesis, increased RBC turnover or diminished erythropoiesis can be problematic. Thus *aplastic crisis* occurs when parvovirus induces transient suppression of erythropoiesis; events that increase splenic RBC destruction (e.g., infectious mononucleosis) trigger *hemolytic crisis.* Half of adults develop gallstones from chronic hyperbilirubinemia.

Hemolytic Disease Due to Red Cell Enzyme Defects: Glucose-6-Phosphate Dehydrogenase Deficiency (p. 634)

Glucose-6-phosphate dehydrogenase (G6PD) is an enzyme in the hexose monophosphate shunt that reduces nicotine adenine dinucleotide phosphate (NAPD) to NADPH; in turn, NADPH reduces RBC glutathione—providing protection against RBC oxidative injury. In G6PD-deficient cells, oxidant stress (e.g., due to inflammation, drugs, or foods, such as fava beans) causes hemoglobin sulfhydryl cross-linking and protein denaturation. The altered hemoglobin precipitates as *Heinz bodies* that can cause direct hemolysis; in addition, the precipitated hemoglobin can attach to the inner cell membrane, reduce deformability, and increase susceptibility to splenic macrophage destruction.

G6PD deficiency is an X-linked disorder; although there are several G6PD variants, only two—G6PD$^-$ and G6PD Mediterranean—lead to clinically significant hemolysis. G6PD$^-$ is present in approximately 10% of American blacks; abnormal protein folding leads to increased proteolytic degradation and thus progressive loss of G6PD in older RBCs. Because younger RBCs are unaffected, hemolytic episodes are usually self-limited. In the Mediterranean form, G6PD levels are much lower and hemolytic episodes are more severe.

Sickle Cell Disease (p. 635)

Sickle cell disease is a hereditary hemoglobinopathy resulting from substitution of valine for glutamic acid at the sixth position of the β-globin chain; the resultant mutant hemoglobin S (HbS) substitutes for the normal β-globin monomer in the hemoglobin tetramer $\alpha_2\beta_2$ (HbA). This is an autosomal recessive disorder; 8% to 10% of African Americans are heterozygous for HbS (*sickle cell trait,* which is largely asymptomatic), whereas 70,000 individuals in the United States are homozygous for the mutant allele ($\alpha_2\beta^s{}_2$) and have *sickle cell disease.*

Pathogenesis (p. 635)

When deoxygenated, HbS polymerizes into long, stiff chains that deform (sickle) RBCs. This in turn causes chronic hemolysis, microvascular occlusion, and tissue damage. Several variables affect the rate and degree of sickling.

- *Interaction of HbS with the other types of hemoglobin within RBC:* In heterozygotes, HbS constitutes only 40% of the hemoglobin with the remainder being HbA; the HbA interferes with HbS polymerization. Consequently in heterozygotes, sickling occurs only with profound hypoxia. β-Globin chains other than HbA also influence sickling. Thus fetal hemoglobin (HbF, with γ-globin chains) also interferes with HbS polymerization, and newborns do not manifest disease complications until 5 to 6 months of age when RBC HbF content is reduced to adult levels. For the fortunate adult patient who has hereditary persistence of HbF, the sickle cell disease is considerably less severe. Another variant hemoglobin is HbC (substituting lysine for the glutamic acid in the β-chain sixth position); in patients with HbSC, HbS constitutes 50% of the hemoglobin, and the HbSC cells have a tendency to lose salt and water, becoming dehydrated—which increases the intracellular HbS concentrations. Both factors increase the tendency of the HbS to polymerize, and thus result in HbSC patients having a symptomatic (albeit milder) sickling disorder called *HbSC disease.*
- *Mean cell hemoglobin concentration (MCHC):* Higher HbS concentrations increase the probability of interaction between individual HbS molecules. Thus dehydration—which increases MCHC—facilitates sickling. Conversely, concurrent diseases that reduce MCHC (e.g., α-thalassemia) lessen sickling severity.
- *Intracellular pH:* Reduced pH reduces hemoglobin oxygen affinity, thereby increasing the proportion of deoxygenated HbS and the propensity to polymerize.
- *Microvascular transit time:* Normally the capillary transit rate is sufficiently high that significant deoxygenation (and therefore sickling) cannot occur. Consequently, sickling is usually confined to tissues with intrinsically sluggish blood flow (e.g., spleen, bone marrow) or those involved by inflammation, where transit rates are retarded.

Although reoxygenation depolymerizes HbS, repeated cycles of sickling eventually result in irreversible RBC damage. This happens because polymerized HbS herniates through the membrane skeleton ensheathed by only a lipid bilayer; such severe membrane derangements cause Ca^{2+} influx, protein cross-linking, and water and potassium efflux. With repeated episodes, RBCs become progressively dehydrated, dense, and rigid, and the most damaged cells eventually become end-stage, nondeformable RBCs that retain the sickle shape even when fully oxygenated. Nondeformable cells are prone to macrophage sequestration and destruction and are also intrinsically more mechanically fragile, undergoing intravascular hemolysis.

Microvascular occlusion with resultant tissue hypoxia and infarction is the most clinically important clinical aspect of sickle cell disease. The propensity to occlude small vessels is not strictly dependent on the percentage of irreversibly sickled cells in the blood; rather it is a function of RBC stickiness (sickled RBCs express increased levels of adhesion molecules), local inflammation, and platelet aggregation. Stagnation of RBCs in inflamed vascular beds likely leads to a vicious cycle of sickling, obstruction, hypoxia, and more inflammation. In addition, free hemoglobin released from ruptured RBC binds and inactivates nitric oxide (NO)—increasing vascular tone and enhancing platelet aggregation.

Morphology (p. 636)

- *Peripheral blood* shows variable numbers of irreversibly sickled cells, reticulocytosis, and target cells due to RBC dehydration.
- In childhood there is *splenomegaly* due to sickled cell trapping in splenic cords. By adulthood repeated episodes of vaso-occlusion have caused progressive fibrosis and shrinkage *(autosplenectomy).*
- *Bone marrow* shows normoblastic hyperplasia. When hyperplasia is severe, expansion of the marrow can cause bone resorption; extramedullary hematopoiesis can occur.
- *Microvascular occlusions* produce damage and infarction in various tissues.

Clinical Features (p. 637)

- Chronic hemolytic anemia (hematocrits from 18% to 30%) is associated with chronic hyperbilirubinemia and a propensity for gallstones. Chronic hypoxia will cause generalized impairment of growth and development.
- *Vaso-occlusive crises* present as painful episodes of ischemic necrosis, most commonly involving bones, lungs, liver, brain, penis, and spleen. Vascular obstruction in the retina can cause loss of visual acuity and even blindness. *Acute chest syndrome* is a particularly serious vaso-occlusive crisis caused by pulmonary inflammation that impedes lung vascular flow; sickling and occlusion compromises pulmonary function and potentially leads to a fatal cycle of worsening pulmonary and systemic hypoxia. Priapism affects almost half of males after puberty, potentially with associated hypoxic injury and erectile dysfunction.
- *Aplastic crisis* due to transient suppression of erythropoiesis is triggered by parvovirus infections. *Sequestration crises* occur in children with intact spleens; massive entrapment of sickled RBCs leads to rapid splenic enlargement, hypovolemia, and occasionally shock.
- Progressive splenic fibrosis and impairment of the alternate complement pathway predispose to infections, particularly involving encapsulated organisms, such as *Streptococcus pneumoniae* and *Haemophilus influenzae.*

Diagnosis is based on clinical findings, sickle cells in the peripheral blood smear, and detection of HbS by hemoglobin electrophoresis. Prenatal detection is possible through fetal DNA analysis. Hydroxyurea is a therapeutic mainstay: it increases HbF levels and also reduces white cell production (reducing inflammation). Some 90% of patients survive to age 20, and over half live to age 60.

Thalassemia Syndromes *(p. 638)*

Thalassemia syndromes *are a heterogeneous group of inherited disorders caused by mutations that reduce α- or β-globin chain synthesis* (Table 14-3). β chains are encoded by a single gene on chromosome 11 (yielding two copies); α chains are encoded by two closely linked genes on chromosome 16 (yielding four copies). Diminished synthesis of one chain has pathologic consequences due to the following: (1) low intracellular hemoglobin (hypochromia) and (2) effects related to a relative excess of the other chain. The syndromes

TABLE 14-3 Clinical and Genetic Classification of Thalassemias

Clinical Syndromes	Genotype	Clinical Features	Molecular Genetics
β-Thalassemias			
β-Thalassemia major	Homozygous β-thalassemia (β^0/β^0, β^+/β^+, β^0/β^+)	Severe; requires blood transfusions	Mainly point mutations that lead to defects in the transcription, splicing, or translation of β-globin mRNA
β-Thalassemia intermedia	Variable (β^0/β^+, β^+/β^+, β^0/β, β^+/β)	Severe but does not require regular blood transfusions	
β-Thalassemia minor	Heterozygous β-thalassemia (β^0/β, β^+/β)	Asymptomatic with mild or absent anemia; red cell abnormalities seen	
α-Thalassemias			
Silent carrier	–/α α/α	Asymptomatic; no red cell abnormality	Mainly gene deletions
α-Thalassemia trait	–/– α/α (Asian) –/α –/α (black African, Asian)	Asymptomatic, like β-thalassemia minor	
HbH disease	–/– –/α	Severe; resembles β-thalassemia intermedia	
Hydrops fetalis	–/– –/–	Lethal in utero without transfusions	

are most common in Mediterranean countries, parts of Africa, and Southeast Asia.

β-Thalassemias (p. 638)

β-*Thalassemias* are characterized by deficient synthesis of β-globin:

- β^0 mutations abrogate β-globin chain synthesis; most commonly these involve chain termination mutations that create premature stop codons.
- β^+ mutations lead to reduced (but detectable) β-globin synthesis; most commonly these involve aberrant RNA splicing, although some are promoter region mutations.

Molecular Pathogenesis *(p. 638).* With decreased β-globin synthesis, there is reduced HbA production; the "under-hemoglobinized" RBCs are hypochromic and microcytic with reduced oxygen-carrying capacity. In addition, excess unbound α chains form highly unstable aggregates that cause cell membrane damage; this leads to precursor destruction in the marrow (ineffective erythropoiesis) and splenic sequestration of mature RBCs. Severe anemia causes marked compensatory expansion of the erythropoietic marrow, ultimately encroaching on cortical bone and causing skeletal abnormalities in growing children. Ineffective erythropoiesis is also associated with excessive absorption of dietary iron; along with repeated blood transfusions this leads to severe iron overload.

Clinical Syndromes *(p. 639).* Classification of β-thalassemia is based on the severity of anemia; severity is based on the genetic defect (β^+ or β^0), as well as gene dosage (homozygous or heterozygous).

- β-*Thalassemia major (p. 640):* Patients with two β-thalassemia alleles (β^+/β^+, β^+/β^0, or β^0/β^0) typically have severe, transfusion-dependent anemia; the manifestations begin 6 to 9 months after birth as hemoglobin synthesis switches from HbF to HbA.
  - Peripheral blood shows marked anisocytosis (variability in cell size) with many microcytic, hypochromic RBCs, target cells, and erythrocyte fragments; poorly hemoglobinized RBC precursors (normoblasts) are also common.
  - There is marked expansion of the hematopoietic marrow, with erosion of existing cortical bone and subsequent new bone formation. Extramedullary hematopoiesis is common with splenomegaly.
  - Without transfusions, death occurs at an early age from profound anemia. Blood transfusions lessen the anemia and suppress the secondary bone deformities. In multiply transfused patients, morbidity and fatality are related to cardiac failure resulting from progressive iron overload and secondary hemochromatosis; iron chelation can slow (but not prevent) these complications. Bone marrow transplant is the only curative therapy.
- β-*Thalassemia minor (p. 641):* Heterozygotes are usually asymptomatic due to sufficient β-globin synthesis.
  - Peripheral blood shows minor abnormalities, including hypochromia, microcytosis, basophilic stippling, and target cells. Hemoglobin electrophoresis shows increased HbA_2 ($\alpha_2\delta_2$ hemoglobin) due to increased ratios of δ- versus β-globin synthesis.
  - Recognition of β-thalassemia trait is important for genetic counseling.
- *Thalassemia intermedia:* Clinical consequences and severity are intermediate between the major and minor forms. These patients are genetically heterogeneous.

α-Thalassemias (p. 641)

α-Thalassemias are due to inherited defects that reduce α-globin synthesis; gene deletion is the most common genetic cause. The clinical consequences are due to imbalanced synthesis of α and non-α chains (γ chains in infancy, β and δ chains after 6 months of age). Free β-chain tetramers (hemoglobin H [HbH]) have extremely high O_2 affinity, and thus cause tissue hypoxia disproportionate to hemoglobin levels. In addition, HbH is prone to oxidation leading to precipitation of intracellular protein aggregates that promote RBC sequestration by macrophages. Free γ chains form stable tetramers (HbBarts) that also bind O_2 with excessive avidity, resulting in tissue hypoxia.

Clinical Syndromes (p. 641).

- *Silent carrier state (p. 641):* Completely asymptomatic, resulting from a single α-globin gene deletion; changes in total α-globin chain synthesis are barely detectable.
- *α-Thalassemia trait (p. 641):* Either one chromosome has both α-globin genes or each chromosome has a deletion of one gene; the clinical picture is comparable to β-thalassemia minor. Although these two genotypes are clinically identical, they differ in whether offspring are at risk for severe α-thalassemia (≥ three α chains deleted).
- *HbH disease (p. 641):* Deletion of three α-globin genes causes marked suppression of α-chain synthesis and formation of unstable HbH tetramers; clinically, it resembles β-thalassemia intermedia.
- *Hydrops fetalis (p. 642):* Deletion of all four α-globin genes. Early fetal development is permitted by embryonic ζ-globin chain synthesis; however, as ζ-globin synthesis ceases and the fetal $\zeta_2\gamma_2$ tetramers are replaced by γ-globin tetramers (HbBarts), the high oxygen affinity of the newly synthesized hemoglobin prevents O_2 release to tissues, and is not compatible with life. Intrauterine (and then lifelong) transfusions can be lifesaving.

Paroxysmal Nocturnal Hemoglobinuria (p. 642)

Paroxysmal nocturnal hemoglobinuria (PNH) is a rare X-linked hemolytic disease resulting from acquired mutations in phosphatidylinositol glycan complementation group A (PIGA) gene; PIGA mutations lead to deficient expression of a family of proteins normally anchored into the cell membrane via glycosylphosphatidylinositol (GPI). Among the GPI-linked proteins affected are several that regulate complement inactivation: decay-accelerating factor (CD55), membrane inhibitor of reactive lysis (CD59), and C8-binding protein. Their deficiency renders RBCs hypersensitive to complement, which is activated spontaneously at low rates. Granulocyte and platelet GPI proteins are also affected, resulting in a predisposition to thrombosis, particularly in portal, cerebral, and hepatic veins. Hemolysis is intravascular but is paroxysmal and nocturnal in only 25% of cases. A monoclonal antibody (eculizumab) that prevents the conversion of complement C5 to C5a dramatically reduces hemolysis, as well as the risk of intravascular thrombosis.

PNH may arise due to an autoimmune response to GPI-linked proteins on hematopoietic stem cells. In this scenario rare clones harboring a mutated *PIGA* gene have a selective advantage and eventually "take over" the marrow. This pathogenic basis explains the association of PNH with aplastic anemia, a marrow failure syndrome with an autoimmune pathogenesis. In 5% to 10% of patients, PNH transforms to acute myeloid leukemia or myelodysplastic syndrome. Hematopoietic stem cell transplantation can be curative.

Immunohemolytic Anemia (p. 643)

Immunohemolytic anemia is caused by antibodies that bind to RBCs and cause their premature destruction; classification is based on the characteristics of the responsible antibody (see later). Diagnosis requires detection of antibodies and/or complement on RBC. This is accomplished by the *direct Coombs test:* patient's RBCs are mixed with antibodies directed against human immunoglobulin (Ig) or complement, with RBC agglutination constituting a positive test. In the *indirect Coombs test* a patient's serum is assayed for its ability to agglutinate test RBCs expressing specific surface antigens.

Warm antibody type (p. 643) is the most common immunohemolytic anemia; half of the cases are idiopathic *(primary),* with the remainder being associated with other autoimmune disorders (e.g., lupus), lymphoid neoplasms, or drug hypersensitivity. Most commonly, IgG anti-RBC antibodies (anti-Rh in most idiopathic cases) coat the RBCs and act as opsonins; erythrocytes become spherocytic due to partial macrophage phagocytosis and are eventually completely destroyed in the spleen. Splenomegaly is characteristic. Drug-induced hemolytic anemias occur through two mechanisms:

- *Antigenic drugs:* Drugs (e.g., penicillin, cephalosporins, quinidine) bind to the RBC surface; antibodies then interact with the drug or an RBC-drug complex.
- *Tolerance-breaking drugs:* Drugs (e.g., α-methyldopa) induce antibodies against intrinsic RBC antigens.

Cold agglutinin type (p. 644) anemia is caused by IgM antibodies that agglutinate RBCs at low temperatures; it accounts for 15% to 30% of immune hemolytic anemias.

- *Acute* hemolysis occurs during recovery from certain infections (e.g., *Mycoplasma,* Epstein-Barr, or human immunodeficiency virus [HIV] infections). It is usually self-limited and rarely induces significant hemolysis.
- *Chronic* hemolysis can be idiopathic or can occur in the setting of B-cell neoplasms. Clinical symptoms result from RBC agglutination and complement fixation in vascular beds ≤30° C; although there is minimal complement-mediated hemolysis, the coated cells are readily phagocytized in spleen, liver, and bone marrow. The hemolytic anemia is of variable severity; vascular obstruction in areas exposed to cold temperatures results in pallor, cyanosis, and Raynaud phenomenon.

Cold hemolysin type (p. 644) anemia occurs in *paroxysmal cold hemoglobinuria,* capable of causing substantial (sometimes fatal) intravascular hemolysis. The autoantibodies are IgG that bind to the P blood group antigen at low temperatures and fix complement; when the temperature is elevated, hemolysis occurs. Most cases occur in children after viral infections and are transient.

Hemolytic Anemia Resulting From Trauma to Red Cells (p. 644)

Turbulent flow and increased shear forces cause RBC fragmentation and intravascular hemolysis; peripheral blood reveals fragmented RBC *(schistocytes).* Causes include the following:

- Prosthetic heart valves (mechanical > bioprosthetic valves)
- Microangiopathic hemolytic anemia with diffuse microvascular narrowing owing to fibrin or platelet deposition (e.g., disseminated intravascular coagulation [DIC]; thrombotic

thrombocytopenic purpura [TTP], hemolytic-uremic syndrome [HUS])

Anemias of Diminished Erythropoiesis (p. 645)

Impaired RBC production can occur due to deficiency of erythropoietin or a vital nutrient (iron, vitamin B_{12}, folate), inherited defects, neoplasia, or stem cell failure.

Megaloblastic Anemias (p. 645)

Megaloblastic anemias are most commonly due to inadequate levels of vitamin B_{12} or folate; multiple pathways can lead to these deficiencies (Table 14-4). Folate and vitamin B_{12} are coenzymes required for the synthesis of thymidine (and are also involved in normal methionine synthesis); in their absence, inadequate DNA synthesis causes defective nuclear maturation of rapidly proliferating cells. The resultant blockade in cell division leads to abnormally large RBC and erythroid precursors (megaloblasts), and also affects granulocyte maturation. Neurologic complications of vitamin B_{12} deficiency (see later) are attributed to abnormal myelin degradation.

TABLE 14-4 Causes of Megaloblastic Anemia

Vitamin B_{12} Deficiency
Decreased Intake
Inadequate diet, vegetarianism
Impaired Absorption
IF deficiency
Pernicious anemia
Gastrectomy
Malabsorption states
Diffuse intestinal disease (e.g., lymphoma, systemic sclerosis)
Ileal resection, ileitis
Competitive parasitic uptake
Fish tapeworm infestation
Bacterial overgrowth in blind loops and diverticula of bowel
Folic Acid Deficiency
Decreased Intake
Inadequate diet, alcoholism, infancy
Impaired absorption
Malabsorption states
Intrinsic intestinal disease
Anticonvulsants, oral contraceptives
Increased Loss
Hemodialysis
Increased Requirement
Pregnancy, infancy, disseminated cancer, markedly increased hematopoiesis
Impaired Utilization
Folic acid antagonists
Unresponsive to Vitamin B_{12} or Folic Acid Therapy
Metabolic inhibitors of DNA synthesis and/or folate metabolism (e.g., methotrexate)

Modified from Beck WS: Megaloblastic anemias. In Wyngaarden JB, Smith LH (eds): *Cecil Textbook of Medicine,* 18th ed. Philadelphia, PA: Saunders, 1988, p 900.

Morphology (p. 645)

- Prominent peripheral blood anisocytosis with abnormally large and oval RBC (macro-ovalocytes).
- In the marrow, erythroid precursor nuclear maturation lags behind cytoplasmic maturation; ineffective erythropoiesis is reflected by increased apoptosis with compensatory megaloblastic hyperplasia.
- Abnormal granulopoiesis with giant metamyelocytes in marrow and hypersegmented neutrophils in peripheral blood.

Normal Vitamin B_{12} Metabolism (p. 645; **Fig. 14-1**)

Microorganisms are the ultimate source of vitamin B_{12} (cobalamin); plants and vegetables contain little cobalamin, and most dietary cobalamin comes from animal products.

- Peptic digestion releases dietary vitamin B_{12}; it is bound to salivary proteins called *R binders.*
- R-B_{12} complexes are digested in the duodenum by pancreatic proteases; released vitamin B_{12} binds to intrinsic factor (IF), a protein secreted by parietal cells of the gastric fundus.
- IF-B_{12} complexes bind to IF receptors in the distal ileum epithelium; absorbed vitamin B_{12} complexes with transcobalamin II and is transported to tissues.
- One percent of ingested vitamin B_{12} can be absorbed through an alternate pathway independent of IF or the terminal ileum.

Except for strict vegans or in chronic alcoholism, most diets contain adequate cobalamin. Thus most deficiencies in vitamin B_{12} result from impaired absorption:

- Achlorhydria (in elderly individuals) impairs vitamin B_{12} release from R binders
- Gastrectomy causes loss of IF
- Pernicious anemia (see following discussion)
- Resection of the distal ileum prevents IF-B_{12} absorption
- Malabsorption syndromes
- Increased requirements (e.g., pregnancy)

Anemias of Vitamin B_{12} Deficiency: Pernicious Anemia (p. 645)

Pernicious anemia is a specific form of megaloblastic anemia caused by autoimmune gastritis and attendant loss of IF production. Gastric injury is likely initiated by autoreactive T cells; secondary autoantibodies against proteins involved in vitamin B_{12} uptake are not the primary cause of disease but can exacerbate the process:

- Type I antibodies (present in 75% of patients) block vitamin B_{12} binding to IF.
- Type II antibodies block IF or IF-B_{12} binding to the ileal receptor.
- Type III antibodies (85% to 90% of patients) directed against parietal proton pump proteins affect acid secretion.

Morphology (p. 648)

- Bone marrow shows megaloblastic erythroid hyperplasia, giant myelocytes and metamyelocytes, hypersegmented neutrophils, and large, multilobed nuclei in megakaryocytes.
- Atrophic glossitis; the tongue is shiny, glazed, and red.
- Gastric fundal atrophy with virtual absence of parietal cells and replacement by mucus-secreting goblet cells ("intestinalization").
- Central nervous system lesions occur in 75% of cases, characterized by demyelination of dorsal and lateral spinal cord tracts.

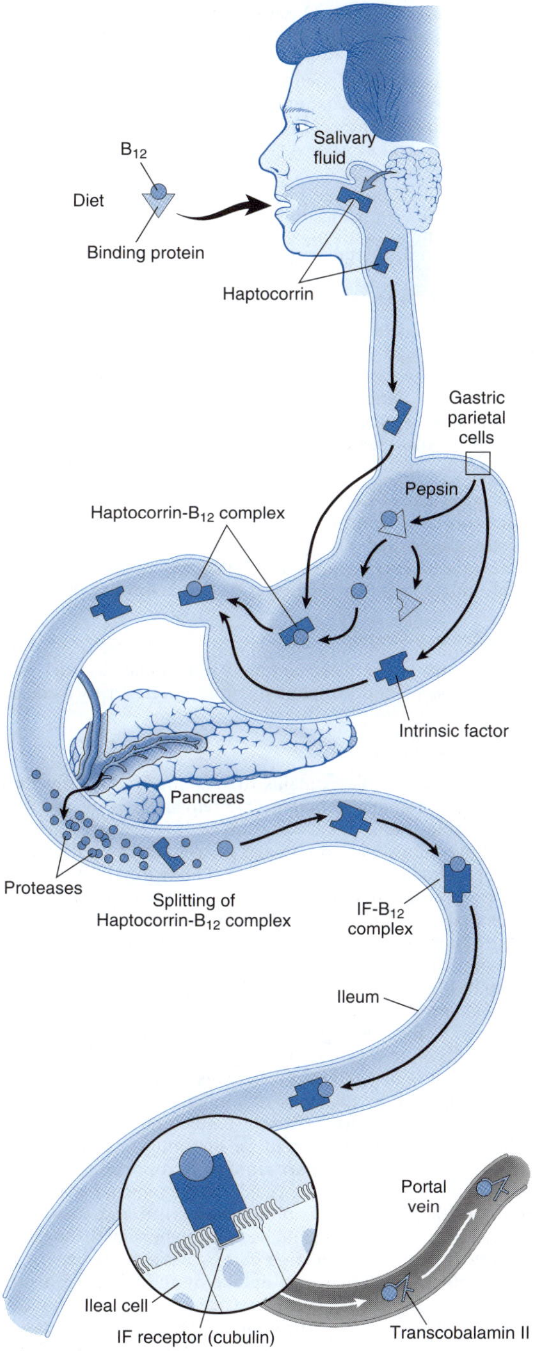

Figure 14-1 Schematic of vitamin B_{12} absorption and metabolism.

***Clinical Features** (p. 648).* Onset is insidious, with symptoms due to anemia and posterolateral spinal tract involvement; the latter includes spastic paresis and sensory ataxia. Diagnosis is based on the presence of megaloblastic anemia, leukopenia with hypersegmented neutrophils, low serum vitamin B_{12} levels, and elevated homocysteine and methylmalonic acid (consequences of diminished thymidine and methionine synthesis). The diagnosis is confirmed by profound reticulocytosis after parenteral vitamin B_{12} administration; serum anti-IF antibodies are highly specific for pernicious anemia. There is a significant association of pernicious anemia with other autoimmune disorders of the adrenal and thyroid glands; patients with pernicious anemia also have an increased risk of gastric cancer.

Anemia of Folate Deficiency *(p. 648)*

Folate is involved in single carbon transfers in a variety of biochemical pathways. Deficiency induces a megaloblastic anemia clinically and hematologically indistinguishable from that seen with vitamin B_{12} deficiency; notably, however, gastric atrophy and the neurologic sequelae of vitamin B_{12} deficiency do not occur. Diagnosis of folate deficiency requires demonstration of reduced serum or RBC folate levels. Deficiency occurs with the following:

- Inadequate intake (e.g., chronic alcoholics, very elderly, or indigents)
- Malabsorption syndromes (e.g., sprue) or diffuse infiltrative disease of the bowel (e.g., lymphoma)
- Increased demand (e.g., pregnancy, infancy, or disseminated cancer)
- Folate antagonists (e.g. methotrexate for chemotherapy)

Iron Deficiency Anemia *(p. 649)*

Iron deficiency is the most common nutritional disorder in the world, with signs and symptoms primarily related to inadequate hemoglobin synthesis.

Iron Metabolism (p. 649)

The normal Western diet contains 10 to 20 mg of iron daily, mostly as heme iron in animal products (the remainder is inorganic iron from vegetables); intake is usually sufficient to balance daily losses of 1 to 2 mg from sloughed skin and gastrointestinal (GI) epithelial cells. Approximately 15% to 20% of total body iron is in *stored form* bound to hemosiderin or ferritin; serum ferritin level is a good indicator of total iron stores. The rest of the body's iron is complexed in a number of functional proteins; 80% is contained in hemoglobin with myoglobin, catalase, and cytochromes making up the rest. Excess iron can be highly toxic, so that uptake must be carefully regulated.

Iron balance is maintained by regulating the absorption of dietary iron across the duodenal epithelium (Fig. 14-2). Heme iron enters mucosal cells directly (approximately 20% is absorbable), whereas nonheme iron is first reduced to ferrous iron (via cytochrome *b*) before transport; only 1% to 2% of nonheme iron is absorbed. Absorbed iron is transported across the basolateral membrane, where it is bound to plasma transferrin for distribution throughout the body; this basolateral transport requires ferroportin, a membrane transporter, and hephaestin to reoxidize the reduced iron. The remaining intracellular iron is bound to ferritin and subsequently lost when the epithelium is sloughed during normal turnover. Iron homeostasis is regulated in large part by hepcidin, a hepatic peptide that blocks duodenal iron uptake by inducing the degradation of ferroportin. As hepcidin levels decrease (e.g., with reduced iron stores or increased erythropoiesis), ferroportin expression is increased, and iron transport into the bloodstream is enhanced. Conversely, as stores become replete, hepcidin levels increase,

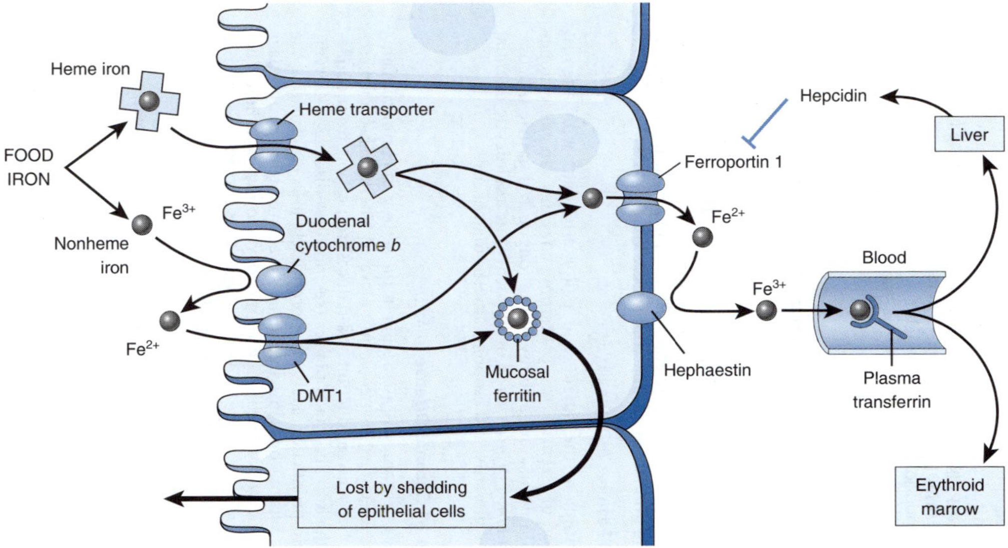

Figure 14-2 Regulation of iron absorption in the duodenum; epithelial cell uptake of both heme and nonheme iron is shown. When the storage sites of the body are replete with iron and erythropoietic activity is normal, plasma hepcidin levels are high. This leads to downregulation of ferroportin and trapping of most of the absorbed iron within the epithelial cells, which is then lost when duodenal epithelial cells are shed into the gut. Conversely, when body iron stores decrease or when erythropoiesis is stimulated, hepcidin levels fall and ferroportin surface expression increases, allowing a greater fraction of the absorbed iron to be transferred to plasma transferrin. *DMT1,* Divalent metal transporter 1.

ferroportin is degraded, and iron transport into the bloodstream is blocked. Hepcidin also blocks the release of iron from macrophages, an important source of iron for heme synthesis in erythropoiesis. Abnormalities in hepcidin levels lead to disturbances in iron metabolism ranging from some forms of anemia to *hemochromatosis* (systemic iron overload).

Etiology (p. 651)

Negative iron balance can result from (1) low dietary intake (rare in the United States); (2) malabsorption; (3) excessive demand (infancy or pregnancy); or (4) chronic blood loss. The latter is the most important cause of iron deficiency anemia in the Western world; blood loss occurs through the GI tract (e.g., peptic ulcers, colonic cancer, hemorrhoids) or the female genital tract (e.g., menstruation).

Pathogenesis (p. 652)

Anemia occurs when iron reserves are depleted; it is accompanied by low serum iron, ferritin, and transferrin saturation levels.

Morphology (p. 652)

Whatever the cause, iron deficiency produces a *hypochromic, microcytic anemia,* with increased RBC central pallor and poikilocytosis. Marrow exhibits mild-moderate erythroid hyperplasia, with loss of stainable iron in marrow macrophages.

Clinical Features (p. 652)

In addition to the fatigue and pallor attendant with anemia, depletion of essential iron-containing enzymes can cause alopecia, koilonychia, and atrophy of the tongue and gastric mucosa. The *Plummer-Vinson triad* of hypochromic microcytic anemia, atrophic glossitis, and esophageal webs may occur.

Anemia of Chronic Disease (p. 652)

Anemia of chronic disease occurs in the setting of chronic inflammation, infections, or neoplasms; elevated interleukin-6 increases hepatic hepcidin production and reduces iron export from duodenal epithelium and macrophages (see previous discussion). Erythropoietin production is also inappropriately low, exacerbating the anemia. Serum iron is low, but ferritin levels are high. The anemia is normocytic or normochromic, or microcytic or hypochromic. Successful treatment of the underlying condition corrects the anemia; erythropoietin therapy is partially effective.

Aplastic Anemia (p. 653)

Aplastic anemia is a syndrome of chronic primary hematopoietic failure; pancytopenia affecting all lineages results.

Pathogenesis (p. 653)

Known causes fall into three broad categories:

- Toxic exposures.
  - Total body irradiation.
  - Drugs or chemicals are the most common causes of secondary aplastic anemia; marrow suppression can be dose related, predictable, and reversible (benzene, alkylating agents, and antimetabolites, such as vincristine) or idiosyncratic, affecting only some exposed individuals in an unpredictable manner (chloramphenicol, chlorpromazine, and streptomycin).

- Viral infections (most commonly non-A, non-B, non-C, and non-G hepatitis).
- Inherited diseases (e.g., Fanconi anemia, defects in telomerase activity).

In idiopathic cases (65% of aplastic anemia), stem cell failure may be due to the following:

- A primary defect in the number or function of stem cells, in some cases due to mutagen exposure; occasionally, genetically damaged stem cells transform to myeloid neoplasms.
- Suppression of antigenically altered stem cells by T cell–mediated immune mechanisms.

Morphology (p. 654)

Hypocellular marrow (hematopoietic cells replaced by fat cells), with secondary effects due to granulocytopenia (infections) and thrombocytopenia (bleeding).

Clinical Features (p. 654)

Onset is insidious with symptoms related to the pancytopenia; splenomegaly is absent. Withdrawal of a potential inciting agent can sometimes lead to recovery; more commonly, bone marrow transplantation or immunosuppression is required.

Pure Red Cell Aplasia (p. 655)

Pure red cell aplasia is a form of marrow failure due to erythroid precursor suppression. Outside of cases associated with B19 parvovirus infections (that infect and destroy RBC precursors), the etiology is likely autoimmune; it can occur in association with drug exposures, autoimmune diseases, and neoplasms (e.g., large granular lymphocytic leukemia or thymoma). In such settings the anemia may remit with immunosuppression, plasmapheresis, or following thymoma resection.

Other Forms of Marrow Failure (p. 655)

- *Myelophthisic anemia:* Space-occupying lesions (e.g., metastatic cancer or granulomatous disease) destroy and/or distort the marrow architecture and depress hematopoiesis; pancytopenia results, often with immature precursors in the peripheral blood.
- *Chronic renal* failure is almost invariably associated with anemia. Although multifactorial, insufficient erythropoietin production is most important; recombinant erythropoietin is usually efficacious.
- *Hepatocellular liver disease* (toxic, infectious, or cirrhotic): Anemia is primarily due to bone marrow failure, often exacerbated by (variceal) bleeding and folate and/or iron deficiency.
- *Endocrine disorders,* especially hypothyroidism.

Polycythemia (p. 656)

Polycythemia denotes an abnormally high RBC count, usually with an associated increase in hemoglobin level. *Relative* increases may be caused by hemoconcentration due to dehydration (e.g., water deprivation, vomiting, or diarrhea) or due to *stress polycythemia* (also called *Gaisböck syndrome*). *Absolute increases* can be the following:

- *Primary* due to *polycythemia vera,* a myeloproliferative disorder in which RBC precursors proliferate in an erythropoietin-independent fashion. Mutations in the erythropoietin receptor can also render its activity erythropoietin-independent.

- *Secondary* due to increased erythropoietin, which may be physiologic (lung disease, high-altitude living, cyanotic heart disease) or pathophysiologic (erythropoietin-secreting tumors, such as renal cell or hepatocellular carcinomas).

Bleeding Disorders: Hemorrhagic Diatheses (p. 656)

Excessive bleeding can result from increased blood vessel fragility, platelet disorders, and/or coagulation defects. Evaluation requires laboratory investigation: prothrombin and partial thromboplastin times (and levels of specific clotting factors and anticoagulants) assess the protein components, whereas platelet number and functional assays (e.g., bleeding time) test the cellular aspects.

Bleeding Disorders Caused by Vessel Wall Abnormalities (p. 656)

Such disorders are relatively common but usually cause only petechiae and purpura without serious bleeding. Platelet counts and coagulation and bleeding times are typically normal. Causes include the following:

- *Infections* (e.g., meningococcus and rickettsia); underlying mechanisms are microvascular damage (vasculitis) or DIC.
- *Drug reactions:* Attributed to immune complex deposition with resulting hypersensitivity vasculitis.
- *Poor vascular support:* Abnormal collagen synthesis (e.g., scurvy or Ehlers-Danlos syndrome), loss of perivascular supporting tissue (e.g., Cushing syndrome), or vascular wall amyloid deposition.
- *Henoch-Schönlein purpura* is a systemic hypersensitivity response due to immune complex deposition and characterized by purpuric rash, abdominal pain, polyarthralgia, and acute glomerulonephritis.
- *Hereditary hemorrhagic telangiectasia (Osler-Weber-Rendu syndrome)* is an autosomal dominant disorder that can be caused by mutations in at least five different genes, most of which modulate transforming growth factor-β (TGF-β) signaling. It is characterized by dilated, thin-walled vessels (often in mucous membranes of the nose and GI tract).
- *Perivascular amyloidosis (often associated with amyloid light chain amyloidosis)* can weaken blood vessel walls; it typically manifests as mucocutaneous petechiae.

Bleeding Related to Reduced Platelet Number: Thrombocytopenia (p. 657)

Thrombocytopenia is defined as counts ≤100,000/μL, but spontaneous bleeding does not occur until platelet numbers ≤20,000/μL; counts between 20,000 and 50,000/μL can exacerbate posttraumatic hemorrhage. Most spontaneous bleeds involve small vessels of the skin and mucous membranes. Causes of thrombocytopenia are as follows:

- *Decreased production* due to ineffective megakaryopoiesis (e.g., HIV, myelodysplastic syndromes) or to generalized marrow disease that also compromises megakaryocyte number (e.g., aplastic anemia, disseminated cancer).
- *Decreased survival* due to increased consumption (e.g., DIC), or to immune-mediated platelet destruction, the latter secondary to antiplatelet antibodies or immune complex deposition on platelets.

- *Sequestration* in the red pulp of enlarged spleens.
- *Dilution* due to massive transfusions. Prolonged storage of whole blood results in prompt subsequent platelet sequestration. Thus although plasma volume and RBC mass are reconstituted by transfusion, the numbers of circulating platelets are relatively reduced.

Chronic Immune Thrombocytopenic Purpura *(p. 658)*

Chronic immune thrombocytopenic purpura (ITP) is caused by autoantibodies to platelets; these can be primary, or arise in the setting of certain exposures or preexisting conditions (e.g., lupus, B-cell neoplasms, or HIV).

Pathogenesis (p. 658)

Platelet autoantibodies are usually directed toward one of two platelet antigens—the platelet membrane glycoprotein complexes IIb-IIIa or Ib-IX. Destruction of antibody-coated platelets occurs in the spleen, and splenectomy can be beneficial.

Morphology (p. 658)

The spleen is normal in size but shows sinusoidal congestion and prominent germinal centers. Bone marrow megakaryocyte numbers are increased.

Clinical Features (p. 658)

Chronic ITP is classically a disease of women <40 years of age; there is often a long history of easy bruising or epistaxis. Cutaneous bleeding often takes the form of petechiae. Initial manifestations can be melena, hematuria, or heavy menses; subarachnoid or intracerebral hemorrhages are rare but serious. The bleeding time is prolonged, whereas prothrombin and partial thromboplastin times are normal; tests for antiplatelet antibody are not reliable. Most patients respond to glucocorticoids (inhibiting macrophage function), but some require splenectomy or immunomodulation (e.g., anti-CD20 antibody).

Acute Immune Thrombocytopenic Purpura *(p. 659)*

Acute ITP is a self-limited disorder seen most often in children after a viral infection; platelet destruction is due to transient production of antiplatelet autoantibodies.

Drug-Induced Thrombocytopenia *(p. 659)*

Drug-induced thrombocytopenia occurs when drugs act as haptens on platelet proteins or participate in the formation of immune complexes that deposit on platelet surfaces; antibodies to the drugs or modified platelet molecules then cause platelet removal via macrophage.

Heparin-induced thrombocytopenia (HIT) has a distinctive pathogenesis. *Type I* thrombocytopenia occurs rapidly after drug administration and is due to a direct platelet-aggregating effect of heparin; it is usually of little clinical significance and spontaneously resolves. *Type II* thrombocytopenia, although less common, has significant potential for adverse clinical consequences. It occurs 5 to 14 days after therapy and is caused by autoantibodies directed against a complex of heparin and platelet factor 4 that activates platelets. This in turn leads to thrombi in arteries and veins—even in the setting of thrombocytopenia—that can be limb- and life-threatening (e.g., from pulmonary embolism of deep venous thromboses). Therapy requires heparin discontinuation and alternate anticoagulation administration.

Human Immunodeficiency Virus-Associated Thrombocytopenia *(p. 659)*

HIV-associated thrombocytopenia is due to both diminished platelet production and increased destruction. Megakaryocytes express both CXCR4 and CD4 and thus can be directly infected by HIV; infected cells are prone to apoptosis and defective platelet production. HIV-mediated dysregulation of B cells leads to antiplatelet autoantibodies that cause their premature destruction.

Thrombotic Microangiopathies: Thrombotic Thrombocytopenic Purpura and Hemolytic-Uremic Syndrome *(p. 659)*

TTP and HUS are related disorders within the spectrum of *thrombotic microangiopathies;* these are characterized by thrombocytopenia, microangiopathic hemolytic anemia, fever, transient neurologic deficits (in TTP), or renal failure (in HUS). Although clinically similar to DIC, activation of the clotting system is not a prominent feature in the thrombotic microangiopathies; rather HUS and TTP are both caused by excessive platelet activation. Most of the clinical manifestations are due to *widespread hyaline microthrombi* in arterioles and capillaries composed of dense aggregates of platelets and fibrin.

- *TTP* is associated with inherited or acquired deficiencies in ADAMTS13, a serum metalloprotease that limits the size of von Willebrand factor (vWF) multimers in the plasma. In its absence, very high-molecular-weight multimers accumulate that are capable of promoting platelet aggregation throughout the microcirculation. In the case of acquired TTP, patients often have antibodies directed against ADAMTS13.
- "Typical" (epidemic) *HUS* most commonly follows GI infections with verotoxin-producing *Escherichia coli;* verotoxin injures endothelial cells and thereby promotes dysregulated platelet activation and aggregation. This form often occurs in children and the elderly during outbreaks of food poisoning.

"Atypical" HUS is associated with defects in proteins that prevent excessive activation of the alternative complement pathway (e.g., complement factor H, membrane cofactor protein, or factor I). Deficiencies can be caused by inherited defects or acquired inhibitory autoantibodies.

Immunosuppression and plasmapheresis are effective in both TTP and atypical HUS, probably due to reduction in the level of causal antibodies. Typical HUS is treated supportively, but some patients will develop permanent renal injury. Endothelial injury mediated by other causes (e.g., toxic drugs, radiation) may cause chronic forms of HUS that are difficult to treat.

Bleeding Disorders Related to Defective Platelet Functions (p. 660)

These disorders are characterized by prolonged bleeding time in association with normal platelet count.

Congenital defects are as follows:

- *Defective platelet adhesion* (e.g., autosomal recessive Bernard-Soulier syndrome caused by deficient platelet membrane glycoprotein complex GpIb-IX [platelet receptor for vWF, necessary for platelet-collagen adhesion]).
- *Defective platelet aggregation* (e.g., Glanzmann thrombasthenia, an autosomal recessive disorder caused by a deficiency of platelet membrane glycoprotein GpIIb-IIIa [involved in binding fibrinogen]).

- *Disorders of platelet secretion* of prostaglandins and/or granule-bound adenosine diphosphate (ADP) that promote further aggregation.

Acquired defects are as follows:

- *Aspirin* irreversibly inhibits cyclooxygenase and can suppress the synthesis of thromboxane A_2, necessary for platelet aggregation.
- *Uremia* causes defects in platelet adhesion, granule secretion, and aggregation.

Hemorrhagic Diatheses Related to Abnormalities in Clotting Factors (p. 661)

The bleeding associated with clotting factor abnormalities differs from that seen with platelet deficiencies:

- Spontaneous petechiae or purpura is uncommon; more often, bleeding manifests as large ecchymoses or hematomas after injury or as prolonged bleeding after laceration or surgery.
- Bleeding into the GI and urinary tracts and particularly into weight-bearing joints *(hemarthrosis)* is common.

Clotting abnormalities can be acquired or hereditary. *Acquired deficiencies* are usually associated with multiple clotting abnormalities. Thus vitamin K deficiency results in depressed synthesis of factors II, VII, IX, and X and protein C, and liver failure of any cause can result in deficient synthesis of multiple coagulation factors. DIC also produces a deficiency of multiple coagulation factors.

Hereditary deficiencies typically affect a single clotting factor. The most common inherited disorders are hemophilia (A and B) and von Willebrand disease.

The Factor VIII-von Willebrand Factor Complex (p. 661)

The factor VIII-vWF complex is a complex made up of two separate proteins—factor VIII and vWF; circulating factor VIII is stabilized by binding to vWF, and deficient levels of vWF thus lead to commensurate reductions in factor VIII (Fig. 14-3).

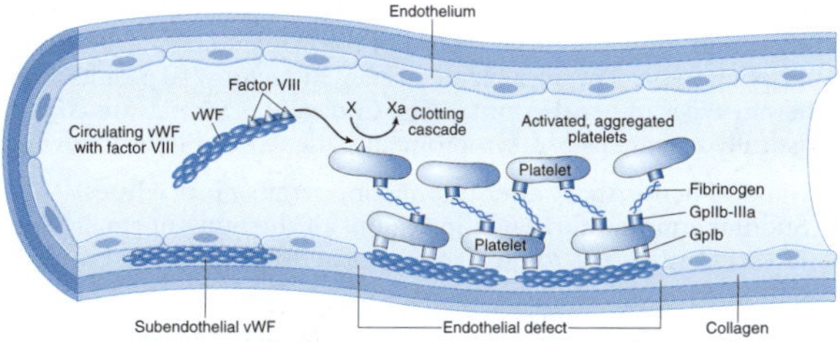

Figure 14-3 Structure and function of factor VIII-vWF complex. Factor VIII is synthesized in the liver and kidney, and vWF is made in endothelial cells and megakaryocytes. The two associate to form a complex in the circulation. vWF is also present in the subendothelial matrix of normal blood vessels and on platelet α-granules. Exposure of subendothelial vWF after endothelial injury causes platelet adhesion via the glycoprotein Ib (GpIb) platelet receptor. Circulating vWF and vWF released from platelet α-granules can also bind exposed subendothelial matrix and contribute to platelet adhesion and activation. Activated platelets form hemostatic aggregates; fibrinogen participates in aggregation through bridging interactions with the glycoprotein IIb-IIIa (GpIIb-IIIa) platelet receptor. Factor VIII takes part in the coagulation cascade as a cofactor in the activation of factor X on the surface of activated platelets.

Factor VIII is an essential cofactor for factor IX in activating factor X (see Chapter 4); factor VIII deficiency causes classic hemophilia (*hemophilia A;* see later).

As described earlier and in Figure 14-3, circulating vWF exists as large multimers. In addition to factor VIII, these multimers interact with other hemostatic proteins; most importantly vWF mediates platelet adhesion to subendothelial matrix by bridging platelet glycoprotein Ib-IX and collagen. vWF also promotes platelet aggregation by binding to factor IIb-IIIa, particularly under high shear stress.

von Willebrand Disease *(p. 662)*

von Willebrand disease is the most common heritable bleeding disorder, affecting 1% of the U.S. population. It is molecularly heterogeneous with several hundred variants (although only a handful are disease-causing); most are autosomal dominant. Symptoms are generally mild (epistaxis, excess bleeding from wounds, etc.) but can be more severe. Therapy can include desmopressin (stimulating vWF release) or infusions of plasma concentrates containing the missing factor(s).

- *Type 1* and *type 3 von Willebrand disease* are associated with reduced levels of vWF. Type 1 is autosomal dominant, with mild-moderate vWF deficiency being most common; it is typically associated with point mutations that affect vWF maturation or result in rapid plasma clearance. Type 3 is an uncommon autosomal recessive variant associated with marked vWF deficiency due to genetic deletions or frameshift mutations on both alleles.
- *Type 2* is an autosomal dominant form caused by qualitative defects in vWF. Type 2A (autosomal dominant) is most common; vWF levels are normal, but the ability to form the most active high-molecular-weight multimers is defective, leading to a functional deficit. Patients have mild-moderate bleeding.

Hemophilia A (Factor VIII Deficiency) *(p. 662)*

Hemophilia A is the most common hereditary disease associated with life-threatening bleeding. It is an X-linked recessive disorder (thus primarily affecting males), characterized by a reduced amount and/or activity of factor VIII; the resulting bleeding diathesis reflects the importance of the factor VIIIa-IXa complex in activating factor X in vivo. Severe disease occurs when factor VIII levels are <1% of normal; patients with 2% to 5% of normal levels have moderately severe disease, and those with 6% to 50% of normal levels typically have a mild phenotype. The variable deficiency in factor VIII results from different types of genetic mutations. Clinically petechiae are characteristically absent; instead, symptomatic patients exhibit the following:

- Massive hemorrhage after trauma or operative procedures.
- Spontaneous hemorrhages in regions of the body normally subject to trauma (e.g. joints); this can lead to progressive, crippling deformities.

The partial thromboplastin time is prolonged (intrinsic pathway defect), and specific diagnosis is made by assay for factor VIII. Treatment consists of replacement therapy with recombinant factor VIII or factor VIII concentrates.

Hemophilia B (Christmas Disease, Factor IX Deficiency) *(p. 663)*

Hemophilia B is an X-linked recessive disease caused by factor IX deficiency; it is clinically indistinguishable from hemophilia A. Identification of hemophilia B requires assay of factor IX levels; treatment involves infusions of recombinant factor IX.

Disseminated Intravascular Coagulation (p. 663)

DIC is a thrombohemorrhagic disorder characterized by excessive activation of coagulation leading to formation of thrombi in the microvasculature. It is a secondary complication in a variety of diseases; DIC symptoms arise from tissue ischemia (due to the thrombosis) and/or bleeding caused by the exuberant consumption of clotting factors or activation of fibrinolytic pathways.

Etiology and Pathogenesis (p. 663)

DIC is triggered by two major mechanisms: (1) release of tissue factor or thromboplastic substances into the circulation or (2) widespread endothelial cell injury (Fig. 14-4).

- *Thromboplastic substances* can be derived from a variety of sources: placenta or amniotic fluid in obstetric complications; damaged tissues following major trauma, burns, or surgery; granules of leukemic cells in acute promyelocytic leukemia; mucus released from certain adenocarcinomas. In sepsis, bacterial endotoxins activate monocytes to release tumor necrosis factor-α, thereby increasing tissue factor expression on endothelial cell membranes while simultaneously decreasing thrombomodulin expression. This results in both activation of the clotting system and inhibition of coagulation control.
- *Endothelial injury* initiates DIC by causing tissue factor release from endothelial cells, promoting platelet aggregation, and activating the intrinsic coagulation pathway by exposing subendothelial connective tissue. Widespread endothelial injury can occur through antigen-antibody complex deposition (e.g., systemic lupus erythematosus), hypoxia, acidosis, temperature extremes (e.g., heatstroke, burns), or infections (e.g., meningococci, rickettsiae).

Morphology (p. 664)

Microthrombi, with infarctions, and in some cases, hemorrhages, are found in many organs and tissues. In lungs, alveolar capillary microthrombi may be associated with histology resembling acute respiratory distress syndrome. In the adrenals, massive hemorrhages due to DIC give rise to the *Waterhouse-Friderichsen syndrome* seen in meningococcemia. Giant hemangiomas can be associated with DIC through the stasis-related formation of thrombi and recurrent blood vessel trauma *(Kasabach-Merritt syndrome).*

Clinical Features (p. 665)

Approximately 50% of DIC occurs in obstetric patients with pregnancy complications; 33% occurs in the setting of carcinomatosis, with sepsis and trauma responsible for most of the remaining cases. In the setting of trauma or obstetric complications, bleeding is the dominant complication, while thrombosis is the major manifestation in malignancy. Onset can be fulminant, as in endotoxic shock or amniotic fluid embolism, or insidious, as in cases of carcinomatosis or retention of a dead fetus. Clinical manifestations include the following:

- Microangiopathic hemolytic anemia
- Respiratory symptoms (e.g., dyspnea, cyanosis)
- Neurologic signs and symptoms, including convulsions and coma
- Oliguria and acute renal failure
- Circulatory failure and shock

Prognosis is highly variable and is heavily impacted by the underlying disorder; the only definitive treatment is to remove the inciting

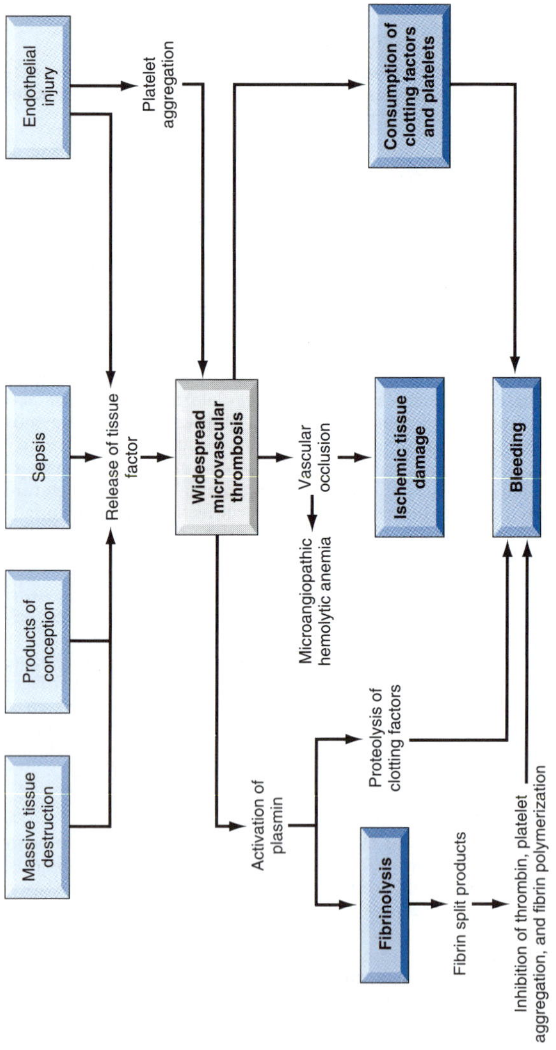

Figure 14-4 Pathophysiology of DIC.

cause. Depending on the clinical picture, anticoagulants (e.g., heparin) or procoagulants (fresh-frozen plasma) can be administered.

Complications of Transfusion (p. 665)

Most transfusion complications are minor and transient. The most common—*febrile nonhemolytic reaction*—results in fever and chills within 6 hours of a transfusion of red cells or platelets. Attributed to the release of donor leukocyte inflammatory mediators, the symptoms respond to antipyretics. Longer storage of blood products leads to more frequent reactions; the frequency of such reactions is decreased by limiting donor leukocyte contamination.

Allergic Reactions (p. 665)

Allergic reactions can occur when blood products containing certain antigens are given to previously sensitized recipients. The most common (1% to 3% of transfusions) are *urticarial allergic reactions* that occur when an allergen in a donated blood product is recognized by recipient IgE antibodies; these are generally mild reactions, and most respond to antihistamines. Potentially fatal allergic reactions can occur in patients with IgA deficiency (frequency of 1:300 to 1:500 people) in which recipient IgG antibodies recognize IgA in the infused blood product.

Acute Hemolytic Reactions (p. 665)

Acute hemolytic reactions are usually due to preformed IgM antibodies in the recipient. The most common scenario involves an error resulting in a patient receiving ABO-incompatible blood. Recipient high-affinity IgM antibodies against polysaccharide blood group antigens A or B lead to intravascular hemolysis and hemoglobinuria, associated with fever, shaking chills, and flank pain. Severe cases can progress to DIC, shock, acute renal failure, and death.

Delayed Hemolytic Reactions (p. 666)

Delayed hemolytic reactions are caused by IgG antibodies to red cell antigens to which the recipient was previously sensitized (e.g., through a previous transfusion); Rh, Kell, and Kidd can cause severe, potentially fatal reactions identical to those resulting from ABO mismatches. Other antibodies that do not fix complement instead cause red cell opsonization, extravascular hemolysis, and spherocytosis, with relatively minor signs and symptoms.

Transfusion-Related Acute Lung Injury (p. 666)

Transfusion-related acute lung injury (TRALI) is a rare (<1 in 10,000) severe, frequently fatal complication caused by the activation of neutrophils in the lung microvasculature. The pathogenesis is proposed to be an initial sequestration and sensitization of neutrophils in lung microvasculature due to endothelial activation by inflammatory mediators, followed by neutrophil activation potentially via antibodies that recognize antigens expressed on neutrophils (e.g., major histocompatibility complex antigens that may be more commonly seen in multiparous women).

Patients with TRALI present dramatically with sudden-onset respiratory failure, fever, hypotension, and hypoxemia, during or soon after a transfusion; chest imaging reveals diffuse bilateral pulmonary infiltrates. The treatment is largely supportive and the outcome is guarded; mortality is 5% in uncomplicated cases and up to 67% in those who are severely ill.

Infectious Complications (p. 666)

Most *bacterial infections* are caused by skin flora, indicating contamination during the blood donation process. Significant bacterial contamination occurs more commonly with platelet preparations (1 in 5000 transfusions) because platelets (unlike red cells) must be stored at room temperature—conditions that favor bacterial growth. Patients present with fever, chills, and hypotension (akin to transfusion reactions), and antibiotics may need to be given while awaiting laboratory results.

Most *viral infections* can be avoided by scrupulous donor selection and screening. However, transfusion-related transmission of HIV, hepatitis C, and hepatitis B can rarely occur when a donor is acutely infected and the virus cannot be detected by nucleic acid testing technology. Rates of transmission of HIV, hepatitis C, and hepatitis B are estimated to be 1 in 2 million, 1 in 1 million, and 1 in 500,000 transfusions, respectively. "Exotic" infectious agents, such as West Nile virus, trypanosomiasis, and babesiosis, can also be rarely transmitted.

15 The Lung

Congenital Anomalies (p. 670)

- *Pulmonary hypoplasia* (small lungs) reflects defective development with diminished weight, volume, and acinar number. This is caused by abnormalities that either compress the lung or impede normal expansion in utero (e.g., congenital diaphragmatic hernia or oligohydramnios).
- *Foregut cysts* are formed by abnormal detachment of primitive foregut; they are typically located in the hilum or mid-mediastinum. Bronchogenic cysts, lined by bronchial-type epithelium, are most common.
- *Pulmonary sequestration* is lung tissue (lobes or segments) lacking connection to the airway system; the vascular supply usually derives from the aorta or its branches (rather than the pulmonary artery).
    - *Extralobar sequestrations* are external to the lungs and occur anywhere in the thorax or mediastinum; commonly found in infants as mass lesions, they are often associated with other congenital anomalies.
    - *Intralobar sequestrations* occur within the lung parenchyma; they typically present in older children associated with recurrent localized infection or bronchiectasis.

Atelectasis (Collapse) (p. 670)

Atelectasis represents incomplete neonatal lung expansion or collapse of previously inflated lung. Significant atelectasis reduces oxygenation and predisposes to infection. Acquired atelectasis is classified as the following:

- *Resorption atelectasis,* following complete airway obstruction and resorption of oxygen in the dependent alveoli. Causes include excessive secretions (mucus plugs), foreign body aspiration, or bronchial neoplasms. The mediastinum shifts toward the atelectatic lung.
- *Compressive atelectasis,* when the pleural space is expanded by fluid (e.g., effusions from cardiac failure or neoplasms or blood from aneurysm rupture) or by air *(pneumothorax)*. The mediastinum shifts away from the atelectatic lung.
- *Contraction atelectasis,* when local or generalized fibrotic changes in the lung or pleura prevent full expansion.

Pulmonary Edema (p. 671)

Pulmonary edema results from either *increased hydrostatic pressure* or *increased capillary permeability* (due to endothelial or alveolar

TABLE 15-1 Classification and Causes of Pulmonary Edema

Hemodynamic Edema
Increased Hydrostatic Pressure (Increased Pulmonary Venous Pressure)
Left-sided heart failure (common)
Volume overload
Pulmonary vein obstruction
Decreased Oncotic Pressure (Less Common)
Hypoalbuminemia
Nephrotic syndrome
Liver disease
Protein-losing enteropathies
Lymphatic Obstruction (Rare)
Edema Due to Alveolar Wall Injury (Microvascular or Epithelial Injury)
Direct Injury
Infections: bacterial pneumonia
Inhaled gases: high concentration oxygen, smoke
Liquid aspiration: gastric contents, near-drowning
Radiation
Indirect Injury
Septicemia
Blood transfusion related
Burns
Drugs and chemicals: chemotherapeutic agents (bleomycin), other medications (methadone, amphotericin B), heroin, cocaine, kerosene, paraquat
Shock, trauma
Edema of Undetermined Origin
High altitude
Neurogenic (central nervous system trauma)

wall injury); therapy and outcome depend on the underlying etiology (Table 15-1). Regardless of cause, lungs become heavy and wet, with dependent fluid accumulation. Histologically capillaries are engorged, and the alveolar spaces exhibit granular pink precipitates. With chronic congestion, the lungs become brown and firm *(brown induration)* due to interstitial fibrosis and hemosiderin-laden macrophages ("heart failure" cells). In addition to impairing normal respiratory function, edema predisposes to infection.

Acute Lung Injury and Acute Respiratory Distress Syndrome (Diffuse Alveolar Damage) (p. 672)

Acute Lung Injury

Acute lung injury (ALI) is characterized by abrupt hypoxemia and diffuse pulmonary infiltrates in the absence of cardiac failure; acute respiratory distress syndrome (ARDS) is at the severe end of the ALI spectrum. Both ALI and ARDS have inflammation-associated increases in pulmonary vascular permeability, associated with endothelial and epithelial cell death; the histologic manifestations are called *diffuse alveolar damage (DAD)*. Causes can be localized to the lungs or systemic; they include infection, trauma, toxic exposures,

TABLE 15-2 Conditions Associated With Development of ARDS

Infection
Sepsis*
Diffuse pulmonary infections*
Viral, *Mycoplasma,* and *Pneumocystis* pneumonia; miliary tuberculosis
Gastric aspiration*
Physical/Injury
Mechanical trauma, including head injuries*
Pulmonary contusions
Near-drowning
Fractures with fat embolism
Burns
Ionizing radiation
Inhaled Irritants
Oxygen toxicity
Smoke
Irritant gases and chemicals
Chemical Injury
Heroin or methadone overdose
Acetylsalicylic acid
Barbiturate overdose
Paraquat
Hematologic Conditions
Transfusion-associated lung injury (TRALI)
Disseminated intravascular coagulation
Pancreatitis
Uremia
Cardiopulmonary Bypass
Hypersensitivity Reactions
Organic solvents
Drugs

*More than 50% of cases of ARDS are associated with these four conditions.

pancreatitis, uremia, and immune reactions (Table 15-2). In the absence of an etiology, similar pathologic changes are termed *acute interstitial pneumonia* (*AIP,* see later).

Pathogenesis (p. 672) (Fig. 15-1)

The integrity of the alveolar wall vascular-air interface is compromised by damage to capillary endothelium and/or alveolar epithelium.

- *Endothelial activation* is an important early event and can occur via circulating inflammatory mediators (resulting from sepsis or severe tissue injury). Alternatively, pneumocyte injury of various types is sensed by resident alveolar macrophages that respond by secreting mediators (e.g., tumor necrosis factor [TNF]) that act on neighboring endothelium.
- Adhesion and extravasation of neutrophils are followed by degranulation and inflammatory mediator release, including proteases, reactive oxygen species, and cytokines. Macrophage migration inhibitory factor (MIF) sustains the ongoing proinflammatory response. The cycle of inflammation and endothelial damage is central to the development of ALI and ARDS.

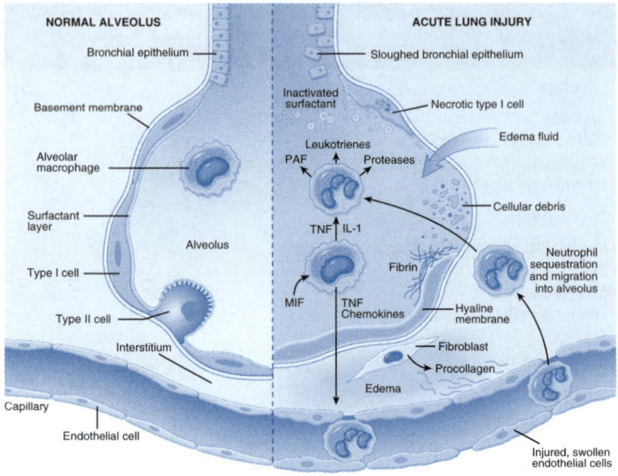

Figure 15-1 The normal alveolus *(left side)* compared with the injured alveolus in the early phase of ALI and ARDS. *IL-1,* Interleukin-1; *MIF,* migration inhibitory factor; *PAF,* platelet-activating factor; *TNF,* tumor necrosis factor. *(Modified with permission from Matthay MA, Ware LB, Zimmerman GA: The acute respiratory distress syndrome.* J Clin Invest *122:2731, 2012.)*

- *Hyaline membranes* are a characteristic feature of ALI and ARDS; these result from a combination of accumulated intra-alveolar fluid from leaky vessels and damage and necrosis of type II alveolar pneumocytes causing surfactant abnormalities.
- Resolution of injury is impeded by epithelial necrosis and inflammatory damage. Eventually, with abatement of the inflammatory stimulus, macrophages remove intra-alveolar debris and release fibrogenic cytokines, such as transforming growth factor-β (TGF-β) and platelet-derived growth factor (PDGF). These factors stimulate fibroblast growth and collagen deposition, leading to fibrosis of alveolar walls.

Morphology (p. 673)

- *Acute:* Lungs are diffusely firm, red, boggy, and heavy; microscopically there is edema, hyaline membranes (composed of necrotic epithelial debris and exuded proteins) and acute inflammation.
- *Organizing:* There is granulation tissue in response to the hyaline membranes with type II pneumocyte hyperplasia; this may resolve or progress to interstitial fibrosis. Fatal cases often have superimposed bacterial infections.

Clinical Course (p. 673)

Dyspnea and tachypnea herald ALI, followed by cyanosis, hypoxemia, and respiratory failure refractory to oxygen therapy; chest x-rays reveal diffuse bilateral infiltrates. The functional abnormalities are not evenly distributed; normal regions of compliance and ventilation are interspersed with consolidation and atelectasis. Poorly aerated regions continue to be perfused, leading to ventilation-perfusion mismatch and hypoxemia. Therapy involves mechanical ventilation and treatment of the underlying cause (e.g., infection); the overall mortality rate is 40%, primarily secondary to sepsis or multiorgan failure. Most survivors recover pulmonary function, but in a minority, diffuse tissue destruction and organization of the exudate lead to scarring, interstitial fibrosis, and chronic pulmonary disease.

Acute Interstitial Pneumonia (p. 674)

AIP is a clinicopathologic entity used to describe widespread ALI of unknown etiology, often with an aggressive course. Mortality is 50%, typically in the first 1 to 2 months; survivors are prone to recurrence and chronic interstitial disease.

Obstructive and Restrictive Lung Diseases (p. 674)

Chronic, noninfectious, diffuse pulmonary disease is physiologically classified as the following:

- *Obstructive disease:* Increased resistance to airflow, at any level from trachea to alveoli
- *Restrictive disease:* Reduced expansion of lung parenchyma, with decreased total lung capacity, generally occurring in two general categories:
  - Chest wall disorders (neuromuscular disease, obesity, pleural disease, etc.)
  - Chronic interstitial and infiltrative diseases

Distinguishing between these two entities is based primarily on pulmonary function tests. *Obstructive diseases* are associated with a decreased maximal airflow rate during forced expiration—the forced expiratory volume in 1 second (FEV_1) divided by the forced vital capacity (FVC) will be a ratio ≤0.7. *Restrictive diseases* are associated with a reduced total lung capacity in association with a reduced FEV_1, so that the FEV_1/FVC ratio is normal.

Obstructive Lung Diseases (p. 674)

The relevant entities—emphysema, chronic bronchitis, asthma, and bronchiectasis—have distinct characteristics (Table 15-3), but can also share some common elements. Emphysema and chronic bronchitis are typically grouped together as *chronic obstructive pulmonary disease* (COPD) because many patients have overlapping features of damage (unsurprising because cigarette smoking is often a common denominator). Asthma is usually distinguished from emphysema and chronic bronchitis by the presence of reversible bronchospasm; however, asthmatic patients can develop an irreversible component. Conversely, typical COPD can also have reversible features.

Emphysema (p. 675)

Emphysema is characterized by irreversible enlargement of airspaces distal to the terminal bronchioles, accompanied by alveolar wall destruction with minimal fibrosis. The fibrosis of small airways also contributes to airflow obstruction. Emphysema is classified according to its anatomic distribution (Fig. 15-2).

- Centriacinar (centrilobular) emphysema (p. 675)
  - Destruction and enlargement of the central or proximal parts of the respiratory unit—the acinus—sparing distal alveoli
  - Predominant involvement of upper lobes and apices
  - Occurs primarily in heavy smokers, often associated with chronic bronchitis

TABLE 15-3 Disorders Associated With Airflow Obstruction: The Spectrum of COPD

Clinical Term	Anatomic Site	Major Pathologic Changes	Etiology	Signs/Symptoms
Chronic bronchitis	Bronchus	Mucous gland hyperplasia, hypersecretion	Tobacco smoke, air pollutants	Cough, sputum production
Bronchiectasis	Bronchus	Airway dilation and scarring	Persistent or severe infections	Cough, purulent sputum, fever
Asthma	Bronchus	Smooth muscle hyperplasia, excess mucus, inflammation	Immunologic or undefined causes	Episodic wheezing cough, dyspnea
Emphysema	Acinus	Airspace enlargement; wall destruction	Tobacco smoke	Dyspnea
Small airway disease, bronchiolitis	Bronchiole	Inflammatory scarring/obliteration	Tobacco smoke, air pollutants, miscellaneous	Cough, dyspnea

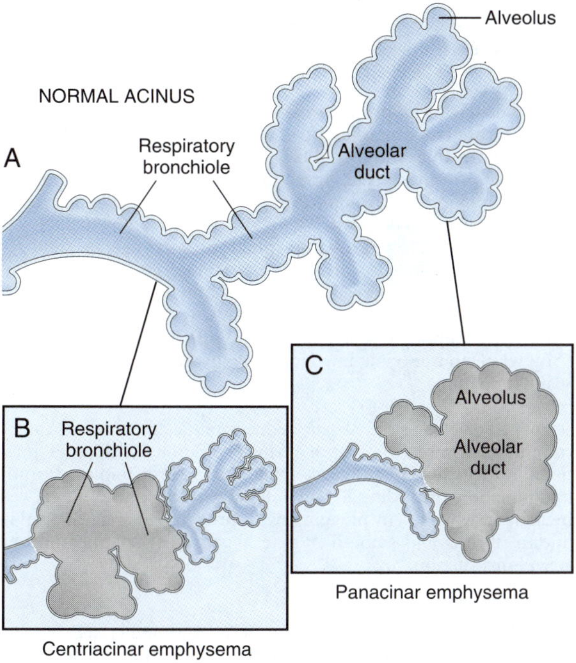

Figure 15-2 Clinically significant patterns of emphysema. A, Structure of the normal acinus. A terminal bronchiole *(not shown)* is immediately proximal to the respiratory bronchiole. **B,** *Centriacinar emphysema* with dilation that initially affects the respiratory bronchioles. **C,** *Panacinar emphysema* with initial distention of the alveolus and alveolar duct; the disease later extends to affect the respiratory bronchioles.

- Panacinar (panlobular) emphysema (p. 675)
  - Uniform destruction and enlargement of the acinus
  - Predominance in lower basal zones
  - Strong association with α_1-antitrypsin deficiency (see Chapter 18)
- Distal acinar (paraseptal) emphysema (p. 675)
  - Involves mostly the distal acinus
  - Typically near the pleura and adjacent to fibrosis or scars
  - Frequently the underlying lesion in spontaneous pneumothorax
- Airspace enlargement with fibrosis (irregular emphysema) (p. 676)
  - Irregular acinar involvement, associated with scarring
  - Most cases are asymptomatic and clinically insignificant

Pathogenesis *(p. 676)*

Inhalation of cigarette smoke and/or other noxious substances causes lung damage and inflammation, leading to the parenchymal destruction of emphysema. Factors that influence the process are as follows:

- *Inflammatory mediators and leukocytes,* including leukotriene B_4, interleukin (IL)-8, and TNF, are released by resident epithelial cells and macrophages; these recruit inflammatory cells, amplify the inflammatory process, and induce structural changes (e.g., through growth factors).

- *Protease-antiprotease imbalance:* Proteases released from inflammatory cells and epithelium can degrade connective tissues. A relative deficiency of protective antiproteases—some of which may be hereditary—can underlie the development of emphysema. Thus individuals with hereditary deficiency of the major protease inhibitor, α_1-antitrypsin, have a marked propensity, compounded by smoking, of developing emphysema; 1% of all emphysema patients have this defect.
- *Oxidative stress* (from tobacco smoke, alveolar damage, and inflammatory cells) also drives tissue damage and inflammation. Genes that sense or regulate oxidant stress are associated with smoking-related lung disease in humans.
- *Infection:* Although infection does not initiate tissue destruction, bacterial and/or viral infections can exacerbate the associated inflammation.

Loss of alveolar elastic tissue reduces radial traction and causes respiratory bronchiole collapse during expiration, resulting in functional obstruction. In addition, small airway (bronchioles <2 mm) inflammation (including T and B lymphocytes) causes goblet cell metaplasia with mucus plugging, with bronchiolar wall thickening due to fibrosis and smooth muscle hyperplasia—augmenting the airway obstruction.

Morphology (p. 677)

With diffuse disease, lungs can become voluminous and overlap the heart. Microscopically alveolar spaces are enlarged, separated by thin septa; septal capillaries are compressed and bloodless. Alveolar wall rupture can produce very large airspaces (*blebs* and *bullae*).

Clinical Course (p. 677)

Symptoms (dyspnea, wheezing, cough) manifest when a third of the pulmonary parenchyma has been lost; there may also be severe weight loss. Patients are classically barrel-chested with obvious prolonged expiration; spirometry is a key diagnostic tool. Classically patients overventilate to compensate for loss of parenchyma and are typically well oxygenated at rest, so-called *pink puffers.* Development of pulmonary hypertension (PH) with heart failure has a poor prognosis; death in severe emphysema is due to the following: (1) respiratory acidosis, (2) right-sided heart failure, or (3) massive pneumothorax.

Other Forms of Emphysema (p. 678)

- *Compensatory hyperinflation* of remaining lung after loss of pulmonary parenchyma (e.g., surgical lobectomy) without septal wall destruction.
- *Obstructive overinflation* due to subtotal obstruction of an airway; this creates a ball-valve that admits air on inspiration but traps it on expiration.
- *Bullous emphysema* is a term for large subpleural blebs or bullae (spaces greater than 1 cm in diameter in the distended state) that can occur in any form of emphysema and can occasionally rupture leading to pneumothorax.
- *Interstitial emphysema* reflects entry of air into connective tissue of lung, mediastinum, or subcutaneous tissues, usually due to alveolar tears after rapid rises in intra-alveolar pressures (e.g., with coughing in the setting of bronchiolar obstruction).

Chronic Bronchitis (p. 678)

Chronic bronchitis is defined as persistent cough with sputum production for at least 3 months in at least two consecutive years, in the absence of any other identifiable cause. It lies on the opposite end of the COPD spectrum from emphysema; most patients fall somewhere between, having features of both. Long-term chronic bronchitis can lead to an acute decline in lung function, cor pulmonale, and heart failure or cause respiratory epithelium dysplasia with malignant transformation.

Pathogenesis (p. 678)

Chronic irritation of the airways by inhaled substances—especially tobacco smoke—is the dominant pathogenic mechanism. In addition to damaging epithelium, smoking (and other inhalants) interferes with the ciliary action of respiratory epithelium, preventing the clearance of mucus and infectious agents. Irritants cause the following:

- *Mucous hypersecretion* with mucus gland hypertrophy is stimulated by inflammatory mediators, such as histamine and IL-13. Goblet cell metaplasia in bronchiolar epithelium contributes to the mucus production and small airway obstruction.
- Inflammation, both acute and chronic, is elicited by inhalants that induce chronic bronchitis. Long-standing inflammation and accompanying fibrosis will cause airway obstruction.
- *Infections* can exacerbate inhalant-initiated injury.

Morphology (p. 679)

- Hyperemia and edema of lung mucous membranes
- Mucinous secretions filling airways
- Mucous gland hyperplasia
- Bronchiolar inflammation and fibrosis
- Bronchial epithelium squamous metaplasia and dysplasia

Clinical Features (p. 679)

Beyond the defining cough and sputum production, dyspnea on exertion eventually develops. In classic cases, patients are hypoxic, cyanotic, and hypercapnic (retain CO_2), so-called *blue bloaters.* Long-standing disease often progresses to cor pulmonale with heart failure; death can also be secondary to infection.

Asthma (p. 679)

This chronic relapsing inflammatory disorder is characterized by paroxysmal reversible bronchospasm due to smooth muscle hyperreactivity; increased mucus production is also a feature. The incidence has increased significantly in the past four decades in the Western world. Asthma can be categorized into two major forms:

- *Atopic (allergic) asthma* (p. 679) is most common. It is caused by a classic type I (immunoglobulin E [IgE])-mediated hypersensitivity reaction triggered by environmental antigens (e.g., dust, pollen, certain foods [see Chapter 6]); a family history of atopy is common.
- *Nonatopic asthma* (p. 679) can be triggered by respiratory tract infections, chemical irritants, or drugs, usually without a family history. Airway hyperirritability is attributed to virally or chemically induced inflammation that reduces the threshold for vagal stimulation by other minor irritants.
- *Drug-induced asthma* (p. 680) can occur with a variety of pharmacologic agents. For example, in some patients, aspirin (and

other nonsteroidal antiinflammatory drugs) can inhibit cyclooxygenase (without affecting lipoxygenase activity) and tip the balance of arachidonic acid metabolism toward bronchoconstrictor leukotrienes.
- *Occupational asthma* (p. 680) can be triggered by fumes (epoxy resins, plastics), organic and chemical dusts (wood, cotton, platinum), gases (toluene), or other chemicals (formaldehyde, penicillin products). The underlying mechanisms vary according to stimulus and include true allergic reactions, direct liberation of bronchoconstrictor substances, and hypersensitivity responses of unknown origin.

Pathogenesis *(p. 680; Fig. 15-3)*

T_H2 responses, IgE, and inflammation (p. 680): T-cell differentiation is skewed to overproduce T_H2-type cells (see Chapter 6) with subsequent IgE- and eosinophil-dominated immune responses; in presensitized patients, repeat antigen exposure causes the following:

- *Acute phase:* Antigen binding to IgE-coated mast cells causes primary (e.g., leukotriene) and secondary (e.g., cytokine) mediator release. Acute-phase mediators cause bronchospasm, edema, mucus secretion, and leukocyte recruitment.
- *Late phase:* Mediated by recruited leukocytes (e.g., eosinophils, lymphocytes, neutrophils, monocytes) and characterized by persistent bronchospasm and edema, leukocytic infiltration, and epithelial damage and loss.

Repeated bouts cause *airway remodeling* with bronchial smooth muscle and mucus gland hypertrophy and hyperplasia, increased vascularity, and increased deposition of subepithelial collagen.

Genetic Susceptibility *(p. 680)*

Multiple susceptibility loci interact with environmental factors to produce asthma; implicated genes can affect primary or secondary immune responses, tissue remodeling, or even patient response to therapy. The strongest genetic associations have been made with certain human leukocyte antigen (HLA) alleles, and polymorphisms in IL-13, CD14 (the monocyte receptor for endotoxin), ADAM-33 (a matrix metalloproteinase that influences smooth muscle and fibroblast proliferation), α_2-adrenergic receptor (influencing airway reactivity), and the IL-4 receptor.

Environmental Factors *(p. 682)*

Asthma occurs at a higher frequency in industrialized societies where the majority of people live in cities: (1) industrialized environments contain many airborne pollutants that can serve as allergens to initiate the T_H2 response, and (2) city life tends to limit the exposure of very young children to certain antigens, particularly microbial antigens. This apparent protective effect of early microbial exposure is encapsulated as the *hygiene hypothesis;* the underlying mechanisms are unclear.

Morphology *(p. 682)*

Lungs are overinflated with patchy atelectasis and mucus plugging of airways. *Microscopically* the lungs exhibit edema, bronchiolar inflammatory infiltrates with numerous eosinophils, subepithelial fibrosis, and bronchial wall smooth muscle and mucosal gland hypertrophy. Whorled mucus plugs *(Curschmann spirals)* and crystalloid eosinophil granule debris *(Charcot-Leyden crystals)* deposit in airways.

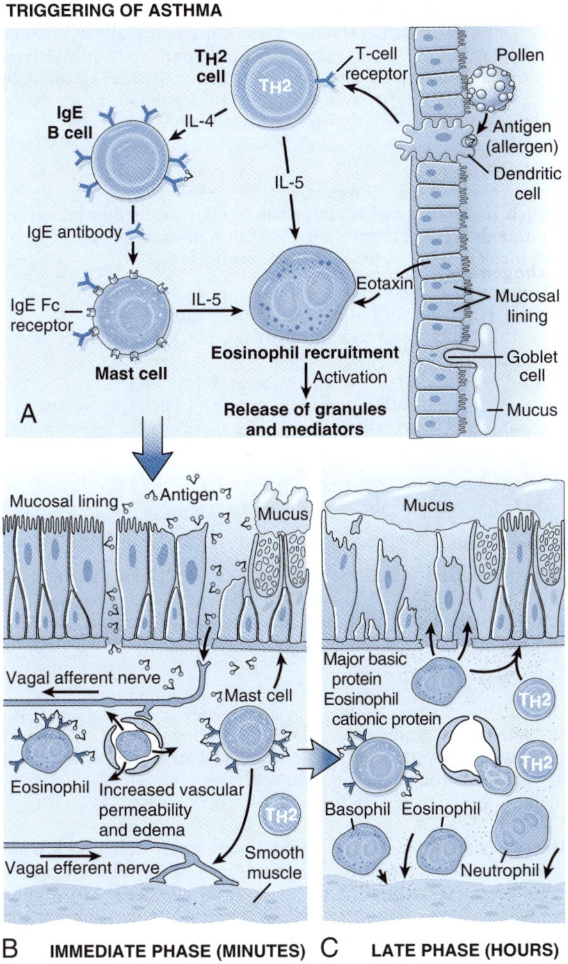

Figure 15-3 Asthma pathogenesis. A, Inhaled allergens (antigen) elicit a T_H2-dominated response favoring IgE production and eosinophil recruitment. **B,** On re-exposure to antigen (Ag), the immediate reaction is triggered by Ag-induced cross-linking of IgE bound to Fc receptors on mast cells; mast cells then release preformed mediators that directly and via neuronal reflexes induce bronchospasm, increased vascular permeability, mucus production, and recruitment of leukocytes. **C,** Leukocytes recruited to the site of reaction (neutrophils, eosinophils, and basophils; lymphocytes and monocytes) release additional mediators that initiate the late phase of asthma. Several factors released from eosinophils (e.g., major basic protein, eosinophil cationic protein) also cause damage to the epithelium.

Clinical Course *(p. 682)*

Classic attacks last up to several hours; symptoms include chest tightness, wheezing, dyspnea, and cough. Diagnosis is based on demonstrating increased airflow obstruction and prolonged exhalation (reducing FEV_1). Over time, repeated bouts of allergen exposure and immune reactions result in structural changes in the bronchial wall, referred to as "airway remodeling," causing a permanent decline in lung function; these include hypertrophy and hyperplasia of bronchial smooth muscle, increased airway vascularity, increased subepithelial mucus gland hypertrophy, and deposition of subepithelial collagen. In severe acute episodes *(status asthmaticus)*, symptoms persist for days to weeks, and significant airflow obstruction can cause cyanosis and even death.

Bronchiectasis (p. 683)

Bronchiectasis represents abnormal *permanent* dilation of airways due to a destructive, necrotizing infection of bronchi and bronchioles; it can develop in the following conditions:

- Congenital or hereditary conditions (e.g., cystic fibrosis, Kartagener syndrome, or pulmonary sequestration)
- Postinfectious (e.g., after necrotizing bacterial, viral, or fungal pneumonia)
- Bronchial obstruction (e.g., by tumor or foreign body)
- Other chronic inflammatory states (e.g., rheumatoid arthritis, chronic graft-versus-host disease, or allergic bronchopulmonary aspergillosis)

Idiopathic bronchiectasis is diagnosed when the other causes are excluded; it accounts for 25% to 50% of cases.

Pathogenesis *(p. 683)*

Obstruction and infection are the major etiologies, and both are likely necessary for full-blown bronchiectasis. Thus bronchial obstruction impedes normal clearing so that infections and inflammation can fester and eventually cause the requisite tissue destruction.

Morphology *(p. 683)*

Most severe changes occur in peripheral lower lobes; airways can be dilated up to 4 times normal size. Histology shows a spectrum of mild-to-necrotizing acute and chronic inflammation of the larger airways with bronchiolar fibrosis.

Clinical Course *(p. 684)*

The presentation is marked by persistent, severe cough, fever, and abundant purulent sputum. Symptoms may be episodic and precipitated by upper respiratory tract infection; alternatively, coughing can be associated with morning rising and positional changes that drain collected pus and secretions into the bronchi. Complications include cor pulmonale, brain abscesses, and amyloidosis.

Chronic Diffuse Interstitial (Restrictive) Diseases (p. 684)

Restrictive lung disorders comprise two general conditions:

- *Chronic interstitial and infiltrative diseases,* such as pneumoconioses and interstitial fibrosis of unknown etiology
- *Chest wall disorders* (e.g., neuromuscular diseases, such as poliomyelitis, severe obesity, pleural diseases, and kyphoscoliosis), which are not discussed here

Chronic interstitial lung diseases are a heterogeneous group of disorders characterized by *inflammation and pulmonary interstitial fibrosis,* particularly involving alveolar walls; many have unknown causes (Table 15-4). The clinical and functional changes are those of *restrictive lung disease;* diffusing capacity,

TABLE 15-4 Major Categories of Chronic Interstitial Lung Disease
Fibrosing
UIP (idiopathic pulmonary fibrosis)
NSIP
COP
Connective tissue disease-associated
Pneumoconiosis
Drug reactions
Radiation pneumonitis
Granulomatous
Sarcoidosis
Hypersensitivity pneumonitis
Eosinophilic
Smoking Related
DIP
Respiratory bronchiolitis–associated interstitial lung disease
Other
Langerhans cell histiocytosis
PAP
Lymphoid interstitial pneumonia

lung volumes, and compliance are all compromised, without evidence of airway obstruction. Secondary PH and cor pulmonale are long-term sequelae. Although the early stages of the different entities can often be distinguished histologically, there is substantial morphologic overlap, and most devolve to a common end stage marked by parenchymal destruction and scarring, so-called *honeycomb lung.*

Fibrosing Diseases (p. 684)

Idiopathic Pulmonary Fibrosis (p. 684)

Idiopathic pulmonary fibrosis is a disorder of unknown cause *characterized by progressive pulmonary interstitial fibrosis.*

Pathogenesis (p. 685)

Cigarette smoking or exposure to various environmental irritants or toxins leads to recurrent cycles of epithelial activation/injury. Such injury triggers abnormal "wound healing" in a susceptible host, with excessive fibroblast proliferation; abnormal telomere shortening (e.g., due to germline loss-of-function mutations in genes that encode telomerase components) is implicated in up to 25% of cases. Injured epithelium may release TGF-β1 inducing both fibrosis as well as further epithelial cell apoptosis.

Morphology (p. 686)

The pathologic pattern of fibrosis is denoted *usual interstitial pneumonia (UIP);* this is nonspecific and can also be seen in connective tissue disorders, chronic hypersensitivity pneumonia, and asbestosis.

- Patchy interstitial fibrosis has a characteristic subpleural and interlobular septal distribution and a lower lobe predominance.
- There is heterogeneity of the histologic changes; new, cellular *fibroblastic foci* with moderate inflammation coexist with older, more densely fibrotic areas.

- Destruction of the alveolar architecture leads to *honeycomb lung* with dense fibrosis and cystic spaces lined by hyperplastic type II pneumocytes or bronchiolar epithelium; arteriolar hypertensive changes are often present.

Clinical Course (p. 686)

The disease typically has an insidious onset between ages 55 and 75 marked by dyspnea on exertion and a dry cough. The course progression is unpredictable in any given patient, but most have a gradual deterioration with hypoxemia and cyanosis despite antiinflammatory and antiproliferative therapies. Mean survival is ≤3 years; lung transplantation is the only definitive therapy.

Nonspecific Interstitial Pneumonia (p. 686)

Nonspecific interstitial pneumonia (NSIP) is a diffusely fibrosing disease of unknown etiology, presenting with chronic dyspnea and cough. The histologic pattern shows either moderate interstitial inflammation or interstitial fibrosis without the temporal heterogeneity seen in UIP. The prognosis for NSIP is better than for UIP.

Cryptogenic Organizing Pneumonia (p. 687)

Formerly called *bronchiolitis obliterans organizing pneumonia (BOOP)*, cryptogenic organizing pneumonia (COP) has an unknown etiology. Patients present with cough and dyspnea, with patchy subpleural or peribronchial consolidation. *Histologically* there are loose fibrous tissue plugs (Masson bodies) within bronchioles, alveolar ducts, and alveoli but no interstitial fibrosis or honeycombing. Patients can spontaneously recover, although most require steroid therapy. Notably the same morphologic changes are seen in response to infections or inflammatory lung injury.

Pulmonary Involvement in Autoimmune Diseases (p. 687)

Pulmonary involvement in autoimmune diseases (e.g., systemic lupus erythematosus, rheumatoid arthritis, and scleroderma) is common; patterns include NSIP, UIP, vascular sclerosis, organizing pneumonia, and bronchiolitis. Prognosis is variable (depending on the underlying disease) but is better than for idiopathic UIP.

Pneumoconioses (p. 687)

Pneumoconioses are the non-neoplastic lung response to inhaled aerosols, including mineral dusts, organic dusts, fumes, and vapors (Table 15-5). In general only a small percentage of an exposed population develops a respiratory disease, suggesting a genetic predisposition in those affected.

Pathogenesis (p. 688)

Pneumoconiosis development depends on the following:

- *Amount of dust retained*, itself a function of the original concentration, duration of exposure, and effectiveness of clearance mechanisms.
- *Size, shape, and particle buoyancy:* Particles between 1 and 5 μm are the most dangerous because they can reach terminal alveoli and settle in their linings.
- *Physicochemical reactivity (toxicity) and particle solubility:* Highly soluble particles may rapidly cause toxicity; insoluble particles may persist and cause a chronic fibrosis.
- *Additional effects of other irritants* (e.g., cigarette smoking).

Certain types of particles cause pathology by *stimulating inflammasome activation* (see Chapter 6) after phagocytosis by pulmonary macrophages.

TABLE 15-5 Lung Diseases Caused by Air Pollutants

Agent	Disease	Exposure
Mineral Dusts		
Coal dust	Anthracosis Macules PMF Caplan syndrome	Coal mining (particularly hard coal)
Silica	Silicosis Caplan syndrome	Metal casting work, sandblasting, hard rock mining, stone cutting, others
Asbestos	Asbestosis Pleural plaques Caplan syndrome Mesothelioma Carcinoma of the lung, larynx, stomach, colon	Mining, milling, manufacturing, and installation and removal of insulation
Beryllium	Acute berylliosis Beryllium granulomatosis Lung carcinoma (?)	Mining, manufacturing
Iron oxide	Siderosis	Welding
Barium sulfate	Baritosis	Mining
Tin oxide	Stannosis	Mining
Organic Dusts That Induce Hypersensitivity Pneumonitis		
Moldy hay	Farmer's lung	Farming
Bagasse	Bagassosis	Manufacturing wallboard, paper
Bird droppings	Bird breeder's lung	Bird handling
Organic Dusts That Induce Asthma		
Cotton, flax, hemp	Byssinosis	Textile manufacturing
Red cedar dust	Asthma	Lumbering, carpentry
Chemical Fumes and Vapors		
Nitrous oxide, sulfur dioxide, ammonia, benzene, insecticides	Bronchitis, asthma Pulmonary edema ARDS Mucosal injury Fulminant poisoning	Occupational and accidental exposure

Coal Workers' Pneumoconiosis *(p. 689).* The spectrum of pulmonary effects of carbon dust varies from (1) asymptomatic *anthracosis* to (2) simple *coal workers' pneumoconiosis (CWP)* without significant pulmonary dysfunction to (3) complicated CWP, or *progressive massive fibrosis (PMF)* with compromised lung function. The factors underlying the progression from simple CWP to PMF are not understood; possibilities include the duration and magnitude of exposure, contaminants in the carbon (e.g., silicates), and the propensity of an individual's coal dust-laden macrophages to produce fibrogenic cytokines.

Morphology (p. 689)

- In *anthracosis,* inhaled carbon is taken up by alveolar and interstitial macrophages, which then accumulate in lymphatics and lymphoid tissues.
- In *simple* CWP, 1- to 2-mm *coal macules* are composed of dust-filled macrophages; slightly larger *coal nodules* also contain delicate networks of collagen. These are located primarily adjacent to respiratory bronchioles.

- In *PMF,* large, blackened collagenous scars (often with central ischemic necrosis) replace substantial portions of the lung.

Clinical Course (p. 689)

CWP usually causes little functional decrement; PMF will develop in <10%, with associated respiratory insufficiency and PH, and may be progressive even without further exposures.

Silicosis *(p. 690).* Prolonged inhalation of silica particles produces a chronic, progressive, nodular fibrosis.

Pathogenesis (p. 690)

Crystalline forms of silica (versus amorphous forms) are most fibrogenic; ingestion by macrophages causes inflammasome activation, with release of oxidants, cytokines (IL-1 and TNF), and growth factors that ultimately cause fibroblast proliferation and collagen deposition. Interestingly silica mixed with a variety of other minerals (e.g., iron) is less fibrogenic.

Morphology (p. 690)

Collagenous nodules start in the upper lung, becoming larger and more diffuse with disease progression. Lesion coalescence forms large areas of dense scar. Calcification or concomitant blackening by coal dust often occurs. Microscopically there are hyalinized whorls of collagen with scant inflammation. Polarized light reveals birefringent silica particles.

Clinical Course (p. 690)

Dyspnea is not usually present until PMF has developed; the disease can progress even after exposure ends. Silicosis is associated with increased susceptibility to tuberculosis, likely due to depressed cell-mediated immunity.

Asbestos-Related Diseases *(p. 690).* Asbestos is a family of fibrous silicates; occupational exposures are linked to the following:

- Localized pleural plaques and effusions or rarely diffuse pleural fibrosis
- Parenchymal interstitial fibrosis *(asbestosis)*
- Lung carcinoma, malignant mesothelioma, and laryngeal and other extrapulmonary neoplasms

Pathogenesis (p. 691)

Different forms of asbestos have different clinical consequences. Straight, stiff *amphiboles* reach the deep lung more readily than flexible, curved *serpentine* fibers, accounting for their greater pathogenicity; serpentine fibers are also more soluble than amphiboles and thus are gradually leached from the tissues.

- Alveolar macrophages ingest inhaled fibers, leading to inflammasome activation and production of mediators (e.g., fibrogenic cytokines and growth factors).
- Asbestos fibers can act as both tumor initiators and promoters. Some oncogenic effects are related to free radical generation, whereas adsorption of potentially toxic substances (e.g., tobacco smoke carcinogens) on fibers also contributes to their tumorigenicity.

Morphology (p. 691)

- *Pleural plaques* are well-circumscribed plaques of dense collagen; although they do not contain asbestos bodies (see later), they only rarely occur in the absence of prior asbestos exposures.

- *Asbestosis* is marked by diffuse interstitial fibrosis that is indistinguishable from similar lesions caused by other disorders (e.g., UIP) *except* for the presence of *asbestos bodies;* these are ingested fibers coated by iron-containing proteinaceous material to form characteristic, beaded, dumbbell-shaped fibers. They occur in the process of attempted macrophage endocytosis; similar iron encrustation can occur with other inorganic particulates and are called *ferruginous bodies.*

Clinical Course (p. 692)

Plaques are typically asymptomatic. Dyspnea is usually the first manifestation of asbestosis, often accompanied by a productive cough; these symptoms typically occur with a lag of 10 to 20 years after exposure. With advanced pneumoconiosis, honeycombing develops, and the course may be static or progress to respiratory failure or cor pulmonale. Asbestosis complicated by pulmonary or pleural malignancy has a grim prognosis.

Complications of Therapies (p. 692)

- *Drug-induced lung diseases* (p. 692) range from acute bronchospasm (aspirin) to cough (angiotensin-converting enzyme inhibitors) to pneumonitis (amiodarone) to fibrosis (bleomycin). Intravenous drug abuse can lead to lung infections, as well as granulomatous and fibrosing responses.
- *Radiation-induced lung disease* (p. 692) occurs in 3% to 44% of patients, beginning as *acute radiation pneumonitis* and DAD 1 to 6 months after therapy; many cases resolve (especially with steroid therapy), but some progress to *chronic radiation pneumonitis* (pulmonary fibrosis).

Granulomatous Diseases (p. 693)

Sarcoidosis (p. 693)

Sarcoidosis is a systemic disease of unknown etiology, characterized by noncaseating granulomas in virtually all tissues; 90% of cases involve hilar lymph nodes or lung. Women are affected more frequently than men, with American blacks affected 10 times more often than whites.

Pathogenesis (p. 693)

Sarcoidosis is likely a disease of disordered immune response in genetically predisposed individuals to certain environmental agents:

- Association with specific HLA genotypes (e.g., HLA-A1 and HLA-B8)
- Accumulation of oligoclonal, activated CD4+ T cells
- Increased T_H1 cytokine production (IL-2 and interferon-γ), causing T-cell expansion and macrophage activation
- Increased macrophage TNF production, leading to granuloma formation
- Impaired dendritic cell function
- Cutaneous anergy to common antigens (e.g., tuberculin or *Candida*)
- Polyclonal hypergammaglobulinemia

Morphology (p. 693)

Granulomas are characteristically noncaseating, with tightly clustered epithelioid histiocytes and frequent multinucleated giant cells. *Schaumann bodies* (laminated, calcified proteinaceous concretions) and *asteroid bodies* (stellate inclusions within giant cells) commonly occur but are not pathognomonic.

- *Lungs exhibit* diffuse, scattered granulomas, forming a reticulonodular pattern on x-rays. Pulmonary lesions tend to heal, and only residual hyalinized scars may be seen.
- *Lymph nodes* are virtually always involved, most commonly in the hilar and mediastinal regions; tonsils are involved in 25% to 33% of cases.
- *Spleen and liver* are microscopically affected in 75% of patients, although gross splenomegaly and hepatomegaly occur in <20%.
- *Bone marrow* involvement is seen in 20%; radiologically visible lesions have a phalangeal predilection.
- *Skin* involvement occurs in 33% to 50% of patients as discrete subcutaneous nodules or erythematous scaling plaques or macules; mucous membrane lesions also occur.
- *Eyes* are affected in 20% to 50% of cases, including iritis, iridocyclitis, or choroid retinitis, often with lacrimal gland inflammation, and reduced lacrimation. Central nervous system involvement occurs in 5% to 15% of patients.
- Bilateral involvement of *salivary glands* constitutes the *Mikulicz syndrome.*

Clinical Course (p. 694)

Because of its varying severity and different patterns of organ involvement, sarcoidosis can be entirely asymptomatic and discovered only incidentally or manifest as isolated cutaneous or ocular lesions, peripheral lymphadenopathy, or hepatosplenomegaly. Patients most commonly present with the insidious onset of respiratory difficulties or constitutional symptoms (fever, night sweats, weight loss).

Diagnosis is established by biopsy demonstrating noncaseating granulomas; other diseases with the same histology (e.g., tuberculosis and fungal infections) are ruled out by culture or special stains. *Sarcoidosis is a diagnosis of exclusion.*

Sarcoidosis follows an unpredictable course and can be a slowly progressive, remitting, and relapsing course (with or without steroid therapy) or can spontaneously resolve. Most patients (65% to 70%) recover with no or only minimal residua; 20% have permanent lung or ocular dysfunction; and 10% to 15% of patients succumb, often to progressive pulmonary fibrosis.

Hypersensitivity Pneumonitis *(p. 694)*

Hypersensitivity pneumonitis is a spectrum of immunologically mediated interstitial disorders caused by inhaled dusts or antigens; as opposed to asthma, these disorders primarily affect the alveoli ("allergic alveolitis"):

- *Farmer's lung: Actinomycetes* spores in hay
- *Pigeon breeder's lung:* Proteins from bird feathers or excreta
- *Humidifier* or *air-conditioner lung:* Bacteria in heated water reservoirs

Morphology (p. 695)

Histologic changes include interstitial pneumonitis and fibrosis centered on bronchioles, and (in two thirds of patients) noncaseating granulomas. Early cessation of exposure to the injurious agent prevents progression to serious chronic fibrosis and honeycombing.

Clinical Features (p. 695)

The clinical manifestations are varied and include cough, dyspnea, fever, diffuse and nodular radiographic densities, and a restrictive pattern of pulmonary dysfunction.

Pulmonary Eosinophilia (p. 695)

These are diverse clinicopathologic conditions characterized by interstitial or alveolar eosinophil infiltrates:

- *Acute eosinophilic pneumonia with respiratory failure:* Unknown etiology; rapid onset of fever, dyspnea, and hypoxia, and prompt response to corticosteroids.
- *Secondary eosinophilia:* Associated with infections, hypersensitivity, asthma, allergic bronchopulmonary aspergillosis, or vasculitis *(Churg-Strauss syndrome)*.
- *Idiopathic chronic eosinophilic pneumonia:* Unknown etiology, manifested by focal lung consolidation with extensive lymphocyte and eosinophil infiltration, as well as interstitial fibrosis; it is steroid responsive.

Smoking-Related Interstitial Diseases (p. 695)

Desquamative Interstitial Pneumonia (p. 695)

Desquamative interstitial pneumonia (DIP) is characterized by an insidious onset of dyspnea and dry cough; histology reveals abundant *intra-alveolar* dusty brown (smokers') macrophages with mild interstitial inflammation and minimal fibrosis. Emphysema is often present. Steroid therapy or smoking cessation yields improvement.

Respiratory Bronchiolitis-Associated Interstitial Lung Disease (p. 696)

Respiratory bronchiolitis-associated interstitial lung disease causes gradual usually mild dyspnea and cough; histology reveals patchy *bronchiolar* accumulations of smokers' macrophages, with peribronchiolar inflammation and mild fibrosis. Smoking cessation yields improvement.

Pulmonary Langerhans Cell Histiocytosis (p. 696)

A rare disease characterized by focal collections of Langerhans cells (immature dendritic cells) that cause progressive fibrosis; the scarring is associated with airway destruction and alveolar damage yielding irregular cystic spaces. More than 95% of affected patients are young adult smoker; smoking cessation leads to improvement in most cases. However, in other cases the Langerhans cells have acquired activating mutations in the serine-threonine kinase BRAF, leading to disease progression.

Pulmonary Alveolar Proteinosis (p. 696)

Pulmonary alveolar proteinosis (PAP) is a rare entity characterized by defects related to granulocyte-macrophage colony-stimulating factor (GM-CSF) or pulmonary macrophage dysfunction that leads to surfactant accumulation in alveoli and bronchioles; there are three distinct pathogenic classes, all with similar histology:

- *Autoimmune PAP* accounts for 90% of cases. Autoantibodies against GM-CSF lead to functional GM-CSF deficiency and to impaired surfactant clearance by pulmonary macrophages.
- *Secondary PAP* follows exposure to irritating dusts or chemicals or occurs in immunocompromised individuals, somehow impairing macrophage maturation or function.
- *Hereditary PAP* occurs in newborns and is caused by mutations involved in either GM-CSF production or signaling.

PAP is characterized *clinically* by respiratory difficulty, cough, and abundant sputum often containing chunks of gelatinous material.

Histologically there is dense, amorphous, periodic acid-Schiff (PAS)-positive, lipid-laden protein exudates filling alveolar spaces. Patients are at risk for developing secondary infections. Whole-lung lavage provides benefit regardless of etiology; GM-CSF therapy is effective in half of patients with autoimmune PAP.

Surfactant Dysfunction Disorders (p. 697)

Surfactant dysfunction disorders are caused by mutations in proteins involved in surfactant trafficking or secretion:

- *ATP-binding cassette protein member 3 (ABCA3)* mutations are most common; these result in an autosomal recessive disorder, usually presenting shortly after birth with rapidly progressive respiratory failure and death.
- *Surfactant protein C* mutations are second most common; these cause an autosomal dominant disorder with variable penetrance and severity.
- *Surfactant protein B* mutations are least common; these cause autosomal recessive disease with rapidly progressive respiratory distress shortly after birth and death within 3 to 6 months.

Diseases of Vascular Origin (p. 697)

Pulmonary Embolism and Infarction (p. 697; see also Chapter 4)

Pulmonary artery occlusions are almost always embolic; in situ thromboses are rare but can occur with PH, pulmonary atherosclerosis, and heart failure. Deep leg veins are the source of over 95% of pulmonary emboli (PE), and the prevalence of PE correlates with predisposition to leg thrombosis.

The pathophysiologic response and clinical significance of PE depend on the extent of pulmonary arterial obstruction, size of occluded vessel(s), number of emboli, overall status of the cardiovascular system, and release of vasoactive factors from platelets at the site of thrombosis. Emboli cause *respiratory compromise* due to lack of perfusion of ventilated lung, and *hemodynamic compromise* due to increased pulmonary arterial resistance.

Clinical Course (p. 698)

Large emboli impact in the major pulmonary arteries or astride the pulmonary artery bifurcation *(saddle embolus)* and can cause sudden death due to *electromechanical dissociation* (no blood in the pulmonary circulation) or acute *cor pulmonale* (right-sided heart failure). Multiple or recurrent small-medium emboli can have the same effect, although more commonly these are clinically silent or only cause transient chest pain and/or hemoptysis from pulmonary hemorrhage. Only 10% of PE cause infarction; this occurs in patients with compromised pulmonary circulation (cardiac failure), and manifest as peripheral, wedge-shaped hemorrhagic areas of necrosis. Uncommonly, multiple small PE (overt or covert) produce PH, vascular sclerosis, and chronic cor pulmonale.

Pulmonary Hypertension (p. 699)

PH is defined as a mean pulmonary artery pressure ≥25 mm Hg at rest; there are five general mechanisms:

- Multiple etiologies that primarily affect pulmonary muscular artery tone (can include autoimmune diseases, such as systemic sclerosis)

- Secondary to left-sided heart failure (ischemic, valvular, congenital, etc.)
- Primary lung parenchymal disease or hypoxia (can include obstructive sleep apnea)
- Chronic pulmonary thromboembolic disease
- Multifactorial

PH is called idiopathic when all other causes are excluded; 80% of these will have a genetic basis.

Pathogenesis *(p. 699)*

Approximately 75% of the familial cases (and 25% of sporadic cases) of PH are caused by mutations in the *bone morphogenetic protein receptor type 2 (BMPR2)* signaling pathway. In vascular smooth muscle cells (SMCs), BMPR2 signaling inhibits proliferation and favors apoptosis; defective signaling therefore results in SMC hyperplasia and increased vascular resistance. Only 10% to 20% of patients with the mutations develop PH, suggesting that the phenotype is influenced by environmental triggers or by modifier genes that affect vascular tone (e.g., endothelin, prostacyclin, nitric oxide, and angiotensin-converting enzyme activities).

Morphology *(p. 700)*

- Atherosclerosis in the pulmonary artery and major branches.
- Medial hypertrophy of muscular and elastic arteries.
- Right ventricular hypertrophy.
- *Plexiform lesions* (tufts within capillary channels creating a vascular plexus) represent the severe end of the spectrum of changes; most prominent in primary PH and with some congenital cardiovascular anomalies.
- Numerous organized thrombi suggest recurrent pulmonary thromboembolism as an etiology.

Clinical Course *(p. 700)*

Clinical signs and symptoms in all forms of PH become evident only with advanced disease. *Idiopathic PH* occurs most often in women 20 to 40 years old; it generally progresses to severe respiratory insufficiency, decompensated cor pulmonale (often with superimposed thromboembolism and pneumonia), and death within 2 to 5 years. Therapy includes vasodilators and lung transplantation.

Diffuse Pulmonary Hemorrhage Syndromes (p. 701)

Goodpasture Syndrome *(p. 701)*

Goodpasture syndrome is caused by autoantibodies directed against the noncollagenous domain of the collagen IV $\alpha3$ chain; these cause basement membrane destruction in renal glomeruli and pulmonary alveoli, giving rise to rapidly progressive glomerulonephritis (see Chapter 20) and necrotizing hemorrhagic interstitial pneumonitis. Most cases occur in the teens or 20s, with a male predominance; the vast majority are smokers. Histology of the lung reveals focal alveolar wall necrosis with intra-alveolar hemorrhage and hemosiderin-laden macrophages; immunofluorescence shows linear immunoglobulin deposition along septal basement membranes. Hemoptysis is a typical presenting feature, followed by symptoms of glomerulonephritis; uremia is the most common cause of death. Therapy involves plasmapheresis and immunosuppression.

Idiopathic Pulmonary Hemosiderosis *(p. 701)*

Idiopathic pulmonary hemosiderosis is a rare disease of children characterized by intermittent diffuse alveolar hemorrhage; it presents with cough and hemoptysis. It responds to immunosuppression, suggesting an underlying immunologic basis.

Polyangiitis With Granulomatosis *(p. 701)*

Previously called *Wegener granulomatosis,* this is an autoimmune disease typically presenting with hemoptysis (see Chapter 11); diagnostically important features are capillaritis and scattered, poorly formed granulomata.

Pulmonary Infections (p. 702)

Pulmonary infections occur when lung or systemic defenses are impaired. Pulmonary defenses include nasal, tracheobronchial, and alveolar mechanisms to filter, neutralize, and clear inhaled organisms and particles. These can be compromised by the following:

- Decreased cough reflex leading to aspiration (e.g., coma, anesthesia, neuromuscular disorders)
- Injury to mucociliary apparatus (e.g., cigarette smoking, viral infection, genetic defects)
- Secretion accumulation (e.g., cystic fibrosis, chronic bronchitis)
- Decreased phagocytic or bactericidal function of alveolar macrophages (e.g., tobacco smoke, oxygen toxicity)
- Edema or congestion (congestive heart failure)
- Inadequate innate immunity (e.g., due to neutrophil and complement defects), germline mutations in MyD88 (adapter protein that links Toll-like receptors to NF-κB activation), humoral immunodeficiency, or congenital and acquired cell-mediated immune defects

Pneumonias are broadly defined as any infection of the lung parenchyma; these are classified by the specific etiologic agent or the clinical setting (Table 15-6). If no pathogen can be isolated (50% of cases), pneumonia is classified according to the clinical setting in which it occurs (e.g., community-acquired, health care-associated), which helps to narrow the possible organisms and thereby direct therapy. Additional points are as follows:

- One type of pneumonia (e.g., viral) often predisposes to another type (e.g., bacterial) due to compromise of systemic or specific pulmonary defenses.
- Although most pneumonias enter via the respiratory tract, hematogenous spread from other sites can occur.
- Many patients with chronic diseases develop terminal infections when hospitalized *(nosocomial infections);* this is due to a combination of antibiotic resistance, invasive procedures, equipment contamination, and a greater chance for exposure.

Community-Acquired Bacterial Pneumonias (p. 702)

Predisposing conditions include extremes of age, chronic disease (e.g., COPD), immune deficiencies, and lack of splenic function. Biomarkers for bacterial infections include hepatic acute-phase reactants, such as C-reactive protein and procalcitonin.

- *Streptococcus pneumoniae* or *pneumococcus* (p. 702) is the most common cause of community-acquired pneumonia.

TABLE 15-6 Pneumonia Syndromes

Community-Acquired Acute Pneumonia

S. pneumoniae
H. influenzae
M. catarrhalis
S. aureus
L. pneumophila
Enterobacteriaceae *(K. pneumoniae)* and *Pseudomonas* spp.
M. pneumoniae
Chlamydia spp. *(Chlamydophila pneumoniae, Chlamydophila psittaci, Chlamydia trachomatis)*
Coxiella burnetii (Q fever)
Viruses: respiratory syncytial virus, parainfluenza virus and human MPV (children); influenza A and B (adults); adenovirus (military recruits);

Health Care-Associated Pneumonia

S. aureus, methicillin-sensitive
S. aureus, methicillin-resistant
P. aeruginosa
S. pneumoniae

Hospital-Acquired Pneumonia

Gram-negative rods, Enterobacteriaceae (*Klebsiella* spp., *Serratia marcescens, Escherichia coli*) and *Pseudomonas* spp.
S. aureus (usually methicillin resistant)

Aspiration Pneumonia

Anaerobic oral flora *(Bacteroides, Prevotella, Fusobacterium, Peptostreptococcus)*, admixed with aerobic bacteria *(S. pneumoniae, S. aureus, H. influenzae, P. aeruginosa)*

Chronic Pneumonia

Nocardia
Actinomyces
Granulomatous: *Mycobacterium tuberculosis* and atypical mycobacteria, *H. capsulatum, C. immitis, B. dermatitidis*

Necrotizing Pneumonia and Lung Abscess

Anaerobic bacteria (extremely common), with or without mixed aerobic infection
S. aureus, K. pneumoniae, Streptococcus pyogenes, and type 3 pneumococcus (uncommon)

Pneumonia in the Immunocompromised Host

Cytomegalovirus
Pneumocystis jiroveci
M. avium-intracellulare
Invasive aspergillosis
Invasive candidiasis
"Usual" bacterial, viral, and fungal organisms (listed herein)

- *Haemophilus influenzae* (p. 703) can cause life-threatening lower respiratory tract infections and meningitis in children and is a common cause of pneumonia in adults, especially those with COPD. It is a pleomorphic gram-negative organism that colonizes the pharynx, occurring as encapsulated and unencapsulated forms; type b (of serotypes a-f) is the most common encapsulated cause of severe invasive disease. Virulence factors include adhesive pili, a factor that dysregulates ciliary beating, and a protease that degrades IgA.
- *Moraxella catarrhalis* (p. 703) causes bacterial pneumonia, especially in the elderly; it exacerbates COPD and is a common cause of pediatric otitis media.

- *Staphylococcus aureus* (p. 703) pneumonia often complicates viral illnesses and has a high risk of abscess formation and empyema. Intravenous drug abusers are at high risk of staphylococcal pneumonia in association with endocarditis.
- *Klebsiella pneumoniae* (p. 703) is the most common cause of gram-negative pneumonia; it afflicts debilitated individuals, especially chronic alcoholics.
- *Pseudomonas aeruginosa* (p. 703) is a common cause of nosocomial infections with a propensity to invade blood vessels and spread systemically; it is also common in cystic fibrosis and neutropenic patients.
- *Legionella pneumophila* (p. 703) is the agent of Legionnaires' disease and Pontiac fever. It flourishes in artificial aquatic environments, such as water-cooling towers, and spreads through aerosolization; infection causes severe pneumonia in the immunocompromised patient.
- *Mycoplasma pneumoniae* (p. 704) infections are common in children and young adults; they occur sporadically as local epidemics (e.g., in schools, military camps, or prisons).

Morphology *(p. 704)*

Bacterial infections—caused by various gram-positive or gram-negative organisms—occur in overlapping morphologic patterns: *bronchopneumonia* and *lobar pneumonia*. Depending on bacterial virulence and host resistance, the same organism can cause bronchopneumonia, lobar pneumonia, or something intermediate.

- *Lobar pneumonia involves essentially an entire lobe.* Four stages of inflammatory response are classically described: after initial *congestion* due to vascular engorgement and alveolar transudates, *red hepatization* marks a stage of massive neutrophilic exudation with hemorrhage (grossly resembling liver). This is followed by *gray hepatization* characterized by red cell disintegration but persistence of fibrinopurulent exudates. The final stage of *resolution* is marked by progressive enzymatic digestion of the exudates and macrophage resorption of the debris, or fibroblast ingrowth. Exudate resolution usually restores normal lung structure and function, but organization with fibrous scarring can occur.
- *Bronchopneumonia is marked by patchy exudative consolidation of lung parenchyma.* Grossly the lungs exhibit focal areas of palpable consolidation. Histologically there is acute (neutrophilic) suppurative exudation filling bronchi, bronchioles, and alveoli; this will also eventually undergo resolution.
- Involvement of the pleura *(pleuritis)* can resolve or result in fibrous thickening and adhesions. Expansion of infection into the pleural space causes a fibrinopurulent *empyema.*

Clinical Course *(p. 705)*

Symptoms include high fever, rigors, and productive cough, occasionally with hemoptysis; a friction rub and pleuritic chest pain herald pleural involvement. The clinical picture is markedly changed by antibiotic administration. Complications include abscess formation, and systemic dissemination causing endocarditis, meningitis, suppurative arthritis, or metastatic abscesses.

Community-Acquired Viral Pneumonia (p. 705)

Common viral infections include influenza types A and B, respiratory syncytial virus, human metapneumovirus (MPV), adenovirus, rhinoviruses, rubeola, and varicella. Manifestations range from relatively mild upper respiratory tract involvements (e.g., the common cold) to severe lower respiratory tract disease. The common pathogenic mechanism is attachment of organisms to epithelial cells, followed by cellular necrosis and inflammation. In alveoli this may cause fluid transudation; in upper airways, loss of the normal mucociliary clearance of the respiratory epithelium predisposes to secondary bacterial infection.

Influenza Infections (p. 706)

Influenza is a single-stranded RNA virus composed of eight strands bound by a nucleoprotein that determines the type of the virus (A, B, or C). Type A influenza viruses infect humans, pigs, horses, and birds and are the major cause of influenza epidemics through viral mutations. Types B and C do not mutate; consequently, childhood infections result in largely lifelong antibody-mediated protection against future disease.

The influenza virus surface is a lipid bilayer studded with viral hemagglutinin (in human-tropic viruses, these are H1, H2, or H3) and viral neuraminidase (N1 or N2) that determine the virus subtype; antibodies to these molecules prevent future infections to the particular viral strain. Clearing an established infection requires cytotoxic T cells and innate immune responses (a macrophage antiinfluenza protein *Mx1*).

Epidemics occur when viruses acquire mutations in their hemagglutinin or neuraminidase proteins that allow escape from most host antibodies *(antigenic drift)*. Pandemics occur when these proteins are replaced altogether by recombination of RNA segments with those of animal viruses *(antigenic shift)*.

Human Metapneumovirus (p. 706)

Human MPV is a paramyxovirus discovered in 2001; it causes bronchiolitis and pneumonia in the very young, very old, and immunocompromised; it is responsible for 5% to 10% of hospitalizations and up to 20% of pediatric outpatient visits for acute respiratory tract infections.

Severe Acute Respiratory Syndrome (p. 707)

Severe acute respiratory syndrome (SARS) is a coronavirus first identified in China in November 2002. Nearly 30% of upper respiratory tract infections are due to coronaviruses, but SARS differs in its ability to infect the lower respiratory tree and spread systemically. Since 2004, the virus has mysteriously disappeared.

Morphology (p. 707)

All viral infections produce similar morphologic changes:

- Patchy or lobar areas of congestion *without* the consolidation of bacterial pneumonias (hence the term *atypical pneumonia*).
- Predominant interstitial pneumonitis with widened, edematous alveolar walls with mononuclear inflammation; some viruses (e.g., herpes simplex, varicella) may be associated with epithelial necrosis and acute inflammation.
- *Hyaline membranes* reflect DAD.
- In some viral infections, characteristic cytopathic changes occur (see Chapter 8).
- Secondary bacterial infections modify the appearance by superimposing ulcerative bronchitis, bronchiolitis, and bacterial pneumonia.

Clinical Course (p. 707)

The clinical manifestations are extremely varied, from severe upper respiratory tract infections *(chest cold)* to nonlocalized systemic illness with myalgias and fever. Edema and exudates may cause ventilation-perfusion mismatches that evoke dyspnea out of proportion to the physical findings. Most viral illnesses are mild and spontaneously resolve.

Health Care-Associated Pneumonia (p. 707)

This is a clinical entity associated with recent hospitalization of ≥2 days; residence in a long-term care facility; attending a hospital or hemodialysis clinic; and recent intravenous antibiotic therapy, chemotherapy, or wound care. The most common organisms are methicillin-resistant *S. aureus* and *P. aeruginosa;* patients have a higher mortality than with community-acquired pneumonia.

Hospital-Acquired Pneumonia (p. 707)

This is defined as a pneumonia acquired during a hospital stay, typically associated with severe underlying disease, immunosuppression, prolonged antibiotic therapy, or invasive devices; mechanical ventilation imparts a high risk. Such infections are serious, often with life-threatening complications, and include gram-positive cocci (mainly *S. aureus* and *S. pneumoniae*) and gram-negative rods (Enterobacteriaceae and *Pseudomonas* species).

Aspiration Pneumonia (p. 708)

Aspiration pneumonia occurs in markedly debilitated or unconscious patients; it results in partly chemical (gastric acid) and partly bacterial (mixed oral flora) pneumonia. The pneumonia is often necrotizing and pursues a fulminant course; lung abscess is a common complication. In contrast, *microaspiration* occurs frequently in almost all people, especially with gastroesophageal reflux disease. It is typically inconsequential resulting in small, poorly formed nonnecrotizing granulomas.

Lung Abscess (p. 708)

This is an infection marked by localized suppurative necrosis of lung tissue.

Etiology and Pathogenesis (p. 708)

Commonly involved are staphylococci, streptococci, numerous gram-negative species, and anaerobes. Mixed infections are frequent, reflecting aspiration of oral contents as a common etiology. Abscesses can be due to the following:

- Aspiration of infective material (e.g., oropharyngeal procedures or secondary to diminished consciousness). Aspiration abscesses are more common on the right, reflecting the more vertical right bronchus.
- Antecedent primary bacterial infection.
- Septic emboli from infected thrombi or right-sided endocarditis.
- Obstructive tumors (10% to 15% of abscesses).
- Direct traumatic punctures or spread of infection from adjacent organs.

Morphology (p. 708)

Abscesses may be single or multiple and vary from microscopic to large cavities. They contain variable mixtures of pus and air, depending on available drainage through airways. Chronic abscesses are often surrounded by a reactive fibrous wall.

Clinical Course (p. 709)

Complications include extension into the pleural cavity, hemorrhage, septic embolization, and secondary amyloidosis.

Chronic Pneumonia (p. 709)

Chronic pneumonia is typically a localized granulomatous inflammation in immunocompetent patients, with or without regional lymph node involvement. In immunocompromised patients the infection may become disseminated. Tuberculosis is described in Chapter 8; the following are fungal causes. Most are asymptomatic and result in only limited granulomatous disease; however, immunocompromise can cause fulminant, widespread dissemination.

Histoplasmosis (p. 709)

Histoplasmosis is an intracellular parasite of macrophages; it is endemic along the Ohio and Mississippi Rivers and in the Caribbean. Infection by *Histoplasma capsulatum* produces granulomas with coagulative necrosis that subsequently undergo fibrosis and concentric calcification. Silver stain identifies the 3- to 5-μm, thin-walled cyst of the fungus, which can persist for years.

Blastomycosis (p. 709)

Blastomycosis occurs in the central and southeastern United States, Canada, Mexico, the Middle East, Africa, and India. It can present as pulmonary, disseminated, and—rarely—primary cutaneous forms. *Blastomyces dermatitidis* is a 5- to 15-μm, thick-walled yeast that divides by broad-based budding; it causes suppurative granulomas.

Coccidioidomycosis (p. 710)

Coccidioidomycosis is endemic in the Southwest and western United States and Mexico, where >80% of the population will have a delayed-type hypersensitivity response to the organism. *Coccidioides immitis* causes lesions varying from pyogenic to granulomatous; silver stains demonstrate a 20- to 60-μm, thick-walled spherule containing small endospores.

Pneumonia in the Immunocompromised Host (p. 711)

Opportunistic infections rarely cause infection in normal hosts but can cause life-threatening pneumonias in the immunocompromised host. Often more than one agent is involved. *Pseudomonas,* mycobacteria, *Legionella,* and *Listeria* are the more common bacterial agents; Cytomegalovirus (CMV) and herpesviruses are the more common viruses; and *Pneumocystis, Candida,* and *Aspergillus* are the most common fungi.

Pulmonary Disease in Human Immunodeficiency Virus Infection (p. 711)

Pulmonary infections account for 30% to 40% of hospitalization in human immunodeficiency virus (HIV)-infected individuals.

- In these patients pulmonary disease may be due to more than one cause, and symptoms may be atypical.
- The absolute CD4+ T-cell count can define the risk of infection with specific organisms:
    - >200/μL: Bacteria, including tuberculosis
    - 50 to 200/μL: *Pneumocystis*
    - <50/μL: CMV and *Mycobacterium avium* complex

- In addition to opportunistic infections, "common" bacterial pathogens also cause severe disease.
- Malignancies (Kaposi sarcoma, lymphoma, lung cancer) also cause pulmonary disease.

Lung Transplantation (p. 711)

Lung transplantation is typically performed in otherwise healthy patients for emphysema, idiopathic pulmonary fibrosis, cystic fibrosis, and primary PH; in most cases, single-lung transplants are performed. Complications include the following:

- Infections (similar to those in other immunocompromised patients).
- Acute rejection (vascular and airway mononuclear cell infiltrates).
- Chronic rejection with variable fibrotic occlusion of small airways *(bronchiolitis obliterans)* is significant in 50% of patients by 3 to 5 years posttransplant.

One-, five-, and ten-year survival rates posttransplant are 79%, 53%, and 30%, respectively.

Tumors (p. 712)

Carcinomas (p. 712)

Carcinomas constitute 90% to 95% of lung tumors; lung cancer is the most frequently diagnosed major cancer in the world (excludes skin cancers) and is the most common cause of cancer death worldwide.

Etiology and Pathogenesis (p. 712)

Etiology and pathogenesis involves a stepwise accumulation of genetic abnormalities; 10 to 20 mutations have occurred by the time a tumor is clinically apparent. Contributory factors are as follows:

- *Tobacco smoking* is the most important etiologic factor, correlating with amount and duration of smoking; 80% of lung cancers occur in active smokers or those who have recently stopped. Risk becomes 60 times greater in habitual smokers (two packs per day for 20 years), although only 11% of heavy smokers develop lung cancer. The mutagenic effect of smoke procarcinogens is modified by genetic variants (e.g., DNA repair efficacy or P-450 polymorphisms that influence conversion to carcinogens). Women have a higher susceptibility to tobacco carcinogens than do men. Cessation of smoking reduces risk after 10 years but never to control levels. *Secondhand smoke* causes 3000 cases of lung cancer annually.
- *Environmental exposures* include radiation (e.g., radon, uranium), air pollution (particulates), and occupational inhaled substances (e.g., nickel, chromates, arsenic). Asbestos increases risk of cancer fivefold (with a latency of 10 to 30 years); when combined with smoking, the risk is fifty-five-fold greater.
- *Molecular genetics.* Smoking-related lung carcinomas arise by a stepwise accumulation of oncogenic "driver" mutations. Some can be found in the "benign" bronchial epithelium of smokers without lung cancers, suggesting that large areas are mutagenized ("field effect"); in this fertile soil, occasional cells accumulate additional complementary driver mutations to become malignant (see Chapter 7).

- *Squamous cell carcinoma* is highly associated with tobacco exposure; it has diverse genetic aberrations, many involving tumor suppressor loci deletions (e.g., 3p, 9p [site of the *CDKN2A* gene], and 17p [site of the *TP53* gene]). p53 protein overexpression is a marker of *TP53* mutations and occurs in 10% to 50% of squamous dysplasias and 60% to 90% of squamous cell carcinoma in situ. Loss of the retinoblastoma (Rb) tumor suppressor occurs in 15% of squamous cell carcinomas. *CDKN2A* is inactivated, and its protein product, p16, is lost in 65% of tumors.
- *Small cell carcinoma* shows the strongest association with smoking; it shares many molecular features with squamous cell carcinoma, including loss-of-function mutations in *TP53* (75% to 90% of tumors), *Rb* (almost 100%), and *MYC* family gene amplification.
- *Adenocarcinomas* commonly have gain-of-function mutations in growth factor receptor signaling pathways, including receptor tyrosine kinases, such as *EGFR, ALK, ROS, MET,* and *RET.* Other tumors often have *KRAS* mutations that code for a protein that lies downstream of receptor tyrosine kinases in various signaling pathways.

Lung cancer in never smokers (p. 714). A quarter of lung cancer worldwide occurs in never smokers, most commonly in women and most commonly adenocarcinomas. These cancers are more likely to have *EGFR* mutations and almost never have *KRAS* mutations.

Precursor (Preinvasive) Lesions

Notably these do not necessarily progress to malignancy:

- Squamous dysplasia and carcinoma in situ
- Atypical adenomatous hyperplasia
- Adenocarcinoma in situ
- Diffuse idiopathic pulmonary neuroendocrine cell hyperplasia

Classification *(p. 714)*

Lung carcinomas are classified by their predominant histologic appearance. However, the most relevant clinical and therapeutic grouping is *small cell carcinomas* (almost always metastatic, high initial response to radiation and chemotherapy) versus *non-small cell carcinomas* (less often metastatic, less responsive).

Morphology *(p. 715)*

- *Adenocarcinoma* is the most common lung cancer (38% of lung cancers). It typically presents as a peripheral mass, with characteristic microscopic gland formation—usually producing mucin—and an adjacent desmoplastic response. These grow more slowly than squamous cell carcinomas but tend to metastasize earlier.
- *Squamous cell carcinoma* (20% of lung cancers) has the closest correlation with smoking. Most arise in or near the lung hilus. Microscopically they vary from well-differentiated keratinizing neoplasms to wildly anaplastic tumors.
- *Small cell carcinoma* (14% of lung cancers) is the most malignant of lung cancers and usually presents as a central or hilar tumor. It is strongly associated with cigarette smoking. The characteristic microscopic features include nests or clusters of small, *oatlike* cells with little cytoplasm, and without squamous or glandular differentiation. Ultrastructurally the cancer cells exhibit neurosecretory granules, and immunohistochemical stains usually demonstrate neuroendocrine markers. These tumors most often produce *paraneoplastic syndromes* (see later).

- *Large cell carcinoma* (3% of lung cancers) probably represents poorly differentiated squamous cell carcinomas or adenocarcinomas.
- Approximately 10% of lung cancers have a combined histology comprising two or more of the types described earlier.

Clinical Course (p. 718)

Presenting symptoms for lung carcinoma include cough, weight loss, chest pain, and dyspnea. Adrenal, brain, liver, and bone are favored metastatic sites. Outcome depends on the type of lung cancer and the stage at presentation. The overall 5-year survival rate is 16% but is 52% for cases detected before metastasis, 22% for cases with only regional metastasis, and 4% with distant metastatic spread. Targeted therapy for patients with adenocarcinoma and activating *EGFR* mutations (15% of patients) prolongs survival. Activating *KRAS* mutations are associated with a worse prognosis. Untreated, small cell carcinoma has a mean survival of 6 to 17 weeks. However, it is usually sensitive to radiation and chemotherapy, and 15% to 25% of patients with limited disease are cured. Nevertheless, small cell carcinoma has almost always metastasized by the time of diagnosis, and mean survival is 1 year.

Secondary pathologies related to lung neoplasm include (1) partial obstruction with distal emphysema and/or postobstructive pneumonia and bronchiectasis, (2) total obstruction with atelectasis, and (3) obstruction of the superior vena cava with impaired head and upper extremity drainage (superior vena cava syndrome). Tumors can also invade neural structures around the trachea, including the cervical sympathic plexus, to give rise to the *Horner syndrome* (ptosis, miosis, and anhidrosis), so-called *Pancoast tumors.*

Paraneoplastic syndromes (p. 718) associated with lung carcinoma (1% to 10% of tumors) result from release of the following:

- Antidiuretic hormone (syndrome of inappropriate antidiuretic hormone)
- Adrenocorticotropic hormone (ACTH; Cushing syndrome)
- Parathormone, parathyroid hormone-related peptide, or prostaglandin E (hypercalcemia)
- Calcitonin (hypocalcemia)
- Gonadotropins (gynecomastia)
- Serotonin (carcinoid syndrome)

Other paraneoplastic syndromes include Lambert-Eaton mysathenic syndrome (due to autoantibody formation), peripheral neuropathy, acanthosis nigricans, and hypertrophic pulmonary osteoarthropathy (finger clubbing).

Neuroendocrine Proliferations and Tumors (p. 719)

A rare disorder called *diffuse idiopathic pulmonary neuroendocrine cell hyperplasia* seems to be a precursor to the development of multiple tumorlets and typical or atypical carcinoids. *Tumorlets* are small, benign hyperplastic nests of neuroendocrine cells, typically seen adjacent to chronic inflammation or scarring.

Carcinoid Tumors (p. 719)

Carcinoid tumors exhibiting neuroendocrine differentiation constitute 1% to 5% of all lung tumors; 20% to 40% of affected patients are nonsmokers. Carcinoid tumors are low-grade malignancies subclassified as typical or atypical; the latter is associated with higher mitotic rates, focal necrosis, increased pleomorphism, and lymphatic invasion.

Morphology (p. 719)

Grossly the tumors are usually intrabronchial, highly vascular, polypoid masses less than 3 to 4 cm. Microscopically there are nests and cords of uniform, small, round cells resembling intestinal carcinoids. Neurosecretory granules are seen ultrastructurally, and neuroendocrine differentiation is confirmed by immunostaining for neuron-specific enolase, serotonin, calcitonin, or bombesin.

Clinical Features (p. 720)

Manifestations relate to intrabronchial obstruction, capacity to metastasize, and the production of vasoactive amines (causing flushing, diarrhea, and cyanosis). Most follow a relatively benign course, with 5-year survivals of 95% for typical carcinoids and 70% for atypical carcinoids.

Miscellaneous Tumors (p. 720)

Hamartomas

Hamartomas are relatively common, benign, nodular neoplasms composed of cartilage and other mesenchymal tissues (e.g., fat, blood vessels, and fibrous tissue).

Mediastinal Tumors

Mediastinal tumors arise from local structures or may represent metastatic disease (Table 15-7); they can invade or compress the lungs. These are discussed elsewhere in appropriate chapters.

Metastatic Tumors (p. 721)

Secondary involvement of the lung by metastatic tumor is common and can occur via direct extension from contiguous organs or via lymphatics or hematogenous routes. Patterns of disease include discrete masses or nodules and growth within peribronchial lymphatics.

Pleura (p. 721)

Most pleural lesions are secondary to underlying lung disease.

TABLE 15-7 Mediastinal Tumors and Other Masses
Anterior Mediastinum
Thymoma
Teratoma
Lymphoma
Thyroid lesions
Parathyroid tumors
Metastatic carcinoma
Posterior Mediastinum
Neurogenic tumors (schwannoma, neurofibroma)
Lymphoma
Metastatic tumor (most are from the lung)
Bronchogenic cyst
Gastroenteric hernia
Middle Mediastinum
Bronchogenic cyst
Pericardial cyst
Lymphoma

Pleural Effusion (p. 721)

Accumulations of transudate (hydrothorax) or serous exudate can occur with the following:

- Increased hydrostatic pressure (e.g., heart failure)
- Increased vascular permeability (e.g., pneumonia)
- Decreased oncotic pressure (e.g., nephrotic syndrome)
- Increased negative intrapleural pressure (e.g., atelectasis)
- Decreased lymphatic drainage (e.g., carcinomatosis)

Inflammatory Pleural Effusions (p. 722)

- *Serofibrinous pleuritis* reflects pulmonary inflammation (e.g., tuberculosis, pneumonia, infarcts, abscesses) or systemic diseases (e.g., rheumatoid arthritis, uremia).
- *Suppurative pleuritis* (empyema) usually reflects pleural space infection leading to pus accumulation.
- *Hemorrhagic pleuritis* occurs with bleeding disorders, neoplastic involvement, and certain rickettsial diseases.

Organization of these exudates with dense fibrous adhesions can affect lung expansion.

Noninflammatory Pleural Effusions (p. 722)

Other pleural fluid accumulations include *hydrothorax* (most commonly due to heart failure but also renal or hepatic failure), *hemothorax* (a fatal complication of a ruptured aortic aneurysm), and *chylothorax* (a collection of milky lymph fluid, usually due to neoplastic lymphatic obstruction).

Pneumothorax (p. 722)

Pneumothorax refers to air or gas in the pleural cavity, usually with associated ipsilateral lung deflation; it can be traumatic (e.g., after rib fractures that puncture the lung) or spontaneous, occurring after peripheral apical bleb rupture. *Tension pneumothorax* occurs when a defect between airways and pleura acts as a one-way valve admitting air during inspiration but failing to release it during expiration. The progressively increasing pleural pressure compresses the contralateral lung and mediastinal structures and represents a serious, potentially fatal complication.

Pleural Tumors (p. 722)

Most common pleural tumors are metastases from lung, breast, ovaries, or other organs. Malignant effusions often contain cytologically detectable tumor cells.

Solitary Fibrous Tumor (p. 723)

These noninvasive, fibrosing, rarely malignant tumors are composed of spindle cells resembling fibroblasts; they also occur in other sites and are not related to asbestos exposure. The tumors are associated with a chromosome 12 inversion creating a *NAB2-STAT6* fusion gene that encodes a chimeric transcription factor that drives tumor development. Resection is usually curative.

Malignant Mesothelioma (p. 723)

This uncommon tumor of mesothelial cells occurs most often in the pleura (less frequently in the peritoneum or other sites). It is associated with asbestos exposure in 90% of cases; the lifetime risk in heavily exposed individuals is 7% to 10%, with a latency period between exposure and tumor development of 25 to 45 years. The most common cytogenetic abnormality (80% of cases) is homozygous deletion of the tumor suppressor gene *CDKN2A/INK4a*, which occurs in about 80% of mesotheliomas. Notably among asbestos workers, *lung carcinoma remains the most common lung tumor.*

Morphology (p. 723)

Tumor spreads diffusely over the lung surface and fissures, forming an encasing sheath. Microscopic patterns are *epithelioid* (60%), *sarcomatoid* (20%), and mixed *(biphasic)* (20%) tumors.

- *Epithelioid pattern* shows epithelium-like cells forming tubules and papillary projections resembling adenocarcinomas. Antigenic (calretinin, WT-1, and CK5/6 positivity) and ultrastructural (long, slender microvilli) features allow distinction from adenocarcinomas (MOC31 and BG8 positivity and short, plump microvilli).
- *Sarcomatoid pattern* shows malignant, spindle-shaped cells resembling fibrosarcoma.

Clinical Course (p. 724)

Patients present with chest pain, dyspnea, and recurrent pleural effusion. Mesotheliomas are highly malignant tumors that invade the lung and can metastasize widely. Few patients survive longer than 2 years.

16

Head and Neck

ORAL CAVITY (p. 727)

Diseases of Teeth and Supporting Structures (p. 727)

Caries (Tooth Decay) (p. 727)

Caries represents focal tooth degradation due to mineral dissolution; it occurs through acids released by oral bacteria during sugar fermentation. Caries is the most common reason for tooth loss before age 35.

Gingivitis (p. 727)

Gingivitis is soft tissue inflammation of the squamous mucosa and soft tissues around teeth, with erythema, edema, bleeding, and gingival degeneration. Inadequate oral hygiene leads to accumulation of *dental plaque* (a biofilm of bacteria, salivary proteins, and desquamated epithelial cells), with subsequent mineralization *(tartar);* plaque bacteria cause caries, and plaque buildup below the gum line leads to gingivitis.

Periodontitis (p. 728)

Periodontitis is inflammation of tooth-supporting structures (e.g., periodontal ligaments, alveolar bone, and cementum); it can progress to complete destruction of the periodontal ligament and alveolar bone, with tooth loss. As opposed to facultative gram-positive colonization of typical plaque, periodontitis-associated plaque contains anaerobic and microaerophilic gram-negative flora. Although typically presenting in isolation, periodontal disease can also occur in several systemic diseases, especially those affecting immunologic function. Periodontal infections can also underlie systemic diseases (e.g., infective endocarditis and brain abscesses).

Inflammatory and Reactive Lesions (p. 728)

Aphthous Ulcers (Canker Sores) (p. 728)

Aphthous ulcers affect up to 40% of the U.S. population; they can have a familial predilection, and recurrent ulcers may be associated with sprue, inflammatory bowel disease, and Behçet disease. Lesions are painful, shallow, hyperemic ulcerations initially infiltrated by mononuclear inflammatory cells; secondary bacterial infection recruits neutrophils.

Fibrous Proliferative Lesions (p. 728)

These are benign reactive lesions, usually cured by surgical excision.

- *Irritation fibromas* typically occur along the "bite line"; these are nodules of fibrous tissue covered by squamous mucosa.
- *Pyogenic granulomas* are rapidly growing, highly vascular lesions similar to granulation tissue. Common in children or during pregnancy, they can regress (particularly after pregnancy), undergo fibrous maturation, or develop into peripheral ossifying fibromas.
- *Peripheral ossifying fibromas* can arise from pyogenic granulomas, although most have unknown etiologies. With a 15% to 20% recurrence rate, surgical excision to the periosteum is the treatment of choice.
- *Peripheral giant cell granulomas* are composed of multinucleated foreign-bodylike giant cells separated by fibroangiomatous stroma.

Infections (p. 729)

Normal oral mucosa resists infection by competitive suppression from low-virulence commensal organisms, high levels of immunoglobulin A (IgA), the antibacterial properties of saliva, and dilution from ingested food and liquids. Alteration in these defenses (e.g., due to immunodeficiency or antibiotic therapy) contributes to infections.

Herpes Simplex Virus Infections (p. 729)

Herpes simplex virus (HSV-1 and -2) infections classically cause "cold sores" with minimal morbidity; 10% to 20% of primary infections present as *acute herpetic gingivostomatitis* with diffuse oral vesicles and ulceration, lymphadenopathy, and fever.

Morphology (p. 729)

Lesions consist of vesicles, large bullae, or shallow ulcerations. Histologically there are intracellular and intercellular edema *(acantholysis),* eosinophilic intranuclear inclusions, and multinucleated giant cells (visualized by microscopic examination of vesicular fluid, so-called *Tzanck test*). Vesicles heal spontaneously in 3 to 4 weeks, but virus treks along regional nerves and becomes dormant in local ganglia; reactivation (driven, e.g., by trauma, infection, or immune suppression) occurs with crops of small vesicles that clear in 4 to 6 days.

Oral Candidiasis (Thrush) (p. 729)

Candida albicans is part of the normal oral flora in half the population; it is the most common fungal infection of the oral cavity. Oral candidiasis can present as erythematous or hyperplastic lesions, but classically manifests as superficial gray-white inflammatory membranes composed of fibrinosuppurative exudates containing fungus. It occurs in the setting of broad-spectrum antibiotics, diabetes, neutropenia, or immunodeficiency.

Deep Fungal Infections (p. 730)

Certain deep fungal infections—histoplasmosis, blastomycosis, coccidioidomycosis, cryptococcosis, zygomycosis, and aspergillosis—have a predilection for the oral cavity and head and neck region. Immunocompromise increases the risk.

Oral Manifestations of Systemic Disease (p. 730)

Some of the more common of these are highlighted in Table 16-1.

Hairy Leukoplakia (p. 730)

Hairy leukoplakia is a distinctive oral lesion seen in immunocompromised patients (80% are human immunodeficiency virus [HIV] infected). Caused by Epstein-Barr virus (EBV), the lesions are white patches of hyperkeratosis on tongue lateral borders; superimposed candidal infections can augment the "hairiness."

Precancerous and Cancerous Lesions (p. 731)

Leukoplakia and Erythroplakia (p. 731)

Tobacco use is the most common antecedent.

- *Leukoplakia* signifies a white plaque on the oral mucosa that cannot be removed by scraping and cannot be classified as another disease entity. Lesions vary from benign epithelial thickenings to highly atypical dysplasia verging on *carcinoma in situ.* Leukoplakia occurs in 3% of individuals; 5% to 25% are premalignant. Thus until proved otherwise, leukoplakia should be considered precancerous.
- *Erythroplakia* is a red, velvety, relatively flat lesion; it is less common than leukoplakia but more ominous because the epithelium is markedly atypical and has greater risk of malignant transformation.

Squamous Cell Carcinoma (p. 731)

Squamous cell carcinoma (SCC) constitutes 95% of oral cancers, with 45,000 new cases annually in the United States; overall 5-year survival is 50%, varying depending on stage (early stage = 80%; late stage = 20%). The high rate of second primaries (3% to 7% per year) suggests "field cancerization" due to diffuse mucosal exposure to carcinogens.

SCC pathogenesis is multifactorial. Tobacco and alcohol are common associations—especially in the oral cavity—although up to 70% of oropharyngeal cancers harbor oncogenic variants of human papillomavirus (HPV, particularly HPV-16). The incidence of HPV-associated oropharyngeal SCC has increased more than twofold since the early 1990s. Patients with HPV-positive tumors do better than those without. Other risk factors are as follows:

- Familial associations related to genomic instability
- Radiation
- Betel nut and paan chewing (India and Asia)

Molecular Biology of SCC (p. 732)

Development of malignancy is a multistage process; although heterogeneous, a general pathway is as follows:

- *p16* inactivation leads to loss of an inhibitor of cyclin-dependent kinase and progression to hyperplasia/hyperkeratosis; these are more common in HPV-associated SCC.
- *p53* mutations lead to progression to dysplasia and can occur in both HPV- and smoking-associated SCC.
- Gross genomic alterations and/or deletions (4q, 6p, 8p, 11q, 13q, or 14q); these typically occur late in the progression to malignancy.
- Cyclin D1 overexpression causes constitutively active cell cycle progression and typically occurs late in the progression to cancer.

TABLE 16-1 Oral Manifestations of Some Systemic Diseases

Systemic Disease	Associated Oral Changes
Infectious Diseases	
Scarlet fever	Fiery red tongue with prominent papillae (raspberry tongue); white-coated tongue through which hyperemic papillae project (strawberry tongue)
Measles	Spotty enanthema in the oral cavity often precedes the skin rash; ulcerations on the buccal mucosa about Stensen duct produce Koplik spots
Infectious mononucleosis	Acute pharyngitis and tonsillitis that may cause coating with a gray-white exudative membrane; enlargement of lymph nodes in the neck, palatal petechiae
Diphtheria	Characteristic dirty white, fibrinosuppurative, tough, inflammatory membrane over the tonsils and retropharynx
HIV	Predisposition to opportunistic oral infections, particularly HSV, *Candida,* and other fungi; oral lesions of Kaposi sarcoma and hairy leukoplakia (described in text)
Dermatologic Conditions*	
Lichen planus	Reticulate, lacelike, white keratotic lesions that sometimes ulcerate and rarely form bullae; seen in more than 50% of patients with cutaneous lichen planus; rarely, is the sole manifestation
Pemphigus	Vesicles and bullae prone to rupture, leaving hyperemic erosions covered with exudates
Bullous pemphigoid	Oral lesions (mucus membrane pemphigoid) resemble those of pemphigus but can be differentiated histologically
Erythema multiforme	Maculopapular, vesiculobullous eruption that sometimes follows an infection elsewhere, ingestion of drugs, development of cancer, or a collagen vascular disease; when there is widespread mucosal and skin involvement, it is referred to as *Stevens-Johnson syndrome*
Hematologic Disorders	
Pancytopenia (agranulocytosis, aplastic anemia)	Severe oral infections in the form of gingivitis, pharyngitis, tonsillitis; may extend to produce cellulitis of the neck *(Ludwig angina)*
Leukemia	With depletion of functioning neutrophils, oral lesions may appear like those in pancytopenia
Monocytic leukemia	Leukemic infiltration and enlargement of the gingivae, often with accompanying periodontitis
Miscellaneous	
Melanotic pigmentation	May appear in Addison disease, hemochromatosis, fibrous dysplasia of bone (Albright syndrome), and Peutz-Jeghers syndrome (gastrointestinal polyposis)
Phenytoin (Dilantin) ingestion	Striking fibrous enlargement of the gingivae
Pregnancy	A friable, red, pyogenic granuloma protruding from the gingiva ("pregnancy tumor")
Rendu-Osler-Weber syndrome	Autosomal dominant disorder with multiple congenital aneurysmal telangiectasias beneath mucosal surfaces of the oral cavity and lips

*See Chapter 25.

Morphology (p. 733)

Tumors occur most commonly in the ventral tongue, mouth floor, lower lip, soft palate, and gingiva; lesions can be raised, firm, ulcerated, or verrucous. Histologically they are typical squamous carcinomas of variable differentiation; the degree of differentiation does not predict clinical behavior. Tumors need not progress to full-thickness SCC in situ before invading the underlying stroma. Local infiltration precedes metastasis; favored sites are cervical lymph nodes, lungs, liver, and bones.

Odontogenic Cysts and Tumors (p. 734)

Epithelium-lined cysts in the mandible and maxilla derive from odontogenic remnants; they may be developmental or inflammatory.

- *Dentigerous cysts* originate near crowns of unerupted teeth and may result from dental follicle degeneration. They are most often associated with impacted third molars. These are unilocular lesions lined by stratified squamous epithelium, with associated chronic inflammation. Complete removal is curative.
- *Odontogenic keratocyst (OKC)* are potentially aggressive; treatment requires complete resection (recurrence rates of 60% for partial resection). They occur most commonly in the posterior mandible of males 10 to 40 years old and are unilocular or multilocular lesions typically lined by parakeratinized stratified squamous epithelium. Patients with multiple OKCs merit evaluation for nevoid basal cell carcinoma syndrome *(Gorlin syndrome),* related to *PTCH* tumor-suppressor gene mutations (see Chapter 25).
- *Periapical cysts* are inflammatory lesions found at tooth apices; these develop from long-standing pulpitis due to caries or tooth trauma. Persistent chronic inflammation leads to granulation tissue and proliferation of quiescent rests of odontogenic epithelium.

Odontogenic Tumors (Table 16-2)

Odontogenic tumors demonstrate diverse histology and clinical behavior. Some are true neoplasms (both benign and malignant); others are hamartomas.

- *Ameloblastoma* is a true neoplasm arising from odontogenic epithelium and showing *no* ectomesenchymal differentiation. It is typically cystic, slow growing, and locally invasive but often has an indolent course.
- *Odontoma* is the most common odontogenic tumor. It is likely a hamartoma, arising from epithelium with extensive enamel and dentin deposition.

UPPER AIRWAYS (p. 735)

Includes nose, pharynx, and larynx; most disorders are more nuisance than threat.

Nose (p. 735)

Inflammations (p. 735)

- *Infectious rhinitis* (p. 735) or "common cold" is caused by adenoviruses, echoviruses, and rhinoviruses. There is erythematous and edematous nasal mucosa with profuse catarrhal discharge; bacterial superinfection can induce mucopurulent exudates.

TABLE 16-2 Histologic Classification of Odontogenic Tumors

Tumors of Odontogenic Epithelium
Benign
Ameloblastoma
Calcifying epithelial odontogenic tumor (Pindborg tumor)
Squamous odontogenic tumor
Adenomatoid odontogenic tumor
Malignant
Ameloblastic carcinoma
Malignant ameloblastoma
Clear-cell odontogenic carcinoma
Ghost cell odontogenic carcinoma
Primary intraosseous SCC
Tumors of Odontogenic Ectomesenchyme
Odontogenic fibroma
Odontogenic myxoma
Cementoblastoma
Tumors of Odontogenic Epithelium and Ectomesenchyme
Benign
Ameloblastic fibroma
Ameloblastic fibro-odontoma
Adenomatoid odontogenic tumor
Odontoameloblastoma
Complex odontoma
Compound odontoma
Calcifying cystic odontogenic tumor (calcifying odontogenic cyst)
Dentinogenic ghost cell tumor
Malignant
Ameloblastic fibrosarcoma

- *Allergic rhinitis* (p. 735) or "hay fever" affects 20% of individuals; it is an IgE-mediated immune reaction (see Chapter 6) with mucosal edema and erythema, and eosinophil-rich infiltrates.
- *Nasal polyps* (p. 735) occur with recurrent rhinitis; these are edematous mucosa infiltrated by neutrophils, eosinophils, and plasma cells. When multiple or large, they obstruct the airway and impair sinus drainage, necessitating removal. Most are *not* due to atopy, and only 0.5% of atopic patients develop polyps.
- *Chronic rhinitis* (p. 735) is the sequel to chronic acute rhinitis. There is superficial mucosal ulceration with variable inflammatory infiltrates that can extend into the sinuses.
- *Sinusitis* (p. 735) is commonly preceded by acute or chronic rhinitis (edema impairs sinus drainage); maxillary sinusitis can occur by extension of a periapical tooth infection. *Kartagener syndrome* is a triad of *sinusitis, bronchiectasis,* and *situs inversus* due to congenitally defective ciliary action. Offending organisms are oral commensals, although diabetics can develop fungal sinusitis (e.g., *mucormycosis*). Although most commonly uncomfortable rather than serious, infections can spread into the orbit or surrounding bone to cause osteomyelitis or dural venous sinus thrombophlebitis.

Necrotizing Lesions of the Nose and Upper Airways (p. 736)

- Spreading fungal infections
- Wegener granulomatosis (see Chapter 11)
- *Lethal midline granuloma,* a lymphoma of natural killer (NK/T) cells infected with EBV (see Chapter 13), often complicated by

ulceration and bacterial superinfection. Asian or Latin American males in their 50s to 60s represent the typical demographic. Radiotherapy can control localized disease, but spread into the cranial vault or necrosis with infection and sepsis can be fatal.

Nasopharynx (p. 736)

Inflammations (p. 736)

Pharyngitis and *tonsillitis* are frequent concomitants of viral upper respiratory infections; there is mucosal edema and erythema with reactive lymphoid hyperplasia. Bacterial superinfection exacerbates the process, particularly in immunocompromised individuals or children without protective immunity.

Tumors of the Nose, Sinuses, and Nasopharynx (p. 737)

- *Nasopharyngeal angiofibroma* (p. 737) is a highly vascularized benign tumor occurring in adolescent boys; serious bleeding can complicate surgical resection. There is a 20% recurrence rate, and in 9% of cases death results from hemorrhage and intracranial extension.
- *Sinonasal (schneiderian) papillomas* (p. 737) are benign neoplasms most commonly seen in males aged 30 to 60 years. These occur in three basic forms: exophytic (most common), endophytic (benign but locally aggressive), and cylindrical. The endophytic and exophytic lesions are associated with HPV types 6 and 11. Complete excision of endophytic lesions is required to prevent recurrence with potential invasion into the orbit or cranial vault; malignant transformation can occur in 10% of cases.
- *Olfactory neuroblastoma (esthesioneuroblastoma)* (p. 737) is an uncommon, highly malignant tumor composed of neuroendocrine cells.
- *NUT midline carcinoma* (p. 737) is an uncommon tumor—often mistaken for SCC—that occurs in the nasopharynx, salivary glands, or other thoracoabdominal midline structures. It is extremely aggressive and resistant to conventional therapy; most patients survive less than a year. It is associated with translocations creating fusion genes encoding chimeric proteins between NUT (a chromatin regulator), and a "chromatin reader" protein, usually BRD4.
- *Nasopharyngeal carcinoma* (p. 737) is characterized by a distinctive geographic distribution, close anatomic relationship to lymphoid tissue, and association with EBV infection. It classically occurs in Africa (in children) and southern China (in adults). Tumors may be keratinizing or nonkeratinizing SCCs or undifferentiated carcinomas with abundant lymphocytic infiltrate. The lesions are often clinically occult for extended periods; 70% have nodal metastases at initial presentation. Most are sensitive to radiotherapy with 50% to 70% 3-year survival rates.

Larynx (p. 738)

Inflammations (p. 738)

Laryngitis can be caused by allergic, viral, bacterial, or chemical injury. In children *Haemophilus influenzae* laryngoepiglottitis can be life threatening due to airway obstruction from rapid-onset, severe mucosal edema; the inspiratory stridor it produces is called *croup*. The most common form of adult laryngitis is caused by heavy smoking and predisposes to squamous epithelial metaplasia and carcinoma.

Reactive Nodules (Vocal Cord Nodules and Polyps) (p. 739)

Reactive nodules occur most often in heavy smokers (unilateral) or singers (*singer's nodules;* bilateral); these are small (millimeters), smooth, rounded excrescences on true vocal cords. These are myxoid, occasionally vascular, connective tissue covered by (occasionally hyperplastic) squamous epithelium. Although causing progressive hoarseness, malignant transformation is rare.

Squamous Papilloma and Papillomatosis (p. 739)

Squamous papillomas are ≤1 cm, benign, squamous epithelium-lined lesions, usually on the true vocal cords; in children they may be multiple *(juvenile laryngeal papillomatosis)* and can spontaneously regress at puberty. Lesions are caused by HPV types 6 and 11; they frequently recur, but cancerous transformation is rare.

Carcinoma of the Larynx (p. 739)

SCC accounts for 95% of laryngeal cancers; it is most common in men in their sixth decade. It usually occurs on the vocal cords but can also develop on the epiglottis or pyriform sinuses. Laryngeal SCC presents as persistent hoarseness but later can produce pain, dysphagia, and hemoptysis. Tobacco smoke is the major cause, although alcohol is also a risk factor; up to the point of frank malignancy, changes typically regress after smoking cessation. HPV, radiation, and asbestos exposure can also contribute. Treatment involves surgery and radiation.

Morphology *(p. 740)*

Epithelial changes range from *hyperplasia* and *atypical hyperplasia* to *dysplasia, carcinoma in situ,* and invasive cancer. The likelihood of developing overt carcinoma is proportional to the atypia seen at first diagnosis.

EARS (p. 740)

The most common aural disorders (in descending order of frequency) are as follows:

- Acute and chronic *otitis* (most often middle ear and mastoid), occasionally leading to a *cholesteatoma*
- Symptomatic *otosclerosis*
- *Polyps*
- *Labyrinthitis*
- *Carcinomas* (mostly external ear)
- *Paragangliomas* (mostly middle ear)

Inflammatory Lesions (p. 740)

- *Acute otitis media* occurs mostly in infants and children. These are typically viral with serous exudates but can have superimposed bacterial infections with suppuration; typical organisms are *Streptococcus pneumoniae, H. influenzae,* and β-hemolytic streptococci. *Chronic disease* is usually caused by *Pseudomonas, Staphylococcus,* or a fungus. Otitis media in diabetics due to

Pseudomonas aeruginosa is especially aggressive and can cause destructive necrotizing lesions.
- *Cholesteatomas* are associated with chronic otitis media; they are 1 to 4 cm cystic lesions with surrounding chronic inflammation, lined by keratinizing squamous epithelium, and filled with amorphous debris, occasionally containing cholesterol spicules.

Otosclerosis (p. 740)

Otosclerosis is *abnormal bone deposition* in the middle ear, hampering stapes footplate mobility. Bone growth occurs through uncoupling of normal resorption and formation, although the cause is obscure; most cases are familial with an autosomal dominant predilection and variable penetrance. The process is slowly progressive, eventually causing marked hearing loss.

NECK (p. 741)

Branchial Cyst (Cervical Lymphoepithelial Cyst) (p. 741)

Branchial cysts are 2- to 5-cm benign lesions with fibrous walls lined by stratified squamous or pseudostratified columnar epithelium accompanied by lymphocytic infiltrates or reactive lymphoid tissue. They arise on the anterolateral neck either from branchial arch remnants; similar lesions can occur in the parotid gland or beneath the tongue.

Thyroglossal Duct Cyst (p. 741)

These cysts arise from remnants of the developmental tract of the embryonic thyroid anlage; thus, they can occur anywhere from the base of the tongue to the anterior neck. Cysts are 1 to 4 cm, lined by squamous or respiratory epithelium, with walls that can exhibit lymphoid follicles and/or thyroid tissue.

Paraganglioma (Carotid Body Tumor) (p. 741)

These are slow-growing tumors typically occurring in individuals 50 to 70 years old; they arise in extra-adrenal paraganglia—either paravertebral or more commonly around the great vessels, including the *carotid bodies.* Paragangliomas consist of nests *(zellballen)* of polygonal neuroendocrine cells enclosed by fibrous trabeculae and elongated sustentacular cells. Sporadic forms are typically single; familial forms (i.e., in multiple endocrine neoplasia 2 syndrome [see Chapter 24]) are usually multiple and bilateral. Carotid body paragangliomas recur after excision in half of cases and can be fatal due to infiltrative growth.

SALIVARY GLANDS (p. 742)

Xerostomia (p. 742)

Xerostomia (dry mouth) is due to lack of salivary secretions; the incidence is as high as 70% of individuals over age 70. It can occur in autoimmune inflammation and fibrosis (e.g., *Sjögren syndrome* [see Chapter 6]) or may be a complication of radiation therapy or a wide variety of pharmacologic agents.

Presentations range from oral dryness to tongue fissuring and ulceration with papillary atrophy to concomitant inflammatory salivary gland enlargement (Sjögren syndrome). Complications include increased caries, candidiasis, and difficulties with swallowing and speaking.

Inflammation (Sialadenitis) (p. 743)

Sialadenitis may be traumatic, viral (*mumps* is most common), bacterial, or autoimmune (e.g., *Sjögren syndrome;* see Chapter 6).

Mucoceles (p. 743) are the most common salivary gland lesions; they result from ductal blockage or rupture with saliva leakage into surrounding stroma. Most often on the lower lip, they typically result from trauma; lesions fluctuate in size, particularly in association with meals. Incomplete excision can result in recurrence. A *ranula* refers specifically to a mucocele of the sublingual gland.

Sialolithiasis (p. 743) is salivary gland ductal obstruction caused by stones (due to edema and/or impacted food debris); *nonspecific sialadenitis* (p. 743) with painful salivary gland enlargement and purulent discharge typically follows ductal obstruction. Dehydration and decreased secretory function predispose to secondary infection by *Staphylococcus aureus* or *Streptococcus viridans.*

Neoplasms (p. 743)

There are 30 benign and malignant tumors of salivary glands (Table 16-3). Parotids account for 65% to 80% (15% to 30% are malignant); 10% occur in the submandibular glands (40% malignant), with the remainder being in the minor salivary glands (70% to 90% malignant).

Pleomorphic Adenoma (p. 744)

These are benign tumors exhibiting mixed epithelial and mesenchymal differentiation; they constitute 60% of all parotid tumors, and lesser percentages in other salivary glands. Tumors are painless, slow-growing, mobile, discrete masses, with epithelial nests

TABLE 16-3 Histologic Classification and Approximate Incidence of Benign and Malignant Tumors of the Salivary Glands

Benign	Malignant
Pleomorphic adenoma (50%) (mixed tumor)	Mucoepidermoid carcinoma (15%)
Warthin tumor (5%-10%)	Adenocarcinoma (NOS) (10%)
Oncocytoma (1%)	Acinic cell carcinoma (5%)
Other adenomas (5%-10%)	Adenoid cystic carcinoma (5%)
Basal cell adenoma	Malignant mixed tumor (3%-5%)
Canalicular adenoma	SCC (1%)
Ductal papillomas	Other carcinomas (2%)

NOS, Not otherwise specified.

Data from Ellis GL, Auclair PL: *Tumors of the Salivary Glands. Atlas of Tumor Pathology,* Third Series. Washington, DC: Armed Forces Institute of Pathology, 1996.

dispersed in a variable matrix of myxoid, hyaline, chondroid, or osseous differentiation.

Recurrence rates approach 25% if not well excised. Malignant transformation (usually as adenocarcinoma or undifferentiated carcinoma) occurs in 10% of tumors of >15 years' duration. Malignant transformation is associated with 30% to 50% 5-year mortality.

Warthin Tumor (Papillary Cystadenoma Lymphomatosum) (p. 745)

Warthin tumor is a benign tumor of unknown histogenesis found almost exclusively in the parotid; 10% are multifocal and 10% are bilateral. The tumor is 8 times more common in smokers. It is well encapsulated, consisting of glandular spaces lined by a double layer of epithelial cells atop a dense lymphoid stroma.

Mucoepidermoid Carcinoma (p. 745)

Mucoepidermoid carcinoma is the most common primary malignant salivary tumor, constituting 15% of all salivary gland neoplasms. Up to 8 cm in size, these lack well-defined capsules. Histologically there are cords, sheets, or cystic arrangements of squamous, mucous, or intermediate cells with mucus-filled vacuoles. Low-grade tumors can invade locally with 15% recurrence rates; high-grade tumors have 25% recurrence rates and 50% 5-year survival rates.

Other Salivary Gland Tumors (p. 746)

- *Adenoid cystic carcinoma* is relatively uncommon; half occur in minor salivary glands. Histologically tumor cells are small with scant cytoplasm; they are arrayed in tubular or cribriform patterns with intercellular spaces filled with excess basement membranelike material. Although slow growing, they are stubbornly recurrent and invasive, eventually becoming metastatic. Five-year survival rates are 60% to 70%.
- *Acinic cell tumors* constitute 2% to 3% of all salivary gland tumors and arise most commonly in the parotid glands; tumor cells resemble normal salivary serous acinar cells. Clinical behavior is dependent on cellular pleomorphism; 10% to 15% metastasize to lymph nodes, and the 5-year survival rate is 90%.

17 The Gastrointestinal Tract

CONGENITAL ABNORMALITIES (p. 750)

Atresia, Fistulas, and Duplications (p. 750)

When present in the esophagus, these usually present shortly after birth with regurgitation during feeding; prompt surgical correction is important. Esophageal atresia is also associated with congenital heart defects, genitourinary malformations, and neurologic disorders.

- *Atresia:* In esophageal atresia a portion of the conduit is replaced by a thin, noncanalized cord, with blind pouches above and below the atretic segment. *Imperforate anus* is the most common form of congenital intestinal atresia, caused by failure of the cloacal membrane to involute.
- *Fistula:* A connection between the esophagus and the trachea or a mainstem bronchus; swallowed material or gastric fluids can enter the respiratory tract.
- *Stenosis* is an incomplete form of atresia; the lumen is reduced by a fibrous thickened wall; this can be congenital or result from inflammatory scarring (e.g., due to chronic reflux, irradiation, or scleroderma).
- *Congenital duplication cysts* are cystic masses with redundant smooth muscle layers; they can occur throughout the gastrointestinal (GI) tract.

Diaphragmatic Hernia, Omphalocele, and Gastroschisis (p. 750)

- *Diaphragmatic* hernia occurs when incomplete formation of the diaphragm allows cephalad displacement of abdominal viscera; when substantial, subsequent pulmonary hypoplasia is incompatible with postnatal life.
- *Omphalocele* occurs when abdominal musculature is incomplete and the viscera herniates into the ventral membranous sac; 40% are associated with other birth defects.
- *Gastroschisis* is similar to omphalocele except that all layers of the abdominal wall (from peritoneum to skin) fail to develop.

Ectopia (p. 750)

Ectopic tissues are common in the GI tract. The most common site for *gastric mucosa* ectopia is the proximal esophagus, leading to dysphagia and esophagitis; it can also occur in the small bowel or colon, presenting with occult blood loss or peptic ulceration. *Pancreatic heterotopia* occurs in esophagus and stomach; in the pylorus it can cause inflammation, scarring, and obstruction.

Meckel Diverticulum (p. 751)

A *true diverticulum* is a blind pouch leading off the alimentary tract, lined by mucosa, and including all three layers of the bowel wall: *mucosa, submucosa,* and *muscularis propria.* Meckel diverticula—the most common of the true diverticula (2% of the population)—result from persistence of the vitelline duct (connecting yolk sac and gut lumen) leaving a solitary outpouching within 85 cm of the ileocecal valve; the male to female ratio is 2:1. Heterotopic gastric mucosa or pancreatic tissue can be present and can cause peptic ulceration.

Pyloric Stenosis (p. 751)

Congenital hypertrophic pyloric stenosis occurs in approximately 1:500 births, with a male to female ratio of 4:1; there is a complex polygenic inheritance and associations with Turner syndrome and trisomy 18. Exposure to erythromycin or its analogues in the first 2 weeks of life is also linked to increased disease incidence. Patients classically present with regurgitation and projectile vomiting within 3 weeks of birth; there is externally visible peristalsis and a palpable firm ovoid mass. Full-thickness, muscle-splitting incision *(myotomy)* is curative.

Acquired pyloric stenosis is a complication of chronic antral gastritis, peptic ulcers close to the pylorus, and malignancy.

Hirschsprung Disease (p. 751)

Also known as congenital aganglionic megacolon, this disorder results from arrested migration of neural crest cells into the gut, yielding an aganglionic segment lacking peristaltic contractions; there is functional obstruction and proximal dilation, progressive dilation, and hypertrophy of unaffected proximal colon. It occurs in approximately 1 in 5000 live births. The rectum is always affected; proximal involvement is more variable.

Pathogenesis (p. 751)

There is a genetic component in most cases. Heterozygous loss-of-function mutations in the RET tyrosine kinase receptor accounts for 15% of sporadic cases and the majority of familial cases; more than seven other genes involved in enteric neurodevelopment have been identified. Penetrance is incomplete, influenced by sex-linked factors (males are 4 times more commonly affected) and other genetic and environmental modifiers.

Clinical Features (p. 752)

Hirschsprung disease presents with neonatal failure to pass meconium or abdominal distention with severely distended *megacolon* (up to several cm diameter); patients risk perforation, sepsis, or enterocolitis with fluid derangement.

Acquired megacolon may occur in Chagas disease, bowel obstruction, inflammatory bowel disease (IBD), and psychosomatic disorders; only in Chagas are ganglia actually lost.

ESOPHAGUS (p. 753)

Esophageal Obstruction (p. 753)

A number of esophageal lesions can cause dysphagia (difficulty swallowing), especially with solid foods. Stenosis is described previously.

- *Spasm* can be short- or long-lived and focal or diffuse; *diffuse esophageal spasm* causes functional obstruction, and increased wall stress can cause diverticula to form.
- *Diverticula* can contain one or more wall layers; if sufficiently large they can accumulate enough food to present as a mass with food regurgitation:
    - Zenker (pharyngeoesophageal) diverticulum occurs immediately above the upper esophageal sphincter.
    - *Traction diverticulum* occurs at the esophageal midpoint.
    - *Epiphrenic diverticulum* occurs immediately above the lower esophageal sphincter (LES).
- *Mucosal webs* are ledgelike protrusions of fibrovascular tissue and overlying epithelium; they are most common in the upper esophagus and typically occur in women over age 40. A constellation of webs, iron deficiency anemia, glossitis, and cheilosis is called the *Plummer-Vinson syndrome* (also called *Paterson–Brown Kelly syndrome*).
- *Esophageal rings (Schatzki rings)* are similar to webs but are circumferential and thicker; they include mucosa, submucosa, and occasionally hypertrophic muscularis propria. Above the gastroesophageal (GE) junction, they are called *A rings* and have squamous epithelium; when located at the squamocolumnar junction, they are *B rings* and can have gastric cardia-type mucosa.

Achalasia (p. 753)

Achalasia is a triad of incomplete relaxation of the LES, increased LES tone (due to cholinergic signaling), and esophageal aperistalsis. *Primary achalasia* is idiopathic and results from failure of distal esophageal neurons to induce LES relaxation during swallowing (normally driven by nitric oxide and vasoactive intestinal peptide signaling); it can also happen with degenerative changes in neural innervation. *Secondary achalasia* can occur with Chagas disease *(Trypanosoma cruzi)*, disorders of the vagal dorsal motor nuclei (polio, surgical ablation), diabetic autonomic neuropathy, in association with Down syndrome, and infiltrative disorders (malignancy, amyloidosis, sarcoidosis). *Allgrove ("triple A") syndrome* is an autosomal recessive disorder characterized by achalasia, alacrima, and adrenocorticotrophic hormone-resistant adrenal insufficiency.

Treatment for achalasia involves myotomy, balloon dilation, and/or botulinum toxin injection to inhibit LES cholinergic neurons.

Esophagitis (p. 754)

Lacerations (p. 754)

Mallory-Weiss tears are longitudinal lacerations (millimeter to centimeter in length) at the GE junction associated with excessive vomiting—often in the setting of alcohol intoxication. Normally, a reflex relaxation of the LES precedes the antiperistaltic wave associated with vomiting; with prolonged vomiting, this relaxation fails, resulting in esophageal stretching and tearing. Patients typically present with hematemesis, and up to 10% of upper GI bleeding is associated with such tears. Mallory-Weiss tears are not usually fatal; healing tends to be prompt, usually without surgery. In contrast, *Boerhaave syndrome* is much less common but more serious; it involves transmural rupture of the distal esophagus with severe mediastinitis; surgical intervention is typically required.

Chemical and Infectious Esophagitis (p. 754)

Esophageal epithelium can be damaged by several agents, including alcohol, corrosive acids or alkalis, excessively hot fluids, and heavy smoking. Pills that lodge and dissolve in the esophagus can also cause esophagitis; irradiation, chemotherapy, or graft-versus-host disease (GVHD) is iatrogenic etiology. Occasionally the esophagus is involved by systemic desquamative disorders (pemphigoid, epidermolysis bullosa) or Crohn disease (CD). Infections occur more frequently in immunocompromised hosts; these include *Herpes simplex* viruses, cytomegalovirus (CMV), or fungal organisms (most commonly *Candida*).

Pain and dysphagia (pain with swallowing) are the chief symptoms; in severe and/or chronic cases, hemorrhage, stricture, or perforation can result.

Morphology *(p. 754)*

The morphology depends on the etiology.

- Dense neutrophilic infiltrates are most common, although chemical injury may initially cause outright necrosis without inflammation.
- Any epithelial ulceration is accompanied by granulation tissue and eventually fibrosis.
- *Candidiasis*—when severe—is associated with adherent gray-white *pseudomembranes* composed of densely matted fungal hyphae and inflammatory cells.
- Herpesviruses typically cause punched-out ulcers, whereas CMV presents with shallower ulcerations with characteristic viral inclusions.
- Lesions associated with esophageal GVHD or blistering disorders resemble their counterparts in skin (see Chapter 25).

Reflux Esophagitis (p. 755)

Reflux of gastric contents is the foremost cause of esophagitis; the clinical condition is called *gastroesophageal reflux disease (GERD).*

Pathogenesis *(p. 755)*

Reflux of gastric juices is the major source of mucosal injury; in severe cases, duodenal bile reflux can exacerbate the damage. Reflux is caused by decreased LES tone and/or increased abdominal pressure and can be caused by alcohol, tobacco use, obesity, central nervous system (CNS) depressants, pregnancy, delayed gastric emptying, or increased gastric volume. *Hiatal hernia* is also a cause of GERD; it occurs when the diaphragmatic crura are separated and the stomach protrudes into the thorax. Hiatal hernias can be congenital or acquired; <10% are symptomatic.

Morphology *(p. 755)*

- Hyperemia and edema
- Basal zone hyperplasia (exceeding 20% of the epithelium) and thinning of superficial epithelial layers
- Neutrophil and/or eosinophil infiltration

Clinical Features (p. 755)

GERD is most common in adults older than 40 years; symptoms include dysphagia, heartburn, and regurgitation of gastric contents into the mouth. Complications of long-standing reflux include ulceration, hematemesis, melena, stricture, or Barrett esophagus. Symptomatic relief (with reduced mucosal damage) is obtained with proton pump inhibitors and/or H_2 histamine receptor antagonists.

Eosinophilic Esophagitis (p. 756)

Adults present with food impaction and dysphagia; children, with feeding intolerance and GERD-like symptoms. The cardinal histologic feature is large numbers of intraepithelial eosinophils. Most patients have one of several atopic disorders (e.g., atopic dermatitis, asthma), and therapy for their esophageal disorder involves dietary restriction and/or steroids.

Esophageal Varices (p. 756)

Pathogenesis (p. 756)

Severe portal hypertension induces collateral bypass channels between the portal and caval circulations (see Chapter 18). These lead to congested subepithelial and submucosal veins in the distal esophagus *(varices)*. In Western societies, alcoholic cirrhosis is the most common cause (90% of cirrhotic patients develop varices); worldwide, hepatic schistosomiasis is the second most common cause.

Morphology (p. 756)

Tortuous, dilated veins are present in the distal esophageal and proximal gastric submucosa; there is irregular luminal protrusion of overlying mucosa, with superficial ulceration, inflammation, or adherent blood clots.

Clinical Features (p. 756)

Varices are present in almost half of patients with cirrhosis; they are clinically silent until they rupture with hematemesis (50% to 80% of patients with varices). Causes of rupture include inflammatory erosion, increased venous pressure, and increased hydrostatic pressure associated with vomiting. Bleeding can be treated with sclerotherapy, balloon tamponade, or band ligation. Up to half die with their first bleed, either due to exsanguinations or following hepatic coma; in survivors there is a 50% chance of recurrence within a year, with the same mortality rate.

Barrett Esophagus (p. 757)

Barrett esophagus is a complication of chronic GERD characterized by *intestinal metaplasia within the esophageal squamous mucosa.* It occurs in an estimated 10% of individuals with chronic GERD; the typical patient is a white male between ages 40 and 60. Barrett esophagus confers an increased risk of esophageal adenocarcinoma; preinvasive *dysplasia* is detected in 0.2% to 2% of patients with Barrett esophagus annually.

Morphology (p. 757)

- *Gross:* Patches of red, velvety mucosa are present above the GE junction.

- *Microscopic:* Intestinal-type columnar epithelium, particularly mucin-secreting goblet cells, is typically required for the diagnosis; gastric cardia-type epithelium that is present above the GE junction may also be acceptable for diagnosis. When present, *dysplasia* is classified as low or high grade. Intramucosal carcinoma is characterized by neoplastic cell invasion into the lamina propria.

Clinical Features (p. 757)

Diagnosis requires both gross (endoscopic) and biopsy confirmation; once identified, periodic surveillance endoscopy is performed to look for dysplasia or frank malignancy. Multifocal high-grade dysplasia (with a high risk for progression) or carcinoma typically requires esophagectomy, although newer modalities (laser ablation, photodynamic therapy) are also used.

Esophageal Tumors (p. 758)

Adenocarcinoma (p. 758)

Esophageal adenocarcinomas largely evolve from dysplastic changes in Barrett mucosa; it occurs most frequently in white males (7:1 male to female ratio) and accounts for half of all U.S. esophageal cancers.

Pathogenesis (p. 758)

There is a stepwise accumulation of genetic and epigenetic alterations from Barrett esophagus to adenocarcinoma. Chromosomal and p53 abnormalities occur early; additional changes include amplification of *c-ERB-B2* and *cyclin D1* and *E genes* and mutations in *Rb* and the *p16/INK4a* cyclin-dependent kinase inhibitor.

Morphology (p. 758)

- *Grossly* lesions range from exophytic nodules to excavated and deeply infiltrative masses, mostly in the distal third of the esophagus.
- *Microscopically* tumors typically produce mucin and form glands, often with intestinal-type morphology; diffusely infiltrative signet-ring tumors are less common, and rarely the histology reveals adenosquamous or small, poorly differentiated cells.

Clinical Features (p. 758)

Although occasionally found during evaluation for GERD or surveillance for Barrett esophagus, esophageal adenocarcinomas typically present with dysphagia, weight loss, hematemesis, chest pain, or vomiting. Because most tumors are detected at advanced stages, the 5-year survival rate is less than 25%.

Squamous Cell Carcinoma (p. 759)

In the United States, esophageal squamous cell carcinoma typically occurs in adults older than 45 years, with men 4 times more frequently than women and blacks 6 times more than whites. Risk factors include alcohol and tobacco use, caustic esophageal injury, previous mediastinal radiation, achalasia, Plummer-Vinson syndrome, and frequent consumption of hot beverages. There is considerable geographic variability, with highest incidences in Iran, central China, Hong Kong, Brazil, and South Africa.

Pathogenesis (p. 759)

The pathogenesis is multifactorial; environment and diet contribute synergistically, modified by genetic factors. Alcohol and tobacco synergize to increase risk, and contribute to the majority of cancers in the United States. Nutritional deficiencies, as well as polycyclic hydrocarbons, nitrosamines, other mutagenic compounds (e.g., from fungal contaminants), and human papillomavirus (HPV) all likely contribute to the geographic variation in incidence. Recurrent genetic abnormalities include amplification of the *SOX2* transcription factor gene, overexpression of the cyclin D1, and loss-of-function mutations in *TP53, E-cadherin,* and *NOTCH1.*

Morphology *(p. 759)*

Half of esophageal squamous cell cancers occur in the middle third of the esophagus.

- They typically begin as in situ gray-white, plaquelike mucosal thickenings.
- Lesions can subsequently expand as exophytic lesions, ulcerate, or become diffusely infiltrative with wall thickening and luminal stenosis.
- A rich submucosal lymphatic network promotes circumferential and longitudinal spread. Tumors can invade deeply into adjacent mediastinal structures.
- Most tumors are moderately to well differentiated; less common variants are verrucous, spindle, and basaloid squamous cell carcinomas.

Clinical Features *(p. 760)*

Onset is insidious, and symptom onset is late; patients develop dysphagia, obstruction, weight loss, hemorrhage, iron deficiency anemia, sepsis secondary to ulceration, or respiratory fistulas with aspiration. Superficial carcinomas have a 5-year survival rate of 75%, but the overall 5-year survival rate is ≤20%.

STOMACH (p. 760)

Gastropathy and Acute Gastritis (p. 760)

Acute gastritis is a transient mucosal inflammatory process; when few inflammatory cells are present (e.g., with nonsteroidal antiinflammatory agents, alcohol, bile, or stress-induced injury), the term *gastropathy* is applied. *Hypertrophic gastropathy* is used for to describe Ménétrier disease or Zollinger-Ellison syndrome. Gastropathy and gastritis can both be asymptomatic or can cause varying degrees of pain, nausea, and vomiting. Severe cases exhibit ulceration with hemorrhage, presenting as hematemesis or melena.

Pathogenesis (p. 761)

Gastropathy and acute gastritis can occur when one or more of the mechanisms that protect gastric mucosa from the acidic environment are overwhelmed or defective (Fig. 17-1). Increased acid production with back-diffusion, decreased bicarbonate or mucin production, or direct mucosal damage can all be pathogenic. Thus chronic use of nonsteroidal antiinflammatory drugs (NSAIDs) reduces bicarbonate production and interferes with the cytoprotective action of prostaglandins (these inhibit acid production, promote mucin synthesis, and increase vascular perfusion); excessive alcohol consumption and heavy smoking can be directly toxic, and hypoxia

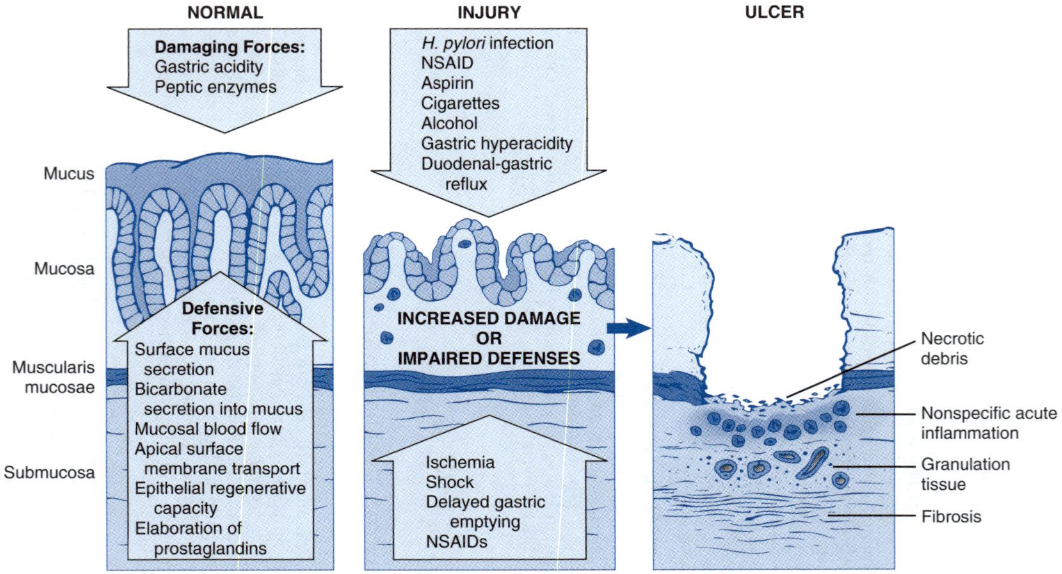

Figure 17-1 Mechanisms of gastric injury and protection. The diagram illustrates the progression from more mild forms of injury to ulceration that may occur with acute or chronic gastritis. Ulcers include layers of necrosis (N), inflammation (I), and granulation tissue (G), but a fibrotic scar (S), which takes time to develop, is present only in chronic lesions.

(e.g., at high altitudes), ischemia, and shock can secondarily injure the mucosa. Gastric injury due to uremia or urease-secreting *Helicobacter pylori* may occur through ammonium ion inhibition of gastric bicarbonate transporters.

Morphology (p. 762)

- *Grossly* there is moderate edema and hyperemia, occasionally with hemorrhage *(acute hemorrhagic erosive gastritis).*
- *Microscopically* neutrophils invade the epithelium, with superficial epithelial sloughing *(erosion)* and a fibrinous luminal exudate.

Stress-Related Mucosal Disease (p. 762)

This refers to focal, acute mucosal defects, typically as a complication of NSAID use or as a consequence of severe physiologic stress:

- *Stress ulcers* occur after shock, sepsis, or severe trauma.
- *Curling ulcers* occur in the proximal duodenum and are associated with burns or trauma.
- *Cushing* ulcers are gastric, duodenal, and esophageal ulcers arising in patients with intracranial disease; they have a high risk of perforation.

Pathogenesis (p. 762)

Hypotension, hypoxia, or stress-induced splanchnic vasoconstriction can cause local ischemia that secondarily leads to gastric mucosal damage. Lesions associated with brain injury are attributed to direct vagal stimulation causing gastric acid hypersecretion. Systemic acidosis may lower the intracellular pH of mucosal cells.

Morphology (p. 762)

Ulcers are usually less than 1 cm in diameter, multiple, and shallow; they may be found anywhere in the stomach. The ulcer base is brown (blood), whereas the adjacent mucosa is normal.

Clinical Features (p. 762)

Most critically ill patients have some evidence of gastric mucosal injury; 1% to 4% will have blood loss sufficient to warrant transfusion. After removal of the injurious factors, healing with complete reepithelialization is the norm. The single most important determinant of outcome is the *ability to correct the underlying conditions.*

Other, non-stress-related causes of gastric bleeding include the following:

- *Dieulafoy lesions* (most common on the lesser curvature near the GE junction); these are caused by abnormal vascular branching leading to a large subepithelial artery that can bleed with minor mucosal erosion.
- *Gastric antral vascular ectasia (GAVE)* is a predominantly idiopathic lesion seen endoscopically as longitudinal stripes of edematous, erythematous mucosa attributed to ectatic mucosal vessels. Histologically the antral mucosa shows reactive gastropathy with dilated capillaries containing fibrin thrombi.

Chronic Gastritis (p. 763)

Chronic gastritis is characterized by ongoing mucosal inflammation with mucosal atrophy; it provides a substrate in which dysplasia (and carcinoma) can arise. Compared to acute gastritis, the symptoms are usually less severe but are more persistent. Causes include

H. pylori infection (most common), autoimmune gastritis (10% of cases; second most common), radiation, bile reflux, mechanical injury (indwelling nasogastric tube), and involvement by systemic disorders, such as amyloid or CD.

Helicobacter pylori Gastritis (p. 763)

Epidemiology (p. 763)

Although *H. pylori* is a widely prevalent gastric infection (colonization rates from 10% to 80% of the population), a much smaller percentage of those infected actually develop gastritis. Nevertheless, *H. pylori* infection is the most common cause of chronic gastritis; organisms are present in up to 90% of individuals with disease. Humans are the only host—spread is via fecal-oral, oral-oral, or environmental routes; consequently, lower socioeconomic status and crowding lead to higher colonization rates.

Pathogenesis (p. 763)

H. pylori induces predominantly an antral gastritis, characterized by increased acid production, and disruption of the normal mucosal protection mechanisms (Fig. 17-1). Virulence factors in *H. pylori* infections include the following:

- *Motility* via flagella
- *Urease production* generating ammonia that raises local pH, enhances bacterial survival, and inhibits gastric bicarbonate transport
- Bacterial *adhesins* to bind surface epithelial cells
- *Toxins* (e.g., cagA and vacA cytotoxins)

Over time, the initial antral gastritis progresses to *multifocal atrophic gastritis* (i.e., mucosal atrophy with reduced acid production) and intestinal metaplasia. Host-pathogen interactions influence whether gastritis results from the initial infection (e.g., polymorphisms in interleukin [IL]-1β and tumor necrosis factor [TNF] genes correlate with the development of chronic disease).

Morphology (p. 763)

- *Grossly,* infected mucosa is erythematous and coarse to nodular.
- *Microscopically H. pylori* are typically found in the antrum; gastric biopsy usually demonstrates organisms concentrated in the superficial mucus overlying surface and neck epithelium. There are variable numbers of intraepithelial and luminal neutrophils (forming *pit abscesses*), and the lamina propria contains abundant plasma cells, macrophages, and lymphocytes.
- Long-standing gastritis is associated with diffuse mucosal atrophy, with intestinal metaplasia and prominent lymphoid aggregates occasionally with germinal centers.

Clinical Features (p. 764)

H. pylori can be diagnosed by antibody serologic test, urea breath test, bacterial culture, direct bacterial visualization in gastric biopsy, or DNA-based tests. *H. pylori* infection is a risk factor for peptic ulcer disease (PUD), gastric adenocarcinoma, and gastric lymphoma.

Autoimmune Gastritis (p. 764)

This form of gastritis typically spares the antrum and is associated with *hypergastrinemia.*

Pathogenesis (p. 765)

CD4+ T cell–mediated autoimmune destruction of parietal cells is the major pathogenic mechanism; there are also circulating and gastric secreted antibodies to parietal cells and intrinsic factor, but these are probably only secondary manifestations of disease and not causal. Parietal cell cytotoxicity leads in turn to defective gastric acid secretion *(achlorhydria)* that triggers hypergastrinemia and antral G-cell hyperplasia. Reduced intrinsic factor production impedes vitamin B_{12} absorption and causes pernicious anemia. Secondary bystander damage to chief cells reduces the pepsinogen I production.

Morphology *(p. 765)*

Rugal folds are lost, and there is diffuse mucosal damage of the acid-producing parietal cells primarily in the body and fundus. The inflammatory infiltrate is predominantly lymphocytes, macrophages, and plasma cells, and lymphoid aggregates can be present.

Clinical Features *(p. 765)*

Autoantibodies are detected early in the course; progression to gastric atrophy occurs over 20 to 30 years. Patients present with symptoms referable to anemia; vitamin B_{12} deficiency can also manifest with atrophic glossitis, malabsorption, peripheral neuropathy, spinal cord lesions, and cerebral dysfunction. A strong genetic underpinning is suggested by the observation that autoimmune gastritis is often associated with other autoimmune diseases such as Hashimoto thyroiditis, type 1 diabetes mellitus, and Addison disease; 20% of relatives of affected patients will also have autoimmune gastritis.

Uncommon Forms of Gastritis (p. 766)

- *Eosinophilic gastritis* (p. 766) is characterized by heavy eosinophilic infiltration of the mucosa or submucosa; it can be infectious, due to allergy to ingested material, or part of a systemic collagen-vascular disease (e.g., scleroderma).
- *Lymphocytic gastritis* (p. 766) is an idiopathic disorder predominantly affecting women; 40% of cases are associated with celiac disease (see later). There is marked accumulation of intraepithelial CD8+ T cells.
- *Granulomatous gastritis* (p. 766) is a diverse group of diseases sharing the presence of granulomas; sarcoid, CD, and infections are causes.

Complications of Chronic Gastritis (p. 766)

Peptic Ulcer Disease (p. 766)

PUD is chronic mucosal ulceration affecting the duodenum or stomach. The most common form occurs in the gastric antrum or duodenum associated with *H. pylori* infection. PUD in the gastric fundus or body is usually accompanied by mucosal atrophy (due to *H. pylori* or autoimmune chronic gastritis).

Epidemiology *(p. 766)*

Nearly all peptic ulcers are associated with *H. pylori* infection, NSAIDs (including low-dose aspirin for cardiovascular benefits), or cigarette smoking; NSAID risk is increased by any concurrent *H. pylori* infection. Other risk factors for PUD include chronic obstructive pulmonary disease (COPD), illicit drugs (that reduce mucosal blood flow), alcoholic cirrhosis, psychological stress, Zollinger-Ellison syndrome, and certain viral infections (CMV, herpes simplex).

Pathogenesis *(p. 766)*

PUD results from imbalances in mucosal damage and defenses (Fig. 17-1). Hyperacidity in PUD can be caused by infection, parietal cell hyperplasia, excessive secretory response, or increased gastrin production (e.g., secondary to hypercalcemia or produced by a tumor). NSAIDs and steroids block the normal prostaglandin cytoprotective effects, and cigarette smoking (and cardiovascular disease) impairs mucosal blood flow and healing.

Morphology *(p. 766)*

Most ulcers are solitary.

- *Grossly* there is a sharply punched-out defect with overhanging mucosal borders and smooth, clean ulcer bases.
- *Microscopically* there are thin layers of fibrinoid debris with underlying inflammation merging into granulation tissue and deep scarring. The surrounding mucosa usually exhibits chronic gastritis.

Clinical Features *(p. 767)*

Classic symptoms include epigastric gnawing, burning, or aching pain, worse at night and 1 to 3 hours after meals. Nausea, vomiting, bloating, belching, and weight loss can also occur. Complications include anemia, hemorrhage, perforation, and obstruction. Malignant transformation is rare and related to underlying gastritis. Treatment is focused on *H. pylori* eradication, removal of offending agents (e.g., NSAIDs), and neutralization or reduced production of gastric acid.

Mucosal Atrophy and Intestinal Metaplasia (p. 768)

Long-standing chronic gastritis can lead to parietal cell loss, associated with intestinal metaplasia, and an increased risk of gastric adenocarcinoma; the risk of malignancy is greatest in autoimmune gastritis. Achlorhydria due to parietal cell deficiency may predispose to cancer by allowing bacterial overgrowth with production of carcinogenic nitrosamines.

Dysplasia (p. 768)

Long-standing chronic gastritis exposes epithelium to inflammation-related free radical damage and proliferative stimuli. Over time, the combination can lead to the accumulation of genetic alterations resulting in carcinoma; preinvasive, in situ lesions can be recognized histologically as *dysplasia*.

Gastritis Cystica (p. 768)

This is an exuberant reactive epithelial proliferation with entrapped epithelium-lined cysts that can exhibit reactive changes that mimic invasive adenocarcinoma. Gastritis cystica is associated with chronic gastritis and partial gastrectomy.

Hypertrophic Gastropathies (p. 768)

These are uncommon conditions featuring giant enlargement of gastric rugal folds due to epithelial hyperplasia; they are linked to excessive growth factor production.

Ménétrier Disease (p. 768)

There is diffuse foveolar cell hyperplasia, with a protein-losing enteropathy that causes systemic hypoproteinemia. It is caused by overexpression of transforming growth factor-α (TGF-α). Risk of gastric adenocarcinoma is increased.

Zollinger-Ellison Syndrome (p. 769)

This is caused by gastrin-secreting tumors *(gastrinomas)* typically in the small bowel or pancreas. Patients classically present with multiple duodenal ulcers and/or chronic diarrhea. Elevated gastrin levels induce a marked (up to fivefold) increase in gastric parietal cells, as well as more modest increases in mucous neck cells and gastric endocrine cells. Gastrinomas are sporadic in 75% of patients; in the remainder they are associated with multiple endocrine neoplasia, type I (MEN-I). Approximately 60% to 90% of gastrinomas are malignant.

Gastric Polyps and Tumors (p. 769)

Polyps are nodules or masses that project above the level of the surrounding mucosa; they can result from epithelial or stromal hyperplasia, inflammation, ectopia, or neoplasia.

Inflammatory and Hyperplastic Polyps (p. 770)

These constitute 75% of gastric polyps; their incidence depends partly on the local prevalence of *H. pylori* infections. They are most common between ages 50 and 60 and typically arise in association with chronic gastritis. The majority are <1 cm and are frequently multiple; they typically have a smooth surface, occasionally with superficial erosions, and histologically show irregular, cystically dilated and elongated glands with variable amounts of acute and chronic inflammation. Risk of dysplasia increases with size; polyps >1.5 cm should be resected.

Fundic Gland Polyps (p. 770)

Fundic gland polyps occur sporadically (typically in women over age 50) or in the setting of familial adenomatous polyposis (FAP); their incidence is also increased by proton pump inhibitors and the consequent increased gastrin secretion. They are single or multiple, smooth, well-circumscribed lesions composed of irregular, cystically dilated glands with minimal inflammation.

Gastric Adenoma (p. 770)

Gastric adenomas comprise 10% of gastric polyps. These almost always occur on a background of FAP or chronic gastritis with atrophy and intestinal metaplasia; the male to female ratio is 3:1 and the incidence increases with age. Usually solitary and <2 cm, gastric adenomas all exhibit some degree of dysplasia; 30% can harbor carcinoma, and lesions >2 cm are particularly concerning.

Gastric Adenocarcinoma (p. 771)

More than 90% of gastric malignancies are adenocarcinomas; they are divided into *intestinal* and *diffuse* forms with different risk factors, genetic perturbations, and clinical and pathologic presentations (see later).

Epidemiology (p. 771)

Worldwide distribution is widely variable; the incidence in Japan, Chile, Costa Rica, and Eastern Europe is twentyfold greater than North America and northern Europe. The U.S. incidence decreased 85% in the twentieth century (mostly due to decreases in the intestinal form that is associated with atrophic gastritis); gastric carcinoma now constitutes <2.5% of all cancer deaths in the United States. The epidemiology suggests a role for environmental factors (e.g., *H. pylori* infections). Diet also influences risk; thus decreased consumption of carcinogens (e.g., N-nitroso compounds and benzo[a]pyrene, associated with some forms of food preservation) and increased intake of antioxidants in green leafy vegetables and fruits reduce gastric cancer incidence. Conversely, *partial gastrectomy* (e.g., for PUD) increases risk by permitting bile reflux and the development of chronic gastritis.

Pathogenesis *(p. 771)*

Loss of intercellular adhesion is a key step in oncogenesis, particularly of *diffuse gastric cancer.* Thus germline mutations in the *CDH1* gene encoding E-cadherin are associated with familial gastric carcinomas and also occur in 50% of sporadic lesions. *Intestinal-type gastric cancers* are associated with FAP, mutations in proteins that associate with E-cadherin (e.g., β-catenin), microsatellite instability, and hypermethylation of *TGFβRII, BAX, IGFRII,* and *p16/INK4a.* In both types of gastric cancer associated with *H. pylori* infections, immune response gene polymorphisms influence risk; *p53* mutations are also present in the majority of sporadic cancers of both types.

Morphology *(p. 772)*

Gastric cancers involve the antrum > lesser curvature > greater curvature.

- Tumors with *intestinal morphology* tend to form bulky exophytic tumors composed of glandular structures. These develop from precursor lesions, including flat dysplasia and adenomas.
- Tumors with a *diffuse infiltrative* pattern of growth tend to be composed of *signet-ring cells* (intracellular mucin vacuoles push the nucleus to the periphery) that are discohesive and do not form glands; these also tend to induce a fibrous desmoplastic response. There are no identified precursor lesions. The gross correlate to these tumors is a rigid thickened gastric wall termed *linitus plastica* (literally "leather bottle").

Clinical Features *(p. 772)*

Gastric carcinoma is an insidious disease; early symptoms resemble those for chronic gastritis (dysphagia, dyspepsia, and nausea). Advanced stages announce themselves with weight loss, anorexia, altered bowel habits, anemia, and hemorrhage. Prognosis critically depends on *depth of invasion* and the *extent of nodal or distant metastases.* After surgical resection, the 5-year survival of early gastric cancer is >90% even with nodal spread; in comparison, advanced gastric cancer has a 5-year survival <20%. Overall 5-year survival in the United States is 30%.

Lymphoma (p. 773)

Extranodal lymphomas can arise in any tissue but do so most commonly in the GI tract and especially the stomach. Patients typically present with dyspepsia and epigastric pain; hematemesis, melena, or weight loss can also occur. *GI lymphomas* (also known as *m*ucosa-*a*ssociated *l*ymphoid *t*issue or *MALTomas*) constitute 5% of gastric malignancies; most are marginal zone B-cell lymphomas. A smaller fraction of primary GI lymphomas are large B-cell lymphomas.

Pathogenesis *(p. 773)*

Extranodal marginal B-cell lymphomas arise at sites of chronic inflammation. In the stomach this is typically associated with chronic

H. pylori infection; interestingly antibiotic treatment and *H. pylori* eradication can induce durable tumor regression. Antibiotic-resistant tumors often harbor a t(11;18) translocation; t(1;14) and t(14;18) translocations are less common but are predictive for response failure. The t(11;18) translocation links the apoptosis inhibitor 2 gene (*API2* on chromosome 11) with the "mutated in MALT lymphoma gene" (*MLT* on chromosome 18); the t(14;18) translocation increases MLT, whereas t(1:14) increases BCL-10 expression. Each of the translocations leads to constitutive NF-κB transcription factor activation, promoting B-cell growth and survival. With time, these MALTomas can transform into the more aggressive diffuse large B-cell lymphomas, often associated with inactivation of *p53* and/or *p16* tumor suppressor genes.

Morphology (p. 773)

Microscopically there is a dense infiltrate of atypical lymphocytes in the lamina propria; focal invasion of the mucosal epithelium forms diagnostic *lymphoepithelial lesions.* Markers are as described for other mature B-cell tumors (see Chapter 13).

Carcinoid Tumor (p. 773)

Carcinoid *(carcinoma-like)* tumors arise from diffusely distributed endocrine cells; they are now properly referred to as *well-differentiated neuroendocrine tumors.* Most arise in the gut (lungs are second in frequency), and 40% occur in the small intestine; the cells of origin in the GI tract are responsible for hormone secretion that coordinate gut function (Table 17-1). Gastric carcinoid tumors may be associated with endocrine cell hyperplasia, autoimmune chronic atrophic gastritis, MEN-I, and Zollinger-Ellison syndrome; gastric endocrine cell hyperplasia has been linked to proton pump inhibitor therapy. Most carcinoid tumors follow a more indolent course than do carcinomas.

Morphology (p. 774)

- *Grossly* carcinoids are yellow-tan intramural or submucosal masses forming small polypoid lesions. An intense desmoplastic response makes them firm and can cause bowel obstruction.
- *Microscopically* the tumors range from islands to sheets of uniform cohesive cells with scant, granular cytoplasm and oval, stippled nuclei; cells are typically positive for neuroendocrine markers (e.g., chromogranin A and synaptophysin).

Clinical Features (p. 774)

Peak incidence is in the sixth decade. Carcinoids are usually indolent, slow-growing malignancies, and symptoms are largely a function of the hormones produced (Table 17-1). Ileal tumors systemically secrete vasoactive products that manifest with cutaneous flushing, bronchospasm, increased bowel motility, and right-sided cardiac valve thickening, so-called *carcinoid syndrome.* Carcinoid syndrome occurs in ≤10% of patients with GI carcinoid due to hepatic metabolism of the secreted products; presence of the syndrome is therefore usually associated with bulky hepatic metastatic disease.

The most important prognostic factor for GI carcinoid is the primary site of the tumor:

- Foregut tumors (esophagus, stomach, and duodenum) rarely metastasize and are cured by resection.
- Midgut carcinoids (jejunum and ileum) are usually multiple and aggressive.

TABLE 17-1 Features of GI Carcinoid Tumors

Feature	Esophagus	Stomach	Proximal Duodenum	Jejunum and Ileum	Appendix	Colorectum
Fraction of GI carcinoids	<1%	<10%	<10%	>40%	<25%	<25%
Mean patient age (yr)	Rare	55	50	65	All ages	60
Location	Distal	Body and fundus	Proximal third, periampullary	Throughout	Tip	Rectum > cecum
Size	Limited data	1-2 cm, multiple; >2 cm, solitary	0.5-2 cm	<3.5 cm	0.2-1 cm	>5 cm (cecum); <1 cm (rectum)
Secretory product(s)	Limited data	Histamine, somatostatin, serotonin	Gastrin, somatostatin, cholecystokinin	Serotonin, substance P, polypeptide YY	Serotonin, polypeptide YY	Serotonin, polypeptide YY
Symptoms	Dysphagia, weight loss, reflux	Gastritis, ulcer, incidental	Peptic ulcer, biliary obstruction, abdominal pain	Asymptomatic, obstruction, metastatic disease	Asymptomatic, incidental	Abdominal pain, weight loss, incidental
Behavior	Limited data	Variable	Variable	Aggressive	Benign	Variable
Disease associations	None	Atrophic gastritis, MEN-I	Zollinger-Ellison syndrome, NF-1, sporadic	None	None	None

- Hindgut tumors (appendix and colon) are usually found only incidentally.
    - *Appendiceal carcinoids* are usually found at the tip, are <2 cm, and are usually benign.
    - *Colonic carcinoids* can be large and can metastasize.
    - Rectal carcinoids can secrete polypeptide hormones and/or cause pain but usually do not metastasize.

Gastrointestinal Stromal Tumor (p. 775)

Gastrointestinal stromal tumor (GIST) is the most common GI mesenchymal tumor; more than half are in the stomach.

Epidemiology (p. 775)

Peak age of GIST diagnosis is in the sixth decade; incidence is increased in patients with neurofibromatosis type I (NF-1) and in children (usually females) with *Carney triad,* a nonhereditary syndrome with GIST, paragangliomas, and pulmonary chondromas.

Pathogenesis (p. 775)

GISTs appear to arise from the interstitial cells of Cajal (pacemakers for gut peristalsis) in the muscularis propria. Approximately 75% to 80% of all GISTs contain *oncogenic gain-of-function mutations in the gene coding for the tyrosine kinase c-KIT* (c-KIT is the stem cell factor receptor); 8% have activating *platelet-derived growth factor receptor-α* (PDGFRA) mutations. Constitutive tyrosine kinase activity leads to downstream activation of RAS and PI3K/AKT pathways promoting tumor cell proliferation and survival. GISTs without mutated c-KIT or PDGFRA can have mutations in other genes that function in these pathways (*NF1, BRAF, HRAS,* or *NRAS*). However, more common are mutations in genes encoding mitochondrial succinate dehydrogenase (SDH) complex proteins; these may cause an accumulation of succinate that dysregulates hypoxia inducible factor-1α (HIF-1α), thereby increasing the transcription of vascular endothelial growth factor *(VEGF)* and insulin-like growth factor-1 *(IGF1R)* genes.

Morphology (p. 776)

- *Grossly* GISTs are usually solitary, well-circumscribed fleshy masses; they can grow as large as 30 cm.
- *Microscopically* tumors are classified as either *epithelioid* (plump and cohesive cells) or *spindle cell type;* c-KIT expression is the most useful diagnostic marker.

Clinical Features (p. 776)

Symptoms are usually related to mass effects or blood loss. Surgical resection is the primary treatment for localized gastric GIST. Metastases are rare when tumors are <5 cm but common when >10 cm. These typically take the form of peritoneal serosal nodules or liver implants; spread outside the abdomen is uncommon. Tumors not amenable to resection can be treated with *imatinib,* a tyrosine kinase inhibitor that inhibits c-KIT and PDGFRA.

SMALL INTESTINE AND COLON (p. 777)

Due to their roles in nutrient and water transport and their interface with diverse food and microbial antigens, the intestines are unsurprisingly involved by an array of malabsorption, infectious, inflammatory, and neoplastic processes.

Intestinal Obstruction (p. 777)

Tumors, infarctions, and strictures (due, e.g., to CD) account for 10% to 15% of obstructions; 80% are attributable to the following four entities (Fig. 17-2):

Hernias (p. 777)

Peritoneal wall defects permit peritoneal sac protrusion *(hernia sac)* in which bowel segments can be trapped *(external herniation)*. Subsequent vascular stasis and edema lead to *incarceration;* vascular compromise leads to *strangulation.* Locations include the femoral and inguinal canals, umbilicus, and surgical scars; there is a lifetime risk of 5%. Hernias are the most common cause of intestinal obstruction worldwide, and the third most common cause in the United States.

Adhesions (p. 777)

Adhesions are residua of localized peritoneal inflammation *(peritonitis)* following surgery, infection, endometriosis, or radiation; healing leads to fibrous bridging between viscera. Congenital adhesions also rarely occur. Adhesions are the most common cause of intestinal obstruction in the United States. Complications include *internal herniation* (within peritoneal cavity), obstruction, and strangulation.

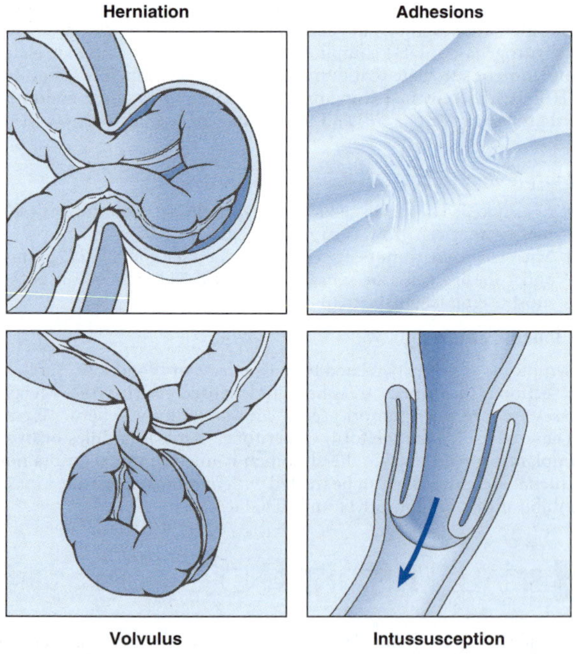

Figure 17-2 Intestinal obstruction. The four major causes of intestinal obstruction are (1) herniation of a segment in the umbilical or inguinal regions, (2) adhesion between loops of intestine, (3) volvulus, and (4) intussusception.

Volvulus (p. 778)

Volvulus is complete twisting of a bowel loop about its mesenteric vascular base, leading to vascular and luminal obstruction with infarction. Volvulus occurs most often in redundant loops of sigmoid colon, followed by cecum and small bowel.

Intussusception (p. 778)

Intussusception occurs when an intestinal segment (usually small bowel) telescopes into the immediately distal segment. Peristalsis propels the invaginated segment, along with its attached mesentery, potentially resulting in obstruction, vessel compression, and infarction. In *infants and children,* intussusception is usually spontaneous or can be associated with rotavirus infection. In older individuals the point of traction is usually a tumor. In children younger than 2 years, intussusception is the most common cause of intestinal obstruction.

Ischemic Bowel Disease (p. 779)

The abundant collateral supply throughout much of the GI tract allows the bowel to usually tolerate slowly progressive loss of blood supply. In comparison, abrupt compromise of any major vessel can cause infarction of several meters of intestine. *Watershed zones* between major vessel branches (e.g., the splenic flexure between superior and inferior mesenteric artery circulations) are most vulnerable. Damage ranges from mucosal infarction to transmural infarction. Because they are at the end of the capillary network, the epithelial cells at the tips of villi are more susceptible to ischemia than are the crypt epithelial cells.

Important causes of ischemia are atherosclerosis, aortic aneurysm, hypercoagulable states, embolization, and vasculitis; hypoperfusion can also be associated with cardiac failure, shock, dehydration, or vasoconstrictive drugs. Mesenteric venous obstruction or thrombosis due to hypercoagulability, masses, or cirrhosis can also cause ischemic disease.

Pathogenesis (p. 779)

An initial *hypoxic injury* occurs at the onset of vascular compromise, although intestinal epithelium is relatively resistant to transient hypoxia. However, subsequent reperfusion leads to an influx of inflammatory cells and mediators (see Chapter 2) causing the majority of damage.

Morphology (p. 779)

- *Mucosal infarction:* Patchy mucosal hemorrhage but with normal serosa.
- *Mural infarction:* Complete mucosal necrosis, with variable necrosis of submucosa and muscularis propria. Distribution is typically segmental, without serositis.
- *Transmural infarction:* Involved bowel segments are usually hemorrhagic, and there is associated serositis. Coagulative necrosis of the muscularis propria with perforation develops within 1 to 4 days.
- *Microscopically* there is atrophy and sloughing of surface epithelium, but preserved crypts can be hyperproliferative. The extent of inflammation and edema depends on the duration of injury. Superimposed bacterial infection can induce pseudomembrane formation.
- Chronic vascular insufficiency results in fibrosis of the lamina propria and occasionally stricture formation.

Clinical Features (p. 779)

Typically occurring in older individuals with coexisting cardiac or vascular disease, ischemic bowel presents with severe abdominal pain, bloody diarrhea or gross melena, abdominal rigidity, nausea, and vomiting. Right-sided colonic disease typically has a more severe course, and coexisting COPD is a poor prognostic indicator. Surgery is indicated in up to 10% of cases; with appropriate management, 30-day mortality is approximately 10% to 20%.

Aangiodysplasia (p. 780)

Lesions of *angiodysplasia* are tortuous, ectatic dilations of mucosal or submucosal veins occurring in approximately 1% of the population; most common in the cecum or ascending colon (usually after age 60), angiodysplasia accounts for 20% of major episodes of lower GI bleeding. Lesions are attributed to partial, intermittent venous occlusion; the cecal or right colonic predilection derives from the greater wall tension in those locations owing to their larger diameter.

Malabsorption and Diarrhea (p. 781)

Malabsorption is characterized by defective absorption of fats, fat- and water-soluble vitamins, proteins, carbohydrates, electrolytes, minerals, and water. General symptoms are diarrhea, flatus, abdominal pain, and muscle wasting; a classic hallmark is *steatorrhea* characterized by excessive fecal fat and greasy, malodorous stools. Clinical consequences (due to various deficiencies) include the following:

- Anemia and mucositis (pyridoxine, folate, or vitamin B_{12})
- Bleeding (vitamin K)
- Osteopenia and tetany (calcium, magnesium, vitamin D)
- Peripheral neuropathy (vitamins A or B_{12})

The most common causes of malabsorption in the United States are celiac disease, pancreatic insufficiency, and CD (Table 17-2). The pathogenesis involves disturbance(s) in the following:

- *Intraluminal digestion:* Emulsification and initial enzymatic breakdown
- *Terminal digestion:* Hydrolysis within the enterocyte brush border
- *Transepithelial transport* through enterocytes
- *Lymphatic transport* of absorbed lipids

Diarrhea is defined as increased stool mass, frequency, or fluidity, usually exceeding 200 g/day. Severe cases can exceed 14 L/day and be fatal without fluid restoration. Painful, bloody, small-volume diarrhea is called *dysentery.* General categories are as follows:

- *Secretory:* Isotonic with plasma and persists during fasting.
- *Osmotic:* Unabsorbed luminal solutes (e.g., due to lactase deficiency) increase osmotic pull of fluid; stool is ≥50 mOsm hyperosmolar relative to plasma and abates with fasting.
- *Malabsorptive:* As described earlier; abates on fasting.
- *Exudative:* Due to inflammatory disease; purulent, bloody stools persist during fasting.

Cystic Fibrosis (p. 782)

The malabsorption associated with cystic fibrosis is due to the absence of the epithelial cystic fibrosis transmembrane conductance regulator (CFTR); this causes defective bicarbonate, sodium, and

TABLE 17-2 Defects in Malabosorptive and Diarrheal Disease

Disease	Intraluminal Digestion	Terminal Digestion	Transepithelial Transport	Lymphatic Transport
Celiac disease		+	+	
Tropical sprue		+	+	
Chronic pancreatitis	+			
Cystic fibrosis	+			
Primary bile acid malabsorption	+		+	
Carcinoid syndrome			+	
Autoimmune enteropathy		+	+	
Disaccharidase deficiency		+		
Whipple disease				+
Abetalipoproteinemia			+	
Viral gastroenteritis		+	+	
Bacterial gastroenteritis		+	+	
Parasitic gastroenteritis		+	+	
IBD	+	+	+	

+ indicates that the process is abnormal in the disease indicated. Other processes are not affected.

water secretion and ultimately results in defective luminal hydration. This occasionally causes intestinal obstruction but more commonly (80% of patients) results in formation of pancreatic intraductal concretions and—in turn—causes pancreatic duct obstruction, low-grade chronic autodigestion of the pancreas, with eventual exocrine pancreatic insufficiency. The resulting failure of nutrient absorption can be treated with oral enzyme supplementation.

Celiac Disease (p. 782)

Also called *gluten-sensitive enteropathy* or *celiac sprue,* celiac disease is an immune-mediated diarrheal disorder triggered by ingestion of gluten-containing foods (e.g., derived from wheat, oat, rye, or barley) in genetically predisposed individuals. The worldwide incidence is 0.6% to 1%.

Pathogenesis (p. 782)

Sprue results from a gluten-mediated delayed-type hypersensitivity—specifically to a 33 amino acid *α-gliadin* polypeptide resistant to digestive enzymes (Fig. 17-3).

- Gliadin induces epithelial IL-15 expression with local activation and proliferation of CD8+ cytotoxic cells that can drive enterocyte apoptosis.
- Gliadin access to the underlying tissue permits increased deamidation by transglutaminase.

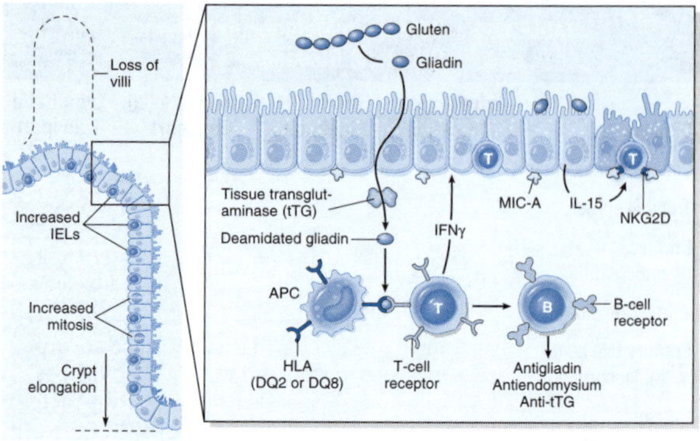

Figure 17-3 Celiac disease pathogenesis and manifestations. *Left:* The morphologic alterations in celiac disease, including villous atrophy, increased numbers of intraepithelial lymphocytes (IELs), and epithelial proliferation with crypt elongation. *Right:* A model for the pathogenesis of celiac disease. Both innate (CD8+ intraepithelial T cells, activated by IL-15) and adaptive (CD4+ T cells, and B cells sensitization to gliadin) immune mechanisms are involved in the tissue responses to gliadin. *NKG2D,* A natural killer cell marker and receptor for MIC-A.

- Deamidated peptide binds to specific MHC on antigen-presenting cells in susceptible individuals (expressing human leukocyte antigen [HLA]-DQ2 or HLA-DQ8), leading to CD4+ T-cell activation and cytokine-mediated epithelial damage.
- Additional factors that influence disease susceptibility include polymorphisms of genes that affect immune regulation and epithelial polarity.

Morphology (p. 783)

Diffusely flattened (atrophic) villi, and elongated regenerative crypts are associated with intraepithelial CD8+ T cells, and exuberant lamina propria chronic inflammation. Severity is greatest in the more proximal intestine.

Clinical Features (p. 783)

Celiac disease occurs in infants to middle age, presenting with diarrhea, flatulence, weight loss, and the effects of anemia. The most sensitive serologic test assesses the presence of immunoglobulin A (IgA) antibodies to tissue transglutaminase or IgA or IgG to deamidated gliadin.

- Celiac disease is often (10% of patients) associated with the pruritic, blistering skin disorder *dermatitis herpetiformis.* Lymphocytic gastritis or colitis is also more common.
- In addition to iron and vitamin deficiencies, there is increased risk of *enteropathy-associated T-cell lymphoma* and small intestine adenocarcinoma.
- Celiac disease usually responds to gluten withdrawal.

Environmental Enteropathy (p. 783)

Also called *tropical enteropathy* or *tropical sprue,* this is a malabsorption and malnutrition syndrome that occurs in areas with poor sanitation; it affects up to 150 million children worldwide. The histology is similar to severe celiac disease. An infectious etiology is implicated, with defective intestinal barrier function; in developing children there may be associated irreversible losses in physical development and cognition. Even with oral antibiotics and nutritional supplementation, the deficits may not be corrected.

Autoimmune Enteropathy (p. 784)

This is an X-linked disorder of children characterized by a persistent autoimmune-driven diarrhea. A severe familial form (IPEX, *i*mmune dysregulation, *p*olyendocrinopathy, *e*nteropathy, and *X*-linked) is due to germline mutations in the *FOXP3* gene, a transcription factor responsible for the differentiation of CD4+ regulatory T cells. Autoantibodies to a variety of GI epithelial cell types may be present.

Lactase (Disaccharidase) Deficiency (p. 784)

Lactase is an apical membrane disaccharidase of surface absorptive cells. With *lactase deficiency*, undigested and unabsorbed lactose exerts an osmotic pull, causing diarrhea and malabsorption; bacterial fermentation of lactose can cause also abdominal distention and flatus. Histologically the mucosa is unremarkable.

- A rare congenital autosomal recessive form is due to mutations in the lactase gene.
- The acquired form is caused by downregulation of lactase gene expression; it is common in Native American, African-American, and Chinese populations.

Abetalipoproteinemia (p. 784)

Abetalipoproteinemia is a rare autosomal recessive disease caused by inability of lipids to egress absorptive epithelial cells. The underlying defect is a mutation in the *microsomal triglyceride transfer protein (MTP)* responsible for transferring lipids to apolipoprotein B within the rough endoplasmic reticulum (ER); thus MTP impacts lipoprotein and fatty acid export from mucosal cells. Affected infants present with failure to thrive, diarrhea, and steatorrhea, as well as complete absence of all lipoproteins containing apolipoprotein B (although the apolipoprotein B gene is unaffected). Failure to absorb essential fatty acids leads to deficiencies of fat-soluble vitamins as well as lipid membrane defects.

- Increased enterocyte triglyceride stores manifest as *lipid vacuolation.*
- Altered erythrocyte lipid membranes manifest as acanthocytes *(burr cells).*

Infectious Enterocolitis (p. 785)

The symptoms of enterocolitis run the gamut from urgency to diarrhea to incontinence and perianal discomfort to abdominal pain; the outcomes can include dehydration, malabsorption, or hemorrhage (Table 17-3). Half of all deaths worldwide before age 5 are due to infectious enterocolitis; in developing countries 2000 children die *daily* as a consequence. Bacterial infections are frequently responsible, but the most common pathogens vary with geography, age, nutrition, and host immune status (see later); pediatric infectious diarrhea is often caused by enteric viruses.

Cholera (p. 785)

Cholera is caused by *Vibrio cholerae,* gram-negative bacteria typically transmitted by drinking contaminated water; humans, shellfish, and plankton are the only reservoirs.

TABLE 17-3 Features of Bacterial Enterocolitides

Infection Type	Geography	Reservoir	Transmission	Epidemiology	Affected GI Sites	Symptoms	Complications
Cholera	India, Africa	Shellfish	Fecal-oral, water	Sporadic, endemic, epidemic	Small intestine	Severe watery diarrhea	Dehydration, electrolyte imbalances
Campylobacter spp.	Developed countries	Chickens, sheep, pigs, cattle	Poultry, milk, other foods	Sporadic; children, travelers	Colon	Watery or bloody diarrhea	Arthritis, Guillain-Barré syndrome
Shigellosis	Worldwide, endemic in developing countries	Humans	Fecal-oral, food, water	Children, migrant workers, travelers, nursing homes	Left colon, ileum	Bloody diarrhea	Reactive arthritis, urethritis, conjunctivitis, hemolytic-uremic syndrome
Salmonellosis	Worldwide	Poultry, farm animals, reptiles	Meat, poultry, eggs, milk	Children, older adults	Colon and small intestine	Watery or bloody diarrhea	Sepsis, abscess
Enteric (typhoid) fever	India, Mexico, Philippines	Humans	Fecal-oral, water	Children. adolescents, travelers	Small intestine	Bloody diarrhea, fever	Chronic infection, carrier state, encephalopathy, myocarditis, intestinal perforation
Yersinia spp.	Northern and central Europe	Pigs, cows, puppies, cats	Pork, milk, water	Clustered cases	Ileum, appendix, right colon	Abdominal pain, fever, diarrhea	Reactive arthritis, erythema nodosum

E. coli							
ETEC	Developing countries	Unknown	Food or fecal-oral	Infants, adolescents, travelers	Small intestine	Severe watery diarrhea	Dehydration, electrolyte imbalances
EPEC	Worldwide	Humans	Fecal-oral	Infants	Small intestine	Watery diarrhea	Dehydration, electrolyte imbalances
EHEC	Worldwide	Widespread, includes cattle	Beef, milk, produce	Sporadic and epidemic	Colon	Bloody diarrhea	Hemolytic-uremic syndrome
EIEC	Developing countries	Unknown	Cheese, other foods, water	Young children	Colon	Bloody diarrhea	Unknown
EAEC	Worldwide	Unknown	Unknown	Children, adults, travelers	Colon	Nonbloody diarrhea, afebrile	Poorly defined
PMC *(C. difficile)*	Worldwide	Humans, hospitals	Antibiotics allow emergence	Immunosuppressed, antibiotic-treated	Colon	Watery diarrhea, fever	Relapse, toxic megacolon
Whipple disease	Rural > urban	Unknown	Unknown	Rare	Small intestine	Malabsorption	Arthritis, CNS disease
Mycobacterial infection	Worldwide	Unknown	Unknown	Immunosuppressed, endemic	Small intestine	Malabsorption	Pneumonia, infection at other sites

Pathogenesis (p. 785)

Vibrio organisms are noninvasive, although flagellar proteins are important for epithelial attachment and efficient bacterial colonization; mucosal biopsies show normal histology. *V. cholerae* causes diarrhea by production of a *cholera toxin* that is internalized after binding enterocyte surface GM1 gangliosides (Fig. 17-4):

- The *toxin A subunit* is processed in the ER to a fragment that enters the cytosol.
- The toxin A fragment interacts with *adenosine diphosphate (ADP) ribosylation factors* to activate the G protein $G_{s\alpha}$.
- Activated $G_{s\alpha}$ stimulates adenylate cyclase (AC).
- The resulting surge in cytosolic adenosine monophosphate (cAMP) opens the cystic fibrosis conductance regulator, CFTR, and releases chloride ions into the lumen.
- Luminal chloride causes secretion of bicarbonate and sodium, with obligate water, leading to massive diarrhea.

Clinical Features (p. 785)

Only a minority of patients develop severe diarrhea; in those unfortunates, up to a liter per hour of "rice water"-like stool can be produced. Without treatment, the mortality is 50% due to dehydration, hypotension, and shock; however, most can be saved with timely rehydration.

Campylobacter Enterocolitis (p. 786)

Campylobacter jejuni is a gram-negative organism; it is the most common bacterial enteric pathogen in developed countries, and an important cause of "traveler's diarrhea." Transmission is often through ingestion of poorly cooked chicken, but water or milk contamination can occur.

Pathogenesis (p. 787)

The major virulence factors are flagellar motility, adherence molecules to facilitate colonization, cytotoxins, and a cholera toxinlike enterotoxin. Infections can also result in extraintestinal complications, such as reactive arthritis and erythema nodosum; 40% of Guillain-Barré syndrome cases are associated with *Campylobacter* infection in the preceding 1 to 2 weeks.

Clinical Features (p. 787)

Diagnosis is primarily through stool cultures; biopsies show only nonspecific neutrophilic colitis with variable epithelial damage. Diarrhea is typically watery; dysentery, associated with invasive strains, occurs in 15% of cases. Antibiotic therapy is usually not required; patients can shed bacteria for a month after symptoms resolve.

Shigellosis (p. 787)

Shigella are nonencapsulated, gram-negative bacilli; they are facultative anaerobes, and one of the most common causes of bloody diarrhea. Humans are the only reservoir; fecal-oral transmission is accomplished with as few as several hundred microbes. Most infections and deaths occur in children under age 5; in endemic areas *Shigella* causes 10% of pediatric diarrhea, and 75% of diarrhea-related deaths.

Pathogenesis (p. 788)

Organisms are highly resistant to gastric acidity; they are taken up by intestinal M cells, escape into the lamina propria, and are ingested by macrophages, which then undergo apoptosis. The subsequent

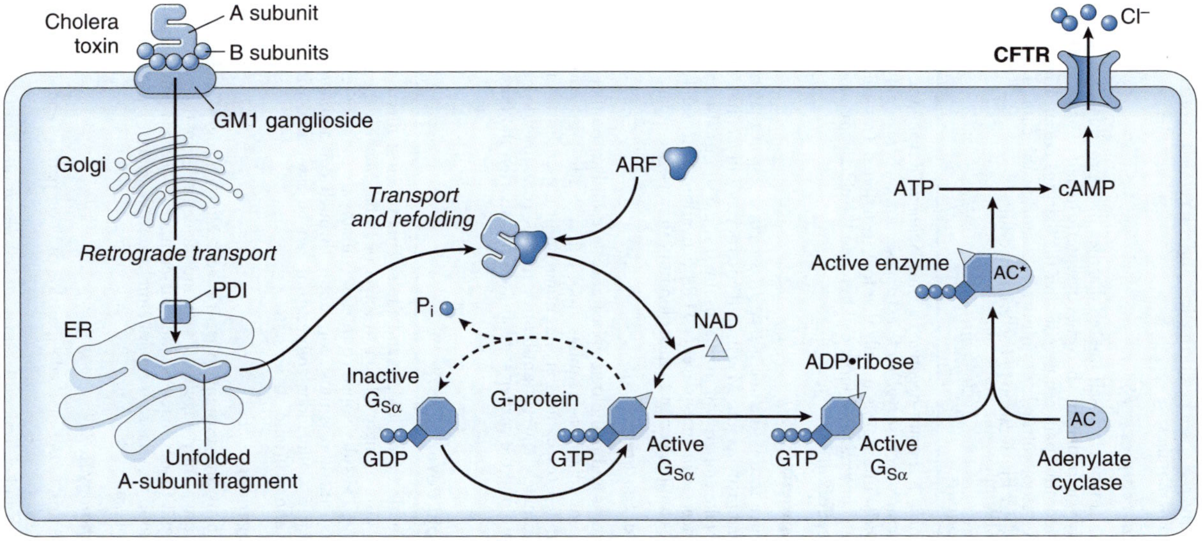

Figure 17-4 Cholera toxin transport and signaling. After retrograde toxin transport to the ER, the A subunit is released by the action of protein disulfide isomerase (PDI) and is then able to access the epithelial cell cytoplasm. In concert with an ADP-ribosylation factor (ARF), the A subunit then ADP-ribosylates $G_{s\alpha}$, which locks it in the active, GTP-bound state. This leads to AC activation, and the cAMP produced opens CFTR to drive chloride secretion and diarrhea. *ATP,* Adenosine triphosphate; GDP, guanosine diphosphate; NAD, nicotine adenine dinucleotide.

inflammation and release of Shiga toxin causes epithelial damage that facilitates even greater bacterial access.

Morphology (p. 788)

The mucosa is hemorrhagic and ulcerated, often with pseudomembranes.

Clinical Features (p. 788)

Shigella is typically a self-limited diarrhea of approximately 6 days. Initially watery diarrhea becomes dysenteric in half of patients; fever and abdominal pain can persist after the diarrhea ceases. Diagnosis requires stool cultures; antibiotics can shorten the clinical course and reduce the duration of bacterial shedding.

Salmonella (p. 788)

Salmonella is a gram-negative bacillus; *Salmonella typhi* and *Salmonella paratyphi* cause *typhoid fever* (next section), whereas nontyphoid *Salmonella* infection is usually due to *S. enteritides*. Transmission is through contaminated food; children and the elderly are most commonly affected.

Pathogenesis (p. 789)

Virulence factors include a *type III secretion system* that transfers bacterial proteins into M cells and enterocytes and facilitates bacterial uptake and growth in phagosomes; some strains also express a virulence factor that prevents TLR4 activation. Mucosal T_H17 responses limit infection to the colon but can cause secondary injury.

Clinical Features (p. 789)

Symptoms and pathologic appearances are similar to other enteric pathogens; diagnosis requires stool cultures. Most infections are self-limited (exceptions are immunocompromised hosts) and last approximately a week; antibiotics are not recommended because they prolong the carrier state and do not shorten the duration of diarrhea.

Typhoid Fever (p. 789)

In endemic areas, children and adolescents are most affected; infection is also strongly related to travel in India, Mexico, the Philippines, and less-developed countries. Humans are the only reservoir, and transmission is most commonly through contaminated food and water. Gallbladder colonization can be associated with gallstones and a chronic carrier state.

Pathogenesis (p. 789)

Organisms are resistant to gastric acid; they invade M cells and are subsequently engulfed by mononuclear cells in the mucosal lymphoid tissues. Bacteria then disseminate widely via lymphatics and blood vessels, causing systemic macrophage and lymph node hyperplasia.

Morphology (p. 789)

- Infection causes marked expansion of Peyer patches and draining nodes.
- Acute and chronic inflammatory cell recruitment to the lamina propria is associated with necrotic debris and overlying mucosal ulceration.
- The liver shows focal hepatocyte necrosis with macrophage aggregates called *typhoid nodules.*

Clinical Features (p. 789)

An initial dysentery is followed by bacteremia (90% of patients), fever, and abdominal pain that can persist for 2 weeks without antibiotic treatment *(typhoid fever)*. Systemic dissemination can cause extraintestinal complications, including encephalopathy, meningitis, endocarditis, myocarditis, pneumonia, and cholecystitis. Patients with sickle cell disease are prone to osteomyelitis.

Yersinia (p. 789)

GI *Yersinia* infections are caused by *Yersinia enterocolitica* and *Yersinia pseudotuberculosis* and typically occur through ingestion of contaminated pork, milk, or water; *Yersinia pestis,* the agent of bubonic plague, is described in Chapter 8.

Pathogenesis (p. 789)

Yersinia invade M cells, using bacterial *adhesions* to bind to host cell β_1 integrins. A bacterial iron uptake system increases *Yersinia* virulence and systemic dissemination; hence patients with hemolytic anemia or hemochromatosis are more likely to become septic and die.

Morphology (p. 790)

Yersinia preferentially invade ileum, appendix, and right colon; organisms proliferate in lymph nodes resulting in regional nodal hyperplasia, and overlying mucosa can become hemorrhagic and ulcerated.

Clinical Features (p. 790)

Abdominal pain, fever, and diarrhea can occur (mimicking appendicitis). Extraintestinal manifestations (pharyngitis, arthralgia, and erythema nodosum) are common, and postinfectious complications include sterile arthritis, Reiter syndrome, myocarditis, glomerulonephritis, and thyroiditis.

Escherichia coli (p. 790)

E. coli are gram-negative bacilli that colonize the normal GI tract; most are nonpathogenic, but a subset (classified by morphology, in vitro characteristics, and pathogenesis) cause disease:

- *Enterotoxigenic E. coli (ETEC)* (p. 790) are spread in contaminated food or water and are the chief cause of traveler's diarrhea. They produce a heat-stable toxin that increases intracellular cyclic guanosine monophosphate (cGMP) or a heat-labile choleralike toxin that increases intracellular cAMP; both cause chloride and water secretion, and inhibit epithelial fluid absorption, leading to a noninflammatory watery diarrhea.
- *Enteropathogenic E. coli (EPEC)* (p.790).
- *Enterohemorrhagic E. coli (EHEC)* (p. 790) are spread in contaminated meat, milk, and vegetables and produce a Shigalike toxin; clinical symptoms and morphology resemble infections with *Shigella dysenteriae.* There are two major serotypes: O157:H7 and non-O157:H7; the former is more likely to cause large outbreaks, dysentery, and hemolytic-uremic syndrome.
- *Enteroinvasive E. coli (EIEC)* (p. 790) are bacteriologically akin to *Shigella.* Although not toxin-producing, they invade epithelial cells and cause an acute, self-limited colitis.
- *Enteroaggregative E. coli (EAEC)* (p. 790) attach to epithelium by adherence fimbriae, aided by a bacterial *dispersin* that neutralizes the negative surface charge of lipopolysaccharide. They produce a Shigalike toxin, but typically cause only a nonbloody diarrhea.

Pseudomembranous Colitis (p. 791)

Pseudomembranous colitis (PMC) is characterized by *formation of adherent inflammatory pseudomembranes overlying sites of mucosal injury;* it is classically caused by overgrowth—and toxin production—by *Clostridium difficile* after competing bowel organisms have been eliminated by antibiotics; *Salmonella, Clostridium perfringens,* or *Staphylococcus aureus* can also cause PMC.

Morphology (p. 791)

There is epithelial denudation with plaquelike adhesion of fibrinopurulent-necrotic, gray-yellow debris and mucus. The pseudomembrane is not specific and can form with any severe mucosal injury (e.g., ischemia or necrotizing infections).

Clinical Features (p. 791)

C. difficile is prevalent in hospitals; 30% of hospitalized patients can be colonized (versus 3% of the general population). Patients present with fever, leukocytosis, crampy abdominal pain, and watery diarrhea; toxin detection in stool yields the definitive diagnosis, and metronidazole or vancomycin are generally effective therapies. There is a 40% incidence of recurrent infection after treatment.

Whipple Disease (p. 791)

This is a rare, systemic condition caused by the gram-positive actinomycete *Tropheryma whipplei.* Patients present with *diarrhea, weight loss, and malabsorption.* Extraintestinal manifestations (due to bacterial spread) include arthritis, fever, lymphadenopathy, and neurologic, cardiac, or pulmonary disease.

Morphology (p. 792)

- *Grossly* there is marked villous expansion in the small bowel, imparting a shaggy appearance to the mucosal surface.
- *Microscopically* the characteristic feature is a dense accumulation of distended foamy macrophages in small intestine lamina propria; these cells are stuffed with periodic acid-Schiff (PAS)-positive bacteria within lysosomes.
- Similarly laden macrophages are present in lymphatics, lymph nodes, joints, and brain.
- Active inflammation is largely absent.

Viral Gastroenteritis (p. 792)

Norovirus (p. 792)

Previously called *Norwalklike virus,* this is a single-stranded RNA virus; it accounts for half of all gastroenteritis outbreaks worldwide. Local outbreaks are due to contaminated food or water, but person-to-person transmission underlies most sporadic cases. Immunocompetent patients develop a self-limited watery diarrhea, often with abdominal pain, nausea, and vomiting. Biopsy morphology is nonspecific.

Rotavirus (p. 793)

An encapsulated segmented double-stranded RNA virus, rotavirus is the most common cause of severe childhood diarrhea (infecting 140 million and causing 1 million deaths worldwide annually). It is readily spread between individuals; the minimal infective inoculum is 10 particles. Rotavirus selectively infects and destroys mature small intestine enterocytes, and the epithelium is repopulated with immature secretory cells; thus a net secretion of water and electrolytes is compounded by malabsorption and an osmotic diarrhea.

Adenovirus (p. 793)

Adenovirus is the second most common cause of pediatric diarrhea; patients present with a self-limited diarrhea, vomiting, and abdominal pain. The histologic findings are nonspecific.

Parasitic Enterocolitis (p. 794)

Parasitic and protozoal infections collectively affect over half of the world's population on a chronic or recurrent basis. Common organisms include the following:

- *Ascaris lumbricoides* (p. 794) infects over a billion individuals worldwide; fecal-oral transmission is followed by an intestine-liver-lung-intestine life cycle. Systemically disseminated larvae can cause hepatic abscesses or pneumonitis; adult worm masses induce an eosinophil-rich inflammation that can physically obstruct the intestine or biliary tract. Diagnosis is made by detecting eggs in the stool.
- *Strongyloides* (p. 794) larvae in fecally contaminated soil penetrate unbroken skin, migrate to the lungs (where they cause inflammation), and then mature into adult worms in the GI tract. Released eggs can hatch in the intestine and luminal larvae can penetrate the mucosa, causing an autoinfection. *Strongyloides* typically incite strong eosinophil responses.
- *Necator duodenale* and *Ancylostoma duodenale (hookworms)* (p. 794) infect more than a billion people worldwide. The life cycle begins with larval penetration through skin and subsequent maturation in the lung; after migration up the trachea, they are swallowed. Worms then attach to duodenal mucosa and extract blood, causing mucosal damage and iron deficiency anemia.
- *Enterobius vermicularis (pinworms)* (p. 794) transmission is principally fecal-oral. Because pinworms do not invade host tissues and their entire life cycle transpires in the intestinal lumen, they rarely cause serious illness. Classically adult worms migrate at night to the anal orifice where eggs are deposited, causing intense irritation and pruritus.
- *Trichuris trichiura (whipworms)* (p. 794) primarily infect children. Although there is no tissue invasion, heavy infestations can cause bloody diarrhea and rectal prolapse.
- *Schistosoma* (p. 794) adult worms can reside within mesenteric veins; trapped eggs in the mucosa and submucosa induce a granulomatous response with bleeding and obstruction.
- *Intestinal cestodes (tapeworms)* (p. 794) infections occur by ingesting raw or undercooked fish, pork, or other contaminated meats. Parasites reside within the lumen without tissue invasion; a scolex attaches to the mucosa, and proglottids contain eggs that are shed in the feces. Occasionally *Diphyllobothrium latum* (a fish tapeworm) compete for host dietary vitamin B_{12} and thereby cause B_{12} deficiency with megaloblastic anemia.
- *Entamoeba histolytica* (p. 794) transmission is fecal-oral. Infection occurs by ingesting acid-resistant cysts; released trophozoites colonize colonic epithelium and reproduce under anaerobic conditions. Dysentery results when amoebae induce colonic epithelial apoptosis, invade into the lamina propria, and attract neutrophils. Subsequent damage yields a classic *flask-shaped ulcer* with a narrow neck and broad base. Amoebae can also embolize to the liver, producing abscesses in over 40% of infected individuals. Metronidazole therapy targets the organism-specific enzyme pyruvate oxidoreductase.

- *Giardia lamblia* (p. 795) is a flagellated protozoan and the most common pathogenic parasitic infection in humans. *Giardia* cysts are ingested from fecally contaminated water or food; duodenal trophozoites exhibit characteristic morphology (pear-shaped and binucleate). *Giardia* does not invade the tissue, but secrete products that damage the microvillus brush border and cause malabsorption. Secretory IgA and mucosal IL-6 are important for clearance; thus immunocompromised individuals are often severely affected. *Giardia* can also persist for prolonged durations in immunocompetent hosts through continuous modification of their major surface antigen.
- *Cryptosporidium* (p. 795) cause a self-limited diarrhea in immunocompetent hosts but can cause chronic diarrhea in immunocompromised individuals. Contaminated drinking water is the most common means of transmission. As few as 10 encysted oocytes can cause disease; stomach acid activates proteases that release motile sporozoites, which are subsequently internalized by absorptive enterocytes. Sodium malabsorption, chloride secretion, and increased epithelial permeability are responsible for the ensuing watery diarrhea.

Irritable Bowel Syndrome (p. 796)

Irritable bowel syndrome (IBS) is characterized by chronic, relapsing abdominal pain, bloating, and changes in stool frequency or form; it is most common in females, aged 20 to 40 years. IBS results from an interplay of psychologic stressors, diet, and abnormal GI motility, perhaps via disruption of signaling in the brain-gut axis.

Inflammatory Bowel Disease (p. 796)

IBD results from inappropriate mucosal immune responses to normal gut flora; it comprises two disorders (Table 17-4):

- *Ulcerative colitis (UC)*—severe ulcerating inflammation extending into the mucosa and submucosa, and limited to the colon and rectum.
- *CD* (also called *regional enteritis*)—typically transmural inflammation, occurring anywhere in the GI tract.

Epidemiology (p. 796)

IBD is more common in women, typically in their teens and 20s. It is also more common in developed countries, leading to the *hygiene hypothesis:* reduced frequency of enteric infections results in inadequate development of mucosal immune regulation.

Pathogenesis (p. 797)

IBD results from *a combination of defects in host interactions with GI flora, intestinal epithelial dysfunction, and aberrant mucosal immunity.* The current prevailing model is that transepithelial flux of microbes activates innate and adaptive immune responses. In a susceptible host, subsequent TNF release and other inflammatory signals increase tight junction permeability. These events establish a self-amplifying cycle of microbial influx and host immune responses that ultimately culminate in IBD (Fig. 17-5).

- *Genetics:* More than 160 IBD-associated genes have been identified, most shared between UC and CD. There is familial clustering, and concordance of monozygotic twins is 50% for CD and

TABLE 17-4 Features That Differ Between Crohn Disease and Ulcerative Colitis

Feature	CD	UC
Macroscopic		
Bowel region	Ileum ± colon	Colon only
Distribution	Skip lesions	Diffuse
Stricture	Yes	Rare
Wall appearance	Thick	Thin
Microscopic		
Inflammation	Transmural	Limited to mucosa
Pseudopolyps	Moderate	Marked
Ulcers	Deep, knifelike	Superficial, broad based
Lymphoid reaction	Marked	Moderate
Fibrosis	Marked	Mild to none
Serositis	Marked	Mild to none
Granulomas	Yes (approximately 35%)	No
Fistulas and sinuses	Yes	No
Clinical		
Perianal fistula	Yes (in colonic disease)	No
Fat and vitamin malabsorption	Yes	No
Malignant potential	With colonic involvement	Yes
Recurrence after surgery	Common	No
Toxic megacolon	No	Yes

Note: All features may not be present in a single case.

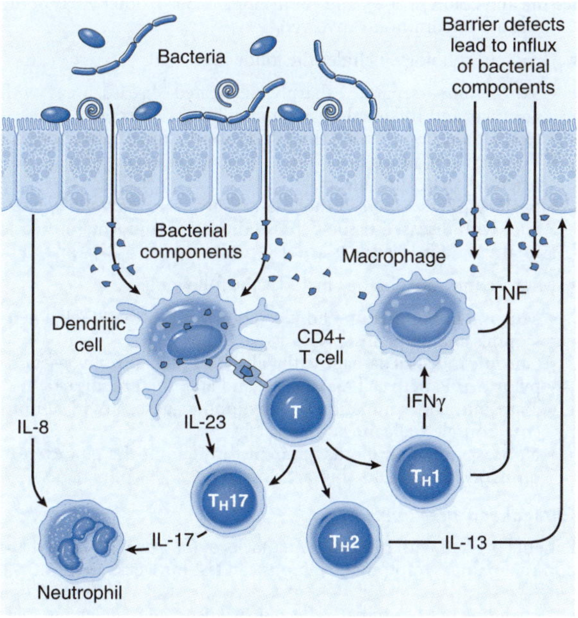

Figure 17-5 One model of IBD pathogenesis. Aspects of both CD and UC are shown. See text for details.

15% for UC. *NOD2* (nucleotide oligomerization binding domain 2) polymorphisms are linked to CD (albeit not absolutely); the gene encodes a protein that binds to intracellular bacterial peptidoglycans and subsequently activates NF-κB. Disease-associated *NOD2* variants are less effective at recognizing and combating microbes, which then enter the lamina propria and trigger greater inflammatory responses. Additional genes uncovered by genome-wide association studies are also related to microbial recognition and/or regulating subsequent immune responses.

- *Mucosal immune responses:* In CD, helper T cells are polarized to produce T_H1 cytokines (see Chapter 6); T_H17 cells may also be contributory, and polymorphisms in the IL-23 receptor (regulating T_H17 cell development) may be protective. Proinflammatory cytokines, such as TNF, interferon-γ (IFN-γ), and IL-13, as well as immunoregulatory molecules, such as IL-10 and TGF-β, also contribute to IBD pathogenesis. Autosomal recessive mutations of the IL-10 and IL-10 receptor genes are linked to severe, early onset IBD.
- *Epithelial defects:* Barrier dysfunction, including defects in epithelial tight junctions, transporter genes, and polymorphisms in extracellular matrix proteins or metalloproteinases are associated with IBD.
- *Microbiota:* The composition of the GI flora, and in particular those organisms that populate the intestinal mucus layer may influence pathogenesis by affecting innate and adaptive immune responses; antibiotics can be helpful in managing IBD.

Crohn Disease (p. 798) (Table 17-2)

Morphology *(p. 799)*

CD involves the small intestine alone in 40% of cases, the small intestine and colon in 30%, and colon alone in 30%; other areas of the GI tract are uncommonly involved.

- Gross morphology includes the following:
  - *Skip lesions*—separate, sharply delineated disease areas with granular and inflamed serosa and adherent "creeping" mesenteric fat; the bowel wall is thick and rubbery and often strictured.
  - Punched-out mucosal *aphthous* ulcers, coalescing into axially oriented serpentine ulcers.
  - Sparing of interspersed mucosa can give a *cobblestone appearance* with diseased tissue depressed relative to normal mucosa; fissures and fistula tracts are also common.

- Microscopic morphology includes the following:
  - Mucosal inflammation and ulceration with intraepithelial neutrophils and crypt abscesses
  - Chronic mucosal damage with villus blunting, atrophy, pseudopyloric or Paneth cell metaplasia, and architectural disarray
  - Transmural inflammation with lymphoid aggregates in submucosa, muscle wall, and subserosal fat
  - Noncaseating granulomas present throughout the gut, even in uninvolved segments (but are seen in only 35% of patients)

Clinical Features *(p. 800)*

Patients present with intermittent attacks of diarrhea, fever, and abdominal pain; asymptomatic periods can last for weeks to months.

- Depending on the segment affected, extensive CD can lead to malabsorption and malnutrition, loss of albumin (protein-losing enteropathy), iron deficiency anemia, and/or vitamin B_{12} deficiency.

- Fibrotic strictures or fistulas to adjacent viscera, abdominal and perineal skin, bladder, or vagina typically require surgical resection; disease often recurs at the anastomosis with 40% of patients requiring additional surgery within a decade.
- Extraintestinal manifestations include migratory polyarthritis, sacroiliitis, ankylosing spondylitis, erythema nodosum, uveitis, cholangitis, and amyloidosis.
- There is increased risk of colonic adenocarcinoma in patients with long-standing colon involvement.
- Anti-TNF antibodies are a potent therapeutic option.

Ulcerative Colitis (p. 800)

Morphology *(p. 800)*

UC is a disease of continuity with no *skip* lesions, involving the rectum and extending proximally in retrograde fashion to involve the entire colon (pancolitis); the distal ileum may also show some inflammation *(backwash ileitis).*

- *Gross:* Mucosa is reddened, granular, and friable with inflammatory *pseudopolyps,* and easy bleeding; there can be extensive ulceration or atrophic and flattened mucosa.
- *Microscopic:* Mucosal inflammation is similar to CD but is generally limited to the mucosa; there are crypt abscesses, ulceration, chronic mucosal damage, glandular architectural distortion, and atrophy, but *no* fissures, aphthous ulcers, or granulomas.

Clinical Features *(p. 800)*

Patients present with intermittent attacks of bloody mucoid diarrhea and abdominal pain that can persist for days to months before subsiding. Although half of patients have clinically mild disease, most patients will relapse within 10 years, and up to 30% will require colectomy within 3 years to control symptoms.

- *Extraintestinal manifestations* include migratory polyarthritis, sacroiliitis, ankylosing spondylitis, uveitis, cholangitis and primary sclerosing cholangitis (up to 7.5% of patients), and skin lesions.
- There is increased *risk of colonic adenocarcinoma* (see later).

Colitis-Associated Neoplasia *(p. 801)*

Risk of malignancy in IBD:

- Increases sharply 8 to 10 years after disease onset
- Is greater with pancolitis versus left-sided only disease
- Increases with the severity and duration of active inflammation
- Patients with long-standing disease are followed by biopsy surveillance; dysplasia is classified histologically as low or high grade and can be multifocal.

Other Causes of Chronic Colitis (p. 802)

Diversion Colitis (p. 802)

Diversion colitis occurs in the blind distal colonic segment created after surgery diverts the fecal stream to an ostomy site. Lack of short-chain fatty acids and other nutrients, and changes in the flora of the segment are implicated. There is mucosal erythema and friability with lymphoplasmacytic inflammation, and a characteristic lymphoid follicular hyperplasia.

Microscopic Colitis (p. 802)

Patients (typically middle-aged women) present as chronic watery diarrhea with abdominal pain. Endoscopic findings are grossly normal, hence the designation "microscopic colitis." There are two forms:

- *Collagenous colitis* is characterized by dense submucosal bandlike collagen with mixed inflammation in the lamina propria.
- *Lymphocytic colitis* is characterized by a prominent intraepithelial infiltrate of lymphocytes without the bandlike collagen; it is associated with autoimmune diseases and sprue.

Graft-Versus-Host Disease (p. 802)

GVHD occurs following hematopoietic stem cell transplantation due to donor T cells targeting antigens on the recipient's GI epithelial cells. It typically presents as a watery diarrhea but may become bloody in severe cases. The small bowel and colon are involved in most cases. Epithelial apoptosis, particularly of crypt cells, is the most common histologic finding.

Sigmoid Diverticular Disease (p. 803)

Acquired *colonic pseudodiverticular outpouchings (diverticulosis)* are uncommon in patients younger than age 30 but occur in 50% of Western populations older than age 60.

Pathogenesis (p. 803)

Focal bowel wall weakness (at sites of penetrating blood vessels) allows mucosal outpouching when there is *increased intraluminal pressure* (e.g., with constipation and exaggerated peristaltic contractions).

Morphology (p. 803)

Multiple flasklike outpouchings, 0.5 to 1 cm in diameter, are more common in the distal colon.

- These occur where the vasculature penetrates the inner circular layer of the muscularis propria at the taeniae coli).
- The diverticulum wall is lined by mucosa and submucosa without significant muscularis propria, although the muscularis between diverticula is hypertrophic.
- Obstruction of diverticula leads to inflammation producing *diverticulitis;* with tissue damage and increased pressure, these can perforate.

Clinical Features (p. 804)

Diverticular disease is usually asymptomatic but may be associated with cramping, abdominal discomfort, and constipation. Diverticulitis can result in pericolic abscesses, sinus tracts, and peritonitis. Even without perforation, diverticulitis can cause fibrotic thickening and stricture formation.

Polyps (p. 804)

Masses that protrude into the gut lumen can be pedunculated or sessile and can be non-neoplastic or neoplastic.

Hyperplastic Polyps (p. 804)

These polyps result from decreased epithelial turnover with delayed shedding; they have no malignant potential. These are usually less than 5 mm and are composed of well-formed mature, albeit crowded, glands.

Inflammatory Polyps (p. 804)

These result from recurrent cycles of injury and healing; there is lamina propria fibromuscular hyperplasia, mixed inflammatory cell infiltrates, and mucosal erosion and/or hyperplasia.

Hamartomatous Polyps (p. 805)

Hamartomatous polyps (tumorlike growths of tissues normally present at the site) are important to recognize because they usually occur in the setting of various genetic or acquired syndromes (Table 17-5).

- *Juvenile polyps* (p. 805) are focal hamartomatous malformations of small intestine and colon mucosa; most occur in children <5 years and involve the rectum (Table 17-5). Mutations in *SMAD4* and *BMPR1A* genes involved in TGF-β signaling are implicated in some cases. Polyps are typically single, large (1 to 3 cm), rounded, and pedunculated, with cystically dilated glands and abundant lamina propria.
- The *juvenile polyposis syndrome* is a rare autosomal dominant disorder characterized by up to 100 hamartomatous polyps. Patients may require colectomy to limit bleeding due to polyp ulceration, and pulmonary arteriovenous malformations are a known extraintestinal manifestation. There is also an increased risk of bowel malignancy; 30% to 50% of patients will develop colonic adenocarcinoma by age 45.
- *Peutz-Jeghers syndrome* (p. 806) is a rare autosomal dominant syndrome (median age of onset is 11 years) associated with multiple GI hamartomatous polyps and mucocutaneous hyperpigmentation. In half of patients, there is a heterozygous loss-of-function mutation in the LKB1/STK11 gene encoding a kinase that regulates cell polarization and growth.

The polyps (small bowel > colon and stomach) are large, pedunculated, and lobulated with arborizing smooth muscle surrounding normal abundant glands; they can initiate intussusception. The hyperpigmentation takes the form of macules around the mouth, eyes, nostrils, buccal mucosa, palms, and genital and perianal regions. Recognition of the syndrome is important because these patients have increased risk of several cancers including colon, pancreas, breast, lung, gonads, and uterus.

Neoplastic Polyps (p. 807)

Colonic adenomas are benign polyp precursors to the majority of colorectal carcinomas; they are characterized by the presence of epithelial dysplasia. The incidence of adenomas approaches 50% by age 50, but it should be emphasized that the majority do *not* progress to malignancy. Most are clinically silent, although large specimens can cause anemia through occult bleeding or rarely protein and potassium loss causes hypoproteinemic hypokalemia.

Risk of malignancy is correlated to size (polyps >4 cm have a 40% risk harboring cancer) and severity of dysplasia.

TABLE 17-5 Gastrointestinal Polyposis Syndromes

Syndrome	Mean Age at Presentation (yr)	Mutated Gene(s); Pathway	GI Lesions	Selected Extra-GI Manifestations
Juvenile polyposis	<5	*SMAD4, BMPR1A;* TGF-β signaling pathway	Juvenile polyps; risk of gastric, small intestinal, colonic, and pancreatic adenocarcinoma	Congenital malformations, digital clubbing
Peutz-Jeghers syndrome	10-15	*STK11;* AMP kinase-related pathways	Arborizing polyps; small intestine > colon > stomach; colonic adenocarcinoma	Pigmented macules; risk of colon, breast, lung, pancreatic, and thyroid cancer
Cowden syndrome, Bannayan-Ruvalcaba-Riley syndrome*	<15	*PTEN:* PI3K/AKT pathway	Hamartomatous or inflammatory intestinal polyps, lipomas, ganglioneuromas	Benign skin tumors, benign and malignant thyroid and breast lesions; no increase in GI cancers
Cronkhite-Canada syndrome	>50	Nonhereditary, unknown cause	Hamartomatous polyps of stomach, small intestine, colon; abnormalities in nonpolypoid mucosa	Nail atrophy, hair loss, abnormal skin pigmentation, cachexia, and anemia. Fatal in up to 50%.
Tuberous sclerosis		*TSC1* (hamartin), *TSC2* (tuberin); mTOR pathway	Hamartomatous polyps	Mental retardation, epilepsy, facial angiofibroma, cortical (CNS) tubers, renal angiomyolipoma
FAP				
Classic FAP	10-15	*APC*	Multiple adenomas	Congenital RPE hypertrophy
Attenuated FAP	40-50	*APC*	Multiple adenomas	
Gardner syndrome	10-15	*APC*	Multiple adenomas	Osteomas, thyroid and desmoid tumors, skin cysts
Turcot syndrome	10-15	*APC*	Multiple adenomas	Medulloblastoma, glioblastoma
MYH-associated polyposis	30-50	*MYH*	Multiple adenomas	

*Also called PTEN hamartoma tumor syndromes.
mTOR, Mammalian target of rapamycin; *RPE,* retinal pigmented epithelium.

Morphology *(p. 808)*

Adenomas range from 0.3 to 10 cm, and can be pedunculated or sessile. Dysplastic changes include hyperplasia, nuclear hyperchromasia, and loss of polarity. Adenomas are classified based on architecture (*tubular, tubulovillous,* and *villous*), although these have little clinical significance.

- In *sessile serrated adenomas* the full gland length exhibits serrated architecture; despite malignant potential, they *do not* have the typical dysplastic changes seen in other adenomas.
- *Intramucosal carcinoma* occurs when dysplastic cells invade the lamina propria or muscularis mucosa. Such polyps will have little metastatic potential because colonic mucosa lacks lymphatic channels.
- Polyps with *invasive adenocarcinoma* are malignant and have metastatic potential because they have crossed into submucosa and can access lymphatics.

Several syndromes characterized by colonic polyps and increased rates of colon cancer may also inform the understanding of the pathogenesis of sporadic colon cancers (Table 17-6).

Adenomatous Polyposis (p. 809)

FAP is an autosomal dominant disorder caused by mutations of the *adenomatous polyposis coli (APC)* gene; 75% of cases are inherited, whereas the remainder represent de novo mutations. Patients in their teens characteristically develop >100 colonic adenomatous polyps, and if untreated colorectal carcinoma will develop in 100% by age 30. Although prophylactic colectomy eliminates the risk of colon cancer, these patients also develop adenomas in the stomach and ampulla of Vater. There are FAP variants:

- *Gardner syndrome* exhibits multiple osteomas (mandible, skull, long bones), epidermal cysts, fibromatosis (desmoid tumors), abnormal dentition (impacted teeth), and increased incidence of duodenal and thyroid cancers.
- *Turcot syndrome* is rarer; besides adenomas, patients develop medulloblastomas.

Some FAP patients without *APC* loss have mutations of the base-excision repair gene *MUTYH.* Moreover, some *APC* and *MUTYH* mutations give rise to attenuated forms of FAP, characterized by delayed polyp development and the appearance of colon carcinoma after age 50.

Hereditary Nonpolyposis Colorectal Cancer *(p. 810)*

Also known as *Lynch syndrome,* hereditary nonpolyposis colorectal cancer (HNPCC) is caused by mutations in genes encoding proteins responsible for the detection, excision, and repair of DNA replication errors (see Chapter 7); it accounts for 2% to 4% of colon cancers. The majority involve mismatch repair genes *MSH2* and *MLH1;* patients inherit one defective copy, and when the second is lost by mutation or epigenetic silencing, mutations accrue at rates up to 1000 times normal, mostly in regions of microsatellite repeats (leading to *microsatellite instability*).

Adenocarcinoma (p. 810)

Colonic adenocarcinoma is the most common GI malignancy and constitutes 15% of all cancer-related deaths in the United States; it is a major cause of morbidity and mortality worldwide with 1.2 million new cases and 600,000 associated deaths each year.

TABLE 17-6 Common Patterns of Sporadic and Familial Colorectal Neoplasia

Etiology	Molecular Defect	Target Gene(s)	Transmission	Predominant Site(s)	Histology
FAP	APC/WNT pathway	*APC*	Autosomal dominant	None	Tubular, villous; typical adenocarcinoma
MYH-associated polyposis	DNA mismatch repair	*MYH*	Autosomal recessive	None	Sessile serrated adenoma; mucinous adenocarcinoma
Hereditary nonpolyposis colorectal cancer	DNA mismatch repair	*MSH2, MLH1*	Autosomal dominant	Right side	Sessile serrated adenoma; mucinous adenocarcinoma
Sporadic colon cancer (70%-80%)	APC/WNT pathway	*APC*	None	Left side	Tubular, villous; typical adenocarcinoma
Sporadic colon cancer (10%-15%)	DNA mismatch repair	*MSH2, MLH1*	None	Right side	Sessile serrated adenoma; mucinous adenocarcinoma
Sporadic colon cancer (5%-10%)	Hypermethylation	*MLH1, BRAF*	None	Right side	Sessile serrated adenoma; mucinous adenocarcinoma

Epidemiology (p. 810)

Dietary factors influence risk; increased rates of colorectal cancer are seen with reduced vegetable fiber intake and increased levels of refined carbohydrates and fat. These may influence the composition of GI flora, as well as the synthesis of carcinogenic by-products that remain in prolonged contact with intestinal mucosa due to diminished stool bulk. Diminished antioxidants (e.g., vitamins A, C, and E) can also influence malignant potential. NSAIDs also have a protective effect—potentially related to inhibition of the formation of prostaglandin E_2 that promotes epithelial proliferation.

Pathogenesis (p. 811)

Multiple genetic and epigenetic events contribute to colorectal carcinogenesis in a now "classic" adenoma-carcinoma sequence that accounts for 80% of sporadic cases (Fig. 17-6). No single event or sequence of events is requisite, but a multihit genetic mechanism appears to be operative.

- *APC/β-catenin pathway* associated with *Wnt* and the classic adenoma-carcinoma sequence. *APC is a key negative regulator of β-catenin;* APC protein normally binds to and promotes β-catenin degradation. With loss of APC, β-catenin accumulates and translocates to the nucleus, where it activates a cassette of genes that promote proliferation.
- In patients with DNA mismatch repair deficiency, mutations accumulate in microsatellite repeats, a condition referred to as microsatellite instability (MSI). Some microsatellite sequences are located in the coding or promoter regions of genes involved in regulation of cell growth, such as those encoding the type II TGF-β receptor and the proapoptotic protein BAX (Fig. 17-7). Because TGF-β inhibits colonic epithelial cell proliferation, mutation of type II TGF-β receptor can contribute to uncontrolled cell growth, whereas loss of *BAX* may enhance the survival of genetically abnormal clones.
- A subset of microsatellite unstable colon cancers without mutations in DNA mismatch repair enzymes have CpG island hypermethylation. In these tumors, the *MLH1* promoter region is typically hypermethylated, reducing MLH1 expression and its repair function. Activating mutations in the oncogene *BRAF* are common in these cancers. Thus the combination of microsatellite instability, *BRAF* activating mutation, and methylation of specific targets, such as *MLH1,* is the signature of this pathway of carcinogenesis.
- Late *KRAS* and *p53* mutations promote growth and prevent apoptosis.
- SMAD mutations reduce TGF-β signaling and thus promote cell cycle progression.
- *Telomerase* reactivation prevents cellular senescence.

Morphology (p. 813)

Tumors are approximately equally distributed along the colon.

- *Grossly:* Polypoid, exophytic masses are characteristic in the cecum and right colon; annular masses with "napkin-ring" obstruction are characteristic of the distal colon. Both forms penetrate the bowel wall over the course of many years.
- *Microscopically* tumors are typically composed of tall, columnar cells resembling adenomatous neoplastic epithelium but with invasion into the submucosa, muscularis propria, or beyond; a minority produce copious extracellular mucin.

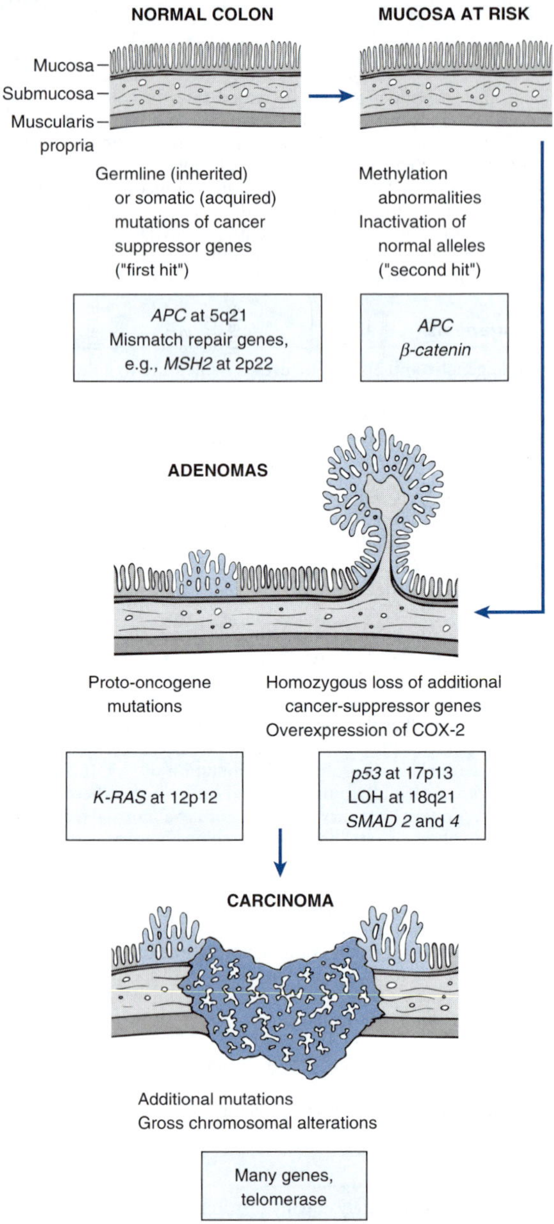

Figure 17-6 Morphologic and molecular changes in the adenoma-carcinoma sequence. Loss of one normal copy of the tumor suppressor gene *APC* occurs early. Individuals born with one mutant allele are therefore at increased risk of developing colon cancer. Alternatively, inactivation of *APC* in colonic epithelium may occur later in life. This is the "first hit" according to the Knudson hypothesis (see Chapter 7). The loss of the intact second copy of *APC* follows ("second hit"). Other changes, including mutation of *KRAS,* losses at 18q21 involving *SMAD2* and *SMAD4,* and inactivation of the tumor suppressor gene *TP53,* lead to the emergence of carcinoma, in which further mutations occur. Although there seems to be a temporal sequence of changes, the accumulation of mutations, rather than their occurrence in a specific order, is most critical.

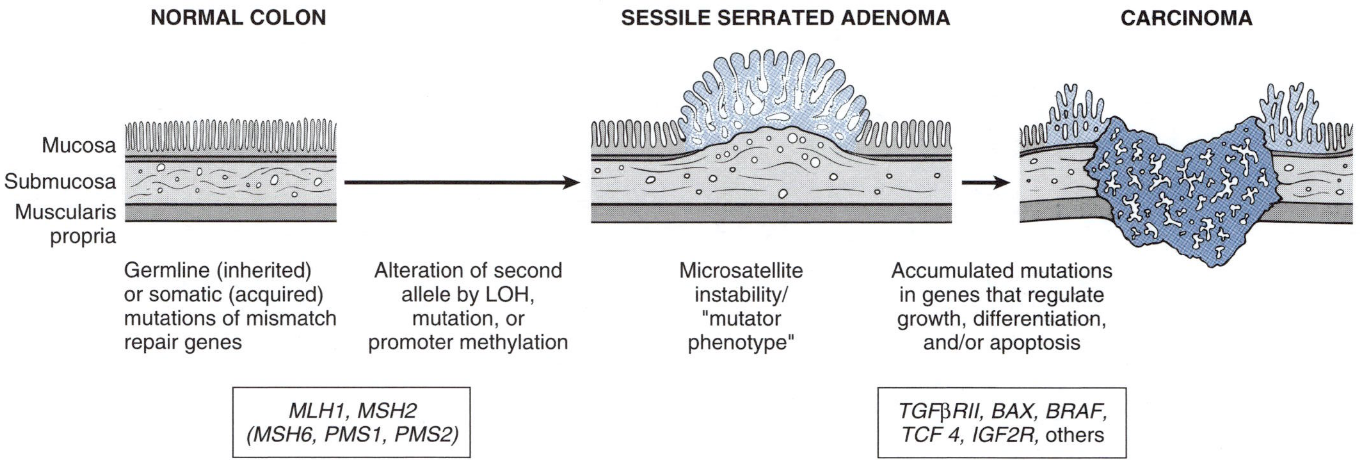

Figure 17-7 Morphologic and molecular changes in the mismatch repair pathway of colon carcinogenesis. Defects in mismatch repair genes result in MSI and permit accumulation of mutations in numerous genes. If these mutations affect genes involved in cell survival and proliferation, cancer may develop. *LOH,* Loss of heterozygosity.

- Carcinomas can also be poorly differentiated, solid tumors without gland formation. Less commonly, foci of neuroendocrine differentiation, signet-ring features, or squamous differentiation occur.
- Invasive tumors characteristically incite a strong *desmoplastic response.*

Clinical Features (p. 813)

Colorectal carcinoma develops insidiously and may go undetected for long periods. Fatigue, weakness, iron deficiency anemia, abdominal discomfort, progressive bowel obstruction, and liver enlargement (metastases) eventually occur. *Prognosis varies with the stage of disease at diagnosis;* 5-year survival rates are related to the depth of tumor penetration and lymph node involvement and range from almost 100% for lesions limited to the mucosa to 40% for extensively invasive tumors; distal metastasis reduces 5-year survival significantly. Overall U.S. 5-year survival is 65%. Currently only surgery can be curative.

Hemorrhoids (p. 815)

Hemorrhoids are variceal dilations of anal and perianal submucosal venous plexi; they affect 5% of adults. Hemorrhoids are causally associated with constipation (straining at stool), venous stasis during pregnancy, and cirrhosis (portal hypertension). *External hemorrhoids* occur with ectasia of the inferior hemorrhoidal plexus below the anorectal line; *internal hemorrhoids* are due to ectasia of the superior hemorrhoidal plexus above the anorectal line. Secondary thrombosis (with recanalization), strangulation, or ulceration with fissure formation can occur.

Acute Appendicitis (p. 816)

Acute appendicitis is the most common acute abdominal condition requiring surgery; the lifetime risk is 7%.

Pathogenesis (p. 816)

Approximately 50% to 80% of appendicitis is associated with obstruction of the appendiceal lumen by a fecalith, tumor, or worms *(Oxyuriasis vermicularis),* causing increased intraluminal pressure. This is followed by ischemia—exacerbated by edema and exudate—and bacterial invasion.

Morphology (p. 816)

- *Early acute appendicitis* exhibits a scant appendiceal neutrophil exudate with subserosal congestion and perivascular neutrophil emigration; the serosa is dull, granular, and red.
- *Advanced acute appendicitis (acute suppurative appendicitis)* involves more severe neutrophilic infiltration with fibrinopurulent serosal exudate, luminal abscess formation, ulceration, and suppurative necrosis. This can progress to *acute gangrenous appendicitis,* followed by perforation.

Clinical Features (p. 816)

Acute appendicitis can occur at any age but mainly affects adolescents and young adults. Classically, there is periumbilical pain migrating to the right lower quadrant, nausea or vomiting, abdominal tenderness, mild fever, and leukocytosis. Other mimics for appendicitis include enterocolitis, mesenteric lymphadenitis, systemic viral infection, acute salpingitis, ectopic pregnancy, mittelschmerz, and Meckel diverticulitis. Complications include pyelophlebitis, portal vein thrombosis, liver abscess, and bacteremia.

Tumors of the Appendix (p. 816)

- *Carcinoid* is the most common tumor of the appendix (see earlier discussion).
- *Mucocele* reflects dilation of the appendiceal lumen by mucinous secretions; it can be due to innocuous obstruction with inspissated mucus, to mucin-secreting adenomas, or to adenocarcinoma.
- *Mucinous cystadenocarcinoma* is indistinguishable from cystadenomas except for *appendiceal wall invasion by neoplastic cells and peritoneal implants.* The peritoneum becomes distended with tenacious, semisolid, mucin-producing anaplastic adenocarcinoma cells, designated *pseudomyxoma peritonei;* it is ultimately fatal.

PERITONEAL CAVITY (p. 817)

Inflammatory Disease (p. 817)

Peritonitis can result from bacterial infection or chemical irritation; the latter can be caused by the following:

- Leakage of bile or pancreatic enzymes (sterile peritonitis).
- Perforation of the biliary system or abdominal viscera usually complicated by bacterial superinfection.
- Acute hemorrhagic pancreatitis; bowel wall damage can lead to secondary bacterial peritonitis.
- Foreign material, inducing granulomas and scarring.
- Endometriosis (ectopic endometrial implants) or ruptured dermoid cysts.
- Ruptured dermoid cysts that release keratins and induce an intense granulomatous reaction.
- Perforation of abdominal viscera.

Peritoneal Infection (p. 817)

Bacterial peritonitis results when GI tract bacteria are released into the abdominal cavity—usually after bowel perforation (e.g., due to appendicitis, peptic ulcer, cholecystitis, diverticulitis, and intestinal ischemia); acute salpingitis, abdominal trauma, or peritoneal dialysis are other potential bacterial sources.

Spontaneous bacterial peritonitis develops without an obvious source of contamination; it occurs in the setting of ascites (e.g., nephrotic syndrome or cirrhosis).

Morphology (*p. 817*)

Peritoneal membranes become dull and gray, followed by exudation and frank suppuration; localized abscesses can develop, although the inflammation tends to remain superficial.

Sclerosing Retroperitonitis (p. 817)

Also known as *Ormond disease,* this disorder is characterized by a dense fibrosis of retroperitoneal tissues; it is likely a primary inflammatory process.

Tumors (p. 817).

Tumors may be primary or secondary; virtually all are malignant.

- *Primary* tumors are rare; they include *mesothelioma* (similar to pleural or pericardial mesotheliomas) and *desmoplastic small round cell tumor*. The latter has a characteristic t(11;22) translocation yielding a fusion of genes associated with Ewing sarcoma and Wilms tumor *(EWS-WT1)*; the tumor morphologically resembles a Ewing sarcoma.
- *Secondary* tumors are common and can derive from any cancer; ovarian and pancreatic adenocarcinomas do so most frequently.

18 Liver and Gallbladder

THE LIVER AND BILE DUCTS (p. 821)

General Features of Liver Disease (p. 822)

Although the liver is vulnerable to a host of insults, the most common primary diseases in the United States are viral hepatitis, alcohol-related liver disease, nonalcoholic fatty liver disease (NAFLD), and hepatocellular carcinoma (HCC). The liver is also secondarily affected by common disorders, such as congestive heart failure and metastatic cancer. Although injury may be apparent through laboratory testing (Table 18-1), an enormous functional hepatic reserve typically masks the clinical impact of early damage. Most liver disease is insidious with symptoms of decompensation developing over weeks to years; nevertheless, disrupted bile flow or progressive disease can be life threatening.

TABLE 18-1 Laboratory Evaluation of Liver Disease

Test Category	Serum Measurement*
Hepatocyte integrity	Cytosolic hepatocellular enzymes†
	Serum aspartate aminotransferase (AST)
	Serum alanine aminotransferase (ALT)
	Serum lactate dehydrogenase (LDH)
Biliary excretory function	Substances normally secreted in bile†
	Serum bilirubin
	Total: unconjugated plus conjugated
	Direct: conjugated only
	Delta: covalently linked to albumin
	Urine bilirubin
	Serum bile acids
	Plasma membrane enzymes (from damage to bile canaliculus)†
	Serum alkaline phosphatase
	Serum GGT
	Serum 5′-nucleotidase
Hepatocyte function	Proteins secreted into the blood
	Serum albumin‡
	Prothrombin time† (factors V, VII, X, prothrombin, fibrinogen)
	Hepatocyte metabolism
	Serum ammonia†
	Aminopyrine breath test (hepatic demethylation)‡
	Galactose elimination (intravenous injection)‡

*The most common tests are in italics.
†An elevation implicates liver disease.
‡A decrease implicates liver disease.

Mechanisms of Injury and Repair (p. 822)

Hepatocyte and Parenchymal Responses (p. 822)

Reversible degenerative changes include fat accumulation *(steatosis)* and bilirubin buildup *(cholestasis)*. When injury is not reversible, hepatocytes die by necrosis or apoptosis:

- *Hepatocyte necrosis* is the predominant mode of death in ischemic-hypoxic injury and responses to oxidative stress: defective osmotic regulation leads to cell swelling and rupture, also marked by local macrophage accumulation.
- *Hepatocyte apoptosis* is typical of cell death associated with acute and chronic hepatitis and is marked by hepatocyte shrinkage, nuclear chromatin condensation *(pyknosis)*, fragmentation *(karyorrhexis)*, and cellular fragmentation into acidophilic *apoptotic bodies* (see Chapter 2).

Even in diseases where hepatocytes are the principal targets of attack (e.g., hepatitis), vascular insults—via inflammation or thrombosis—lead to confluent zones of parenchymal necrosis. The resultant cirrhosis is a common form of liver disease.

Hepatocyte regeneration occurs primarily by proliferation of hepatocytes adjacent to those that have died; *stem cell replenishment is usually not a significant part of parenchymal repair.* In severe liver injury, the canal of Hering—the primary intrahepatic stem cell niche—can be activated, but how much these cells contribute to healing is unclear. With chronic disease, hepatocytes can reach replicative senescence, at which point, stem cell activation leads to the formation of *ductular reactions* that can contribute significantly to parenchymal restoration.

Scar Formation and Regression (p. 823)

The hepatic *stellate cell,* a lipid (vitamin A) storing cell, is primarily responsible for liver scar deposition. Stellate cells can be activated by (1) inflammatory cytokines, such as tumor necrosis factor (TNF), lymphotoxin, and interleukin-1β (IL-1β), and lipid peroxidation products; (2) cytokine and chemokine production by Kupffer cells, endothelial cells, hepatocytes, and bile duct epithelial cells; (3) in response to disruption of the extracellular matrix (ECM); and (4) direct stimulation of stellate cells by toxins. Such activation causes stellate cells to develop into highly fibrogenic and contractile myofibroblasts; subsequent fibrogenesis is driven by cytokines released by Kupffer cells and lymphocytes (e.g., transforming growth factor-β [TGF-β]), and stellate cell contraction is stimulated by endothelin-1 (ET-1) (Fig. 18-1). Portal fibroblasts also contribute to scar deposition, with ductular reactions leading to the activation and recruitment of such fibrogenic cells.

If the chronic injury leading to scar formation is interrupted (e.g., clearance of hepatitis virus infection, cessation of alcohol use), then stellate cell activation ceases, and the fibrosis can be fragmented by metalloproteinases produced by hepatocytes. In this way, scar formation can be reversed.

Inflammation and Immunity (p. 824)

Innate and adaptive immune systems are involved in liver injury and repair. Toll-like receptors detect molecules derived from foreign invaders, such as bacteria and viruses. These processes lead to elaboration of proinflammatory cytokines. Adaptive immunity plays a critical role in viral hepatitis, largely by destroying infected hepatocytes.

Liver Failure (p. 825)

Liver failure occurs when greater than 80% to 90% of hepatic function is lost; without liver transplantation, the mortality rate is 80%.

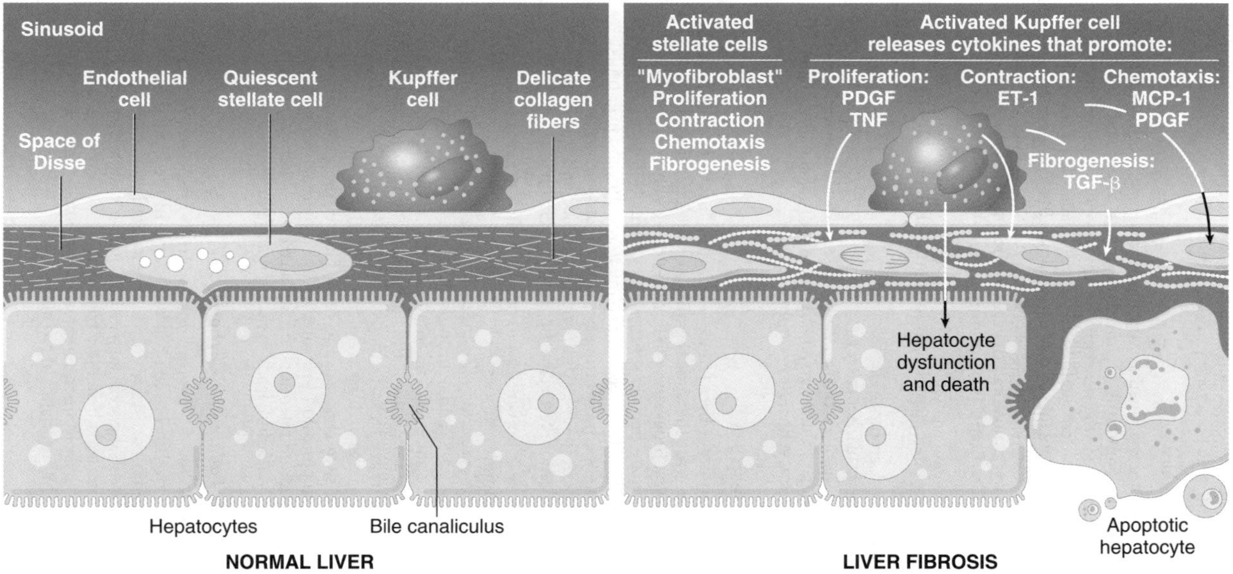

Figure 18-1 Stellate cell activation and liver fibrosis. Kupffer cell activation leads to secretion of multiple cytokines. Platelet-derived growth factor (PDGF) and TNF activate stellate cells, and contraction of the activated stellate cells is stimulated by ET-1. Fibrosis is stimulated by TGF-β. Chemotaxis of activated stellate cells to areas of injury is promoted by PDGF and monocyte chemotactic protein-1 (MCP-1). See text for details.

Although occasionally caused by massive acute destruction *(fulminant hepatic failure),* it is more commonly a consequence of successive waves of injury or progressive chronic damage. Patients with marginal hepatic function can also be tipped into frank failure when intercurrent disease places a greater demand on hepatic function.

Acute Liver Failure *(p. 825)*

Acute liver failure is defined as liver illness associated with encephalopathy within 6 months of initial diagnosis; fulminant hepatic failure is designated when encephalopathy develops within 2 weeks of jaundice onset. Most acute liver failure is caused by massive hepatic necrosis attributable to drugs or toxins, often compounded by immune-mediated hepatocyte destruction; acetaminophen overdose accounts for almost half of cases in the United States, whereas in Asia, hepatitis B and E predominate. A useful mnemonic is as follows:

- A: Acetaminophen, hepatitis A, autoimmune hepatitis (AIH)
- B: Hepatitis B
- C: Hepatitis C, cryptogenic
- D: Drugs or toxins, hepatitis D
- E: Hepatitis E, esoteric causes (Wilson disease, Budd-Chiari disease)
- F: Fatty change of the microvesicular type (fatty liver of pregnancy, valproate, tetracycline, Reye syndrome)

Clinical Course (p. 826)

The manifestations of liver failure—reflecting loss of normal hepatocyte function—are the same regardless of etiology: nausea, vomiting, and jaundice, progressing to encephalopathy and coagulopathy (due to inadequate hepatic synthesis of coagulation factors). The liver initially swells due to edema and inflammation, and liver transaminases are elevated, reflecting hepatocyte destruction. With ongoing destruction, the liver dramatically shrinks, and transaminase levels decline because few viable hepatocytes remain.

- Portal hypertension can lead to ascites, which is exacerbated by reduced albumin synthesis.
- *Hepatic encephalopathy,* a life-threatening disorder of central nervous system (CNS) and neuromuscular transmission is caused by portosystemic shunting and loss of hepatocellular function. Resulting excess ammonia in the blood impairs neuronal function and causes brain edema, leading to disturbances in consciousness (confusion to coma), limb rigidity, hyperreflexia, and asterixis.
- *Hepatorenal syndrome,* causing renal failure; the etiology is decreased renal perfusion pressure, followed by renal vasoconstriction, with sodium retention and impaired free-water excretion.
- Unabated, liver failure leads to multiorgan failure and death.

Chronic Liver Failure and Cirrhosis *(p. 827)*

Chronic liver failure—often (but not uniformly) associated with cirrhosis—is the twelfth leading cause of death in the United States. The most common causes worldwide are alcohol abuse, viral hepatitis, and nonalcoholic steatohepatitis (NASH), with biliary disease and hemochromatosis being less frequent. In 20% of cases, an etiology cannot be ascertained *(cryptogenic cirrhosis).* There are three morphologic characteristics of cirrhosis:

- *Bridging fibrosis* linking portal tracts to each other and to central veins
- *Parenchymal nodules* resulting from hepatocyte regeneration when encircled by fibrosis
- Disruption of hepatic parenchymal architecture

Clinical Features (p. 828)

Cirrhosis can be clinically silent until far advanced (40% of patients); it ultimately presents with anorexia, weight loss, weakness, and debilitation. Hyperestrogenemia, due to impaired estrogen metabolism, can manifest with palmar erythema, spider angiomata, hypogonadism, and gynecomastia. Overt hepatic failure can be precipitated by intercurrent infection or gastrointestinal (GI) hemorrhage. Death can be due to the following:

- Progressive liver failure with encephalopathy and coagulopathy
- Complications of portal hypertension, such as variceal bleeding (see later)
- Bacterial infections due to gut mucosal damage and Kupffer cell dysfunction
- HCC (see later discussion)

Portal Hypertension (p. 828)

Portal hypertension results from a combination of increased flow into the portal circulation and/or increased resistance to portal blood flow; causes are as follows (Table 18-2):

- *Prehepatic:* Thrombosis, portal vein narrowing, increased splanchnic arterial circulation, or massive splenomegaly with increased splenic vein blood flow.
- *Intrahepatic:* Cirrhosis (most common), schistosomiasis, massive fatty change, granulomatous disease, or nodular regenerative hyperplasia.
- *Posthepatic:* Right-sided heart failure, constrictive pericarditis, or hepatic vein obstruction

Major clinical consequences of portal hypertension are as follows (Fig. 18-2):

- *Ascites* (p. 829), a collection of excess serous fluid in the peritoneal cavity. Most often a consequence of cirrhosis, the pathogenesis involves the following:
  - Hepatic sinusoidal hypertension (exacerbated by hypoalbuminemia)
  - Percolation of hepatic lymph into the peritoneal cavity

TABLE 18-2 Location and Causes of Portal Hypertension

Prehepatic Causes

Obstructive thrombosis of portal vein
Structural abnormalities such as narrowing of the portal vein before it ramifies in the liver

Intrahepatic Causes

Cirrhosis from any cause
Nodular regenerative hyperplasia
PBC (even in the absence of cirrhosis)
Schistosomiasis
Massive fatty change
Diffuse, fibrosing granulomatous disease (e.g., sarcoid)
Infiltrative malignancy, primary or metastatic
Focal malignancy with invasion into portal vein (particularly HCC)
Amyloidosis

Posthepatic Causes

Severe right-sided heart failure
Constrictive pericarditis
Hepatic vein outflow obstruction

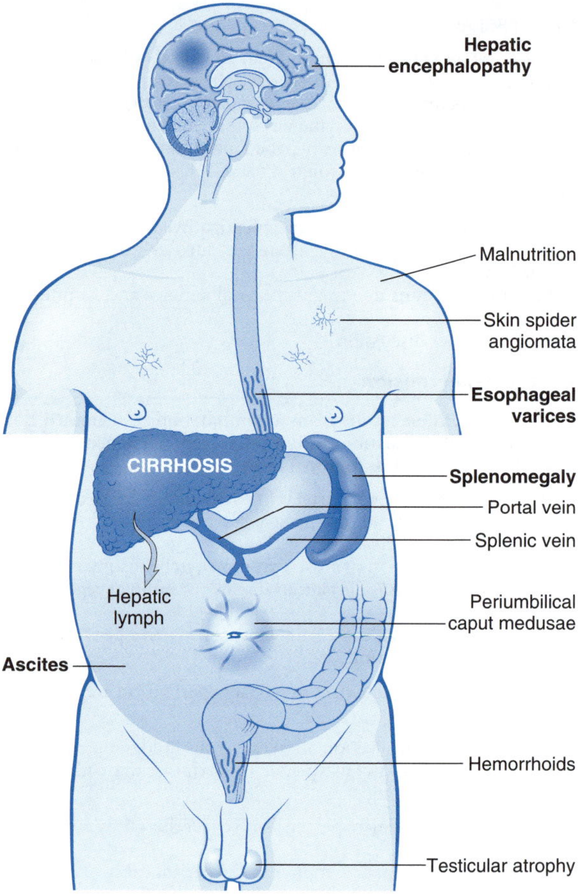

Figure 18-2 Major clinical consequences of portal hypertension in the setting of cirrhosis, shown for the male. In women, oligomenorrhea, amenorrhea, and sterility as a result of hypogonadism are frequent. Clinically significant findings are boldfaced.

    - Splanchnic vasodilation causes systemic hypotension that triggers vasoconstrictor responses (e.g., renin-angiotensin), with renal retention of sodium and water, and subsequent intestinal capillary transudation

- *Portosystemic shunts* (p. 830) arise as portal pressures rise; flow is reversed from the portal into the systemic circulation where there are shared capillary beds.
    - *Esophagogastric varices* are the most significant; they occur in 40% of patients with advanced cirrhosis. These rupture and can cause massive hematemesis; each bleed has a 30% mortality.
    - Rectum (hemorrhoids).
    - Falciform ligament and umbilicus *(caput medusae).*
- *Splenomegaly* (p. 830) is caused by long-standing congestion and can cause thrombocytopenia (or even pancytopenia) due to hypersplenism.

- *Hepatopulmonary syndrome* occurs in up to a third of patients with cirrhosis and portal hypertension; patients develop intrapulmonary vascular dilation (perhaps due to increased nitric oxide [NO] production) with accelerated flow that reduces the time for oxygen diffusion and leads to ventilation-perfusion mismatch and hypoxia.
- *Portopulmonary hypertension* results from excessive pulmonary vasoconstriction and vascular remodeling, perhaps due to inadequate liver clearance of circulating ET-1.

Acute-on-Chronic Liver Failure (p. 830)

Advanced chronic liver disease may be well compensated despite cirrhosis with extensive vascular shunting. However, large volumes of liver have borderline vascular supply, and sepsis or cardiac failure may lead to hypotension that tips the balance into acute liver failure. Similarly, otherwise minor superimposed drug or toxic injury can also precipitate failure. The short-term mortality of such patients is approximately 50%.

Patients with chronic hepatitis B infection who become superinfected with hepatitis D can also undergo sudden decompensation, as can patients with medically suppressed hepatitis B who develop resistant viral mutants.

Malignancy can also induce acute failure in a compensated patient, either due to hepatic metastases of a secondary, unrelated tumor, or secondary to the liver disease itself, particularly HCC or cholangiocarcinoma (CCA).

Infectious Disorders (p. 830)

Viral Hepatitis (p. 830)

Several systemic viral infections can involve the liver (e.g., Epstein-Barr virus, cytomegalovirus, and yellow fever virus). Less commonly—usually in children and immunosuppressed individuals—rubella, adenovirus, enterovirus, and herpesvirus also cause hepatic infections. Nevertheless, unless specified, the term *viral hepatitis refers only to infection of the liver by the hepatotropic viruses A, B, C, D, or E.* All produce similar clinical and morphologic patterns of acute hepatitis but vary in their routes of transmission and potential to induce carrier states or chronic disease (Table 18-3).

Hepatitis A Virus *(p. 831)*

Hepatitis A virus (HAV) is a single-stranded RNA virus that causes a benign, self-limited disease; fulminant HAV is rare (fatality rate 0.1% to 0.3%). It is not directly cytopathic; hepatocyte damage is due to CD8+ T-cell responses. HAV accounts for 25% of acute hepatitis worldwide; it has a fecal-oral route of spread. Acute infection is marked by anti-HAV immunoglobulin M (IgM) in serum; IgG appears as IgM declines (within a few months) and persists for years, conferring long-term immunity. An effective vaccine is available.

Hepatitis B Virus *(p. 831)*

Hepatitis B virus (HBV) can cause the following (Fig. 18-3):

- Acute, self-limited hepatitis
- Nonprogressive chronic hepatitis
- Progressive chronic disease culminating in cirrhosis (and increased risk of HCC)
- Fulminant hepatitis with massive liver necrosis
- Asymptomatic carrier state

TABLE 18-3 The Hepatitis Viruses

Virus	Hepatitis A	Hepatitis B	Hepatitis C	Hepatitis D	Hepatitis E
Type of virus	ssRNA	Partially dsDNA	ssRNA	Circular defective ssRNA	ssRNA
Viral family	Hepatovirus; related to picornavirus	Hepadnavirus	Flaviviridae	Subviral particle in Deltaviridae family	Hepevirus
Route of transmission	Fecal-oral (contaminated food or water)	Parenteral, sexual contact, perinatal	Parenteral; intranasal cocaine use is a risk factor	Parenteral	Fecal-oral
Mean incubation period	2-6 wk	2-26 wk (mean 8 wk)	4-26 wk (mean 9 wk)	Same as HBV	4-5 wk
Frequency of chronic liver disease	Never	5%-10%	>80%	10% (coinfection); 90%-100% for superinfection	In immunocompromised hosts only
Diagnosis	Detection of serum IgM antibodies	Detection of HBsAg or antibody to HBcAg; PCR for HBV DNA	Third-generation ELISA for antibody detection; PCR for HCV RNA	Detection of IgM and IgG antibodies; HDV RNA serum; HDAg in liver	Detection of serum IgM and IgG antibodies; PCR for HEV RNA

dsDNA, Double-stranded DNA; *ELISA,* enzyme-linked immunosorbent assay; *HBcAg,* hepatitis B core antigen; *HDAg,* hepatitis D antigen; *IV,* intravenous; *PCR,* polymerase chain reaction; *ssRNA,* single-stranded RNA.
From Washington K: Inflammatory and infectious diseases of the liver. In Iacobuzio-Donahue CA, Montgomery EA (eds): *Gastrointestinal and Liver Pathology.* Philadelphia, PA, Churchill Livingstone; 2005, p 503.

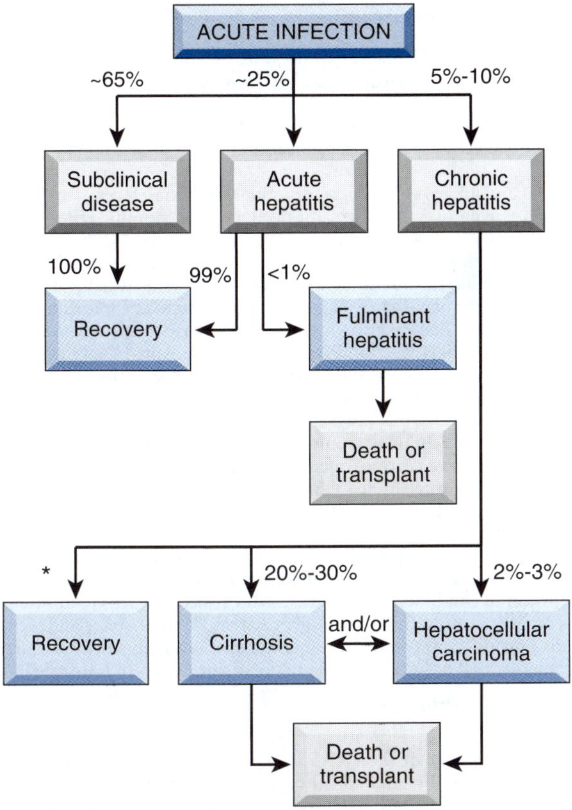

Figure 18-3 Potential outcomes of hepatitis B infection in adults, with their approximate frequencies in the United States. *Spontaneous HBsAg clearance occurs during chronic HBV infection at an estimated annual incidence of 1% to 2% in Western countries. Fulminant hepatitis and acute hepatic failure are used interchangeably.

The host immune response to the virus is the major determinant of the outcome of infection. Younger age at infection has a higher probability of chronicity. Innate immunity is protective during the initial phases of infection, and strong responses by virus-specific CD4+ and CD8+ interferon (IFN)-γ-producing cells are associated with resolution. Antibodies prevent subsequent reinfection and form the basis of effective vaccines. HBV is not cytopathic; rather, hepatocyte killing is mediated by cytotoxic CD8+ T lymphocytes directed against virus-infected cells. Viral DNA sequences can also integrate into host genomes, constituting a pathway for cancer development.

HBV is a circular, partially double-stranded DNA virus; mature virus exists as a spherical "Dane particle" with an outer surface protein and lipid envelope encasing an electron-dense core. There are eight viral genotypes with distinct global distributions. The HBV genome has four open reading frames:

- Nucleocapsid core antigen (HBcAg), plus a longer polypeptide transcript (HBeAg) that is secreted into the bloodstream.
- Hepatitis B surface antigen (HBsAg) envelope glycoproteins (large, middle, and small); infected hepatocytes can synthesize

and secrete massive quantities of noninfective HBsAg (mostly small HBsAg).
- Polymerase with both DNA polymerase and reverse transcriptase activity; viral replication occurs through an intermediate RNA template: DNA→RNA→DNA.
- Hbx protein, a transcriptional transactivator of host and viral genes, necessary for viral replication.

HBsAg appears before symptoms (anorexia, fever, jaundice), peaks during overt disease, and declines over months. HBeAg and HBV DNA appear soon after HBsAg and before disease onset; HBeAg is detectable in serum during viral replication, although some mutant strains do not produce it. HBeAg usually declines within weeks; persistence suggests progression to chronic disease.

IgM anti-HBcAg is usually the first antibody to appear, followed shortly by anti-HBeAg and IgG anti-HBcAg. Anti-HBsAg signifies the end of acute disease and persists for years, conferring immunity. A chronic carrier is defined by the presence of HBsAg in serum for 6 months.

More than 2 billion people worldwide have been infected, and 400 million have chronic infections; there are 46,000 new cases annually in the United States. Chronic disease is difficult to cure due to the development of resistant mutant strains. The mode of transmission varies geographically; in high-prevalence areas (Africa, Asia), transmission during childbirth accounts for 90%. In intermediate-prevalence regions (southern and eastern Europe), horizontal transmission in childhood by minor cuts or breaks in mucus membranes is most common. In low-prevalence areas (United States and western Europe), intravenous drug abuse and unprotected intercourse (heterosexual or homosexual) are the major modes of transmission.

Hepatitis C Virus *(p. 833)*

Hepatitis C virus (HCV) is a single-stranded RNA, enveloped virus. Low fidelity of the HCV RNA polymerase causes substantial genomic variability and constitutes a major obstacle to vaccine development; indeed any given individual can harbor a population of related but divergent *quasispecies,* and the presence of high titers of anti-HCV IgG does not confer effective immunity. Viral replication begins with translation of a single polypeptide that is processed into nucleocapsid protein, envelope proteins, and seven nonstructural proteins; the E2 envelope protein is a target of several anti-HCV antibodies but is also the most variable region of the genome, allowing escape from otherwise neutralizing titers. Thus anti-HCV antibodies do not confer protection, and a characteristic feature of HCV infection is repeated bouts of damage. *As opposed to HBV, progression to chronic disease occurs in most (80% to 90%) HCV-infected patients, and cirrhosis occurs in 20%.* Like HBV, hepatocellular damage is immune-mediated, although the cellular immune responses are largely unable to completely eradicate HCV infections.

In the United States 1.3% of the population (3.6 million individuals) have antibodies to HCV, and 2.7 million individuals are chronically infected (accounting for half of the U.S. burden of chronic liver disease); the incidence has significantly declined as a result of blood supply screening. Primary risk groups are intravenous drug abusers and individuals with multiple sexual partners. HCV RNA is detectable in blood for 1 to 3 weeks during active infection, coincident with transaminase elevations; anti-HCV antibodies occur in only 50% to 70% of patients in the acute setting, although 90% of patients with chronic disease will eventually develop such antibodies. Chronic HCV infection is potentially curable; older treatment includes IFN-α and ribovarin, whereas newer drugs that target viral protease and polymerase can achieve undetectable levels of virus in the vast majority of patients.

Hepatitis D Virus (p. 835)

Hepatitis D virus (HDV) is a defective RNA virus that can replicate and cause infection only when encapsulated by HBsAg. Thus *HDV infection can develop only when there is concomitant HBV infection.* Acute coinfection by HDV and HBV leads to hepatitis that ranges from mild to fulminant, but chronicity rarely develops. In comparison, HDV *superinfection* of an unrecognized HBV carrier or in a patient with chronic HBV leads to eruption of acute hepatitis, with frequent conversion to chronic disease and cirrhosis (Table 18-3). Worldwide, 5% of 300 million HBV-infected individuals (15 million) are coinfected with HDV; there is a high prevalence (20% to 40%) in Africa, the Middle East, Italy, and the Amazon basin; it is uncommon in the United States, Southeast Asia, and China.

HDV has an HBV envelope; the only protein produced by the virus is an internal polypeptide assembly called the *delta antigen* (HDAg), associated with a small circular single-stranded RNA. Viral replication requires host RNA polymerase activity.

HDV RNA appears in blood and liver before and during early acute symptomatic infection. IgM anti-HDV indicates recent HDV exposure; IgM anti-HbcAg suggests acute HBV coinfection, whereas serum HBsAg implies a superinfection. Vaccination against HBV can prevent HDV infection.

Hepatitis E Virus (p. 835)

Hepatitis E virus (HEV) is a nonenveloped single-stranded RNA virus; it is an enterically transmitted, water-borne infection with several animal reservoirs (monkeys, cats, pigs, and dogs). HEV epidemics have occurred in Asia, Mexico, and Africa; HEV is also endemic in India, where 30% to 60% of cases of acute hepatitis are HEV related. Although HEV is typically a self-limiting disease with no tendency to chronicity, *there is a high rate (20%) of fatal fulminant hepatitis in pregnant women.* HEV antigen is found in hepatocytes during active infection, and virions and RNA can be detected in stool and serum before symptom onset. The subsequent development of IgG anti-HEV confers long-lived protection against reinfection.

Clinicopathologic Syndromes of Viral Hepatitis (p. 835; Table 18-3)

Infection by any of the hepatotropic viruses can be asymptomatic or symptomatic; a fulminant course is uncommon. Serologic and molecular studies are essential for viral hepatitis diagnosis and to distinguish the different types.

- *Acute asymptomatic infection with recovery (p. 836):* Patients are identified only incidentally based on elevated transaminases or by antiviral antibody titers. HAV and HBV infections are frequently subclinical.
- *Acute symptomatic infection with recovery (p. 836):* Acute symptomatic infections are all similar, with a variable incubation period, asymptomatic preicteric phase, symptomatic icteric phase, and convalescence. Peak infectivity occurs during the last asymptomatic days of the incubation period and the early days of acute symptoms.
- *Acute liver failure (p. 836):* Viral hepatitis causes 10% of cases of acute hepatic failure; globally hepatitis A and E are the most common causes, whereas HBV is more common in Asian and Mediterranean countries. Survival for more than a week may allow residual hepatocyte replication, and activation of stem and progenitor cells yields prominent ductular reactions; recovery

depends on restoration of missing parenchyma. Care is supportive, and liver transplantation is the only option when the disease does not resolve.

- *Chronic hepatitis (p. 836):* This is defined as symptomatic (fatigue, malaise, jaundice), biochemical, or serologic evidence of ongoing hepatic disease for >6 months. Acute HCV infection progresses to chronic hepatitis in 80% of cases, a third of which may develop cirrhosis. In addition to ongoing liver injury and the risk of cirrhosis and/or HCC, immune complex disease (due to circulating antibody-antigen complexes) may develop with vasculitis and glomerulonephritis; 35% of chronic hepatitis C patients develop cryoglobulinemia.
- *The carrier state (p. 836):* A *carrier* harbors and can transmit hepatitis but has no manifest symptoms. This includes patients with chronic disease but few or no symptoms, and those with little or no adverse effects *(healthy carriers);* for HBV, healthy carriers lack HBeAg but have anti-HBeAg, normal serum aminotransferase levels, low serum HBV DNA, and a liver biopsy without significant necrosis or inflammation. In the United States adult HBV infections rarely produce a healthy carrier state; in contrast, >90% of HBV infections acquired early in life in endemic areas result in healthy carrier states.
- *HIV and chronic viral hepatitis (p. 837):* Similar transmission modes and risks result in frequent HIV and hepatitis virus coinfections; 10% of HIV patients are infected with HBV and 30% with HCV, often resulting in more aggressive liver disease. Chronic hepatitis is a major cause of morbidity and mortality in HIV-infected patients, and liver disease is the second most common cause of death in acquired immunodeficiency syndrome (AIDS).

Morphology of Acute and Chronic Hepatitis (p. 837)

Most of the morphologic changes are shared by all the hepatotropic viruses; these features are largely nonspecific and can be mimicked by drug reactions or autoimmune liver disease. Nevertheless, a few histologic changes can suggest a specific virus: in HBV, infected hepatocytes can show a finely granular "ground glass" cytoplasm packed with HBsAg; in HCV there are often portal lymphoid aggregates, bile duct reactive changes, and lobular regions of macrovesicular steatosis.

- *Acute hepatitis*
  - Injured hepatocytes are eosinophilic and rounded with shrunken or fragmented nuclei *(apoptosis)* or swollen *(ballooning degeneration)*. In severe hepatitis, confluent damage causes *bridging necrosis* between portal and central regions of adjacent lobules. Cholestasis can occur.
  - There is Kupffer cell hyperplasia, and macrophage aggregates mark the site of hepatocyte loss. Portal tracts exhibit mononuclear cell inflammation often with spillover into the adjacent parenchyma associated with periportal apoptosis *(interface hepatitis)*.
- *Chronic hepatitis*
  - Histology ranges from exceedingly mild to severe to cirrhosis.
  - In mild disease the inflammatory infiltrates are limited to portal tracts.
  - Progressive disease is marked by extension of chronic inflammation from portal tracts with *interface hepatitis;* linking of portal-portal and portal-central regions constitutes *bridging necrosis.*
  - *Continued loss of hepatocytes results in fibrous septum formation; associated hepatocyte regeneration results in cirrhosis.*

Bacterial, Parasitic, and Helminthic Infections (p. 839)

- Extrahepatic infections (especially sepsis) can induce hepatic inflammation and varying degrees of cholestasis.
- Biliary obstruction and intrabiliary bacterial proliferation can cause a severe acute inflammatory response *(ascending cholangitis).*
- Parasitic infections (e.g., amebic, echinococcal, malarial, or helminthic organisms) are common causes of hepatic abscesses in developing countries (see Chapter 8). Liver flukes, most common in Southeast Asia, cause a high rate of CCA.
- Abscesses occurring in developed countries are rare and are usually bacterial or candidal; sources are intra-abdominal (via portal vein), systemic (via arterial supply), biliary tree, direct extension, and penetrating injuries. Abscesses are associated with fever, right upper-quadrant pain, tender hepatomegaly, and possibly jaundice. Mortality without drainage is 90%; survival is dramatically improved by early treatment. Rupture of echinococcal cysts can precipitate systemic spread of the organism with severe immune-mediated shock.

Autoimmune Hepatitis (p. 839)

AIH is a chronic, progressive hepatitis often with a strong genetic predisposition (in Caucasians there is a frequent DRB1 allele association). AIH can be triggered by viral infections or drugs or may be a component of other autoimmune disorders (e.g., rheumatoid arthritis, Sjögren syndrome, or ulcerative colitis). The entire histologic spectrum of hepatitis can be seen in AIH, but *clusters of periportal plasma cells are characteristic.*

There is a female predominance (78%), with elevated serum IgG levels but no serum markers of viral infection. AIH is classified on the basis of the patterns of autoantibodies (in the United States, type 1 is much more common):

- *Type 1 AIH* shows autoantibodies to nuclear (ANA), smooth muscle (SMA), actin (AAA), and soluble liver antigen–liver-pancreas (SLA-LP) antigens; it is associated with the HLA-DR3 haplotype.
- *Type 2 AIH* exhibits autoantibodies directed against the liver kidney microsome-1 (ALKM-1) and liver cytosol-1 (ACL-1) antigens.

Acute onset of symptoms of liver failure occurs in 40% of patients; symptomatic patients tend to show substantial liver destruction and scarring at the time of diagnosis. Untreated, 6-month mortality can reach 40%, and 40% of survivors will develop cirrhosis. Immunosuppression is a mainstay of therapy, with transplantation for end-stage disease; AIH recurs in 20% of transplants.

Drug- and Toxin-Induced Liver Injury (p. 840)

Damage from toxin or drug should be considered in the differential diagnosis of any form of liver disease (e.g., *hepatocyte necrosis, hepatitis, cholestasis, fibrosis,* or *insidious onset of liver dysfunction*) (Table 18-4). Injury due to drugs or toxins can be immediate or develop over weeks to months; mechanisms include direct toxicity, hepatic conversion to an active toxin, or immune-mediated injury.

Some compounds are predictably toxic, whereas others can idiosyncratically cause injury. Thus *acetaminophen* in sufficiently high doses is uniformly injurious due to the production of a toxic metabolite by the cytochrome P-450 system. Conversely, *chlorpromazine* causes cholestasis only in patients that are slow to metabolize it, and *halothane* in particular individuals can induce a fatal AIH.

TABLE 18-4 Patterns of Drug- and Toxin-Induced Hepatic Injury

Pattern of Injury	Morphologic Findings	Examples of Associated Agents
Cholestatic	Bland hepatocellular cholestasis, without inflammation	Contraceptive and anabolic steroids, antibiotics, HAART
Cholestatic hepatitis	Cholestasis with lobular necroinflammatory activity; may show bile duct destruction	Antibiotics, phenothiazines, statins
Hepatocellular necrosis	Spotty hepatocyte necrosis	Methyldopa, phenytoin
	Massive necrosis	Acetaminophen, halothane
	Chronic hepatitis	Isoniazid
Fatty liver disease	Large and small droplet fat	Ethanol, corticosteroids, methotrexate, total parenteral nutrition
	"Microvesicular steatosis" (diffuse small droplet fat)	Valproate, tetracycline, aspirin (Reye syndrome), HAART
	Steatohepatitis with Mallory-Denk bodies	Ethanol, amiodarone
Fibrosis and cirrhosis	Periportal and pericellular fibrosis	Alcohol, methotrexate, enalapril, vitamin A and other retinoids
Granulomas	Noncaseating epithelioid granulomas	Sulfonamides, amiodarone, isoniazid
	Fibrin ring granulomas	Allopurinol
Vascular lesions	SOS (veno-occlusive disease): obliteration of central veins	High-dose chemotherapy, bush teas
	Budd-Chiari syndrome	Oral contraceptives
	Peliosis hepatitis: blood-filled cavities, not lined by endothelial cells	Anabolic steroids, tamoxifen
Neoplasms	Hepatocellular adenoma	Oral contraceptives, anabolic steroids
	HCC	Alcohol, Thorotrast
	CCA	Thorotrast
	Angiosarcoma	Thorotrast, vinyl chloride

HAART, Highly active anti-retroviral therapy.

Adapted from Washington K: Metabolic and toxic conditions of the liver. In Iacobuzio-Donahue CA, Montgomery EA (eds): *Gastrointestinal and Liver Pathology.* Philadelphia, PA, Churchill Livingstone; 2005, p. 503.

Alcoholic Liver Disease (p. 842)

Alcoholic liver disease (ALD) is the leading cause of liver pathology in most Western countries; globally it accounts for 3.8% of deaths. There are three (overlapping) forms of ALD:

Morphology (p. 842)

- *Hepatic steatosis (fatty liver)* is marked by microvesicular lipid droplets within hepatocytes and can occur with even moderate alcohol intake. With chronic alcohol intake, lipid accumulates in *macrovesicular* droplets, displacing the nucleus. The liver becomes enlarged, soft, greasy, and yellow. There is little-to-no fibrosis (at least initially), and the condition is reversible.

- *Alcoholic hepatitis* is characterized by ballooning degeneration and hepatocyte necrosis. There is also *Mallory-Denk body* formation (intracellular eosinophilic aggregates of intermediate filaments), *neutrophilic reaction* to degenerating hepatocytes, portal and periportal mononuclear inflammation, and *fibrosis.*
- *Alcoholic steatofibrosis* is often accompanied by stellate cell activation. Regenerative nodules can be prominent or obliterated by dense fibrous scar. End-stage alcoholic cirrhosis resembles cirrhosis of virtually any other cause.

Pathogenesis *(p. 843)*

- Only 10% to 15% of alcoholics develop cirrhosis, suggesting other factors in the development and severity of ALD:
  - *Gender:* Women are more susceptible to alcohol-related damage. This is partly related to gender-related alcohol pharmacokinetics and metabolism; however, estrogen also increases gut permeability to endotoxin, with subsequent Kupffer cell activation and increased proinflammatory cytokine production.
  - *Ethnic and genetic differences:* African Americans have higher cirrhosis rates than Caucasian Americans, independent of alcohol consumption levels. Polymorphisms in metabolizing enzymes (e.g., aldehyde dehydrogenase) or cytokine promoters are associated with higher frequencies of alcoholic cirrhosis.
  - *Comorbid conditions:* Iron overload or viral hepatitis increases the severity of ALD.
- *Steatosis* results from the following:
  - Impaired lipoprotein assembly and secretion
  - Increased peripheral catabolism of fat
  - Shunting of substrates away from catabolism and toward lipid biosynthesis
- Alcoholic hepatitis results from the following:
  - Acetaldehyde generated from alcohol catabolism, inducing lipid peroxidation and acetaldehyde-protein adduct formation.
  - Induction of cytochrome P-450 generating reactive oxygen species (ROS) and augmenting catabolism of other drugs to form potentially toxic metabolites
  - Impaired metabolism of methionine resulting in reduced glutathione levels that are protective for oxidative injury
  - Alcohol stimulating ET release from sinusoidal endothelium and causing vasoconstriction with diminished hepatic perfusion
  - Alcohol-mediated release of bacterial endotoxin from the GI tract, causing increasing inflammatory responses

Clinical Features *(p. 844)*

- *Hepatic steatosis* is associated with hepatomegaly and mild elevations of serum bilirubin and alkaline phosphatase. Abstention and adequate diet are sufficient treatments.
- *Alcoholic hepatitis* usually manifests acutely after a bout of heavy drinking; manifestations range from minimal to fulminant hepatic failure, and include malaise, anorexia, and tender hepatomegaly. Bilirubin and alkaline phosphatase are elevated, accompanied by neutrophilic leukocytosis. Each bout incurs a 10% to 20% mortality, and repeated incidents lead to cirrhosis in a third of patients. Typically, adequate nutrition and abstention leads to a slow resolution; occasionally the hepatitis persists and progresses to cirrhosis.
- *Alcoholic cirrhosis* is irreversible; its manifestations are similar to any other form of cirrhosis.

Five-year survival for patients with ALD approaches 90% for abstainers but drops to 50% to 60% for those who continue to drink. Death can result from hepatic coma, GI hemorrhage, intercurrent infection, hepatorenal syndrome, and/or HCC.

Metabolic Liver Disease (p. 845)

Nonalcoholic Fatty Liver Disease (p. 845)

NAFLD is a group of conditions characterized by hepatic steatosis in the absence of heavy alcohol consumption. At the most pathologic end of this group, *NASH* involves steatosis plus hepatocyte damage and inflammation. The rising incidence of NAFLD (3% to 5% of Americans) is attributed to the increasing prevalence of obesity; NAFLD is strongly associated with the metabolic syndrome of dyslipidemia, hyperinsulinemia, and insulin resistance.

Pathogenesis (p. 845)

NAFLD is probably a consequence of hepatocyte fat accumulation and increased hepatic oxidative stress leading to increased lipid peroxidation and ROS generation. Increased visceral adipose tissue also becomes dysfunctional, with reduced adiponectin production, and the increased synthesis of proinflammatory cytokines, such as TNF-α and IL-6.

Morphology (p. 846)

Hepatocytes are filled with fat vacuoles in the absence of inflammatory infiltration (steatosis) or with inflammatory infiltrates (steatohepatitis). Varying degrees of fibrosis are present.

Clinical Features (p. 846; Fig. 18-4)

Patients with simple steatosis are generally asymptomatic with little risk of progression to cirrhosis. With NASH, individuals can

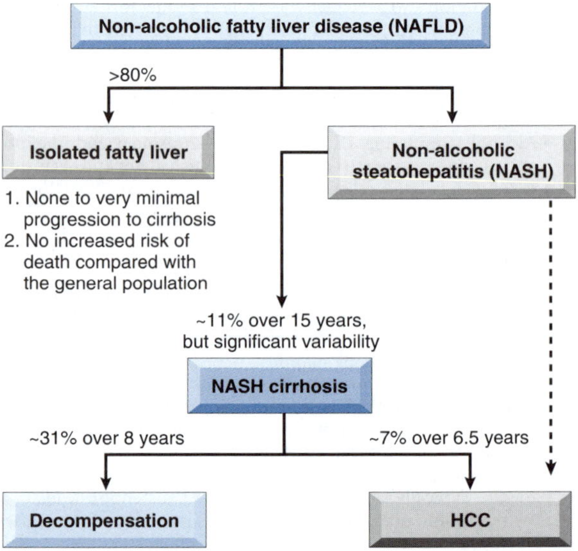

Figure 18-4 Natural history of NAFLD phenotypes. Isolated fatty liver shows minimal risk for progression to cirrhosis or increased mortality, whereas NASH shows increased overall mortality as well as increased risk for cirrhosis and HCC.

be symptom free, although many report fatigue, malaise, and/or right upper-quadrant discomfort; serum transaminase levels are elevated in 90% of patients, and there is increased risk for cirrhosis and HCC. Because of the association between NASH and the metabolic syndrome, cardiovascular disease is a frequent cause of morbidity and mortality. Treatment is therefore targeted at correcting the associated obesity, hyperlipidemia, and insulin resistance.

Hemochromatosis (p. 847)

Hemochromatosis is characterized by excessive iron accumulation in the parenchymal cells of various organs, particularly liver and pancreas.

- *Hereditary hemochromatosis (primary hemochromatosis)* is a homozygous recessive heritable disorder caused by excessive iron absorption.
- *Hemosiderosis (secondary hemochromatosis)* denotes disorders associated with parenteral iron administration (e.g., repetitive transfusions, ineffective erythropoiesis, increased iron intake, or chronic liver disease).

Pathogenesis (p. 847)

Tissue damage in hemochromatiosis is attributed to direct iron toxicity, presumably via free radical formation with lipid peroxidation, stimulation of collagen formation by hepatocyte stellate cells, and/or iron- and ROS-DNA interactions.

Total body iron content is regulated by intestinal absorption (see Chapter 14). *Hepcidin* exerts the greatest effect by controlling the expression of ferroportin, an iron efflux channel on intestinal epithelium and macrophages; *hepcidin lowers plasma iron, whereas hepcidin deficiency causes iron overload.* Other proteins involved in iron metabolism (e.g., hemojuvelin [HJV], transferrin receptor 2 [TFR2], and HFE) do so largely by modulating hepcidin levels (Fig. 18-5).

The adult form of hemochromatosis is almost always caused by mutations of the *HFE* gene. More than 70% of patients have a cysteine-to-tyrosine substitution at amino acid 282 (C282Y) that inactivates HFE and reduces hepcidin expression. The frequency of C282Y heterozygosity is 11% (homozygosity occurs with a frequency of 0.45%). However, disease penetrance is low, and the genetic condition alone does not invariably lead to hemochromatosis.

Morphology (p. 848)

Iron accumulates as hemosiderin in various tissues—in decreasing order of severity: liver, pancreas, myocardium, endocrine glands, joints, and skin. Cirrhosis and pancreatic fibrosis are the chief additional morphologic changes.

Clinical Features (p. 849)

Fully developed cases of hemochromatosis uniformly exhibit micronodular cirrhosis; diabetes mellitus and skin pigmentation occurs in 75% to 80% of these individuals. Iron accumulation is lifelong, but the injury caused by excessive iron is gradual, so that symptoms usually appear after age 40. Males predominate (6:1) owing to physiologic iron loss in women (e.g., menstruation, pregnancy) that delays the iron accumulation.

Death can result from cirrhosis (and/or HCC) and cardiac involvement. Regular phlebotomy is sufficient treatment; early diagnosis can therefore enable normal life expectancy, and screening of genetic probands is therefore important.

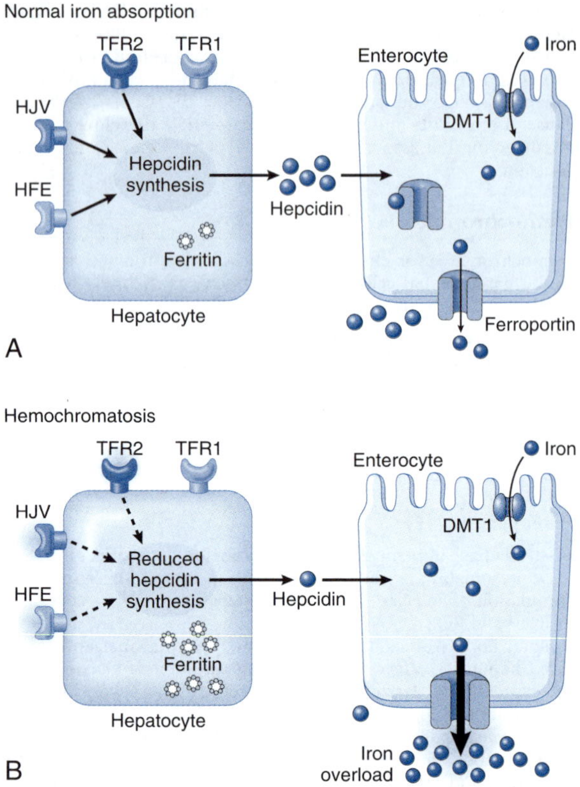

Figure 18-5 **A,** *Normal iron absorption:* HFE (protein product of the *HFE* gene), HJV, and TFR2 regulate hepatocyte hepcidin synthesis. Hepcidin then binds to ferroportin on enterocytes leading to internalization of the complex and ferroportin degradation. Ferroportin degradation reduces iron efflux from enterocytes. Through these regulatory interactions normal iron absorption is maintained. **B,** *Hemochromatosis:* In hereditary hemochromatosis, HFE, HJV, or TFR2 gene mutations lead to reduced hepcidin synthesis. The resulting decreased hepcidin-ferroportin interaction allows for increased ferroportin activity and increased iron efflux from enterocytes, giving rise to systemic iron overload. *DMT1,* Divalent metal transporter 1.

Wilson Disease (p. 849)

This autosomal recessive disorder is caused by mutations of the *ATP7B* gene coding for a canalicular copper-transporting ATPase; copper absorption and delivery to the liver is normal, but (1) copper excretion into the bile is reduced, (2) copper is not incorporated into ceruloplasmin, and (3) ceruloplasmin secretion into the blood is inhibited. This causes copper accumulation in the liver that results in hepatic injury through ROS generation. In addition, spillover into the circulation of nonceruloplasmin-bound copper causes hemolysis and pathology in other sites, especially cornea and brain.

Morphology *(p. 850)*

Liver damage ranges from minor to severe, manifested by fatty change, acute and chronic hepatitis (with Mallory-Denk bodies), cirrhosis, and/or (rarely) massive necrosis. CNS toxicity predominantly affects the basal ganglia, with atrophy and even cavitation. Nearly all patients with neurologic involvement develop eye lesions called *Kayser-Fleischer rings*—green-brown copper deposits in Descemet membrane of the corneal limbus.

Clinical Features (p. 850)

Age at onset and clinical presentation are extremely variable; acute or chronic liver disease before age 40 is the most common initial manifestation. Neuropsychiatric disorders also occur, including mild behavioral changes, frank psychosis, and Parkinson-like symptoms. The biochemical diagnosis is based on decreased serum ceruloplasmin, *increased hepatic copper content,* and increased urinary copper excretion. *Serum copper levels are of no diagnostic value.* Copper chelation is standard therapy; liver transplantation may be necessary.

α_1-Antitrypsin Deficiency (p. 850)

α_1-Antitrypsin (α_1-AT) deficiency is an autosomal recessive disorder marked by very low serum levels of this protein; α_1-AT normally inhibits neutrophil proteases released at sites of acute inflammation (e.g., elastase, cathepsin G, and proteinase 3). Deficiency leads primarily to emphysema because the activity of destructive proteases is not curtailed (see Chapter 15), as well as hepatic disease caused by the hepatocellular accumulation of misfolded protein.

Pathogenesis (p. 851)

α_1-AT is synthesized primarily by hepatocytes. The gene is extremely polymorphic with more than 75 isoforms designated alphabetically based on gel migration mobilities; the most common genotype (>90% of people) is designated as protease inhibitor (Pi) MM. Most mutations result in no or only moderate reductions in α_1-AT levels and have no clinical manifestations. However, PiZZ homozygotes (the most common disease genotype) have circulating α_1-AT levels below 10% of normal. This occurs because PiZ has a single glutamic acid to lysine substitution, resulting in protein misfolding and preventing egress from the endoplasmic reticulum (ER). This triggers the ER stress response including autophagy, mitochondrial dysfunction, and proinflammatory NF-κB activation, all causing hepatocyte damage. Additional genetic or environmental factors modify the pathogenesis because only 10% to 15% of PiZZ homozygotes develop overt liver disease.

Morphology (p. 851)

α_1-AT deficiency is characterized by periodic acid-Schiff (PAS)-positive (diastase-resistant) cytoplasmic globules in periportal hepatocytes. Hepatic manifestations range from cholestasis to hepatitis to cirrhosis.

Clinical Features (p. 851)

Neonatal hepatitis with cholestatic jaundice occurs in 10% to 20% of newborns with α_1-AT deficiency; later presentation may be attributable to acute hepatitis or complications of cirrhosis. HCC develops in 2% to 3% of PiZZ homozygous adults. Smoking accentuates lung emphysematous damage. Treatment is liver transplantation.

Cholestatic Diseases (p. 852)

Bile serves two functions: (1) emulsification of dietary fat and (2) elimination of bilirubin, excess cholesterol, and other hydrophobic waste products that cannot be excreted into urine. Excess bilirubin (the end product of heme degradation) leads to *jaundice* and *icterus* (yellow skin and sclera discoloration, respectively); common causes are bilirubin overproduction, hepatitis, and bile outflow obstruction. *Cholestasis* denotes systemic retention of all bile solutes, including bilirubin, bile salts, and cholesterol.

Bilirubin and Bile Formation (p. 852)

The degradation of heme (>85% derived from hemoglobin) throughout the body progresses from biliverdin to bilirubin; the latter is bound to albumin and delivered to the liver. After carrier-mediated uptake, bilirubin is conjugated with 1 to 2 molecules of glucuronic acid by the hepatic endoplasmic transferase UGT1A1. The resulting water-soluble bilirubin glucuronides are excreted in the bile and subsequently deconjugated by gut bacteria and degraded to urobilinogens that are primarily fecally eliminated; 20% of urobilinogens are resorbed and recycled to the liver, with a small fraction excreted in the urine.

Bile acids are water-soluble modifications of cholesterol (mostly cholic acid and chenodeoxycholic acid) that act as detergents to solubilize dietary and biliary lipids. Bile salts (bile acids conjugated to taurine or glycine) constitute two thirds of bile organic compounds. More than 95% of bile acids and salts are reabsorbed from the gut and recirculate back to the liver *(enterohepatic circulation).*

Pathophysiology of Jaundice (p. 853)

Jaundice occurs when bilirubin production exceeds hepatic uptake, conjugation, and/or excretion. Excess production or diminished uptake and/or conjugation causes *unconjugated hyperbilirubinemia;* defective excretion (intrahepatic or bile flow-related) causes mostly *conjugated hyperbilirubinemia.*

- *Unconjugated bilirubin* is virtually insoluble in water; it normally circulates tightly bound to albumin and cannot be excreted in urine. A small amount of unconjugated bilirubin circulates as a free anion that can diffuse into tissues (especially neonatal brain) and cause injury; this unbound fraction can increase with severe hemolysis or when drugs displace bilirubin from albumin.
- *Conjugated bilirubin* is water-soluble, nontoxic, and only loosely bound to albumin; excess conjugated bilirubin can be renally excreted.

Neonatal Jaundice (Physiologic Jaundice of the Newborn; p. 853)

Because hepatic metabolic machinery does not mature until approximately 2 weeks of age, almost every newborn develops transient, mild unconjugated hyperbilirubinemia. This can be exacerbated by breast-feeding due to bilirubin-deconjugating enzymes in breast milk.

Hereditary Hyperbilirubinemias (p. 853)

- *Unconjugated hyperbilirubinemia*
  - *Crigler-Najjar syndrome type I (autosomal recessive):* Total absence of UGT1A1 causes jaundice with high serum levels of unconjugated bilirubin and a histologically normal liver. Without liver transplantation, fatal neurologic damage *(kernicterus)* will ensue.
  - *Crigler-Najjar syndrome type II (autosomal dominant):* Less severe UGT1A1 deficiency. Although kernicterus can occur, the condition is not usually lethal.
  - *Gilbert syndrome (autosomal recessive):* Mild, fluctuating unconjugated hyperbilirubinemia, with 30% reduction in UGT1A1 activity attributable in most cases to a mutation that affects gene transcription. Affecting 6% to 10% of the population, the hyperbilirubinemia (and jaundice) may be exacerbated by infection, strenuous exercise, or fasting.

- *Conjugated hyperbilirubinemia*
  - *Dubin-Johnson syndrome (autosomal recessive):* Defective hepatocyte secretion of bilirubin conjugates due to absent bilirubin glucuronide transport protein (multidrug resistance protein 2). The liver is brown, with accumulated pigment granules (polymers of epinephrine metabolites, *not* bilirubin pigment). Patients are jaundiced but have normal life expectancy.
  - *Rotor syndrome (autosomal recessive):* Defective hepatocellular bilirubin uptake or excretion. The liver is not pigmented; patients are jaundiced with normal life spans.

Cholestasis (p. 853)

Cholestasis denotes impaired bile formation or flow, leading to the accumulation of intrahepatic bile pigments. Cholestasis can be extrahepatic (due to duct obstruction) or intrahepatic (due to hepatocellular dysfunction or canalicular obstruction). Consequences include jaundice, *pruritus* from bile salt retention, *xanthomas* (skin accumulations of cholesterol), and intestinal malabsorption with nutritional deficiencies due to poor uptake of fat-soluble vitamins (A, D, and K). Serum alkaline phosphatase and γ-glutamyl transpeptidase (GGT) are characteristically elevated.

Morphology (p. 854)

Whether intrahepatic or extrahepatic cholestasis, bile pigment accumulates within the hepatic parenchyma, leading to dilated bile canaliculi and hepatocyte degeneration.

Large Bile Duct Obstruction (p. 854)

Bile duct obstruction in adults is most commonly due to extrahepatic cholelithiasis (gallstones), followed by pancreatic or biliary malignancies and postsurgical strictures. In children, causes include biliary atresia, cystic fibrosis, choledochal cysts, or insufficient intrahepatic bile duct formation. The initial morphologic features of cholestasis are entirely reversible with correction of the obstruction. Prolonged obstruction can lead to biliary cirrhosis.

Subtotal or intermittent obstruction may promote *ascending cholangitis* with secondary bacterial infection of the biliary tree that manifests with fever, chills, abdominal pain, and jaundice.

Morphology (p. 854)

Obstruction, either intrahepatic or extrahepatic, causes distention of upstream bile ducts, with ductule proliferation, edema, and acute inflammation. If unresolved, chronic inflammation will initiate periportal fibrosis, eventually leading to hepatic scarring and regenerative nodule formation—biliary cirrhosis. Cholestasis may lead to feathery degeneration of periportal hepatocytes, cytoplasmic swelling with Mallory-Denk bodies, and infarcts caused by the detergent effects of extravasated bile.

Cholestasis of Sepsis (p. 854)

Sepsis may affect the liver through the following:

- Direct effects of intrahepatic infection (e.g., abscess formation or cholangitis)
- Ischemia due to hypotension
- Response to circulating microbial products
  - *Canalicular cholestasis,* with canalicular bile plugs, is associated with activated Kupffer cells and mild portal inflammation.
  - *Ductular cholestasis* is a more ominous finding with dilated canals of Hering and bile ductules, and often accompanies septic shock.

Primary Hepatolithiasis (p. 855)

This is a disorder of intrahepatic gallstone formation causing recurrent ascending cholangitis, progressive inflammatory destruction of hepatic parenchyma, and increased incidence of biliary neoplasia. The disease has a high prevalence in east Asia. The stones are pigmented calcium bilirubinate.

Neonatal Cholestasis (p. 856)

Neonatal cholestasis (prolonged conjugated hyperbilirubinemia) affects 1 in 2500 live births; infants present with jaundice, dark urine, light stools, and hepatomegaly. The major causes are cholangiopathies (20% of cases; primarily biliary atresia) and a variety of disorders collectively referred to as *neonatal hepatitis* (although not all are inflammatory). Neonatal infections, α_1-AT deficiency, toxic exposures, and metabolic diseases (e.g., Niemann-Pick) may be responsible; no cause is identified in 10% to 15% of cases. Establishing an etiology is important because biliary atresia requires surgical intervention.

Biliary Atresia (*p. 857*)

Biliary atresia causes a third of neonatal cholestasis occurring in 1 in 12,000 live births; it is defined as extrahepatic biliary tree obstruction within the first 3 months of life. It is the single most frequent cause of death from liver disease in early childhood and accounts for the majority of children referred for liver transplantation.

Pathogenesis (p. 857)

- The severe early *fetal form* (20% of cases) is due to aberrant intrauterine development of the biliary tree and is frequently associated with other anomalies.
- The *perinatal form,* presumed secondary to viral infections and/or autoimmunity, results from postnatal destruction of a normal biliary tree.

Morphology (p. 857)

In both forms, there is inflammation and fibrosing stricture of the extrahepatic biliary tree, progressing into the intrahepatic biliary system. The liver shows florid features of duct obstruction:

- Marked bile duct proliferation
- Portal tract edema
- Fibrosis progressing to cirrhosis within 6 months

Clinical Features (p. 858)

Neonatal cholestasis is seen in an infant of normal birth weight and postnatal weight gain. If untreated (liver transplantation), death occurs within 2 years of birth.

Autoimmune Cholangiopathies (p. 858)

This section discusses the two main autoimmune disorders of intrahepatic bile ducts: primary biliary cirrhosis (PBC) and primary sclerosing cholangitis (PSC). These disorders are summarized in Table 18-5.

Primary Biliary Cirrhosis (p. 858)

PBC is a disorder causing nonsuppurative inflammatory destruction of small- and medium-sized intrahepatic bile ducts. It is primarily

TABLE 18-5 Main Features of Primary Biliary Cirrhosis and Primary Sclerosing Cholangitis

Parameter	PBC	PSC
Age	Median age 50 years (30-70)	Median age 30 years
Gender	90% female	70% male
Clinical course	Progressive	Unpredictable but progressive
Associated conditions	Sjögren syndrome (70%) Scleroderma (5%) Thyroid disease (20%)	Inflammatory bowel disease (70%) Pancreatitis (≤25%) Idiopathic fibrosing diseases (retroperitoneal fibrosis)
Serology	95% AMA-positive 50% ANA-positive 40% ANCA-positive	0%-5% AMA-positive (low titer) 6% ANA-positive 65% ANCA-positive
Radiology	Normal	Strictures and beading of large bile ducts; pruning of smaller ducts
Duct lesion	Florid duct lesions and loss of small ducts only	Inflammatory destruction of extrahepatic and large intrahepatic ducts; fibrotic obliteration of medium and small intrahepatic ducts

AMA, Antimitochondrial antibody; *ANA*, antinuclear antibody; *ANCA*, antineutrophil cytoplasmic antibody.

a disease of middle-aged women and does not lead inexorably to cirrhosis. PBC is thought to be an autoimmune disorder. Antimitochondrial antibodies that recognize the E2 component of the pyruvate dehydrogenase complex (PDC-E2) occur in 90% to 95% of patients and are the most characteristic laboratory finding; PDC-E2-specific T cells and antibodies against other cellular components (nuclear pore proteins and centromeric proteins) are also present.

Morphology *(p. 858)*

Lesions exhibit varying degrees of severity throughout the liver.

- Dense chronic portal tract inflammation with focal noncaseating granulomas is associated with interlobular bile duct destruction and generalized cholestasis.
- Intrahepatic biliary obstruction leads to progressive secondary upstream damage, with ductular proliferation, and inflammation and necrosis of periportal hepatocytes, often with prominent Mallory-Denk bodies.
- At end stage, PBC is indistinguishable from other forms of cirrhosis.

Clinical Features *(p. 859)*

Onset is insidious, with pruritus, hepatomegaly, jaundice, and xanthomas (from retained cholesterol); with progression to cirrhosis, variceal bleeding and encephalopathy occur. Serum alkaline phosphatase, γ-glutamyltransferase, and cholesterol levels are increased. Patients can have extrahepatic autoimmune manifestations (e.g., Sjögren syndrome, scleroderma, thyroiditis, Raynaud phenomenon, and membranous glomerulonephritis). Untreated, patients follow one of two pathways to end-stage disease—either hyperbilirubinemia or portal hypertension. Treatment of early-stage disease with oral ursodeoxycholic acid greatly slows progression presumably through altering the biochemical composition of bile.

Primary Sclerosing Cholangitis (p. 859)

PSC is chronic cholestatic disease distinguished by inflammation and obliterative fibrosis of both the extrahepatic and intrahepatic biliary tree; dilation of the preserved segments yields a characteristic "beading" of injected radiologic contrast material. Patients with PSC also typically have ulcerative colitis (70% of patients); that association and the presence of circulating autoantibodies (ANA, anti-SMA, rheumatoid factor, and an atypical p-antineutrophil cytoplasmic antibody (p-ANCA) against a nuclear envelope protein) all suggest an autoimmune-mediated pathogenesis.

Morphology (p. 860)

Bile ducts exhibit periductular inflammation and concentric (onionskin) fibrosis, with progressive atrophy and eventual luminal obliteration; obstruction culminates in biliary cirrhosis and hepatic failure.

Clinical Features (p. 860)

PSC is most common in middle-aged men. It follows a protracted course (5 to 15 years); severe disease is associated with weight loss, ascites, variceal bleeding, and encephalopathy. There is an increased incidence of chronic pancreatitis and HCC; 7% of patients will develop CCA. Liver transplant is the definitive therapy for end-stage disease.

Structural Anomalies of the Biliary Tree (p. 861)

Choledochal Cysts (p. 861)

These congenital dilations of the common bile duct present most often in children <10 years with nonspecific symptoms of jaundice and recurrent colicky abdominal pain; the female to male ratio is 3 to 4:1. The cysts predispose to stone formation, stenosis and stricture, pancreatitis, obstructive biliary complications, and bile duct carcinoma in the adult.

Fibropolycystic Disease (p. 861)

Fibropolycystic disease of the liver is a heterogeneous group of lesions in which the primary abnormalities are congenital malformations of the biliary tree. Lesions may be found only incidentally or can present as hepatosplenomegaly and portal hypertension. All the lesions are related to abnormal development of the biliary tree representing *ductal plate malformations* associated with persistence of the fetal periportal ductal plate. The caliber of involved portal tracts determines the different size, morphology, and distributions of lesions. Fibropolycystic liver disease often occurs with autosomal recessive polycystic renal disease, involving the protein polycystin (see Chapter 20). Persons with fibropolycystic liver disease have an increased risk for CCA.

- *Von Meyenberg complexes* ("bile duct hamartomas"; p. 861) are small clusters of dilated bile ducts or cysts within a fibrous stroma; they are extremely common but usually clinically insignificant.
- *Intrahepatic or extrahepatic biliary cysts* (p. 861): In isolation these may lead to ascending cholangitis, so-called *Caroli disease.* When biliary cysts occur in association with congenital hepatic fibrosis, the lesion is called *Caroli syndrome.*
- *Congenital hepatic fibrosis* (p. 861) is caused by incomplete involution of embryonic ductal structures with ensuing portal tract fibrosis, which can cause portal hypertension.

Circulatory Disorders (p. 862)

Impaired Blood Flow Into the Liver (p. 862)

Hepatic Artery Compromise (p. 862)

Infarction is rare due to the dual hepatic blood supply. However, thrombosis or compression of intrahepatic arterial branches can infrequently result in localized pale infarct, occasionally made hemorrhagic by portal blood suffusion.

Portal Vein Obstruction and Thrombosis (p. 862)

Manifestations of extrahepatic portal vein obstruction can range from insidious and well tolerated to catastrophic and potentially lethal (e.g., due to variceal bleeding). Causes include neonatal umbilical vein infection or catheterization, intra-abdominal sepsis causing pylephlebitis in the splanchnic circulation, acquired or heritable coagulopathies, trauma, pancreatic lesions that initiate splenic vein thromboses, and cirrhosis.

Impaired Blood Flow Through the Liver (p. 863)

Cirrhosis is the most important cause. Sinusoidal occlusion can also be caused by sickle cell disease, disseminated intravascular coagulation, eclampsia, and diffuse intrasinusoidal metastatic tumor.

Peliosis Hepatitis (p. 863)

Peliosis hepatitis is a reversible hepatic sinusoid dilation associated with impeded efflux of hepatic blood. It can occur in the setting of malignancy, tuberculosis, posttransplantation immunodeficiency, and sex hormone administration (e.g., anabolic steroids, oral contraceptives, danazol). *Bartonella* species have been seen in the sinusoidal endothelial cells in AIDS-associated peliosis. The etiology is unknown; lesions typically regress after correction of the underlying causes.

Hepatic Venous Outflow Obstruction (p. 863)

Hepatic Vein Thrombosis (p. 863)

Budd-Chiari syndrome occurs when two or more major hepatic veins are obstructed; hepatic damage is a consequence of increased intrahepatic blood pressure. Hepatic vein thrombosis occurs in the setting of primary myeloproliferative disorders (e.g., polycythemia vera), heritable coagulopathies, pregnancy, antiphospholipid antibody syndrome, paroxysmal nocturnal hemoglobinuria, and intra-abdominal cancers.

The mortality of untreated acute hepatic vein thrombosis is high; prompt surgical portosystemic shunting improves the prognosis. Subacute or chronic cases are considerably less lethal but can develop superimposed fibrosis.

Sinusoidal Obstruction Syndrome (Veno-Occlusive Disease; p. 864)

Sinusoidal obstruction syndrome (SOS)—originally described in Jamaican drinkers of pyrrolizidine alkaloid-containing bush tea—now occurs primarily as a consequence of toxic injury to sinusoidal endothelium by chemotherapy; mortality approaches 30%. Patients present with tender hepatomegaly, ascites, weight gain, and jaundice.

Morphology (p. 863)

SOS is characterized by patchy obliteration of smaller hepatic vein radicles by endothelial swelling and collagen deposition. Acute SOS shows centribolular congestion with hepatocellular necrosis, whereas progressive disease exhibits venule lumen obliteration with dense perivenular fibrosis and hemosiderin deposition.

Passive Congestion and Centrilobular Necrosis (p. 864)

Systemic hypoperfusion (e.g., shock) leads to hepatocyte necrosis around the central vein *(centrilobular necrosis)*. With superimposed passive congestion (e.g., right-sided heart failure or constrictive pericarditis), there is hemorrhage as well, producing *centrilobular hemorrhagic necrosis,* with the liver taking on a variegated mottled appearance ("nutmeg liver"). Protracted right-sided heart failure causes chronic passive congestion and pericentral fibrosis *(cardiac sclerosis),* eventually culminating in cirrhosis.

Hepatic Complications of Organ or Hematopoietic Stem Cell Transplantation (p. 865)

Graft-Versus-Host Disease and Liver Graft Rejection (p. 865)

- Graft-versus-host disease (GVHD) occurs in the setting of bone marrow or stem cell transplantation and is characterized by *direct lymphocyte attack on liver cells, particularly bile duct epithelium.*
  - *Acute GVHD* is characterized by hepatitis (parenchymal inflammation and hepatocyte necrosis), chronic vascular inflammation and intimal proliferation *(endothelialitis),* and *bile duct destruction.*
  - *Chronic GVHD* exhibits portal tract inflammation, bile duct destruction (or complete loss), and fibrosis.
- *Acute rejection* of liver allografts exhibits portal tract inflammation (frequently including eosinophils), bile duct damage, and endothelialitis. *Chronic rejection,* occurring months or years after transplantation, is characterized by bile duct loss and arteriopathy, with eventual graft failure.

Hepatic Disease Associated With Pregnancy (p. 865)

Abnormal liver tests occur in 3% to 5% of pregnancies. Viral hepatitis is the most common cause of jaundice in pregnancy; with the exception of HEV (20% mortality rates in pregnancy), these infections are not typically influenced by pregnancy. Rarely (0.1%) pregnancies cause direct hepatic complications (that are usually nonfatal): acute fatty liver of pregnancy (AFLP) and intrahepatic cholestasis of pregnancy (ICP).

Preeclampsia and Eclampsia (p. 866)

Preeclampsia affects 3% to 5% of pregnancies; it is characterized by hypertension, proteinuria, peripheral edema, coagulation abnormalities, and varying degrees of disseminated intravascular coagulation. With onset of hyperreflexia and convulsion, the condition is called *eclampsia,* and severe cases can require termination of the pregnancy. The *HELLP* syndrome (*h*emolysis, *e*levated *l*iver enzymes, and *low* *p*latelets) can be the primary manifestation of preeclampsia.

Morphology (p. 866)

Grossly there are small, red, hemorrhagic patches, with occasional yellow-white areas of infarction. Microscopically there is periportal sinusoidal fibrin deposition, periportal necrosis, and hemorrhage. Coalescence of bleeding can form hepatic hematomas capable of fatal rupture.

Acute Fatty Liver of Pregnancy (p. 866)

AFLP is a rare entity (1 in 13,000 deliveries) that can present along a spectrum from subclinical hepatocyte dysfunction to hepatic failure, coma, and death. Mitochondrial dysfunction is generally implicated; in particular, congenital fetal deficiency in long-chain 3-hydroxyacyl coenzyme A dehydrogenase results in toxic levels of fetal metabolites that can cause maternal hepatotoxicity. Microscopically there is *microvesicular steatosis;* in severe cases portal inflammation and hepatocyte dropout and lobular disarray can occur. Definitive treatment is termination of pregnancy.

Intrahepatic Cholestasis of Pregnancy (p. 866)

ICP is attributed to the altered hormonal state of pregnancy; it is characterized by pruritus and jaundice in the third trimester, with mild cholestasis. Although generally benign, pruritus can be severe, and maternal gallstones or malabsorption can also occur.

Nodules and Tumors (p. 867)

Nodular Hyperplasias (p. 867)

Nodular hyperplasias are solitary or multiple benign hepatocellular nodules in the absence of cirrhosis; the putative cause is focal hepatic vascular obliteration, with compensatory hypertrophy of adjacent well-vascularized lobules.

- *Focal nodular hyperplasia* occurs in young to middle-aged adults and is an irregular, unencapsulated mass containing a central stellate fibrous scar.
- *Nodular regenerative hyperplasia* is a diffuse nodular transformation of the liver *without fibrosis,* occurring as a consequence of conditions affecting intrahepatic blood flow (e.g., in solid-organ transplants [especially kidney], bone marrow transplants, and vasculitis).

Benign Neoplasms (p. 867)

- *Cavernous hemangiomas* are the most common benign liver tumors; they are identical to blood vessel tumors seen in other locations (see Chapter 11).
- *Hepatocellular adenomas* (p. 867) are benign hepatocyte neoplasms up to 30 cm in diameter; they occur commonly in young women, usually associated with oral contraceptive use. Three subtypes are described with different risks of malignant transformation:
    - *HNF1-α-inactivated hepatocellular adenomas:* HNF1-α encodes a transcription factor, and germline mutations are responsible for autosomal dominant maturity-onset diabetes of the young, type 3. These lesions are most commonly found in women.

- *β-Catenin-activated hepatocellular adenomas:* Activating mutations of β-catenin are considered at very high risk for malignant transformation and should be resected even when asymptomatic. They are associated with oral contraceptive and anabolic steroid use in both men and women.
- *Inflammatory hepatocellular adenomas:* These lesions are found in both men and women and are associated with NAFLD. They have activating mutations in gp130, a coreceptor for IL-6, leading to constitutive JAK-STAT signaling and overexpression of acute phase reactants. They have a small risk of malignant transformation.

Malignant Tumors (p. 869)

- In the United States, the vast majority of tumors involving the liver are *metastatic.*
- *HCC* is the most common *primary* liver cancer; CCAs are much less common.

Hepatoblastoma (p. 869)

Hepatoblastoma is the most common liver tumor of early childhood. A characteristic feature is activation of the Wnt-β-catenin signaling pathway; hepatoblstomas are also associated with familial polyposis syndrome and Beckwith-Wiedemann syndrome.

- The *epithelial type* vaguely recapitulates liver development.
- The *mixed epithelial and mesenchymal type* contains foci of mesenchymal differentiation including osteoid, cartilage, or striated muscle.

Hepatoblastomas are usually fatal if untreated, but resection and chemotherapy yield 80% 5-year survival rates.

Hepatocellular Carcinoma (p. 870)

HCC accounts for approximately 5% of all cancers worldwide, with a 3 to 8:1 male predominance. It occurs most commonly in developing countries with high rates of HBV infection, particularly where infection starts in infancy and there is a high associated carrier rate. Half of such cases are not associated with cirrhosis; rather there may be important adjunct exposure to aflatoxin (a mycotoxin produced by *Aspergillus* species that contaminates staple food crops). In Western populations, increased rates of hepatitis C infection are also driving HCC incidence.

Pathogenesis (p. 870)

HCC usually arises in the background of chronic liver disease. Major etiologic factors are chronic viral infection (HBV or HCV), chronic alcoholism, NASH, and food contaminants (e.g., aflatoxins); lesser causes include hemochromatosis, tyrosinemia, and α_1-AT deficiency. Activating mutations of β-catenin occur in 40% of HCC, and p53 inactivation is present in 60% of HCC. Chronic inflammation is associated with genotoxic products, cytokine production, and hepatocyte regeneration; such changes—along with an underlying genetic susceptibility—presumably underlie tumorigenesis. IL-6 can suppress hepatocyte differentiation and promote hepatocyte proliferation by regulating the function of the transcription factor HNF4-α.

Morphology (p. 872)

HCC can present as a solitary mass, multifocal nodules, or a diffusely infiltrative cancer with massive liver enlargement, often (although not necessarily) in a background of cirrhosis; intrahepatic spread and vascular invasion are common. Histologically lesions may range from well differentiated to highly anaplastic and undifferentiated.

- A distinctive variant is *fibrolamellar carcinoma.* Constituting 5% of HCC, it usually presents as a single scirrhous, hard tumor occurring in 20- to 40-year-olds *in the absence of chronic liver disease.* The cells are well-differentiated cells in cords or nests separated by dense lamellar collagen bundles.

Clinical Features (p. 873)

Features include hepatomegaly, right upper-quadrant pain, weight loss, and elevated serum α-fetoprotein. Prognosis depends on the resectability of the tumor; mortality is secondary to cachexia, GI or esophageal variceal bleeding, liver failure with hepatic coma, or tumor rupture and fatal hemorrhage.

Cholangiocarcinoma *(p. 874)*

CCA arises from elements of the intrahepatic and extrahepatic biliary tree; 50% to 60% are perihilar (so-called *Klatskin tumors*), 20% to 30% are distal, and 10% are intrahepatic. CCA accounts for 3% of U.S. cancer deaths and 7.6% of cancer deaths worldwide. Clinical outlook is dismal because CCA is rarely resectable at diagnosis.

Although most cases arise without apparent antecedent conditions, chronic inflammation and cholestasis increase risk. CCA can be associated with PSC, congenital fibropolycystic lesions, hepatolithiasis, NAFLD, and HBV or HCV. In Southeast Asia, protracted biliary tree parasitic infection by *Opisthorchis sinensis* is a major risk factor.

Morphology (p. 874)

CCA can manifest as a single large mass, as multifocal nodules, or can be diffusely infiltrative. In contrast to HCC, CAA is typically pale because biliary epithelium does not secrete bilirubin pigment. Microscopically there are variably differentiated bile duct elements that resemble adenocarcinomas elsewhere in the alimentary tract; most CAA are markedly desmoplastic with dense collagenous stroma.

Other Primary Hepatic Malignant Tumors *(p. 875)*

Some tumors show *combined hepatocellular and CCA,* suggesting an origin from a multipotent stem cell. *Angiosarcomas* of the liver resemble those occurring elsewhere and are associated with exposures to vinyl chloride, arsenic, or Thorotrast. Hepatic *lymphomas* (mostly diffuse large B-cell lymphomas) occur primarily in middle-aged men and can occur in association with hepatitis B and C, HIV, and PBC.

Metastasis *(p. 875)*

Any cancer in the body—including those of the blood-forming elements—can spread to the liver; colon, breast, lung, and pancreas primaries are most common. Typically, multiple implants are present, with massive hepatic enlargement. Large implants tend to have defective vascular supplies and become centrally necrotic. Massive involvement of the liver is usually present before hepatic failure develops.

GALLBLADDER (p. 875)

Congenital Anomalies (p. 875)

The gallbladder can be congenitally absent or exist in aberrant locations (e.g., embedded in hepatic substance); other variants include a folded fundus *(phrygian cap)* or a duplicated or bilobed gallbladder. There can be agenesis of the common or hepatic bile ducts, or hypoplastic narrowing of the biliary channels.

Cholelithiasis (Gallstones) (p. 875)

More than 95% of biliary tract disease is attributable to cholelithiasis. Gallstones afflict 10% to 20% of adult populations in developed countries; 90% of calculi are *cholesterol stones* (>50% cholesterol monohydrate), with the remainder being pigmented (bilirubin calcium salts). The vast majority of stones remain asymptomatic for decades.

Risk factors for cholesterol gallstones relate to increased hepatic cholesterol uptake or synthesis, or increased biliary cholesterol secretion (p. 876):

- Native Americans; 75% prevalence among Hopi, Navajo, and Pima groups
- Industrialized countries
- Increasing age, female more than male (2:1 ratio)
- Estrogenic influences, including oral contraception and pregnancy
- Obesity, metabolic syndromes, hypercholesterolemia, and rapid weight loss
- Gallbladder stasis, as in spinal cord injury
- Heritable conditions related to hepatic biliary transport (e.g., common variants of the adenosine triphosphate [ATP]-binding cassette sterol transporter encoded by the *ABCG8* gene)

Pathogenesis

- *Cholesterol stones (p. 876):* When cholesterol concentrations exceed the solubilizing capacity of bile salts *(supersaturation)*, cholesterol nucleates into solid cholesterol monohydrate crystals. Four conditions contribute to cholesterol stone formation:
  - Bile must be supersaturated with cholesterol.
  - Gallbladder hypomotility promotes crystal nucleation.
  - Cholesterol nucleation in bile is accelerated by microprecipitates of calcium salts (inorganic or bilirubin salts).
  - Mucus hypersecretion in the gallbladder traps the crystals, permitting aggregation into stones.
- *Pigment stones (p. 876):* Pigment stones form in the setting of unconjugated bilirubin *(most commonly due to chronic hemolytic conditions)* and precipitation of calcium bilirubin salts. In underdeveloped countries, pigmented stones are often formed because biliary infections (e.g., with *Escherichia coli, Ascaris lumbricoides,* or *O. sinensis*) promote bilirubin glucuronide deconjugation.

Morphology (p. 877)

- *Cholesterol stones* arise exclusively in the gallbladder and are classically hard and pale yellow; bilirubin salts can impart a black color. When composed predominantly of cholesterol, they are radiolucent; calcium carbonate deposition in 10% to 20% of stones is sufficient to render them radiopaque. Single stones are ovoid; multiple stones tend to be faceted.
- *Pigmented stones* can be black (sterile gallbladder bile) or brown (with infection); both are soft and usually multiple and 50% to 75% of pigmented stones are radiopaque.

Clinical Features (p. 877)

Approximately 70% to 80% of gallstone patients are asymptomatic throughout life; patients with stones become symptomatic at the rate of 1% to 4% per year, with risk diminishing with time. *Symptoms* include spasmodic, colicky pain, due to passing stones in the bile ducts (smaller stones more commonly cause symptoms than large stones). Associated gallbladder inflammation *(cholecystitis)* generates right upper-abdominal pain. More severe complications include empyema, perforation, fistulas, biliary tree inflammation *(cholangitis)*, obstructive cholestasis or pancreatitis, and erosion of a gallstone into adjacent bowel *(gallstone ileus)*. Clear mucinous secretions in an obstructed gallbladder distend the gallbladder *(mucocele)*. There is also increased risk for gallbladder carcinoma.

Cholecystitis (p. 877)

Acute Cholecystitis (*p. 877*)

Acute cholecystitis is an acute inflammation of the gallbladder precipitated most frequently by gallstone obstruction. The 10% of cases without gallstone obstruction usually occur in severely ill patients.

Pathogenesis (p. 878)

- *Acute calculous cholecystitis* (*with* gallstones) is initiated by chemical irritation of the gallbladder by retained bile acids; there is subsequent release of inflammatory mediators (lysolecithin, prostaglandins), and the gallbladder develops dysmotility. In severe cases distention and increased luminal pressures compromise mucosal blood flow causing ischemia; bacterial contamination can be a late complication.
- *Acute acalculous cholecystitis* results from ischemia due to diminished flow in the end-arterial cystic artery circulation; it occurs in the setting of sepsis with hypotension and multiorgan failure, immunosuppression, major trauma or burns, diabetes mellitus, or infections.

Morphology (p. 878)

In acute cholecystitis there is an enlarged, tense, bright red to blotchy green-black gallbladder with a serosal fibrinous exudate. Luminal contents range from turbid to purulent. In severe cases the gallbladder is transformed into a green-black necrotic organ *(gangrenous cholecystitis)* with multiple perforations. In milder cases there is only gallbladder wall edema and hyperemia.

Clinical Features (p. 878)

Acute cholecystitis may be mild and intermittent or may be a surgical emergency. *Symptoms* include right upper-quadrant or epigastric pain, fever, anorexia, tachycardia, diaphoresis, and nausea and vomiting. Jaundice suggests common bile duct obstruction.

Self-limited attacks subside over several days; up to 25% of patients develop more severe symptoms and require surgical intervention. In severely ill patients with acalculous cholecystitis, symptoms may not be evident due to the comorbid conditions, and the mortality rate is higher.

Chronic Cholecystitis (*p. 878*)

Chronic cholecystitis can be a consequence of repeated bouts of acute cholecystitis but often develops without antecedent attacks. Although gallstones are usually present (90%), they may not play a direct role in initiating inflammation. Rather, chronic bile supersaturation with cholesterol permits cholesterol suffusion of the gallbladder wall and initiation of inflammation and gallbladder dysmotility. Patient populations and symptoms are the same as for the acute cholecystitis.

Morphology (p. 878)

Gallbladders can be contracted (from fibrosis), normal in size, or enlarged (from obstruction). The wall is variably thickened and gray-white. The mucosa is generally preserved but may be atrophied. Cholesterol-laden macrophages in the lamina propria are common *(cholesterolosis)* and gallstones are frequent. Inflammation is variable with occasional mucosal outpouchings *(Rokitansky-Aschoff sinuses)*. Rarely there is mural dystrophic calcification *(porcelain gallbladder)* or a fibrosed, nodular gallbladder with marked histiocytic inflammation *(xanthogranulomatous cholecystitis)*.

Clinical Features (p. 879)

Recurrent attacks of steady or colicky epigastric or right upper-quadrant pain occur. Complications are the same as for acute cholecystitis, including bacterial superinfection, gallbladder perforation and abscess formation or peritonitis, and the formation of biliary-enteric fistulas.

Carcinoma (p. 879)

Carcinoma of the gallbladder is slightly more common in women, typically presenting over age 70. Gallstones coexist in 95% of U.S. patients; chronic gallbladder inflammation (with or without stones) is a critical risk factor. Gallstones are less common precursors in Asian populations, where pyogenic and parasitic diseases dominate as causes. Gallbladder cancers harbor recurrent molecular alterations: ERBB2 (Her-2/neu) is overexpressed in 30% to 60% of cases and mutations of chromatin remodeling genes (*PBRM1* and *MLL3*) occur in a quarter of cases.

Morphology (p. 880)

Tumors may be *infiltrating*, with diffuse gallbladder thickening and induration, or *exophytic*—growing into the lumen as an irregular, cauliflower-like mass. Most gallbladder carcinomas are adenocarcinomas; the histologic appearance can vary from papillary to infiltrating and can range from moderately differentiated to undifferentiated. Rarely there are squamous, adenosquamous, carcinoid, or mesenchymal variants. Tumors spread by local invasion of liver, extension to cystic duct and portohepatic lymph nodes, and metastatic seeding of peritoneum, viscera, and lungs.

Clinical Features (p. 880)

Symptoms are insidious and indistinguishable from those caused by cholelithiasis. Tumors are usually unresectable when discovered.

19

The Pancreas

Congenital Anomalies (p. 883)

Pancreas Divisum (p. 883)

The most common of pancreatic congenital anomalies (3% to 10% incidence). Failure of the ventral and dorsal fetal duct systems to fuse causes the bulk of pancreatic secretions to drain through the smaller minor papilla (rather than the large-caliber papilla of Vater); the relative stenosis predisposes to chronic pancreatitis.

Annular Pancreas (p. 883)

A bandlike ring of normal pancreatic tissue completely encircles the second portion of the duodenum and can cause duodenal obstruction.

Ectopic Pancreas (p. 883)

Pancreatic parenchyma in an abnormal location is common (2% incidence); sites include stomach, duodenum, jejunum, Meckel diverticulum, and ileum. These are typically submucosal, can be single or multiple, and measure several millimeters to a few centimeters. Although mostly asymptomatic, they can cause inflammation and pain or rarely mucosal bleeding.

Agenesis (p. 884)

Some cases of congenital pancreatic absence are associated with homozygous germline mutations of the *PDX1* gene, encoding a homeobox transcription factor.

Pancreatitis (p. 884)

The pancreas protects itself from enzymatic autodigestion through the following mechanisms:

- Digestive enzymes are synthesized as inactive proenzymes *(zymogens)*, packaged within secretory granules.
- Zymogens are typically cleaved to become functional enzymes by trypsin, which itself is not activated until the precursor trypsinogen encounters duodenal enteropeptidase (enterokinase) in the small bowel.
- Acinar and ductal cells secrete trypsin inhibitors, including *serine protease inhibitor Kazal type l (SPINK1)*, that limit intrapancreatic trypsin activation.
- Low calcium induces trypsin to cleave and inactivate itself.

Pancreatitis occurs when these protective mechanisms are unbalanced. Pancreatitis is divided into two forms, *acute* and *chronic;*

although both are initiated by injuries causing pancreatic autodigestion, they have different characteristic pathologic and clinical features.

Acute Pancreatitis (p. 884)

Acute pancreatitis is reversible parenchymal damage associated with inflammation; 80% of cases are associated with biliary tract disease (mostly gallstones) or alcoholism (Table 19-1).

Pathogenesis (p. 884)

Acute pancreatitis results from inappropriate release and activation of pancreatic enzymes, which digest parenchyma and elicit inflammation; in particular, untimely activation of trypsinogen is a key triggering event.

- Proelastase and prophospholipase are proteolytically activated, damaging blood vessels and adipose tissue, respectively.
- Trypsin converts prekallikrein to kallikrein, which activates both kinin and factor XII, the latter initiating the complement and coagulation pathways.
- Pancreatic inflammation and thrombosis damage acinar cells and amplify intraparenchymal enzyme activation.

Mechanisms underlying pancreatic enzyme activation are as follows:

- *Pancreatic duct obstruction* can occur through gallstones or sludge in the ampulla of Vater, periampullary neoplasms, choledochoceles (congenital cystic dilations of the common bile duct), parasites (e.g., *Ascaris lumbricoides*), or congenital anomalies, such as pancreas divisum. Such obstruction leads to interstitial accumulation of enzyme-rich fluid; lipase in this fluid (synthesized in an activated form) causes fat necrosis, with subsequent parenchymal release of proinflammatory cytokines. The resulting inflammation and interstitial edema compromises vascular flow, adding ischemia to the ongoing parenchymal injury.

TABLE 19-1 Etiologic Factors in Acute Pancreatitis
Metabolic
Alcoholism
Hyperlipoproteinemia
Hypercalcemia
Drugs (e.g., azathioprine)
Genetic
Mutations in genes encoding trypsin, trypsin regulators, or proteins that regulate calcium metabolism
Mechanical
Gallstones
Trauma
Iatrogenic injury
Operative injury
Endoscopic procedures with dye injection
Vascular
Shock
Atheroembolism
Vasculitis
Infectious
Mumps

- *Primary acinar cell injury* can occur through oxidative stress, leading to the generation of NF-κB transcription factors that induce cytokines that drive inflammatory responses. Increased calcium levels by any mechanism increases enzyme activation by abrogating the autoinhibition of trypsin self-digestion.
- *Defective intracellular transport of proenzymes within acinar cells:* Exocrine enzymes that are misdirected toward lysosomes rather than toward secretion pathways result in lysosomal hydrolysis of the proenzymes with enzyme activation and release.
- *Alcohol* has a direct toxic effect on pancreatic acinar cells and also increases oxidative stress. Alcohol can also result in functional obstruction by (1) contracting the sphincter at the ampulla of Vater and (2) increasing pancreatic protein secretion, leading to inspissated protein plugs that block small ducts.
- *Metabolic disorders* can result in hypertriglyceridemia and hypercalcemic states (e.g., due to hyperparathyroidism).
- *Medications:* Agents ranging from furosemide to estrogens to chemotherapeutic agents; most mechanisms are unknown.
- *Physical injury of acinar cells* (e.g., through blunt abdominal trauma or during surgery or endoscopic retrograde cholangiopancreatography).
- *Ischemic injury of acinar cells* (e.g., due to shock, vascular thrombosis, embolism, or vasculitis).
- *Infections* (e.g., mumps) can cause direct acinar cell injury.
- *Cystic fibrosis* (see Chapter 10) is associated with pancreatitis, particularly in patients with concurrent *SPINK1* mutations. Mutations in the cystic fibrosis conductance regulator gene (CFTR) decrease bicarbonate secretion by pancreatic ductal cells, promoting protein plugging and duct obstruction.
- *Hereditary pancreatitis* (p. 886) is characterized by recurrent bouts of pancreatitis typically beginning in childhood. Most cases have autosomal dominant gain-of-function mutations in the cationic trypsinogen gene *(PRSS1)*, rendering activated trypsin resistant to its own self-inactivation. Others have inactivating autosomal recessive mutations in *SPINK1;* altered proteins fail to inhibit trypsin activity. Patients with hereditary pancreatitis have a 40% lifetime risk of developing pancreatic cancer.

Morphology *(p. 887)*

Acute pancreatitis can range from mild interstitial edema and inflammation to extensive necrosis and hemorrhage. Basic features include the following:

- Vascular leakage causing edema
- Necrosis of regional fat by lipolytic enzymes
- Acute inflammation
- Proteolytic destruction of the pancreatic substance
- Vascular injury with subsequent interstitial hemorrhage

Mild (acute interstitial) pancreatitis shows only the first three of these. *Acute necrotizing pancreatitis* exhibits gray-white parenchymal necrosis and chalky white fat necrosis. In acute hemorrhagic pancreatitis there is patchy red-black hemorrhage interspersed with fat necrosis.

Clinical Features *(p. 887)*

Patients typically present with abdominal pain, nausea, and anorexia, along with elevated plasma levels of pancreatic enzymes (amylase and lipase). Full-blown acute pancreatitis is a medical emergency presenting with "acute abdomen" (intense abdominal pain), peripheral vascular collapse, and shock from explosive activation of the systemic inflammatory response. Death (5% of patients) can occur from shock, acute respiratory distress syndrome, or acute renal failure.

Laboratory findings include marked serum amylase (and later, lipase) elevations; glycosuria occurs occasionally. Hypocalcemia results from precipitation of calcium soaps in the fat necrosis. In approximately half of cases the necrotic debris becomes secondarily infected.

Treatment involves restricting oral intake to "rest" the pancreas, with analgesia, nutrition, and volume support. The pancreas can return to normal function if the acute pancreatitis resolves. Possible sequelae include sterile *pancreatic abscesses* from tissue liquefaction and *pancreatic pseudocysts*—localized collections of necrotic, hemorrhagic material rich in pancreatic enzymes.

Chronic Pancreatitis (p. 888)

Chronic pancreatitis is defined as inflammation with *irreversible parenchymal destruction and fibrosis;* in late stages the endocrine parenchyma is also destroyed. Incidence ranges from 0.04% to 5% of the population; the typical patient is a middle-aged male. Causes overlap with those of acute pancreatitis, but long-term alcohol abuse is most common; approximately a quarter of chronic pancreatitis has a genetic basis. Long-standing pancreatic duct obstruction (calculi or neoplasm) and autoimmune injury are other etiologies.

Pathogenesis *(p. 888)*

Most patients with recurrent bouts of acute pancreatitis develop chronic pancreatitis.

- *Acute pancreatitis* causes perilobular fibrosis, duct distortion, and altered pancreatic secretions.
- *Local inflammatory mediator production* causes acinar cell death; fibrogenic cytokines (e.g., transforming growth factor-β [TGF-β]) and platelet-derived growth factor (PDGF) promote fibrosis by activating periacinar myofibroblasts (Fig. 19-1)
- *Autoimmune pancreatitis* is associated with immunoglobulin (Ig) G4-secreting plasma cells and is a manifestation of IgG4-related disease (see Chapter 6)

Morphology *(p. 888)*

There is replacement of pancreatic acinar tissue by dense, fibrous connective tissue, with relative sparing of the islets of Langerhans until late stage. The pancreas is hard with focal calcification. Chronic pancreatitis associated with alcohol abuse displays ductal dilation with intraluminal calcifications and protein plugs. *Autoimmune pancreatitis* is characterized by a mixed inflammatory cell infiltrate, venulitis, and increased numbers of IgG4-producing plasma cells.

Clinical Features *(p. 889)*

Chronic pancreatitis can be silent or heralded by recurrent attacks of pain and/or jaundice. Episodes can be precipitated by alcohol abuse, overeating (increasing pancreatic demand), and opiates (or other drugs) that increase the tone of the sphincter of Oddi. Late complications relate primarily to the loss of exocrine and endocrine function:

- Malabsorption
- Diabetes mellitus
- Pseudocysts

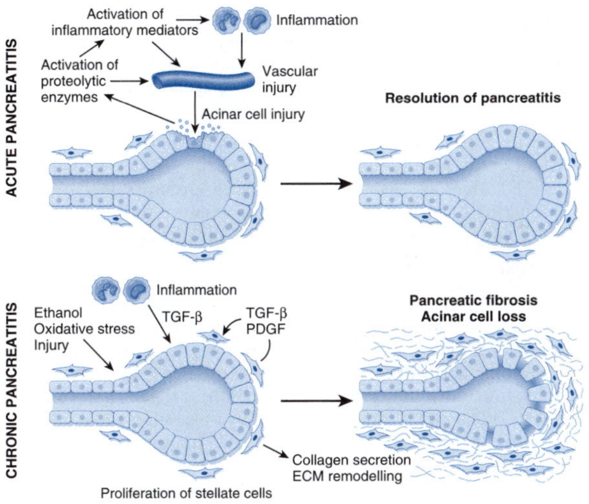

Figure 19-1 Comparison of the mediators in acute and chronic pancreatitis. In *acute pancreatitis (top),* acinar injury results in release of proteolytic enzymes, leading to activation of the clotting cascade, acute and chronic inflammation, vascular injury, and edema. In most cases, complete resolution occurs with restoration of acinar cell mass. In *chronic pancreatitis (bottom),* repeated episodes of acinar cell injury induce profibrogenic cytokines, such as TGF-β and PDGF. These drive myofibroblast proliferation, collagen secretion, and extracellular matrix (ECM) remodeling. Repeated injury produces irreversible fibrosis, with loss of acinar cell mass and ultimately pancreatic insufficiency.

The long-term outlook is poor, with mortality rates of 50% within 20 to 25 years.

Non-Neoplastic Cysts (p. 889)

Congenital Cysts (p. 889)

Congenital cysts are caused by anomalous development of the pancreatic ducts; in *congenital polycystic disease* (see Chapter 20), they frequently coexist with kidney and liver cysts. In *von Hippel-Lindau disease* (see Chapter 28), pancreatic cysts and angiomas of the central nervous system are seen. They are usually unilocular and thin-walled with a cuboidal epithelial lining.

Pseudocysts (p. 889)

Pseudocysts are collections of necrotic, hemorrhagic material rich in pancreatic enzymes; formed by walling off areas of fat necrosis, they account for 75% of pancreatic cysts. They are not lined by epithelium (thus "pseudocysts") but rather are encircled by fibrosed granulation tissue. They occur after bouts of acute pancreatitis or following trauma. Although many spontaneously resolve, they can become secondarily infected or compress adjacent structures.

Neoplasms (p. 890)

Neoplasms of the pancreas are broadly grouped as cystic or solid.

Cystic Neoplasms (p. 890)

Only 5% to 15% of pancreatic cysts are neoplasms, and cystic tumors constitute fewer than 5% of pancreatic neoplasms; they typically present as painless, slow-growing masses.

- *Serous cystic neoplasms (serous cystadenomas):* Constituting 25% of all cystic neoplasms, these are typically seen in women over age 60; they are usually solitary, well-circumscribed nodules occurring in the pancreatic tail with a central stellate scar. *VHL* tumor suppressor gene inactivation is the most common genetic abnormality. These are almost always benign and resection is curative.
- *Mucinous cystic neoplasm:* Almost 95% occur in women, and most arise as slow-growing, painless masses in the pancreatic tail. These multiloculated cystic neoplasms are lined by mucin-producing columnar cells within a dense stroma, and the cysts are filled with thick mucinous material. One third of these lesions harbor an invasive adenocarcinoma; when noninvasive, surgical resection is curative. *KRAS* and the *TP53* and *RNF43* tumor suppressor genes are frequently mutated.
- *Intraductal papillary mucinous neoplasm (IPMN):* These are intraductal, mucin-producing neoplasms, more common in men than women. Most arise in the head of the gland, and 10% to 20% are multifocal. They differ from mucinous cystic neoplasms by lacking an associated dense stroma and by involving a larger pancreatic duct but have a similar malignant potential. These are frequently associated with *KRAS, GNAS, TP53, SMAD4,* and *RNF43* mutations.
- *Solid-pseudopapillary tumor:* These round, well-circumscribed neoplasms have solid and cystic regions; they occur mainly in young women and cause abdominal discomfort due to their large size. These tumors are almost always associated with hyperactivation of the Wnt signaling pathway due to activating mutations of the *CTNNB1* (β-catenin) oncogene. Although some are locally aggressive, complete resection is usually curative.

Pancreatic Carcinoma (p. 892)

Pancreatic cancer is an *infiltrating ductal adenocarcinoma;* it is the fourth leading cause of cancer deaths in the United States.

Precursors to Pancreatic Cancer (p. 892)

There is a progression from non-neoplastic epithelium to small ductal noninvasive lesions to invasive carcinoma (Fig. 19-2). The precursor lesions are called pancreatic intraepithelial neoplasms (PanINs); these show characteristic genetic and epigenetic alterations, as well as dramatic telomere shortening that may predispose to additional progressive chromosomal aberrations.

Pathogenesis (p. 892)

Multiple genes are somatically mutated or epigenetically silenced in pancreatic carcinoma; the patterns of genetic alterations in pancreatic carcinoma as a group differ from those seen in other malignancies (Table 19-2).

- *KRAS* (p. 892) is the most frequently altered oncogene in pancreatic cancer (90% to 95% of cases), resulting in a constitutively active protein and augmented proliferation and cell survival via the MAP kinase and PI3 kinase-AKT pathways (see Chapter 7).

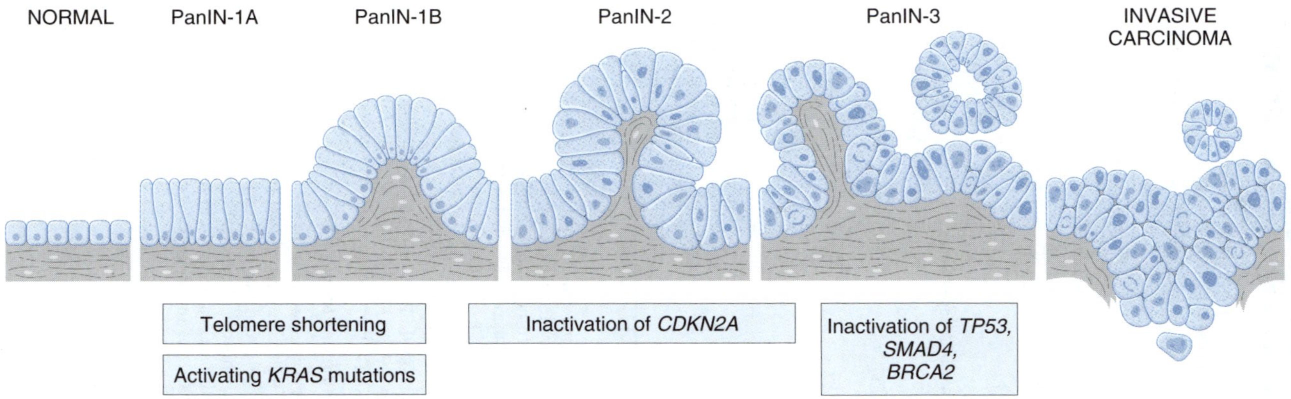

Figure 19-2 Model for the progression from normal duct epithelium *(far left)* through PanINs *(center)* to invasive carcinoma *(far right)*. It is postulated that telomere shortening and mutations of the oncogene *KRAS* occur early, that inactivation of the *CDKN2A* tumor suppressor gene that encodes the cell cycle regulator p16 occurs in intermediate grade lesions, and that the inactivation of the *TP53*, *SMAD4*, and *BRCA2* tumor suppressor genes occur in higher grade (PanIN-3) lesions. Although there is a general temporal sequence of changes, the buildup of multiple mutations is more important than the specific order of their accumulation. *(Adapted from Wilentz RE, Iacobuzio-Donahue CA, Argani P, et al: Loss of expression of DPC4 in pancreatic intraepithelial neoplasia: evidence that DPC4 inactivation occurs late in neoplastic progression.* Cancer Res *2000;60:2002.)*

TABLE 19-2 Somatic Molecular Alterations in Invasive Pancreatic Adenocarcinoma

Gene	Chromosomal Region	Percentage of Carcinoma With Genetic Alteration	Gene Function
Oncogenes			
KRAS	12p	90	Growth factor signal transducer
AKT2	19q	10-20	Growth factor signal transducer
MYB	6q	10	Transcription factor
NCOA3/AIB1	20q	10	Chromatin regulator
MAP2K4/MKK4	17p	5	Growth factor signal transducer
Tumor Suppressor and DNA Repair Genes			
p16/CDKN2A	9p	95	Negative cell cycle regulator
TP53	17p	50-70	Response to DNA damage
SMAD4	18q	55	TGF-β pathway
GATA-6	18q	10	Transcription factor
RB	13q	5	Negative cell cycle regulator
STK11	19p	5	Regulation of cellular metabolism
ATM	11q	5	DNA damage response
ARID1A	1p	4	Chromatin regulator
TGFBR1	9q	2	TGF-β pathway
TGFBR2	3p	2	TGF-β pathway

- *CDKN2A* (p. 893) is inactivated in 95% of cases, resulting in loss of an important cell cycle checkpoint.
- *SMAD4* (p. 893) is a tumor suppressor gene that is inactivated in more than half of pancreatic cancers; it encodes a protein critical for TGF-β receptor signal transduction.
- *TP53* (p. 893) inactivation occurs in 70% to 75% of pancreatic cancers; it leads to loss of a cell cycle checkpoint and loss of a protein that induces apoptosis and cell senescence.
- *DNA methylation abnormalities* (p. 893) with hypermethylation (and thus silencing) of several tumor suppressor genes.

Epidemiology and Inheritance (p. 893)

Approximately 80% of cases occur in individuals aged 60 to 80 and is more common in blacks than whites; smoking increases the risk approximately twofold. Chronic pancreatitis, consumption of a diet rich in fats, a family history of pancreatic cancer (*BRCA2* mutations account for 10% of pancreatic cancer in Ashkenazi Jews), germline mutations in CDKN2A, and diabetes mellitus impose a modestly increased risk.

Morphology (p. 893)

Approximately 60% of pancreatic cancers arise in the head of the gland, 15% occur in the body, 5% in the tail, and 20% diffusely involve the organ. These are typically highly invasive and elicit an intense host scarring response ("desmoplasia"). Most carcinomas in the head of the pancreas obstruct the distal common bile duct bile leading to jaundice; conversely, cancers of the body and tail can remain clinically silent for long periods of time and are often large or widely metastatic when initially discovered. Extensive perineural and vascular invasion are common. *Microscopically* the neoplastic cells commonly form moderately differentiated glandular patterns resembling ductal epithelium.

Clinical Features (p. 894)

Weight loss and pain are typical presenting symptoms; obstructive jaundice develops with tumors in the head of the gland. Metastases are common, and >80% of pancreatic adenocarcinomas are unresectable at presentation; massive liver metastasis frequently develops. The outlook is dismal: first-year mortality rate exceeds 80% and the 5-year survival rate is <5%. Migratory thrombophlebitis (*Trousseau syndrome;* see Chapter 4) can occur with pancreatic neoplasms (as well as other adenocarcinomas).

Acinar Cell Carcinoma (p. 895)

These tumors exhibit acinar cell differentiation, with zymogen granules and the production of exocrine enzymes (e.g., trypsin; lipase release causes metastatic fat necrosis in 15% of patients).

Pancreatoblastoma (p. 895)

These are rare malignant tumors, primarily seen in childhood; microscopically these consist of squamous islands admixed with acinar cells.

20 The Kidney

More than a half million in the United States have end-stage renal disease (ESRD); two thirds require dialysis, costing over $40 billion annually. One-year mortality for ESRD exceeds that of most newly diagnosed cancers. Globally, acute kidney injury occurs in more than 2 million people; it is a major risk factor for chronic kidney disease (CKD) and ESRD.

Renal diseases can be categorized based on the four basic anatomic compartments affected:

- Glomeruli (often immunologically mediated injury)
- Tubules (frequently toxic or infectious injury)
- Interstitium
- Blood vessels

Many disorders affect more than one structure; the anatomic interdependence of these compartments means that damage to one will usually secondarily affect the others. Whatever the initial insult, all forms of *chronic renal disease* ultimately destroy all four kidney elements, culminating in end-stage disease.

Clinical Manifestations of Renal Diseases (p. 898)

Important terms include the following:

- *Azotemia:* Elevation of the blood urea nitrogen (BUN) and creatinine levels, largely due to decreased glomerular filtration rate (GFR).
- *Prerenal azotemia* occurs with kidney hypoperfusion (e.g., with congestive heart failure, shock, volume depletion, or hemorrhage).
- *Postrenal azotemia* occurs when urinary outflow is obstructed after exiting the kidney.
- *Uremia* is the constellation of clinical signs and symptoms associated with azotemia; these include metabolic, hematologic, endocrine, gastrointestinal (GI), neural, and cardiovascular effects.

Renal diseases typically manifest as clinically recognizable syndromes; many—but not all—primarily affect glomeruli:

- *Nephritic syndrome* (hematuria, mild-to-moderate proteinuria, and hypertension) is due to glomerular injury.
- *Rapidly progressive glomerulonephritis* (RPGN) is a nephritic syndrome with a rapid (hour to days) decline in GFR.
- *Nephrotic syndrome* (>3.5 g/day proteinuria, hypoalbuminemia, edema, hyperlipidemia, and lipiduria) is also due to glomerular injury.
- *Asymptomatic hematuria or proteinuria* is usually a manifestation of mild glomerular injury.
- The progression from normal renal function to symptomatic CKD progresses through stages defined by measures of creatinine that allow estimation of GFR.
- *Acute tubular injury (ATI)* is manifested by rapid (hours to days) decline in GFR and resulting azotemia; it can result from injury to any kidney anatomic compartment.

- *CKD* is characterized by significant reduction in GFR lasting >3 months and/or prolonged albuminuria; it is the end stage of all chronic renal diseases (with diabetes and hypertension being the major causes) and affects 11% of all adults in the United States.
- *ESRD* (<5% of normal GFR).

Other forms of kidney injury include the following:

- *Renal tubular defects*—due to disorders of tubules and/or interstitium—manifest with polyuria and electrolyte abnormalities.
- *Urinary tract obstruction* and *renal tumors* have varied clinical manifestations based on the specific anatomic location and nature of the lesion.
- *Urinary tract infections* (UTIs) can affect the kidney *(pyelonephritis)* or bladder *(cystitis).*
- *Nephrolithiasis (renal stones)* is manifested by renal colic and hematuria.

Glomerular Diseases (p. 899)

- *Primary glomerulonephritis (GN):* Renal glomeruli are the principal target of injury.
- *Secondary glomerular disease:* Glomeruli are damaged by a systemic disease (e.g., hypertension, vasculitis, diabetes, amyloidosis).

Clinical manifestations and glomerular histologic changes can be similar in primary and secondary forms of injury.

Table 20-1 lists the most common forms of glomerular diseases. The clinical manifestations of such disorders can be organized into the five major glomerular syndromes summarized in Table 20-2.

TABLE 20-1 Glomerular Diseases
Primary Glomerulopathies
Acute proliferative GN
Postinfectious
Other
Rapidly progressive (crescentic) GN
MGN
MCD
FSGS
MPGN
Dense deposit disease
IgA nephropathy
Chronic GN
Systemic Diseases With Glomerular Involvement
SLE
Diabetes mellitus
Amyloidosis
Goodpasture syndrome
Microscopic polyarteritis/polyangiitis
Wegener granulomatosis
Henoch-Schönlein purpura
Bacterial endocarditis
Hereditary Disorders
Alport syndrome
Thin basement membrane disease
Fabry disease

Pathologic Responses of the Glomerulus to Injury (p. 902)

Hypercellularity: Glomerular inflammatory diseases exhibit increased cellularity due to (1) proliferation of mesangial and endothelial cells, (2) infiltration of leukocytes, and (3) proliferation of glomerular epithelial cells to form *crescents.*

Basement Membrane Thickening: Capillary wall thickening is visualized by light microscopy using the periodic acid-Schiff stain; electron microscopy (EM) shows this is to be composed of subendothelial or subepithelial depositions of immune complexes, fibrin, amyloid, and cryoglobulins, in addition to increased synthesis of basement membrane components.

Hyalinosis and Sclerosis: Hyalinosis results from injury to endothelium and capillary walls leading to plasma proteins insudating in extravascular spaces; *sclerosis* reflects deposition of extracellular collagenous matrix.

Lesions may be *diffuse* (involving all glomeruli) or *focal* (involving a fraction of glomeruli). They can also be *global* (involving the entire glomerulus) or *segmental* (involving just a part of any given glomerulus). Finally, lesions can be classified as *capillary loop* or *mesangial,* meaning they only affect those.

Pathogenesis of Glomerular Injury (p. 903)

Although nonimmune factors can initiate GN or influence its progression, *immune mechanisms underlie most forms of glomerular injury* (Table 20-3). Thus immunoglobulin (Ig) deposition—either

TABLE 20-2 Glomerular Syndromes

Syndrome	Manifestations
Nephritic syndrome	Hematuria, azotemia, variable proteinuria, oliguria, edema, and hypertension
RPGN	Acute nephritis, proteinuria, and acute renal failure
Nephrotic syndrome	>3.5 g/day proteinuria, hypoalbuminemia, hyperlipidemia, lipiduria
Chronic renal failure	Azotemia → uremia progressing for months to years
Isolated urinary abnormalities	Glomerular hematuria and/or subnephrotic proteinuria

TABLE 20-3 Immune Mechanisms of Glomerular Injury

Antibody-Mediated Injury

In Situ Immune Complex Deposition

Fixed intrinsic tissue antigens
NC1 domain of type IV collagen antigen (anti-GBM nephritis)
PLA2R antigen (membranous glomerulopathy)
Mesangial antigens
Others
Planted antigens
Exogenous (infectious agents, drugs)
Endogenous (DNA, nuclear proteins, Igs, immune complexes, IgA)

Circulating Immune Complex Deposition

Endogenous antigens (e.g., DNA, tumor antigens)
Exogenous antigens (e.g., infectious products)

Cell-Mediated Immune Injury

Activation of Alternative Complement Pathway

directly or as antigen-antibody complexes—along with activated complement and/or recruited inflammatory cells is found in the glomeruli of the majority of GN patients (Fig. 20-1).

Diseases Caused by in Situ Formation of Immune Complexes (p. 903)

Antibodies can react directly with intrinsic matrix or cellular (endothelial, mesangial, or epithelial) antigens or with circulating antigens that have been "trapped" in the glomerulus.

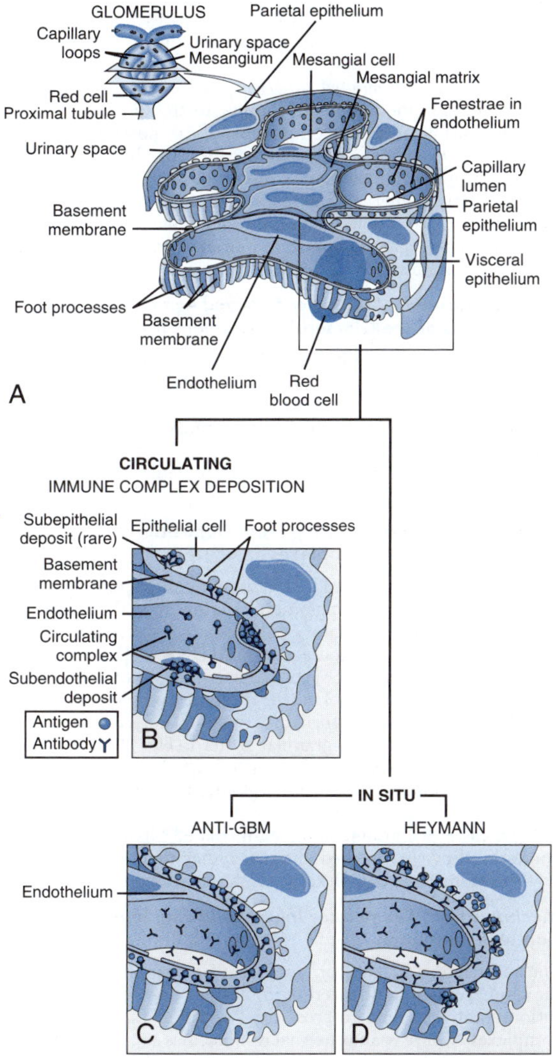

Figure 20-1 **A,** Schematic representation of a portion of a glomerulus. **B-D,** Antibody-mediated glomerular injury can result either from the deposition of circulating immune complexes **(B)** or from in situ formation of complexes exemplified by anti-GBM disease **(C)** or Heymann nephritis **(D)**.

Heymann nephritis is an experimental rat model of GN that involves immunization with renal tubular proteins (Fig. 20-1, *D*); immunized animals develop antibodies to a *megalin* protein antigen expressed on the basal surface of visceral epithelial cells. Antibody binding to megalin results in localized immune complex formation.

In the majority of human membranous GN the antigen that drives a similar process is *M-type phospholipase A_2 receptor (PLA2R);* antibody binding to PLA2R leads to complement activation and subsequent shedding of immune complexes that deposit along the subepithelial aspect of the basement membrane. This is reflected as a thickened membrane by light microscopy, a *granular* pattern of immunofluorescence staining for Ig and activated complement, and subepithelial electron dense deposits by EM.

Antibodies against planted antigens (p. 904) cause similar pathology. Circulating molecules can localize to the kidney by interaction with various intrinsic components of the glomerulus; cationic molecules (DNA, nucleosomes, microbial products, drugs, and aggregated proteins, including immune complexes) all have affinity for the anionic glomerular basement membrane (GBM) and can become trapped. Antibodies that bind to these planted antigens often induce a discrete, granular pattern of Ig and complement immunofluorescence staining (Fig. 20-1, *B*).

Disease Caused by Antibodies Directed Against Normal Components of the Glomerular Basement Membrane *(p. 905)*

Anti-GBM antibody-induced GN is an autoimmune disease in which antibodies are directed against intrinsic, fixed antigens of the GBM; the classic anti-GBM disorder is Goodpasture syndrome, in which the autoantibody binds the noncollagenous domain of the $\alpha3$ chain of type IV collagen. Such autoantibodies typically yield a linear immunofluorescence staining pattern (Fig. 20-1, *C*).

Glomerulonephritis Resulting From Deposition of Circulating Immune Complexes *(p. 905)*

Glomerular injury is caused by the trapping of circulating antigen-antibody complexes within glomeruli, followed by the activation of complement and inflammatory cells bearing Fc receptors. Antigens can be endogenous (e.g., double-stranded DNA [dsDNA] in systemic lupus erythematosus [SLE]) or exogenous (e.g., infectious agents) but in most cases are not known. Immune complex deposits can be subendothelial, subepithelial, or mesangial, and immunofluorescence staining shows a granular pattern (Fig. 20-1, *A*); the site of localization in the glomerulus depends on the charge and size of the immune complexes, as well as glomerular hemodynamics and mesangial function.

Most cases of immune complex-mediated GN are due to antibodies binding to adsorbed antigen, rather than to deposition of preformed immune complexes from the circulation.

Mechanisms of Glomerular Injury Following Immune Complex Formation *(p. 905)*

The localization of antigen, antibody, or immune complexes in the glomerulus is influenced by molecular charge and size. Thus cationic antigens tend to cross the GBM and form subepithelial complexes, whereas anionic macromolecules are trapped subendothelially; molecules with neutral charge tend to accumulate in the mesangium. Large complexes are not usually nephritogenic because mononuclear phagocytes clear them before they can access the kidney. The pattern of localization also influences the type of subsequent injury and the histologic features that develop. Thus subendothelial immune complexes are accessible to the circulation and more likely to involve leukocytes. Conversely, immune complexes confined to subepithelial locations (where the basement membrane prevents interaction with circulating leukocytes) typically have a noninflammatory pathology.

Cell-Mediated Immunity in Glomerulonephritis (p. 906)

Although antibody-mediated mechanisms underlie many forms of GN, sensitized T cells can potentially contribute (e.g., direct cytotoxicity or released cytokines may cause foot process effacement or epithelial detachment leading to proteinuria).

Activation of Alternative Complement Pathway (p. 906)

Activation of the alternative complement pathway occurs in dense deposit disease and in diseases termed C3 glomerulopathies.

Mediators of Glomerular Injury (p. 907)

Activated complement fragments are chemotactic, and Ig localized in glomeruli binds Fc-receptor-bearing cells; activated T cells also secrete a host of chemokines that recruit cellular effectors. Injury ensues through the following mechanisms (Fig. 20-2):

Cells (p. 907)

- *Neutrophils and monocytes* release proteases, oxygen-derived free radicals, and arachidonic acid metabolites.
- *Macrophages and T lymphocytes* release cytokines and growth factors.
- *Platelets* aggregate and release eicosanoids and growth factors.
- *Resident glomerular cells (particularly mesangial cells)* produce cytokines, growth factors, chemokines, oxygen free radicals, eicosanoids, and endothelin.

Soluble Mediators (p. 907)

- *Complement activation: C5b-C9* (membrane attack complex) causes cell lysis and induces mesangial cell activation.
- *Eicosanoids, nitric oxide (NO), angiotensin, and endothelin* affect vascular flow.

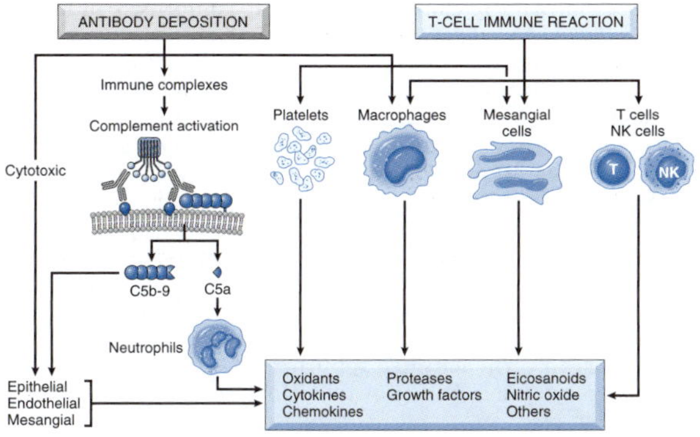

Figure 20-2 Mediators of immune glomerular injury.

- *Cytokines* (especially *interleukin [IL]-1* and *tumor necrosis factor [TNF]*) and *chemokines* (e.g., *CCL5*) influence inflammatory cell adhesion and recruitment.
- *Chemokines: Platelet-derived growth factor (PDGF)* influences mesangial cell proliferation; *transforming growth factor-β* and *fibroblast growth factor* affect matrix deposition; and *vascular endothelial growth factor (VEGF)* maintains endothelial integrity and regulates capillary permeability.
- *Coagulation proteins,* especially fibrin, can stimulate parietal epithelial cell proliferation *(crescent formation).*

Epithelial Cell Injury *(p. 908)*

Podocytes have very limited capacity to regenerate, and their injury is a common feature of virtually any form of glomerular disease. Such *podocytopathy* can be caused by antibodies to podocyte antigens, toxins, cytokines, or infections; it is manifested initially by loss of normal slit diaphragms and progresses to foot process effacement, vacuolization, and podocyte detachment from the GBM; functionally this results in proteinuria. Mutations in slit diaphragm components, such as nephrin and podocin, can also underlie hereditary forms of nephrotic syndrome without any glomerular inflammatory damage.

Mechanisms of Progression in Glomerular Diseases *(p. 908)*

Regardless of etiology, once GFR is reduced to 30% to 50% of normal, progression to end-stage renal failure proceeds at a relatively constant rate. There are two major features of progressive renal damage:

- *Focal segmental glomerulosclerosis (FSGS)* (p. 908) is initiated as an *adaptive change* in the relatively unaffected glomeruli of diseased kidneys. *Compensatory hypertrophy* of the remaining glomeruli putatively preserves renal function; however, proteinuria and segmental glomerulosclerosis soon develop, followed by total glomerular scarring and uremia. Glomerular hypertrophy is driven by *hemodynamic changes,* including increased glomerular blood flow, filtration, and transcapillary pressure *(glomerular hypertension),* often with systemic hypertension. In this setting, endothelial and epithelial injury lead to protein accumulation, followed by macrophage recruitment, mesangial cell activation, and increased matrix synthesis. This is compounded by the fact that mature visceral epithelial cells (podocytes) cannot proliferate after injury, and loss leads to either abnormal stretching of neighbors to compensate or uncovered (leaky) basement membrane. Ultimately a vicious cycle of glomerular scarring supervenes; as glomeruli sclerose and drop out, the remaining glomeruli undergo the same compensatory changes that will ultimately result in *their* fibrosis.
- *Tubulointerstitial fibrosis* (p. 909). Tubulointerstitial injury is a component of many forms of acute and chronic GN; indeed renal function generally correlates better with the extent of tubulointerstitial damage than with the severity of glomerular injury. Tubulointerstitial injury results from ischemia (diminished perfusion downstream of sclerotic glomeruli or damaged capillaries) and inflammation in the surrounding interstitium. Proteinuria also causes direct injury to and activation of tubular cells. In turn, activated tubular cells elaborate proinflammatory cytokines and growth factors that drive interstitial fibrosis.

Table 20-4 summarizes the main clinical and pathologic features of the major forms of primary glomerulonephritides.

TABLE 20-4 Summary of Major Primary Glomerulonephritides

			Glomerular Pathology		
Disease	**Most Frequent Clinical Presentation**	**Pathogenesis**	**Light Microscopy**	**Fluorescence Microscopy**	**EM**
Postinfectious GN	Nephritic syndrome	Immune complex mediated; circulating or planted antigen	Diffuse endocapillary proliferation; leukocytic infiltration	Granular IgG and C3 in GBM and mesangium; granular IgA in some cases	Primarily subepithelial humps; subendothelial deposits in early disease stages.
Goodpasture syndrome	RPGN	Anti-GBM COL4-A3 antigen	Extracapillary proliferation with crescents; necrosis	Linear IgG and C3; fibrin in crescents	No deposits; GBM disruptions; fibrin
Chronic GN	Chronic renal failure	Variable	Hyalinized glomeruli	Granular or negative	
MGN	Nephrotic syndrome	in situ immune complex formation; PLA2R antigen in most cases of primary disease mostly unknown	Diffuse capillary wall thickening	Granular IgG and C3; diffuse	Subepithelial deposits
MCD	Nephrotic syndrome	Unknown; loss of glomerular polyanion; podocyte injury	Normal; lipid in tubules	Negative	Loss of foot processes; no deposits
FSGS	Nephrotic syndrome; non-nephrotic proteinuria	Unknown, ablation nephropathy plasma factor (?); podocyte injury	Focal and segmental sclerosis and hyalinosis	Focal; IgM + C3 in many cases	Loss of foot processes; epithelial denudation

Continued

TABLE 20-4 Summary of Major Primary Glomerulonephritides—cont'd

			Glomerular Pathology		
Disease	**Most Frequent Clinical Presentation**	**Pathogenesis**	**Light Microscopy**	**Fluorescence Microscopy**	**EM**
MPGN type I	Nephrotic syndrome	Immune complex	Mesangial proliferative or membranoproliferative patterns of proliferation; GBM thickening; splitting	IgG + C3; C1q + C4	Subendothelial deposits
Dense deposit disease (MPGN type II)	Hematuria Chronic renal failure	Autoantibody; alternative complement pathway	Mesangial proliferative or membranoproliferative patterns of proliferation; GBM thickening; splitting	C3; no C1q or C4	Dense deposits
IgA nephropathy	Recurrent hematuria or proteinuria	Unknown	Focal mesangial proliferative GN; mesangial widening	IgA ± IgG, IgM, and C3 in mesangium	Mesangial and paramesangial dense deposits

Nephritic Syndrome (p. 909)

Acute Proliferative (Poststreptococcal, Postinfectious) Glomerulonephritis (p. 909)

Poststreptococcal GN (PSGN) (p. 909) is caused by immune complexes formed in situ from the deposition of streptococcal antigens (principally streptococcal pyogenic exotoxin B) and subsequent binding of specific antibodies.

Morphology (p. 910)

- There is *diffuse* GN with *global* hypercellularity due to neutrophil and monocyte infiltration and endothelial, mesangial, and epithelial cell proliferation.
- Immunofluorescence shows granular mesangial and GBM IgG, IgM, and C3 deposition.
- EM shows subepithelial, *humplike* deposits.

Clinical Course (p. 911)

Patients present with *nephritic syndrome* 1 to 4 weeks after a pharyngeal or cutaneous streptococcal infection (other infections can do this as well); only certain strains (types 1, 4, and 12) of group A β-hemolytic streptococci are nephritogenic, likely associated with expression of certain cationic proteins. Antistreptococcal antibody titers are elevated, and serum complement C3 concentrations are decreased. More than 95% of children recover quickly; <1% develop a rapidly progressive disease, with the remainder progressing to chronic renal failure. In adults with sporadic PSGN, only 60% recover quickly; the remainder develop rapidly progressive disease, chronic renal failure, or delayed (but eventual) resolution.

Nonstreptococcal Acute Glomerulonephritis (Postinfectious Glomerulonephritis) (p. 912)

Nonstreptococcal acute GN is a similar form of immune complex GN but is associated with other infections, including bacterial, viral, and parasitic; occasionally immune deposits contain IgA rather than IgG.

Rapidly Progressive (Crescentic) Glomerulonephritis (p. 912)

RPGN is characterized clinically by a rapid, progressive renal decline. RPGN is divided into three broad groups based on immunologic findings, with a common denominator of severe glomerular injury; in each group, diseases can be idiopathic or associated with known disorders (Table 20-5).

TABLE 20-5 Rapidly Progressive Glomerulonephritis
Type I RPGN (Anti-GBM Antibody)
Renal limited
Goodpasture syndrome
Type II RPGN (Immune Complex)
Idiopathic
Postinfectious
SLE
Henoch-Schönlein purpura (IgA)
Others
Type III RPGN (Pauci-Immune)
ANCA-associated
Idiopathic
Wegener granulomatosis
Microscopic polyarteritis nodosa/microscopic polyangiitis

Classification and Pathogenesis (p. 912)

- *Type I RPGN* (20% of RPGN) *is an anti-GBM disease* characterized by linear IgG (and C3) GBM deposits. In some cases the anti-GBM antibodies cross-react with pulmonary alveolar basement membranes to produce pulmonary hemorrhages *(Goodpasture syndrome)*. The reason for autoantibody formation is unknown, although a high prevalence of certain HLA haplotypes suggests a genetic predilection; solvent exposures or virus infections have been implicated as the inciting trigger in susceptible hosts.
- *Type II RPGN* (25% of RPGN) *is an immune complex-mediated disease.* It can be a complication of any of the immune complex nephritides, including postinfectious GN. Immunofluorescence shows characteristic granular staining; besides crescent formation, there is often glomerular cellular proliferation.
- *Type III RPGN (pauci-immune type)* (>50% of RPGN) is characterized by the absence of anti-GBM antibodies or immune complexes. Instead, patients typically have circulating *antineutrophil cytoplasmic antibody (ANCA),* associated with a systemic vasculitis (see Chapter 11). In idiopathic cases, more than 90% of patients have elevated ANCA titers. It is not yet clear that the ANCAs are causal in any of the type III RPGN.

Morphology (p. 913)

- RPGN histology is characterized by distinctive *crescents* formed by parietal cell proliferation and inflammatory cell migration into Bowman space. With time, crescents can undergo sclerosis.
- Immunofluorescence reveals linear staining in anti-GBM disease, granular deposits in immune complex disease, and little to no staining for pauci-immune disease.
- EM in RPGN classically exhibits distinct *ruptures in the GBM;* subepithelial electron-dense deposits can also occur in type II disease.

Clinical Course (p. 913)

All forms of RPGN typically present with hematuria, red cell casts, moderate proteinuria, and variable hypertension and edema. In Goodpasture syndrome the course may be dominated by recurrent hemoptysis. Serum analyses for anti-GBM, antinuclear antibodies, and ANCA are diagnostically helpful. Renal involvement is usually progressive over the course of a few weeks, culminating in severe oliguria. Functional recovery can occur with intensive plasmapheresis combined with steroids and cytotoxic agents.

Nephrotic Syndrome (p. 914)

Nephrotic syndrome is characterized by excessive glomerular permeability to plasma proteins (proteinuria >3.5 g/day). Depending on the lesions, the proteinuria can be highly selective (e.g., primarily low-molecular-weight proteins [chiefly albumin]). With more severe injury, nonselective proteinuria includes higher-molecular-weight proteins in addition to albumin. Heavy proteinuria leads to hypoalbuminemia, decreased colloid osmotic pressure, and systemic edema. There are also *sodium and water retention, hyperlipidemia, lipiduria, vulnerability to infection, and thrombotic complications* (the later due to loss of serum anticoagulants and antiplasmins). The diseases causing nephrotic syndrome are listed in Table 20-6.

Membranous Nephropathy *(p. 915)*

Membranous nephropathy (MGN) is a common cause of adult nephrotic syndrome; it is primary (idiopathic) in 75% of patients,

TABLE 20-6 Causes of Nephrotic Syndrome

Causes	Approximate Prevalence (%)*	
	Children	Adults
Primary Glomerular Disease		
MGN	3	30
MCD	75	8
FSGS	10	35
MPGN and dense deposit disease†	10	10
Other proliferative glomerulonephritides (focal, "pure mesangial," IgA nephropathy)†	2	17
Systemic Diseases		
Diabetes mellitus		
Amyloidosis		
SLE		
Drugs (nonsteroidal antiinflammatory, penicillamine, heroin)		
Infections (malaria, syphilis, hepatitis B and C, HIV)		
Malignant disease (carcinoma, lymphoma)		
Miscellaneous (bee-sting allergy, hereditary nephritis)		

*Approximate prevalence of primary disease = 95% of nephrotic syndrome in children, 60% in adults. Approximate prevalence of systemic disease = 5% in children, 40% in adults.
†Membranoproliferative and other proliferative glomerulonephritides may result in mixed nephrotic/nephritic syndromes.

whereas the remainder occurs in association with malignancy, SLE, drug exposures (e.g., nonsteroidal antiinflammatory drugs [NSAIDs], penicillamine, captopril), infections, or autoimmune disorders (e.g., thyroiditis).

Pathogenesis (p. 915)

MGN is a form of chronic immune complex–mediated disease. Antibodies can be against self-antigens (SLE) or exogenous proteins (infections) or haptens (drugs). Two common endogenous antigens are as follows:

- Neutral endopeptidase, a membrane protein recognized by placentally transferred maternal antibodies in neonatal MGN
- PLA2R, with lesions similar to those seen in Heymann nephritis

Capillary leakiness results from complement activation that in turn activates epithelial and mesangial cells to liberate damaging proteases and oxidants.

Morphology (p. 915)

- By light microscopy there is diffuse thickening of the capillary wall (hence the term *membranous*). Tubular epithelial cells contain protein reabsorption droplets, and there is interstitial chronic inflammation. With progressive disease, glomeruli sclerose.
- Immunofluorescence reveals diffuse GBM granular staining for Ig and complement.
- EM shows *subepithelial* GBM deposits, which eventually incorporate into the GBM and assume an intramembranous location.

Clinical Features (p. 915)

MGN usually manifests by insidious onset of nephrotic syndrome; hypertension and/or hematuria also occur in 15% to 35% of cases. The course of disease is variable but usually indolent. Proteinuria persists in 60% of patients, but only 10% die or progress to renal failure in 10 years; 40% eventually progress to renal insufficiency. Secondary causes of membranous GN should be excluded in any new case.

Minimal Change Disease *(p. 917)*

Minimal change disease (MCD) is the major cause of nephrotic syndrome in children, with a peak incidence between ages 2 and 6. The disease occasionally follows a respiratory infection or routine immunization but is also associated with atopic disorders and Hodgkin lymphoma (and other lymphomas and leukemias).

Etiology and Pathogenesis (p. 917)

The current favored hypothesis is that MCD results from immune dysfunction and elaboration of a circulating cytokine(s) that affects visceral epithelial cells; this causes loss of glomerular polyanions that form part of the normal permeability barrier and results in increased leakiness.

Morphology (p. 917)

- *Light microscopy* shows normal glomeruli (hence *minimal change*).
- *Immunofluorescence* shows no immune deposits.
- *EM* reveals diffuse effacement of the foot processes ("fusion") of visceral epithelial cells.

Clinical Features (p. 917)

The most characteristic feature of this condition is the dramatic response to corticosteroid therapy. Despite the heavy proteinuria (mostly albumin), the long-term prognosis is excellent.

Focal Segmental Glomerulosclerosis *(p. 918)*

FSGS occurs as follows:

- As a primary (idiopathic) disorder; this is the most common cause of adult nephrotic syndrome in the United States.
- Secondary to other known disorders (e.g., heroin abuse, human immunodeficiency virus [HIV] infection, sickle cell disease, obesity).
- After glomerular necrosis due to other causes (e.g., IgA nephropathy).
- As an adaptive response to loss of renal tissue (see previous discussion; e.g., chronic reflux, analgesic abuse, or unilateral renal agenesis).
- Secondary to mutations of proteins that maintain the glomerular filtration barrier (e.g., podocyte proteins, such as podocin, and α-actinin 4, or slit diaphragm proteins, such as nephrin).

Idiopathic Focal Segmental Glomerulosclerosis

Idiopathic FSGS accounts for 10% and 35% of pediatric and adult nephrotic syndrome, respectively. Although it may fall on the spectrum of MCD, it differs by the following:

- A greater incidence of hematuria, reduced GFR, and hypertension.
- Proteinuria is typically nonselective.
- Poor response to corticosteroids.
- Higher rate of progression to ESRD (50% within 10 years).

Pathogenesis (p. 918)

The primary glomerular lesion in all FSGS is *visceral epithelial damage* (effacement or detachment) in affected glomerular segments. Some cases of FSGS have a genetic basis related to proteins that localize to the slit diaphragm or adjacent podocyte cytoskeleton and regulate glomerular permeability:

- *Nephrin* or *podocin* in the slit diaphragm
- Podocyte actin-binding protein α-actinin
- *TRPC6*, a podocyte protein that affects calcium flux

In other cases circulating cytokine(s) or genetic defects of the slit diaphragm complex are implicated. The ensuing glomerular sclerosis and hyalinosis stem from entrapment of plasma proteins and increased matrix synthesis.

Morphology (p. 919)

- *Light microscopy* is characterized by *sclerosis* of some but not all glomeruli (thus *focal*); in affected glomeruli, only a portion of the capillary tuft is involved (thus *segmental*).
- *Immunofluorescence* can show IgM and C3 in sclerotic areas or mesangium.
- *EM*—in both sclerotic and nonsclerotic areas—reveals diffuse foot process effacement with focal epithelial detachment.

Clinical Course (p. 919)

In addition to proteinuria (which is relatively nonselective), FSGS patients often present with hematuria, reduced GFR, and hypertension. Idiopathic FSGS responds variably to steroids, and progression to chronic renal failure occurs in more than 20%; FSGS recurs in 25% to 50% of renal allograft recipients; proteinuria can occur within 24 hours of transplant, emphasizing the potential role of circulating factors.

Human Immunodeficiency Virus-Associated Nephropathy *(p. 919)*

HIV-associated nephropathy occurs in 5% to 10% of HIV-infected individuals, often manifesting as a severe *collapsing glomerulopathy variant* of FSGS. There is retraction and/or collapse of the entire glomerular tuft and striking cystic dilation of tubular segments with associated inflammation and fibrosis. Proliferation and hypertrophy of glomerular visceral epithelium is associated with *endothelial tubuloreticular inclusions* (visualized by EM) caused by interferon-α-induced changes in the endoplasmic reticulum. The cause is unclear.

Membranoproliferative Glomerulonephritis *(p. 920)*

Membranoproliferative glomerulonephritis (MPGN) accounts for 10% of nephrotic syndrome; it can be idiopathic or secondary to another disorder or agent.

Pathogenesis (p. 920)

MPGN is categorized into two forms:

- *Type I* (most common) is most likely a consequence of antigen-antibody complex deposition and complement activation; the antigens in the complexes can originate from infection (e.g., hepatitis B or C, endocarditis, HIV), SLE, or malignancy, but in most cases the source is unknown. Type I MPGN can also be associated with α_1-antitrypsin deficiency or can be idiopathic.
- *Type II (dense deposit disease)* is due to activation of the alternate complement pathway; most such patients have *C3 nephritic factor* in the serum, an autoantibody against C3 convertase that stabilizes C3 convertase activity.

Morphology (p. 920)

- *Type I:* Light microscopy reveals both thickened capillary loops and glomerular cell proliferation; glomeruli appear "lobular" due to mesangial proliferation. Capillary walls often have a *double-contour* appearance due to interposition of cellular elements (mesangial, endothelial, or leukocyte) between reduplicated capillary basement membranes. In type I MPGN, EM is characterized by subendothelial electron-dense deposits; by immunofluorescence there is granular deposition of IgG, C3, C1q, and C4.
- *Type II:* There is a broader spectrum of light microscopic changes, from predominantly mesangial proliferation to inflammation with crescents. The defining feature is an electron-dense deposition of unknown material in the GBM; irregular glomerular C3 immunofluorescence can be seen outside of the dense deposits.

Clinical Features (p. 921)

Most patients present in adolescence or young adulthood with nephrotic syndrome, occasionally with hematuria. Although steroids may slow the progression, approximately 50% of patients develop chronic renal failure within 10 years. There is a high recurrence rate in transplant recipients, particularly in patients with type II disease.

Isolated Glomerular Abnormalities (p. 923)

IgA Nephropathy (Berger Disease) *(p. 923)*

IgA nephropathy is probably the most common type of GN worldwide; it is a major cause of recurrent hematuria.

Pathogenesis (p. 923)

IgA nephropathy is associated with genetic or acquired defects in the O-linked glycosylation of mucosal IgA (mainly IgA1 isotypes). Such qualitative alterations in the IgA molecule lead to augmented deposition in the mesangium and can also elicit autoantibodies that form immune complexes. Immune deposits directly activate mesangial cells, inducing proliferation, matrix synthesis, and cytokine and growth factor production. They also recruit inflammatory cells and can activate the alternate complement pathway. Increased IgA synthesis can occur secondary to respiratory or GI exposures to environmental agents (viruses, bacteria, food proteins, etc.). IgA nephropathy also occurs with increased frequency in patients with *celiac disease* or with liver pathology (due to diminished IgA clearance capacity).

Morphology (p. 923)

By light microscopy, glomeruli can appear nearly normal, showing only subtle mesangial hypercellularity, or can have focal proliferative or sclerotic lesions. Immunofluorescence reveals IgA, C3, and properdin deposition, and EM shows mesangial electron-dense deposits.

Clinical Features (p. 924)

Patients typically present with gross hematuria following a respiratory, GI, or urinary infection. The hematuria typically lasts for several days, then subsides, only to recur. Chronic renal failure develops in 15% to 40% over a period of 20 years. Older age of onset, heavy proteinuria, hypertension, crescents, and vascular sclerosis portend a poorer prognosis. Recurrence of IgA deposits is common in allografts, and 15% will redevelop clinical disease.

Hereditary Nephritis (p. 924)

Hereditary nephritis is a heterogeneous group of renal diseases associated with glomerular injury.

Alport Syndrome (p. 924)

Alport syndrome is manifested by hematuria progressing to chronic renal failure, associated with nerve deafness, lens dislocation, cataracts, and corneal dystrophy.

Pathogenesis (p. 924)

There is defective assembly of type IV collagen in the GBM, normally composed of a trimeric complex of α3, α4, and α5 subunits. The X-linked form (85% of cases) is due to mutations in the α5 chain; 90% of affected males progress to ESRD by age 40. Autosomal forms are due to mutations in the α3 or α4 subunits. Abnormal type IV collagen affects the function of GBM, eye lens, and cochlea. Because the α3 chain also includes the Goodpasture antigen, Alport patients with the X-linked form do not express that molecule.

Morphology (p. 924)

By EM there is alternating thickening and thinning of the GBM, with splitting and laminations of the lamina densa, producing a basket-weave appearance. With disease progression, FSGS, tubular atrophy, and interstitial fibrosis supervene.

Thin Basement Membrane Lesion (Benign Familial Hematuria) (p. 925)

Thin basement membrane lesion is a fairly common (1% of the population) entity manifesting as familial asymptomatic hematuria. Although proteinuria can be present, renal function is normal, and the prognosis is excellent; ocular abnormalities and hearing loss do not occur. The disorder is due to mutations in the type IV collagen α3 or α4 chains resulting in the GBM being only 150 to 250 nm thick (normal is 300 to 400 nm).

Chronic Glomerulonephritis (p. 925)

Chronic GN is the common end stage of a number of different entities. Although PSGN rarely progresses to chronic GN (except in adults), crescentic GN frequently does, and membranous GN, MPGN, IgA nephropathy, and FSGS are variable in their rates of progression.

Morphology (p. 925)

- *Grossly* the kidneys are symmetrically contracted with diffusely granular surfaces and a thinned cortex.
- *Microscopically* glomeruli are completely effaced by hyalinized connective tissue, making it impossible to identify the cause of the antecedent lesion; there is marked tubular atrophy. Associated hypertension leads to marked arteriolar sclerosis.

Clinical Course (p. 925)

Patients with chronic end-stage GN frequently develop hypertension; other secondary manifestations of uremia include pericarditis, uremic gastroenteritis, and secondary hyperparathyroidism with nephrocalcinosis and renal osteodystrophy.

Glomerular Lesions Associated With Systemic Diseases (p. 926)

Henoch-Schönlein Purpura (p. 926)

Henoch-Schönlein purpura can occur at any age but typically presents in children aged 3 to 8 years; findings include purpuric skin lesions (due to a vasculitis), abdominal symptoms (pain, vomiting, bleeding), arthralgia, and GN with some combination of hematuria, nephritic syndrome, and/or nephrotic syndrome. Glomerular lesions vary from focal mesangial proliferation to crescentic GN but are always associated with *mesangial IgA deposition.* Although the course is variable, the overall prognosis is usually excellent; recurrent hematuria can persist for years.

Glomerulonephritis Associated With Bacterial Endocarditis and Other Systemic Infections (p. 926)

This is due to immune complex (bacterial antigens and host antibodies) deposition. Presentations typically involve hematuria, although nephritic syndrome and even RPGN can occur. Renal lesions fall on a morphologic continuum from focal necrotizing GN to diffuse GN to crescentic GN; immunofluorescence and EM studies show granular immune complex deposition.

Diabetic Nephropathy (p. 926)

Diabetic nephropathy is the leading cause of chronic kidney failure in the United States; ESRD occurs in 40% of type 1 and type 2 diabetics (see also Chapter 24).

Fibrillary Glomerulonephritis (p. 926)

Fibrillary GN is a morphologic GN variant characterized by fibrillar deposits in the mesangium and glomerular capillary walls resembling amyloid but ultrastructurally distinct. Immunofluorescence microscopy reveals deposition of polyclonal IgG (often IgG4), light chains, and C3. Patients develop nephrotic syndrome, hematuria, and progressive renal insufficiency. The disease recurs in kidney transplants. The pathogenesis of this entity is unknown.

Other Systemic Disorders (p. 926)

Other systemic disorders associated with glomerular lesions include *Goodpasture syndrome* (see Chapter 15), *microscopic polyangiitis,* and *granulomatosis with polyangiitis* (see Chapter 11); all produce similar forms of GN ranging from focal segmental necrotizing GN to crescentic GN. *Essential mixed cryoglobulinemia* can induce cutaneous vasculitis, synovitis, and MPGN. *Plasma cell dyscrasias* can be associated with amyloidosis.

Tubular and Interstitial Diseases (p. 927)

Acute Tubular Injury (p. 927)

Because tubular necrosis is not a consistent feature of tubule injury, ATI is preferred over the older term acute tubular necrosis (ATN). ATI is the most common cause of acute renal failure and accounts for 50% of acute renal failure in hospitalized patients. Causes include the following:

- *Ischemia:* For example, shock, circulatory collapse, dehydration, malignant hypertension, vasculitis, and hypercoagulable states
- *Direct toxic injury:* For example, drugs, radiocontrast dyes, myoglobin, hemoglobin, and radiation

Pathogenesis (p. 927)

Reversible and irreversible tubular damage and persistent, severe vascular disturbances are the underlying etiologies for ATI (Fig. 20-3). Tubular epithelial cells are particularly sensitive to ischemia (high metabolic demand) as well as toxins (active transport system for ions and organic acids and capacity for drug concentration).

- Ischemia causes a reversible *loss of cell polarity* with redistribution of membrane proteins (e.g., sodium-potassium ATPase) from the basolateral to the luminal surface of the tubular cells.
- Abnormal ion transport leads to *increased sodium delivery to distal tubules* causing vasoconstriction through activation of the renin-angiotensin axis.
- Vasoconstriction also occurs secondary to endothelial dysfunction with increased endothelin and decreased NO and prostacyclin production.
- Ischemic tubular cells express cytokines and adhesion molecules that recruit leukocytes.
- Injured tubular cells detach from the basement membranes and cause *luminal obstruction,* increased intratubular pressure, and decreased GFR.
- Glomerular filtrate in the lumen of the damaged tubules leaks back into the interstitium, resulting in interstitial edema, increased interstitial pressure, and further tubule damage.
- Glomerular ultrafiltration is also directly affected by ischemia and toxins, attributed to mesangial contraction.

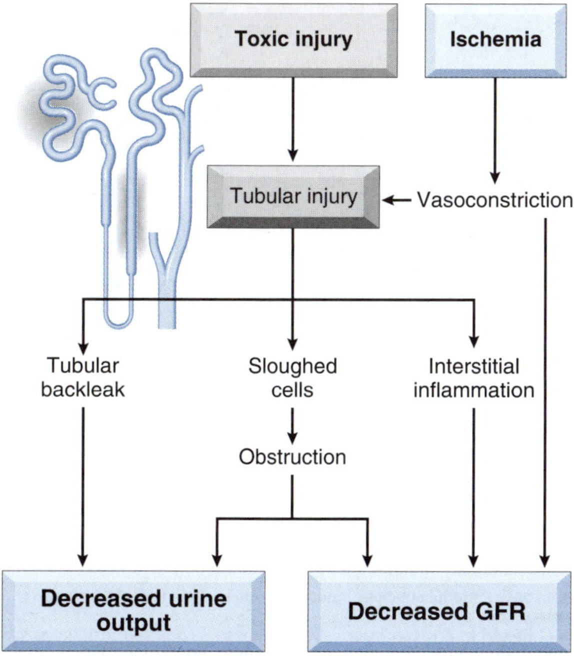

Figure 20-3 Postulated sequence in ischemic or toxic ATI.

Morphology (p. 928)

Findings include the following (Fig. 20-4):

- *Ischemic ATI:* Patchy tubular necrosis alternates with lesser degrees of tubular cell injury; the proximal tubule straight segments (PST) and thick ascending loop of Henle (HL) are most affected.
- *Nephrotoxic ATI:* Variable degrees of tubular injury and necrosis, mostly in proximal tubules.
- Distal tubules and collecting ducts (CDs) contain cellular and protein casts, and there is interstitial edema with a variable inflammatory infiltrate. The recovery phase shows epithelial regeneration (i.e., tubular cells with hyperchromatic nuclei and mitotic figures).

Clinical Course (p. 929)

The clinical course of ATI is highly variable but classically proceeds through three stages:

- *Initiation phase (up to 36 hours):* Dominated by the inciting event, there is a slight decline in urine output and a rise in BUN.
- *Maintenance phase:* Marked by oliguria (40 to 400 mL/day), salt and water overload, hyperkalemia, metabolic acidosis, and rising BUN.
- *Recovery phase:* Heralded by rising urine volumes (up to 3 L/day), with water, sodium, and especially potassium losses (hypokalemia becomes a concern). Eventually renal tubular function is restored, and the concentrating ability improves.

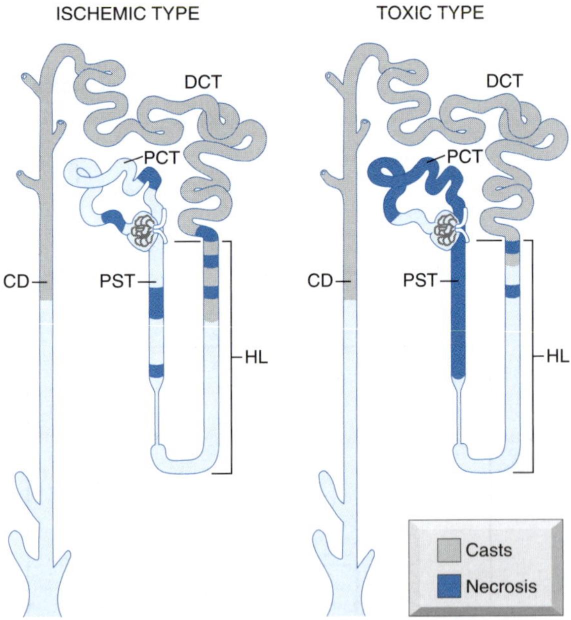

Figure 20-4 Patterns of tubular damage in ischemic and toxic ATI. In ischemia, tubular necrosis is patchy, and segments of PSTs and ascending limbs of HL are most vulnerable. With toxic injury, extensive necrosis is present along the proximal convoluted tubule (PCT) segments with many toxins (e.g., mercury), but necrosis of the distal tubule, particularly ascending HL, also occurs. In both types, lumens of the distal convoluted tubules (DCT) and CDs contain casts.

- Prognosis depends in part on the cause; it is *good* (>95% survival) in most cases of nephrotoxic ATI but is poor (>50% mortality) for ATI secondary to overwhelming sepsis or other causes of multiorgan failure.

Tubulointerstitial Nephritis (p. 929)

Tubulointerstitial nephritis (TIN) can be distinguished from primary glomerular diseases by the absence of nephritic or nephrotic syndromes. It typically presents with azotemia, but patients may also have polyuria (due to inability to concentrate urine), salt wasting, or defective acid excretion (metabolic acidosis). TIN can result from the progression of primary glomerular diseases, as well as from ischemia or systemic disorders, such as diabetes. There are also a number of primary etiologies (Table 20-7).

Pyelonephritis and Urinary Tract Infection *(p. 930)*

UTI denotes infection of the bladder *(cystitis),* the urethra or ureter, the kidneys *(pyelonephritis),* or all of the above. The most common organisms (85% of cases) are the normal gram-negative bacilli inhabitants of the GI tract. UTIs are much more common in women, due to the shorter urethra, hormonal changes affecting mucosal bacterial adherence, and the absence of prostatic fluid antibacterial compounds; other UTI risk factors include long-term

TABLE 20-7 Causes of Tubulointerstitial Nephritis
Infections
Acute bacterial pyelonephritis
CPN (including reflux nephropathy)
Other infections (e.g., viruses, parasites)
Toxins
Drugs
Acute-hypersensitivity interstitial nephritis
Analgesics
Heavy metals
Lead, cadmium
Metabolic Diseases
Urate nephropathy
Nephrocalcinosis (hypercalcemic nephropathy)
Acute phosphate nephropathy
Hypokalemic nephropathy
Oxalate nephropathy
Physical Factors
Chronic urinary tract obstruction
Neoplasms
Multiple myeloma (light chain cast nephropathy)
Immunologic Reactions
Transplant rejection
Sjögren syndrome
Sarcoidosis
Vascular Diseases
Miscellaneous
Balkan nephropathy
Nephronophthisis-medullary cystic disease complex
"Idiopathic" interstitial nephritis

catheterization, vesicoureteral reflux, pregnancy, diabetes mellitus, immunosuppression, and lower urinary tract obstructions from congenital defects, benign prostatic hypertrophy, tumors, or calculi. *Hematogenous spread* of bacteria to the renal parenchyma occurs much less commonly.

Etiology and Pathogenesis (p. 930)

In either gender pyelonephritis is most commonly the result of *ascending infection* from the bladder. The typical sequence of events is as follows:

- Colonization of the distal urethra and introitus (females) through expression of adherence molecules (*adhesins* on pili).
- Multiplication of bacteria in the bladder, facilitated by adhesion virulence factors and urinary tract obstruction or stasis.
- Vesicoureteral reflux through an incompetent vesicoureteral orifice allowing retrograde seeding of the renal pelvis and renal papillae. Vesicoureteral reflux is most often due to congenital defects in the intravesicular portion of the ureter (1% to 2% of otherwise normal individuals) and may be accentuated by cystitis.
- Intrarenal reflux through open papillae to renal tissue.
- UTIs can be clinically silent (i.e., asymptomatic bacteriuria with or without *pyuria* [leukocytes in the urine]). More often UTIs cause dysuria and frequency and—in pyelonephritis (see later)—flank pain, fever, and urine leukocyte *casts.*

Acute Pyelonephritis *(p. 931)*

Acute pyelonephritis is marked by patchy, suppurative inflammation, tubular necrosis, and intratubular neutrophil casts.

Morphology (p. 931)

More advanced changes include abscesses, *papillary necrosis* (especially with sickle cell disease, in diabetics, and in cases of obstruction), *pyonephrosis* (pelvis filled with pus), *perinephric abscesses,* and eventually renal scars with fibrotic deformation of the cortex and underlying calyx and pelvis.

Clinical Features (p. 933)

Uncomplicated pyelonephritis follows a benign course with antibiotic therapy but can recur or progress in the presence of vesicoureteral reflux, obstruction, immunocompromise, diabetes, and other conditions.

Polyomavirus is an emerging viral etiology for renal infections in kidney allografts. Latent infections (common in the general population) get reactivated in immunosuppressed hosts, causing tubular epithelial infections and associated inflammation that can result in allograft failure in 1% to 5% of infected patients.

Chronic Pyelonephritis and Reflux Nephropathy *(p. 933)*

Chronic pyelonephritis (CPN) is characterized by tubulointerstitial inflammation, renal scarring, and dilated, deformed calyces. It can be divided into two forms:

- *Reflux nephropathy* (p. 934) is most common. It begins in childhood, as a result of infections superimposed on congenital vesicoureteral reflux and intrarenal reflux; it can be unilateral or bilateral.
- *Chronic obstructive pyelonephritis* (p. 934) occurs when chronic obstruction (e.g., with *hydronephrosis*) predisposing the kidney to infections; the effects of chronic obstruction also contribute to parenchymal atrophy.

Morphology (p. 934)

Both major types of CPN are associated with broad scars, deformed calyces, and significant tubulointerstitial inflammation and fibrosis. Secondary FSGS (due to loss of glomerular mass) and vascular hypertensive changes can also be present.

Clinical Features (p. 934)

Both forms of CPN can manifest with the symptoms of acute pyelonephritis or can have a silent, insidious onset, sometimes presenting only very late in their course with hypertension or evidence of renal dysfunction in the absence of persisting infection. The development of proteinuria and FSGS is a poor prognostic sign.

Tubulointerstitial Nephritis Induced by Drugs and Toxins (*p. 935*)

Drug- and toxin-induced TIN is the second most common cause of ATI (after pyelonephritis); injury occurs through direct toxicity or by eliciting an immunologic response.

- *Acute drug-induced interstitial nephritis* (p. 935) results from an idiosyncratic hypersensitivity reaction to a variety of drugs (e.g., sulfonamides, synthetic penicillins, diuretics, and NSAIDs); *analgesic nephropathy* is usually caused by excessive intake of phenacetin-containing analgesic *mixtures.* Drug-induced interstitial nephritis begins approximately 2 weeks after exposure with the offending agent(s) acting as immunizing haptens. Drugs covalently bind to tubular cellular or matrix components, become immunogenic, and induce antibody (IgE) and T cell–mediated immune reactions.

Morphology (p. 935)

Biopsy exhibits edema, patchy tubular necrosis, and tubulointerstitial infiltrates, with variable combinations of lymphocytes, histiocytes, eosinophils, neutrophils, plasma cells, and occasionally well-formed granulomas.

Clinical Features (p. 936)

Recognition of a drug etiology is important because withdrawal usually leads to full recovery. Fever, eosinophilia, skin rash, hematuria, mild proteinuria, sterile pyuria, azotemia, and acute renal failure can be variably present. Excreted necrotic papillae (due to ischemia from microvascular compression caused by interstitial edema) will cause gross hematuria or renal colic due to ureteric obstruction.

- *Nephropathy associated with NSAIDs* (p. 936) occurs as some combination of the following:

  Cyclo-oxygenase inhibitors cause decreased synthesis of vasodilatory prostaglandins
  Hypersensitivity interstitial nephritis (see earlier discussion)
  Cytokine elaboration leading to podocyte foot process effacement (MCD)
  MGN of uncertain etiology

Other Tubulointerstitial Diseases (p. 936)

Urate Nephropathy (*p. 936*)

Urate nephropathy can cause acute or chronic renal failure, depending on the tempo of uric acid deposition.

- *Acute urate nephropathy* occurs when uric acid crystals precipitate in tubules and CDs, leading to obstruction. This may be a consequence of *tumor lysis syndrome* following chemotherapy for hematologic malignancy.

- *Chronic urate nephropathy* occurs with more prolonged hyperuricemia (e.g., with gout). The acidic environment of the collecting system leads to deposition of monosodium urate, ultimately obstructing the tubules (with cortical atrophy) or forming *tophi* consisting of foreign body giant cells and fibrosis.
- *Nephrolithiasis:* Uric acid stones are present in 22% of patients with gout and 42% of patients with secondary hyperuricemia.

Hypercalcemia and Nephrocalcinosis *(p. 937)*

Disorders associated with hypercalcemia induce renal calcium deposition *(nephrocalcinosis)* and calcium stone formation. Both can cause renal failure through tubular obstruction; nephrocalcinosis can also cause renal insufficiency through direct tubular epithelial effects. Calcium phosphate deposition can also be a consequence of consuming high quantities of phosphate solutions (e.g., for colonoscopic bowel preps).

Light Chain Cast Nephropathy ("Myeloma Kidney") *(p. 937)*

Renal insufficiency occurs in 50% of patients with *multiple myeloma.* Several factors contribute to renal insufficiency:

- *Bence Jones proteinuria and cast nephropathy.* Some light chains are directly toxic to epithelial cells. In addition, under acidic conditions, Bence Jones proteins combine with *Tamm-Horsfall* urinary glycoproteins to form large casts that obstruct the tubular lumens and induce a peritubular inflammatory reaction *(cast nephropathy).* Bence Jones proteinuria occurs in 70% of patients with myeloma.
- *Amyloidosis* occurs in 6% to 24% of myeloma patients.
- *Light chain deposition disease* occurs when light chains deposit in GBM or mesangium, causing a glomerulopathy, or in tubular basement membranes, causing a TIN.
- *Hypercalcemia and hyperuricemia* are common features of myeloma.

Bile Cast Nephropathy *(p. 938)*

Hepatorenal syndrome refers to impairment of renal function in patients with liver failure; markedly elevated serum bilirubin is associated with tubular bile cast formation *(cholemic nephrosis)* that can have direct tubular toxic effects as well as obstruct the nephron.

Vascular Diseases (p. 938)

Nearly all kidney diseases and many systemic disorders secondarily affect the renal vasculature. In particular, hypertension affects renal vessels; conversely, any renal vascular changes tend to amplify the hypertension.

Nephrosclerosis (p. 938)

Nephrosclerosis denotes the kidney pathology associated with renal arteriolar sclerosis. The arteriolar lumens are stenosed by wall thickening and hyalinization from deposition of insudated proteins and increased basement membrane matrix synthesis. Larger muscular arteries show *fibroelastic hyperplasia,* with both medial and intimal thickening. The vascular lesions cause diffuse ischemic atrophy of nephrons; as a result the kidneys are relatively small and exhibit diffuse granular surfaces due to scarring and contraction of individual glomeruli.

Benign nephrosclerosis rarely causes renal failure but can cause mild proteinuria. The severity of nephrosclerosis is associated with increasing age, black more so than white people, hypertension, and diabetes; progression to renal failure is correlated to the severity of hypertension, the presence of comorbid disease (e.g., diabetes), and African origin.

Malignant Nephrosclerosis (p. 939)

Malignant nephrosclerosis is associated with accelerated hypertension. Although this can occur in previously normotensive people, most cases are superimposed on preexisting benign essential hypertension (1% to 5% of such patients), chronic renal disease (particularly GN or reflux nephropathy), or scleroderma.

Pathogenesis (p. 939)

Following an initial vascular insult (e.g., long-standing benign hypertension, arteritis, coagulopathy), endothelial injury, platelet deposition, and increased vascular permeability lead to *fibrinoid necrosis* and intravascular thrombosis. These cause renal ischemia, with stimulation of the renin-angiotensin and other vasoconstrictive systems (e.g., endothelin), as well as aldosterone-driven salt (and water) retention, perpetuating an ever-increasing cycle of escalating blood pressures.

Morphology (p. 939)

Pathologic changes include fibrinoid necrosis of arterioles, hyperplastic arteriopathy (onion-skinning), necrotic glomeruli, and a glomerular thrombotic microangiopathy.

Clinical Features (p. 940)

Patients have systolic pressures >200 mm Hg and diastolic blood pressures >120 mm Hg; there is also proteinuria, hematuria, papilledema, encephalopathy, cardiovascular abnormalities, and eventually renal failure. Plasma renin, angiotensin, and aldosterone levels are all increased. With prompt antihypertensive intervention, 75% of patients survive 5 years, and half recover precrisis renal function.

Renal Artery Stenosis (p. 940)

Unilateral renal artery stenosis accounts for 2% to 5% of patients with renal hypertension; the vascular narrowing induces excessive renin secretion by the involved kidney. Obstructive *atheromatous plaque* at the renal artery take-off underlies 70% of cases; others are caused by *fibromuscular dysplasia.* The latter is a heterogeneous group of disorders, usually occurring in young women (ages 20 to 40) and characterized by nonarteriosclerotic *intimal, medial,* or *adventitial* hyperplasia. If performed before arteriolosclerosis develops in the contralateral kidney, revascularization surgery cures 70% to 80% of cases.

Thrombotic Microangiopathies (p. 941)

This group of diseases has overlapping clinical manifestations (e.g., microangiopathic hemolytic anemia, thrombocytopenia, renal failure, and manifestations of intravascular coagulation [see Chapter 14]). *Endothelial injury* and *platelet activation and aggregation* are shared pathogenic mechanisms, leading to increased leukocyte adhesion, increased endothelin and decreased NO production (favoring vasoconstriction) and endothelial lysis. *Hemolytic uremic syndrome* (HUS; p. 941) is largely due to endothelial injury, whereas platelet activation underlies *thrombotic thrombocytopenic purpura* (TTP; p. 942).

- *Typical (childhood) HUS* is associated with consumption of food contaminated with bacteria (e.g., *Escherichia coli* strain O157:H7) that synthesize Shigalike toxins.
- *Atypical HUS* is associated with mutations of complement-regulatory proteins, antiphospholipid antibodies, contraceptives, complications of pregnancy, certain drugs, radiation, and scleroderma.
- *TTP* is caused by inherited or acquired deficiencies of ADAMTS13, a plasma metalloproteinase that regulates von Willebrand factor function.

Morphology (p. 943)

Although they have diverse causes, these disorders are characterized morphologically by thromboses in the interlobular arteries, afferent arterioles, and glomeruli, together with necrosis and thickening of the vessel walls. The morphologic changes are similar to those in malignant hypertension, but the changes can precede the development of hypertension or be seen in its absence.

Other Vascular Disorders (p. 943)

Atheroembolic Renal Disease (p. 943)

Cholesterol crystals and debris embolize from atheromatous plaques after manipulation of severely diseased aortas (e.g., during aortic cannulation). They lodge in intrarenal vessels, causing arterial narrowing and focal ischemic injury. Rarely, renal function becomes compromised.

Sickle Cell Nephropathy (p. 943)

Sickle cell nephropathy occurs in both sickle cell heterozygotes and homozygotes; accelerated sickling in the hypertonic, hypoxic renal medulla leads to vascular occlusion with hematuria, diminished concentrating ability, and even proteinuria. Patchy *papillary necrosis* with cortical scarring can also result.

Diffuse Cortical Necrosis (p. 944)

Diffuse cortical necrosis is an uncommon but potentially fatal complication of obstetric emergency (e.g., abruptio placentae), septic shock, or extensive surgery. Patients develop diffuse glomerular and arteriolar microthrombi (morphologically akin to disseminated intravascular coagulopathy) leading to renal necrosis. The etiology is unknown.

Renal Infarcts (p. 944)

Renal infarcts are common occurrences because kidneys receive 25% of cardiac output (and a substantial number of any systemic atheroemboli) and because of their "end organ" arterial blood supply without significant collateral circulation. Left atrial or ventricle mural thrombi (secondary to atrial fibrillation or myocardial infarction) are a major source of emboli, followed by left-sided valvular vegetations, aortic aneurysms, and aortic atherosclerosis. Most renal infarcts are asymptomatic but can cause pain and/or hematuria. Large infarcts of one kidney can cause hypertension.

Congenital and Developmental Anomalies (p. 944)

Approximately 10% of newborns have potentially significant malformations of the urinary system; renal dysplasias and hypoplasias account for 20% of pediatric chronic renal failure. Most arise from acquired developmental defects rather than as heritable lesions.

- *Agenesis of the kidney* (p. 944). *Bilateral* absence of renal development is incompatible with life. *Unilateral* agenesis is associated with compensatory hypertrophy of the remaining kidney; with time, the hypertrophied kidney can develop glomerulosclerosis and renal failure.
- *Hypoplasia* (p. 944) refers to failure to develop to normal size, usually as a unilateral defect. A truly hypoplastic kidney shows no scars and possesses a reduced number (≤6) of renal lobes and pyramids.
- *Ectopic* kidneys (p. 945) lie either just above the pelvic brim or sometimes within the pelvis. Kinking or tortuosity of the ureters may cause urinary obstruction, predisposing to bacterial infection.
- *Horseshoe kidneys* (p. 945) result from renal fusion—upper poles in 10% of cases, and lower poles in 90%—producing a U-shaped structure continuous across the midline and anterior to the aorta and inferior vena cava.

Cystic Diseases of the Kidney (p. 945)

Table 20-8 summarizes the genetics, pathologic findings, and clinical consequences of the various cystic diseases.

Autosomal Dominant (Adult) Polycystic Kidney Disease (p. 945)

Autosomal dominant (adult) polycystic kidney disease (ADPKD) occurs in 1 of 400 to 1000 persons and accounts for 5% to 10% of chronic renal failure; it has high penetrance and is universally bilateral.

Genetics and Pathogenesis (p. 946)

ADPKD is caused in most cases by mutations in one of two genes:

- *PKD1* mutations account for about 85% of cases. *PKD1* encodes *polycystin 1,* a large (460 kD) protein that localizes to tubular epithelial cells and has domains involved in cell-cell and cell-matrix interactions.
- *PKD2* mutations are responsible for most of the remaining cases. *PKD2* encodes *polycystin 2,* a cation channel; mutations disrupt the regulation of intracellular calcium.

The pathogenesis for ADPKD is hypothesized to involve the sensing and transduction of mechanical signals. Thus a single, apical, nonmotile primary cilium in tubular epithelial cells functions as a mechanosensor to monitor changes in fluid flow and shear stress, whereas intercellular junctional complexes and focal adhesions monitor forces between cells and extracellular matrix (ECM). In response to external forces, these sensors regulate ion flux that in turn modulate cell polarity and proliferation. Polycystin 1 and 2 are both localized to the primary cilium and potentially form a complex that regulates intracellular calcium in response to fluid flow. Mutated proteins could conceivably affect intracellular second messengers and thereby influence proliferation, apoptosis, ECM interactions, and secretory function leading to the progressive formation of tubular cysts.

Morphology (p. 947)

Kidneys are massively enlarged and composed almost entirely of cysts up to 3 to 4 cm in diameter. Cysts arise anywhere along the

TABLE 20-8 Summary of Renal Cystic Diseases

	Inheritance	Pathologic Features	Clinical Features or Complications	Typical Outcome	Diagrammatic Representation
Adult polycystic kidney disease	Autosomal dominant	Large multicystic kidneys, liver cysts, berry aneurysms	Hematuria, flank pain, UTI, renal stones, hypertension	Chronic renal failure beginning at age 40-60 yr	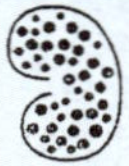
Childhood polycystic kidney disease	Autosomal recessive	Enlarged, cystic kidneys at birth	Hepatic fibrosis	Variable, death in infancy or childhood	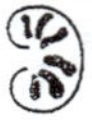
Medullary sponge kidney	None	Medullary cysts on excretory urography	Hematuria, UTI, recurrent renal stones	Benign	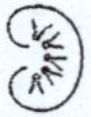
Familial juvenile nephronophthisis	Autosomal recessive	Corticomedullary cysts, shrunken kidneys	Salt wasting, polyuria, growth retardation, anemia	Progressive renal failure beginning in childhood	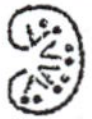
Adult-onset medullary cystic disease	Autosomal dominant	Corticomedullary cysts, shrunken kidneys	Salt wasting, polyuria	Chronic renal failure beginning in adulthood	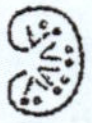
Simple cysts	None	Single or multiple cysts in normal-sized kidneys	Microscopic hematuria	Benign	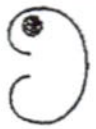
Acquired renal cystic disease	None	Cystic degeneration in end-stage kidney disease	Hemorrhage, erythrocytosis, neoplasia	Dependence on dialysis	

nephron and compress adjacent parenchyma. In late disease there is interstitial inflammation and fibrosis.

Clinical Features (p. 947)

Although most patients are asymptomatic until renal insufficiency supervenes, cystic dilation or hemorrhage can cause pain and/or hematuria, and hypertension, polyuria, and proteinuria also occur. For *PKD1* mutations, renal failure is present in 35% by age 50, 70% by age 60, and 95% by age 70; the corresponding figures for *PKD2* mutations are 5%, 15%, and 45%. Progression is accentuated in the presence of hypertension. Approximately 40% of patients have scattered liver biliary cysts *(polycystic liver disease)*, and *mitral valve prolapse* occurs in 20% to 25%. Approximately 40% of patients die of hypertensive or coronary heart disease, 25% of infections, 15% from ruptured *berry aneurysms* in the circle of Willis (causing subarachnoid hemorrhages) or hypertensive brain hemorrhage, and the rest of other causes.

Autosomal Recessive (Childhood) Polycystic Kidney Disease (p. 947)

Autosomal recessive (childhood) polycystic kidney disease (ARPKD) is genetically distinct from ADPKD; it is categorized by age of presentation (*perinatal* through *juvenile*) and the presence of associated hepatic lesions. In most cases the disease is caused by mutations of *PKHD1* (chromosome 6p21-p23), encoding for *fibrocystin*, a large transmembrane protein that localizes to the primary cilium of tubular epithelial cells. Kidneys are enlarged by multiple, cylindrically dilated CDs oriented at right angles to the cortex and filling both the cortex and medulla. The liver almost always has cysts and proliferating bile ducts; in the infantile and juvenile forms patients develop *congenital hepatic fibrosis.*

Cystic Diseases of Renal Medulla (p. 948)

Medullary Sponge Kidney (p. 948)

Medullary sponge kidney presents in adults with multiple cystic dilations in the medullary CDs. Although typically an innocuous lesion discovered incidentally by radiographic studies, it can predispose to renal calculi.

Nephronophthisis and Adult-Onset Medullary Cystic Disease (p. 948)

These constitute a family of progressive renal disorders characterized by small medullary cysts typically concentrated at the corticomedullary junction. There are four variants:

- Sporadic, nonfamilial (20%)
- Familial juvenile nephronophthisis (50%); autosomal recessive
- Renal-retinal dysplasia (15%); autosomal recessive
- Adult-onset medullary cystic disease (15%); autosomal dominant

Affected children present with polyuria, sodium wasting, and tubular acidosis, followed by progression to renal failure over 5 to 10 years. These disorders should be strongly considered in children with otherwise unexplained chronic renal failure, a positive family history, and chronic TIN on biopsy.

Genetics and Pathogenesis (p. 948)

At least 16 gene loci have been identified; *NPH1, NPH2,* and *NPH3* underlie the juvenile form of nephronophthisis. The gene products of *NPH1* and *NPH3* are called *nephrocystins* and are associated with the primary cilia; *NHP2* codes for *inversin,* which mediates right-left embryologic patterning. Initial injury to the distal tubules with basement membrane disruption leads to chronic progressive tubular atrophy and interstitial fibrosis.

Multicystic Renal Dysplasia (p. 949)

This is a sporadic disorder and can be unilateral or bilateral. Affected kidneys are enlarged and multicystic with abnormal lobar organization; histologically there are immature ducts surrounded by undifferentiated mesenchyme, often with cartilage formation. Most cases are associated with obstructive abnormalities of the ureter and lower urinary tract.

Acquired (Dialysis-Associated) Cystic Disease (p. 949)

End-stage kidneys of patients undergoing prolonged renal dialysis develop multiple cortical and medullary cysts due to obstruction from calculi and/or interstitial fibrosis. The cysts often contain calcium oxalate crystals and are commonly lined by atypical, hyperplastic epithelium that can undergo malignant transformation; 7% of patients will develop renal cell carcinoma within 10 years.

Simple Cysts (p. 949)

Commonly encountered, single or multiple cysts of the cortex (rarely medulla) are lined by low cuboidal epithelium and can range from 1 to 10 cm in size. They have smooth walls and are filled with clear serous fluid; occasionally, hemorrhage can cause flank pain, and calcification with irregular contours can mimic renal carcinoma.

Urinary Tract Obstruction (Obstructive Uropathy) (p. 950)

Obstruction increases susceptibility to infection and to stone formation, and unrelieved obstruction almost always leads to permanent renal atrophy. *Hydronephrosis is the term for pelvis and calyceal dilation associated with progressive renal atrophy of the kidney following outflow obstruction.* Causes include the following:

- Congenital anomalies (urethral valves or strictures, meatal stenosis, bladder neck obstruction, ureteropelvic junction obstruction, severe vesicoureteral reflux)
- Urinary calculi
- Benign prostatic hypertrophy
- Tumors of prostate, bladder, cervix, or uterus
- Inflammation (prostatitis, ureteritis, urethritis, retroperitoneal fibrosis)
- Sloughed papillae or blood clots
- Normal pregnancy
- Uterine prolapse and cystocele
- Functional disorders (neurogenic bladder)

Morphology (p. 950)

When obstruction is sudden and complete, GFR reduction leads to relatively modest pelvis and calyceal dilation, with only mild parenchymal atrophy. When the obstruction is subtotal or intermittent, GFR is not suppressed, and progressive dilation ensues. Obstruction also triggers interstitial inflammation and fibrosis.

Clinical Features (p. 950)

Most early symptoms are the consequence of the underlying obstruction (e.g., renal colic from a stone). Unilateral obstruction can remain silent for long periods because the unaffected kidney can usually compensate. In bilateral partial obstruction, manifestations include polyuria, distal tubular acidosis, salt wasting, renal calculi, TIN, atrophy, and hypertension. Complete bilateral obstruction results in oliguria or anuria; relief of such blockade is accompanied by a brisk postobstructive diuresis.

Urolithiasis (Renal Calculi, Stones) (p. 951)

Calculi can arise at any level in the urinary tract, although most form in the kidney. In the United States there is a 5% to 10% lifetime risk of urolithiasis, with men affected more commonly than women, and a peak incidence between ages 20 and 30. Hereditary associations are characterized by excessive production or secretion of stone-forming substances (e.g., gout, cystinuria, and primary hyperoxaluria).

Etiology and Pathogenesis (p. 951)

Increased concentrations of stone constituents, changes in urinary pH, decreased urine volume, and bacteria all play a role in stone formation. In addition, *loss of inhibitors* of crystal formation (e.g., citrate, pyrophosphate, glycosaminoglycans, osteopontin, and a glycoprotein called *nephrocalcin*) can also contribute.

There are four types of calculi; all also contain an organic matrix of mucoprotein (1% to 5% by weight):

- Approximately 70% are *calcium-containing stones* composed of calcium oxalate and/or calcium phosphate. These are usually associated with hypercalcemia or hypercalciuria (60%); hyperoxaluria and hyperuricosuria are contributory in others, and in 15% to 20%, there is no demonstrable metabolic abnormality.
- Approximately 5% to 10% of calculi are *triple phosphate* or *struvite* stones composed of magnesium ammonium phosphate. Struvite stones precipitate in alkaline urine generated by bacterial infections that convert urea to ammonia (e.g., *Proteus*). *Staghorn calculi*—occupying large parts of the renal pelvis—are struvite stones usually associated with infections.
- Approximately 5% to 10% are *uric acid stones;* more than half of such patients are neither hyperuricemic nor hyperuricosuric and instead make exceptionally acidic urine (pH < 5.5) that causes uric acid to precipitate.
- Between 1% and 2% of calculi are composed of *cystine* and are caused by genetic defects in renal amino acid resorption.

Clinical Features (p. 952)

Stones frequently cause clinical symptoms, including obstruction, ulceration, bleeding, and pain *(renal colic);* they also predispose to renal infection.

Neoplasms of the Kidney (p. 952)

Benign Neoplasms (p. 952)

Renal Papillary Adenoma (p. 952)

Renal papillary adenoma is a common (7% to 22% of autopsies), usually small (0.5 cm), yellow cortical tumor. Histologically most consist of vacuolated epithelial cells forming tubules and complex branching papillary structures. Adenomas are histologically indistinguishable from low-grade papillary renal cell carcinomas, and they share some of their cytogenetic features; 3 cm is the size cutoff separating those that metastasize from those that rarely do.

Angiomyolipoma (*p. 952*)

Angiomyolipoma is a hamartomatous lesion composed of vessels, smooth muscle, and fat; these are present in 25% to 50% of patients with tuberous sclerosis. They are clinically significant primarily for their susceptibility to spontaneously hemorrhage.

Oncocytoma (*p. 953*)

Oncocytoma is an epithelial tumor composed of eosinophilic cells arising from CD intercalated cells; on EM the cells are packed with mitochondria. They are common (5% to 15% of resected renal neoplasms) and can be large (up to 12 cm).

Malignant Neoplasms (p. 953)

Renal Cell Carcinoma (Adenocarcinoma of the Kidney) (*p. 953*)

Renal cell carcinoma represents 3% of all visceral cancers and 85% of renal cancers in adults; they usually occur in patients 50 to 70 years old and show a 2:1 male preponderance. There are approximately 65,000 new cases each year, with 13,000 deaths annually. Tobacco is the most significant risk factor, although obesity, hypertension, unopposed estrogens, and exposures to asbestos, petroleum products, and heavy metals are also implicated. ESRD and CKD also increase risk. Most renal cancer is sporadic, but autosomal dominant familial cancers account for 4% of cases.

- *von Hippel-Lindau (VHL) syndrome:* 50% to 70% of patients with certain *VHL* mutations develop renal cysts, as well as bilateral, frequently multicentric renal cell carcinomas. A host of mutations in the *VHL* gene (see later) are implicated in carcinogenesis of both familial and sporadic clear cell tumors; these do not necessarily induce the other manifestations of the syndrome.
- *Hereditary leiomyomatosis* and renal cell cancer syndrome is an autosomal dominant disease caused by mutations of the FH gene encoding fumarate hydratase; patients have cutaneous and uterine leiomyomata and an aggressive type of papillary carcinoma.
- *Hereditary papillary carcinoma* is ascribed to mutations in the *MET* proto-oncogene; it is an autosomal dominant entity manifesting with multiple bilateral papillary tumors.
- *Birt-Hogg-Dube syndrome* is an autosomal dominant disorder caused by mutations of the *BHD* gene encoding folliculin. Patients have constellation of skin (fibrofolliculomas, trichodiscomas, and acrochordons), pulmonary (cysts or blebs), and renal tumors.

Classification of Renal Cell Carcinoma: Histology, Cytogenetics, and Genetics

- *Clear cell (nonpapillary) carcinoma* is the most common type (70% to 80%); 95% are sporadic, and in 98% of these tumors—*whether familial, sporadic, or associated with VHL*—there is a loss of sequences on chromosome 3p at a locus that harbors *VHL*. *VHL* is a tumor suppressor gene that encodes part of a ubiquitin ligase complex involved in targeting proteins for degradation. When *VHL* is mutated, hypoxia-inducible factor-1 levels remain high, and this constitutively active protein increases the production of growth and angiogenic factors that promote tumorigenesis.

- *Papillary carcinoma* accounts for 10% to 15% of renal cell cancers and occurs in both familial and sporadic forms. The familial form is associated with mutations of the *MET* proto-oncogene that serves as a tyrosine kinase receptor for *hepatocyte growth factor.*
- *Chromophobe carcinoma* constitutes 5% of renal cell cancers; they derive from CD intercalated cells. Although they exhibit multiple chromosome losses and extreme hypodiploidy, they have an excellent prognosis.
- *Xp11 translocation carcinoma* occurs in young patients; it is defined by translocations of the TFE3 gene (at Xp11.2), all resulting in TFE3 transcription factor overexpression.
- *CD (Bellini duct) carcinoma* make up only 1% of renal cancers; they arise from medullary CD cells.

Morphology (p. 954)

- *Clear cell carcinomas* are usually solitary, large (>3 cm), spherical, bright yellow-gray masses that distort the renal outline. They exhibit large areas of ischemic opaque, gray-white necrosis, foci of hemorrhagic discoloration, and areas of softening. Tumors can bulge into the calyces and pelvis and invade the renal vein to grow as a solid column of cells within this vessel. Histologically they can be solid, trabecular, or tubular growths; individual cells are polygonal with abundant clear cytoplasm, and there is a delicate arborizing vasculature.
- *Papillary carcinomas* can be multifocal and bilateral. These are typically hemorrhagic and cystic. Microscopically these are composed of cuboidal cells arranged in papillary formations, often with interstitial foam cells and psammoma bodies.
- *Chromophobe renal carcinoma* is composed of pale, eosinophilic cells with perinuclear halos arranged of sheets around blood vessels.

Clinical Features (p. 955)

Patients classically (but only 10% of the time) present with flank pain, palpable mass, and hematuria. More commonly tumors declare at a larger size (10 cm) with fever, malaise, and weight loss. Renal cell carcinomas also produce a host of paraneoplastic syndromes attributable to hormone production: polycythemia, hypercalcemia, hypertension, feminization or masculinization, Cushing syndrome, eosinophilia, leukemoid reaction, and amyloidosis. *Prognosis* depends on tumor size and the extent of spread at diagnosis. Renal cell carcinoma tends to metastasize before symptoms are felt; in 25% of patients, there is radiographic evidence of metastases at presentation. In the absence of metastases, 5-year survivals are 70% to 95%.

Urothelial Carcinoma of the Renal Pelvis *(p. 955)*

Approximately 5% to 10% of renal tumors originate from renal pelvic urothelium; they tend to manifest relatively early due to hematuria or obstruction. Their histologic type is the same as for urothelial tumors in the bladder (see Chapter 21), ranging from well-differentiated papillary lesions to anaplastic, invasive carcinomas. They are often multifocal, and in 50% of cases there is a concomitant bladder tumor. Five-year survival rate varies from 50% to 100% for low-grade superficial tumors to 10% with high-grade infiltrating tumors.

21 The Lower Urinary Tract and Male Genital System

THE LOWER URINARY TRACT (p. 959)

Ureters (p. 960)

Congenital Anomalies (p. 960)

Congenital anomalies are seen in 2% to 3% of autopsies; most have no clinical significance although occasionally can cause obstruction:

- *Double ureters* are usually unilateral and are associated with double renal pelves or with the anomalous development of a large kidney having a partially bifid pelvis. Double ureters may pursue separate courses to the bladder but are commonly joined within the bladder wall.
- Congenital or acquired *ureteropelvic junction obstruction* can be an important cause of hydronephrosis, especially in children. The obstruction is typically secondary to disorganized junctional smooth muscle or excess stromal matrix.
- *Diverticula* are saccular outpouchings of the ureteral wall, and *hydroureter* reflects tortuous, dilated ureters; both can be congenital or acquired and lead to urinary stasis that can underlie recurrent infections.

Tumors and Tumorlike Lesions (p. 960)

Primary ureteral tumors are rare. *Benign ureteral neoplasms* are usually mesenchymal; *fibroepithelial polyps* present as small intraluminal projections, most commonly in children. *Malignant ureteral neoplasms* are primarily urothelial carcinomas comparable to similar tumors in the renal pelvis and bladder.

Obstructive Lesions (p. 960)

Ureteral obstruction can be secondary to calculi or clots, strictures (either extrinsic or due to congenital or postinflammatory narrowing), tumors, or neurogenic bladder dysfunction (Table 21-1). Ureteral dilation (hydroureter) is less important than the secondary renal hydrophrosis and/or pyelonephritis (see Chapter 20).

Sclerosing retroperitoneal fibrosis (p. 961) is an uncommon cause of obstruction characterized by retroperitoneal inflammation and fibrosis that encases the ureters and leads to hydronephrosis. A subset is caused by immunoglobulin (Ig)G4-related disease (see Chapter 6), but various drugs, inflammatory processes, and neoplasms can also be causal; most cases have no obvious cause *(Ormond disease)*.

TABLE 21-1 Major Causes of Ureteral Obstruction

Type of Obstruction	Cause
Intrinsic	
Calculi	Of renal origin, rarely more than 5 mm in diameter Larger renal stones cannot enter ureters Impact at loci of ureteral narrowing—ureteropelvic junction, where ureters cross iliac vessels and where they enter bladder—and cause excruciating "renal colic"
Strictures	Congenital or acquired (inflammation)
Tumors	Transitional cell carcinomas arising in ureters Rarely benign tumors or fibroepithelial polyps
Blood clots	Massive hematuria from renal calculi, tumors, or papillary necrosis
Neurogenic	Interruption of the neural pathways to the bladder
Extrinsic	
Pregnancy	Physiologic relaxation of smooth muscle or pressure on ureters at pelvic brim from enlarging fundus
Periureteral inflammation	Salpingitis, diverticulitis, peritonitis, sclerosing retroperitoneal fibrosis
Endometriosis	With pelvic lesions, followed by scarring
Tumors	Cancers of the rectum, bladder, prostate, ovaries, uterus, cervix; lymphomas, sarcomas

Urinary Bladder (p. 961)

Congenital Anomalies (p. 961)

- *Vesicoureteral reflux* (p. 961) is a major contributor to renal infections and scarring (see Chapter 20). Abnormal congenital connections may lead to fistulas between bladder and vagina, rectum, or uterus.
- *Diverticula* (p. 961) are outpouchings of the bladder wall that can arise as congenital defects but more commonly are acquired in the setting of persistent urethral obstruction (e.g., with prostatic enlargement). Urinary stasis in the diverticula predisposes to infection and calculi formation, as well as vesicoureteral reflux; carcinomas arising within them tend to be more advanced due to thinning of the underlying wall.
- *Exstrophy* (p. 962) of the bladder is due to developmental failure of the anterior abdominal wall; the bladder communicates directly with the overlying skin or lies as an exposed sac. Complications include chronic infection and an increased incidence of adenocarcinoma.
- *Urachal fistulas* (p. 962) arise from persistent remnant tracts of the *urachus* between fetal bladder and allantois. Occasionally only the central portion of the tract persists as a *urachal cyst;* such cysts can be a nidus for carcinoma development.

Inflammation (p. 962)

Acute and Chronic Cystitis (p. 962)

Urinary tract infections (UTIs) are extensively discussed in Chapter 20; they typically take the form of nonspecific acute and/or chronic inflammation. In addition to the typical bacterial causes (mostly coliforms), infectious cystitis can be caused by *Mycobacterium tuberculosis* (secondary to renal tuberculosis), fungi (mostly *Candida*), viruses, *Chlamydia,* and *Mycoplasma;* Schistosomiasis cystitis is common in the Middle East. Radiation and chemotherapies can also precipitate bladder inflammation and/or hemorrhage. Cystitis symptoms include urinary frequency, lower abdominal pain, and *dysuria* (pain on urination).

Special Forms of Cystitis *(p. 962)*

- *Interstitial cystitis (chronic pelvic pain syndrome)* (p. 962) is a form of chronic cystitis, occurring usually in women, and causing pain and dysuria in the absence of infection. Punctate hemorrhages characterize early lesions, followed classically in late-stage disease by localized ulceration *(Hunner ulcer)* with inflammation and transmural fibrosis. Mast cells are characteristically seen but are of uncertain significance.
- *Malakoplakia* (p. 963) occurs in chronic bacterial cystitis (mostly due to *Escherichia coli* or *Proteus* species) and is more common in immunosuppressed patients. Lesions are characterized by 3- to 4-cm soft, yellow, mucosal plaques, composed primarily of foamy macrophages stuffed with bacterial debris; the macrophages also display intralysosomal laminated calcified concretions called *Michaelis-Gutmann bodies;* their presence suggests defective macrophage phagocytic or degradative function.
- *Polypoid cystitis* (p. 963) is an inflammatory lesion caused by irritation of the bladder mucosa, most commonly due to indwelling catheters. The urothelium forms broad bulbous polypoid projections with marked submucosal edema.

Metaplastic Lesions (p. 963)

- *Cystitis glandularis and cystitis cystica* (p. 963) are common lesions in the setting of chronic cystitis but also occur in normal bladders. These are composed of nests of transitional epithelium *(Brunn nests)* that grow downward into the lamina propria and transform into cuboidal epithelium (*cystitis glandularis,* occasionally with intestinal metaplasia) or flattened cells lining fluid-filled cysts *(cystitis cystica).* They do not increase the risk of developing adenocarcinoma.
- *Squamous metaplasia* (p. 963) can occur as a response to injury.
- *Nephrogenic adenoma* (p. 963) results when shed tubular cells implant and proliferate at sites of injured urothelium. Although there can be extension into the superficial detrusor muscle, and lesions can be sizable, these are benign.

Neoplasms (p. 964)

In the United States bladder cancer accounts for 7% of all malignancies and 3% of cancer deaths; 95% are of epithelial origin, the remainder being mesenchymal.

Urothelial Tumors *(p. 964)*

Urothelial tumors run the gamut from small benign lesions to aggressive cancers with a high mortality; these can occur anywhere from the renal pelvis to the distal urethra, and many are multifocal at presentation.

Precursor lesions to malignancy fall into two categories:

- *Noninvasive papillary tumors* are most common, with lesions exhibiting a range of atypia that can reflect biologic behavior.
- *Carcinoma in situ* (CIS) represents a high-grade lesion of cytologically malignant cells present within a flat urothelium; the cells often lack cohesiveness and shed into the urine (detectable on urine cytology).

In half of patients, tumor has already invaded the bladder wall at the time of initial presentation. The absence of precursor lesions in such cases suggests obliteration by the high-grade invasive component. Although lamina propria invasion worsens prognosis, involvement of the muscularis propria (detrusor muscle) is the major determinant of outcome; at that stage there is a 30% 5-year mortality.

Epidemiology and Pathogenesis (p. 964)

Bladder cancer has a male to female ratio of 3:1 and is more common in industrialized nations, affecting urban populations more than rural dwellers; 80% of patients are aged 50 to 80 years. Risk factors include the following:

- Cigarette smoking increases risk threefold to sevenfold; 50% to 80% of bladder cancers in men are associated with cigarette smoking.
- Industrial exposure to arylamines, particularly 2-naphthylamine.
- *Schistosoma haematobium* infections (70% will be squamous), causing chronic inflammatory response to ova within the bladder wall.
- Chronic analgesic use.
- Long-term cyclophosphamide exposure (causes hemorrhagic cystitis).
- Bladder radiation.

The cytogenetic and molecular alterations are heterogeneous, but most tumors, even when multicentric, are clonal. Chromosome 9 deletions or monosomy are common (30% to 60% of tumors); 9p deletions involve the tumor suppressor genes *p16 (INK4a)* and *p15.* Low-grade superficial papillary tumors are characterized by gain-of-function mutations in fibroblast growth factor receptor 3 (FGFR3), *RAS* mutations, and chromosome 9 deletions; a minority may then lose *TP53* and/or *Rb* function and progress to invasion. Other, more aggressive, high-grade flat or papillary lesions can be initiated by *TP53* mutations; with loss of chromosome 9 and acquisition of other mutations, these become invasive.

Morphology (p. 965)

Urothelial malignancy ranges from papillary to nodular or flat.

- Most *papillary* lesions are low grade (<10% risk of invasion); they appear as red excrescences from 0.5 to 5 cm in size:
  - *Exophytic papillomas* (urothelium over fingerlike papillae with loose fibrovascular cores) have an extremely low incidence of progression or recurrence.
  - *Inverted papillomas* (bland urothelium extending into the lamina propria) are uniformly benign.
  - *Papillary urothelial neoplasms of low malignant potential* are slightly larger than papillomas with thicker urothelium and enlarged nuclei, but rare mitoses and infrequent invasion.
  - *Low-grade papillary urothelial carcinomas* characteristically have orderly cytology and architecture, with minimal atypia; they can invade but are rarely fatal lesions.
  - *High-grade papillary urothelial cancers* contain discohesive cells with anaplastic features and architectural disarray; these have a high risk (80%) for progression and metastases.
- CIS usually appears as an area of mucosal reddening, granularity, or thickening without producing an evident intraluminal mass. CIS is commonly multifocal; if untreated, 50% to 75% progress to invasive cancer.

Other Epithelial Bladder Tumors (p. 967)

- *Squamous cell carcinomas* are associated with chronic bladder infection and inflammation; these represent 3% to 7% of bladder cancers in the United States but occur much more frequently in countries endemic for urinary schistosomiasis.
- *Mixed urothelial carcinomas with areas of squamous carcinoma* are invasive, fungating, and/or ulcerating tumors; they are more common than purely squamous cell bladder cancers.
- *Adenocarcinomas* of the bladder are rare; they can arise from urachal remnants or in the setting of intestinal metaplasia.

Clinical Course of Bladder Cancer (p. 967)

Bladder tumors classically manifest with *painless hematuria;* frequency, urgency, and dysuria can also occur. At presentation 60% of neoplasms are single and 70% are localized to the bladder.

Patients tend to develop new tumors (occasionally of higher grade) after primary excision; recurrences can either reflect new tumors or (because they share the same genetic changes as the initial tumor) represent shedding and implantation of the original tumor cells.

Prognosis depends on the histologic grade and stage at diagnosis. Papillomas, papillary urothelial neoplasms of low malignant potential, and low-grade papillary urothelial cancer carry a 98% 10-year survival rate regardless of the number of recurrences. In contrast, an initial high-grade cancer portends a 25% mortality. After initial diagnosis, routine follow-up involves surveillance cystoscopies to look for tumor recurrence. Cytologic examination of cells obtained from urine samples can use fluorescence in situ hybridization (FISH) to detect chromosomal abnormalities (aneuploidy of chromosome 3, 7, and 17 and 9p deletions). A major limitation of both FISH and cytologic screening is poor sensitivity in detecting low-grade neoplasms.

Therapy depends on the grade and stage and whether the lesion is flat or papillary. For small, low-grade papillary tumors, primary transurethral resection is sufficient (followed by lifelong periodic cystoscopic and urine cytologic examinations). After primary resection, patients with higher-grade but still focal lesions can receive topical instillation of an attenuated strain of tuberculous bacillus (bacillus Calmette-Guérin [BCG]) that induces a therapeutic inflammatory response. Radical cystectomy is indicated for tumor invading the muscularis propria, CIS or high-grade papillary cancer refractory to immunotherapy, or CIS extending into the prostatic urethra and prostatic ducts. Metastatic bladder cancer requires chemotherapy.

Mesenchymal Tumors (p. 968)

Mesenchymal tumors are rare.

Benign tumors (p. 968) resemble their counterparts elsewhere, with *leiomyomas* being most common.

Sarcomas (p. 968) typically produce large (10 to 15 cm) exophytic masses; *embryonal rhabdomyosarcoma* is most common in children, and *leiomyosarcoma* is most common in adults.

Obstruction (p. 969)

Bladder outlet obstruction can eventually impact renal function. Prostate nodular hyperplasia is the most common cause in men; bladder cystocele is the most common cause in women. Infrequent causes include congenital urethral strictures, inflammatory urethral strictures, inflammatory fibrosis, bladder tumors, invasion of the bladder neck by contiguous tumors, calculi or foreign body obstructions caused by foreign bodies and calculi, and neurogenic bladder.

Urethra (p. 969)

Inflammation (p. 969)

Urethritis is classically denoted as either *gonococcal* or *nongonococcal* and is often accompanied by cystitis (women) or prostatitis (men). The most common nongonococcal organisms are *E. coli* and other enterics; *Chlamydia* is responsible for 25% to 60% of nongonococcal urethritis in men and 20% in women, with *Mycoplasma* being a less frequent cause. Noninfectious urethritis can also be one component of a *reactive arthritis* triad including arthritis and conjunctivitis.

Tumors and Tumorlike Lesions (p. 969)

- *Caruncles* are painful, small, red inflammatory lesions (essentially polyps of inflamed granulation tissue) of the external urethral meatus in women; they are exquisitely friable and bleed easily. Excision is curative.
- *Benign epithelial tumors* include squamous and urothelial papillomas, inverted urothelial papillomas, and condylomas.
- *Primary carcinoma of the urethra* is uncommon; in the proximal urethra, these are analogous to bladder urothelial malignancy, whereas in the distal urethra, they are more commonly squamous cell carcinomas.

THE MALE GENITAL TRACT (p. 970)

Penis (p. 970)

Congenital Anomalies (p. 970)

Hypospadias and Epispadias (p. 970)

Malformations of the urethral canal can produce aberrant openings either on the *ventral* aspect of the penis *(hypospadias)* or on the *dorsal* surface *(epispadias)*. These can be associated with other urogenital malformations, including *undescended testes.* Constriction can predispose to UTIs, and severe displacement of the orifice can be a cause of sterility.

Phimosis (p. 970)

Phimosis is the designation for a prepuce (foreskin) orifice too small to permit normal retraction; it can be a primary developmental defect but is more often secondary to inflammation. Phimosis predisposes to secondary infections and carcinoma from chronic accumulation of secretions and other debris *(smegma).*

Inflammation (p. 970)

Inflammations characteristically involve both the glans penis and the prepuce.

- The *sexually transmitted* causes of inflammation (e.g., syphilis, gonorrhea, chancroid, lymphopathia venereum, genital herpes, and granuloma inguinale) are discussed in Chapter 8.
- *Balanoposthitis* refers to nonspecific infection by other organisms (e.g., *Candida,* anaerobic or pyogenic bacteria, and *Gardnerella*). Most are a consequence of poor local hygiene in uncircumcised males due to accumulated smegma and can lead to phimosis.

Tumors (p. 970)

Benign Tumors (p. 970)

- *Condyloma acuminatum* (p. 970) is a benign sexually transmitted epithelial proliferation caused by *human papillomavirus* (HPV), especially types 6 and 11. After excision they tend to recur but rarely transform to malignancy.

Morphology (p. 970)

- *Gross:* Single or multiple sessile or pedunculated red papillary excrescences 1 to 5 mm in size, often involving the coronal sulcus or inner prepuce.
- *Microscopic:* Branching papillae covered by hyperplastic (but orderly) stratified squamous epithelium, often with hyperkeratosis; epithelial cell vacuolation *(koilocytosis)* is common.
- *Peyronie disease* (p. 971) causes fibrosis of the penile corpus cavernosum, resulting in curvature and pain during intercourse.

Malignant Tumors (p. 971)

- *CIS* (p. 971) lesions are strongly associated with HPV infection, especially type 16.
    - *Bowen disease* can involve either male or female genitalia, generally in patients over age 35. Men typically present with solitary or multiple thickened, gray-white or red, shiny plaques over the penile shaft. Histology reveals marked epithelial atypia with lack of orderly maturation but *no invasion.* Over the span of years transition to invasive squamous cell carcinoma occurs in approximately 10% of cases.
    - *Bowenoid papulosis* presents as multiple, pigmented papular lesions on external genitalia in younger sexually active patients. The lesions are histologically indistinguishable from Bowen disease, but evolution into invasive carcinoma is rare, and they frequently spontaneously regress.
- *Invasive carcinoma* (p. 971). Penile squamous cell carcinoma accounts for <1% of cancers in U.S. men; most cases occur between ages 40 and 70. The prevalence is higher in regions where circumcision is not routinely practiced and is also related to carcinogens within smegma accumulating under the foreskin, as well as HPV types 16 and 18. Cigarette smoking also increases risk.

Clinical Features (p. 972)

The clinical course is characterized by slow growth; metastases can occur in regional (inguinal and iliac) lymph nodes, but distant metastases are uncommon. The 5-year survival rate is 66% for lesions confined to the penis and 27% with regional node involvement.

Testis and Epididymis (p. 972)

Congenital Anomalies (p. 972)

Cryptorchidism (p. 972)

Cryptorchidism affects 1% of 1-year-old boys and represents *failure of descent;* it is usually unilateral and an isolated anomaly but can be bilateral in 25% of patients and occur with other genitourinary malformations. Although testes can be found anywhere along the normal abdomen-to-scrotal sac pathway, defects in transabdominal descent (under the control of *müllerian inhibiting substance*) account for only 5% to 10% of cases; most cryptorchidism involves abnormalities in the descent through the inguinal canal into the scrotal sac (under the control of androgens), and in most patients the cryptorchid testis is palpable in the inguinal canal.

Morphology (p. 972)

Histologic changes in maldescended testes can manifest as early as age 2; these include *decreased germ cell development, thickening* and *hyalinization* of seminiferous tubule basement membrane, and interstitial *fibrosis,* with relative sparing of Leydig cells. Histologic deterioration in the contralateral *descended* testis suggests an intrinsic defect in testicular development.

Beyond sterility, cryptorchidism is associated with *inguinal hernias* (10% to 20% of cases) and an increased incidence of *testicular malignancy.* Most cryptorchid testes spontaneously descend in the first year of life; for those that do not, surgical correction *(orchiopexy)* before the second birthday improves (but does not guarantee) fertility and reduces cancer risk.

Regressive Changes (p. 973)

Atrophy and Decreased Fertility (p. 973)

Atrophy and decreased fertility can be the following:

- Primary, due to a developmental abnormality (e.g., *Klinefelter syndrome*).
- Secondary to cryptorchidism, vascular disease (e.g., atherosclerosis), inflammatory disorders, hypopituitarism, malnutrition, persistently elevated levels of follicle-stimulating hormone, exogenous androgenic or antiandrogenic hormones, radiation, and chemotherapy.

The morphologic alterations are identical to those seen in cryptorchidism.

Inflammation (p. 973)

Inflammatory conditions are generally more common in the epididymis than in the testis; the exception is syphilis, which begins in the testis and secondarily progresses to involve the epididymis.

Nonspecific Epididymitis and Orchitis (p. 973)

Nonspecific epididymitis and orchitis typically result from a primary UTI that reaches the epididymis via the vas deferens or spermatic cord lymphatics. Causes vary with the age of the patient:

- *Childhood epididymitis* is usually associated with congenital genitourinary abnormalities and gram-negative rod infections.
- In sexually active men younger than age 35, *Chlamydia trachomatis* and *Neisseria gonorrhoeae* are the common culprits.
- In men over 35 years, common UTI agents (e.g., *E. coli* and *Pseudomonas*) are usually causal.

Granulomatous (Autoimmune) Orchitis (p. 974)

Granulomatous (autoimmune) orchitis presents in middle age as a painless to moderately tender testicular mass of sudden onset; the histology reveals spermatic tubule granulomas. An autoimmune pathogenesis is suspected.

Specific Inflammations (p. 974)

- *Gonorrhea* (p. 974): Most cases represent *retrograde extension* of infection from the posterior urethra to the prostate, seminal vesicles, and epididymis; untreated, the infection can produce suppurative orchitis.

- *Mumps* (p. 974): Mumps orchitis is uncommon in children but develops in 20% to 30% of postpubertal males infected with mumps. Acute interstitial orchitis typically develops approximately 1 week after onset of parotid inflammation.
- *Tuberculosis* (p. 974): Tuberculosis almost always begins in the *epididymis,* with secondary involvement of the testis; the histology of caseating granulomas is identical to that seen in other sites.
- *Syphilis* (p. 974): Syphilis can occur in both congenital and acquired syphilis and can present as isolated orchitis without involvement of adnexal structures. Histologically there can be nodular *gummas* or *diffuse interstitial inflammation* with edema, lymphoplasmacytic inflammation, and obliterative endarteritis.

Vascular Disorders (p. 974)

Torsion (*p. 974*)

Twisting of the spermatic cord cuts off the testicular *venous drainage;* because the thick-walled arteries typically remain patent, there is intense vascular engorgement potentially followed by hemorrhagic infarction.

- *Neonatal torsion* occurs either in utero or shortly after birth; it lacks any associated anatomic defect.
- *Adult torsion* typically presents in adolescence as sudden dramatic testicular pain; it is associated with a *bilateral anatomic defect* giving the testis increased mobility *(bell clapper abnormality).*

Torsion often occurs without any inciting injury and can even occur during sleep. Torsion is a true urologic emergency; surgical untwisting within 6 hours of onset can preserve testicular viability. To prevent a recurrence or a similar fate in the contralateral testis, both testes are surgically fixed to the scrotum *(orchiopexy).*

Spermatic Cord and Paratesticular Tumors (p. 975)

- *Lipomas* commonly involve the proximal spermatic cord; however, in some cases fat around the cord may only represent retroperitoneal adipose tissue that has been pulled into the inguinal canal with a hernia sac.
- *Adenomatoid tumors* are the most common benign paratesticular neoplasms. These are small nodules of mesothelial cells usually near the upper epididymal pole.
- Of malignant tumors in this location, *rhabdomyosarcomas* are most common in children, and *liposarcomas* are most common in adults.

Testicular Tumors (p. 975)

Testicular tumors are generally divided into two major categories (Table 21-2):

- *Germ cell tumors* (95% of cases) are generally malignant; these are further divided into *seminomas* and *nonseminomas.*
- *Sex cord-stromal tumors* are generally benign.

Seminomatous tumors are composed of cells that resemble primordial germ cells or early gonocytes. The *nonseminomatous tumors* can resemble undifferentiated embryonic stem cells *(embryonal carcinoma)* or differentiate along other lineages, generating *yolk sac tumors, choriocarcinomas,* and *teratomas.* Although germ cell tumors may be composed of a single tissue component, approximately 60% of cases contain mixtures of seminomatous and nonseminomatous components.

TABLE 21-2 Pathologic Classification of Common Testicular Tumors

Germ Cell Tumors
Seminomatous tumors
Seminoma
Spermatocytic seminoma
Nonseminomatous tumors
Embryonal carcinoma
Yolk sac (endodermal sinus) tumor
Choriocarcinoma
Teratoma
Sex Cord-Stromal Tumors
Leydig cell tumor
Sertoli cell tumor

Germ Cell Tumors (*p. 975*)

Germ cell tumors have an incidence of 6 in 100,000 in the United States, and involve whites 5 times more often than blacks; they constitute the most common malignancy in men aged 15 to 34 and account for 10% of cancer deaths in that group.

Pathogenesis (p. 975)

Several risk factors are implicated:

- *Cryptorchidism* is the most important; it is associated with 10% of cases.
- *Testicular dysgenesis syndrome (TDS),* including cryptorchidism, hypospadias, and poor sperm quality; TDS has been related to pesticide and nonsteroidal estrogen exposures in utero.
- *Genetic factors:* There is familial clustering and an increased incidence of testicular carcinoma among brothers and sons of affected individuals; many of the cancer susceptibility loci are thought to be involved in gonadal development.

Most tumors arise from a focus of *intratubular germ cell neoplasia (ITGCN),* which occurs in utero but remains dormant until puberty. These cells retain expression of transcription factors *OCT3/4* and *NANOG* associated with totipotentiality; they also share some of the genetic alterations found in many germ cell tumors (e.g., additional copies of chromosome 12p and/or activating mutations of c-KIT). The neoplastic ITGCN cells then give rise to *seminomas* or transform into a *totipotential* neoplastic cell (e.g., *embryonal carcinoma*) capable of further differentiation.

Seminoma (p. 976)

Seminoma accounts for 50% of all testicular germ cell tumors; it has a peak incidence between ages 30 and 40.

Morphology (p. 976)

- *Gross:* Homogeneous, lobulated, gray-white mass, generally devoid of hemorrhage or necrosis; the tunica albuginea usually remains intact.
- *Microscopic:* This germ cell neoplasm is the one most likely to exhibit a single histologic pattern.
    - The mass is composed of large polyhedral *seminoma cells* containing abundant clear cytoplasm (due to glycogen), large nuclei, and prominent nucleoli.
    - A fibrous stroma of variable density divides the neoplastic cells into irregular *lobules,* and there is a lymphocytic (and occasionally granulomatous) infiltrate.

- Tumor cells are diffusely positive for c-KIT, OCT4, and placental alkaline phosphatase (PLAP).
- Approximately 15% contain syncytiotrophoblasts; human chorionic gonadotropin (hCG) is present in such cells.

Spermatocytic Seminoma (p. 976)

Spermatocytic seminoma is an uncommon neoplasm (1% to 2% of all germ cell tumors), typically occurring in older patients (>65 years old). These are usually indolent tumors with little tendency to metastasize; they are *not* associated with ITGCN.

Morphology (p. 977)

- *Gross:* Soft, gray cut surface sometimes with mucoid cysts.
- *Microscopic:* Lesions are composed of a *mixture* of three cell populations—small cells resembling secondary spermatocytes, medium-sized cells with a round nucleus and eosinophilic cytoplasm, and scattered giant cells.

Embryonal Carcinoma (p. 977)

Embryonal carcinoma has a peak incidence between ages 20 and 30; these cancers are more *aggressive* than seminomas.

Morphology (p. 977)

- *Gross:* Most are poorly demarcated, small, gray-white masses punctuated by hemorrhage and/or necrosis. Extension through the tunica albuginea into the epididymis or cord is common.
- *Microscopic:* Lesions are composed of primitive epithelial cells with indistinct cell borders, forming irregular sheets, tubules, alveoli, and papillary structures. Mitoses and giant cells are common; tumor cells are positive for OCT3/4, PLAP, cytokeratin, and CD30 but are negative for c-KIT.

Yolk Sac Tumor (Endodermal Sinus Tumor) (p. 977)

Yok sac tumor is the most common testicular neoplasm below the age of 3 years; the prognosis is very good. Most adult cases occur as a component of embryonal carcinoma.

Morphology (p. 977)

- *Gross:* This is typically an infiltrative, homogeneous, yellow-white mucinous tumor.
- *Microscopic:* Lesions are composed of cuboidal neoplastic cells arrayed in a lacelike (reticular) network; solid areas and papillae may also be seen. Structures resembling primitive glomeruli *(Schiller-Duval bodies)* are seen in half. Eosinophilic, hyaline globules containing immunoreactive *α-fetoprotein (AFP)* and α_1-*antitrypsin* are associated with neoplastic cells.

Choriocarcinoma (p. 978)

Choriocarcinoma is a highly malignant neoplasm composed of both cytotrophoblastic and syncytiotrophoblastic elements; it comprises <1% of all germ cell tumors.

Morphology (p. 978)

- *Gross:* The neoplasm is often small, even in the presence of widespread systemic metastases; it ranges from a hemorrhagic mass to an inconspicuous lesion replaced by a fibrous scar.

- *Microscopic:* Lesions are composed of polygonal, comparatively uniform cytotrophoblastic cells growing in sheets and cords, admixed with multinucleated syncytiotrophoblastic cells; hCG is readily demonstrable.

Teratoma (p. 978)

Teratoma is a neoplasm showing differentiation along endodermal, mesodermal, and ectodermal lines; these occur at any age. Although pure teratomas are rare, the frequency of teratomas mixed with other germinal cell tumors approaches 50%. In children, mature teratomas behave as benign tumors, and patients have an excellent prognosis. In the postpubertal male all teratomas are regarded as malignant regardless of the maturity or immaturity of the various elements.

Morphology (p. 978)

- *Gross:* Tumors are usually large (5 to 10 cm), with a heterogeneous appearance; hemorrhage and necrosis suggest admixture with embryonal and/or choriocarcinoma.
- *Microscopic:* Teratomas are composed of a haphazard array of *differentiated* mesodermal (e.g., muscle, cartilage, adipose tissue), ectodermal (e.g., neural tissue, skin), and endodermal (e.g., gut, bronchial epithelium) elements. Elements may be mature (resembling adult tissues) or immature (sharing histologic features with embryonic or fetal tissues).

Teratoma with malignant transformation signifies a nongerm cell malignancy developing within a teratoma. When the nongerm cell component spreads outside the testis, it usually does not respond to chemotherapy; therefore cure depends on tumor resectability.

Mixed Tumors *(p. 979)*

Clinical Features of Testicular Germ Cell Tumors (p. 979)

In 60% of cases, testicular germ cell tumors contain mixtures of multiple cell types; prognosis is a function of the most aggressive element. Although most germ cell tumors are capable of rapid, wide dissemination, they usually respond to current therapies.

- Most cases present with *painless enlargement of the testis;* clinical evaluation does not reliably distinguish between the various types.
- Because testicular biopsy could cause "tumor spillage" necessitating scrotal excision *in addition to* orchiectomy, standard management is radical orchiectomy based on a presumption of malignancy.
- Lymphatic metastases typically first involve *retroperitoneal para-aortic* nodes but can then spread more widely; *hematogenous* metastases predominantly involve the lung, followed by liver, brain, and bone. Because of the histologic mixtures present in many of these tumors, metastases need not be identical to the primary tumors and can contain other germ cell elements (e.g., teratomatous metastases from an "apparent" embryonal carcinoma primary).
- Nonseminomatous germ cell tumors (NSGCTs) are generally more aggressive than seminomas, and patients do slightly worse.
    - *Seminomas* are typically radiosensitive, and 70% present with localized (clinical stage I) disease. More than 95% of patients with stage I or stage II disease (extension to retroperitoneal nodes) are cured.

- *NSGCTs* are relatively radioresistant, and 60% present with advanced disease (stage II, or stage III = metastases above the diaphragm); 90% can achieve remission with chemotherapy.
- *Pure choriocarcinomas* are particularly aggressive, and extensive hematogenous metastases can be present even with small primary lesions. They have a poor prognosis.

Biomarkers

- Germ cell neoplasms often produce hormones or enzymes that can be used for diagnosis and monitoring:
  - *AFP* is markedly elevated in endodermal sinus tumors but present at lower levels in other germ cell tumors.
  - High *hCG* is typical of choriocarcinomas but also present at lower levels in 15% of seminomas, as well as other NSGCT.
  - Lactate dehydrogenase, although nonspecific, can provide an approximate measure of tumor burden.

Tumors of Sex Cord-Gonadal Stroma (p. 979)

Classification is based on Leydig versus Sertoli cell differentiation.

Leydig Cell Tumors (p. 980)

Leydig cell tumors account for only 2% of all testicular tumors; most occur between the ages of 20 and 60 years. Tumors can produce androgens, estrogens, and/or corticosteroids; patients typically present with a *testicular mass* but can also exhibit changes referable to hormone elaboration (e.g., gynecomastia or sexual precocity). Most are benign, although 10% invade or metastasize.

Sertoli Cell Tumors (p. 980)

Sertoli cell tumors typically present only as a testicular mass and are hormonally silent; 10% pursue a malignant course.

Testicular Lymphoma (p. 980)

Testicular lymphomas account for 5% of all testicular neoplasms and are the most common testicular tumor in patients older than 60 years. Most are diffuse large B-cell non-Hodgkin lymphomas and disseminate widely, with a high incidence of central nervous system (CNS) involvement.

Miscellaneous Lesions of Tunica Vaginalis (p. 980)

- *Hydrocele:* Accumulation of serous fluid within the mesothelial-lined tunica vaginalis, usually due to generalized edema.
- *Hematocele:* Accumulation of blood secondary to trauma, torsion, or a generalized bleeding diathesis.
- *Chylocele:* Accumulation of lymphatic fluid, secondary to lymphatic obstruction (e.g., elephantiasis).
- *Spermatocele:* Local cystic accumulation of semen in dilated ductuli efferentes or rete testis.
- *Varicocele:* Dilated vein in the spermatic cord; may be asymptomatic or contribute to infertility.
- *Malignant mesothelioma* rarely arises in the tunica vaginalis.

Prostate (p. 980)

Prostatic parenchyma can be divided into four biologically and anatomically distinct zones; the proliferative lesions are different for each region (Fig. 21-1).

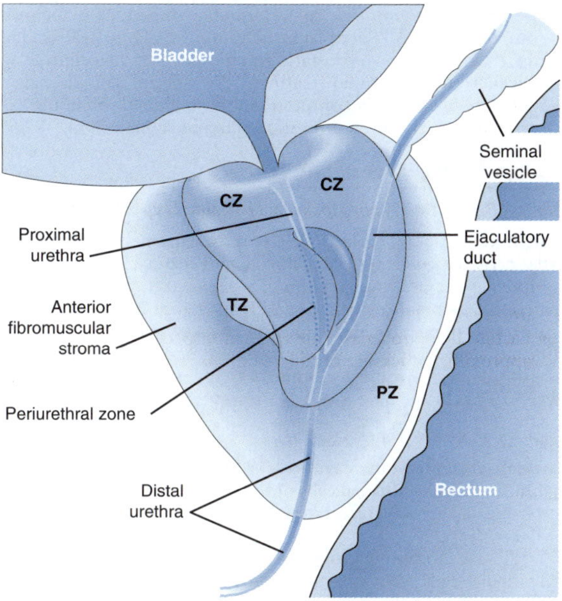

Figure 21-1 Normal adult prostate. Four zones include a central zone (CZ), a peripheral zone (PZ), a transitional zone (TZ), and a periurethral zone. Most carcinomas arise in the PZ and may be palpable during digital examination of the rectum. Nodular hyperplasia arises from the more centrally situated TZ typically leading to urinary obstruction.

Inflammation (p. 981)

- *Acute bacterial prostatitis* (p. 981) is typically caused by organisms associated with UTI (e.g., *E. coli*, other gram-negative rods, enterococci, and staphylococci).
    - Prostatic infection occurs through urinary reflux or lymphohematogenous seeding from more distant sites; it can also follow catheterization or surgical manipulation.
    - Patients present with fever, chills, dysuria, and a boggy, markedly tender prostate; diagnosis is based on clinical features and urine culture.
- *Chronic bacterial prostatitis* (p. 981) is an insidious disorder that can be asymptomatic or associated with low back pain, suprapubic and perineal discomfort, and dysuria. It is frequently associated with a history of *recurrent UTI* but without previous acute prostatitis; the organisms are those typically involved in acute prostatitis.
    - Because antibiotics penetrate the prostate poorly, bacteria find safe haven and can recurrently seed the urinary tract.
    - Diagnosis is based on finding leukocytes and positive bacterial cultures in prostatic secretions.
- *Chronic abacterial prostatitis* (p. 981) is the most common form of prostatitis.
    - Manifestations are similar to chronic bacterial prostatitis but *without* recurrent UTIs.
    - Prostatic secretions contain >10 leukocytes per high-power field, but cultures are uniformly negative.

- *Granulomatous prostatitis* (p. 981). In the United States the most common cause is related to instillation of BCG to treat bladder cancer; in this setting, prostatic granulomas are of no clinical significance and require no treatment. Nonspecific granulomatous prostatitis is relatively common and represents a reaction to secretions from ruptured prostatic ducts and acini.

Benign Enlargement (p. 982)

Benign Prostatic Hyperplasia or Nodular Hyperplasia (p. 982)

Benign prostatic hyperplasia (BPH) is an extremely common disorder caused by periurethral epithelial and stromal hyperplasia that compresses the urethra; symptoms are related to urinary flow obstruction. Histologic evidence of BPH is present in 20% of men by age 40, 70% of men by age 60, and 90% by age 70; only half will have clinically detectable prostate enlargement, and of those, only 50% develop clinical symptoms. Some 30% of white American males over 50 years of age have moderate-to-severe symptoms.

Etiology and Pathogenesis (p. 982)

The critical mediator in this process is dihydrotestosterone (DHT)—synthesized by the stromal cells of the prostate from circulating testosterone via 5α-reductase, type 2 (Fig. 21-2).

- DHT binds to the nuclear androgen receptor (AR) in stromal and epithelial cells, activating the transcription of androgen-dependent genes.
- DHT is not a direct mitogen but does increase the production of secondary growth factors and their receptors, in particular fibroblast growth factor (FGF)-7 by stromal cells.
- FGF-7 acts in a paracrine manner to stimulate *stromal cell proliferation and inhibits epithelial apoptosis.*

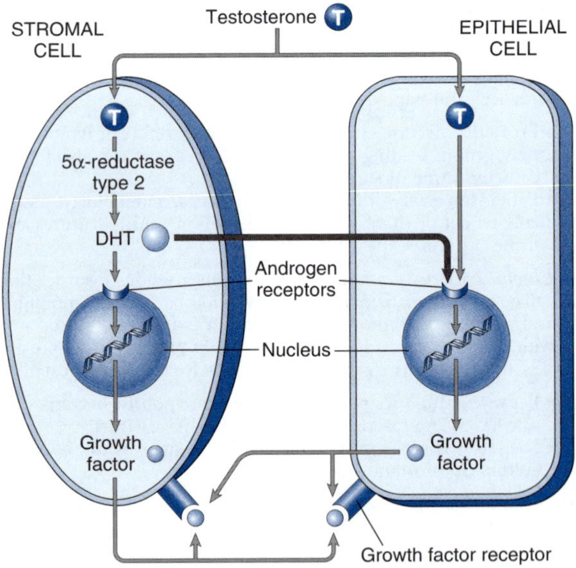

Figure 21-2 Simplified scheme of the pathogenesis of prostatic hyperplasia, emphasizing the central role of stromal cells in generating DHT; DHT may also be produced in skin and liver by both type 1 and 2 5α-reductase.

- Augmented FGF-1 and -2, and TGF-β production also contribute by driving fibroblast proliferation.

Morphology (p. 982)

- *Gross:* The gland is enlarged by nodules primarily in the transitional and periurethral zones (Fig. 21-1); the cut surface demonstrates well-demarcated nodules that can vary from firm and pale-gray (predominantly fibromuscular stromal) to yellow-pink and soft (mostly glands).
- *Microscopic:* Nodules are composed of variable mixtures of proliferating glands and fibromuscular stroma; glands are lined by two layers of cells—a basal layer of low cuboidal epithelium covered by a layer of columnar secretory cells. Other changes include *squamous metaplasia* and *infarcts.*

Clinical Features (p. 983)

The symptoms of lower urinary tract obstruction are due to the increased size of the prostate, the extrinsic compression of the urethra, and smooth muscle-mediated contraction of the prostate. In turn the increased resistance to urinary outflow leads to bladder hypertrophy and distention, with urinary retention. Patients manifest with the following:

- Urinary frequency, nocturia, and difficulty starting and stopping the stream of urine.
- Chronic urinary stasis with resultant bacterial overgrowth and UTIs.
- Urinary bladder diverticula and hydronephrosis.

Therapy can include α-blockers that inhibit the α_1-adrenergic receptors mediating prostate smooth muscle tone. In addition, 5α-reductase inhibitors can reduce the underlying DHT-mediated stimulation, and—for recalcitrant prostates—surgical (e.g., transurethral resection of the prostate [TURP]) and various other debulking approaches are available.

Tumors (p. 983)

Adenocarcinoma (p. 983)

Prostatic carcinoma is the *most common* form of cancer in men (29% of U.S. cancers) with a one in six lifetime risk; it is responsible for 9% of cancer deaths. Prostatic carcinoma occurs predominantly in men over age 50; the incidence increases from 20% in men >50 years to 70% for men in their 70s. It is uncommon in Asians and is more common in blacks than in whites. The clinical behavior ranges from aggressively lethal to indolent and incidental.

Etiology and Pathogenesis (p. 984)

Clinical and epidemiologic data implicate advancing age, race, hormonal influences, genetic factors, and environmental factors (e.g., diet).

- *Androgens:* Prostate cancer cells depend on androgen interactions with AR to activate progrowth and prosurvival genes.
  - The X-linked AR gene contains a polymorphic sequence composed of CAG (glutamine) repeats. AR with shorter glutamine repeats (common in blacks) are more sensitive to androgens, whereas AR with fewer repeats (common in Asians) are less sensitive; whites typically have intermediate-length repeats.
  - Castration and antiandrogen therapies slow tumor progression, although most tumors eventually become resistant to androgen

blockade (e.g., through mutations that allow activation by low-level androgens or nonandrogen ligands or that bypass the need for AR).

- *Germline genes:* Risk increases with the number of first-degree relatives with prostate cancer (one relative = twofold increased risk; two relatives = fivefold increased risk), and the onset of disease occurs at an earlier age.
  - *BRCA2* mutations increase risk twentyfold, but most familial prostate cancers are associated with loci that only modestly affect risk.
  - Mutations in *HOXB13* (a homeobox gene encoding a transcription factor that regulates prostate development) confer substantially increased risk.
  - Several risk loci are associated with innate immunity, suggesting that inflammation can underlie prostate cancer development.
- Acquired mutations and epigenetic changes include the following:
  - Chromosomal rearrangements that juxtapose an *ETS* family transcription factor gene next to the androgen-regulated *TMPRSS2* promoter lead to overexpression of the ETS transcription factors that make prostate epithelial cells more invasive.
  - Hypermethylation of the glutathione *S*-transferase gene down-regulates its expression and leads to increased susceptibility to a variety of carcinogens normally modified by the enzyme.
  - Common genetic alterations in prostate cancer include amplification of the 8q24 locus containing the *MYC* oncogene and deletions involving the *PTEN* tumor suppressor. In late-stage disease, loss of *TP53* (by deletion or mutation) and deletions involving *Rb* are common, as are amplifications of the AR gene locus.
- *Diet:* Risk is associated with increased fat consumption; dietary products that appear to prevent, inhibit, or delay progression of prostate cancer include lycopenes (found in tomatoes), vitamin D, selenium, and soy products.
- *Precursor lesions: Prostatic intraepithelial neoplasia (PIN)* is now identified as a precursor on the spectrum to prostatic carcinoma; it contains many of the molecular changes seen in malignancy (e.g., *ETS* rearrangements).

Morphology (p. 985)

Most cases (70%) arise in the peripheral zone of the prostate, usually in the posterior prostate.

- *Gross:* Primary lesions characteristically are poorly demarcated, gritty, firm, and yellow. Locally advanced cases may infiltrate the seminal vesicles and urinary bladder; invasion of the rectum is uncommon.
- *Microscopic:* Most are well-differentiated *adenocarcinomas* with small, crowded glands lined by a single layer of epithelium *(lacking the outer basal layer of cells);* nuclei are large and often exhibit nucleoli. Perineural invasion is a sign of malignancy.
  - High-grade PIN consisting of architecturally benign but cytologically atypical cells is associated with 80% of prostate carcinomas.
  - The *Gleason system* stratifies prostate cancers into five grades based on their glandular patterns (1 = closest to normal; 5 = no glandular differentiation), without regard to cytologic features. The scores of the dominant grade and the second most common grade are added (e.g., Gleason grade 3 + 4; the most

well-differentiated tumor has a score of 2 [1 + 1], and the least well-differentiated tumor has a score of 10 [5 + 5]). Low-to-moderate-grade Gleason scores (2 to 6) suggest treatable disease, whereas higher-grade scores portend a grave prognosis.

Clinical Course (p. 988)

- The treatment and prognosis of prostatic carcinoma are influenced primarily by the stage and Gleason grade of the disease. Localized (clinical stage T1 or T2) disease is treated primarily with *surgery or radiotherapy* with a 15-year survival rate of 90%.
- Many prostate cancers have a relatively indolent course; thus it may take 10 years to see benefit from surgery or radiotherapy, and watchful waiting is an appropriate treatment for many older men (or those with significant comorbidity).
- *Metastases* occur initially in obturator nodes, followed by spread to other nodal groups. *Hematogenous dissemination* occurs primarily to bone, most often in the form of *osteoblastic* metastases.
- External beam radiotherapy can be used to treat prostate cancer that is too locally advanced to be cured by surgery. Hormonal therapy for metastatic disease can include orchiectomy, administration of synthetic analogues of luteinizing hormone-releasing hormone, or pharmacologic blockade of the AR; tumors often become refractory to antiandrogen therapies.

Prostate-Specific Antigen (p. 988)

Prostate-specific antigen (PSA) is the most important test used in the diagnosis and management of prostate cancer. PSA is a product of prostatic epithelium and is normally secreted in the semen; serum levels are elevated to a lesser extent in BPH than prostate cancer, although there is considerable overlap. Important points include the following:

- *PSA is organ-specific yet not cancer-specific.* Other factors such as BPH, prostatitis, infarct, and instrumentation of the prostate can increase serum PSA levels. As men age, their prostates tend to enlarge with BPH, with corresponding higher serum PSA levels. Furthermore, 20% to 40% of patients with organ-confined prostate cancer have PSA below the thresholds usually set for screening for malignancy.
- *PSA velocity (rate of change of PSA)* may be a more useful measurement than just a single PSA value. This reflects the finding that PSA levels rise faster in prostate cancer than for age-related hyperplasia. Multiple measurements need to be made over a period of 1 to 2 years.
- In the setting of known prostatic carcinoma, PSA monitoring is useful in assessing response to therapy or progression of disease.

In addition to PSA, *PCA3* is a noncoding RNA which is overexpressed in 95% of prostate cancers and can be quantified in urine, serving as an additional biomarker. The combination of urinary PCA3 plus urine *TMPRSS2-ERG* fusion DNA may have increased sensitivity and specificity compared to PSA screening alone.

22 The Female Genital Tract

Infections (p. 992)

Many common infections of the female genital tract (e.g., *Candida, Trichomonas,* and *Gardnerella*) typically cause discomfort but do not have serious sequelae. Others (e.g., *Neisseria gonorrhoeae* and *Chlamydia*) are major causes of female infertility; *Ureaplasma urealyticum* and *Mycoplasma hominis* infections are implicated in preterm deliveries. Herpes simplex viruses (HSVs) can cause painful genital ulcerations, whereas human papillomaviruses (HPVs) are involved in the pathogenesis of cervical, vaginal, and vulvar cancers.

Many of these infections are sexually transmitted, including trichomoniasis, gonorrhea, chancroid, granuloma inguinale, lymphogranuloma venereum, syphilis, *Mycoplasma, Chlamydia,* HSV, and HPV. Most of the sexually transmitted infections are discussed in Chapter 8; the following are highlighted specifically for their role in female genital tract pathology.

Infections of the Lower Genital Tract (p. 993)

- *HSV:* Although HSV-1 usually causes an oropharyngeal infection and HSV-2 typically involves genital mucosa and skin, either virus can instigate lesions in either site.
  By age 40, 30% of women are seropositive for antibodies against HSV-2. Only a third of newly infected individuals are symptomatic. Infections present with red papules 3 to 7 days after contact; these progress to vesicles and painful, coalescent ulcers, associated with fever, malaise, and tender lymphadenopathy. Although lesions spontaneously heal within 1 to 3 weeks, HSV establishes a latent infection in lumbosacral nerve ganglia and can be reactivated by stress, trauma, immunosuppression, or hormonal changes. Diagnosis is made on the basis of clinical findings and viral cultures.
  Antiviral agents can shorten the duration of symptomatic lesions but do not eliminate latent infections. The most important consequence of HSV infection is transmission to the neonate during birth.
- *Molluscum contagiosum* is a poxvirus infection of skin and mucous membranes; of the four types, type I is most common, and type II is most often sexually transmitted. After a 6-week incubation, characteristic dimpled dome-shaped lesions erupt; these contain cells with intracytoplasmic viral inclusions.
- *Fungal infections* (especially *candidiasis*) are common; yeasts form part of the normal vaginal microflora and can expand to cause symptomatic infections when the normal host microbial ecosystem is disrupted (e.g., by diabetes, antibiotics, pregnancy, or immunosuppression).
- *Trichomonas vaginalis* is a flagellated protozoan transmitted by sexual contact; patients can be asymptomatic or present with

yellow, frothy vaginal discharge, vulvovaginal discomfort, dysuria, or dyspareunia.

- *Gardnerella vaginalis* is a gram-negative bacillus and the major cause of bacterial vaginitis; patients present with a thin, green-gray, fishy-smelling discharge. Such infections can precipitate premature labor.
- *Chlamydia trachomatis* infections mainly take the form of cervicitis; occasional infections can ascend to the uterus and fallopian tubes, resulting in endometritis and salpingitis (and thus are a cause of pelvic inflammatory disease [PID]; see later).

Infections Involving the Lower and Upper Genital Tract (p. 994)

Pelvic Inflammatory Disease (p. 994)

PID results from infections that arise in the vulva or vagina and ascend to involve the other genital tract structures (e.g., cervix, uterus, fallopian tubes, and ovaries); symptoms include pelvic pain, adnexal tenderness, fever, and vaginal discharge. *Gonococcus* is the most common cause, followed by *Chlamydia* and postabortal or postpartum polymicrobial infections (e.g., staphylococci, streptococci, coliforms, and/or *Clostridium perfringens*). Ascending *gonococcal* infections tend to spread via the mucosal surfaces, eliciting an acute suppurative reaction; nongonococcal infections—after abortion or other therapeutic procedures—are typically distributed through lymphatics and veins. Peritonitis and bacteremia (with systemic seeding) are acute complications; chronic sequelae include tubal scarring and obstruction, infertility, increased risk of ectopic pregnancy, pelvic pain, and gastrointestinal (GI)-pelvic adhesions that can cause intestinal obstruction.

Vulva (p. 995)

Bartholin Cyst (p. 996)

Bartholin gland cysts are common lesions resulting from inflammatory occlusion of the draining ducts; they are typically lined by flattened epithelium and can be large (3 to 5 cm) and painful. Treatment involves excision or permanent opening *(marsupialization)*. Bartholin gland infections can also produce abscesses, requiring drainage.

Non-Neoplastic Epithelial Disorders (p. 996)

A heterogeneous group of lesions—clinically designated as *leukoplakia*—manifest as opaque, white, plaquelike thickenings and are often accompanied by pruritus and scaling. Inflammatory etiologies must be distinguished from neoplastic causes.

Lichen Sclerosus (p. 996)

Lesions begin as papules or macules that eventually coalesce into smooth, white parchmentlike areas. Microscopically there is epidermal thinning, superficial hyperkeratosis, and dermal fibrosis with a scant mononuclear perivascular infiltrate. The labia can become atrophic and stiffened, with constriction of the vaginal orifice. An autoimmune response is implicated.

Squamous Cell Hyperplasia (p. 996)

This is a nonspecific response to recurrent rubbing or scratching to relieve pruritus; it is characterized by white plaques that histologically reveal thickened epithelium, hyperkeratosis, and dermal inflammation. Although there is no epithelial atypia and no increased predisposition to malignancy, squamous cell hyperplasia is often present at the margins of vulvar carcinoma.

Benign Exophytic Lesions (p. 996)

As opposed to *condyloma acuminatum* (due to HPV infection; see later) or *condyloma latum* (due to syphilis; see Chapter 8), vulvar *fibroepithelial polyps* (skin tags) and *squamous papillomas* are not related to any infectious agent. The latter are benign exophytic proliferations lined by nonkeratinizing squamous epithelium and can be single or numerous *(vulvar papillomatosis).*

Condyloma Acuminatum (p. 997)

These are verrucous lesions on the vulva, perineum, vagina, and (rarely) cervix that are sexually transmitted by HPV types 6 or 11. Histologically they comprise sessile branching epithelial proliferations of stratified squamous epithelium; mature superficial cells exhibit characteristic perinuclear cytoplasmic clearing with nuclear atypia *(koilocytotic atypia).* Condyloma acuminatum is not considered precancerous.

Squamous Neoplastic Lesions (p. 997)

Vulvar Intraepithelial Neoplasia and Vulvar Carcinoma (p. 997)

Vulvar carcinoma is relatively uncommon, representing only 3% of female genital cancers; most occur in women over age 60. A third of cases are *basaloid* or *warty carcinomas* related to HPV infections (typically HPV-16); two thirds are keratinizing squamous cell carcinoma unrelated to HPV. Prognosis of vulvar carcinomas depends on size, depth of invasion, and lymph node status; patients with lesions <2 cm in diameter have a 90% 5-year survival after vulvectomy and lymphadenectomy, whereas regional lymph node metastasis portends a poor prognosis.

- *Basaloid* and *warty carcinomas* arise from precancerous in situ lesions called *classic vulvar intraepithelial neoplasia (VIN)* (previously designated *carcinoma in situ* or *Bowen disease*); most are positive for HPV-16 and are often associated with vaginal and/or cervical HPV-related lesions. Cancer risk increases with age and immunosuppression.
- *Keratinizing squamous cell carcinomas* typically arise in the setting of long-standing lichen sclerosus or squamous cell hyperplasia; the immediately premalignant lesions are called *differentiated VIN,* distinguished by basal atypia with apparently normal superficial epithelial maturation and differentiation. Risk of cancer development is a function of age, extent, and immune status.

Glandular Neoplastic Lesions (p. 999)

Papillary Hidradenoma (p. 999)

This benign tumor arises from modified apocrine sweat glands. It presents as a sharply circumscribed nodule of tubular ducts lined by nonciliated columnar cells atop a layer of flattened myoepithelial cells.

Extramammary Paget Disease (p. 999)

This malignant lesion appears as a red, crusted, sharply demarcated, maplike area. Histologically there are large, anaplastic, mucin-containing tumor cells lying singly or in small clusters within the epidermis and its appendages; most lesions are confined to the epidermis, and invasion is rare, but even with wide excision, there is a high recurrence rate.

Vagina (p. 1000)

Developmental Anomalies (p. 1000)

- *Septate (double) vagina* accompanies a double uterus and arises from failure of complete fusion of the müllerian ducts. Causes include genetic syndromes, in utero exposure to diethylstilbestrol (DES), or abnormalities of epithelial-stromal signaling in fetal development.
- *Vaginal adenosis* represents red, granular patches of remnant endocervical-type columnar epithelium that have not undergone the normal replacement by squamous epithelium characteristic of adult vaginal mucosa. It occurs at low frequency in normal women but is present in 35% to 90% of women exposed in utero to DES; in that latter setting vaginal adenosis can be a substrate for clear cell carcinoma.
- *Gartner duct cysts* are relatively common lesions derived from wolffian (mesonephric) duct rests and found along the lateral walls of the vagina. These are 1- to 2-cm fluid-filled submucosal cysts.

Premalignant and Malignant Neoplasms of the Vagina (p. 1000)

Most *benign* vaginal tumors occur in reproductive-age women; these include stromal polyps, leiomyomas, and hemangiomas.

Vaginal Intraepithelial Neoplasia and Squamous Cell Carcinoma (p. 1000)

Primary vaginal carcinomas are rare; virtually all are *squamous cell carcinomas* associated with high-risk HPV infection. These arise from *vaginal intraepithelial neoplasia,* analogous to malignant precursor lesions in cervical carcinoma. The upper posterior vagina is the site most commonly affected.

Embryonal Rhabdomyosarcoma (p. 1001)

This is an uncommon, highly malignant vaginal tumor in infants and children consisting of embryonal rhabdomyoblasts. The tumors are polypoid, bulky masses with grapelike clusters (hence the alternate name, *sarcoma botryoides*) that can protrude from the vagina. Tumor cells are small, with oval nuclei and small eccentric cytoplasmic protrusions. Tumors tend to invade locally and cause death by penetration into the peritoneal cavity or through urinary tract obstruction.

Cervix (p. 1001)

The cervix consists of the *ectocervix* and the *endocervical canal;* the ectocervix is covered by a mature squamous epithelium continuous with the vaginal wall. At the *external os,* the ectocervix converges into the endocervix, lined by columnar, mucus-secreting epithelium. This transition is called the *squamocolumnar junction;* its position is variable but trends upward over time into the endocervical canal. The progressive replacement of glandular epithelium by advancing squamous epithelium is called *squamous metaplasia.* The site where columnar epithelium abuts the squamous epithelium is termed the "transformation zone" and is a unique environment that is highly susceptible to infections with HPV due to the presence of immature squamous metaplastic epithelial cells; as a result this zone is the site where cancers and precursor lesions develop.

Inflammations (p. 1001)

Acute and Chronic Cervicitis (p. 1001)

Lactobacilli dominate the cervical and vaginal microbial ecosystem; their production of lactic acid (keeping the pH below 4.5) and hydrogen peroxide largely suppresses the growth of other saprophytic and pathogenic species. However, higher pH (associated with douching, bleeding, or sexual intercourse) can reduce hydrogen peroxide production, and antibiotic therapy can decimate the bacteria, potentially leading to overgrowth by pathogenic species (*acute cervicitis* or *vaginitis*).

Chronic cervicitis is found at a low level in virtually all women and is of little clinical significance. However, infections with gonococci, chlamydiae, mycoplasmas, and HSV can produce significant acute and/or chronic cervicitis and can lead to upper genital tract disease and/or complications of pregnancy. Marked cervical inflammation produces reactive and reparative epithelial changes that can lead to abnormal cytologic smears.

Endocervical Polyps (p. 1002)

Endocervical polyps are benign exophytic growths; they can present with irregular vaginal "spotting." They are composed of a loose connective tissue stroma with dilated glands and inflammation, covered by endocervical epithelium.

Premalignant and Malignant Neoplasms of the Cervix (p. 1002)

Worldwide, cervical cancer is the third most common malignancy in women with more than 500,000 new cases annually and a 50% mortality. By comparison, although cervical cancer was the leading cause of cancer deaths in the United States only 50 years ago, there are now only approximately 12,000 new cases of cervical carcinoma each year, leading to 4000 deaths. The difference-maker has been the *Pap test,* indicating that widespread screening permits the detection and eradication of preinvasive lesions that can progress to cancer if left untreated.

Pathogenesis (p. 1002)

HPV types of high oncogenic risk are the most important factor in cervical oncogenesis (types of low oncogenic risk are associated with condyloma acuminatum); HPV-16 (60% of cases of cervical cancer) and HPV-18 (10% of cases) are most important. Additional risk factors relate to the likelihood of exposure (e.g., multiple sexual partners) and host immune responses. Most HPV infections are asymptomatic and do not cause any tissue changes; 50% are cleared within 8 months and 90% by 2 years. Persistent infection (as with high-risk types or immunocompromise) increases the risk of developing malignancy.

HPV are DNA viruses that infect only immature basal cells of the squamous epithelium (through a break in the epithelium) or metaplastic squamous cells at the cervical squamocolumnar junction. However, HSVs *replicate* in the maturing nonproliferating squamous cells (such viral proliferation is reflected in koilocytotic change of the cells). In order for HSV to induce DNA replication in these cells, it must therefore reactivate the cellular mitotic cycle; HSV does so primarily by interfering with the function of the p53 and Rb tumor suppressors. Thus viral E6 and E7 proteins do the following:

- Upregulate cyclin E expression (E7 induces Rb degradation)
- Interrupt apoptotic pathways (E6 induces p53 degradation)
- Induce centrosome duplication and genomic instability (E6, E7)
- Upregulate telomerase expression (E6)

It is important to note that *all* HPV types increase the proliferation and lifespan of infected cells; the relative oncogenic risk of the different virus types may be related to whether the viral DNA is integrated (cancers) or episomal (condylomas and precancerous lesions), or whether the high-risk viruses induce additional genetic changes (e.g., 3p deletions). HPV infections alone are not sufficient to cause cancer. Definitive development of malignancy likely also depends on effects related to other coinfections, inflammatory responses, hormonal influences, and carcinogenic exposures.

Cervical Intraepithelial Neoplasia (Squamous Intraepithelial Lesions; *p. 1003)*

Precancerous cervical epithelial histologic changes are classified as *low-grade* or *high-grade squamous intraepithelial lesions*—LSILs and HSILs, respectively. More than 80% of LSIL and 100% of HSIL lesions are associated with high-risk HPV; HPV-16 is the most common type associated with both.

- *LSILs* show only mild dysplasia, involving the more basal layers of the epithelium. Although associated with productive HPV infection, there is no significant alteration of the host cell cycle. Approximately 60% of LSILs spontaneously regress within 2 years, whereas another 30% will persist over that period; only 10% progress to HSIL, and LSIL does not proceed directly to invasive carcinoma. It is therefore not treated like a premalignant lesion.
- *HSILs* exhibit moderate-to-severe dysplasia and involve progressively more of the epithelial thickness; this category also includes *carcinoma in situ.* There is further HPV-driven deregulation of the cell cycle, with increased proliferation, decreased epithelial maturation, and diminished viral replication. Approximately 30% of HSIL will regress over 2 years, 60% will persist, and 10% will progress to carcinoma within a 2- to 10-year period.

Morphology (p. 1003)

Lesions are classified according to distribution of cellular and nuclear atypia, including nuclear enlargement, hyperchromasia, chromatin granularity, size variation, and koilocytosis:

- In *LSILs,* the atypia is confined to the basal third of the epithelium.
- In *HSILs,* the atypia extends to two thirds (or more) of the epithelial thickness.

Cervical Carcinoma *(p. 1004)*

Squamous cell carcinoma constitutes 80% of cervical cancers, whereas adenocarcinoma comprises 15%, and adenosquamous and neuroendocrine carcinomas collectively amount to 5%; all are associated with high-risk HPV. Peak incidence of invasive cervical cancer is age 45; increasingly, cervical cancers are detected at subclinical stages by routine Pap smear screening.

Morphology (p. 1005)

- *Gross:* Lesions can be exophytic or infiltrative.
- *Microscopic:* Squamous lesions can be keratinizing or nonkeratinizing; adenocarcinomas tend to be glandular but relatively

mucin-depleted; adenosquamous lesions are composed of intermixed malignant squamous and glandular elements; neuroendocrine tumors resemble small cell malignancy of the lung.

- Staging is based on depth of invasion, involvement of adjacent structures, and/or metastatic spread.

Clinical Features (p. 1006)

Although early invasive cancers may be treated by cervical cone biopsy, most are managed by hysterectomy and lymph node dissection, with irradiation for advanced disease. Prognosis and survival depend on stage more than grade; 5-year survival for microinvasive carcinoma is 100% ranging to <50% for the most advanced disease; neuroendocrine tumors have a particularly poor prognosis.

Cervical Cancer Screening and Prevention (p. 1006)

Adjunct HPV DNA testing can be added to the routine cytology screening; positivity in an individual for high-risk HPV types—even with normal cytology—mandates more frequent testing. An abnormal Pap smear is typically followed by a colposcopic exam with selected biopsies; LSILs can be followed conservatively, whereas HSIL pathology is usually treated by cervical conization and lifelong follow-up. Prophylactic vaccines directed against HPV types 6 and 11 (condylomas) and 16 and 18 (70% of cervical cancers) can markedly reduce the incidence of HSILs but do not eliminate cancer risk from other HPV types.

Body of Uterus and Endometrium (p. 1007)

Endometrial Histology in the Menstrual Cycle (p. 1007)

The endometrium undergoes dynamic physiologic and morphologic changes during the menstrual cycle in response to ovarian sex steroid hormones; the ovary is influenced by hormones produced by the pituitary responding to hypothalamic inputs. Ovarian hormones affect the endometrium by binding to nuclear receptors. For example, estrogen drives glandular and stromal proliferation in the *proliferative phase;* interestingly, much of the effect on glandular proliferation occurs through estrogen induction of stromal cell growth factors (e.g., insulin-like growth factor 1 and epidermal growth factor) that bind receptors expressed on the epithelial cells. During the *secretory phase,* progesterone downregulates the expression of estrogen receptor in both the glands and the stroma, suppressing endometrial proliferation; at the same time, progesterone promotes glandular and stromal differentiation. Endometrial stem cells play a central role in endometrial regeneration after menses and can also contribute to the development of ectopic endometrial tissue and endometrial cancer.

Functional Endometrial Disorders (Dysfunctional Uterine Bleeding) (p. 1008)

The most common gynecologic problem during active reproductive life is excessive bleeding during or between menstrual periods. The various causes differ depending on the age of the individual (Table 22-1). Although bleeding can result from a well-defined organic lesion (e.g., submucosal leiomyoma, endometrial polyp, or chronic endometritis), the most common etiology is *dysfunctional uterine bleeding (DUB),* defined as *abnormal bleeding in the absence of an organic (structural) lesion.* Disturbances in the finely tuned

TABLE 22-1 Causes of Abnormal Uterine Bleeding by Age Group

Age Group	Causes
Prepuberty	Precocious puberty (hypothalamic, pituitary, or ovarian origin)
Adolescence	Anovulatory cycle, coagulation disorders
Reproductive age	Complications of pregnancy (abortion, trophoblastic disease, ectopic pregnancy) Organic lesions (leiomyoma, adenomyosis, polyps, endometrial hyperplasia, carcinoma) Anovulatory cycle Ovulatory dysfunctional bleeding (e.g., inadequate luteal phase)
Perimenopausal	DUB Anovulatory cycle Irregular shedding Organic lesions (carcinoma, hyperplasia, polyps)
Postmenopausal	Organic lesions (carcinoma, hyperplasia, polyps) Endometrial atrophy

hormonal regulation of endometrial proliferation, differentiation, and shedding are the most common causes.

- *Anovulatory cycle* (p. 1009): Lack of ovulation causes prolonged, excessive estrogen without the counteractive progestational phase; most anovulatory cycles have no obvious explanation and are attributed to subtle hormonal imbalances. DUB associated with menopause may be related to ovarian insufficiency and anovulatory cycles.
- *Inadequate luteal phase* (p. 1010) results in low progesterone output with early menses and is often associated with infertility.

Inflammatory Disorders (p. 1010)

- *Acute endometritis* (p. 1010) is uncommon, usually limited to bacterial infections occurring after delivery or miscarriage and related to retained products of conception. Curettage and antibiotics are usually sufficient therapy.
- *Chronic endometritis* (p. 1010) can present with abnormal bleeding, pain, discharge, and/or infertility; histologically there is endometrial plasma cell and macrophage infiltration. It occurs in patients with the following:
    - Chronic PID (*Chlamydia* is a common culprit)
    - Retained gestational tissue postabortion or postpartum
    - Intrauterine contraceptive devices
    - Disseminated tuberculosis (rare)
    - 15% have no obvious cause

Endometriosis and Adenomyosis (p. 1010)

Endometriosis is the presence of endometrial tissue *outside* the uterus; it involves (in descending order) ovaries, uterine ligaments, rectovaginal septum, cul de sac, pelvic peritoneum, GI tract, mucosa of the cervix, vagina, or fallopian tube, and laparotomy scars. These ectopic foci of endometrium are under the influence of ovarian hormones and therefore undergo cyclic menstrual changes with periodic bleeding but have no means of sloughing externally like normal endometrial lining.

The pathogenesis of endometriosis is proposed to involve either (1) retrograde menstruation through the fallopian tubes, allowing diffuse seeding of endometrial tissue, or (2) metaplasia of coelomic epithelium or differentiation from bone marrow–derived stem cells. Endometriotic tissue differs from normal endometrium by exhibiting marked activation of inflammatory cascades and increased stromal aromatase activity (and thus estrogen production). Overproduction of prostaglandins and estrogen (and relative progesterone resistance) enhances the survival and persistence of endometriotic foci.

Morphology *(p. 1012)*

- *Gross:* Endometriosis manifests as red-blue to yellow-brown mucosal or serosal nodules. Extensive disease can be marked by organizing hemorrhage and fibrosis. Large cystic masses in the ovaries can be filled with brown fluid from previous hemorrhage forming "chocolate cysts" or endometriomas.
- *Microscopic:* Foci classically exhibit endometrial glands and stroma, with or without hemosiderin.

Clinical Features *(p. 1012)*

Endometriosis typically manifests in the third and fourth decades, affecting 6% to 10% of women; symptoms include infertility, *dysmenorrhea* (painful menstruation), *dyspareunia* (pain with intercourse), pain on defecation (due to involvement of the rectal wall), *dysuria* (from bladder wall involvement), and pelvic pain (due to periuterine adhesions). Uncommonly, malignancy can develop from the ectopic foci. *Adenomyosis* is a related disorder characterized by nests of endometrial tissues in the uterine myometrium. These are continuous with the endometrial lining, suggesting downgrowth; 20% of women are affected.

Endometrial Polyps (p. 1012)

Endometrial polyps are exophytic masses of endometrial glands and stroma that project into the endometrial cavity; they may be associated with elevated estrogens or tamoxifen therapy. The stromal cells in endometrial polyps have chromosomal rearrangements similar to those in other benign mesenchymal tumors, suggesting that the polyp stroma is neoplastic and that the associated glands are just reactive. The glands can thus be hyperplastic or atrophic and may even occasionally demonstrate secretory changes *(functional polyps).* Endometrial polyps are usually benign and manifest primarily with abnormal bleeding, but can occasionally develop into adenocarcinoma.

Endometrial Hyperplasia (p. 1012)

Endometrial hyperplasia—defined as an increased proliferation of endometrial glands relative to the stroma—is an important cause of abnormal uterine bleeding; it is also clinically important as a precursor lesion in the continuum to endometrial carcinoma. This lesion is associated with prolonged estrogen stimulation of the endometrium; causes range from exogenous administration to anovulation, obesity, polycystic ovarian disease, and functioning estrogen-producing tumors. Endometrial hyperplasia is often associated with inactivation of the *PTEN* tumor suppressor gene (20% of cases), leading to enhanced AKT phosphorylation with increased proliferation and diminished apoptosis.

Morphology *(p. 1013)*

- *Nonatypical hyperplasia* exhibits benign, cystically dilated glands in response to persistent estrogen stimulation; these rarely progress to adenocarcinoma.

- *Atypical hyperplasia (endometrial intraepithelial neoplasia)* shows gland crowding and cytologic changes; there is substantial overlap with endometrial adenocarcinoma, and 23% to 48% of patients with such changes have concurrent malignancy.

Atypical hyperplasia is managed by hysterectomy or a trial of progestin therapy and close follow-up; lack of regression prompts removal of the uterus.

Malignant Tumors of the Endometrium (p. 1013)

Carcinoma of the Endometrium *(p. 1013)*

Endometrial carcinoma accounts for 7% of all invasive cancers in women, with a peak incidence at age 55 to 65 years; there are more than 47,000 new cases annually in the United States, with more than 8000 associated deaths each year. Two epidemiologic and pathophysiologic categories are described (Table 22-2; Fig. 22-1):

Type I (Endometrial) Carcinomas (p. 1014)

Type I (endometrial) carcinomas are the most common (80%); these are well differentiated *(endometrioid carcinoma)* and typically arise in the setting of *endometrial hyperplasia* (with the same overall risk associations). *PTEN* mutations are seen in 30% to 80% of endometrioid carcinomas; in addition, tumors often exhibit microsatellite instability, as well as mutations involving components of the PI3 kinase complex, and *KRAS* and β-catenin oncogenes. Loss-of-function mutations in *ARID1A,* a regulator of chromatin structure, occur in approximately one third of tumors. Defects involving *DNA mismatch repair genes* occur in 20% of sporadic tumors; these are particularly prevalent in endometrial carcinomas in families with hereditary nonpolyposis colorectal carcinoma. *P53* loss-of-function mutations may be late events.

Morphology (p. 1016)

- *Gross:* These can be localized polypoid tumors or diffuse spreading lesions.
- *Microscopic:* Most (85%) are endometrioid adenocarcinomas with epithelium resembling normal endometrium; grading depends on the mix of well-differentiated glands and more poorly differentiated solid tumor. Foci of squamous differentiation are seen in 20% of cases.

Type II (Serous) Carcinomas (p. 1017)

Type II (serous) carcinomas typically arise a decade later than type I tumors and occur in the setting of *endometrial atrophy;* these are poorly differentiated tumors. The most common subtype is *serous carcinoma* due to biologic overlaps with similar ovarian lesions; *p53* mutations are present in at least 90% and appear to be early oncogenic events. Endometrial intraepithelial carcinoma (EIC) without invasion is a precursor to serous carcinoma.

TABLE 22-2 Natural History of Squamous Intraepithelial Lesions With Approximate 2-Year Follow-up

Lesion	Regress	Persist	Progress
LSIL	60%	30%	10% to HSIL
HSIL	30%	60%	10% to carcinoma*

*Progression within 2-10 yr.

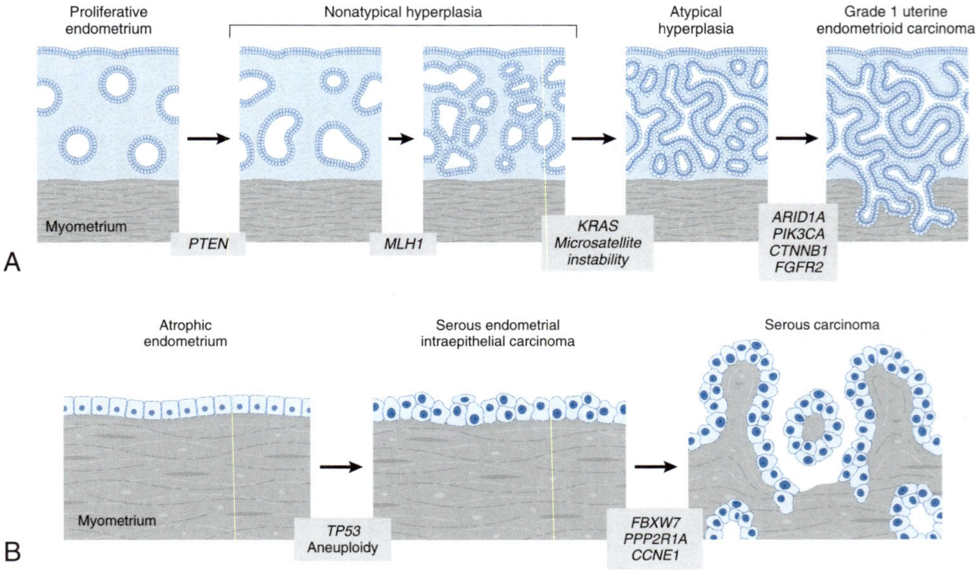

Figure 22-1 **A,** Schematic depicting the development of type I endometrial carcinoma arising in the setting of hyperplasia. **B,** Schematic diagram of the development of type II endometrial carcinoma. The most common molecular genetic alterations are shown at the time they are most likely to occur during the progression of the disease. *CCNE1,* Cyclin E gene; *CTNNB1,* beta-catenin gene; *PPP2R1A,* PP2A gene.

Morphology *(p. 1018)*

- *Gross:* Tumors are usually large and bulky or deeply invasive.
- *Microscopic:* Invasive lesions exhibit a papillary or glandular growth pattern characteristically with marked cellular atypia.

Clinical Features *(p. 1018).* Patients typically present with uterine bleeding or an abnormal Pap smear. Prognosis depends largely on disease stage and grade; it is excellent (90% 5-year survival) when cancer is confined to the uterine corpus and is well differentiated. However, serous tumors have a propensity for extensive extrauterine spread even when apparently confined to the endometrium, and 5-year survivals are 18% to 27%; serous carcinoma occurs more frequently in black women.

Malignant Mixed Müllerian Tumors *(p. 1018)*

Malignant mixed müllerian tumor (MMMT) are endometrial adenocarcinomas associated with concurrent malignant stroma changes attributable to a common neoplastic precursor for both lineages. The stromal component tends to differentiate into a variety of malignant mesodermal components. Mutations are typically found in *PTEN, TP53,* and PIK3CA. MMMT are highly malignant; 5-year survival rates = 25% to 30%.

Morphology (p. 1018)

- *Gross:* Tumors are bulky, fleshy, and polypoid.
- *Microscopic:* Lesions consist of malignant glandular and stromal elements; the stromal sarcomatous elements may show muscle, cartilage, and osteoid differentiation.

Tumors of Endometrial Stroma (p. 1019)

These are relatively uncommon tumors, comprising <5% of endometrial cancers.

Adenosarcomas *(p. 1019)*

These characteristically occur in the fourth and fifth decades of life; they are estrogen-sensitive tumors exhibiting *stromal neoplasia with benign glands.* Grossly they are large polypoid growths, generally considered as low-grade malignancies, although a quarter of cases recur after hysterectomy.

Stromal Tumors *(p. 1019)*

- *Benign stromal nodules* are discrete lumps of stromal neoplasia within the myometrium.
- *Endometrial stromal sarcomas* are lesions composed of malignant stroma interposed between myometrial bundles; they are distinguished by diffuse infiltration and/or lymphatic invasion. A recurrent translocation involving *JAZF1* (encoding a transcriptional repressor) and *SUZ12* (encoding a protein that participates in repressive histone marking) leads to aberrant expression of oncogenes. Five-year survival rates approach 50%.

Tumors of the Myometrium (p. 1019)

Leiomyomas *(p. 1019)*

Commonly called "fibroids," these are *benign masses of uterine smooth muscle cells;* they are the most common tumor in women. Although most have a normal karyotype, approximately 40% have a balanced t(12;14) translocation or rearrangements of 6p; these involve *HMGIC* and *HMGIY* genes that encode DNA-binding factors that regulate chromatin structure. Approximately 70% of leiomyomas also have mutations in *MED12,* involving a component of the multiprotein Mediator complex that stimulates gene expression by bridging promoters and enhancers. Leiomyomas may be asymptomatic or can present with abnormal uterine bleeding, pain, urinary bladder disorders, and impaired fertility. Malignant transformation is extremely rare.

Morphology (p. 1020)

- *Gross:* Tumors are sharply circumscribed, discrete, round, firm, gray-white nodules that occur within the myometrium (intramural), beneath the serosa (subserosal), or immediately beneath the endometrium (submucosal).
- *Microscopic:* Lesions show characteristically whorled bundles of relatively uniform smooth muscle cells, with rare mitoses; variants can exhibit increased cellularity or atypical, bizarre cells.

Leiomyosarcomas (p. 1020)

Leiomyosarcomas are uncommon malignancies that form bulky, fleshy masses in the uterine wall or projecting into the lumen. These tumors have complex, highly variable karyotypes, and a subset expresses *MED12* mutations akin to those that occur in leiomyomas. Histologic features that distinguish these from benign leiomyomas include increased numbers of mitoses (5 to 10 per 10 high-power fields), accompanied by a wide range of cellular atypia and/or necrosis.

These tumors disseminate throughout the abdominal cavity and aggressively metastasize. The overall 5-year survival rate is 40%, although anaplastic tumors have 5-year survivals of only 10% to 15%.

Fallopian Tubes (p. 1021)

Inflammations (p. 1021)

Suppurative salpingitis is typically a component of PID; gonococcal infections account for 60% of cases although any of the pyogenic organisms can be involved; *Chlamydia* is less often a factor. *Tuberculous salpingitis* is rare in the United States but is an important cause of infertility worldwide.

Tumors and Cysts (p. 1021)

- The most common primary lesions are benign *paratubal cysts*—1- to 2-mm translucent cysts filled with serous fluid; larger versions near the fimbria are called *hydatids of Morgagni.*
- Benign neoplasms include *adenomatoid tumors,* comprising small nodules of mesothelial cells.
- Primary tubal *adenocarcinoma* is rare. Even early-stage tumors have a 40% 5-year mortality; prognosis worsens with higher stages.

Ovaries (p. 1022)

Non-Neoplastic and Functional Cysts (p. 1022)

Follicle and Luteal Cysts (p. 1022)

Extremely common findings, these are typically multiple and usually <2 cm; they are lined by follicular or luteinized cells with a clear, serous fluid. Cysts derive from unruptured graafian follicles or follicles that have resealed after rupture. Although typically asymptomatic, they can rupture with ensuing peritoneal inflammation and pain.

Polycystic Ovaries and Stromal Hyperthecosis (p. 1022)

Polycystic ovary syndrome (PCOS; Stein-Leventhal syndrome) affects 6% to 10% of reproductive-age women; it presents with numerous cystic follicles, often with associated oligomenorrhea, persistent anovulation, obesity, hirsutism, and insulin resistance. Disturbances in androgen biosynthesis are causally implicated. The ovaries are enlarged with innumerable subcortical cysts. Due to increased estrone levels, PCOS also increases the risk for endometrial hyperplasia and carcinoma.

Stromal hyperthecosis is a disorder of ovarian stroma typically in postmenopausal women; it is reflected by stromal hypercellularity and luteinization visible as discrete nests of cells with vacuolated cytoplasm. The clinical manifestations are similar to PCOS, although virilization can be profound.

Ovarian Tumors (p. 1022)

Ovarian tumors can arise from the epithelium, germ cells, or sex cord-stroma; overall, 80% are benign, and most occur in women 20 to 45 years old (Table 22-3). Malignant tumors typically occur in older women (45 to 65 years) and represent 3% of all female cancers; because most are detected only after spreading beyond the ovary, they account for a disproportionate number of cancer deaths.

Epithelial Tumors (p. 1023)

Most primary ovarian neoplasms are epithelial; *most arise from müllerian epithelium.* Classification is based on the extent of proliferation and type of differentiation; greater proliferation generally connotes greater malignant potential. Proliferation patterns are classified as *benign, borderline,* and *malignant,* and the differentiation patterns are *serous, mucinous,* or *endometrioid.* Benign lesions are further subclassified based on the components of the tumor: *cystic (cystadenomas), fibrocystic (cystadenofibromas),* and *predominantly fibrous (adenofibromas).* A cystic component in malignant tumors can lead to a designation of *cystadenocarcinoma.*

Ovarian carcinomas are categorized as shown in Figure 22-2. *Type I carcinomas* are low-grade tumors arising in association with

TABLE 22-3 Frequency of Major Ovarian Tumors

Type	Percentage of Malignant Ovarian Tumors	Percentage That Are Bilateral
Serous		
Benign (60%)		25
Borderline (15%)	47	30
Malignant (25%)		65
Mucinous		
Benign (80%)		5
Borderline (10%)	3	10
Malignant (10%)		<5
Endometrioid carcinoma	20	40
Undifferentiated carcinoma	10	—
Clear Cell carcinoma	6	40
Granulosa cell tumor	5	5
Teratoma		15
Benign (96%)	1	Rare
Malignant (4%)		
Metastatic	5	>50
Others	3	—

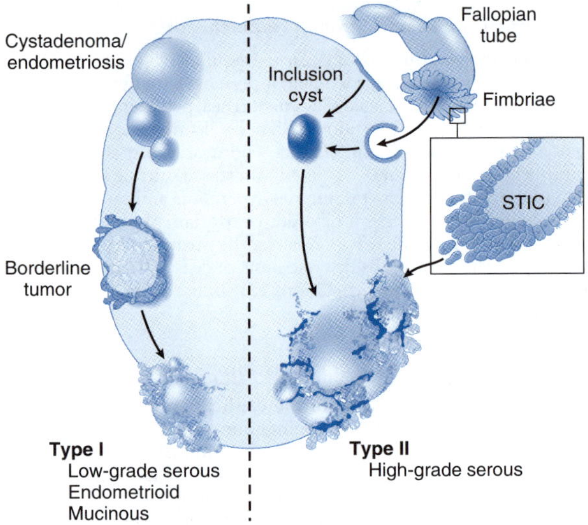

Figure 22-2 Schematic diagram of the pathogenesis of ovarian epithelial tumors. Type I tumors progress from benign tumors through borderline tumors that may give rise to a low-grade carcinoma. These include low-grade serous, endometrioid, and mucinous carcinomas. Type II tumors arise from inclusion cysts or fallopian tube epithelium via intraepithelial precursors that are often not identified. They demonstrate high-grade features and are most commonly of serous histology. *STIC,* Serous tubal intraepithelial carcinoma.

borderline tumors or endometriosis; these include low-grade serous, endometrioid, and mucinous tumors. *Type II carcinomas* are most often high-grade serous tumors arising from serous intraepithelial carcinoma.

Serous Tumors (p. 1024)

Serous tumors account for 30% of all ovarian tumors; 70% are benign or borderline. Serous carcinomas are the most common ovarian malignancy (40% of the total). Prognosis is linked to stage and tumor grade; even with extensive extraovarian spread, low-grade tumors can progress relatively slowly. Five-year survivals for borderline and malignant tumors confined to the ovary are 100% and 70%, respectively; 5-year survivals for similar tumors involving the peritoneum are 90% and 25%.

Pathogenesis *(p. 1024).* Nulliparity, gonadal dysgenesis, family history, and heritable mutations are important risk factors. *BRCA1* and *BRCA2* mutations incur a risk of ovarian cancer developing by age 70 in 20% to 60% of patients; most will be high grade. Low-grade tumors tend to arise in serous borderline tumors and have *KRAS* and *BRAF* mutations; conversely, high-grade tumors have a high frequency of *TP53* mutations. Many of these tumors appear to arise from the fimbriated end of the fallopian tube.

Morphology *(p. 1025)*

- *Gross:* These are typically large cystic masses filled with serous fluid; intracystic loculations can occur. Benign cystadenomas have a smooth and glistening inner lining. The *cystadenocarcinomas* can have small mural nodularities or papillary projections. Bilaterality is common.

- *Microscopic features include the following:*
  - Benign lesions are lined by a single layer of tall, columnar, ciliated epithelial cells, occasionally forming microscopic papillae.
  - Frankly malignant cystadenocarcinomas have multilayered epithelium with many papillary areas and large, solid epithelial masses focally invading the stroma.
  - Borderline tumors demonstrate mild atypia with complex micropapillary epithelial architecture without invasion.

Mucinous Tumors (p. 1026)

Mucinous tumors account for approximately 20% to 25% of all ovarian neoplasms. The vast majority are benign or borderline; primary mucinous carcinomas amount to only 3% of all ovarian malignancies. *KRAS* mutations are a common feature, even in the benign lesions. These tumors can seed the peritoneum with numerous implants that produce extensive mucinous ascites, so-called *pseudomyxoma peritonei* (although this condition is more commonly due to primary appendiceal tumors). Ten-year survival rates for noninvasive stage I disease are >95%; frankly invasive malignant tumors have a 10-year survival of >90%.

Morphology *(p. 1026)*

- *Gross:* Tumors tend to produce large, multiloculated, cystic masses filled with sticky, gelatinous fluid. Only 5% are bilateral.
- *Microscopic features include the following:*
  - Benign lesions are lined by tall, columnar nonciliated epithelium akin to benign cervical or intestinal epithelium with apical mucin.
  - Borderline mucinous tumors exhibit complex growth similar to tubular or villous adenomas in the GI tract.
  - Mucinous carcinomas usually exhibit confluent glandular growth representing a form of expansile invasion.

Endometrioid Ovarian Tumors (p. 1027)

Endometrioid carcinomas account for 10% to 15% of all ovarian cancers; they exhibit epithelium resembling benign or malignant endometrium. Approximately 15% to 20% of cases occur in the setting of concurrent endometriosis, although direct origin from the ovarian surface is also possible. In 15% to 30% of cases, independent endometrial carcinomas also occur. *PTEN, KRAS,* and β-catenin mutations occur frequently, and *TP53* mutations are common in poorly differentiated tumors. Five-year survival for stage I disease is 75%.

Morphology *(p. 1027)*

- *Gross:* Lesions are a combination of solid and cystic masses; 40% are bilateral.
- *Microscopic:* The glandular patterns bear a strong resemblance to endometrial adenocarcinoma.

Clear Cell Carcinoma (p. 1028)

Clear cell carcinoma is uncommon; it is considered a variant of endometrioid adenocarcinoma. Tumors can be cystic or solid; the large epithelial cells contain abundant clear cytoplasm. Patients with cancer confined to the ovary have 5-year survivals of 90%; however, extraovarian spread portends a poor prognosis.

Transitional Cell Tumors (p. 1028)

Also called Brenner tumors, these comprise 10% of ovarian epithelial tumors. They are a variably sized (1 to 30 cm), solid tumor *(adenofibroma)* characterized by dense fibrous stroma and nests of epithelium resembling urinary transitional or rarely columnar epithelium. They are usually unilateral; the vast majority are benign.

Clinical Course, Detection, and Prevention of Ovarian Epithelial Tumors (p. 1028)

- Ovarian epithelial tumors tend to have similar manifestations: Lower abdominal pain and enlargement, with symptoms secondary to bowel or bladder compression. Benign lesions are readily resected; malignant lesions are associated with progressive cachexia, and dissemination beyond the capsule can cause massive ascites and/or diffuse peritoneal studding. Most patients are diagnosed only after the tumor has become large or disseminated, leading to poor overall survival statistics.
- CA-125 is a serum marker for ovarian carcinomas but lacks sensitivity and specificity. It is thus most useful as a tool in monitoring disease progression than in primary diagnosis.
- Screening to identify at-risk patients (e.g., patients with *BRCA* mutations) can identify candidates for prophylactic salpingo-oophorectomy.

Germ Cell Tumors *(p. 1029)*

Germ cell tumors represent 15% to 20% of all ovarian tumors; most are *benign cystic teratomas.* They are similar to male germ cell tumors and arise from neoplastic transformation of totipotential germ cells capable of differentiating into the three germ cell layers (Fig. 22-3).

Teratomas (p. 1029)

- *Mature (benign) teratomas* (*dermoid cysts;* p. 1029) typically arise in young women during their active reproductive years. The karyotype of virtually all benign teratomas is 46,XX, and they likely arise from an ovum after the first meiotic division. Mature teratomas are characteristically cystic masses lined by squamous epithelium with adnexal structures, including hair shafts and sebaceous glands; tooth structures and tissues from other germ cell layers can often also be identified (e.g., cartilage, bone, thyroid, and neural tissues). Tumors are bilateral in 10% to 15% of cases. The vast majority are cured by excision; 1% undergo malignant transformation, most commonly as squamous cell carcinoma.
- *Monodermal or specialized teratomas* (p. 1030) differentiate along the line of a single abnormal tissue. The most common is *struma ovarii,* composed entirely of mature thyroid tissue; ovarian carcinoid is another variant.

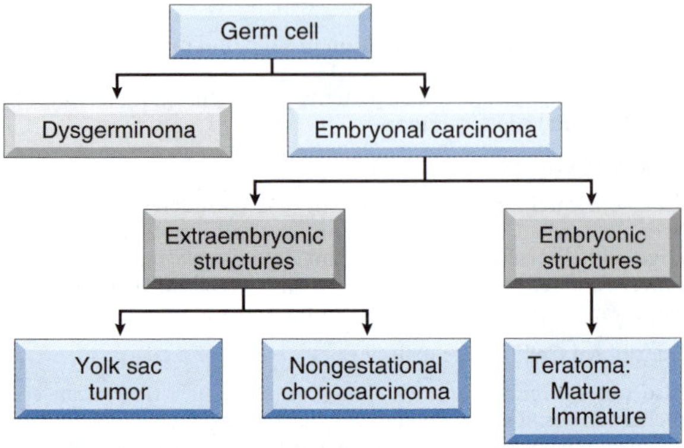

Figure 22-3 Histogenesis and interrelationships of tumors of germ cell origin.

- *Immature (malignant) teratomas* (p. 1030) are rare tumors composed of embryonic (rather than adult) elements resembling immature fetal tissues. These occur chiefly in adolescents and young women. Although they grow rapidly and frequently penetrate the capsule, low-grade tumors have an excellent prognosis, and even high-grade malignancies can respond well to chemotherapy.

Dysgerminoma (p. 1030)

Dygerminoma is the ovarian counterpart of testicular seminoma. These account for 2% of all ovarian cancers, but approximately half of the malignant germ cell tumors. Most occur between ages 20 and 40, and most have no endocrine function. Oct3, Oct4, and Nanog transcription factor expression by dygerminomas maintain pluripotency; the tumors also express the c-KIT receptor tyrosine kinase. All dysgerminomas are malignant, but only approximately one third are highly aggressive; because they are chemosensitive, overall survival exceeds 80%.

Yolk Sac Tumor (p. 1031)

Yolk sac tumor (also called *endodermal sinus tumor*) is a rare malignancy resulting from differentiation of germ cells towards yolk sac structures. Histologically there are glomerulus-like structures with a central vessel enveloped by germ cells within a cystic space lined by additional germ cells *(Schiller-Duval body)*. Intracellular and extracellular hyaline droplets are conspicuous and can contain α-fetoprotein. The tumors occur in children and young women and grow aggressively, although they are chemoresponsive and survival is >80%, independent of disease stage.

Choriocarcinoma (p. 1031)

Choriocarcinoma is another example of extraembryonic differentiation of malignant germ cells; most such tumors exist in combination with other germ cell tumors. Histologically they are identical to placental malignancies and elaborate chorionic gonadotropins. Ovarian choriocarcinomas are highly malignant, metastasize widely, and are much more resistant to chemotherapy than their placental counterparts.

Sex Cord-Stromal Tumors *(p. 1032)*

These tumors originate from ovarian stroma, which in turn derives from the sex cords of the embryonic gonad. The tumors frequently produce estrogens or androgens.

Granulosa Cell Tumors (p. 1032)

Granulosa cell tumors constitute 5% of all ovarian tumors; they are composed of various combinations of theca and granulosa cells. Mutations in *FOXL2* that encode a granulosa cell transcription factor are present in virtually all adult granulosa cell tumors, and two thirds of cases occur in postmenopausal women. Inhibin produced by granulosa cells can be a useful biomarker to diagnose and monitor tumors.

- These tumors can elaborate large amounts of estrogen and thus induce precocious sexual development and endometrial hyperplasia; they predispose to endometrial carcinoma. Occasionally granulosa cell tumors produce masculinizing androgens.
- Although 5% to 25% of granulosa cell tumors are malignant, most have an indolent course, with 10-year survival rates of 85%. Pure thecomas are virtually always benign.

Morphology *(p. 1032)*

- *Gross:* Tumors are usually unilateral, solid, and white-yellow.
- *Microscopic:* The granulosa cell component consists of small cuboidal-to-polygonal cells growing in cords, sheets, or strands; there can be occasional glandlike structures with acidophilic material

(Call-Exner body). The thecal cell components are composed of sheets of plump spindle cells often containing lipid droplets.

Fibromas, Thecomas, and Fibrothecomas (p. 1033)

Fibromas, thecomas, and fibrothecomas account for 4% of all ovarian neoplasms; the vast majority are benign. They are usually unilateral, solid, hard, gray-white masses. The fibroma component is composed of well-differentiated fibroblasts and scant collagenous connective tissue; the thecoma portion contains plump spindle cells with lipid droplets.

Curiously, 40% of tumors are associated with ascites and less often right-sided hydrothorax *(Meigs syndrome)*. They can also be associated with basal cell nevus syndrome (see Chapter 25).

Sertoli-Leydig Cell Tumors (p. 1033)

Sertoli-Leydig cell tumors recapitulate the cells of the testes and commonly produce masculinization or defeminization. They are usually unilateral and consist of tubules composed of Sertoli cells and/or Leydig cells interspersed with stroma. More than 50% of cases have mutations in *DICER1*, a gene encoding an endonuclease that is essential for microRNA processing.

Other Sex Cord-Stromal Tumors (p. 1033)

- *Hilus cell tumors (pure Leydig cell tumors)* are rare, unilateral tumors formed from Leydig cells; these produce testosterone and cause virilization.
- *Pregnancy luteoma* is a rare tumor resembling the corpus luteum of pregnancy; these cause virilization in pregnant patients and their female fetuses.
- *Gonadoblastoma* is an uncommon tumor composed of germ cells and sex-cord stromal derivatives; it occurs in patients with abnormal sexual development and in gonads of indeterminate nature (e.g., phenotypic males with undescended testicles and female internal organs). Half of cases also have a dysgerminoma.

Metastatic Tumors (p. 1034)

Metastatic tumors of the ovary most commonly derive from tumors of müllerian origin (e.g., uterus, fallopian tube, contralateral ovary, or pelvic peritoneum); the sources of the most common extramüllerian metastases are carcinomas of the breast and GI tract. *Krukenberg tumors* are ovarian neoplasms (often bilateral) caused by metastatic mucin-producing signet cells, usually originating from the stomach.

Gestational and Placental Disorders (p. 1034)

Disorders of Early Pregnancy (p. 1035)

Spontaneous Abortion (p. 1035)

Spontaneous abortion ("miscarriage") is defined as pregnancy loss before 20 weeks of gestation; 10% to 15% of clinically recognized pregnancies (and a significant number of unrecognized pregnancies) terminate spontaneously. Causes are the following:

- Maternal (e.g., diabetes, luteal-phase defects, and other endocrine disorders)
- Fetal, with 50% having chromosomal abnormalities and additional numbers with more subtle genetic defects
- Uterine defects (e.g., leiomyomas, polyps, or malformations)

- Systemic disorders affecting the maternal vasculature (e.g., antiphospholipid antibody syndrome, coagulopathies, or hypertension)
- Infections (e.g., Toxoplasmosis, *Mycoplasma, Listeria,* and several viruses)

Ectopic Pregnancy (p. 1036)

Ectopic pregnancy denotes embryo implantation at a site other than the uterus—often fallopian tubes (90%) but also the ovary or abdominal cavity; it occurs in 2% of pregnancies. Predisposing factors include PID with scarring (35% to 50% of patients), intrauterine devices (twofold increased risk), and peritubal adhesions related to endometriosis or prior surgery; 50% occur in apparently normal tubes.

Clinical Features (p. 1036)

Tubal pregnancy has one of four outcomes:

- Intratubal hemorrhage with the formation of *hematosalpinx*
- Tubal rupture with intraperitoneal hemorrhage
- Spontaneous regression with resorption of the products of conception
- Extrusion into the abdominal cavity (tubal abortion)

Tubal rupture is a medical emergency characterized by acute abdomen and shock; diagnosis is suggested by high human chorionic gonadotropin (hCG) levels, ultrasonographic findings, and an endometrial biopsy showing decidual changes and absent chorionic villi. Ectopic pregnancy still accounts for 4% to 10% of pregnancy-related deaths.

Disorders of Late Pregnancy (p. 1036)

Placental pathologies can have outcomes that range from mild intrauterine growth retardation to fetal demise and can also precipitate maternal preeclampsia.

Twin Placentas (p. 1036)

Twin pregnancies arise from fertilization of two ova (dizygotic) or division of one fertilized ovum (monozygotic). The resulting placentas can be monochorionic or dichorionic; a single chorion indicates monozygotic twins, and depending on the time of splitting these can be monoamniotic or diamniotic. Dichorionic placentas are always diamniotic and can occur with either monozygotic or dizygotic twins (Fig. 22-4).

In monochorionic twin pregnancies, vascular anastomoses can allow sharing of the fetal circulations. *Twin-twin transfusion syndrome* occurs if imbalanced flow occurs through an arteriovenous shunt; subsequent disparities in blood volume can lead to death of one or both fetuses.

Abnormalities of Placental Implantation (p. 1037)

- *Placenta previa* denotes placental implantation in the lower uterine segment or cervix and is associated with severe third-trimester bleeding. Complete coverage of the cervical os requires a cesarean delivery to avert the placental rupture and maternal exsanguination of a vaginal delivery.
- *Placenta accreta* occurs when there is absence of decidua and the placenta adheres directly to the myometrium; at delivery the placenta fails to separate, and there is potentially life-threatening hemorrhage.

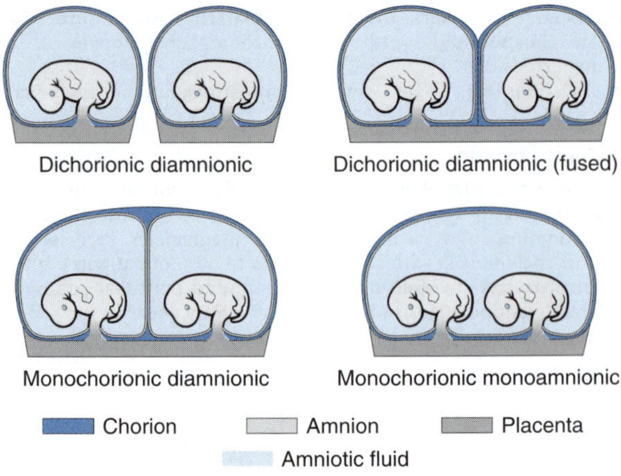

Figure 22-4 Diagrammatic representation of the various types of twin placentation and their membrane relationships. *(Adapted from Gersell DJ, Kraus FT: Diseases of the placenta. In Kurman R (ed):* Blaustein's Pathology of the Female Genital Tract. *New York, NY: Springer, 1994, p. 975-1048.)*

Placental Infections (p. 1037)

- Ascending (usually bacterial) infections via the birth canal are most common; these can cause infection of the chorionic membranes *(acute chorioamnionitis)* that then produces premature membrane rupture and preterm delivery. Inflammation involves the chorion-amnion and fetal umbilical and chorionic plate vessels.
- Hematogenous infections can result from a maternal septicemia, including *Listeria*, streptococcus, and TORCH (*to*xoplasmosis, *r*ubella, *c*ytomegalovirus, *h*erpes) organisms. These are characterized by villous chronic inflammation *(villitis)*.

Preeclampsia and Eclampsia (p. 1037)

Preeclampsia is a syndrome characterized by hypertension, proteinuria, and edema; it occurs in 3% to 5% of pregnancies, usually in the third trimester. *Eclampsia* is a more severe form associated with seizures and coma. Patients can also present with hypercoagulability, renal failure, and pulmonary edema; 10% develop HELLP syndrome (see Chapter 18)—hemolysis, elevated liver enzymes, and low platelets.

Pathogenesis (p. 1038)

The syndromes are associated with systemic endothelial dysfunction, vasoconstriction, and increased vascular permeability driven by placental-derived factors.

- *Abnormal placental vasculature:* In normal pregnancy, fetal trophoblast cells convert the maternal high-resistance decidual spiral arteries into high capacitance uteroplacental vessels lacking a smooth muscle coat. In preeclampsia the remodeling does not occur, and the placenta cannot meet the perfusion demands of late pregnancy. Placental vessel thrombosis or fibrinoid necrosis can have a similar outcome.
- *Endothelial dysfunction and angiogenesis or antiangiogenesis imbalance:* In response to hypoxia the ischemic placenta releases copious amounts of antiangiogenic factors (sFlt-1 and endoglin) that reduce placental vascular development. Placental sFlt-1 and

endoglin in the circulation also lead to widespread maternal endothelial dysfunction by inhibiting vascular endothelial growth factor (VEGF) and transforming growth factor-β (TGF-β)-dependent nitric oxide and prostacyclin production. The consequences include systemic hypertension, and the ensuing endothelial dysfunction leads to proteinuria, edema, and hypercoagulability.

- *Coagulation abnormalities:* Hypercoagulability is likely related to reduced endothelial production of PGI_2 (prostacyclin), and increased release of procoagulant factors, attributable to the antagonism of VEGF by sFlt-1.

Morphology (p. 1039)

The placenta exhibits numerous small, peripheral infarcts, with accelerated villous maturation indicative of chronic ischemia and retroplacental hematomas.

Clinical Features (p. 1039)

Preeclampsia usually occurs after the thirty-fourth week of pregnancy; onset is typically insidious. Delivery is the only definitive treatment, but mild preterm disease can be managed conservatively with monitoring and bed rest. In severe disease, antihypertensive therapy does not affect the course or outcome. In most cases preeclampsia has no permanent sequelae, although 20% of patients will eventually develop hypertension and microalbuminuria, and there is a twofold increase in risk for heart or central nervous system (CNS) vascular disease.

Gestational Trophoblastic Disease (p. 1039)

Gestational trophoblastic disease is a spectrum of tumors and tumor-like conditions, characterized by proliferation of trophoblastic tissue.

Hydatidiform Mole (p. 1039)

Hydatidiform moles are characterized by cystic swelling of chorionic villi, accompanied by variable trophoblastic proliferation; these can be precursors of choriocarcinoma. Risk of a mole is highest at either extreme of the reproductive years; the incidence in the United States is 1 per 1000 to 2000 pregnancies. Benign noninvasive moles are classified as *complete* and *partial,* based on histologic, cytogenetic, and flow cytometric studies (Fig. 22-5; Table 22-4).

- *Complete mole* (p. 1039) occurs when an egg that has lost its chromosomes is fertilized by one or two sperm; all genetic material is therefore paternally derived. Approximately 90% of complete moles derive from the duplicated genetic material of one sperm and are 46,XX; the remainder derive from two sperm and are 46,XX or 46,XY. There is a 2.5% risk of choriocarcinoma and 15% risk of persistent or invasive mole.
- *Partial mole* (p. 1040) occurs when an egg with normal chromosomal content is fertilized by two sperm to get a triploid complement of genetic material; the karyotype is 69,XXX or 69,XXY. There is no increased risk of choriocarcinoma.

Morphology (p. 1040)

- *Gross:* Moles consist of masses of thin-walled, translucent, cystic, grapelike structures. Fetal parts are rarely seen in complete moles and are more common in partial moles.
- *Microscopic:* Complete moles show hydropic swelling of villi, inadequate vascularization of villi, and significant trophoblastic proliferation. Partial moles show only focal edema and focal and slight trophoblastic proliferation.

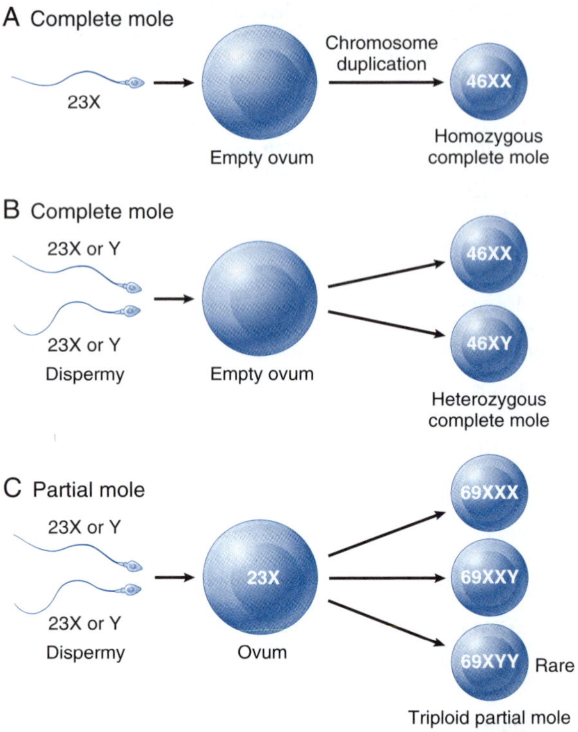

Figure 22-5 Origin of complete and partial hydatidiform moles. A, Complete moles most commonly arise from fertilization of an empty ovum by a single sperm that undergoes duplication of its chromosomes. **B,** Less commonly, complete moles arise from dispermy in which two sperm fertilize an empty ovum. **C,** Partial moles arise from two sperm fertilizing a single ovum.

TABLE 22-4 Features of Complete Versus Partial Hydatidiform Mole

Feature	Complete Mole	Partial Mole
Karyotype	46,XX (46,XY)	Triploid
Villous edema	All villi	Some villi
Trophoblast proliferation	Diffuse, circumferential	Focal; slight
Atypia	Often present	Absent
Serum hCG	Elevated	Less elevated
hCG in tissue	++++	+
Behavior	2% choriocarcinoma	Rare choriocarcinoma

hCG, Human chorionic gonadotropin.

Clinical Features (p. 1040)

Moles can be diagnosed by ultrasound examination and by serum hCG, revealing levels exceeding those produced by a normal pregnancy of similar age. Thorough curettage is adequate therapy for most moles; follow-up hCG determinations can identify potential invasive moles or choriocarcinomas.

Invasive Mole *(p. 1041)*

An invasive mole penetrates and may even perforate the uterine wall, associated with proliferating cytotrophoblasts and syncytiotrophoblasts; villi can embolize to distant sites but do not grow. Invasive moles are associated with persistently elevated hCG. The tumor responds well to chemotherapy.

Choriocarcinoma *(p. 1041)*

Choriocarcinoma is a malignant tumor arising in 1:20,000 to 1:30,000 pregnancies in the United States. Half arise in hydatidiform moles, 25% in previous abortions, 22% in normal pregnancies, and the rest in ectopic pregnancies.

Morphology (p. 1041)

- *Gross:* Tumors are large, soft, yellow-white fleshy masses with areas of necrosis and hemorrhage.
- *Microscopic:* Lesions consist of mixed cytotrophoblast and syncytiotrophoblast proliferations. The tumor invades the underlying endometrium, penetrates blood vessels and lymphatics, and can metastasize widely.

Clinical Features (p. 1041)

Choriocarcinomas manifest with vaginal bleeding and discharge that can appear in the course of an apparently normal pregnancy, after a miscarriage, or after curettage; hCG titers are elevated to levels above those seen in hydatidiform mole. Widespread metastases are already commonly present at the time of initial discovery. Gestational choriocarcinomas are highly sensitive to chemotherapy, with 100% remission rates and high cure rates.

Placental-Site Trophoblastic Tumor *(p. 1041)*

Placental-site trophoblastic tumor (PSTT) comprises <2% of gestational trophoblastic tumors; it represents neoplastic proliferation of extravillous (intermediate) trophoblasts. The lesion differs from choriocarcinoma because syncytiotrophoblastic and cytotrophoblastic elements are absent and the tumors make lower levels of hCG. Most are only locally invasive, but 10% to 15% result in metastases and death.

23 The Breast

Breast pathology is best understood in the context of its normal anatomy (Fig. 23-1). Breasts are composed of specialized epithelium and stroma, either of which can develop benign or malignant lesions. It is worth noting that two cell types (derived from the same precursor stem cells) line the ducts and lobules—*myoepithelial cells* on the basement membrane and overlying luminal *epithelial cells.* The stroma also takes two forms—*interlobular stroma* composed of intermixed adipose and dense fibrous connective tissue and *intralobular stroma* around acini composed of hormone-responsive, breast-specific, fibroblast-like cells. Stroma and epithelial interactions promote normal breast structure and function.

During pregnancy the breast architecture becomes almost completely composed of lobules with scant stroma. Although epithelial cells undergo some degree of apoptosis after cessation of lactation, the lobules only partially regress, and these permanent changes in lobular size and number may explain the reduction in breast cancer risk seen in women who have children at a young age.

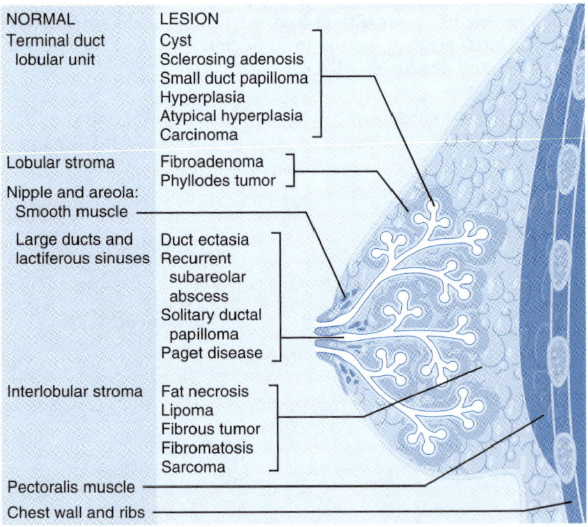

Figure 23-1 Anatomic origins of common breast lesions.

Disorders of Development (p. 1044)

- *Milk line remnants* (p. 1044) can produce hormone-responsive supernumerary nipples or breast tissue from the axilla to the perineum. These mainly come to attention secondary to painful premenstrual enlargement.
- *Accessory axillary breast tissue* (p. 1045): Occasionally, normal ductal tissue extends into subcutaneous tissue of the axilla or chest wall. This can present as a lump in the setting of lactational hyperplasia or can give rise to carcinoma outside the breast proper.
- *Congenital nipple inversion* (p. 1045) is common and usually spontaneously corrects during pregnancy or with traction; *acquired nipple inversion* is concerning for carcinoma or inflammatory conditions.

Clinical Presentation of Breast Disease (p. 1045)

- *Pain (mastalgia or mastodynia)* is a common breast symptom. Diffuse cyclic pain may be related to premenstrual edema. Noncyclic pain is usually localized and can occur secondary to infection, trauma, or ruptured cysts. Almost all painful masses are benign, although 10% of breast cancer presents with pain.
- *Palpable masses* are generally >2 cm and are common; normal breast "lumpiness" must be differentiated from a discrete mass. Most palpable lesions are cysts, fibroadenomas, and carcinoma, with the likelihood of malignancy increasing with age; 10% of dominant masses in women under age 40 are cancer, whereas in women over age 50, 60% are malignant.
- *Nipple discharge* is less common but is worrisome for cancer when unilateral and spontaneous—cancer-associated discharge occurs in 7% of malignancies in women under 60, and in 30% of cancers in women over 60. Bloody or serous discharges are most commonly due to cysts or intraductal papillomas, and benign bloody discharge can also occur during pregnancy. Milky discharge (galactorrhea) outside of pregnancy can be related to prolactin-producing pituitary adenomas, hypothyroidism, anovulatory cycles, or certain medications.
- The principal *mammographic signs* associated with carcinoma are *densities* and *calcifications*. Most neoplasms (benign and malignant) are radiologically denser than normal breast tissue; the value of mammography is the ability to detect lesions as small as 1 cm. Calcifications form on secretions, necrotic debris, or hyalinized stroma and are associated with both benign and malignant lesions. Calcifications associated with malignancy are typically small, irregular, numerous, and clustered; *ductal carcinoma in situ (DCIS)* is most commonly detected as calcifications.
- The sensitivity and specificity of mammography increase with age, due to the progressive replacement of radiodense, fibrous, youthful breast tissue with fatty, radiolucent stroma. At age 40 mammographic lesions are carcinoma in only 10% of cases; this increases to 25% in patients over age 50. Although earlier diagnosis through routine mammographic screening has been attributed to decreasing breast cancer mortality, the benefits have not been as great as anticipated. Approximately 10% of invasive carcinomas are not detected by mammography. Moreover, 70% to 80% of cancers that are detected by mammography are already invasive and many have metastasized. Ironically the cancers most likely to kill are the least likely to be detected by mammography because they typically occur in young women who are not

routinely screened or are rapidly growing malignancies that blossom between mammograms. Finally, many cancers detected by mammography (10% to 30%) are clinically indolent and would not cause the patient any harm (reminiscent of many prostate cancers).

Inflammatory Disorders (p. 1046)

Breast inflammation *(mastitis)* is rare except during lactation. "Inflammatory carcinoma" mimics inflammation by obstructing dermal lymphatics; it should be suspected in a nonlactating woman with the clinical appearance of mastitis.

Acute Mastitis (p. 1046)

Almost all cases occur during the first month of lactation when the breast is vulnerable to bacterial infections (*Staphylococcus* and *Streptococcus*) through nipple cracks and fissures. Acute mastitis usually resolves with antibiotic treatment and continued breastfeeding.

Squamous Metaplasia of Lactiferous Ducts (p. 1046)

This condition results in keratin shedding and subsequent ductal plugging; duct dilation and rupture then lead to intense chronic and granulomatous inflammation that presents as a painful subareolar mass in both sexes (synonymous terms: *recurrent subareolar abscess, squamous metaplasia of lactiferous ducts,* and *Zuska disease*). Smoking is associated with 90% of cases, as is vitamin A deficiency. Secondary bacterial infections can occur, and recurrent cases may be complicated by periareolar fistulous tracts and/or nipple inversion. Treatment includes surgical excision of the involved ducts.

Duct Ectasia (p. 1046)

Mammary duct ectasia usually presents as an ill-defined, usually painless periareolar mass with viscous, white nipple secretions. It tends to occur in multiparous women 50 to 70 years old; there is no association with smoking. The lesion is characterized by inspissation of secretions, duct dilation without squamous metaplasia, and periductal inflammation that can lead to fibrosis and skin retraction.

Fat Necrosis (p. 1047)

Fat necrosis presents as a painless palpable mass, skin thickening or retraction, or mammographic density and/or calcifications. It is associated with prior trauma or surgery. Histologically lesions progress from hemorrhage with acute inflammation and liquefactive fat necrosis to chronic inflammation with giant cells and hemosiderin to scar tissue.

Lymphocytic Mastopathy (Sclerosing Lymphocytic Lobulitis; p. 1047)

Lesions present as single or multiple rock-hard palpable masses; histology reveals collagenized stroma around atrophic ducts, with a prominent lymphocytic infiltrate. An association with type 1 diabetes mellitus and autoimmune thyroid disease suggests an autoimmune etiology.

Granulomatous Mastitis (p. 1047)

This can be associated with systemic diseases (sarcoidosis, granulomatosis with polyangiitis), foreign bodies (e.g., piercings), or granulomatous infections (e.g., mycobacteria or fungi). *Granulomatous lobular mastitis* is a rare entity occurring in parous women, attributed to hypersensitivity responses to antigens expressed during lactation.

Benign Epithelial Lesions (p. 1048)

These lesions are categorized according to the risk of developing breast malignancy (Table 23-1); in the vast majority of cases *breast cancer does not develop.*

Nonproliferative Breast Changes (Fibrocystic Changes) (p. 1048)

These lesions have essentially no malignant potential; they represent the common findings seen in "lumpy bumpy" breasts.

Morphology (p. 1048)

- *Cysts* form by lobular dilation and unfolding and can coalesce to form larger lesions; they are lined by flattened atrophic epithelium or metaplastic apocrine cells and frequently exhibit calcifications.
- *Fibrosis* occurs secondary to cyst rupture and inflammation.
- *Adenosis* is defined as increased numbers of acini per lobule; it occurs normally during pregnancy and can be a focal finding in nonpregnant breasts. Acini are often enlarged but are not distorted and are lined by columnar epithelium that can exhibit atypia

TABLE 23-1 Epithelial Breast Lesions and the Risk of Developing Invasive Carcinoma

Pathologic Lesion	Relative Risk (Absolute Lifetime Risk)*
Nonproliferative Breast Changes (Fibrocystic Changes) Duct ectasia Cysts Apocrine change Mild hyperplasia Adenosis Fibroadenoma without complex features	1.0 (3%)
Proliferative Disease Without Atypia Moderate or florid hyperplasia Sclerosing adenosis Papilloma Complex sclerosing lesion (radial scar) Fibroadenoma with complex features	1.5-2.0 (5%-7%)
Proliferative Disease With Atypia ADH ALH	4.0-5.0 (13%-17%)
Carcinoma In Situ LCIS DCIS	8.0-10.0 (25%-30%)

*Relative risk is the risk compared with women without any risk factors. Absolute lifetime risk is the percentage of patients expected to develop invasive carcinoma if untreated.

(such "flat epithelial atypia" is a clonal proliferation associated with deletions on chromosome 16q); calcification is occasionally present.

- *Lactational adenomas* are palpable masses in pregnant or lactating women. These are normal-appearing breast tissue with lactational changes; they are not neoplastic but rather an exaggerated local response to gestational hormones.

Proliferative Breast Disease Without Atypia (p. 1048)

These lesions are characterized by epithelial or stromal proliferation but without cytologic or architectural atypia. They are not clonal and do not commonly have any genetic changes but nevertheless are associated with a small increase in risk for subsequent carcinoma.

Morphology (p. 1049)

- *Epithelial hyperplasia* is defined by more than two cell layers around ducts and lobules.
- *Sclerosing adenosis* is reflected by increased numbers of acini per lobule, with central distortion and compression and peripheral dilation.
- *Complex sclerosing lesions* have components of sclerosing adenosis, papillomas, and epithelial hyperplasia.
- *Papillomas* reflect epithelial growth and associated fibrovascular cores within dilated ducts; more than 80% of large duct papillomas produce a nipple discharge.

Gynecomastia (p. 1049)

Gynecomastia can be unilateral or bilateral and presents as a button-like subareolar enlargement; it is significant primarily as an indicator of estrogen and androgen imbalance. Gynecomastia can occur during puberty, in Klinefelter syndrome, due to hormone-producing tumors, in men with cirrhosis, or as a side effect of drugs. Histologically there is ductal epithelial and stromal hyperplasia; lobule formation is rare.

Proliferative Breast Disease With Atypia (p. 1050)

Lesions are clonal proliferations with some—but not all—of the histologic features of *carcinoma in situ.* These include atypical ductal and atypical lobular hyperplasia (ALH), occasionally associated with radiologic calcifications. Chromosomal aberrations include loss of 16q or gain of 17p; ALH also shows loss of E-cadherin expression.

Morphology (p. 1050)

- *Atypical ductal hyperplasia (ADH)* shares some morphologic features with DCIS but is limited in extent.
- *ALH* shares features with lobular carcinoma in situ (LCIS), but cells do not distend more than 50% of acini within a lobule.

Clinical Significance of Benign Epithelial Changes (p. 1051)

Table 23-1 highlights the epidemiologic relationship between benign histologic changes and the subsequent development of invasive cancer:

- Nonproliferative changes do not increase the risk of cancer.
- Proliferative disease is associated with a one and a halffold to twofold increased risk.
- Proliferative disease with atypia confers a fourfold to fivefold increased risk, although only 20% of such women develop breast cancer.

Carcinoma of the Breast (p. 1051)

Breast carcinoma is the most common nonskin malignancy in women; a female living to age 90 has a one in eight chance of developing breast cancer. However, <20% of women with invasive breast cancer die of it.

Most breast malignancies are adenocarcinomas; they are divided into three major biologic subgroups, with different treatment responses and outcomes:

- Estrogen receptor (ER)-positive, HER2-negative (50% to 65%)
- HER2-positive (10% to 20%; tumors can be ER-positive or ER-negative)
- ER-negative, HER2-negative (10% to 20% of tumors)

Incidence and Epidemiology (p. 1052)

Breast cancer is rare in women younger than 25; after age 30 the incidence of ER-positive cancers increases with age, whereas ER-negative and HER2-positive cancer rates are relatively constant (Fig. 23-2). Due to mammographic screening, breast cancer incidence increased in the 1980s; however, this was accompanied by a downward trend in the clinical stage at presentation—now predominantly DCIS or stage I disease without nodal metastases—and declining mortality rates. Breast cancer incidence is 4 to 7 times higher in the United States and Europe than in other countries. However, worldwide rates are rising—attributed to delayed pregnancies, fewer pregnancies, and decreased breastfeeding—and by 2020 approximately 70% of cases are predicted to occur in developing countries.

Risk Factors

- *Gender:* Only 1% of breast cancers occur in men.
- *Germline mutations:* 5% to 10% of breast cancers occur in patients with germline mutations; lifetime risk in such individuals exceeds 90%.

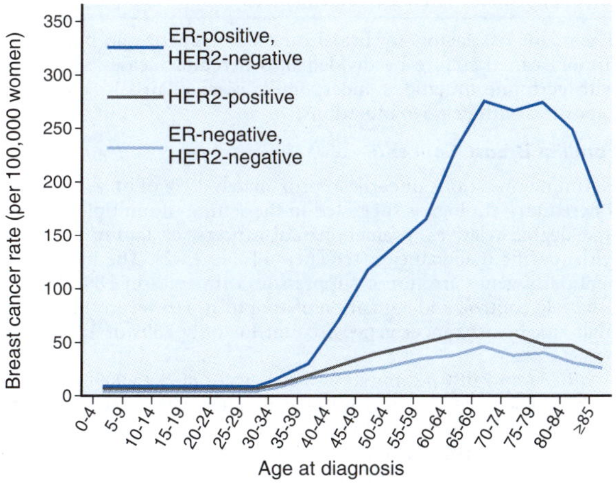

Figure 23-2 Incidence of ER-positive, ER-negative, and HER2-positive breast cancers according to age; rates are per 100,000 women. ER-negative and HER2-positive cancers have a relatively constant incidence after age 40 years. In contrast, ER-positive cancers show a marked increase in incidence starting at around age 40 and peaking at age 70 to 80.

- *First-degree relatives with breast cancer:* 15% to 20% of women with breast cancer have an affected first-degree relative (mother, sister, or daughter) but do not have an identified genetic mutation. Most such family risk is probably due to the interaction of low-risk susceptibility genes and shared environmental factors.
- *Race or ethnicity:* NonHispanic white women have the highest incidence, whereas Native American women have the lowest rates of breast cancer in the United States. Black women tend to present with more advanced malignancy and have higher mortality rates, in part related to variation in cancer risk genes.
- *Age:* Risk peaks at 70 to 80 years (Fig. 23-2).
- *Age at menarche:* Early menarche (<11 years) and late menopause increase risk.
- *Age at first live birth:* Earlier full-term pregnancy (<20 years) halves the risk relative to nulliparous women or women with a first birth over age 35.
- *Benign breast disease:* Proliferative changes or atypical hyperplasia increase risk (Table 23-1).
- *Estrogen exposure:* Menopausal hormone replacement therapy increases risk, whereas oral contraceptives do not increase risk. Reducing endogenous estrogens through oophorectomy or hormonal blockade decreases breast cancer risk up to 75%.
- *Breast density, radiation exposure,* and *carcinoma of the contralateral breast or endometrium* (likely reflecting prolonged estrogen exposures) all increase risk.
- *Diet:* Heavy alcohol consumption increases risk, but cancer risk is not associated with any specific type of food.
- *Obesity:* Obesity below age 40 reduces risk by increasing anovulatory cycling, whereas postmenopausal obesity increases risk through augmented estrogen synthesis.
- *Exercise:* Physical activity confers a small protective effect.
- *Breastfeeding:* The greater the duration of breastfeeding, the greater the reduction in overall risk; lactation suppresses ovulation and can drive terminal differentiation of luminal cells.

Etiology and Pathogenesis (p. 1054)

The major risk factors for breast cancer are genetic and hormonal; tumors can therefore be divided into hereditary cases associated with germline mutations and sporadic cases related to hormonal exposures with de novo mutations.

Familial Breast Cancer *(p. 1054)*

Germline mutations underlie approximately 12% of breast cancers; a hereditary etiology is suggested in the setting of multiple affected first-degree relatives, premenopausal cancers, or family members with specific malignancies (see later) (Table 23-2). The major susceptibility genes are tumor suppressors with roles in DNA repair, cell cycle control, and regulation of apoptosis. However, the known high-risk breast cancer genes account for only 25% of all familial breast cancers.

BRCA1 and *BRCA2* mutations account for 80% to 90% of breast malignancies that can be attributed to single gene mutations and approximately 3% of all breast cancers. Penetrance varies from 30% to 90%, depending on the specific mutation, and these tumors tend to be poorly differentiated; most are ER-positive and HER2-negative. BRCA mutations also increase the risk of ovarian, prostatic, and pancreatic cancers. Mutations in *CHEK2, TP53, PTEN,* and *LKB1/STK11* collectively account for fewer than 10% of hereditary breast carcinomas.

TABLE 23-2 Most Common "Single Gene" Mutations Associated With Hereditary Susceptibility to Breast Cancer

Gene (Location) Syndrome (Incidence)*	% of "Single Gene" Hereditary Cancers†	Breast Cancer Risk by Age 70‡	Changes in Sporadic Breast Cancer	Other Associated Cancers	Functions	Comments
BRCA1 (17q21) Familial breast and ovarian cancer (1 in 860)	52% (approximately 2% of all breast cancers)	40%-90%	Mutations rare; inactivated in 50% of some subtypes (e.g., medullary and metaplastic) by methylation	Ovarian, male breast cancer (but lower than *BRCA2*), prostate, pancreas, fallopian tube	Tumor suppressor, transcriptional regulation, repair of double-stranded DNA breaks	Breast carcinomas are commonly poorly differentiated and triple negative (basal-like), and have *p53* mutations.
BRCA2 (13q12-13) Familial breast and ovarian cancer (1 in 740)	32% (approximately 1% of all breast cancers)	30%-90%	Mutations and loss of expression rare	Ovarian, male breast cancer, prostate, pancreas, stomach, melanoma, gallbladder, bile duct, pharynx	Tumor suppressor, transcriptional regulation, repair of double-stranded DNA breaks	Biallelic germline mutations cause a rare form of Fanconi anemia (see Chapter 7)
p53 (17p13.1) Li-Fraumeni (1 in 5000)	3% (<1% of all breast cancers)	>90%	Mutations in 20%, LOH in 30%-42%; most frequent in triple negative cancers	Sarcoma, leukemia, brain tumors, adrenocortical carcinoma, others	Tumor suppressor with critical roles in cell cycle control, DNA replication, DNA repair, and apoptosis	*p53* is the most commonly mutated gene in sporadic breast cancers
CHEK2 (22q12.1) Li-Fraumeni variant (1 in 100)	5% (approximately 1% of all breast cancers)	10%-20%	Mutations rare (<5%); loss of protein expression in at least one third by unknown mechanism(s)	Prostate, thyroid, kidney, colon	Cell cycle checkpoint kinase, recognition and repair of DNA damage, activates *BRCA1* and *p53* by phosphorylation	May increase risk for breast cancer after radiation exposure

*Frequency of heterozygotes in the U.S. population; the incidence of gene mutations is higher in some ethnic populations (e.g., *BRCA1* and *BRCA2* mutations occur at high frequencies in Askenazi Jews).
†Defined as familial breast cancers showing a pattern of inheritance consistent with a major effect of a single gene.
‡Risk varies with specific mutations and is likely modified by other genes.
LOH, Loss of heterozygosity.

Sporadic Breast Cancer *(p. 1055)*

Hormone exposure is the major risk factor for sporadic cancers; moreover, most of these tumors are ER-positive and occur in postmenopausal women. Hormone exposure increases the number of target cells by stimulating breast growth; by driving proliferation, hormones also place cells at risk for DNA mutations. Metabolites of estrogen can also directly cause mutations or generate DNA-damaging free radicals.

Molecular Mechanisms of Carcinogenesis and Tumor Progression *(p. 1055)*

The most common driver mutations involve *PIK3CA* (encoding phosphoinositide-3 kinase, a component of signaling pathways downstream of growth factor receptors), *HER2, MYC,* and *CCND1* (encoding cyclin D1), *TP53,* and (in familial cancers) *BRCA1* and *BRCA2.* Three major genetic pathways are identified, leading to distinct types of malignancy (Fig. 23-3):

- *ER-positive, HER2-negative cancers* constitute 50% to 65% of cases. These are often associated with 1q gains, 16q losses, and activating mutations in *PIK3CA.* ER-positive cancers are termed "luminal"; they resemble normal breast luminal cells in terms of their mRNA expression patterns, with several genes that are regulated by estrogen.
- *HER2-positive cancers* constitute 20% of cases; they are associated with amplifications of the HER2 gene on chromosome 17q and may be either ER-positive or -negative. The gene expression pattern is dominated by proliferation-related genes regulated by signaling pathways downstream of the HER2 receptor tyrosine kinase.
- *ER-negative, HER2-negative cancers* comprise 15% of cases and occur through pathways independent of ER-regulated gene expression and *HER2* gene amplifications. This is the most common tumor type in patients with germline *BRCA1* mutations and also occur with increased frequency in black women. Sporadic tumors of this type often have loss-of-function mutations in *TP53;* mutations in *BRCA1* are uncommon, but *BRCA1* may be silenced in sporadic tumors through epigenetic mechanisms. These tumors have a "basal-like" pattern of mRNA expression, including many genes expressed in normal myoepithelial cells.

The development of breast epithelial neoplasia also depends on stromal cell interactions; increased amounts of fibrous stroma is both a marker of risk and biologically important for tumorigenesis, likely by creating a microenvironment conducive to tumor development and growth. Angiogenesis and tumor-associated inflammation are commonly associated with carcinoma, starting at the in situ stage.

Types of Breast Carcinoma (p. 1057)

More than 95% are adenocarcinomas; these may be "in situ" (proliferation limited to ducts and lobules by the basement membrane), but 70% will be invasive (penetrating the basement membrane with metastatic capacity) at the time of clinical detection. Different histologic types have characteristic clinical, biologic, and prognostic implications.

The terms *ductal* and *lobular* describe subsets of both in situ and invasive carcinomas, but breast cancers actually arise from cells in the terminal duct lobular unit. *Carcinoma in situ* was originally classified as DCIS or LCIS based on the resemblance of the involved spaces to normal ducts or lobules; however, these growth patterns are not related to the cell of origin but rather reflect differences in tumor cell genetics and biology.

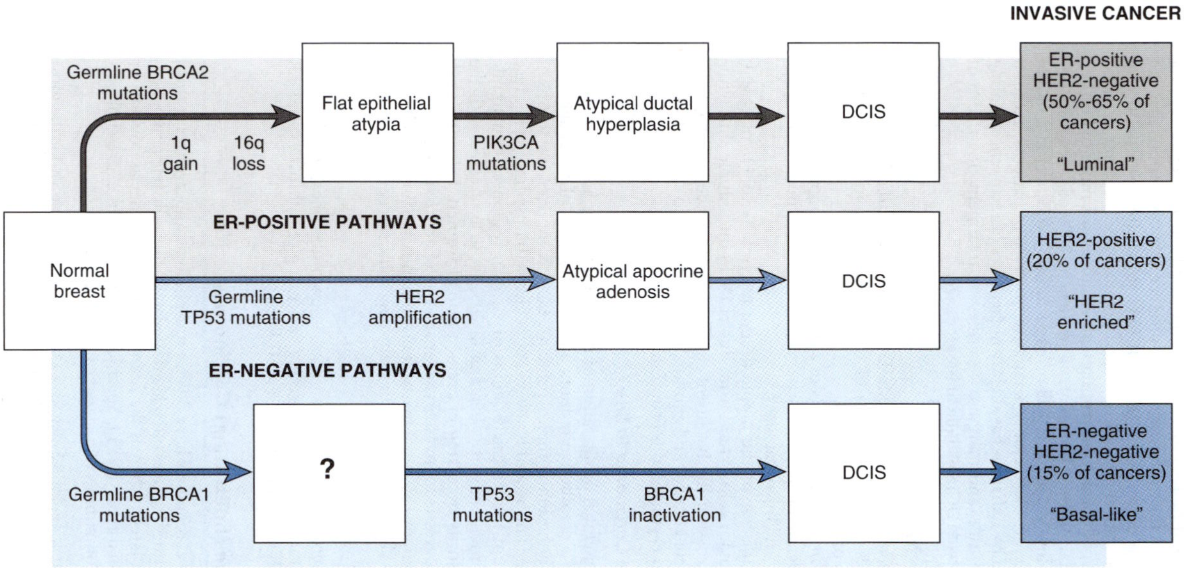

Figure 23-3 Major pathways of breast cancer development. The most common pathway *(top)* leads to ER-positive carcinomas. Recognizable precursor lesions include flat epithelial atypia and atypical hyperplasia. A less common pathway *(bottom)* leads to carcinomas that are negative for ER and HER2. The box with the question mark indicates that no precursor lesions have been identified—perhaps because lesions progress quickly to carcinoma. The third pathway *(middle)* consists of HER2-positive cancers, which may be ER-positive or ER-negative. Amplification of the *HER2* gene is also present in a subset of atypical apocrine lesions, which may represent a precursor lesion. Each molecular subtype has a characteristic gene expression profile termed luminal, HER2 enriched, and basal-like, respectively. See text for other details.

Carcinoma In Situ (p. 1057)

Ductal Carcinoma In Situ (p. 1057)

DCIS is a malignant clonal proliferation of epithelial cells limited to ducts and lobules by the basement membrane; DCIS can spread throughout the ductal system and produce extensive lesions that can involve an entire breast sector. It now constitutes 15% to 30% of all breast cancers in well-screened populations; most are detected mammographically, presenting with calcifications more often than periductal fibrosis. It is bilateral in 10% to 20% of cases. Left untreated, low-grade DCIS will progress to invasive cancer at a rate of 1% per year. Mastectomy is curative in >95% of patients; excision followed by radiation has slightly higher rates of recurrence relating to grade, size, and margins. Regardless of treatment, 1% to 3% of women with DCIS will die of breast cancer.

Morphology (p. 1057)

- *Comedocarcinoma* (comedo DCIS) is characterized by ducts and lobules dilated by sheets of high-grade pleomorphic cells with zones of central necrosis.
- *Noncomedo DCIS* consists of a monomorphic population of cells of varying nuclear grades; patterns include cribriform, solid, papillary, and micropapillary.
- *Paget disease* of the nipple occurs rarely (1% to 4% of cases); malignant cells extend from ductal DCIS into nipple skin without crossing the basement membrane. These cells disrupt the epithelial barrier and allow extracellular fluid to seep out, creating an erythematous eruption with a scaly crust.

Lobular Carcinoma In Situ (p. 1059)

LCIS is a clonal proliferation of cells within ducts and lobules that grow in a discohesive fashion, attributed to loss of E-cadherin or catenin adhesion complex proteins. LCIS comprises 1% to 6% of all breast cancers and is always an incidental biopsy finding because it does not induce calcifications or stromal responses visualizable by mammography; it is bilateral in 20% to 40% of cases, with the vast majority occurring in premenopausal women. Left untreated, LCIS progresses to invasive cancer at a rate of approximately 1% per year. Therapy can entail mastectomy or tamoxifen but typically now involves close follow-up with mammographic screening.

Morphology (p. 1059)

Lesions consist of a uniform population of discohesive cells, often with intracellular mucin forming signet ring cells. Most express ER and PR but do not overexpress HER2.

Invasive (Infiltrating) Carcinomas (p. 1060)

Invasive carcinomas have diverse morphologic appearances; a third have distinct features often associated with clinically relevant behaviors (see later), whereas the rest are lumped together as "ductal" or "no special type" (NST). Specific gene and protein expression patterns allow a molecular classification (Table 23-3):

- ER-positive, HER2-negative ("luminal," 50% to 65%) is the most common form of invasive breast cancer; it is divided into two subgroups based on proliferation rates:
  - Low proliferation (40% to 55%) comprises the majority of breast cancers in older individuals and is the most common type detected by mammography. The gene expression signature is dominated by genes regulated by the ER, and accordingly they

TABLE 23-3 Molecular Subtypes of Invasive Breast Cancer

Defining Features	ER-Positive, HER2-Negative		HER2-Positive (ER-Positive or Negative*)	ER-Negative,† HER2-Negative
Frequency	Approximately 40%-55% (Low proliferation)	Approximately 10% (High proliferation)	Approximately 20%	Approximately 15%
Included special histologic types	Well or moderately differentiated lobular, tubular, mucinous	Poorly differentiated lobular	Some apocrine	Medullary,‡ adenoid cystic,‡ secretory,‡ metaplastic
Typical patient groups	Older women, men; cancers detected by mammographic screening	*BRCA2* mutation carriers	Young women, nonwhite women, *TP53* mutation carriers (ER-positive)	Young women, *BRCA1* mutation carriers, black and Hispanic women
Metastatic pattern	Bone (70%), more common than visceral (25%) or brain (<10%)	Bone (80%) more common than visceral (30%) or brain (10%)	Bone (70%), visceral (45%), and brain (30%) are all common	Bone (40%), visceral (35%), brain (25%) are all common
Relapse pattern	Late, >10 yr, long survival possible with metastases	Intermediate	Usually short, <10 yr, survival with metastases rare	Usually short, <5 yr, survival with metastases rare
Complete response to chemotherapy	<10%	Approximately 10%	ER-positive—15% ER-negative—>30%	Approximately 30%

*Approximately half of HER2-positive cancers are ER-positive and half ER-negative. ER and PR levels tend to be low in this group.
†This group is also referred to as "triple negative" carcinoma.
‡Some special histologic types have a more favorable prognosis than this group as a whole.

respond well to hormonal therapy (without substantial benefit from adjunct chemotherapy). They have the lowest incidence of local recurrence, are often cured by surgery, and metastasize infrequently—often after a long lag-time (over 6 years).
  - High-proliferation (10%) tumors are often associated with *BRCA2* germline mutations, with an associated higher burden of chromosomal aberrations. Unlike low-grade, ER-positive cancers, 10% of these carcinomas show a complete response to chemotherapy.

- HER2-positive (approximately 20% of cancers) is the second most common form of invasive breast cancer; HER2-positive cancers are more common in young and in nonwhite women. Half of HER2-positive cancers are also ER-positive; 50% of cancers arising in the context of germline *TP53* mutations (Li-Fraumeni syndrome) are both ER- and HER2-positive. These cancers characteristically have complex interchromosomal translocations, high-level amplifications of *HER2,* and a high mutational load. More than a third of these carcinomas respond completely to antibodies that block HER2 activity (trastuzumab). Primary or acquired resistance to these antibodies can occur through expression of a truncated form of HER2—lacking the trastuzumab-binding site but retaining kinase activity—or can occur through upregulation of downstream pathways, such as the PI-3 kinase pathway. HER2-positive cancers can metastasize when small and early in their course, often to viscera and brain.
- ER-negative, HER2-negative tumors ("basal-like" triple negative carcinoma; 15% of cancers) are the third major subtype. These typically occur in younger premenopausal women, in blacks, and in women with *BRCA1* mutations. Due to high proliferation rates, these cancers can present as new masses occurring in the interval between mammographic screenings. They share a number of genetic similarities with serous ovarian carcinomas, including the association with germline *BRCA1* mutations. These cancers can metastasize when small. However, 30% completely respond to chemotherapy. Local recurrence is common (usually within 5 years), even after mastectomy. Distant metastasis portends a poor prognosis.

Morphology *(p. 1062)*

The mammographic and gross appearance of invasive carcinoma varies depending on the stromal reaction:

- Most commonly they are hard, irregular, radiodense masses due to desmoplasia.
- Less commonly they are composed of sheets of tumor cells with scant stromal reaction, or scattered neoplastic glands or single tumor cells infiltrating fibrofatty tissue (difficult to visualize on mammography).
- Invasive carcinomas presenting on mammography as calcifications without an associated density are generally <1 cm in size.

Larger carcinomas can invade the pectoralis muscle, invade into the dermis, and cause skin dimpling, or retraction of the nipple.

Grading uses the *Nottingham Histologic Score,* evaluating tubule formation, nuclear pleomorphism, and mitotic rate:

- Grade I (well differentiated): Tubular pattern with small, round nuclei and have a low proliferative rate.
- Grade II (moderately differentiated): Some tubule formation, but solid clusters or single infiltrating cells are also present, with mitoses and greater nuclear pleomorphism.

- Grade III (poorly differentiated): Invade as ragged nests or solid sheets of cells with enlarged irregular nuclei, a high proliferative rate, and areas of tumor necrosis.
    - *ER-positive, HER2-negative carcinoma:* Many morphologic patterns are possible, with grades ranging from well to poorly differentiated.
    - *HER2-positive carcinoma:* The majority are poorly differentiated, and there is no specific morphologic pattern.
    - *ER-negative, HER2-negative carcinoma:* Almost all are poorly differentiated; many have pushing borders with a central fibrosis or necrosis.

Special Histologic Types of Invasive Carcinoma *(p. 1064)*

There are multiple subtypes of invasive carcinoma with distinctive morphologies and relatively unique biologic characteristics; these often harbor unique genetic aberrations.

Lobular carcinoma usually presents as a palpable mass or mammographic density; however, in 25% of cases the tumor invades with little desmoplasia making detection difficult. The histologic hallmark is the presence of discohesive infiltrating tumor cells (often with signet ring morphology), without tubule formation. Most cases have biallelic loss of *CDH1* (encoding E-cadherin). Metastases often involve the peritoneum and retroperitoneum, leptomeninges (carcinomatous meningitis), GI tract, ovaries, and uterus. Germline *CDH1* mutations also increase the risk of gastric signet ring cell carcinoma.

Medullary carcinomas are typically ER-negative, HER2-negative, presenting as well-circumscribed masses with minimal desmoplasia. They often have features characteristic of *BRCA1*-associated carcinomas (in cancers in *BRCA1* carriers, 13% are of medullary type, and 60% having medullary features [Table 23-3]). Although most medullary carcinomas do not have germline *BRCA1* mutations, two thirds have *BRCA1* promoter hypermethylation leading to reduced *BRCA1* expression. This subtype has a relatively better prognosis compared to other poorly differentiated carcinomas; intratumor lymphocyte infiltrates are associated with higher survival rates and a greater response to chemotherapy.

Inflammatory carcinoma refers to tumors that present with a swollen, erythematous breast due to extensive lymphatic invasion and destruction; the overall prognosis is poor.

Male Breast Cancer *(p. 1066)*

Carcinoma of the male breast is rare (1% of all breast cancers). Risk factors and prognostic factors are similar to those for women (e.g., first-degree relatives, increased estrogen exposures). Male breast cancer is strongly associated with *BRCA2* (*BRCA2* mutations will be present in 60% to 76% of families with a male having breast cancer); *BRCA1* mutations are less frequently associated. The same histologic types of breast cancer are found in men and women. Because of the scant amount of male breast tissue, carcinomas tend to invade skin and chest wall earlier and present at higher stages. However, matched by stage, prognosis is similar in men and women.

Prognostic and Predictive Factors *(p. 1066)*

Prognostic factors include extent of cancer (tumor stage) and the underlying cancer biology. The five stages (0 to IV) defined by the American Joint Committee on Cancer (AJCC) and Union Contre Le Cancer (UICC) are highly correlated with survival (Table 23-4). The molecular biology of breast cancers has improved outcome prediction (Fig. 23-4).

TABLE 23-4 Survival Rate by Cancer Stage

Stage*	T: Primary Cancer	N: Lymph Nodes	M: Distant Metastasis	10-Yr Survival (%)
0	DCIS or LCIS	No metastases	Absent	92
I	Invasive carcinoma ≤2 cm	No metastases or only micrometastases	Absent	87
II	Invasive carcinoma >2 cm	1-3 positive LNs	Absent	65
	Invasive carcinoma >2 cm but ≤5 cm	0-3 positive LNs	Absent	
III	Invasive carcinoma >5 cm	Negative or positive LNs	Absent	40
	Any size invasive carcinoma	≥4 positive LNs	Absent	
	Invasive carcinoma with skin or chest wall involvement or inflammatory carcinoma	Negative or positive LNs	Absent	
IV	Any size invasive carcinoma	Negative or positive LNs	Present	5

*AJCC Cancer Staging Manual, 7th Edition, Chapter 32, Breast, pp. 347-369, New York, Springer, 2010. The groups listed in the table are based on the characteristics of the primary carcinoma and the axillary lymph nodes. For rare women with involved internal mammary lymph nodes or supraclavicular LNs, there are additional staging criteria.

DCIS, Ductal carcinoma in situ; *LCIS,* lobular carcinoma in situ; *LN,* lymph nodes.

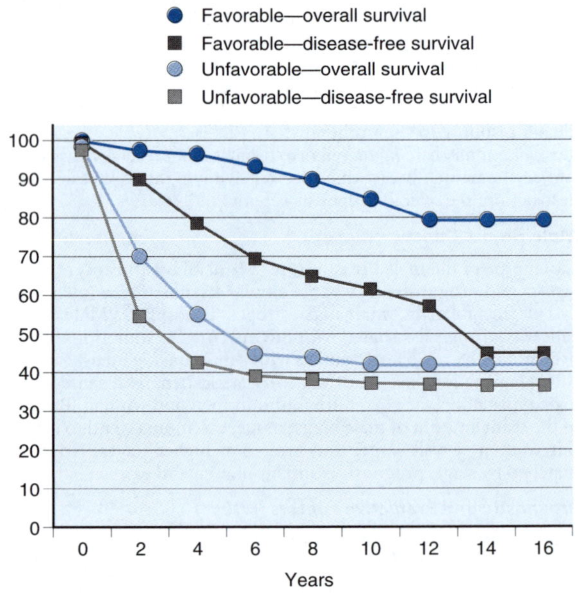

Figure 23-4 Biologic breast cancer type predicts outcome. Overall survival and disease-free survival are shown for the most favorable biologic type (well-differentiated, ER-positive, HER2-negative, low proliferation) and least favorable biologic type (poorly differentiated, ER-negative and/or HER2-positive).

- *Invasive carcinoma versus carcinoma in situ:* By definition, carcinoma in situ cannot metastasize; thus adequate DCIS treatment is usually curative. Deaths associated with DCIS are attributed to subsequent invasive carcinoma or occult areas of invasion.
- *Distant metastases:* Once distant metastases are present, cure is unlikely, although long-term remissions and palliation can be achieved.
- *Lymph node metastases:* In the absence of distant metastases, axillary lymph node status is the most important prognostic factor. If nodes are cancer free, the 10-year disease-free survival rate is 70% to 80%; that falls to 35% to 40% with one to three positive nodes and 10% to 15% with >10 positive nodes. Most breast cancers drain to one to two "sentinel nodes" in the ipsilateral axilla identifiable by colored dye or radioactive tracer. Women with negative sentinel nodes can be spared the morbidity of a full axillary dissection. Notably 10% to 20% of patients without nodal metastases ultimately develop distant metastatic disease, perhaps due to hematogenous spread or to internal mammary nodal metastasis.
- *Tumor size:* Tumor size is an independent prognostic factor and also predicts the likelihood of metastasis. Women with node-negative carcinomas <1 cm in size have a 10-year survival rate >90%; survival drops to 77% for cancers >2 cm.
- *Locally advanced disease:* Carcinomas invading into skin or skeletal muscle are usually large and have a worse prognosis.
- *Inflammatory carcinoma:* Dermal lymphatic involvement portends a very poor prognosis with 3% to 10% 3-year survivals.
- *Lymphovascular invasion (LVI):* This is a poor prognostic factor in women without lymph node metastases, and a risk factor for local recurrence.

Other prognostic factors related to tumor biology include the following:

- *Molecular subtype* based on proliferation and ER and HER2 expression.
- *Special histologic types:* In general, carcinomas classified as a special type (e.g., tubular, mucinous, or medullary) have a better prognosis than NST carcinomas. Metaplastic or micropapillary carcinoma portends a poorer prognosis.
- *Histologic grade.*
- *Proliferative rate:* A high proliferative rate is a poor prognostic factor, although such tumors may be more chemoresponsive. Proliferation is more important for ER-positive, HER2-negative cancers because the ER-negative and/or HER2-positive tumors generally have high proliferative rates.
- *ERs and progesterone receptors (PRs):* Hormone receptor expression predicts hormone responsiveness but also lack of sensitivity to conventional chemotherapy. Conversely, tumors lacking hormone receptors do not usually respond to hormones but are more susceptible to chemotherapy.
- *Her2/neu:* Overexpression connotes a worse prognosis but predicts response to trastuzumab.

Current therapeutic approaches include combinations of surgery (mastectomy or breast-conserving surgery) and postoperative radiation, with systemic hormonal treatment, chemotherapy, or both.

Stromal Tumors (p. 1068)

Breast-specific intralobular stroma gives rise to biphasic (stroma and epithelium) breast tumors, fibroadenomas, and phyllodes tumors; interlobular stroma gives rise to the same benign and malignant tumors that occur in other stroma (e.g., lipomas and sarcomas).

Fibroadenomas *(p. 1069)*

Fibroadenomas are the most common benign tumor of the female breast, occurring most often during the reproductive period and regressing and calcifying after menopause; no consistent cytogenetic changes have been demonstrated. Fibroadenomas present clinically as rubbery, well-circumscribed palpable masses, ovoid mammographic densities, or mammographic calcifications. Fibroadenoma epithelium is hormone responsive, and tumors can grow during pregnancy. Some fibroadenomas are polyclonal hyperplasias of lobular stroma, responding to specific stimuli (e.g., cyclosporine).

Phyllodes Tumors *(p. 1069)*

Phyllodes tumors occur most commonly after age 60, typically presenting as palpable masses. The stroma frequently overgrows the epithelial component, forming clefts and slits, and creating bulbous protrusions; increased cellularity, mitotic activity, stromal overgrowth, and infiltrative borders differentiate them from fibroadenomas. Gains in chromosome 1q is the most common cytogenetic alteration; the frequency of chromosomal changes and overexpression of the HOXB13 homeobox transcription factor increases with grade and is generally associated with more aggressive behavior. Most phyllodes tumors can be cured by wide local excision; nodal or distant metastases are rare.

Lesions of Interlobular Stroma *(p. 1070)*

Tumors of interlobular stroma are composed of stromal cells without an epithelial component. These include *pseudoangiomatous stromal hyperplasia* and *fibromatosis* (fibroblasts and myofibroblasts), *myofibroblastoma* (myofibroblasts), and lipomas.

Malignant Tumors of Interlobular Stroma *(p. 1070)*

Malignant tumors of interlobular stroma are rare; the most common is angiosarcoma, arising as a primary tumor in young women, after radiation therapy for breast cancer. Primary angiosarcomas are usually high grade and carry a poor prognosis.

Other Malignant Tumors of the Breast (p. 1070)

Malignant tumors (identical to their counterparts elsewhere) can arise from breast skin or adnexal structures. Breast can be a primary site of lymphomas or can be involved by a systemic lymphoma; most are diffuse large B-cell type. Metastases to the breast are rare and typically arise from a contralateral breast carcinoma; nonmammary metastases are most commonly melanomas and ovarian cancers.

24 The Endocrine System

Endocrine signaling occurs through secreted hormones acting on target cells distant from the site of synthesis; target tissue responses also typically include *feedback inhibition* of the original hormone production.

Endocrine disorders result from either of the following:

- Hormone underproduction or overproduction
- Mass lesions that can be nonfunctional or associated with abnormal hormone levels

Pituitary Gland (p. 1074)

The pituitary gland—along with the hypothalamus—plays a critical role in the regulation of most other endocrine glands. It is composed of two morphologically and functionally distinct components:

- *Anterior lobe (adenohypophysis; 80% of the pituitary):* Hypothalamic factors carried to the anterior pituitary by a portal circulation influence hormone production by the six basic anterior lobe cell types (Fig. 24-1):
  - *Somatotrophs:* Growth hormone (GH)
  - *Mammosomatotrophs:* GH and prolactin (PRL)
  - *Lactotrophs:* PRL
  - *Corticotrophs:* Adrenocorticotropic hormone (ACTH), pro-epiomelanocortin (POMC), and melanocyte-stimulating hormone (MSH)
  - *Thyrotrophs:* Thyroid-stimulating hormone (TSH)
  - *Gonadotrophs:* Follicle-stimulating hormone (FSH) and luteinizing hormone (LH)
- *Posterior lobe (neurohypophysis)* comprises modified glial cells *(pituicytes)* and axonal processes extending from the hypothalamus; oxytocin and vasopressin (antidiuretic hormone [ADH]) synthesized by the hypothalamus are stored in the axon terminals. Oxytocin stimulates smooth muscle cell contraction in the gravid uterus and around mammary lactiferous ducts; ADH participates in water regulation.

Clinical Manifestations of Pituitary Disease (p. 1075)

- *Hyperpituitarism* (increased hormone production) results from anterior pituitary adenomas (most common), hyperplasia, or malignancy or hormone secretion by nonpituitary tumors, or hypothalamic disorders.
- *Hypopituitarism* (decreased hormone production) can be caused by ischemic injury, surgery, radiation, inflammation, or nonfunctional (but compressive) pituitary adenomas.

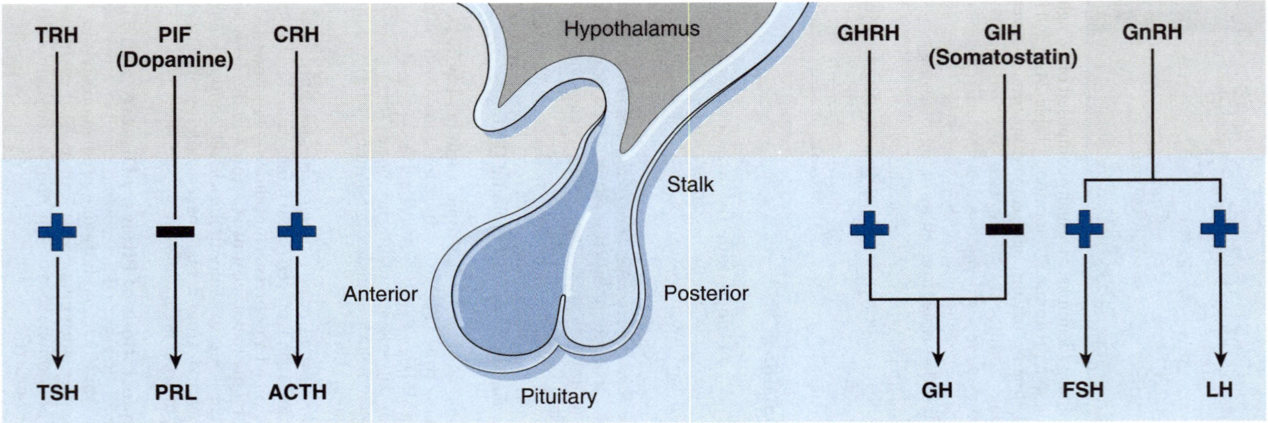

Figure 24-1 Anterior pituitary hormones. The adenohypophysis (anterior pituitary) releases six hormones under the control of various stimulatory and inhibitory hypothalamic releasing factors: TSH (thyrotropin), PRL, ACTH (corticotropin), GH (somatotropin), FSH, and LH. The stimulatory releasing factors are TRH, CRH, GHRH, and GnRH. The inhibitory hypothalamic influences comprise PIF and GIH. *CRH,* Corticotropin-releasing hormone; *GHRH,* growth hormone-releasing hormone; *GIH,* growth hormone inhibitory factor or somatostatin; *GnRH,* gonadotropin-releasing hormone; *PIF,* prolactin inhibitory factor or dopamine.

- *Local mass effects* include optic nerve compression, diplopia, and visual field abnormalities (classically *bitemporal hemianopsia*) and increased intracranial pressure with headache, nausea, and vomiting. Mass effects can arise gradually or abruptly; the latter occurs with enlargement due to acute hemorrhage into an adenoma *(pituitary apoplexy).*
- *Posterior pituitary lesions* typically manifest due to elevated or depressed ADH.

Pituitary Adenomas and Hyperpituitarism (p. 1075)

Functional pituitary adenomas are usually composed of a single cell type, producing one predominant hormone (Table 24-1); GH and PRL constitute the most common dual combination. Conversely, pituitary adenomas can be nonfunctional and cause hypopituitarism by destroying normal parenchyma. *Microadenomas* are <1 cm, and *macroadenomas* are >1 cm; nonfunctional tumors are usually macroadenomas coming to attention primarily due to mass effects (e.g., visual field abnormalities or elevated intracranial pressure). The prevalence of pituitary adenomas is 14%, with a peak incidence from age 35 to 60 years; the vast majority are clinically silent microadenomas.

Pathogenesis (p. 1076; Table 24-2)

Most adenomas involve sporadic mutations; 5% arise from inherited genetic defect.

- Spontaneous mutations of the α-subunit of the G_s stimulatory G protein (encoded by the *GNAS* gene) occur in 40% of somatotroph adenomas (and a smaller fraction of corticotroph adenomas); such mutations result in constitutive activation of $G_s\alpha$ with persistent cyclic adenosine monophosphate (cAMP) generation and unchecked proliferation. *GNAS* mutations are not seen in thyrotroph, lactotroph, and gonadotroph adenomas because their proliferation is not driven through cAMP-dependent pathways.

TABLE 24-1 Classification of Pituitary Adenomas

Pituitary Cell Type	Hormone	Associated Syndrome*
Corticotroph	ACTH and other POMC-derived peptides	Cushing syndrome Nelson syndrome
Somatotroph	GH	Gigantism (children) Acromegaly (adults)
Lactotroph	PRL	Galactorrhea and amenorrhea (in females) Sexual dysfunction, infertility
Mammosomatotroph	PRL, GH	Combined features of GH and PRL excess
Thyrotroph	TSH	Hyperthyroidism
Gonadotroph	FSH, LH	Hypogonadism, mass effects, and hypopituitarism

*Note that the nonfunctional adenomas in each category typically present with mass effects accompanied by hypopituitarism due to destruction of normal parenchyma.

ACTH, Adrenocorticotropic hormone; *FSH,* follicle-stimulating hormone; *GH,* growth hormone; *LH,* luteinizing hormone; *POMC,* proepiomelanocortin; *TSH,* thyroid-stimulating hormone.

Adapted from Ezzat S, Asa L: Mechanisms of disease: the pathogenesis of pituitary tumors. *Nat Clin Prac Endocrinol Metab* 2:200-230, 2006.

TABLE 24-2 Genetic Alterations in Pituitary Tumors

Gene	Protein Function	Mechanism of Alteration	Most Commonly Associated Pituitary Tumor
Gain of Function			
GNAS	GNAS encodes for α subunit of stimulatory G-protein, $G_s\alpha$. Oncogenic mutation of GNAS constitutively activates $G_s\alpha$, leading to upregulation of intracellular cAMP activity	Activating mutation	GH adenomas
*PRKAR1A**	*PRKAR1A* encodes for a negative regulator of protein kinase A (PKA), a downstream mediator of cAMP signaling. Loss of PKA regulation leads to inappropriate cAMP activity	Germline inactivating mutations of *PRKAR1A* are present in autosomal dominant Carney complex	GH and PRL adenomas
Cyclin D1	Cell cycle regulatory protein; promotes G1-S transition	Overexpression	Aggressive adenomas
HRAS	Ras regulates multiple oncogenic pathways including proliferation, cell survival, and metabolism	Activating mutation	Pituitary carcinomas
Loss of Function			
*MEN1**	MEN1 encodes for menin, a protein with protean roles in tumor suppression, including repression of oncogenic transcription factor JunD, and in histone modification	Germline inactivating mutations of *MEN1* (MEN, type 1)	GH, PRL, and ACTH adenomas
CDKN1B (p27/KIP1)*	The p27 protein is a negative regulator of the cell cycle	Germline inactivating mutations of *CDKN1B* ("MEN-1-like" syndrome)	ACTH adenomas
Aryl hydrocarbon receptor interacting protein (AIP)*	Receptor for aryl hydrocarbons and a ligand-activated transcription factor	Germline mutations of *AIP* cause pituitary adenoma predisposition (PAP) syndrome	GH adenomas (especially in patients younger than 35 years of age)
Rb	Rb protein is a negative regulator of the cell cycle (see Chapter 7)	Methylation of *Rb* gene promoter	Aggressive adenomas

*Genetic alterations associated with *familial* predisposition to pituitary adenomas.

Partially adapted from Boikos SA, Stratakis CA: Molecular genetics of the cAMP-dependent protein kinase pathway and of sporadic pituitary tumorigenesis. *Hum Mol Genet* 16:R80-R87, 2007.

- Germline mutations associated with familial adenomas include the following:
  - *MEN1* mutations (affecting the tumor suppressor protein *menin*) underlie the multiple endocrine neoplasia-1 (MEN-1) syndrome (see later).
  - *CDKN1B* encodes the cell-cycle checkpoint regulator p27; mutations give rise to an "MEN-1-like syndrome."
  - *Protein kinase A regulatory subunit 1α (PRKAR1A)* encodes a tumor suppressor that regulates protein kinase A activity, downstream of cAMP-mediated signaling. It is mutated in *Carney syndrome,* an autosomal dominant disorder associated with pituitary and other endocrine tumors.
  - *AIP* codes for the tumor suppressor *aryl hydrocarbon receptor-interacting protein;* mutations often lead GH-producing adenomas and acromegaly.

Morphology *(p. 1077)*

- *Gross:* Tumors are usually solitary, forming discrete soft masses within the sella turcica. Larger adenomas can compress or infiltrate adjacent structures *(invasive adenomas).*
- *Microscopic:* Adenomas are generally composed of uniform, monomorphous cell populations arrayed in sheets, cords, or nests with scant extracellular matrix. Immunohistochemistry can be used to identify the hormone product. Nuclear atypia, necrosis, and hemorrhage can occur but do not imply malignancy; however, a subset of adenomas with increased mitotic activity (>3%) are associated with *p53* mutations, cyclin D1 overexpression, or epigenetic silencing of *retinoblastoma (Rb),* and have a greater propensity for aggressive behavior.

Lactotroph Adenoma *(p. 1078)*

Prolactinomas are the most common functional pituitary tumor (30%). Even microadenomas can secrete sufficient PRL to cause hyperprolactinemia; moreover, serum PRL concentrations tend to correlate with adenoma size. Hyperprolactinemia can produce amenorrhea (25% of cases), galactorrhea, loss of libido, and infertility.

Hyperprolactinemia is normal during pregnancy. In addition to adenomas, pathologic hyperprolactinemia can be caused by *lactotroph hyperplasia,* occurring when the normal dopamine inhibition of PRL secretion is blocked. This can result from damage to the hypothalamic dopaminergic neurons, pituitary stalk transsection (e.g., head trauma), or drugs that block dopamine receptors; any suprasellar mass can potentially disturb the normal hypothalamic inhibitory pathways. Consequently, mild PRL elevations—even in the presence of a pituitary adenoma—do not necessarily indicate a PRL-secreting tumor.

Somatotroph Adenomas *(p. 1079)*

GH-secreting tumors are the second most common functioning adenoma. Hypersecretion of GH stimulates hepatic production of insulin-like growth factor 1 (IGF-1), which causes many of the clinical manifestations; the effects depend on the age of onset. If somatotroph adenomas appear *before* epiphyseal closure, elevated GH results in *gigantism* characterized by a generalized increase in body size and disproportionately long arms and legs. If increased GH appears *after* epiphyseal closure, patients develop *acromegaly,* with enlargement of head, hands, feet, jaw, tongue, and soft tissues. GH excess is also associated with gonadal dysfunction, diabetes mellitus, muscle weakness, hypertension, arthritis, congestive heart failure, and increased risk of gastrointestinal (GI) cancers.

Diagnosis relies on documenting elevated serum GH and IGF-1 levels; failure to suppress GH production by an oral glucose load is the most sensitive assay. Tumors can be surgically removed, or GH secretion can be reduced by drug therapy with somatostatin analogues or GH receptor antagonists. Effective control of GH levels leads to gradual recession of the tissue overgrowth and resolution of the metabolic abnormalities.

Corticotroph Adenomas *(p. 1079)*

Corticotroph cell adenomas are typically microadenomas at the time of diagnosis because ACTH production leads to early symptoms related to adrenal hypercortisolism *(Cushing disease)*. In addition to adenomas, a wide variety of conditions can also cause elevated cortisol levels (*Cushing syndrome,* discussed under adrenal pathology). Surgical removal of the adrenals results in loss of inhibitory feedback to the pituitary corticotrophs and can induce the formation of large, destructive adenomas *(Nelson syndrome);* these can also cause hyperpigmentation through effects on melanocytes of other products of the ACTH precursor.

Other Anterior Pituitary Adenomas *(p. 1080)*

- *Gonadotroph adenomas* (10% to 15% of pituitary adenomas) typically occur in middle-aged men and women. Because they produce hormones somewhat variably and the secretory products do not cause recognizable symptoms, most tumors are detected only when they become large enough to cause neurologic symptoms. Impaired LH production is the most common gonadotroph deficiency; in men the resulting low serum testosterone manifests as decreased energy and libido, whereas in premenopausal women the outcome is amenorrhea.
- *Thyrotroph adenomas* (1% of pituitary adenomas) are rare causes of hyperthyroidism.
- *Nonfunctioning pituitary adenomas* (25% to 30% of pituitary adenomas) include nonsecretory ("silent") variants of functioning adenomas, as well as true hormone-negative adenomas; the latter are unusual. Patients with nonfunctioning adenomas typically present with mass effects.
- *Pituitary carcinomas* are quite rare (<1%); most are functional (secreting PRL or ACTH most commonly). Diagnosis of carcinoma requires the demonstration of metastases.

Hypopituitarism (p. 1080)

Hypopituitarism can result from diseases of the hypothalamus and/or pituitary. Hypofunction occurs when 75% of the parenchyma is lost. Manifestations depend on which hormone(s) are lacking. Causes include the following:

- *Tumors and other mass lesions* in the sella (adenomas, metastases, or cysts) can cause damage by compression of adjacent normal pituitary.
- *Traumatic brain injury* and/or *subarachnoid hemorrhage.*
- *Pituitary surgery or radiation:* Surgical excision of a pituitary adenoma may inadvertently remove sufficient normal tissue to cause hypopituitarism; radiation to prevent regrowth of residual tumor can damage nonadenomatous tissue.
- *Pituitary apoplexy* can present dramatically with sudden onset of excruciating headache, diplopia, and hypopituitarism; it is a neurosurgical emergency because in severe cases it can precipitate cardiovascular collapse and sudden death.
- *Sheehan syndrome* results from sudden infarction of the anterior lobe occurring in the setting of obstetric hemorrhage or shock.

This occurs because the pituitary enlarges to almost twice its normal size during pregnancy but does so without accompanying increases in vascular perfusion; it can then become frankly ischemic with any substantial blood loss or diminished perfusion pressure. Ischemic pituitary necrosis can also be encountered in other conditions, such as disseminated intravascular coagulation or sickle cell anemia, elevated intracranial pressure, traumatic injury, or shock.

- *Rathke cleft cysts* can accumulate proteinaceous fluid and expand.
- *Empty sella syndrome* can occur with any condition that destroys part or all of the pituitary gland:
  - In *primary empty sella,* defects in the diaphragma sellae allow arachnoid mater and cerebrospinal fluid to herniate into the sella, causing pituitary compression. Classically, affected individuals are obese multigravida women. In addition to hypopituitarism, patients can present with visual field defects and hyperprolactinemia due to loss of inhibitory hypothalamic tracts.
  - In *secondary empty sella,* surgery or radiation leaves behind a vacant space; hypopituitarism results from the treatment or spontaneous infarction.
- *Genetic defects* are rare; the best described are mutations in the pituitary-specific homeobox gene *PIT1,* causing deficiencies in GH, PRL, and TSH.
- *Hypothalamic lesions* interfere with the delivery of pituitary hormone-releasing factors, and can also lead to reduced ADH secretion, resulting in diabetes insipidus (see later). Such hypothalamic lesions include *tumors,* which may be benign (e.g., craniopharyngioma) or malignant; most of the latter are metastases from tumors, such as breast and lung carcinoma.
- *Inflammatory disorders and infections.*

Posterior Pituitary Syndromes (p. 1081)

- Inappropriate *oxytocin* secretion has not been associated with clinical abnormalities.
- *ADH deficiency (diabetes insipidus)* results in *hypernatremia* due to ineffective renal water resorption; patients present clinically with polyuria and polydipsia. It can result from head trauma, tumors, inflammatory disorders, or surgery involving the hypothalamus or pituitary.
- *Syndrome of inappropriate ADH secretion (SIADH)* results in *hyponatremia* due to excessive renal water resorption; patients present clinically with cerebral edema and resultant neurologic dysfunction. The most frequent causes include ectopic ADH secretion by malignancies (especially small cell lung carcinoma), non-neoplastic pulmonary diseases (e.g., tuberculosis, pneumonia), and hypothalamus and/or posterior pituitary injury.

Hypothalamic Suprasellar Tumors (p. 1082)

Such tumors can induce anterior pituitary hypofunction or hyperfunction and/or diabetes insipidus; the most common lesions are gliomas (see Chapter 28) and craniopharyngiomas. *Craniopharyngiomas* derive from Rathke pouch remnants, are slow growing, and account for 1% to 5% of intracranial tumors. There is a bimodal age distribution with one peak between ages 5 and 15 years and the second after age 65. Children usually present with endocrine deficiencies (e.g., growth retardation, whereas adults present with visual disturbances and headaches). Even with local invasion, these tumors have an excellent prognosis; malignant transformation is rare.

Morphology (p. 1082)

- *Gross:* Craniopharyngiomas average 3 to 4 cm in diameter and are characteristically cystic or multiloculated.
- *Microscopic:* Lesions are composed of a mixture of squamous epithelial elements and stroma; two variants are recognized:
  - *Adamantinomatous craniopharyngioma* is more common in children. These lesions commonly calcify. There is a "spongy" reticulum with peripheral palisading of the epithelium and compact, lamellar keratin ("wet keratin"). Cysts in these tumors contain cholesterol-rich, thick, brownish-yellow fluid likened to "machinery oil."
  - *Papillary craniopharyngioma* is more common in adults. These lesions rarely calcify; they are composed of sheets and papillae of well-differentiated squamous epithelium lacking keratin or cysts.

Thyroid Gland (p. 1082)

- TSH binding to thyroid epithelial receptors leads to activation of a coupled G_s protein and increased intracellular cAMP.
- Elevated cAMP promotes epithelial proliferation, thyroglobulin synthesis, and systemic thyroxine (T_4) release (with lesser amounts of triiodothyronine [T_3]).
- T_4 and T_3 circulate bound to thyroxine-binding globulin (TBG).
- Most free T_4 is deiodinated to T_3, which binds to nuclear thyroid receptors (TRs) in target cells with tenfold greater affinity than T_4 and has proportionately greater activity.
- Thyroid hormone-TR complexes regulate target gene transcription by binding to thyroid hormone response elements (TREs); the result is a globally augmented basal metabolic rate with broadly increased protein synthesis and carbohydrate and lipid catabolism.
- *Goitrogens* diminish T_4/T_3 synthesis, which increases TSH release, and in turn causes hyperplastic thyroid enlargement *(goiter).*
- Propylthiouracil blocks iodide oxidation (blocking thyroid hormone production) and inhibits T_4 deiodination to T_3; high-dose iodide inhibits thyroglobulin proteolysis.
- Thyroid *parafollicular (C) cells* secrete *calcitonin;* this blocks calcium resorption by osteoclasts and augments skeletal calcium deposition.

Hyperthyroidism (p. 1083)

Thyrotoxicosis is a hypermetabolic state caused by elevated circulating levels of free T_3 and T_4; it is most commonly due to primary hyperactivity of the thyroid *(hyperthyroidism).* Causes include the following:

- Thyroid hyperplasia (Graves disease; 85% of cases)
- Hyperfunctional multinodular goiter
- Hyperfunctional thyroid adenoma

Secondary causes include pituitary thyrotroph adenomas, excess exogenous thyroid hormone (e.g., as treatment for hypothyroidism), and thyroid inflammatory diseases.

Clinical Course (p. 1083)

Symptoms and signs of hyperthyroidism relate to the resulting hypermetabolic state and overactivity of the sympathetic nervous system:

- *Cardiac:* Increased cardiac contractility and increased peripheral oxygen requirements can cause cardiomegaly, tachycardia, palpitations, and arrhythmias (particularly atrial fibrillation); congestive failure may supervene, particularly with preexisting cardiac disease.

- *Ocular:* Wide, staring gaze and lid lag are due to sympathetic overstimulation of the levator palpebrae superioris; patients with Graves disease can also have a deposition ophthalmopathy (see later).
- *Neuromuscular:* Sympathetic nervous system overactivity (with increased β-adrenergic tone) causes tremor, hyperactivity, emotional lability, anxiety, inability to concentrate, and insomnia. Proximal muscle weakness and diminished mass are also common.
- *Cutaneous:* Increased blood flow and peripheral vasodilation lead to warm, moist, and flushed skin; Graves patients can also develop an infiltrative dermopathy.
- *GI:* Hypermotility, malabsorption, and diarrhea are due to sympathetic hyperstimulation.
- *Sketelal:* Enhanced bone resorption leads to osteoporosis and increased risk of fractures.
- *Thyroid storm* designates abrupt onset of severe hyperthyroidism; it usually occurs in Graves patients due to acute elevation in circulating catecholamines (e.g., secondary to injury, surgery, infection, or any exogenous stress) and is a medical emergency due to the risk of fatal arrhythmia.
- Thyrotoxicosis in the elderly may be blunted by various comorbidities, leading to so-called *apathetic hyperthyroidism;* diagnosis is made during laboratory evaluation for unexplained weight loss or cardiovascular deterioration.

Serum TSH levels are the most useful single screening test for hyperthyroidism; TSH is decreased even at the earliest stages and is usually associated with increased free serum T_4. Treatments include β-blockade to reduce adrenergic tone, propylthiouracil or similar agents to block hormone synthesis and peripheral T_4 to T_3 conversion, and iodine to block thyroglogulin proteolysis; radioiodine can ablate thyroid epithelium over a period of 6 to 18 weeks.

Hypothyroidism (p. 1085)

Hypothyroidism is caused by any structural or functional derangement that interferes with adequate thyroid hormone production or rarely the ability of the end organ to respond to thyroid hormone (Table 24-3); overt hypothyroidism affects 0.3% of the population, and subclinical disease occurs in >4%. Adult hypothyroidism

TABLE 24-3 Causes of Hypothyroidism
Primary
Genetic defects in thyroid development (*PAX8, FOXE1,* TSH receptor mutations) (rare)
Thyroid hormone resistance syndrome (*THRB* mutations) (rare)
Postablative
Surgery, radioiodine therapy, or external irradiation
Autoimmune hypothyroidism
Hashimoto thyroiditis*
Iodine deficiency*
Drugs (lithium, iodides, *p*-aminosalicylic acid)*
Congenital biosynthetic defect (dyshormonogenetic goiter) (rare)*
Secondary (Central)
Pituitary failure (rare)
Hypothalamic failure (rare)

*Associated with enlargement of thyroid ("goitrous hypothyroidism"). Hashimoto thyroiditis and postablative hypothyroidism account for the majority of cases of hypothyroidism in developed countries.

FOXE1, Forkhead box E1; *PAX8,* paired box 8; *THRB,* thyroid hormone receptor β.

is associated with insidious slowing of physical and mental activity, associated with fatigue, cold intolerance, and apathy; decreased sympathetic activity reduces sweating and causes constipation. Hypothyroidism during the neonatal period can have profound developmental effects (*cretinism;* see later). Older children with hypothyroidism exhibit signs and symptoms intermediate between those of the cretin and those of the hypothyroid adult.

- *Primary hypothyroidism* (vast majority of cases) can be accompanied by thyroid enlargement (goiter).
  - In iodine-sufficient areas of the world, the most common cause of hypothyroidism is *autoimmune thyroiditis* (most frequently, *Hashimoto thyroiditis*); patients typically have circulating antimicrosomal, antithyroid peroxidase, and antithyroglobulin autoantibodies. It can occur in isolation or as part of *autoimmune polyendocrine syndrome* (APS; see discussion under "adrenal glands").
  - Other causes of primary hypothyroidism include dietary iodine deficiency-associated endemic goiter and goitrogens.
  - Genetic causes include mutations in genes that affect thyroid development (e.g., *PAX8*), or inactivating mutations of the TSH receptor.
  - Following thyroid surgery or radiation or due to infiltrative disorders.
- *Secondary hypothyroidism* is caused by TSH deficiency—or more rarely—by thyrotropin-releasing hormone (TRH) deficiency.

An elevated TSH level is the most sensitive screening test for primary hypothyroidism, owing to a loss of feedback inhibition of TRH and TSH production; T_4 levels are reduced in any cause of hypothyroidism. Clinical manifestations are *cretinism* if thyroid deficiency develops in utero through early childhood and *myxedema* in older children and adults.

Cretinism *(p. 1085)*

Cretinism is associated with dietary iodine deficiency and goiter (endemic form) and rarely with defects in hormone synthesis (sporadic form). There is impaired skeletal and central nervous system (CNS) development, with mental retardation, short stature, umbilical hernia, and coarse facial features, wide-set eyes, and an enlarged, protruding tongue. Maternal thyroid hormones cross the placenta and are critical for normal fetal brain development in the period before fetal thyroid development. Thus the severity of mental impairment depends on the timing of any in utero deficiency; maternal thyroid hormone deficiency in late pregnancy may allow normal brain development.

Myxedema *(p. 1086)*

Myxedema is a term applied to hypothyroidism developing in adolescence or adulthood. In addition to slowing of mental and physical activity, findings include periorbital edema, coarsening of skin and facial features, cardiomegaly with congestive failure, and lipid profiles that promote atherogenesis; patients can also have pericardial effusion, hair loss, and accumulation of mucopolysaccharide-rich ground substance within the dermis *(myxedema)* and other tissues.

Thyroiditis (p. 1086)

Thyroid inflammation *(thyroiditis)* manifestations vary from severe pain (e.g., infectious thyroiditis) to thyroid dysfunction with little inflammation *(subacute lymphocytic thyroiditis)*.

Hashimoto Thyroiditis *(p. 1086)*

Hashimoto thyroiditis is an autoimmune disease, resulting in parenchymal destruction and progressive thyroid failure. It is the most common cause of hypothyroidism in locations where iodine levels are sufficient and is a major cause of nonendemic goiter in children. It is most prevalent between ages 45 and 65, with a 10 to 20:1 female predominance. There is a 40% concordance of disease in monozygotic twins, and half of asymptomatic siblings of Hashimoto thyroiditis patients have circulating antithyroid antibodies.

Pathogenesis (p. 1086)

Hashimoto thyroiditis occurs secondary to a loss of self-tolerance to thyroid antigens; the inciting events are unknown, but the disease is linked to genetic polymorphisms in proteins that negatively regulate T-cell responses (cytotoxic T lymphocyte–associated antigen-4 [CTLA-4] and protein tyrosine phosphatase-22 *[PTPN22]*), potentially leading to regulatory T-cell abnormalities. Autoimmune injury is mediated by circulating antibodies to thyroglobulin and thyroid peroxidase, CD8+ cytotoxic T cells, and/or T_H1 cytokine activation of macrophages. Injury is accompanied by progressive thyroid epithelium depletion, mononuclear cell infiltration, and fibrosis.

Morphology (p. 1087)

- *Gross:* The thyroid is typically diffusely enlarged with pale parenchyma and an intact capsule.
- *Microscopic:* Lesions exhibit an exuberant infiltrate of lymphocytes, plasma cells, and macrophages, occasional germinal centers, atrophic follicles with eosinophilic granular cytoplasm in residual follicular cells (*Hürthle cells,* a metaplastic response). Fibrosis can be abundant.

Clinical Course (p. 1087)

Hashimoto thyroiditis presents with painless thyroid enlargement usually associated with some degree of hypothyroidism. Hyperthyroidism *(hashitoxicosis)* can be seen early but is transient. Patients have an increased risk of developing other autoimmune diseases (e.g., type 1 diabetes, autoimmune adrenalitis, systemic lupus erythematosus, and Sjögren syndrome). There is a small risk of subsequent B-cell nonHodgkin lymphoma.

Subacute Lymphocytic (Painless) Thyroiditis *(p. 1088)*

This is an uncommon cause of hyperthyroidism, occurring most commonly in middle-aged women; a similar process occurs in up to 5% of postpartum women. Both entities have antithyroid antibodies and are variants of autoimmune thyroiditis.

Morphology (p. 1088)

The thyroid appears grossly normal. Histology demonstrates lymphocyte infiltrates with germinal centers and follicular disruption, but no fibrosis or Hürthle cell metaplasia.

Clinical Course (p. 1088)

Patients present with painless goiter and/or hyperthyroidism; a third can progress to overt hypothyroidism.

Granulomatous Thyroiditis *(p. 1088)*

Also called *de Quervain thyroiditis,* this occurs much less frequently than Hashimoto thyroiditis. It most commonly affects women (4:1) between the ages of 40 and 50.

Pathogenesis (p. 1088)

Subacute thyroiditis is attributed to a viral infection or postviral inflammatory process, resulting in cytotoxic T cell–mediated follicular epithelial damage. Because the immune response is virus-initiated, it is self-limited.

Morphology (p. 1088)

- *Gross:* There is variable symmetric or irregular glandular enlargement.
- *Microscopic:* Early lesions include thyroid follicular disruption with a neutrophilic infiltrate. Later features include lymphocyte, macrophage, and plasma cell infiltrates around damaged thyroid follicles, with fibrosis and occasional multinucleated giant cells.

Clinical Course (p. 1088)

Granulomatous thyroiditis is the most common cause of thyroid pain. Any hyperthyroidism is transient and fades in 2 to 6 weeks; normal thyroid function usually recovers after 6 to 8 weeks.

Riedel thyroiditis is an uncommon fibrosing process of unknown etiology associated with replacement of thyroid parenchyma by dense fibrous tissue penetrating the capsule and extending into contiguous neck structures. There can be fibrosis in other sites (e.g., retroperitoneum), and Riedel thyroiditis is likely a manifestation of systemic autoimmune immunoglobulin (Ig)G4-related disease (see Chapter 6).

Graves Disease (p. 1089)

This is the most common cause of endogenous hyperthyroidism; a clinical triad includes the following:

- Hyperthyroidism due to hyperfunctional, diffuse thyroid enlargement
- Infiltrative ophthalmopathy with resultant exophthalmos
- Localized, infiltrative dermopathy present in a minority of patients

Women are affected 10 times more frequently than men; peak incidence is between ages 20 and 40 with the disease affecting up to 2% of U.S. women. There is a 30% to 40% concordance rate among identical twins, and genetic susceptibility is linked to CTLA-4 and PTPN22 polymorphisms; patients are at risk of developing other autoimmune disorders.

Pathogenesis (*p. 1089*)

Graves disease is an autoimmune disorder caused predominantly by autoantibodies directed against the TSH receptor (TSHR). *Thyroid-stimulating Ig* binds to the TSHR and mimics the action of TSH, leading to T_3 and T_4 release; it is relatively specific for Graves disease and occurs in 90% of cases. Some patients have TSHR *blocking antibodies* that can potentially cause hypothyroidism.

Autoimmunity also contributes to the characteristic *infiltrative ophthalmopathy* with *exophthalmos* (eye protrusion); orbital preadipocyte fibroblasts express TSHR and thus become another target of the autoimmune attack. Retro-orbital connective tissues and extraocular muscles expand due to the following:

- Marked mononuclear cell infiltration (predominantly T cells)
- Inflammatory edema and swelling of extraocular muscles
- Increased extracellular matrix, including hyaluronic acid and chondroitin sulfate
- Increased adipocyte number

Morphology *(p. 1089)*

- *Gross:* The gland is symmetrically enlarged, with an intact capsule and soft parenchyma.
- *Microscopic:* Lesions show diffuse follicular epithelial hyperplasia, manifested by crowding into irregular papillary folds. Colloid is substantially decreased. Interfollicular parenchyma contains hyperplastic lymphoid tissue and increased numbers of blood vessels.

Changes in extrathyroidal tissue include generalized lymphoid hyperplasia. Both ophthalmopathy and dermopathy (most common over the shins; so-called *pretibial myxedema*) are characterized by lymphocyte infiltration and accumulation of hydrophilic glycosaminoglycans.

Clinical Course *(p. 1090)*

T_4 and T_3 levels are elevated and TSH is depressed. Clinical manifestations are referable to thyrotoxicosis, diffuse thyroid hyperplasia, ophthalmopathy, and dermopathy. Ophthalmopathy may be self-limited or can progress to severe proptosis despite control of the hyperthyroidism. Patients are treated with β-blockade and measures to diminish thyroid hormone synthesis (e.g., propylthiouracil).

Diffuse and Multinodular Goiters (p. 1090)

Thyroid enlargement *(goiter)* is the most common manifestation of thyroid disease; it reflects impaired synthesis of thyroid hormone with resultant TSH production and follicular hyperplasia to restore a euthyroid state. If the compensatory hyperplasia cannot overcome the impairment in hormone synthesis, *goitrous hypothyroidism* results.

Diffuse Nontoxic (Simple) Goiter *(p. 1091)*

This form diffusely involves the entire gland without producing nodularity; enlarged follicles are filled with colloid, hence the alternate term *colloid goiter.*

- *Endemic goiters* occur in geographic areas with low iodine levels (e.g., Alps, Andes, and Himalayas). With dietary iodine supplementation, the frequency and severity have declined significantly. However, diets with high goitrogen content (e.g., cruciferous vegetables like cassava and cabbage) can also precipitate simple goiters.
- *Sporadic goiters* occur less frequently; there is a striking preponderance of young females. Causes include goitrogen ingestion or hereditary defects in thyroid hormone synthesis.

Morphology (p. 1091)

Two stages can be identified in the evolution of diffuse goiter:

- Hyperplastic stage
  - *Gross:* The thyroid gland is diffuse and symmetrically enlarged.
  - *Microscopic:* There is follicular epithelium hypertrophy and hyperplasia; some follicles are hugely distended while others remain small.
- *Colloid involution stage* (as thyroid hormone demand is met)
  - *Gross:* The cut surface is glassy, brown, and translucent.
  - *Microscopic:* There is variable involution of follicular epithelium to form an enlarged, colloid-rich gland.

Clinical Course (p. 1091)

Most patients with simple goiters are clinically euthyroid; thus clinical manifestations are primarily related to mass effects. TSH levels are elevated.

Multinodular Goiter (p. 1091)

Recurrent episodes of stimulation and involution of diffuse goiters result in irregularly enlarged *multinodular goiters* and can produce extreme thyroid enlargements. Multinodular goiters occur due to variations in follicular cell responses to hormonal stimulation; acquired mutations in the TSH signaling pathway (leading to constitutive activation) can also eventually result in formation of nodules with autonomous growth.

Morphology (p. 1092)

- *Gross:* Multinodular goiters are multilobulated, asymmetrically enlarged glands and can be massively enlarged (>2000 g). Irregular expansion can produce lateral pressure on the trachea and esophagus or can present as a single dominant mass. Cut section reveals variable amounts of brown gelatinous colloid, focal hemorrhage, fibrosis, calcification, and cystic change.
- *Microscopic:* There is a variable degree of colloid accumulation, inactive flattened epithelium interspersed with follicular epithelial hyperplasia, and focal intervening areas of scarring and hemorrhage.

Clinical Course (p. 1092)

- Mass effects (occasionally complicated by acute expansion by hemorrhage) dominate the clinical picture: cosmetic deformity, esophageal compression with dysphagia, tracheal compression, and superior vena cava obstruction can occur.
- Most patients are euthyroid or subclinically hyperthyroid (evidenced by reduced TSH). However, in 10% of patients, a hyperfunctioning nodule can develop and cause hyperthyroidism (toxic multinodular goiter, or *Plummer syndrome*); this is not accompanied by the infiltrative ophthalmopathy and dermopathy of Graves disease.

Neoplasms of the Thyroid (p. 1092)

Solitary thyroid nodules occur in 1% to 10% of the U.S. population (with significantly higher rates in endemic goitrous regions); female to male ratio = 4:1, and the incidence increases throughout life. Although less than 1% of solitary thyroid nodules are malignant, this represents 15,000 new U.S. cases of thyroid carcinoma annually; most are indolent with 90% survival at 20 years. Risk of malignancy increases with the following:

- Solitary nodules more than multiple nodules
- Nodules in younger patients (<40 years old)
- Nodules in men more than women
- A history of head or neck radiation treatment
- Nodules that do not take up radioactive iodine in imaging studies *(cold nodules)*

Adenomas (p. 1093)

Thyroid adenomas are discrete, solitary masses derived from follicular epithelium *(follicular adenomas).* Most are nonfunctional, and they are not usually precursors to malignancy.

Pathogenesis (p. 1093)

Gain-of-function somatic mutations of components of the TSH receptor signaling pathway (commonly TSHR or GNAS) lead to autonomous proliferation and underlie approximately 50% of toxic adenomas; these changes are rare in thyroid malignancy. *RAS* or phoshphatidylinositol-3-kinase subunit *(PIK3CA)* mutations occur in 20% of nonfunctioning adenomas; these mutations are also common in follicular carcinomas.

Morphology (p. 1093)

- *Gross:* Most adenomas are gray-white to red-brown (depending on cellularity and colloid content), well-demarcated, solitary encapsulated lesions, occasionally with fibrosis, hemorrhage, or calcification.
- *Microscopic:* Constituent cells typically form uniform-appearing follicles containing colloid; the epithelium shows little nuclear variability or mitotic activity, and the follicular growth pattern is usually distinct from adjacent non-neoplastic thyroid. *Hürthle cell (oxyphil) adenomas,* exhibiting granular, eosinophilic cells, behave like conventional adenomas. Follicular adenomas are distinguished by an intact well-formed capsule; follicular carcinomas demonstrate capsular and/or vascular invasion.

Clinical Features (p. 1094)

Most lesions present as dominant painless masses. Nonfunctioning adenomas take up less radioactive iodine than adjacent normal thyroid ("cold nodule"), but <10% of cold nodules eventually prove to be malignant. Because capsular integrity is a critical distinguishing feature, definitive diagnosis can be made only after careful histologic examination of the resected specimen.

Carcinomas (p. 1094)

Thyroid carcinoma accounts for 1.5% of all U.S. malignancies. Most occur in adults, with a slight female predominance; the vast majority are well-differentiated lesions derived from thyroid follicular epithelium.

- Papillary carcinoma (>85%)
- Follicular carcinoma (5% to 15%)
- Anaplastic (undifferentiated) carcinomas (<5%)
- Medullary carcinoma (5%; not derived from follicular epithelium)

Pathogenesis (p. 1094)

- *Genetic factors:* The epithelial-derived thyroid malignancies are associated with gain-of-function mutations in the mitogen-activated protein (MAP) kinase and the PI3 kinase/AKT pathways; these lead to constitutive cell activation in the absence of TSH ligand binding (Fig. 24-2).
- *Papillary carcinomas* are associated with MAP kinase pathway mutations:
    - Rearrangements of RET or NTRK1 tyrosine kinase receptors place the kinase domain of these receptors under the transcriptional control of genes that are constitutively active in thyroid epithelium. RET has more than 15 potential fusion partners; novel RET/papillary thyroid cancer (RET/PTC) fusion proteins are present in 20% to 40% of papillary thyroid cancers, whereas similar NTRK1 fusion proteins occur in 5% to 10%. Constitutive expression of these proteins leads to ongoing MAP kinase activation.

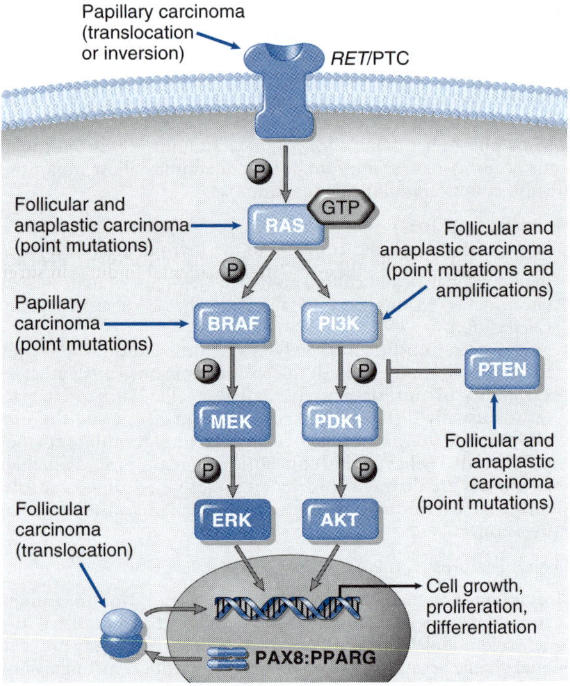

Figure 24-2 Genetic alterations in follicular cell-derived malignancies of the thyroid gland.

  - Gain-of-function *BRAF* mutations occur in 30% to 50% of papillary thyroid cancers and also result in constitutive MAP kinase activation.

- *Follicular carcinomas* are associated with the following:
  - Gain-of-function mutations in *RAS* or *PIK3CA,* amplification of *PIK3CA,* or loss-of-function mutations in the *PTEN* tumor suppressor gene (PTEN negatively regulates the pathway) lead to constitutive activation of the PI3 kinase/AKT pathway and are associated with up to 50% of follicular carcinomas.
  - A t(2;3)(q13;p25) translocation fuses *PAX8* (a thyroid homeobox gene) with *PPARG* (a peroxisome proliferator-activated receptor gene) coding for a nuclear hormone receptor implicated in cellular differentiation cells. These are associated with 30% to 50% of follicular carcinomas.
- *Anaplastic (undifferentiated) carcinomas* exhibit *RAS* or *PIK3CA* mutations, as well as mutations in *p53* or β-catenin that can portend aggressive behavior.
- *Medullary thyroid carcinomas* arise from thyroid parafollicular C cells. Familial versions occur in MEN type 2 (see later), associated with germline activating mutations of the *RET* proto-oncogene mutations; similar *RET* mutations occur in half of sporadic medullary thyroid cancers.
- *Environmental factors:* The major risk factor is *ionizing radiation exposure,* particularly in the first two decades of life. *Iodine deficiency* is linked to a higher frequency of follicular carcinomas.

Papillary Carcinoma (p. 1095)

Papillary carcinoma occurs most commonly between ages 25 and 50; these account for the vast majority of thyroid carcinomas associated with previous radiation exposure.

Morphology (p. 1096)

- *Gross:* Tumors are solitary or multifocal lesions; they may be circumscribed or infiltrate adjacent parenchyma. Calcification, fibrosis, and cystic changes are common. Conventional papillary carcinomas <1 cm and confined to the thyroid, are called *papillary microcarcinomas;* these are often incidental findings in surgical resections.
- *Microscopic:* There are more than a dozen histologic variants often associated with particular mutations; lesions vary from papillary (with dense fibrovascular cores) to follicular (*follicular variant* of papillary carcinoma) to sclerosing and can have slightly different clinical behaviors. *Psammoma bodies* (concentric calcifications) and foci of lymphatic invasion variably occur. Definitive diagnosis is based on nuclear features even in the absence of papillary architecture:
  - Hypochromatic empty nuclei ("Orphan Annie eyes") and nuclear grooves
  - Eosinophilic intranuclear inclusions (cytoplasmic invaginations)

Clinical Course *(p. 1097).* Most papillary carcinomas present as isolated asymptomatic "cold" thyroid nodules, although the first manifestation may be cervical node metastasis. Thyroid lesions move freely during swallowing and are grossly indistinguishable from benign nodules; hoarseness, dysphagia, cough, or dyspnea suggests advanced disease. Ten-year survivals exceed 95%; unfavorable factors include age >40, extrathyroidal extension, and distant metastases.

Follicular Carcinoma (p. 1097)

Follicular carcinoma is threefold more common in women, with a peak incidence between ages 40 and 60; there is an increased prevalence in areas of dietary iodine deficiency.

Morphology (p. 1097)

- *Gross:* Tumors are single nodules that may be well circumscribed or infiltrative. Distinguishing minimally invasive follicular carcinomas from follicular adenomas requires extensive sampling of the thyroid-tumor interface.
- *Microscopic:* The nuclear features noted in papillary carcinomas are absent. Most tumors exhibit a microfollicular pattern with relatively uniform, colloid-filled follicles reminiscent of normal thyroid. Other patterns include a trabecular or sheetlike architecture and histologic variants containing large numbers of Hürthle cells.

Clinical Course *(p. 1098).* Most present as slowly growing, painless "cold" nodules. Lymphatic invasion is rare, but hematogenous metastasis to bone, lungs, and liver is common. Prognosis depends on the stage and extent of invasion: minimally invasive follicular carcinoma has a 10-year survival rate >90%, whereas invasive carcinoma with metastases has a 50% 10-year mortality. Therapy involves resection, radioactive iodine to ablate metastatic lesions, and thyroid hormone administration to reduce TSH that could be potentially stimulatory for malignant epithelium.

Anaplastic (Undifferentiated) Carcinoma (p. 1098)

Anaplastic (undifferentiated) carcinoma is an aggressive variant (mortality rates approaching 100%); it occurs most commonly in patients over age 65 and is associated with prior or concurrent well-differentiated thyroid cancer.

Morphology *(p. 1098). Microscopically* these neoplasms are composed of highly anaplastic cells, including large, pleomorphic giant cells and spindle cells with a sarcomatous appearance.

Clinical Course *(p. 1099).* Tumors usually present as rapidly enlarging bulky masses that have already invaded neck structures or metastasized to lung at the time of original diagnosis. Death is usually secondary to aggressive local growth.

Medullary Carcinoma (p. 1099)

Medullary carcinoma is a neuroendocrine neoplasm derived from parafollicular C cells; these secrete *calcitonin* (and can also produce serotonin, ACTH, and vasoactive intestinal peptide [VIP]). Most (70%) cases are sporadic; the remainder occur with MEN-2 syndromes or familial medullary thyroid carcinoma (FMTC). *RET* proto-oncogene activating mutations are involved in both sporadic and familial cases.

Morphology *(p. 1099)*

- *Gross:* Sporadic tumors are usually solitary; bilaterality and multicentricity are typical of familial cases. Tumors are firm, gray-tan, and infiltrative, occasionally with hemorrhage and focal necrosis.
- *Microscopic:* Cells are polygonal to spindle-shaped arrayed in nests, trabeculae, and occasionally follicles. Stromal *amyloid deposits* (derived from calcitonin) are often present. C-cell hyperplasia in the surrounding parenchyma is typical in familial cases but is usually absent in sporadic cases.

Clinical Course *(p. 1099)*

- Sporadic cases usually present as a thyroid mass, sometimes associated with dysphagia, or hoarseness. Initial manifestations may be paraneoplastic related to hormone secretion (e.g., diarrhea due to VIP, or Cushing syndrome due to ACTH); hypocalcemia is uncommon despite elevated calcitonin levels. Secretion of carcinoembryonic antigen is also a useful biomarker to assess tumor burden or follow therapeutic efficacy.
- Familial cases can present with thyroid or extrathyroidal neoplasms or through screening of asymptomatic relatives of affected patients.
- Medullary carcinomas arising in the context of MEN-2B are more aggressive and metastasize more often than those arising sporadically or with other familial syndromes.

Congenital Anomalies *(p. 1100)*

Thyroglossal duct cysts are developmental remnants of thyroid migration from the tongue foramen cecum. They can present at any age, primarily as midline masses anterior to the trachea. Cysts high in the neck are lined by stratified squamous epithelium; those more inferior are lined by thyroidal acinar epithelium. Lymphocytic infiltrates are often conspicuous. Superimposed infections can generate abscess cavities; rarely they can give rise to carcinoma.

Parathyroid Glands (p. 1100)

Parathyroid activity is controlled by the level of free (ionized) circulating calcium; elevated calcium levels inhibit parathyroid hormone (PTH) synthesis and secretion, whereas hypocalcemia stimulates PTH production. PTH increases calcium levels by the following:

- Driving osteoclast differentiation (and thereby bone resorption) by increasing osteoblast. expression of receptor activator of NF-κB ligand (RANKL) that binds to RANK on osteoclast precursors.
- Increasing renal tubular reabsorption of calcium.
- Increasing renal vitamin D conversion to the active 1,25 dihydroxylated form.
- Increasing urinary phosphate excretion.
- Augmenting GI calcium absorption.

Malignancy—secondary to paraneoplastic production of PTH-related protein (PTHrP)—is the most common cause of clinically apparent hypercalcemia; primary hyperparathyroidism is a more common cause of asymptomatic hypercalcemia. In addition to increasing osteoblast RANKL expression, PTHrP also inhibits the expression of osteoprotegerin, a "decoy receptor" that normally binds to RANKL and blocks its interactions with RANK (Table 24-4).

Hyperparathyroidism (p. 1101)

- *Primary hyperparathyroidism:* Autonomous PTH overproduction, usually from an adenoma or parathyroid hyperplasia
- *Secondary hyperparathyroidism:* Compensatory PTH hypersecretion secondary to prolonged hypocalcemia (e.g., due to chronic renal failure)
- *Tertiary hyperparathyroidism:* Persistent PTH hypersecretion after hypocalcemia is corrected (e.g., after renal transplant)

Primary Hyperparathyroidism (*p. 1101*)

A common endocrine disorder (25 cases per 100,000 population in the United States) and an important etiology of hypercalcemia; most cases are sporadic, occurring in patients over age 50, with a 4:1 female predominance. Causes include the following:

- Adenoma: 85% to 95% (most are monoclonal)
- Primary hyperplasia: 5% to 10% (most are monoclonal, as well)
- Parathyroid carcinoma: 1%

TABLE 24-4 Causes of Hypercalcemia

Raised [PTH]	Decreased [PTH]
Hyperparathyroidism	Hypercalcemia of malignancy*
Primary (adenoma > hyperplasia)*	Vitamin D toxicity
Secondary†	Immobilization
Tertiary†	Thiazide diuretics
FHH	Granulomatous disease (sarcoidosis)

*Primary hyperparathyroidism is the most common cause of hypercalcemia overall. Malignancy is the most common cause of *symptomatic* hypercalcemia. Primary hyperparathyroidism and malignancy account for nearly 90% of cases of hypercalcemia.

†Secondary and tertiary hyperparathyroidism are most commonly associated with progressive renal failure.

PTH, Parathyroid hormone concentration.

Solitary adenomas are the most common cause of primary hyperparathyroidism; two acquired defects have a role in pathogenesis:

- *Cyclin D1 overexpression* is associated with 40% of sporadic parathyroid adenomas; approximately half of these occur through relocation of the *cyclin D1* gene adjacent to the 5′ flanking region of the *PTH* gene.
- *MEN1* (a tumor suppressor gene) mutations leading to homozygous inactivation occur in 20% to 30% of sporadic adenomas.

Familial syndromes are a much less common cause of primary hyperparathyroidism:

- *MEN-1 syndrome:* Parathyroid adenomas and hyperplasia can be associated with germline *MEN1* mutations.
- *MEN-2 syndrome* is due to activating mutations of the *RET* tyrosine kinase receptor.
- *Familial hypocalciuric hypercalcemia (FHH)* is an autosomal dominant disorder resulting from loss-of-function mutations in the parathyroid *calcium-sensing receptor gene (CASR).*

Morphology (p. 1102)

Morphologic changes involve the parathyroid glands as well as all other organs affected by hypercalcemia.

- Parathyroid adenomas
  - *Gross:* Tumors are almost all solitary, well-circumscribed, tan-brown nodules, averaging 0.5 to 5 g and surrounded by a delicate capsule; remaining glands are usually normal or smaller in size secondary to hypercalcemic feedback inhibition.
  - *Microscopic:* Lesions are composed predominantly of *chief cells* (source of PTH) arrayed in uniform sheets, trabeculae, or follicles; foci of *oxyphil cells* (packed with mitochondria) may be present, and bizarre atypia is not uncommon. Adipose tissue is inconspicuous.
- Primary hyperplasia
  - *Gross:* All glands are typically involved although not necessarily uniformly; combined weights rarely exceed 1 g.
  - *Microscopic:* Chief cell hyperplasia typically involves glands in a diffuse or multinodular pattern. Adipose tissue is inconspicuous.
- *Parathyroid carcinoma* may be grossly and microscopically difficult to distinguish from an adenoma.
  - *Gross:* Typically one gland is enlarged by a gray-white, irregular mass sometimes exceeding 10 g.
  - *Microscopic:* Lesional cells are usually uniform and not too dissimilar from normal parathyroid cells; diagnosis of malignancy is based on the presence of local invasion and/or metastases.
- Other organs:
  - Skeletal changes include osteoclast activation with bone resorption. In severe cases, affected bones show thinned cortices with increased marrow fibrous tissue accompanied by foci of hemorrhage and cyst formation *(osteitis fibrosa cystica).*
  - Hypercalcemia promotes *nephrolithiasis,* renal interstitial and tubular calcification *(nephrocalcinosis),* and *metastatic calcifications* elsewhere.

Clinical Course (p. 1103)

- *Asymptomatic hyperparathyroidism* is typically discovered by routine serum calcium measurements; serum PTH levels are inappropriately elevated for the level of serum calcium (conversely, PTH levels are low in the hypercalcemia resulting from nonparathyroid diseases).

Cancer is a less common etiology of hypercalcemia; it can occur with both solid tumors and hematologic malignancies, especially multiple myeloma. In 80% of cases, osteolytic tumors induce hypercalcemia by secreting PTHrP (functions similar to PTH in inducing osteoclastic bone resorption); the remaining 20% induce hypercalcemia through bony metastases and subsequent cytokine-induced bone resorption.

- *Symptomatic primary hyperparathyroidism* is traditionally associated with a constellation of symptoms: painful bones, renal stones, abdominal groans, and psychic moans:
  - Bone disease and pain with fractures secondary to osteoporosis and osteitis fibrosa cystica.
  - Nephrolithiasis (renal stones) occurs in 20% of patients; pain is secondary to obstructive uropathy. Chronic renal insufficiency can cause polyuria and polydipsia.
  - GI disturbances include constipation, nausea, peptic ulcers, pancreatitis, and gallstones.
  - CNS alterations include depression, lethargy, and eventually seizures.
  - Other findings include weakness, fatigue, and cardiac valve calcifications.

Secondary Hyperparathyroidism (p. 1103)

Secondary hyperparathyroidism results from any condition that causes chronic hypocalcemia, thereby driving compensatory parathyroid overactivity; *renal failure is the most common etiology.* Renal failure triggers phosphate retention and hyperphosphatemia; elevated phosphate levels directly depress serum calcium causing a compensatory hypersecretion of PTH. Renal disease also leads to reduced 1-hydroxylation of vitamin D, which impairs GI calcium absorption; reduced vitamin D also removes normal feedback mechanisms that inhibit PTH secretion. Parathyroid glands and bones exhibit the same morphologic features (albeit usually less severe) as for other causes of hyperparathyroidism. Metastatic calcifications in vessels can lead to significant ischemic damage to skin and other organs *(calciphylaxis).* Secondary hyperparathyroidism responds to correction of the underlying renal disease or to vitamin D supplementation with phosphate binders to reduce the hyperphosphatemia.

Occasionally, autonomous parathyroid activity develops after long-term hyperparathyroidism *(tertiary hyperparathyroidism),* requiring surgical resection to treat.

Hypoparathyroidism (p. 1104)

Causes of hypoparathyroidism include the following:

- Surgical (e.g., thyroidectomy or treatment of hyperparathyroidism)
- Autoimmune hypoparathyroidism associated with APS, type I (see later)
- Autosomal dominant hypoparathyroidism due to gain-of-function mutations in the *CASR* gene (causing increased sensitivity of the calcium receptor)
- Familial isolated hypoparathyroidism, due either to primary PTH mutations that affect its precursor processing (autosomal dominant) or to loss-of-function mutations in the *GCM2* gene responsible for parathyroid development (autosomal recessive)
- Congenital absence of all glands (e.g., DiGeorge syndrome)

Manifestations are related to the chronicity and severity of the hypocalcemia:

- *Tetany* (characterized by neuromuscular irritability) is the hypocalcemic hallmark: symptoms range from muscle cramps and carpopedal spasms to laryngeal stridor and convulsions.
- *Mental status changes* (e.g., anxiety, depression, or psychosis).
- *Intracranial manifestations,* including basal ganglia calcifications, parkinsonian-like movement disorders, and elevated intracranial pressure.
- *Ocular changes* with lens calcification and cataract formation.
- *Cardiac conduction defects,* producing a characteristic prolongation of the QT interval.
- *Dental developmental defects* (when hypoparathyroidism is present early in development), including hypoplasia and defective enamel and root formation.

Pseudohypoparathyroidism (p. 1105)

Pathogenesis is related to *GNAS1* mutations that code for a defective G protein normally responsible for mediating PTH activity. Target tissues are relatively resistant to PTH, resulting in hypocalcemia, compensatory parathyroid hyperfunction, and a variety of skeletal and developmental abnormalities. Because the same G protein mediates the action of TSH and LH or FSH, hypothyroidism and hypogonadism can also occur.

The Endocrine Pancreas (p. 1105)

There are approximately one million *islets of Langerhans* in each pancreas, containing four major and two minor types of cells.

- Major types:
  - *β-Cells produce insulin* that regulates tissue glucose utilization.
  - *α-Cells secrete glucagon* that stimulates lipolysis and hepatic glycogenolysis and gluconeogenesis, as well as counter-regulating insulin release.
  - *δ-Cells secrete somatostatin* that suppresses both insulin and glucagon release.
  - *PP cells secrete pancreatic polypeptide* that stimulates gastric and intestinal enzyme secretion and inhibits intestinal motility.
- Minor types:
  - *D1 cells* elaborate *VIP* that induces glycogenolysis and hyperglycemia and stimulates GI fluid secretion.
  - *Enterochromaffin cells synthesize serotonin* that stimulates bowel motility.

Diabetes Mellitus (p. 1105)

Diabetes mellitus is a group of metabolic disorders sharing the *common underlying feature of hyperglycemia.* The net effect is a chronic disorder of carbohydrate, fat, and protein metabolism with long-term complications affecting blood vessels, kidneys, eyes, and nerves; it is the leading cause of end-stage renal disease, adult-onset blindness, and nontraumatic lower extremity amputation. In the United States >25 million people (8% of the population) are diabetic, with 1.9 million new cases diagnosed annually; it costs approximately $174 billion annually and is one of the "top ten" causes of death. Worldwide, 346 million people are affected, with a 40% to 80% mortality rate, depending on health care resources.

Diagnosis *(p. 1106)*

Blood glucose is normally maintained between 70 and 120 mg/dL. Diabetes mellitus is diagnosed by demonstrating blood glucose elevations by any one of three criteria:

- Random glucose level ≥200 mg/dL, with classical signs and symptoms (see later)
- Fasting glucose level ≥126 mg/dL on more than one occasion
- Abnormal oral glucose tolerance test (OGTT) (i.e., glucose ≥200 mg/dL 2 hours after a standard carbohydrate load)
- A glycated hemoglobin (Hb_{A1C}) level ≥6.5% (Hb_{A1C} is a glycated modification of hemoglobin that occurs nonenzymatically in the presence of glucose metabolites)

Individuals with fasting glucose of 100 to 126 mg/dL, OGTT values of 140 to 200 mg/dL, or Hb_{A1C} levels of 5.7% to 6.4% have impaired glucose tolerance and are considered to be "prediabetic." Such patients have a 25% risk of progressing to overt diabetes within 5 years and have a significant risk of developing cardiovascular complications.

Classification *(p. 1107)*

The causes of diabetes mellitus are listed in Table 24-5; the vast majority of cases fall into one of two basic etiologies (Table 24-6):

- *Type 1 diabetes mellitus* is an autoimmune disease characterized by pancreatic β-cell destruction and an absolute insulin deficiency. It accounts for 5% to 10% of all cases and is the most common cause in patients under age 20.
- *Type 2 diabetes mellitus* is caused by a combination of peripheral insulin resistance and inadequate compensatory responses by pancreatic β-cells ("relative insulin deficiency"). It accounts for 90% to 95% of cases; the vast majority of patients are overweight.

Glucose Homeostasis *(p. 1107)*

Normal glucose homeostasis is tightly regulated by three interrelated processes: hepatic glucose production, glucose uptake by peripheral tissues (chiefly skeletal muscle), and the actions of insulin and counter-regulatory hormones (e.g., glucagon). During fasting, low insulin and high glucagon maintain peripheral glucose levels by facilitating hepatic gluconeogenesis and glycogenolysis, and by decreasing glycogen synthesis. After feeding, rising insulin and diminished glucagon lead to glucose uptake and use (primarily in skeletal muscle), as well as hepatic glycogen synthesis.

Regulation of Insulin Release (p. 1108)

In the *immediate phase* of insulin release a rise in glucose leads to increased uptake into β-cells through the GLUT-2 insulin-independent glucose transporter (Fig. 24-3); as glucose is metabolized, intracellular adenosine triphosphate (ATP) increases. This inhibits the activity of an ATP-sensitive K^+ channel, leading in turn to membrane depolarization, influx of extracellular Ca^{2+}, and insulin release from preformed stores. Persistent stimulus also results in increased insulin synthesis.

Oral food intake also induces the release of *incretin* hormones (glucose-dependent insulinotropic polypeptide [GIP] and glucagon-like peptide-1 [GLP-1]; see later) that increase β-cell insulin secretion,

TABLE 24-5 Classification of Diabetes Mellitus

1. *Type 1 diabetes* mellitus (β-cell destruction, usually leading to absolute insulin deficiency)
   Immune-mediated
   Idiopathic
2. *Type 2 diabetes* mellitus (combination of insulin resistance and β-cell dysfunction)
3. *Genetic defects of β-cell function*
   MODY, caused by mutations in the following:
      Hepatocyte nuclear factor 4α *(HNF4A),* MODY1
      Glucokinase *(GCK),* MODY2
      Hepatocyte nuclear factor 1α *(HNF1A),* MODY3
      Pancreatic and duodenal homeobox 1 *(PDX1),* MODY4
      Hepatocyte nuclear factor 1β *(HNF1B),* MODY5
      Neurogenic differentiation factor 1 *(NEUROD1),* MODY6
   Neonatal diabetes (activating mutations in *KCNJ11* and *ABCC8,* encoding Kir6.2 and SUR1, respectively)
   MIDD due to mitochondrial DNA mutations (m.3243A→G)
   Defects in proinsulin conversion
   Insulin gene mutations
4. *Genetic defects in insulin action*
   Type A insulin resistance
   Lipoatrophic diabetes, including mutations in *PPARG*
5. *Exocrine pancreatic defects*
   Chronic pancreatitis
   Pancreatectomy or trauma
   Neoplasia
   Cystic fibrosis
   Hemochromatosis
   Fibrocalculous pancreatopathy
6. *Endocrinopathies*
   Acromegaly
   Cushing syndrome
   Hyperthyroidism
   Pheochromocytoma
   Glucagonoma
7. *Infections*
   Cytomegalovirus
   Coxsackie B virus
   Congenital rubella
8. *Drugs*
   Glucocorticoids
   Thyroid hormone
   Interferon-α
   Protease inhibitors
   β-Adrenergic agonists
   Thiazides
   Nicotinic acid
   Phenytoin (Dilantin)
   Vacor
9. *Genetic syndromes associated with diabetes*
   Down syndrome
   Klinefelter syndrome
   Turner syndrome
   Prader-Willi syndrome
10. *Gestational diabetes mellitus*

American Diabetes Association: Position statement from the American Diabetes Association on the diagnosis and classification of diabetes mellitus, *Diabetes Care* 31(Suppl. 1):S55-S60, 2008.

TABLE 24-6 Type 1 Versus Type 2 Diabetes Mellitus

Type 1 Diabetes Mellitus	Type 2 Diabetes Mellitus
Clinical	
Onset: usually childhood and adolescence	Onset: usually adult; increasing incidence in childhood and adolescence
Normal weight or weight loss preceding diagnosis	Vast majority are obese (80%)
Progressive decrease in insulin levels	Increased blood insulin (early); normal or moderate decrease in insulin (late)
Circulating islet autoantibodies (antiinsulin, anti-GAD, anti-ICA512)	No islet autoantibodies
Diabetic ketoacidosis in absence of insulin therapy	Nonketotic hyperosmolar coma more common
Genetics	
Major linkage to MHC class II genes; also linked to polymorphisms in *CTLA4* and *PTPN22*, and insulin gene VNTRs	No HLA linkage; linkage to candidate diabetogenic and obesity-related genes (*TCF7L2, PPARG, FTO*, etc.)
Pathogenesis	
Dysfunction in T-cell selection and regulation leading to breakdown in self-tolerance to islet autoantigens	Insulin resistance in peripheral tissues, failure of compensation by β-cells
	Multiple obesity-associated factors (circulating nonesterified fatty acids, inflammatory mediators, adipocytokines) linked to pathogenesis of insulin resistance
Pathology	
Insulitis (inflammatory infiltrate of T cells and macrophages)	No insulitis; amyloid deposition in islets
β-Cell depletion, islet atrophy	Mild β-cell depletion

HLA, Human leukocyte antigen; *MHC*, major histocompatibility complex; *VNTRs*, variable number of tandem repeats.

decrease glucagon secretion, and delay gastric emptying (promoting satiety):

- *GIP*, secreted by enteroendocrine "K cells" in the proximal small bowel.
- *GLP-1*, secreted by "L cells" in the distal ileum and colon.

Circulating GIP and GLP-1 are degraded by dipeptidyl peptidases (DPPs), especially DPP-4.

The "incretin effect" is significantly blunted in patients with type 2 diabetes mellitus, hence the development of two new classes of drugs for such individuals: *GLP-1 receptor agonists* and DPP-4 inhibitors.

Insulin Action and Insulin Signaling Pathways (p. 1109)

The principal metabolic function of insulin is to increase glucose transport into target cells—primarily skeletal muscle and adipocytes; glucose uptake into most other cell types is insulin-independent. Once internalized, glucose is either stored as glycogen (skeletal muscle) or lipid (adipose tissue) or oxidized to generate ATP. Insulin inhibits lipid catabolism by adipocytes, inhibits glycogen breakdown, and promotes amino acid uptake and protein synthesis while diminishing protein degradation; it is also mitogenic for several cell types (Fig. 24-4).

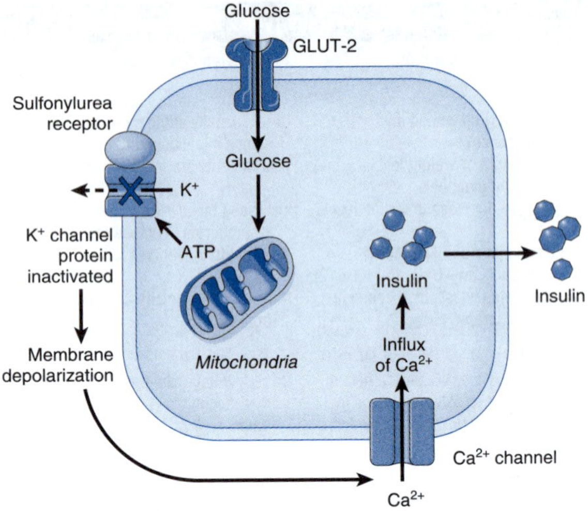

Figure 24-3 Immediate phase of insulin secretion. Glucose enters β-islet cells via the GLUT-2 insulin-independent glucose transporter. Resulting ATP production leads to inhibition of a K^+ channel receptor (a heterodimer of the sulfonylurea receptor [SUR1] and the Kir6.2 K^+-channel protein) and membrane depolarization with Ca^{2+} influx. Increased intracellular calcium leads to release of stored insulin. The sulfonylurea class of oral hypoglycemic agents binds to the SUR1 receptor protein and mediates membrane depolarization and subsequent insulin release.

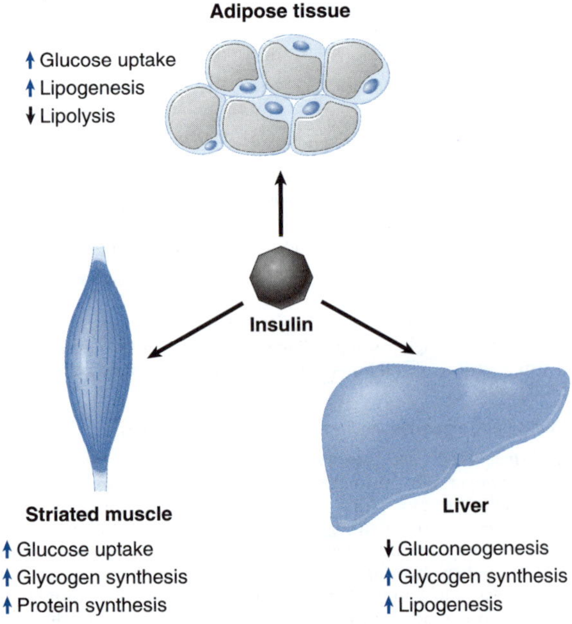

Figure 24-4 Metabolic actions of insulin in striated muscle, adipose tissue, and liver.

Insulin acts through a heterodimeric insulin receptor; binding stimulates receptor kinase activity and induces phosphorylation of several insulin receptor substrate (IRS) proteins with activation of downstream cascades including the PI3 and MAP kinase pathways. These lead eventually to AKT pathway activation, culminating in movement of the GLUT-4 glucose transporter protein to the plasma membrane; the outcome is increased glucose transport. A variety of phosphatases (e.g., protein tyrosine phosphatase 1B and PTEN) can negatively regulate this activation cascade.

Pathogenesis of Type I Diabetes Mellitus (p. 1109)

This form of diabetes results from autoimmune β-islet cell destruction. Although the clinical onset is typically abrupt (occurring after >90% of β-cells have been destroyed), the autoimmune process starts many years before the disease becomes evident. Pathogenesis involves a combination of genetic susceptibility and environmental insults.

- *Genetic susceptibility:* By far the most important genetic association (50%) is with the class II major histocompatibility complex (MHC) human leukocyte antigen (HLA) locus. Approximately 90% to 95% of whites with type 1 diabetes mellitus have HLA-DR3 or DR4 haplotypes (compared with 40% of normal subjects), and an associated DQ8 haplotype incurs the greatest inherited risk. Non-MHC polymorphisms associated with disease susceptibility include the insulin gene itself, CTLA-4, and PTPN22; mutations in the *autoimmune regulator (AIRE)* gene encoding an immune regulator cause autoimmune polyendocrinopathy syndrome, type I (APS1).
- *Environmental factors:* Several viral agents have been implicated as potential triggers for an autoimmune attack, including coxsackieviruses, mumps, cytomegalovirus, and rubella. A postulated mechanism is "molecular mimicry," in which viruses produce proteins that elicit host immune responses that cross-react with self-tissues.
- *Mechanisms of β-cell destruction* (p. 1110): The fundamental immune abnormality is failure of T-cell self-tolerance:
  - CD4+ T_H1 cells cause tissue injury by releasing cytokines (e.g., IFN-γ and TNF) and activating macrophages.
  - CD8+ cytotoxic T lymphocytes directly kill β-cells.
  - Autoantibodies against islet cells and insulin may also participate; β-cell antigens include the enzyme glutamic acid decarboxylase (GAD) and islet cell autoantigen 512. In susceptible children who have not developed diabetes, islet cell autoantibodies can be predictive of diabetes development.

Pathogenesis of Type 2 Diabetes Mellitus (p. 1111)

This form of diabetes is a complex multifactorial disease; there is no evidence to suggest an autoimmune etiology.

- *Genetic factors:* These are important as evidenced by a >90% disease concordance in monozygotic twins; first-degree relatives have fivefold to tenfold higher risk than those without a family history. At least 30 loci—many associated with *insulin secretion*—increase lifetime risk for type 2 diabetes mellitus.
- *Environmental factors:* The most important risk factor is obesity, particularly central or visceral obesity; >80% of individuals with type 2 diabetes mellitus are obese. Sedentary lifestyle is another independent risk factor. Weight loss and exercise improve insulin sensitivity; they are the usual nonpharmacologic measures attempted for milder type 2 diabetes mellitus patients.

- *Metabolic defects in diabetes;* two cardinal findings are as follows:
  - Insulin resistance (decreased responses of muscle, fat, and liver to insulin)—this predates the development of hyperglycemia and is usually accompanied by compensatory β-cell hyperfunction and hyperinsulinemia
  - Inadequate insulin secretion in the face of insulin resistance and hyperglycemia (β-cell dysfunction)

Insulin Resistance (p. 1111)

Insulin resistance is reflected by diminished skeletal muscle glucose uptake, reduced hepatic glycolysis and fatty acid oxidation, and the inability to suppress hepatic gluconeogenesis. Defects in the insulin signaling pathway are implicated, including reduced tyrosine phosphorylation of the insulin receptor and IRS proteins in peripheral tissues, reducing cell-surface glucose transporter GLUT-4.

- *Obesity and insulin resistance* (p. 1112): Diabetes risk increases as the body mass index increases; central obesity (abdominal fat) is more closely linked to insulin resistance than is peripheral obesity (gluteal and subcutaneous fat).
  - *Free fatty acids (FFAs)* are markedly increased in muscle and liver of obese; these can overwhelm the fatty acid oxidation pathways leading to accumulation of potentially "toxic" intermediates, such as ceramide and diacylglycerol, that can drive aberrant serine-threonine *(not tyrosine)* phosphorylation of the insulin receptor and IRS proteins that *attenuate* insulin signaling responses. FFAs can also compete with glucose for substrate oxidation, leading to feedback inhibition of glycolysis.
  - *Adipokines:* Fat is a source of cytokines, including those that are proglycemic (e.g., resistin and retinol binding protein 4) and antiglycemic (e.g., leptin and adiponectin). The latter improve tissue insulin sensitivity by enhancing AMP-activated protein kinase (AMPK) activity, thus promoting fatty acid oxidation (notably AMPK is the target of the oral hypoglycemic agent metformin). Adiponectin levels are reduced in obesity.
  - *Inflammation:* Excess FFAs within macrophages and β-cells can activate inflammasomes—multiprotein cytoplasmic complexes that generate interleukin (IL)-1β (see Chapter 6). IL-1β then mediates the production of additional proinflammatory cytokines that are released into the circulation and promote insulin resistance.

β-Cell Dysfunction (p. 1112)

Increased β-cell function occurs early in type 2 diabetes as a compensatory measure to counter insulin resistance and maintain euglycemia. However, eventually this increased capacity is "exhausted," and the hyperinsulinemic state gives way to a state of relative insulin deficiency. Mechanisms include excess FFAs ("lipotoxicity") and chronic hyperglycemia ("glucotoxicity") that compromise β-cell function. Reduced GIP and GLP-1 secretion also underlie an "incretin effect" with reduced insulin secretion. Amyloid deposition within islets is present in more than 90% of diabetic islets, although whether it is a cause or an effect of β-cell "burnout" is unknown.

Monogenic Forms of Diabetes *(p. 1112)*

These are uncommon, resulting from either a primary defect in β-cell function or insulin-receptor signaling (Table 24-5).

- *Genetic defects in β-cell function* (p. 1112) affect β-cell mass and/or insulin production (without β-cell loss) and are responsible for

1% to 2% of diabetes cases. The causes are heterogeneous but are typified by the following:

- Autosomal dominant inheritance with high penetrance
- Early onset, usually before age 25 and even in the neonatal period
- Absence of obesity
- Absence of β-cell autoantibodies

Maturity-onset diabetes of the young (MODY) is the largest subgroup in this category. Six distinct loss-of-function genetic defects have been identified (Table 24-5), including glucokinase mutations that block glucose entry into the glycolytic cycle—and thus raise the glucose threshold necessary to trigger insulin release.

Permanent neonatal diabetes results from gain-of-function mutations of the subunits of the β-cell ATP-sensitive K^+ channel (Fig. 24-3); these cause constitutive channel activation, and membrane hyperpolarization, and thus prevent insulin release leading to hypoinsulinemic diabetes.

Maternally inherited diabetes and deafness (MIDD) results from mitochondrial DNA mutations; impaired ATP synthesis in β-cells results in diminished insulin release. Patients also have bilateral sensorineural deafness.

- *Genetic defects in insulin responses* (p. 1113). Rarely insulin receptor mutations affecting synthesis, ligand binding, or intracellular signaling can result in severe insulin resistance and diabetes. Such patients may also exhibit *acanthosis nigricans* (velvety hyperpigmented cutaneous macules), and—in women—polycystic ovaries and elevated androgens. *Lipoatrophic diabetes* is hyperglycemia accompanied by loss of subcutaneous adipose tissue.

Diabetes and Pregnancy *(p. 1113)*

Diabetes in pregnancy occurs when women with preexisting diabetes become pregnant or when previously euglycemic women develop impaired glucose tolerance during pregnancy ("gestational" diabetes); approximately 5% of U.S. pregnancies are complicated by hyperglycemia, with rates rising in parallel with the overall incidence of obesity and diabetes. Pregnancy is a "diabetogenic" state; the hormonal milieu favors insulin resistance, so that otherwise susceptible individuals (due to genetic and environmental factors) can develop de novo gestational diabetes. When hyperglycemia is already present in the periconception period, fetuses have an increased risk of *stillbirth* and *congenital malformations.* Poorly controlled diabetes during pregnancy can cause excessive birth weight *(macrosomia),* as well as long-term sequelae, such as obesity and diabetes. Although gestational diabetes typically resolves following delivery, most affected women develop overt diabetes within 10 to 20 years.

Clinical Features of Diabetes *(Table 24-6; p. 1113)*

Type 1 diabetes mellitus can occur at any age; initially the exogenous insulin requirements may be minimal, due to endogenous insulin secretion *(honeymoon period).* Thereafter any residual β-cell reserve is exhausted and insulin requirements increase dramatically. The transition from impaired glucose tolerance to overt diabetes can be abrupt and may be triggered in some cases by increased insulin requirements (e.g., an infection).

Although type 2 diabetics are typically >40 years old and frequently obese, obesity and sedentary lifestyles are increasing the frequency of type 2 diabetes in children and adolescents. Symptoms can include unexplained fatigue, dizziness, or blurred vision, but the diagnosis is most commonly made by routine blood testing in asymptomatic persons.

- The *classic triad of diabetes* (p. 1113) is polyuria, polydipsia, and polyphagia; diabetic ketoacidosis (DKA) can also occur (Fig. 24-5). All are due to the *catabolic* state resulting from insufficient insulin (and unopposed glucagon, GH, and epinephrine) affecting glucose, fat, and protein metabolism:
  - Glucose cannot be taken up into fat or muscle, and hepatic and muscle glycogen reserves are depleted (glycogenolysis) while glycogen synthesis also ceases. The resulting hyperglycemia

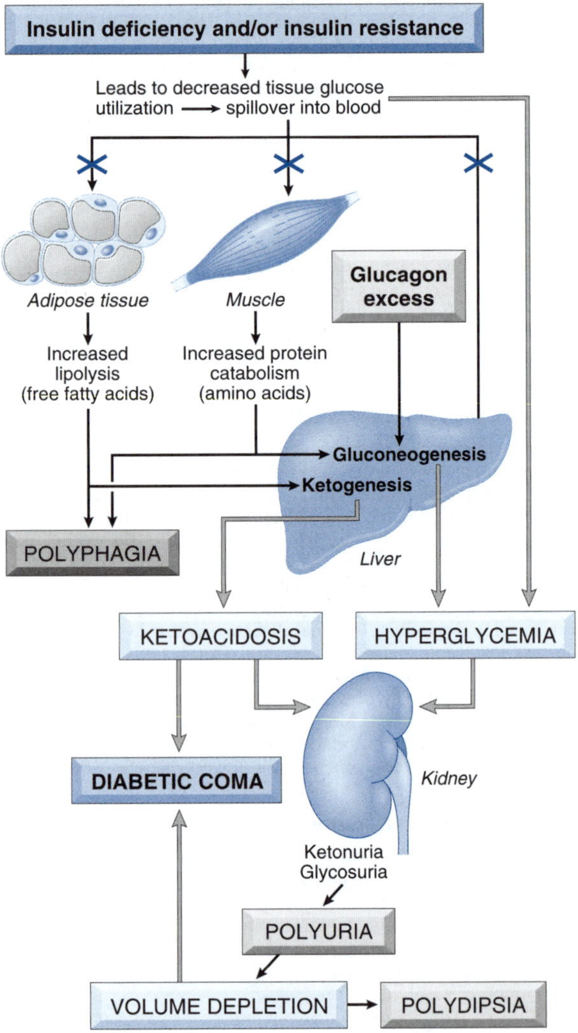

Figure 24-5 Sequence of metabolic derangements underlying the clinical manifestations of diabetes. Absolute insulin deficiency leads to a catabolic state, culminating in ketoacidosis and severe volume depletion. Left untreated, these can cause sufficient central nervous system compromise to lead to coma and eventual death.

exceeds the renal threshold for reabsorption, and glycosuria ensues, inducing an osmotic diuresis causing water and electrolyte loss *(polyuria)* and a secondary triggering of thirst via brain osmoreceptors *(polydipsia);* protein and fat catabolism provides building blocks for gluconeogenesis but causes a negative energy balance that leads to increased appetite *(polyphagia).*

- Despite the increased appetite, catabolic effects prevail, resulting in weight loss and muscle weakness. The combination of polyphagia and weight loss is paradoxical and should always raise the suspicion of diabetes.

- *Acute metabolic complications of diabetes* (p. 1113): *DKA* is a severe complication of type 1 diabetes mellitus (Fig. 24-5); it occurs less frequently and less severely in type 2 diabetes (due to residual low-level insulin). The most common precipitating factor for DKA is lack of insulin, although other stressors can increase epinephrine production that blocks insulin action and stimulates glucagon secretion. Insulin deficiency—coupled with glucagon excess—results in the following:
  - Decreased peripheral glucose utilization with increased gluconeogenesis, causing severe hyperglycemia, osmotic diuresis, and dehydration.
  - Activation of ketogenic pathways, with lipoprotein lipase degrading adipose stores to generate FFAs and protein degradation leading to increased ketogenic amino acids; subsequent hepatic metabolism produces *ketone bodies* (acetoacetic acid and β-hydroxybutyric acid) that cause *ketonemia* and *ketonuria.* If the urinary excretion of ketones is compromised by dehydration, the result is a systemic *metabolic ketoacidosis.*
  - Clinical manifestations include fatigue, nausea and vomiting, severe abdominal pain, a characteristic fruity odor (due to acetone), and deep, labored breathing (also known as *Kussmaul breathing*). Prolonged DKA can cause altered consciousness and coma; reversal requires insulin administration, correction of the acidosis, and treatment of any underlying precipitating factor (e.g., infection).

Although type 2 diabetics do not typically develop DKA, they can develop *hyperosmolar hyperosmotic syndrome (HHS)* due to severe dehydration from sustained osmotic diuresis. The absence of ketoacidosis and its symptoms (nausea, vomiting, Kussmaul breathing) can delay medical intervention until severe dehydration and impairment of mental status occur.

Ironically *hypoglycemia* is the most common acute metabolic complication in either type of diabetes. This can occur due to a missed meal, excessive physical exertion, an excess insulin administration, or during medication dose adjustment. Signs and symptoms include dizziness, confusion, sweating, palpitations, and tachycardia; if hypoglycemia persists, loss of consciousness may occur.

Chronic Complications of Diabetes (p. 1115)

The morbidity associated with long-standing diabetes of any cause is attributable to *macrovascular disease* (accelerated atherosclerosis) precipitating myocardial infarction, stroke, or extremity gangrene, and *microvascular disease* (capillary dysfunction) causing nephropathy, retinopathy, and neuropathy. Hyperglycemia is the major factor, although insulin resistance and dyslipidemia can contribute.

- *Formation of advanced glycation end products (AGEs)* (p. 1115) occurs through nonenzymatic interactions between protein amino groups and glucose-derived metabolites; a natural baseline rate of AGE formation is markedly accelerated by hyperglycemia. AGEs bind to a specific receptor (RAGE) expressed on vascular wall and inflammatory cells; this leads to proinflammatory cytokine release, generation of reactive oxygen species, increased procoagulant activity, and enhanced vascular smooth muscle proliferation and matrix synthesis. AGEs can also directly cross-link matrix proteins, leading to protein deposition, loss of vascular wall elasticity, poor endothelial adhesion, leaky basement membranes, and persistence of poorly degradable cross-linked adducts.

- *Activation of protein kinase c* (p. 1115): Intracellular hyperglycemia stimulates the de novo synthesis of diacylgylcerol, which in turn activates protein kinase C (PKC); PKC activation leads to the following:
    - Production of vascular endothelial growth factor (VEGF)
    - Increased endothelin-1 and diminished nitric oxide (increased vascular tone)
    - Increased fibrosis due to transforming growth factor-β (TGF-β) production
    - Production of plasminogen-activator inhibitor-1, reducing fibrinolysis, and promoting thrombosis
    - Production of proinflammatory cytokines by endothelium
- *Oxidative stress and disturbances in polyol pathways* (p. 1116): In tissues that do not require insulin for glucose transport (e.g., nerves, lens, kidney, blood vessels), hyperglycemia leads to increased intracellular glucose. This glucose is metabolized to sorbitol and then fructose (using nicotinamide adenine dinucleotide phosphate [NADPH] reducing equivalents), so that an equilibrium with extracellular solute is not achieved. The accompanying osmotic load leads to water influx and osmotic cell injury. Reductions in NADPH also lead to reduced glutathione regeneration and increased cellular susceptibility to oxidative stress.
- *Hexosamine pathways and generation of fructose-6-phosphate* (p. 1116): Hyperglycemia-induced flux through the hexosamine pathway increases intracellular levels of *fructose-6-phosphate,* which is a substrate for glycosylation of proteins, leading to generation of excess proteoglycans, and abnormal expression of TGF-β and plasminogen activator inhibitor-1 (PAI-1).

Morphology and Clinical Features of Chronic Complications of Diabetes (p. 1116)

***Morphology** (p. 1117).*

- *Pancreas:* Findings are variable.
    - *Type 1:* Islet number and size are reduced, and a lymphocytic infiltrate *(insulitis)* may be present.
    - *Type 2:* Subtle reduction in islet cell mass may be accompanied by amyloid deposition, occasionally effacing the islets.

- *Diabetic macrovascular disease* is manifested as accelerated or exacerbated atherosclerosis in the aorta and large and medium-sized arteries; hyaline arteriolosclerosis is more prevalent and severe.
- *Diabetic microangiopathy* is reflected by diffuse basement membrane thickening, most evident in the capillaries of the skin, skeletal muscle, retina, renal glomeruli, and renal medulla. Such capillaries are more leaky than normal to plasma proteins. Basement membrane thickening can also affect nonvascular structures, such as renal tubules, Bowman capsule, peripheral nerves, and placenta.

- Diabetic nephropathy:
  - Glomerular involvement includes diffuse basement membrane thickening, mesangial sclerosis, nodular glomerulosclerosis *(Kimmelstiel-Wilson lesion)*, and/or exudative lesions.
  - Vascular effects include renal artery atherosclerosis and arteriolosclerosis, including benign nephrosclerosis with hypertension.
  - There is increased incidence of infections, including pyelonephritis and sometimes necrotizing papillitis.
  - *Diabetic ocular complications* take the form of retinopathy (see Chapter 29), cataracts (lens opacification), or glaucoma (increased intraocular pressure) with optic nerve damage.
  - *Diabetic neuropathy* is a combination of direct neural injury as well as microvascular ischemia (see Chapter 27).

Clinical Manifestations of Chronic Diabetes (p. 1119)

Complications of long-standing diabetes (p. 1113) include the following:

- *Cardiovascular events* (e.g., myocardial infarction, renal vascular insufficiency, and stroke) are the most common causes of death. Diabetics have a fourfold greater risk of dying of cardiovascular causes compared with the nondiabetic population. In most instances these occur 15 to 20 years after hyperglycemic onset; diabetes-associated hypertension, dyslipidemia, and hypercoagulability are frequent associated conditions.
- *Diabetic nephropathy* is a leading cause in the United States of end-stage renal disease; 30% to 40% of all diabetics develop some degree of nephropathy, with the frequency influenced by ethnic makeup (blacks and Native Americans have greater risk than whites). Microalbuminuria is the earliest manifestation (between 30 and 300 mg/day); without intervention, 80% of type 1 diabetics and 20% to 40% of type 2 diabetics will develop overt nephropathy with macroalbuminuria (>300 mg/day) and 75% and 20%, respectively, will progress to end-stage renal disease within 20 years.
- *Diabetic retinopathy* develops in 60% to 80% of patients within 15 to 20 years of diagnosis. The fundamental lesion is neovascularization attributable to hypoxia-induced overexpression of VEGF in the retina.
- *Diabetic neuropathy* typically presents with extremity *distal symmetric polyneuropathy*, affecting both sensory and motor function. *Autonomic neuropathy* can produce bladder, bowel, or sexual dysfunction, and *diabetic mononeuropathy* can manifest with sudden cranial nerve palsy or foot or hand drop.
- *Enhanced susceptibility to infections* is attributable to compromised tissue perfusion, diminished neutrophil function, and impaired macrophage cytokine production.
- *In patients with long-standing diabetes*, glycemic control is monitored by measuring the circulating levels of hemoglobin A1C (Hb_{A1C}); normal levels in nondiabetics are 4% to 6% of the total hemoglobin content. Unlike blood glucose levels, Hb_{A1C} allows the integration of glucose levels over the 120-day lifespan of an erythrocyte; in diabetics with good glycemic control, it should constitute <7%.

Pancreatic Neuroendocrine Neoplasms (p. 1121)

Pancreatic neuroendocrine tumors (PanNETs) are also known as islet cell tumors. Constituting only 2% of all pancreatic neoplasms, they may be single or multiple, may be benign or malignant, and can secrete hormones or be nonfunctional. Insulinomas are the most common islet cell tumor, and 90% are benign; 60% to 90% of other pancreatic endocrine neoplasms are malignant. Unequivocal criteria for malignancy include metastases, vascular invasion, and/or local infiltration.

Sporadic PanNETs exhibit recurrent somatic alterations in *MEN1* (also causes familial MEN syndrome, type 1), loss-of-function mutations in tumor suppressor genes, such as *PTEN* and *TSC2* (see Chapter 7), and inactivating mutations in α-thalassemia or mental retardation syndrome, X-linked *(ATRX)* or death-domain associated protein *(DAXX)*.

Hyperinsulinism (Insulinoma) *(p. 1121)*

β-Cell tumors can elaborate sufficient insulin to cause hypoglycemia; symptoms (confusion, stupor, or loss of consciousness) occur with serum glucose <50 mg/dL.

Morphology (p. 1121)

Most are solitary lesions, <2 cm and well encapsulated, composed of cords and nests of well-differentiated β-cells; carcinomas (approximately 10% of cases) are diagnosed based on metastasis or invasion.

Clinical Features (p. 1121)

Hypoglycemic symptoms are mild in all but 20% of cases; surgical resection yields prompt normalization of glycemia. Hyperinsulinism can also be caused by diffuse islet hyperplasia (in neonates and infants in the setting of maternal diabetes), Beckwith-Wiedemann syndrome, and rare metabolic disorders.

Zollinger-Ellison Syndrome (Gastrinomas) *(p. 1121)*

Gastrin hypersecretion is usually due to gastrin-producing *gastrinomas;* these can occur in the pancreas, duodenum, or peripancreatic soft tissue. The classic "Z-E" syndrome comprises a triad of severe peptic ulcer disease, gastric hypersecretion, and pancreatic islet lesions.

Clinical Features (p. 1122)

The majority of patients present with diarrhea, and duodenal and gastric ulcers are often multiple. Although the ulcers are identical to those found in the general population, they are often intractable to therapy; they may also occur in unusual locations, such as the jejunum. More than half of the gastrinomas have metastasized or are locally invasive at the time of diagnosis; approximately 25% arise in conjunction with other endocrine tumors, as part of the MEN-1 syndrome.

Other Rare Pancreatic Endocrine Neoplasms *(p. 1122)*

- *α-Cell tumors (glucagonomas)* are associated with elevated glucagon and a syndrome that includes mild diabetes, necrolytic migratory erythema (a skin rash), and anemia.
- *δ-Cell tumors (somatostatinomas)* exhibit high somatostatin levels and a syndrome comprising diabetes mellitus, cholelithiasis, steatorrhea, and hypochlorhydria.
- *VIPoma* causes a *watery diarrhea, hypokalemia, achlorhydria syndrome (WDHA syndrome);* neural crest tumors (e.g., neuroblastomas) can present with the same syndrome.
- *Pancreatic carcinoid tumors* produce serotonin.
- *Pancreatic polypeptide-secreting endocrine tumors* are rare and usually asymptomatic.

Adrenal Glands (p. 1122)

Adrenal Cortex (p. 1122)

Adrenocortical Hyperfunction (Hyperadrenalism) (p. 1123)

Adrenal hyperfunction syndromes are related to overproduction of one or more of the three basic adrenal cortical steroids:

- Cushing syndrome (excess glucocorticoids)
- Hyperaldosteronism (excess mineralocorticoids)
- Adrenogenital syndromes (excess androgens)

Hypercortisolism (Cushing Syndrome) (p. 1123)

Hypercortisolism occurs with the following:

- Administration of *exogenous* glucocorticoids (most common cause)
- Primary hypothalamic-pituitary disorders associated with ACTH hypersecretion
- Cortisol hypersecretion by adrenal adenoma, carcinoma, or nodular hyperplasia
- Ectopic ACTH production by a nonendocrine neoplasm

Pituitary ACTH hypersecretion (Cushing disease) typically occurs in women (4:1 ratio) and accounts for 70% of cases of *endogenous* hypercortisolism. Most cases are associated with an ACTH-producing pituitary adenoma. Serum ACTH is elevated and is not suppressed by low-dose dexamethasone challenge but is reduced by high-dose challenge.

Ectopic ACTH secretion by nonpituitary tumors accounts for 10% of cases of endogenous *Cushing syndrome.* It occurs most commonly in men aged 40 to 60 associated with small cell lung carcinoma, although carcinoid tumors, thyroid medullary carcinoma, and islet cell tumors can also be ACTH sources. Serum ACTH is elevated and its secretion is completely insensitive to either low-dose or high-dose dexamethasone. Rarely, Cushing syndrome can be associated with ectopic secretion of corticotropin-releasing factor (CRF), with resultant ACTH overproduction and hypercortisolism.

Primary adrenal neoplasms (e.g., adenoma [10% of cases] or carcinoma [5%]) are the most common causes for *ACTH-independent* Cushing syndrome. ACTH levels are quite low (feedback inhibition), and dexamethasone challenge has no effect on cortisol levels.

ACTH-independent primary cortical hyperplasia is uncommon; it is often reflected by adrenal cortical *macronodular hyperplasia.* Although macronodular hyperplasia is ACTH-autonomous, cortisol production can instead be driven by *non-ACTH hormones* (e.g., LH, ADH, or serotonin) for which the epithelium has overexpressed the corresponding receptors. Macronodular hyperplasia also occurs in the setting of the *McCune-Albright syndrome* (due to activating mutations in *GNAS*), and when genes controlling intracellular cAMP are mutated.

***Morphology** (p. 1124).*

- *Pituitary:* Regardless of etiology, elevated glucocorticoid levels induce *Crooke hyaline change*—the normal granular, basophilic cytoplasm of ACTH-producing cells becomes pale and homogeneous due to keratin filament deposition.
- *Adrenals:* Morphology depends on the cause of hypercortisolism.
    - *Exogenous glucocorticoids* suppress endogenous ACTH and result in cortical atrophy; the zona glomerulosa will be of normal thickness because it functions independently of ACTH.

- *Endogenous elevations of ACTH* cause bilateral cortical hyperplasia.
- *Macronodular hyperplasia* exhibits almost complete replacement of the cortex by nodules ≤3 cm, containing an admixture of lipid-poor and lipid-rich cells.
- *Primary neoplasms* resemble nonfunctional cortical neoplasms (see later); adenomas are generally small (<30 g), yellow, and well circumscribed, whereas carcinomas tend to be larger and unencapsulated. There is atrophy of the adjacent residual cortex and the contralateral gland.

Clinical Course *(p. 1125).* Cushing syndrome develops slowly and early manifestations (hypertension and weight gain) are nonspecific. However, the full-blown syndrome complex has a number of characteristic features, including the following:

- Adipose tissue redistribution with central obesity, moon facies, and fat accumulation on the posterior neck and back ("buffalo hump")
- Atrophy of type 2 fast-twitch myofibers with decreased muscle mass and proximal muscle weakness
- Hyperglycemia, glucosuria, and polydipsia *(secondary diabetes)* due to cortisol-induced gluconeogenesis and inhibition of glucose uptake
- Poor wound healing and abdominal striae due to catabolic effects on collagen
- Bone resorption and osteoporosis with increased risk of fractures
- Increased risk of infection due to immunosuppression
- Hirsutism and menstrual abnormalities
- Mental disturbances including depression and frank psychosis

Primary Hyperaldosteronism (p. 1125)

Primary hyperaldosteronism is characterized by autonomous aldosterone secretion; this leads to sodium retention and potassium excretion, with resultant hypertension and hypokalemia. The renin-angiotensin system is suppressed, and thus plasma renin activity is low. Causes include the following:

- *Primary idiopathic hyperaldosteronism* accounts for 60% of cases; etiology is unknown.
- *Adrenocortical neoplasm* (35% of cases); these are usually solitary aldosterone-secreting adenomas *(Conn syndrome)*, typically arising in middle age with a female to male ratio = 2:1. Adrenocortical carcinoma is a rarer cause, except in children.
- *Glucocorticoid-remediable hyperaldosteronism* is a rare heritable form caused by fusion between *CYP11B1* (the 11β-hydroxylase gene) and *CYP11B2* (the aldosterone synthase gene); aldosterone secretion is regulated by ACTH and is thus suppressible by exogenous glucocorticoids.

In *secondary hyperaldosteronism,* aldosterone release occurs through activation of the renin-angiotensin system; it is encountered in conditions such as congestive heart failure, decreased renal perfusion, and pregnancy (due to increased angiotensinogen synthesis).

Morphology *(p. 1126).*

- *Gross: Aldosterone-producing adenomas* are usually solitary, small, yellow encapsulated lesions; they occur more commonly on the left side. Adjacent normal cortex is not atrophic.
- *Microscopic:* Cells in adenomas are lipid-laden and usually resemble zona fasciculata cells; they frequently exhibit periodic acid-Schiff

stain (PAS)-reactive, eosinophilic, laminated cytoplasmic inclusions *(spironolactone bodies).*

- *Primary idiopathic hyperplasia* is characterized by hyperplasia of cells resembling normal zona glomerulosa.

Clinical Course *(p. 1126). Hypertension is the major feature;* sodium retention increases the total body sodium and expands the extracellular fluid volume. Aldosterone also contributes to endothelial dysfunction leading to reduced nitric oxide synthesis and increased oxidative stress. Hypokalemia, when present, results from renal potassium wasting and can cause a variety of neuromuscular manifestations, including weakness, paresthesias, visual disturbances, and occasionally tetany. Therapy involves resection of adenomas, aldosterone antagonists (e.g., spironolactone) for primary idiopathic aldosteronism, and correction of the underlying cause in cases of secondary hyperaldosteronism.

Adrenogenital Syndromes (p. 1127)

Disorders of sexual differentiation (e.g., female virilization or male precocious puberty) can be caused by primary gonadal or adrenal disorders. Unlike gonadal androgens, ACTH regulates adrenal androgen formation; thus oversecretion can be primary or a component of Cushing disease (Fig. 24-6).

- *Androgen-secreting adrenal cortical neoplasms* are more likely to be carcinomas than adenomas.
- *Congenital adrenal hyperplasia (CAH)* is a group of autosomal recessive metabolic disorders affecting enzymes involved in adrenal steroid synthesis; cortisol production is mainly affected, although certain defects are also associated with salt wasting due to impaired aldosterone synthesis. Steroidogenesis is then channeled into other pathways (Fig. 24-6), leading to increased production of androgens; in all cases, adrenals exhibit bilateral cortical hyperplasia.

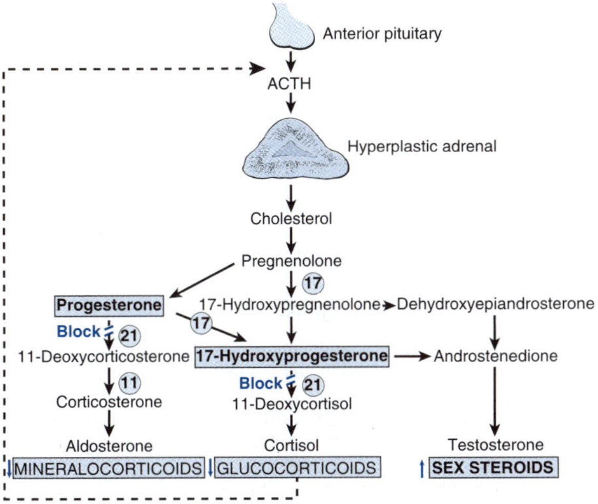

Figure 24-6 Consequences of 21-hydroxylase deficiency. Absence of the enzyme impairs both cortisol and aldosterone synthesis. Subsequent loss of feedback inhibition *(dashed line)* leads to increased ACTH production with cortical hyperplasia and steroidogenesis being funneled into testosterone synthesis. The sites of action of 11-, 17-, and 21-hydroxylase are shown by the circled numbers.

21-Hydroxylase Deficiency (p. 1128)

21-Hydroxylase deficiency is caused by mutations in CYP21A and results in defective conversion of progesterone to 11-deoxycorticosterone; it accounts for >90% of CAH and depending on the nature of the mutation can manifest as three different syndromes:

- *Salt-wasting syndrome* is associated with a complete deficiency of 21-hydroxylase activity and thus absent aldosterone or cortisol production. It is recognized shortly after birth, by salt wasting, hyponatremia, and hyperkalemia—leading to acidosis, hypotension, and cardiovascular collapse; females exhibit virilization.
- *Simple virilizing adrenogenital syndrome without salt wasting* is associated with incomplete loss of hydroxylase activity (approximately a third of patients). Patients have sufficient aldosterone to avoid a salt-wasting crisis, but reduced cortisol production still drives ACTH secretion and ultimately increased testosterone synthesis.
- *Nonclassic (late onset) adrenal virilism* is more common than the other syndromes; partial 21-hydroxylase deficiency in this case results in either no symptoms or only subtle features of androgenic excess later in life (e.g., hirsutism, acne, or menstrual irregularities).

Clinical Course *(p. 1128).* Clinical consequences are determined by the specific enzyme deficiency; effects are related to either androgen excess and/or aldosterone and glucocorticoid deficiency. CAH should be suspected in any neonate with ambiguous genitalia; severe enzyme deficiency in infancy can be life threatening. CAH patients are treated with exogenous glucocorticoids and/or mineralocorticoid supplementation for salt-wasting variants.

Adrenocortical Insufficiency *(p. 1129)*

Insufficiency can occur through either acute or chronic primary loss of adrenal function or secondary to diminished ACTH production.

Primary Acute Adrenocortical Insufficiency (p. 1129)

Primary acute adrenocortical insufficiency can occur due to the following:

- A sudden increase in glucocorticoid requirements in patients with chronic insufficiency *(adrenal crisis)*
- Rapid withdrawal of steroids—or failure to increase steroid doses in periods of stress—in patients with adrenal suppression secondary to long-term glucocorticoid therapy
- Massive adrenal hemorrhage (e.g., neonatal adrenal hemorrhage, postsurgical disseminated intravascular coagulation, Waterhouse-Friderichsen syndrome)

Waterhouse-Friderichsen Syndrome (p. 1129)

Waterhouse-Friderichsen syndrome is an uncommon but catastrophic event, characterized by the following:

- Overwhelming septicemic infection, classically due to meningococcus (although other virulent bacterial infections can also be responsible).
- Rapidly progressive hypotension and shock.
- Disseminated intravascular coagulation with purpura.
- Massive adrenal hemorrhage with adrenal insufficiency; the clinical course can be devastatingly abrupt unless recognition is prompt and appropriate antibiotic therapy is provided.

Primary Chronic Adrenocortical Insufficiency (Addison Disease) (p. 1130)

Primary chronic adrenocortical insufficiency is an uncommon condition associated with destruction of at least 90% of the adrenal cortex. Causes include the following:

- *Autoimmune adrenalitis* (60% to 70% of cases)
  - *APS1* is caused by mutations in the *AIRE* gene. *AIRE* codes for a thymic transcription factor that drives the expression of many peripheral tissue antigens; thymic expression of these antigens allows self-reactive T cells to undergo clonal deletion. In the absence of normal AIRE function, central tolerance is compromised and autoimmunity develops. APS1 patients develop autoantibodies against IL-17 and IL-22, principal effector cytokines in the defense against fungal infections. APS1 is characterized by chronic mucocutaneous candidiasis and abnormalities of skin, dental enamel, and nails (ectodermal dystrophy), occurring in association with a combination of organ-specific autoimmune disorders (autoimmune adrenalitis, autoimmune hypoparathyroidism, idiopathic hypogonadism, pernicious anemia).
  - *Autoimmune polyendocrinopathy syndrome type 2 (APS2)* usually presents in early adulthood as a combination of adrenal insufficiency and autoimmune thyroiditis or type 1 diabetes; mucocutaneous candidiasis, and ectodermal dysplasia do not occur.
- *Infectious processes,* particularly tuberculosis and those caused by fungi, such as *Histoplasma capsulatum* and *Coccidioides immitis.* Patients with AIDS are at risk for developing adrenal insufficiency from complications of their disease (cytomegalovirus, *Mycobacterium avium-intracellulare,* Kaposi sarcoma).
- *Metastatic neoplasms;* most common are lung and breast carcinomas.
- Rare genetic disorders, including *adrenal hypoplasia congenita* (an X-linked disorder caused by mutations in a transcription factor involved in adrenal development) and *adrenoleukodystrophy* (see Chapter 28).

***Clinical Course** (p. 1131).* Features of Addison disease include insidious onset of weakness, fatigue, and anorexia; patients also develop hyperkalemia, hyponatremia, and hypotension due to mineralocorticoid insufficiency. Cutaneous hyperpigmentation can result from elevation of POMC (due to loss of cortisol feedback on the pituitary), which is the precursor peptide to both ACTH and MSH. Acute stresses (e.g., trauma or infection) can precipitate acute adrenal crisis, with rapid progression to death unless corticosteroid therapy is promptly initiated.

Secondary Adrenocortical Insufficiency (p. 1131)

Secondary adrenocortical insufficiency occurs with any hypothalamic or pituitary disorder leading to diminished ACTH production (e.g., tumor, infection, infarction); it can be an isolated deficiency or associated with decreased levels of other pituitary hormones *(panhypopituitarism).* It is distinguished from primary hypoadrenalism by the following:

- Absence of hyperpigmentation.
- Near-normal aldosterone levels because production is largely independent of ACTH; thus hyponatremia and hyperkalemia are not features of secondary adrenocortical insufficiency.

Adrenocortical Neoplasms (p. 1132)

Most adrenal cortical neoplasms are sporadic, although *Li-Fraumeni syndrome* (associated with germline *p53* mutations) and *Beckwith-Wiedemann syndrome* (an imprinting disorder) are associated with a predilection for adrenal cortical carcinomas. Adrenal cortical carcinomas are highly malignant neoplasms (mean survival is 2 years) and are usually large infiltrative lesions at the time of primary diagnosis; they tend to invade the adrenal vein, inferior vena cava, and lymphatics. Functional adenomas are commonly associated with hyperaldosteronism and Cushing syndrome; functional carcinomas tend to be virilizing. Functioning and nonfunctioning tumors cannot be distinguished morphologically; differentiation requires laboratory measurement of hormones or relevant metabolites.

Morphology (p. 1132)

- Adenomas
  - *Gross:* Tumors are typically well-circumscribed, yellow-brown lesions up to 2.5 cm. In nonfunctioning adenomas, the adjacent cortex is normal thickness; in functioning neoplasms, the adjacent cortex is typically atrophic.
  - *Microscopic:* Lesions resemble the normal cortical cells, although nuclear atypia is not uncommon.
- Adrenal cortical carcinomas
  - *Gross:* Tumors are typically variegated with areas of hemorrhage, cystic change, and necrosis.
  - *Microscopic:* Cells range from well differentiated to markedly anaplastic.

Other Adrenal Lesions (p. 1133)

The prevalence of "adrenal incidentalomas" discovered by CT scans is approximately 4%, with an age-dependent increase in prevalence; the vast majority are nonsecreting cortical adenomas. Other lesions include adrenal cysts and *adrenal myelolipomas;* the latter is a benign lesion composed of mature fat and hematopoietic elements.

Adrenal Medulla (p. 1133)

Most adrenal medullary disorders are neoplasms; neuroblastomas and other neuroblastic tumors are discussed in Chapter 10.

Pheochromocytoma (p. 1134)

Pheochromocytomas are relatively uncommon tumors of chromaffin cells. The tumors produce catecholamines and typically present with hypertension; they are therefore significant as surgically correctable causes of high blood pressure. They are memorable for obeying a "rule of 10s":

- 10% are extra-adrenal (e.g., organ of Zuckerkandl or carotid body), where they are designated *paragangliomas.*
- 10% of sporadic adrenal pheochromocytomas are bilateral (50% in cases associated with familial syndromes).
- 10% are biologically malignant (i.e., associated with metastasis); malignancy occurs in 20% to 40% in familial syndromes or in extra-adrenal pheochromocytomas.
- 10% are *not* associated with hypertension.
- As many as 25% (not 10% unfortunately) of phenochromocytomas arise in familial syndromes associated with germline mutations in at least one of six different genes, including MEN-2A and -2B syndromes (*RET* mutations, described later), type I

neurofibromatosis (*NF1* mutations; see Chapter 7), von Hippel-Lindau (VHL) syndrome (*VHL* mutations; see Chapter 7), and familial paraganglioma syndromes (mutations in the subunits of the succinate dehydrogenase complex).

Morphology (p. 1134)

- *Gross:* Tumors range from 1 g to 4 kg. Tumors are highly vascular; the cut surface is usually yellow-tan and associated with hemorrhage, necrosis, or cystic change. Incubation of fresh tissue with potassium dichromate turns the tumor dark black due to catecholamine oxidation (hence the term *chromaffin*).
- *Microscopic:* Tumors are composed of clusters ("zellballen") of polygonal to spindle-shaped chief cells (exhibiting neuroendocrine markers) admixed with sustentacular cells (expressing S-100), all delimited by a rich vascular network. Cellular and nuclear pleomorphism is common. Metastasis is the sole criterion of malignancy.

Clinical Consequences (p. 1135)

The dominant clinical consequence in patients with pheochromocytoma is hypertension; this is typically paroxysmal (due to sudden catechol release) with abrupt blood pressure elevations, tachycardia, palpitations, headache, sweating, tremor, and a sense of foreboding. The acute hypertension can precipitate congestive heart failure, myocardial infarcts, cardiac arrhythmia, and/or cerebral hemorrhage. Cardiac complications are also attributed to ischemic myocardial damage secondary to catecholamine-induced vasoconstriction. Laboratory diagnosis is based on increased urinary catecholamines and their metabolites (e.g., vanillylmandelic acid). Surgical excision requires on-board adrenergic blockade to prevent hypertensive crisis; therapy for metastatic disease requires long-term blood pressure control.

Multiple Endocrine Neoplasia Syndromes (p. 1136)

MEN are a group of heritable diseases resulting in proliferative lesions (hyperplasia, adenomas, and carcinomas) of multiple endocrine organs (Table 24-7). Relative to sporadic tumors, those associated with MEN, are as follows:

- Occur at a younger age than their sporadic counterparts
- Arise in multiple organs, either synchronously (at the same time) or sequentially
- Are often multifocal
- Are usually preceded by asymptomatic endocrine hyperplasia
- Are usually preceded by an asymptomatic stage of endocrine hyperplasia involving the cell of origin (e.g., C-cell hyperplasia adjacent to medullary thyroid cancers)
- Are usually more aggressive and recur in a higher proportion of cases

Multiple Endocrine Neoplasia, Type 1 (*p. 1136*)

MEN-1 (Wermer syndrome) is classically characterized by 3 "Ps":

- *Parathyroid: Primary hyperparathyroidism*—due to hyperplasia or adenomas—occurs in 80% to 95% of cases and is often the initial manifestation.
- *Pancreas:* Endocrine tumors are typically aggressive (presenting with metastases) and are often functional. Pancreatic peptide is the most common hormone produced so that there is not necessarily an accompanying hypersecretory syndrome; insulinomas and gastrinomas are next in frequency.
- *Pituitary:* Anterior adenomas are most commonly prolactinomas.

TABLE 24-7 Multiple Endocrine Neoplasia Syndromes

	MEN-1	MEN-2A	MEN-2B
Pituitary	Adenomas		
Parathyroid	Hyperplasia +++ Adenomas +	Hyperplasia +	
Pancreatic islets	Hyperplasia ++ Adenomas ++ Carcinomas +++		
Adrenal	Cortical hyperplasia	Pheochromocytoma ++	Pheochromocytoma +++
Thyroid		C-cell hyperplasia +++ Medullary carcinoma +++	C-cell hyperplasia +++ Medullary carcinoma +++
Extraendocrine changes			Mucocutaneous ganglioneuromas Marfanoid habitus
Mutant gene locus	*MEN1*	*RET*	*RET*

Relative frequency: +, Uncommon; +++, common.

Notably the duodenum (*not* a "P") is the most common source of gastrinomas in MEN-1; these patients can also develop carcinoid tumors, thyroid and adrenocortical adenomas, and lipomas.

MEN-1 is caused by germline mutations in the *MEN1* tumor suppressor gene, encoding the protein *menin*—a component of several different transcription factor complexes. Peptide hormone overproduction dominates the clinical picture, with malignant behavior by one of the tumors often being the cause of death.

Multiple Endocrine Neoplasia, Type 2 *(p. 1137)*

MEN-2 is divided into three distinct syndromes:

- *MEN-2A (Sipple syndrome)* is characterized by thyroid medullary carcinoma (almost 100%), pheochromocytoma (40% to 50%), and parathyroid hyperplasia with hypercalcemia (10% to 20%). It is caused by germline gain-of-function *RET* proto-oncogene mutations (see Chapter 7).
- *MEN-2B* is characterized by thyroid medullary carcinoma and pheochromocytomas but does not develop hyperparathyroidism; instead patients develop neuromas or ganglioneuromas of multiple sites and exhibit a marfanoid habitus, with long axial skeletal features and hyperextensible joints. The syndrome is caused by a unique single amino acid substitution in RET leading to constitutive activation of its tyrosine kinase activity.
- *Familial medullary thyroid cancer* is a variant of MEN-2A, with a strong predisposition to thyroid malignancy but without the other clinical manifestations.

Although MEN-1 genetic screening has questionable long-term value, screening of at-risk family members in the MEN-2 syndromes can be lifesaving because early thyroidectomy can potentially mitigate the fatal complications of medullary thyroid carcinoma.

Pineal Gland (p. 1137)

The principal pineal secretory product is melatonin, involved in control of circadian rhythms, including sleep-wake cycles.

Pineal tumors are exceptionally rare; most (50% to 70%) arise from sequestered embryonic germ cells and commonly take the form of *germinomas* resembling testicular seminomas.

Pinealomas (p. 1137)

Pinealomas are true tumors of pineocytes (as opposed to germ cell tumors). They are classified based on their degree of differentiation (pineoblastomas versus pineocytomas); less differentiated tumors (pineoblastomas) are typically more aggressive.

25 The Skin

The Skin: More Than a Mechanical Barrier (p. 1141)

- *Squamous epithelial cells (keratinocytes)* constitute the majority of epidermal cells, are tightly adherent to each other through desmosomes, and synthesize the keratin mechanical barrier; they also produce cytokines that regulate the cutaneous environment, as well as antimicrobial *defensins.*
- *Melanocytes* produce *melanin* pigment to absorb ultraviolet (UV) radiation in sunlight.
- *Dendritic cells* (*Langerhans cells* in the epidermis) and *dendrocytes* process and present antigen to activate the immune system.
- *T lymphocytes* (helper, cytotoxic, and regulatory) specifically home to the skin through the expression of cutaneous lymphocyte-associated antigen (CLA) and CCR4 and CCR10 chemokine receptors; small numbers of B lymphocytes are also present.
- The *cutaneous microbiome* of symbiotic-commensal organisms prevents colonization and "educates" the cutaneous immune system to enhance responses to potential pathogens.
- *Neural end organs*
    - *Afferent nerve fibers* detect pain, temperature, vibration, and touch.
    - *Autonomic efferent fibers* regulate adnexal sweat glands and piloerector muscles and can also influence cutaneous immune responses.
    - *Merkel cells* may have neuroendocrine and/or mechanoreceptor functions.
- *Sweat glands* permit cooling.
- *Hair follicles* elaborate hair shafts and are repositories for epithelial stem cells.
- *Gross and microscopic nomenclature* for skin lesions (Table 25-1).

Disorders of Pigmentation and Melanocytes (p. 1143)

Freckles (Ephelis) (p. 1143)

Freckles are common childhood pigmented lesions, 1- to 10-mm tan-red to brown macules, fading and recurring depending on the amount of sun exposure. Melanocyte density is normal; the hyperpigmentation of the lesions reflects focal melanin overproduction, and/or enhanced pigment donation to basal keratinocytes. *Café au lait* spots in neurofibromatosis (see Chapter 27) are histologically similar but are larger, arise independent of sun exposure, and contain aggregated melanosomes (macromelanosomes).

TABLE 25-1 Nomenclature of Skin Lesions

	Definition
Macroscopic Lesions	
Excoriation	Traumatic lesion breaking the epidermis and causing a raw linear area (i.e., deep scratch); often self-induced
Lichenification	Thickened, rough skin (similar to a lichen on a rock); usually the result of repeated rubbing
Macule, Patch	Circumscribed, flat lesion distinguished from surrounding skin by color. Macules are 5 mm in diameter or less; patches are greater than 5 mm
Onycholysis	Separation of nail plate from nail bed
Papule, Nodule	Elevated, dome-shaped or flat-topped lesion. Papules are 5 mm or less across, whereas nodules are greater than 5 mm in size.
Plaque	Elevated, flat-topped lesion, usually greater than 5 mm across (may be caused by coalescent papules)
Pustule	Discrete, pus-filled, raised lesion
Scale	Dry, horny, platelike excrescence; usually the result of imperfect cornification
Vesicle, Bulla, Blister	Fluid-filled, raised lesion 5 mm or less across (vesicle) or greater than 5 mm across (bulla). Blister is the common term for either.
Wheal	Itchy, transient, elevated lesion with variable blanching and erythema formed as the result of dermal edema
Microscopic Lesions	
Acanthosis	Diffuse epidermal hyperplasia
Dyskeratosis	Abnormal, premature keratinization within cells below the stratum granulosum
Erosion	Discontinuity of the skin showing incomplete loss of the epidermis
Exocytosis	Infiltration of the epidermis by inflammatory cells
Hydropic swelling (ballooning)	Intracellular edema of keratinocytes, often seen in viral infections
Hypergranulosis	Hyperplasia of the stratum granulosum, often due to intense rubbing
Hyperkeratosis	Thickening of the stratum corneum, often associated with a qualitative abnormality of the keratin
Lentiginous	A linear pattern of melanocyte proliferation within the epidermal basal cell layer
Papillomatosis	Surface elevation caused by hyperplasia and enlargement of contiguous dermal papillae
Parakeratosis	Keratinization with retained nuclei in the stratum corneum. On mucous membranes, parakeratosis is normal.
Spongiosis	Intercellular edema of the epidermis
Ulceration	Discontinuity of the skin showing complete loss of the epidermis, revealing dermis or subcutis
Vacuolization	Formation of vacuoles within or adjacent to cells; often refers to basal cell-basement membrane zone area

Lentigo (p. 1144)

Lentigo (plural, *lentigines*) is a benign, hyperpigmented macule (5 to 10 mm) common in infancy and childhood; these can involve both skin and mucous membranes. Lentigines do not darken with sun exposure; lesions characteristically exhibit hyperpigmented, non-nested basal melanocyte hyperplasia, often with rete ridge elongation and thinning.

Melanocytic Nevus (Pigmented Nevus, Mole) (p. 1144)

Melanocytic nevi are congenital or acquired *melanocyte neoplasms;* common acquired moles are well-demarcated, uniformly tan-brown papules (≤6 mm), but there are several variants (Table 25-2).

Pathogenesis (p. 1144)

Many nevi have acquired mutations in *BRAF* or *NRAS,* genes involved in RAS signaling (see later). These changes cause a limited period of proliferation, followed—in most cases—by permanent growth arrest due to accumulation of p16/INK4a (an inhibitor of cyclin-dependent kinases).

Morphology (p. 1144)

Moles arise from basal melanocytes—rounded cells exhibiting uniform nuclei and inconspicuous nucleoli (Fig. 25-1); nevi mature through characteristic stages:

- *Junctional nevi*—nests of nevus cells at the dermoepidermal junction—are the earliest lesions.
- *Compound nevi* develop as nests or cords of melanocytes that extend into the underlying dermis.
- In *dermal nevi* the epidermal component is lost.
- As nevus cells enter the dermis they undergo maturation, becoming smaller and nonpigmented, resembling neural tissue *(neurotization).*

  In comparison, melanomas exhibit little to no maturation.

TABLE 25-2 Variant Forms of Nevocellular Nevi

Nevus Variant	Diagnostic Architectural Features	Diagnostic Cytologic Features	Clinical Significance
Congenital nevus	Deep dermal and sometimes subcutaneous growth around adnexa, neurovascular bundles, and blood vessel walls	Identical to ordinary acquired nevi	Present at birth; large variants have increased melanoma risk
Blue nevus	Nonnested dermal infiltration, often with associated fibrosis	Highly dendritic, heavily pigmented nevus cells	Black-blue nodule; often confused with melanoma clinically
Spindle and epithelioid cell nevus (Spitz nevus)	Fascicular growth	Large, plump cells with pink-blue cytoplasm; fusiform cells	Common in children; red-pink nodule; often confused with hemangioma clinically
Halo nevus	Lymphocytic infiltration surrounding nevus cells	Identical to ordinary acquired nevi	Host immune response against nevus cells and surrounding normal melanocytes
Dysplastic nevus	Large, coalescent intraepidermal nests	Cytologic atypia	Potential precursor of malignant melanoma

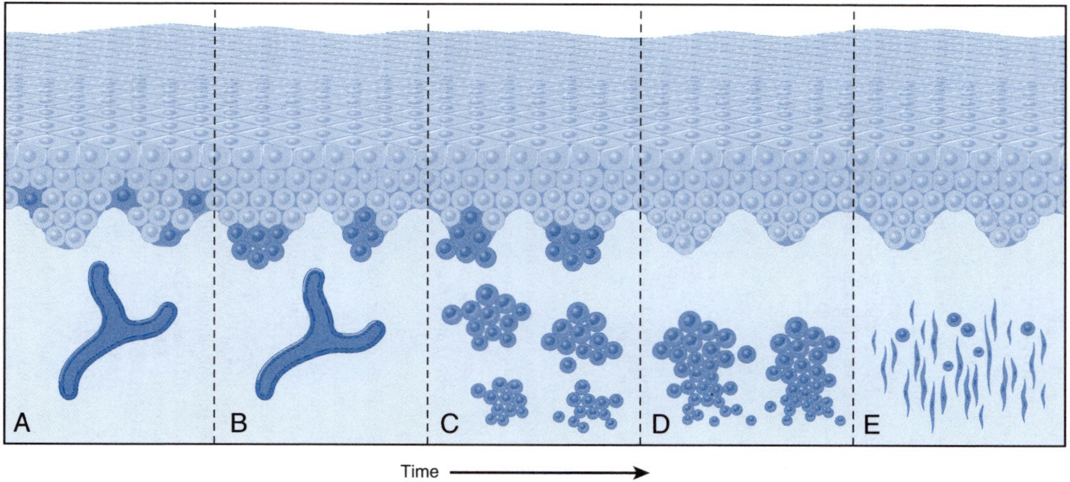

Figure 25-1 Maturation sequence of nondysplastic melanocytic nevi; nevi typically progress through the entire sequence but can "pause" at any stage for variable lengths of time. **A,** Normal skin shows only scattered basal melanocytes. **B,** Junctional nevus. **C,** Compound nevus. **D,** Dermal nevus. **E,** Mature dermal nevus with *neurotization.*

Dysplastic Nevi (p. 1145)

Dysplastic nevi are larger (>5 mm) than most acquired nevi; they are flat macules to slightly raised plaques with variegated pigmentation and irregular borders occurring in both sun-exposed and protected skin. They can number in the hundreds in individuals with the *dysplastic nevus syndrome*—half of such patients develop melanomas by age 60, some of which arise within a dysplastic nevus. However, most dysplastic nevi are clinically stable and sporadic isolated lesions have a low risk of malignant transformation.

Pathogenesis *(p. 1146)*

Dysplastic nevus syndrome is an autosomal dominant disorder often associated with mutations in proteins associated with cell cycling (e.g., *CDKN2A* encoding p16/INK4a or cyclin-dependent kinase CDK4); acquired *NRAS* and *BRAF* mutations are also common. Because not all germline mutations in *CDKN2A* or *CDK4* result in dysplastic nevi and not all dysplastic nevi have mutations in those genes, other modifier genes are implicated, including *TERT* overexpression (encoding the catalytic subunit of telomerase).

Morphology *(p. 1146)*

Histologically most dysplastic nevi are compound nevi exhibiting cytologic and architectural atypia: enlarged and fused nests of nevus cells, lentiginous melanocyte hyperplasia, linear papillary dermal fibrosis, and pigment incontinence (release of melanin from dead melanocytes into the dermis).

Melanoma (p. 1147)

This malignant tumor most commonly arises in skin but can also occur in oral and anogenital mucosal surfaces, esophagus, meninges, and eye. The incidence of cutaneous malignant melanoma is increasing, with approximately 76,000 cases and more than 9700 deaths annually in the United States (as of 2014).

Pathogenesis *(p. 1147)*

Sun exposure and inherited genes are most important.

- Most melanomas arise in sun-exposed areas, with lightly pigmented individuals at greater peril; severe sunburns early in life are the most important risk factor.
- Ten to fifteen percent of melanomas are familial and often occur in the setting of dysplastic nevus syndrome.
- Polymorphisms linked to reduced melanin production modestly increase risk in light-skinned individuals.
- Mutations that increase RAS and PI3K/AKT proliferation pathways are strongly associated with sporadic melanomas; activating *BRAF* mutations (encoding a serine-threonine kinase downstream of RAS) occur in 40% to 50% of melanomas, and activating *NRAS* mutations occur in an additional 15% to 20% of cases (Fig. 25-2).
- Mutations that reduce retinoblastoma (Rb) protein activity or affect genes encoding CDK inhibitors (e.g., p16/INK4a) are strongly associated with both familial and sporadic melanomas and are probably important in the loss of cellular senescence in melanomas.
- Mutations in the promoter for *TERT* (encoding the catalytic subunit of telomerase) occur in 70% of tumors, providing binding sites for Ets family transcription factors (upregulated by BRAF signaling), and acting to prevent replicative senescence in these tumors.

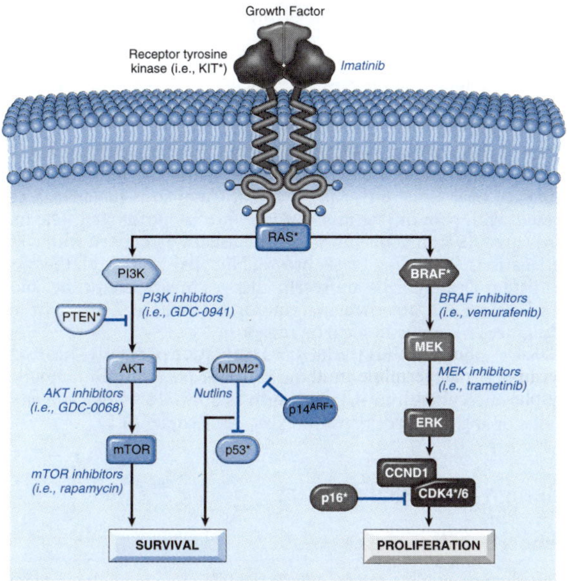

Figure 25-2 Intracellular mechanisms (and therapeutic targets) in the pathway to melanoma. Growth factors activate signaling circuits to drive receptor tyrosine kinases (e.g., KIT), RAS, and two key downstream pathways: the serine-threonine kinase BRAF and the phospholipid kinase PI3K. Proteins indicated by asterisks are mutated in melanoma. Components of these pathways that have been targeted by drugs are indicated.

Morphology *(p. 1149)*

Melanomas are composed of large cells with expanded, irregular nuclei containing peripherally clumped chromatin and prominent eosinophilic nucleoli. Melanomas progress from *radial* to *vertical growth patterns:*

- *Radial growth* describes horizontal spread within the epidermis and superficial dermis; tumor cells typically lack the capacity to metastasize. Lesions include the following:
    - *Lentigo maligna:* An indolent lesion on the face that may not progress for decades.
    - *Superficial spreading:* The most common form of melanoma, usually involving sun-exposed skin.
    - *Acral and mucosal lentiginous* melanoma unrelated to skin exposure.
- *Vertical growth* occurs unpredictably and is characterized by dermal invasion of an expanding clonal mass of cells, lacking cellular maturation. These cells often have the capacity to metastasize, with the probability of distal spread correlating with the depth of invasion; the distance—called the *Breslow thickness*—is measured from the epidermal granular layer to the deepest intradermal tumor cells.

Prognostic Factors *(p. 1150)*

Prognostic factors predict the risk of metastatic spread; these include the following (more favorable determinants are in parentheses):

- Breslow thickness (thinner is better)
- Number of mitoses (<1 per mm^2)
- Evidence of regression (absent)
- Ulceration (absent)

- Presence of tumor-infiltrating lymphocytes (many)
- Gender (female)
- Location (extremity)
- Sentinel node micrometastasis (absent)

Clinical Features *(p. 1150)*

The ABCDE warning signs of melanoma are *A*symmetry, irregular *B*orders, variegated *C*olor, increasing *D*iameter, and *E*volution (change) over time, especially if rapid. Cutaneous melanoma can present with pain or pruritus, but most are asymptomatic. The majority are >10 mm at diagnosis and are usually associated with color variegations (including black, brown, blue, red, and gray); the most consistent clinical signs are recent changes in size, shape, or color. The borders are often irregular and/or notched, with zones of hypopigmentation due to focal regression.

Newer therapies target the RAS and PI3K-AKT pathways (Fig. 25-2). In addition, the recognition that melanoma is inherently immunogenic has spawned interest in therapies such as anti-CTLA4 blocking antibodies or anti-PD1 blocking antibodies (see Chapter 6).

Benign Epithelial Tumors (p. 1151)

Seborrheic Keratoses (p. 1151)

Seborrheic keratoses typically arise in middle-aged and older individuals, most commonly on the trunk; similar, smaller facial lesions in non-whites are called *dermatosis papulosa nigra.* When seborrheic keratoses occur explosively in large numbers, they may represent a paraneoplastic syndrome *(Leser-Trélat sign),* due to tumor elaboration of transforming growth factor (TNF)-α. Activating mutations in fibroblast growth factor receptor-3 (FGFR3) likely drive the growth of many sporadic lesions.

Morphology *(p. 1151)*

- *Gross:* Lesions are uniform, tan-brown, velvety or granular, round plaques millimeters to several centimeters in diameter; keratin-filled plugs may be evident.
- *Microscopic:* Lesions are sharply demarcated and exophytic, with hyperplasia of variably pigmented basaloid cells and *hyperkeratosis;* keratin-filled *horn cysts* are common features. When irritated and inflamed, the basaloid cells undergo squamous differentiation.

Acanthosis Nigricans (p. 1151)

Lesions are thickened, velvety hyperpigmented plaques typically occurring in flexural areas (axilla, groin, neck, anogenital region); they can be a marker of benign or malignant conditions:

- The *benign* type makes up 80% of all cases; it develops gradually, usually arising in childhood through puberty, and can be an autosomal dominant trait with variable penetrance (associated with activating *FGFR3* mutations), associated with obesity or endocrine disorders (especially diabetes), or a component of several rare congenital disorders.
- The *malignant* type arises in middle-aged and older individuals, often in association with an occult adenocarcinoma (possibly due to tumor elaboration of epidermal growth factors).

Morphology *(p. 1152)*

Lesions exhibit hyperkeratosis, with prominent rete ridges and basal hyperpigmentation (without melanocyte hyperplasia).

Fibroepithelial Polyp (p. 1152)

Also called *acrochordon, squamous papilloma,* or *skin tag,* fibroepithelial polyps are found on the neck, trunk, face, or intertriginous zones and are exceptionally common benign lesions in middle-aged and older individuals. These are soft, flesh-colored tumors attached by a slender fibrovascular stalk covered by benign epidermis. The vast majority are sporadic, but they can be associated with pregnancy, diabetes, or intestinal polyposis.

Epithelial Cyst (Wen) (p. 1152)

Epithelial cysts are common lesions presenting as well-circumscribed, firm, subcutaneous nodules; these develop through downgrowth and cystic expansion of epidermal or follicular epithelium. Traumatic rupture can spill keratin into the dermis, leading to often painful granulomatous inflammation.

Adnexal (Appendage) Tumors (p. 1152)

These are typically nondescript, flesh-colored, benign papules or nodules; some have a predilection for specific body surfaces (e.g., *eccrine poromas* on palms and soles). Although most are localized and not aggressive, a subset can be malignant (e.g., *sebaceous carcinoma* arising in eyelid meibomian glands); others have a mendelian pattern of inheritance and occur as multiple disfiguring lesions. Some can serve as markers for visceral malignancies (e.g., multiple trichilemmomas in *Cowden syndrome* [due to germline mutations in the tumor suppressor gene *PTEN*] are associated with increased risk of breast cancer).

- *Cylindromas* usually occur on the scalp and forehead; lesions are composed of islands of basaloid cells with apocrine or eccrine differentiation that may coalesce to form hatlike growths *(turban tumor)*. Lesions can be dominantly inherited associated with inactivating mutations of the *CYLD* tumor suppressor gene.
- *Syringomas* usually occur as multiple, small, tan papules near the lower eyelids, composed of basaloid epithelium with eccrine differentiation.
- *Sebaceous adenomas* exhibit lobular proliferations of sebocytes with frothy, lipid-filled cytoplasm. They can be associated with internal malignancy in the Muir-Torre syndrome (a subset of the hereditary nonpolyposis colorectal cancer [HNPCC] syndrome; see Chapter 17), linked to germline deficits in DNA mismatch repair proteins.
- *Trichoepitheliomas* are proliferations of basaloid cells that form hair follicle-like structures.
- *Pilomatrixomas* are proliferations of basaloid cells that show hairlike differentiation; they are associated with activating mutations of the *CTNNB1* gene encoding β-catenin.
- *Apocrine carcinomas* occur in the axilla and scalp and exhibit ductal differentiation showing prominent apocrine secretion.

Premalignant and Malignant Epidermal Tumors (p. 1154)

The molecular causes of skin cancers in rare hereditary cancer syndromes also contribute to the pathogenesis of more common acquired lesions (Table 25-3).

TABLE 25-3 Survey of Familial Cancer Syndromes With Cutaneous Manifestations

Disease	Inheritance	Chromosomal Location	Gene or Protein	Function and Manifestation
Ataxia-telangiectasia	AR	11q22.3	*ATM*/ATM*	DNA repair after radiation injury; p53 signaling and neurologic and vascular lesions
NBCCS	AD	9q22.3	*PTCH*//PTCH	Developmental gene and multiple BCCs; jaw cysts, etc.
Cowden syndrome	AD	10q23	*PTEN, MMAC1*/PTEN, TEP1, MMAC1	Lipid phosphatase and benign follicular appendage tumors (trichilemmomas); internal adenocarcinoma (often breast)
Familial melanoma syndrome	AD	9p21	*CDKN2*/p16INK4 *CDKN2*/p14ARF	Inhibits CDKs from phosphorylating Rb, thus arresting cell cycle and melanoma Binds MDM2 and thus, preserves p53 and melanoma
Muir-Torre syndrome	AD	2p22	*hMSH2*/hMSH2	Involved in DNA mismatch repair and benign and malignant sebaceous tumors; internal adenocarcinoma
Neurofibromatosis I	AD	17q11.2	*NF1*/neurofibromin	Negatively regulates Ras family of signal molecules and neurofibromas
Neurofibromatosis II	AD	22q12.2	*NF2*/merlin	Integrates cytoskeletal signaling and neurofibromas and acoustic neuromas
Tuberous sclerosis	AD	9q34 16p13.3	*TSC1*/hamartin *TSC2*/tuberin	Interacts with tuberin; function unknown Interacts with hamartin; may regulate Ras proteins and angiofibromas, mental retardation
Xeroderma pigmentosum	AR	9q22 and others	*XPA*/XPA and others	Nucleotide excision repair and melanoma and nonmelanoma skin cancers

*By convention, genes are italicized and proteins are not italicized.
AD, Autosomal dominant; *AR*, autosomal recessive; *CDK*, cyclin-dependent kinase.

Actinic Keratosis (p. 1154)

This is a premalignant dysplastic lesion associated with chronic sun exposure, especially in light-skinned individuals; ionizing radiation, hydrocarbons, and arsenicals can induce similar lesions. Because many undergo malignant transformation, local eradication is indicated. Imiquimod can be used to eradicate the abnormal cells through activation of innate immunity via Toll-like receptor stimulation.

Morphology (p. 1154)

- *Gross:* Lesions are usually <1 cm, tan-brown, red, or flesh-colored, with a rough consistency; exuberant keratin production can form "cutaneous horns."
- *Microscopic:* Lesions exhibit cytologic atypia in the lower epidermis, frequently with basal cell hyperplasia and dyskeratosis; intercellular bridges are present. *Hyperkeratosis* and *parakeratosis* are common, although epidermal atrophy can occur. The dermis exhibits thickened, blue-gray elastic fibers *(elastosis),* due to aberrant synthesis by sun-damaged fibroblasts.

Squamous Cell Carcinoma (p. 1155)

Squamous cell carcinoma is the second most common tumor of sun-exposed skin of older individuals (basal cell carcinoma [BCC] holds the dubious distinction of being first); it occurs more frequently in men than in women, with the exception of lower leg lesions, and <5% of lesions metastasize to regional nodes.

Pathogenesis (p. 1155)

UV radiation is the greatest predisposing factor, primarily by inducing DNA damage, but also by dampening the immune functioning of Langerhans cells; immunosuppression (e.g., by chemotherapy) also reduces host surveillance and increases keratinocyte susceptibility to infection and transformation by oncogenic viruses (especially human papillomavirus [HPV] subtypes 5 and 8). Other risks include industrial carcinogens (tars), chronic skin ulcers, old burn scars, draining osteomyelitis, ionizing radiation, and (for oral mucosa) tobacco or betel nut chewing. Acquired or germline (e.g., xeroderma pigmentosum) *p53* mutations may allow cell-cycle progression despite low-fidelity DNA repair of UV-induced damage; this leads to rapid accumulation of mutations and eventual carcinogenesis. Driver mutations that increase RAS signaling or that decrease Notch signaling also contribute to the transformation process.

Morphology (p. 1155)

- *Gross:* In situ squamous cell carcinomas are well-demarcated, red, scaling plaques; invasive lesions are nodular, variably hyperkeratotic, and prone to ulceration.
- *Microscopic: In situ carcinoma* has full-thickness epidermal atypia; invasive tumors vary from well differentiated (with prominent keratinization) to highly anaplastic with necrosis.

Basal Cell Carcinoma (p. 1155)

BCC is the most common invasive human cancer (1 million cases in the United States annually); they are slow growing and rarely metastasize. Immunosuppression and defects in DNA repair (e.g., xeroderma pigmentosum) increase the incidence.

Pathogenesis *(p. 1155)*

Most BCCs have mutations resulting in unfettered Hedgehog signaling. This was discovered through investigation of *nevoid basal cell carcinoma syndrome (NBCCS or Gorlin syndrome)*, a rare autosomal dominant disorder characterized by multiple BCCs usually manifesting before age 20; patients also develop medulloblastomas, ovarian fibromas, odontogenic keratocysts, pits of the palms and soles and can have multiple developmental abnormalities.

The responsible *PTCH* gene on chromosome 9q22.3 is the human homologue for the *Drosophila* developmental gene *patched;* it encodes the receptor for the *sonic hedgehog (SHH)* gene product. In the absence of SHH, PTCH binds to another transmembrane protein (SMO) and blocks its activation of downstream signals. When SHH and PTCH interact, SMO is released and can trigger a signal cascade that involves the GLI1 transcription factor. Absence of *PTCH* (as in NBCCS) or acquired *PTCH* or *SMO* mutations (sporadic tumors) lead to constitutive SMO activation and the development of BCC; 30% of sporadic BCCs have *PTCH* mutations (Fig. 25-3). Additional *p53* mutations are present in 40% to 60% of BCCs.

Morphology *(p. 1157)*

- *Gross:* Tumors typically present as pearly papules, often with prominent telangiectatic vessels; some are melanin pigmented. Advanced lesions ulcerate and can show extensive local invasion, hence the term *rodent ulcer.*
- *Microscopic:* Lesions exhibit monotonous basal cell proliferation, either as *multifocal superficial growths* over a large area (several centimeters) of skin or as *nodules* extending deeply into the dermis.

Tumors of the Dermis (p. 1158)

Benign Fibrous Histiocytoma (Dermatofibroma) (p. 1158)

Benign fibrous histiocytomas are a heterogeneous group of indolent neoplasms of dermal fibroblasts and histiocytes usually occurring in adults; they frequently occur on the legs of young women. Antecedent trauma and aberrant healing are often causally implicated.

Morphology *(p. 1158)*

- *Gross:* Lesions are firm, tan-brown, occasionally tender papules occasionally as large as several centimeters; lateral compression causes inward dimpling.
- *Microscopic: Dermatofibromas* are most common; these exhibit spindle-shaped fibroblasts in a well-defined, middermal, nonencapsulated mass, occasionally extending into subcutaneous fat. Many cases have overlying epidermal hyperplasia.

Dermatofibrosarcoma Protuberans (p. 1158)

This well-differentiated, slow-growing fibrosarcoma is locally aggressive but rarely metastasizes.

Pathogenesis *(p. 1158)*

The molecular hallmark is a balanced translocation between the collagen 1A1 and platelet-derived growth factor-β genes; this juxtaposes the *COL1A1* promoter and the coding region of *PDGFβ* leading to PDGFβ overexpression and tumor cell proliferation. Treatment involves inhibition of the PDGF receptor tyrosine kinase.

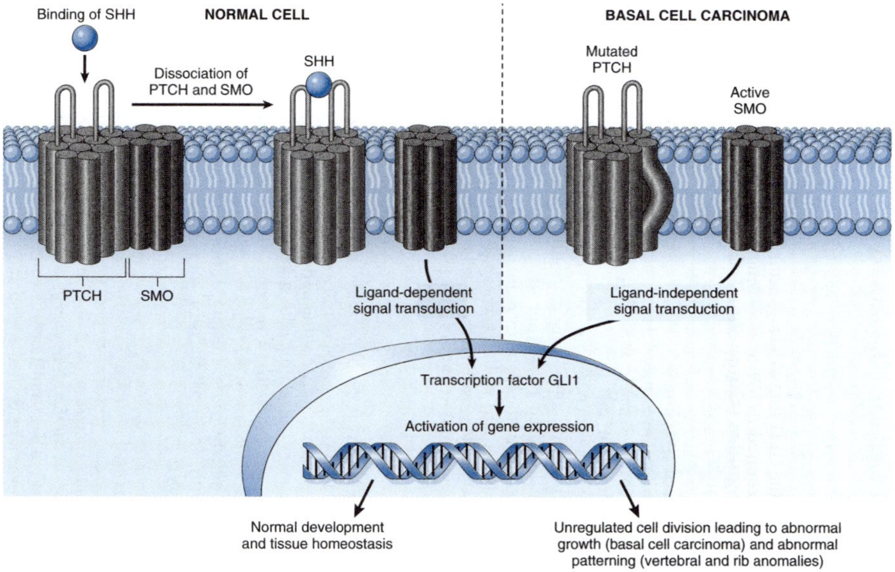

Figure 25-3 Normal and oncogenic hedgehog signaling. *Left,* Normally PTCH and SMO form a receptor complex that can bind SHH. In the absence of SHH, PTCH blocks SMO activity. When SHH binds PTCH, SMO is released to trigger a signal transduction cascade that leads to activation of GLI1 and other transcription factors. *Right,* Mutations in *PTCH,* and less often in *SMO,* allow SMO to signal without SHH binding and produce constitutive activation of GLI1. GLI signaling is a characteristic feature of sporadic BCCs and tumors associated with the NBCCS.

Morphology *(p. 1159)*

- *Gross:* Tumors are firm nodules arising as protuberant, occasionally ulcerated aggregates within an indurated plaque, typically on the trunk.
- *Microscopic:* Lesions are cellular and composed of radially oriented fibroblasts; mitoses are rare. The overlying epidermis is thinned, and there often is microscopic extension into subcutaneous fat.

Tumors of Cellular Migrants to the Skin (p. 1159)

These are proliferative disorders of cells that arise elsewhere but home to skin (e.g., Langerhans cells, T lymphocytes, and mast cells).

Mycosis Fungoides (Cutaneous T-Cell Lymphoma) (p. 1159)

Cutaneous T-cell lymphoma (CTCL) represents a spectrum of T-cell lymphoproliferative disorders of the skin; *mycosis fungoides* is a chronic process, whereas *mycosis fungoides d'emblée* is a more aggressive nodular variant.

Mycosis fungoides is a cutaneous T-cell lymphoma that can evolve into a generalized lymphoma; most cases afflict individuals over age 40 and remain localized to skin for many years. *Sézary syndrome* occurs with seeding of the blood by malignant T cells, accompanied by diffuse erythema and scaling *(erythroderma).* The proliferating cells in CTCL are CD4+, with clonal T-cell receptor gene rearrangements; CLA expression is responsible for the cutaneous homing behavior.

Morphology *(p. 1160)*

- *Gross:* Early lesions resemble eczema and typically arise on the trunk; these progress to scaly, red-brown patches, scaling plaques (similar to psoriasis), or fungating nodules (up to 10 cm) on various body surfaces, correlating with systemic spread.
- *Microscopic:* The *hallmark* of mycosis fungoides is the *Sézary-Lutzner cell,* a malignant CD4+ (T-helper) cell with a hyperconvoluted or *cerebriform* nucleus; these form bandlike dermal infiltrates with single cell invasion into the epidermis *(Pautrier microabscesses).*

Mastocytosis (p. 1160)

Mastocytosis is a spectrum of rare disorders characterized by increased numbers of cutaneous mast cells. Symptoms reflect the consequences of mast cell degranulation; histamine release causes pruritus, flushing, rhinorrhea, or dermal edema and erythema. *Wheal* formation when lesional skin is rubbed is termed the *Darier sign; dermatographism* indicates wheal formation evoked by rubbing normal skin. Rarely mast cell heparin release can cause epistaxis or gastrointestinal bleeding; bone pain can occur secondary to osteoclastic and osteoblastic involvement.

Urticaria pigmentosa (50% of all cases) is an exclusively cutaneous form of mastocytosis occurring mainly in children, with a generally favorable prognosis. Systemic mastocytosis occurs in 10% of patients, usually adults, and carries a much poorer prognosis. Many cases of mastocytosis are caused by acquired point mutations of the c-KIT receptor tyrosine kinase, leading to mast cell proliferation and survival.

Morphology (p. 1161)

- *Gross:* Skin lesions are multiple, round-oval, nonscaling, red-brown papules and plaques.
- *Microscopic:* Lesions exhibit variable dermal fibrosis, edema, eosinophils, and numerous mast cells.

Disorders of Epidermal Maturation (p. 1161)

Ichthyosis (p. 1161)

Ichthyosis is a spectrum of disorders of epidermal maturation leading to chronic excessive keratin accumulation *(hyperkeratosis)* resembling fish scales (hence the name). There are X-linked, autosomal recessive, and autosomal dominant forms; acquired variants (e.g., *ichthyosis vulgaris*) can be associated with various malignancies. The primary defect in most forms is increased cell-cell adhesion resulting in abnormal (insufficient) desquamation. For example, X-linked disease is caused by steroid sulfatase deficiency, leading to increased amounts of proadhesive cholesterol sulfate in intercellular spaces, and persistent cell-cell adhesion in the stratum corneum.

Morphology (p. 1162)

Microscopically lesions exhibit compacted stratum corneum, with minimal inflammation; the thickness of the epidermis or stratum granulosum is used to subclassify the disorders.

Acute Inflammatory Dermatoses (p. 1162)

This is an enormous family of conditions, characterized by short-lived (days to weeks) mononuclear inflammatory infiltrates associated with edema and variable tissue damage.

Urticaria (p. 1162)

Urticaria ("hives") is characterized by focal mast cell degranulation, with histamine-mediated dermal edema and pruritus (*wheal* formation). Individual lesions develop and regress within hours, but sequential lesions can occur for months. *Angioedema* is distinguished by the presence of both *dermal* and *subcutaneous fat* edema.

Pathogenesis (p. 1162)

Most lesions are driven by antigen-specific cross-linking of immunoglobulin (Ig)E bound to mast cells (see Chapter 6). *IgE-independent urticaria* can occur through chemical-induced mast cell degranulation (e.g., opiates, certain antibiotics, curare, or radiocontrast materials) or by suppression of prostaglandin synthesis (i.e., with aspirin). Persistent urticaria may reflect an inability to clear the inciting antigen or can reflect cryptic collagen vascular disorders or Hodgkin lymphoma. *Hereditary angioneurotic edema* is caused by deficient C1 esterase inhibitor and subsequent unregulated activation of the early complement components.

Morphology (p. 1162)

- *Gross:* Lesions vary from small, pruritic papules to large edematous plaques. Areas exposed to pressure (e.g., trunk, distal extremities, and ears) are more prone to urticaria.
- *Microscopic:* Sparse mononuclear perivascular infiltrates are associated with edema and occasional dermal eosinophils.

Acute Eczematous Dermatitis (p. 1163)

These are a family of disorders of differing etiology—but common immune-driven morphology. Eczematous dermatitis is subdivided based on the initiating factors:

- Allergic contact dermatitis (e.g., poison ivy)
- Atopic dermatitis
- Drug-related eczematous dermatitis
- Photoeczematous dermatitis
- Primary irritant dermatitis

Pathogenesis *(p. 1163)*

Many forms of *eczema* constitute a cutaneous delayed-type hypersensitivity response driven by Langerhans cell presentation of antigens acquired at the epidermal surface. The subsequent pathogenesis is attributed to cytokine release by recruited memory cells and nonspecific accumulation of additional inflammatory cells. UV exposures and neuropeptides released near the epidermis can affect Langerhans cell function.

Morphology *(p. 1163)*

- *Gross:* Lesions range from pruritic, red, and papulovesicular to blistered, oozing, and crusted. With chronic exposure, these can evolve into psoriasis-like scaling plaques. Bacterial superinfection produces a yellow crust *(impetiginization).*
- *Microscopic:* Early *spongiosis* progresses to frank fluid accumulation, splaying keratinocytes apart and forming intraepidermal vesicles. Dermal perivascular lymphocytic infiltrates are associated with mast cell degranulation and papillary dermal edema. Drug hypersensitivity lesions may have eosinophils. In chronic lesions the vesicular phase is replaced with progressive *acanthosis* and *hyperkeratosis.*

Erythema Multiforme (p. 1164)

Erythema multiforme is an uncommon, self-limited hypersensitivity response; triggers can be certain drugs, infections, malignancy, or collagen vascular disorders. Patients present with an array of "multiform" lesions, including the characteristic targetoid lesion.

- *Stevens-Johnson syndrome* is a severe, febrile form typically occurring in children; there are erosions and hemorrhagic crusting of the lips, oral mucosa, conjunctiva, urethra, and anogenital regions. Bacterial superinfection may be life threatening.
- *Toxic epidermal necrolysis* is another variant, characterized by diffuse mucocutaneous epithelial necrosis and sloughing; it is clinically analogous to extensive third-degree burns.

Pathogenesis *(p. 1164)*

The etiology shares similarities to other immunologic cutaneous disorders (e.g., graft-versus-host disease and skin allograft rejection). Epithelial cells are injured by skin-homing (CLA+) CD8+ cytotoxic T cells (CTLs) responding to as yet uncharacterized antigens; these cells are prominent in the central portion of lesions, whereas CD4+ T cells and Langerhans cells localize to the raised erythematous periphery.

Morphology *(p. 1164)*

- *Gross: Multiform* lesions include macules, papules, vesicles, and bullae; *targets* are red maculopapular lesions with central pallor. Symmetric involvement of the extremities is common.

- *Microscopic:* Early lesions show dermoepidermal and perivascular lymphocytic infiltrates with dermal edema and focal basal keratinocyte degeneration and necrosis. Exocytosis is associated with epidermal necrosis, blistering, and shallow erosions. *Target lesions* show central necrosis with associated perivenular inflammation.

Chronic Inflammatory Dermatoses (p. 1165)

These are persistent inflammatory disorders (months to years) characterized by excessive scaling due to defective desquamation.

Psoriasis (p. 1165)

Psoriasis affects 1% to 2% of the U.S. population and can be associated with other disorders (e.g., arthritis, myopathy, enteropathy, spondylitic joint disease, or acquired immunodeficiency syndrome [AIDS]). It most commonly affects the elbows, knees, scalp, lumbosacral area, intergluteal cleft, and glans penis; occasionally the entire body can be affected *(erythroderma).* Nail changes (30% of cases) consist of yellow-brown discoloration with onycholysis, thickening, and crumbling. Rarely, small pustules form on erythematous plaques *(pustular psoriasis);* when localized to hands and feet, this is benign, but systemic involvement can be life threatening.

Pathogenesis *(p. 1165)*

An association with certain HLA types suggests a genetic component; the genesis of new lesions at sites of trauma *(Koebner phenomenon)* suggests a role for exogenous stimuli. Sensitized CD4+ T_H1 and T_H17 cells and activated CTLs accumulate in the epidermis and may drive keratinocyte proliferation by elaborating cytokines (e.g., interleukin [IL]-12, interferon-γ, and IL-17; TNF in particular is a major pathogenic mediator).

Morphology *(p. 1165)*

- *Gross:* Classic lesions are well-demarcated, salmon-pink plaques with silvery scaling. *Annular, linear, gyrate,* or *serpiginous* variations occur.
- *Microscopic:* Lesions exhibit marked acanthosis with downward rete elongation, and mitoses well above the basal layer. The stratum granulosum is thinned or absent, with extensive overlying parakeratosis. The epidermis adjacent to the acanthotic rete is markedly thinned; dilated vessels in the underlying dermal papillae yield pinpoint bleeds when the overlying scale is removed *(Auspitz sign).* Aggregates of epidermal neutrophils occur within small spongiotic foci in the stratum spinosum *(spongiform pustules)* or within the parakeratotic stratum corneum *(Munro microabscesses).* Larger, abscesslike accumulations may also occur in pustular psoriasis.

Seborrheic Dermatitis (p. 1166)

Seborrhea affects up to 5% of the general population; although it typically involves skin with high densities of sebaceous glands (e.g., scalp, forehead, nasolabial folds, and presternum), it is an inflammatory disease of the epidermis and is *not* a disease of sebaceous glands.

Pathogenesis *(p. 1166)*

Although the precise etiology is unknown, increased sebum production in response to androgens (or due to dopamine deficiency in the case of Parkinson patients) is likely contributory. Nevertheless, sebum overproduction may be necessary but not sufficient to cause the disorder. Thus colonization of the skin by certain fungal species of the genus *Malassezia* is also implicated. A severe form of seborrheic dermatitis is also seen in many human immunodeficiency virus (HIV)-infected individuals with low CD4 counts.

Morphology *(p. 1166)*

- *Gross:* Lesions are macules or papules on a greasy, yellow erythematous base, often with scaling and crusting. Dandruff is the common expression of scalp lesions.
- *Microscopic:* Early lesions resemble spongiotic dermatitis, whereas later lesions are more reminiscent of acanthotic psoriasis. Mounds of perakeratosis admixed with acute inflammatory cells accumulate around hair follicles; there is also a superficial perivascular infiltrate of neutrophils and lymphocytes.

Lichen Planus (p. 1166)

Lichen planus is usually a self-limited disease that resolves after 1 to 2 years, leaving only postinflammatory hyperpigmentation; oral lesions may persist longer and occasionally become malignant.

Pathogenesis *(p. 1166)*

The etiology is unknown, but T-cell infiltrates with Langerhans cell hyperplasia suggest cell-mediated immune injury to altered antigens in basal cells; notably, the Koebner phenomenon also occurs in lichen planus.

Morphology *(p. 1167)*

- *Gross:* Lesions are *pruritic, purple, polygonal planar papules* that may coalesce into *plaques;* lesions are often highlighted by white dots or lines (areas of hypergranulosis) called *Wickham striae.* Lesions are typically multiple and symmetrically distributed, often on the wrists and elbows and on the glans penis; oral mucosal lesions are generally white and netlike. A form with preferential involvement of hair follicle epithelium is called *lichen planopilaris.*
- *Microscopic:* There is a dense, bandlike dermoepidermal junction, lymphocytic infiltrate with basal cell degeneration and necrosis, and jagged rete sawtoothing. Necrotic basal cells may be sloughed into inflamed papillary dermis, forming *colloid* or *Civatte bodies.* Chronic changes include acanthosis, hyperkeratosis, and thickening of the granular cell layer.

Blistering (Bullous) Diseases (p. 1167)

These are *primary* blistering disorders, as opposed to vesicles and bullae that occur as a *secondary* phenomenon in a variety of unrelated conditions. The level within the skin where the blister occurs is important for diagnosis and is understandable based on knowledge of intercellular and cell-matrix attachments (Fig. 25-4).

Inflammatory Blistering Disorders (p. 1167)

Pemphigus *(p. 1167)*

Pemphigus is an uncommon and potentially life-threatening autoimmune disorder typically affecting patients 30 to 60 years old; treatment involves immunosuppression to reduce the titers of the

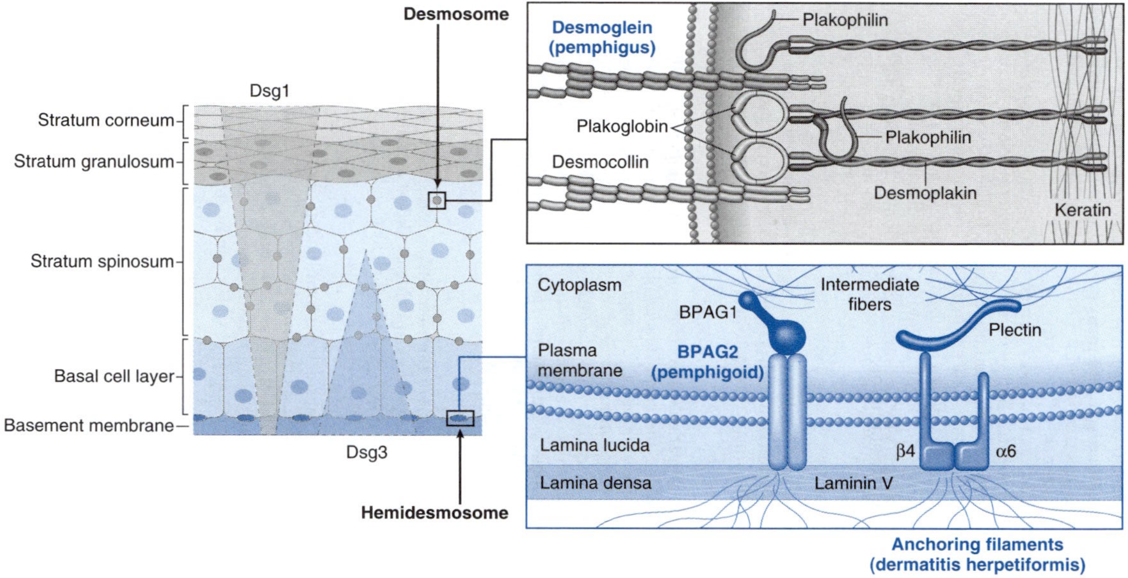

Figure 25-4 Squamous cell adhesion molecules. Desmogleins 1 and 3 (Dsg1 and Dsg3) are desmosome components with different distributions within the epidermis *(left panel)*. Thus in *pemphigus vulgaris*, autoantibodies to Dsg1 *and* Dsg3 lead to blisters just above the basal layer; however, in *pemphigus foliaceus,* the autoantibodies are against only Dsg1, and the blister occurs in the stratum granulosum. In *bullous pemphigoid,* the autoantibodies bind BPAG2 in hemidesmosomes, leading to blisters within the lamina lucida in the basement membrane; in *dermatitis herpetiformis,* IgA autoantibodies against the hemidesmosome-anchoring fibrils also cause sub-basal blisters. The various forms of *epidermolysa bullosa* are caused by genetic defects in the proteins that form desmosomes or hemidesmosomes.

pathogenic autoantibodies. There are multiple variants, depending on the level of the blister and the clinical manifestations:

- *Pemphigus vulgaris* accounts for 80% of cases; it involves oral mucosa, scalp, face, intertriginous zones, trunk, and pressure points. Lesions are superficial, easily ruptured blisters that leave shallow, crusted erosions. If untreated, it is almost uniformly fatal.
- *Pemphigus vegetans* is a rare form presenting with large, moist verrucous plaques studded with pustules, typically in flexural and intertriginous zones.
- *Pemphigus foliaceus* is a more benign form occurring epidemically in South America and sporadically elsewhere. Lesions occur mainly on the face, scalp, and upper trunk. Bullae are extremely superficial, leaving only slight erythema and crusting after rupture.
- *Pemphigus erythematosus* is a localized, milder variant of pemphigus foliaceus, typically involving only a malar distribution.
- *Paraneoplastic pemphigus* occurs in association with various malignancies, most commonly non-Hodgkin lymphoma.

Pathogenesis (p. 1169)

Patients have circulating IgG directed against desmoglein components (Fig. 25-4). Binding of these autoantibodies directly disrupts intercellular adhesion and also activates intercellular proteases.

Morphology (p. 1169)

Microscopically all variants are characterized by *acantholysis* with intercellular clefting and *intraepithelial* blisters, with a variable dermal inflammatory infiltrate. For pemphigus vulgaris and vegetans, the separation occurs immediately above the basal layer *(suprabasal blister),* leaving an intact layer of "tombstone"-like basal cells; in the vegetans variant, there is also overlying epidermal hyperplasia. In the foliaceus variant, only the stratum granulosum is involved. With anti-Ig or anticomplement immunofluorescence, netlike *(reticular)* staining may be seen in the epidermis, outlining each keratinocyte.

Bullous Pemphigoid *(p. 1170)*

Bullous pemphigoid is an autoimmune blistering disease of skin and mucosa typically affecting elderly individuals. Bullae do not rupture as easily as in pemphigus and, if uninfected, heal without scarring.

Pathogenesis (p. 1170)

Bullous pemphigoid is caused by autoantibodies against hemidesmosome proteins (bullous pemphigoid antigen, BPAG) that attach epidermal cells to the basal membrane; only antibodies against BPAG2 cause blistering. Bound autoantibodies cause injury via complement activation and granulocyte recruitment.

Morphology (p. 1170)

- *Gross:* Lesions are 2- to 8-cm tense bullae containing clear fluid; inner thigh, forearm flexor surfaces, lower abdomen, and intertriginous zones are common sites, and oral mucosa is involved in 10% to 15% of patients.
- *Microscopic:* Subepidermal nonacantholytic blister with *linear* dermoepidermal junction staining for Ig and complement. There is a variable, superficial, perivascular dermal inflammatory cell infiltrate, and degranulated eosinophils are typically seen directly beneath the basal epithelial cells.

Dermatitis Herpetiformis (p. 1170)

Dermatitis herpetiformis is an uncommon disorder, characterized by intensely pruritic urticaria and grouped vesicles; typically occurring in young men, it can be associated with celiac disease (see Chapter 17) and responds to a gluten-free diet.

Pathogenesis (p. 1171)

Dermatitis herpetiformis is presumably mediated either by immune complex deposition in the skin or by gliadin (a gluten protein) antibodies cross-reacting with junction-anchoring components (e.g., reticulin).

Morphology (p. 1171)

- *Gross:* Plaques and grouped vesicles are typically bilateral and symmetric, involving the extensor surfaces, upper back, and buttocks.
- *Microscopic:* Neutrophils and fibrin accumulate in the tips of dermal papillae *(microabscesses)* with overlying basal vacuolization coalescing to large subepidermal blisters. Immunofluorescence shows granular IgA deposits at the dermal papillae tips.

Noninflammatory Blistering Disorders (p. 1171)

Epidermolysis Bullosa (p. 1171)

Epidermolysis bullosa is a large (ten or so) group of noninflammatory disorders that have in common blistering at pressure sites or trauma due to defects in the structural proteins forming the dermoepidermal junction.

- *Simplex type* results from mutations in keratins 5 or 14, leading to structural defects in the epidermal basal cell layer.
- *Junctional type* is caused by defects in either BPAG2 or *laminin;* the latter is a protein that links hemidesmosomes and anchoring fibrils; the result is blistering at the lamina lucida in otherwise histologically normal skin.
- *Dystrophic type* shows blistering beneath the lamina densa due to type VII collagen mutations; this form typically leads to cutaneous scarring.

Porphyria (p. 1171)

Porphyria is a group of inborn or acquired disturbances of porphyrin metabolism (there are five major types based on biochemical and clinical features); porphyrins are the ring structures that bind metal ions in hemoglobin, myoglobin, and cytochromes. The cutaneous lesions consist of urticaria and vesicles that are exacerbated by sun exposure and heal without scarring. Histologically there are subepidermal vesicles with marked thickening of the walls of superficial dermal vessels. The pathogenesis is unknown.

Disorders of Epidermal Appendages (p. 1172)

Acne Vulgaris (p. 1172)

Acne vulgaris is a common chronic lesion of hair follicles (particularly the sebaceous glands), typically occurring in the middle-late teens and in males more than females. It is associated with hormonal changes and alterations in hair follicle maturation and can be induced by sex hormones, corticosteroids, occupational exposure (coal tars), or occlusive conditions (heavy clothes). There may be a heritable component.

Pathogenesis (p. 1173)

Acne likely involves bacterial *(Propionibacterium acnes)* lipase degradation of sebaceous oils to form highly irritating fatty acids that incite inflammatory responses. Keratinization of the follicle and development of a keratin plug that blocks sebum outflow is also contributory. Antibiotics (e.g., tetracyclines) may be effective by eliminating the bacteria and/or inhibiting the lipase activity, and vitamin A derivatives (13-*cis*-retinoic acid) have efficacy through their antisebaceous action.

Morphology *(p. 1173)*

- *Gross:*
  - *Noninflammatory acne* is characterized by *open comedones*—follicular papules with central black keratin plugs (the color is due to oxidized melanin)—and *closed comedones*—follicular papules with central plugs trapped beneath the epidermis. The latter can rupture and cause inflammation.
  - *Inflammatory acne* presents with erythematous papules, nodules, and pustules.
- *Microscopic:* Comedones are composed of expanding masses of lipid and keratin at the midportion of hair follicles, with follicular dilation and epithelial and sebaceous gland atrophy. There is a variable lymphohistiocytic infiltrate, but with rupture there is extensive acute and chronic inflammation, occasionally with ensuing scar formation.

Rosacea (p. 1173)

Rosacea affects up to 3% of the U.S. population, with a predilection for middle-aged females.

Pathogenesis *(p. 1174)*

Inappropriate activation of the innate immune system (characterized by increased cathelicidin production) is implicated. The cathelicidin peptides in patients with rosacea are qualitatively distinct from those in individuals without the disease, due to alternative processing by proteases, such as kallikrein 5 (which is in turn upregulated through activation of the Toll-like receptor 2).

Morphology *(p. 1174)*

- *Gross:* The disorder has four characteristic stages: (1) flushing, (2) persistent erythema and telangiectasia, (3) pustules and papules, and (4) *rhinophyma*—permanent thickening of the nasal skin by confluent papules and follicles.
- *Microscopic:* Lesions exhibit a nonspecific perifollicular lymphocyte infiltrate with dermal edema and telangiectasia. In the pustular phase, neutrophilic infiltrates and follicular rupture can elicit a dermal granulomatous response. Rhinophyma is associated with sebaceous hyperplasia and follicular plugging by keratotic debris.

Panniculitis (p. 1174)

Panniculitis is inflammation of subcutaneous fat; it may be acute or chronic and commonly involves the lower extremities.

Erythema Nodosum (p. 1174)

Erythema nodosum is the most common form of panniculitis; it typically has an acute onset and may be idiopathic or occur in association with specific drugs, infections (especially β-hemolytic streptococcus), sarcoidosis, inflammatory bowel disease, or visceral malignancy. It presents with ill-defined, exquisitely tender erythematous nodules, occasionally with fever and malaise. With time, old lesions flatten and become ecchymotic without scarring, whereas new lesions develop. Deep wedge biopsy shows distinctive early septal widening (edema, fibrin deposition, and neutrophil infiltration) and lymphohistiocytic infiltration (occasionally with giant cells and eosinophils) without vasculitis.

Erythema Induratum (p. 1174)

Erythema induratum is an uncommon form of panniculitis, typically affecting adolescents and menopausal women. It may represent a primary vasculitis of subcutaneous fat with subsequent inflammation and necrosis of adipose tissue. It presents as an erythematous, slightly tender nodule that eventually ulcerates and scars. Early lesions show necrotizing vasculitis in small to medium-sized vessels in deep dermis and subcutis. Eventually the fat lobules develop granulomatous inflammation and necrosis.

Weber-Christian disease (relapsing febrile nodular panniculitis) is a rare, lobular form of panniculitis; it presents as crops of erythematous plaques or nodules (mainly on the legs), associated with deep lymphohistiocytic infiltrates and occasional giant cells.

Factitial panniculitis (from self-administered foreign substances), deep mycotic infections in immunocompromised hosts, and occasionally disorders, such as systemic lupus erythematosus (SLE), can mimic the clinical and histologic appearance of primary panniculitis.

Infection (p. 1175)

Verrucae (Warts) (p. 1175)

Verrucae are common, spontaneously regressing (6 months to 2 years) lesions, typically seen in children and adolescents. They are caused by papillomaviruses, transmitted by direct contact.

Verrucae are classified by appearance and anatomic location:

- *Verruca vulgaris* is most common, typically found on the hand dorsum; lesions are gray-white to tan, flat to convex, <1-cm papules with a rough surface.
- *Verruca plana (flat wart)* usually present on the face or hand dorsum as flat, smooth, tan papules smaller than verruca vulgaris.
- *Verruca plantaris (soles) or palmaris (palms)* are rough, scaly 1- to 2-cm lesions; these can coalesce and be confused with calluses.
- *Condyloma acuminatum (anogenital and venereal warts)* are soft, tan, cauliflower-like masses measuring up to many centimeters in diameter.

Pathogenesis (p. 1175)

More than 150 HPVs have been identified, many capable of causing lesions; the clinical variants of warts are often associated with specific HPV subtypes. Thus anogenital warts are caused predominantly by HPV 6 and 11, and type 16 is associated with lesion dysplasia and in situ squamous cell carcinoma.

Morphology (p. 1175)

Microscopically all variants have undulant *(verrucous)* epidermal hyperplasia and superficial keratinocyte perinuclear vacuolization *(koilocytosis)*. Electron microscopy reveals numerous intranuclear viral particles.

Molluscum Contagiosum (p. 1175)

This is a common, self-limited poxvirus infection transmitted by direct contact.

Morphology (p. 1175)

- *Gross:* Firm, pruritic, pink to skin-colored, umbilicated papules (0.2 to 2 cm) are seen on the trunk or anogenital regions; cheesy material containing diagnostic molluscum bodies can be expressed from the central umbilications.

- *Microscopic:* Lesions exhibit cuplike verrucous epidermal hyperplasia with pathognomonic *molluscum bodies*—eosinophilic cytoplasmic inclusions in the stratum granulosum or stratum corneum containing numerous virions.

Impetigo (p. 1176)

Impetigo is a common superficial bacterial infection; *Staphylococcus aureus* is the most common agent, although β-hemolytic streptococci can also cause lesions. It is highly contagious; infection typically involves exposed skin, particularly the face and hands. A bullous form mainly occurs in children.

Pathogenesis (p. 1177)

Epidermal bacterial infections provoke a destructive innate immune response with a serous exudate. Blister formation is driven by bacterial production of a toxin that cleaves Dsg1.

Morphology (p. 1177)

- *Gross:* Lesions begin as erythematous macules that progress to small pustules and eventually to shallow erosions with a honey-colored crust.
- *Microscopic:* Characteristically there are subcorneal pustules filled with neutrophils and gram-positive cocci accompanied by nonspecific dermal inflammation. The crust is formed by superficial layering of serum, neutrophils, and cellular debris.

Superficial Fungal Infections (p. 1177)

Superficial fungal infections are confined to the nonviable stratum corneum; they are caused by dermatophytes derived from soil or animal contacts.

- *Tinea capitis* typically occurs in children. It causes asymptomatic hairless patches on the scalp, associated with mild erythema, crusting, and scale.
- *Tinea barbae* affects the beard area in adult men.
- *Tinea corporis* is a common superficial dermatophytosis of the body, especially in children. Predisposing factors are excessive heat or humidity, exposure to infected animals, and chronic foot or nail dermatophytosis. It typically presents with an expanding erythematous plaque with an elevated scaling border.
- *Tinea cruris* is typically found in the inguinal areas; obesity, heat, friction, and maceration are predisposing factors. It presents as moist red patches with raised scaling borders.
- *Tinea pedis (athlete's foot)* affects 30% to 40% of the population at some point; it is characterized by erythema and scaling, beginning in the webbed spaces between the digits. Most of the inflammation is due to secondary bacterial superinfection.
- *Tinea versicolor* (due to the yeast *Malassezia furfur*) typically presents on the upper trunk as groups of various-sized hyperpigmented or hypopigmented macules with a peripheral scale.
- *Onychomycosis* is a nail dermatophytosis characterized by discoloration, thickening, and deformity of the nail plate.

Morphology (p. 1177)

There is histologic variability depending on the organism, host response, and extent of bacterial superinfection; nevertheless, lesions characteristically exhibit reactive epidermal changes similar to mild eczematous dermatitis. Fungal organisms in the stratum corneum are revealed by special stains and can be cultured from scrapings of affected areas.

26

Bones, Joints, and Soft Tissue Tumors

BONES (p. 1180)

Matrix (p. 1180)

Bone matrix is 65% inorganic mineral (hydroxyapatite = $Ca_{10}(PO_4)_6(OH)_2$) and 35% *osteoid*—mainly type I collagen with smaller amounts of *osteonectin* (a calcium-binding glycoprotein) and *osteocalcin* (also called osteopontin, involved in bone mineralization). Several cytokines and growth factors are also embedded and are responsible for regulating cell proliferation, maturation, and metabolism. In addition to providing strength, hydroxyapatite serves as a repository for 99% of the body's calcium and 85% of its phosphorus. Matrix is synthesized in two histologic forms:

- *Woven bone* is produced rapidly (e.g., in fetal development or fracture repair), but the haphazard arrangement of collagen fibers imparts less structural integrity.
- *Lamellar bone* is more slowly produced and has parallel collagen fibers.

In an adult the presence of woven bone is always abnormal but is nonspecific and can be found in a variety of pathologic settings (discussed later).

Cells (p. 1180)

- *Osteoblasts* are responsible for bone matrix synthesis and initiating mineralization; they derive from *osteoprogenitor cells*—pluripotent mesenchymal stem cells.
- *Osteocytes* are long-lived cells responsible for local bone calcium and phosphate homeostasis and for translating mechanical forces into biologic activity *(mechanotransduction)*; they derive from osteoblasts.
- *Osteoclasts* are short-lived (2 weeks) multinucleated cells responsible for bone resorption; macrophage colony-stimulating factor (M-CSF), interleukin-1 (IL-1), and tumor necrosis factor (TNF) drive their differentiation from the same hematopoietic precursors as monocytes and macrophages (Fig. 26-1).

Development (p. 1181)

- *Enchondral ossification:* During embryogenesis, most bones are generated by conversion of a cartilage mold synthesized by mesenchymal precursor cells. The central portion of the mold is digested by *chondroclasts,* creating the medullary canal; simultaneously, at midshaft *(diaphysis),* osteoblasts deposit cortical bone beneath the nascent periosteum (so-called *primary center of ossification*), producing *radial*

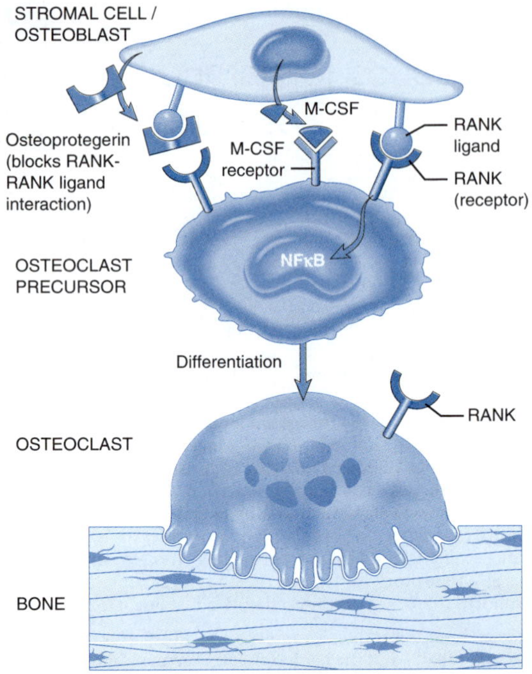

Figure 26-1 Molecular mechanisms regulating osteoclast formation and function. Osteoclasts are derived from the same mononuclear cells that differentiate into macrophages. Osteoblast or stromal cell membrane-associated RANKL binds to RANK on the surface of osteoclast precursors. This interaction *plus* M-CSF induces precursor cells to become functional osteoclasts. Stromal cells also secrete OPG, which acts as a "decoy" receptor for RANKL, preventing it from binding the RANK receptor on osteoclast precursors. Consequently, OPG prevents bone resorption by inhibiting osteoclast differentiation. *RANK,* Receptor activator for NF-κB; *RANKL,* RANK ligand.

bone growth. At each longitudinal end *(epiphysis),* endochondral ossification proceeds in a centrifugal fashion *(secondary center of ossification).* Eventually a plate of cartilage is sandwiched between the two expanding centers of ossification, forming the *physis* or *growth plate.* The chondrocytes within the growth plate undergo sequential proliferation, hypertrophy, and apoptosis; in the apoptotic zone the matrix mineralizes and is invaded by capillaries, providing the nutrients for osteoblasts to be activated and synthesize osteoid. Remnant struts of cartilage act as scaffolding for the deposition of bone, forming the first bony trabeculae; new bone progressively deposits at the bottom of the growth plate, resulting in longitudinal bone growth.

- *Intramembranous ossification:* Flat bones (e.g., in the cranium) are formed by osteoblasts directly adherent to a fibrous layer of tissue derived from mesenchyme, without a cartilage mold; bone enlargement occurs by additional deposition on the preexisting surface. This mechanism of appositional growth is instrumental in bone development and modeling.
- *Bone development* is controlled by the following:
  - Growth hormone (GH) acting on resting chondrocytes to induce and maintain proliferation.
  - Thyroid hormone (T_3) acting on proliferating chondrocytes to induce hypertrophy.

- Indian hedgehog (Ihh), made by prehypertrophic chondrocytes, coordinating chondrocyte proliferation and differentiation and osteoblast proliferation.
- Parathyroid hormone-related protein (PTHrP), made by perichondrial stromal cells and early proliferating chondrocytes, activating the PTH receptor and maintaining chondrocyte proliferation.
- Wnt is a family of secreted factors promoting both proliferation and maturation of chondrocytes.
- SOX9 is a transcription factor expressed by proliferating chondrocytes driving precursor differentiation into chondrocytes.
- RUNX2 is a transcription factor expressed in early hypertrophic chondrocytes and immature mesenchymal cells, controlling terminal chondrocyte and osteoblast differentiation.
- Fibroblast growth factors (FGFs, most notably FGF3) acting on hypertrophic chondrocytes to inhibit proliferation and promote differentiation.
- Bone morphogenic proteins (BMPs, members of the transforming growth factor [TGF]-β family) affecting chondrocyte proliferation and hypertrophy.

Homeostasis and Remodeling (p. 1182)

The adult skeleton is constantly remodeling; approximately 10% is replaced annually, allowing response to structural and mechanical demands. Beginning in the fourth decade, resorption exceeds formation, so there is a steady decline in skeletal mass. Remodeling occurs through an orderly sequence of osteoclast attachment, resorption, osteoblast attachment and proliferation, and then matrix synthesis.

The balance between bone formation and resorption is modulated by osteoprotegerin (OPG) and RANKL (Fig. 26-1); these are influenced by hormones (PTH, estrogen, testosterone, and glucocorticoids), vitamin D, inflammatory cytokines (e.g., IL-1), and growth factors (e.g., bone morphogenetic factors). PTH, IL-1, and glucocorticoids promote osteoclast differentiation and bone turnover; BMPs and sex hormones generally block osteoclast differentiation or activity by favoring OPG expression.

Breakdown of matrix by osteoclasts liberates and activates matrix proteins, growth factors, cytokines, and enzymes (e.g., collagenase), including some that stimulate osteoblasts. Thus as bone is broken down, substances are released that initiate renewal (Fig. 26-2).

Developmental Disorders of Bone and Cartilage (p. 1183)

Although acquired bone disorders usually present in adulthood, most developmental anomalies are caused by genetic mutations and typically manifest during early stages of bone formation (Table 26-1). Different point mutations in the same gene can result in different phenotypes, whereas mutations in diverse genes can have a similar clinical presentation.

- *Dysostoses:* Developmental anomalies due to abnormal mesenchymal cell migration or differentiation; they can occur in isolation or part of a syndrome complex. They often result from mutations in homeobox transcription factor genes, cytokines, or cytokine receptors. Common forms of dysostoses are as follows:
    - Complete absence of a bone or digit *(aplasia)*
    - Extra bones or digits *(supernumerary digit)*
    - Abnormal bone fusion (*syndactyly, craniostosis,* etc.)

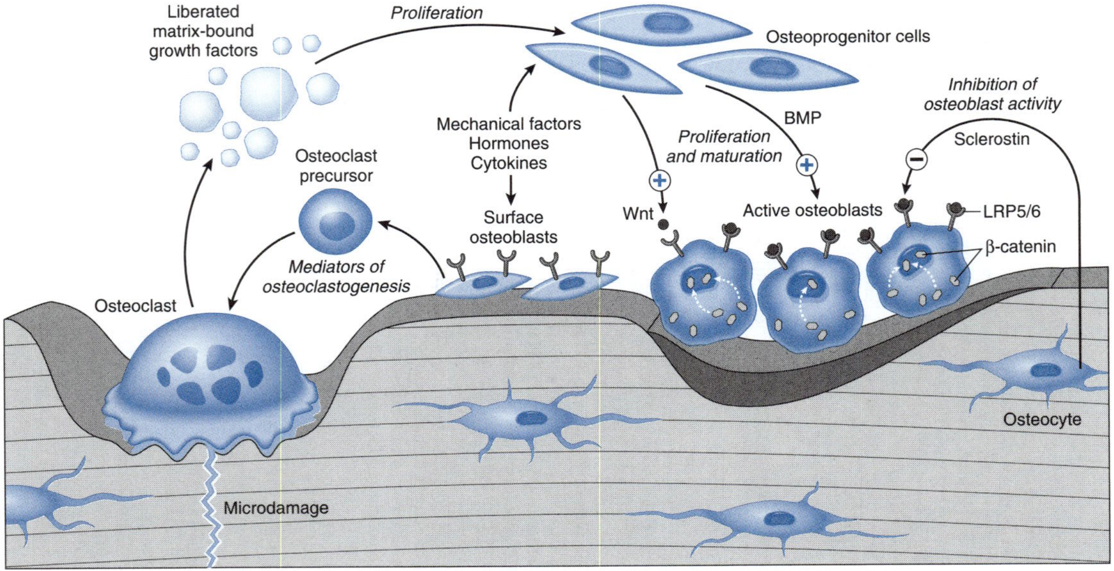

Figure 26-2 Bone cells and their interrelated activities. Hormones, cytokines, growth factors, and signal-transducing molecules allow communication between osteoblasts and osteoclasts. Bone resorption and formation in remodeling are coupled processes that are controlled by systemic factors and local cytokines, some of which are deposited in the bone matrix. *BMP,* Bone morphogenic protein; *LRP5/6,* LDL receptor-related proteins 5 and 6.

TABLE 26-1 Diseases of the Skeleton With Identified Genetic Defects

Disorder	Gene Symbol	Affected Molecule	Clinical Phenotype
Defects in Transcription Factors Producing Abnormalities in Mesenchymal Condensation and Related Cell Differentiation			
Brachydactyly types D and E	*HOXD13*	Transcription factor	Short, broad terminal phalanges of first digits
Camptomelic dysplasia	*SOX9*	Transcription factor	Sex reversal, abnormal skeletal development
Cleidocranial dysplasia	*RUNX2*	Transcription factor	Abnormal clavicles, wormian bones, supernumerary teeth
Holt-Oram syndrome	*TBX5*	Transcription factor	Congenital abnormalities, forelimb anomalies
Nail-patella syndrome	*LMX1B*	Transcription factor	Hypoplastic nails, hypoplastic or aplastic patellas, dislocated radial head, progressive nephropathy
Waardenburg syndrome types 1 and 3	*PAX3*	Transcription factor	Hearing loss, abnormal pigmentation, craniofacial abnormalities
Defects in Hormones and Signal Transduction Proteins Producing Abnormal Proliferation or Maturation of Osteoblasts, Osteoclasts, or Chondrocytes			
Achondroplasia	*FGFR3*	Receptor	Short stature, rhizomelic shortening of limbs, frontal bossing, midface deficiency
Hypochondroplasia	*FGFR3*	Receptor	Disproportionately short stature, micromelia, relative macrocephaly
Osteopetrosis, autosomal dominant	*LRP5*	Receptor	Increased bone density, hearing loss, skeletal fragility
Osteopetrosis, infantile form	*RANKL*	Receptor ligand	Increased bone density
Osteoporosis-pseudoglioma syndrome	*LRP5*	Receptor	Congenital or infant-onset loss of vision, skeletal fragility
Thanatophoric dysplasia	*FGFR3*	Receptor	Severe limb shortening and bowing, frontal bossing, depressed nasal bridge
Defects in Extracellular Structural Proteins			
Achondrogenesis type 2	*COL2A1*	Type II collagen	Short trunk
Metaphyseal dysplasia, Schmid type	*COL10A1*	Type X collagen	Mildly short stature
Osteogenesis imperfecta types 1-4	*COL1A1, COL1A2*	Type I collagen	Bone fragility
Defects in Metabolic Enzymes and Transporters			
Osteopetrosis with renal tubular acidosis	*CA2*	Carbonic anhydrase	Increased bone density, fragility, renal tubular acidosis
Osteopetrosis, late onset type 2	*CLCN7*	Chloride channel	Increased bone density, fragility

Modified from Mundlos S, Olsen BR: Heritable diseases of the skeleton. Part I: Molecular insights into skeletal development—transcription factors and signaling pathways. *FASEB J* 11:125-132, 1997; Mundlos S, Olsen BR: Heritable diseases of the skeleton. Part II: Molecular insights into skeletal development—matrix components and their homeostasis. *FASEB J* 11:227-233, 1997; Superti-Furga A, Bonafé L, Rimoin DL: Molecular-pathogenetic classification of genetic disorders of the skeleton. *Am J Med Genet* 106:262-293, 2001; Krakow D, Rimoin DL: The skeletal dysplasias. *Genet Med* 12(6):327-341, 2010.

- *Dysplasias:* Mutations in signal molecules or matrix constituents that control development or remodeling of the entire skeleton, causing more global effects.

Defects in Nuclear Proteins and Transcription Factors (p. 1184; Table 26-1)

Defects in Hormones and Signal Transduction Proteins (p. 1184)

- *Achondroplasia* is the most common form of dwarfism; some cases are familial, but 90% involve new mutations, most arising in the paternal allele. All cases are caused by autosomal dominant gain-of-function mutations in the fibroblast growth factor receptor-3 (FGFR3), leading to FGFR3 constitutive activation that inhibits endochondral growth. Anatomically the growth plates are shortened and disordered, resulting in abnormally short extremity bones; because appositional growth is not affected, bones are of normal width and the skull appears comparatively enlarged.
- *Thanatophoric dysplasia* is the most common lethal form of dwarfism (1 in 20,000 live births); it is also caused by gain-of-function mutations in FGFR3 (different from those in achondroplasia). Growth plates show reduced chondrocyte proliferation and disorganization; an underdeveloped thoracic cavity leads to respiratory insufficiency and frequently perinatal death.
- *Abnormal bone density* (*osteoporosis* = too little bone, or *osteopetrosis* = too much bone) can result from mutations that affect osteoclast differentiation or function. Depending on the gene defect, mutations in the LPR5 receptor on osteoblasts. *LPR5* can manifest as either osteoporosis or osteopetrosis. Mutations of *RANKL* leading to decreased or absent osteoclasts can cause osteopetrosis.

Defects in Extracellular Structural Proteins (p. 1185)

Type I Collagen Diseases (Osteogenesis Imperfecta, Brittle Bone Disease) (p. 1185)

Type I collagen diseases represent a group of related genetic disorders caused by qualitatively or quantitatively abnormal type I collagen synthesis. These are typically due to autosomal dominant mutations in type I collagen $\alpha 1$ or $\alpha 2$ chains; glycines are replaced by other amino acids, leading to defective triple helix formation, including the proper assembly of wild-type collagen chains (a *dominant negative* effect). Morphologically there is *osteopenia* (too little bone), with marked cortical thinning and trabecular rarefaction, leading to increased fracture susceptibility. The classic "blue sclera" is due to decreased collagen content causing translucent sclera that permits visualization of the underlying choroid; hearing loss is related in part to impeded conduction due to abnormalities of bones of the middle and inner ear; dental imperfections are due to dentin deficiency. There are four major subtypes based on the specific biosynthetic abnormality and the clinical manifestations. Syndromes range from *type II* that is uniformly fatal in the perinatal period (from multiple bone fractures) to other variants with increased risk of fractures but compatible with long-term survival.

Diseases Associated With Mutations of Types II, IX, X, and XI Collagen (p. 1185)

Diseases associated with mutations of types II, IX, X, and XI collagen are related to abnormal hyaline cartilage synthesis (Table 26-1). Absence of type II collagen synthesis leads to a severe phenotype due to insufficient bone formation; reduced synthesis results in milder forms of disease.

Defects in Metabolic Pathways (Enzymes, Ion Channels, and Transporters) (p. 1186)

Osteopetrosis (p. 1186)

Osteopetrosis *(marble bone disease, Albers-Schönberg disease)* is a group of genetic disorders characterized by reduced osteoclastic activity; although there is increased mass, the bone is abnormally brittle and fractures like chalk. Diffuse skeletal sclerosis also impinges on the medullary cavity and impairs hematopoiesis.

Pathogenesis (p. 1186)

Most mutations interfere with osteoclast acidification of the resorptive pit, a step required to dissolve matrix calcium hydroxyapatite before bone resorption. Thus mutations in carbonic anhydrase II reduce the formation of protons from CO_2 and water (they also block renal tubular acidification of urine). *CLCN7* mutations interfere with the function of the osteoclast H^+-ATPase proton pump.

Clinical Features (p. 1187)

Fractures and anemia are common; patients can also have hydrocephaly and cranial nerve defects (optic atrophy, deafness, and facial paralysis) due to abnormal skull bone remodeling. Recurrent infections (inadequate white cell production) and hepatosplenomegaly (due to extramedullary hematopoiesis) are also features. The disease can be treated with bone marrow transplantation because osteoclasts derive from monocyte precursors.

Diseases Associated With Defects in Degradation of Macromolecules (p. 1187)

Mucopolysaccharidoses (p. 1187)

Mucopolysaccharidoses are lysosomal storage diseases caused by deficiencies in enzymes that degrade mucopolysaccharides (e.g., dermatan sulfate, heparan sulfate, and keratan sulfate). Because chondrocytes are responsible for mucopolysaccharide metabolism, hyaline cartilage (e.g., growth plates, costal cartilages, and articular surfaces) is typically most affected; patients are frequently short with malformed bones and chest abnormalities.

Acquired Disorders of Bone and Cartilage (p. 1187)

Osteopenia and Osteoporosis (p. 1187)

Osteopenia simply means decreased bone mass; *osteoporosis* is osteopenia severe enough to significantly increase fracture risk. Radiographically osteopenia is defined as bone mass 1 to 2.5 standard deviations below the mean peak bone mass in young adults; osteoporosis is bone mass ≥2.5 standard deviations below the mean or with atraumatic or vertebral compression fracture. Osteoporosis can be localized to a specific site (e.g., disuse osteoporosis of a limb) or can be a generalized disorder of primary (senile) or secondary causes (i.e., due to endocrine abnormalities, malabsorption, or neoplasia). Osteoporosis occurs most commonly in aged individuals and is most pronounced in postmenopausal women.

Pathogenesis (p. 1187)

Senile and postmenopausal osteoporosis are multifactorial disorders (Fig. 26-3).

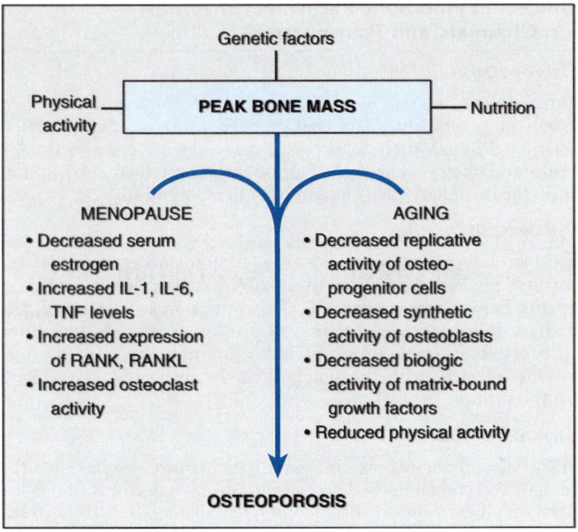

Figure 26-3 Pathophysiology of postmenopausal and senile osteoporosis. *IL,* Interleukin; *RANK,* receptor activator for nuclear factor κB; *RANKL,* RANK ligand; *TNF,* tumor necrosis factor.

- Genetic factors are the major determinant of peak bone density; polymorphisms in RANKL, RANK, OPG, LRP5, and the estrogen and vitamin D receptors have all been implicated. Physical activity, muscle strength, diet (e.g., calcium and vitamin D), and hormonal status also influence bone deposition. After achieving peak bone mass in young adulthood, each cycle of bone turnover accrues a predictable shortfall in bone formation relative to absorption, averaging a 0.7% deficit each year regardless of gender.
- Age-related changes diminish osteoblast proliferation and biosynthetic potential; osteogenic growth factors bound to the extracellular matrix also show diminished activity with increasing age.
- Decreased physical activity accelerates bone loss because mechanical forces stimulate normal bone remodeling; the magnitude of bone loading influences bone density more than the number of load cycles.
- In postmenopausal women, decreased estrogen levels promote increased osteoclastic activity by increasing monocyte production of IL-1, IL-6, and TNF; these cytokines recruit and activate osteoclasts by increasing RANKL expression while reducing OPG synthesis. Compensatory osteoblastic activity occurs, but it does not keep pace with the bone loss. Following menopause, cortical bone may be lost at a rate of 2% per year and cancellous bone at 9% per year.

Morphology *(p. 1189)*

The entire skeleton is involved in postmenopausal and senile osteoporosis, but increased osteoclast activity mainly affects bone with increased surface area (e.g., the cancellous compartment of vertebral bodies). Progressive thinning of trabeculae leads to progressive microfractures and eventual bony collapse. Cortical bone is thinned by subperiosteal and endosteal resorption, and haversian systems are widened.

Clinical Course (p. 1189)

Microfractures cause pain and loss in height and stability of the vertebral column. Osteoporosis also predisposes to fractures of pelvis, femoral neck, and spine; complications—including pulmonary embolism and pneumonia—are responsible for 50,000 deaths per year. Osteoporosis cannot be reliably identified on standard radiograms until 30% to 40% of bone mass has been lost; early detection requires bone densitometry measurements. Therapy involves exercise, calcium and vitamin D supplementation, and osteoclast inhibition with bisphosphonates.

Paget Disease (Osteitis Deformans) (p. 1189)

This is a disease of excess disordered and architecturally unsound bone mass.

Pathogenesis (p. 1190)

Both environmental and genetic factors are implicated; mutations in the *SQSTM1* gene (enhancing RANK signaling) increase susceptibility and are present in 40% to 50% of familial cases and 5% to 10% of sporadic cases. A contributory role for paramyxovirus infection remains unproven.

Morphology (p. 1190)

Paget disease progresses through three stages:

- The *osteolytic phase* is marked by resorption by numerous, large osteoclasts (some containing >100 nuclei).
- The *mixed phase* exhibits osteoclasts and osteoblasts lining bone surfaces with disordered woven and lamellar bone formation; adjacent marrow spaces are replaced by loose connective tissue. The lamellar bone assumes a pathognomonic *mosaic* pattern.
- The *burnt-out phase* is marked by bone sclerosis composed of coarsely thickened trabeculae and cortices; the bone is soft and porous and lacks structural stability.

Clinical Course (p. 1190)

Paget disease has an average age of onset of 70 years; the prevalence is high in the United States (1%) and Europe but low in China, Japan, and Africa. It is monostotic in 15% of cases (polyostotic in the remainder), and the axial skeleton or proximal femur are involved in 80% of patients. Pain is a common feature, associated with fractures, nerve compression, osteoarthritis (OA), and skeletal deformities (e.g., tibial bowing, skull enlargement). Less commonly, the vascularity of polyostotic lesions can cause high-output heart failure. In 1% of patients, secondary sarcoma develops. Most affected individuals have mild symptoms that respond to calcitonin and bisphosphonate treatment.

Rickets (Children) and Osteomalacia (Adults) (p. 1191)

These are disorders characterized by defective matrix mineralization; most often secondary to vitamin D deficiency or other calcium metabolic disturbance (see Chapter 9). In children there is defective bone deposition in growth plates; in adults, bone formed during remodeling is undermineralized and therefore prone to fracture.

Hyperparathyroidism (p. 1191)

PTH regulates calcium levels through osteoclast activation (by increasing RANKL expression on osteoblasts), renal tubule calcium resorption and phosphate excretion, and active vitamin D synthesis. Excessive

PTH can result from autonomous parathyroid production *(primary hyperparathyroidism)* or from underlying renal disease (*secondary hyperparathyroidism;* see Chapter 24), driving unabated osteoclast activity.

Morphology *(p. 1191)*

- The entire skeleton is affected, although some sites more so than others; cortical bone is affected more than cancellous bone.
- Increased bone resorption is also associated with increased osteoblast activity; fibrovascular tissues replace the surrounding marrow spaces.
- Microfractures and associated hemorrhages elicit an influx of macrophages and reparative fibrous tissue (so-called *brown tumors*) and the designation *osteitis fibrosa cystica* (also known as *von Recklinghausen disease of bone*).

Renal Osteodystrophy (p. 1192)

Chronic renal failure leads to increased osteoclastic activity and reduced matrix mineralization *(osteomalacia);* the results include osteoporosis and/or osteopenia and growth retardation. Patients exhibit some combination of *high-turnover osteodystrophy* (characterized by increased bone resorption and formation) and *low-turnover disease* (manifested by largely quiescent bone).

Pathogenesis *(p. 1192; Fig. 26-4)*

- *Tubular dysfunction:* Renal tubular acidosis leads to acidemia that leaches bone hydroxyapatite, causing matrix demineralization (osteomalacia).
- *Generalized renal failure* leads to reduced phosphate excretion, with chronic hyperphosphatemia and hypocalcemia that drives *secondary hyperparathyroidism.*
- *Decreased production of secreted factors:* Chronic renal failure leads to diminished renal production of the following:
  - 1,25-OH_2-vitamin D_3, causing reduced calcium absorption and increased osteoclast activity
  - BMP-7, causing reduced osteoblast differentiation and proliferation
  - Klotho, a membrane-bound protein that interacts with osteocyte-produced FGF-23 to regulate phosphate homeostasis and vitamin D production

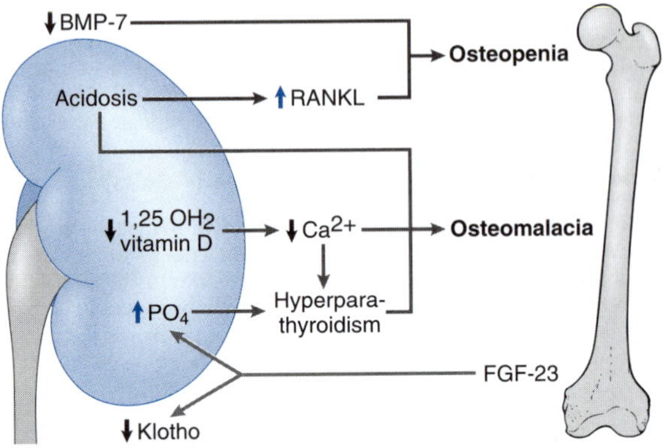

Figure 26-4 Mechanisms of renal osteodystrophy involve electrolyte levels and endocrine signaling between bone and kidney.

Fractures (p. 1193)

Fractures are classified as the following:

- Complete or incomplete
- Closed (simple) when the overlying tissue is intact; compound when the fracture communicates with the skin
- Comminuted when the bone is splintered
- Displaced when the ends of the fractured bone are not aligned
- Pathologic fractures are breaks in bones altered by a disease process (e.g., tumor)
- Stress fractures are slowly developing breaks associated with repetitive physical loading
- "Greenstick" when the fracture extends only partially through the bone; common in soft bones of infancy

Healing of Fractures (p. 1193)

Fracture healing—regulated by cytokines and growth factors—involves reactivating bone formation pathways that normally occur during embryogenesis:

- *Procallus formation:* Within a week of breaking, fracture site hematomas are organized by an influx of inflammatory cells, fibroblasts, and new vessels; platelets and inflammatory cells release platelet-derived growth factor (PDGF), TGF-β, FGF, and ILs that trigger osteoprogenitor cells and stimulate osteoclast and osteoblast activity.
- The procallus is converted to a *fibrocartilaginous callus* composed of reactive mesenchymal cells; the new cartilage along the fracture line undergoes enchondral ossification (analogous to bone formation at a growth plate), eventually forming a *bony callus.* Progressive mineralization increases callus stiffness and strength.
- The osseous callus is eventually remodeled along lines of weight bearing to complete the repair.

If fractures are well aligned and the original weight-bearing strains are restored, virtually perfect repair is accomplished. Imperfect results are seen with malalignment, comminution, inadequate immobilization, infection, and superimposed systemic abnormality (e.g., dietary deficiency, osteoporosis). Nonunion with excessive motion along the fracture gap can cause callus cystic degeneration; the luminal surface can then become synovium-lined to create a false joint *(pseudoarthrosis).*

Osteonecrosis (Avascular Necrosis) (p. 1194)

Bone and marrow infarction is relatively common; traumatic fracture (which causes vascular interruption) is the most common cause, with the remaining majority of osteonecrosis being either idiopathic or associated with corticosteroid administration. Other, less frequent causes include infection, radiation therapy, vasculitis, sickle cell and other anemias, Gaucher disease, and air embolism *(caisson disease).*

Morphology (p. 1194)

Medullary infarcts are geographic and involve cancellous bone and marrow. Cortical bone is usually not affected because of collateral blood flow, and articular cartilage over subchondral infarcts remains viable by virtue of nutrient diffusion from synovial fluid.

Necrotic bone shows empty lacunae; ruptured adipocytes can have associated fat saponification. *Creeping substitution* with new bone occurs from the margin of the infarct. In subchondral infarcts the articular cartilage may collapse into the necrotic bone.

Clinical Course (p. 1195)

Patients may be asymptomatic, but subchondral lesions often cause joint pain and predispose to subsequent OA. More than 10% of the half million joint replacements in the United States annually are for complications of osteonecrosis.

Osteomyelitis (p. 1195)

Osteomyelitis denotes inflammation of bone and marrow, virtually always secondary to infection; bacteria, fungi, viruses, and parasites can all be causes. Osteomyelitis can occur with any systemic infection but is typically a primary solitary focus of disease.

Pyogenic Osteomyelitis (p. 1195)

Pyogenic osteomyelitis is almost always bacterial; seeding occurs by the following:

- Hematogenous spread (common in children, typically involving long bones)
- Extension from a contiguous infection (e.g., diabetic foot ulcer)
- Open fracture or surgical procedure

In half of cases, no organism can be identified. *Staphylococcus aureus* is responsible for 80% to 90% of the remainder, largely related to receptors that enhance adherence to bone matrix; patients with sickle cell anemia are prone to *Salmonella* infections.

The location of infection is influenced by the osseous circulation, which varies with age. In the neonate, metaphyseal vessels penetrate the growth plate, resulting in infections of the metaphysis, epiphysis, or both; localization of infections in the metaphysis is typical in children. After growth plate closure, the metaphyseal and epiphyseal vessels merge, allowing potential seeding of the epiphyses and subchondral regions.

Morphology (p. 1195)

Changes are dependent on the chronicity and location of the infection. Once in bone, bacteria engender an acute inflammatory response.

- Entrapped bone undergoes necrosis within the first 48 hours; bacteria and inflammation percolate within the shaft and along haversian systems to involve the periosteum.
- Lifting of the periosteum compromises vascular supply, leading to a zone of bone necrosis *(sequestrum)*; rupture of the periosteum can lead to a soft tissue abscess and a *draining sinus*.
- After the first week, chronic inflammatory infiltrates stimulate osteoclastic bone resorption, ingrowth of fibrous connective tissue, and deposition of reactive bone.
- The subperiosteal new bone encasing the inflammatory focus is called an *involucrum*. A small walled-off intracortical abscess is called a *Brodie abscess*.

Clinical Course (p. 1196)

Pyogenic osteomyelitis is classically an acute febrile illness associated with local pain; subtle lesions can present in infants as unexplained fever or in adults as focal pain without fever. Antibiotics and surgical drainage are usually curative, although 5% to 25% of cases persist as chronic infections (due to extensive bone necrosis, inadequate therapy, or immunocompromise). Complications include pathologic fracture, amyloidosis, endocarditis, and development of squamous cell carcinoma in the sinus tract or sarcoma in the infected bone.

Mycobacterial Osteomyelitis (p. 1196)

Tuberculous osteomyelitis occurs in 1% to 3% of patients with tuberculosis; organisms are typically bloodborne, although direct extension or lymphatic seeding can occur. The spine is involved in 40% of cases *(Pott disease)* with frequent invasion into soft tissues and abscess formation. Lesions exhibit typical granulomatous reaction with caseous necrosis.

Skeletal Syphilis (p. 1196)

Treponema pallidum (syphilis) and *Treponema pertenue* (yaws) can both involve bone. In congenital syphilis the bone lesions are fully developed at birth, with spirochetes localizing to areas of active enchondral ossification *(osteochondritis)* and in the periosteum *(periostitis); saber shin* is produced by massive reactive periosteal bone deposition on the tibia. In acquired syphilis, bone disease usually occurs 2 to 5 years after initial infection (tertiary stage). Syphilitic bone infections exhibit edematous granulation tissue containing numerous plasma cells, necrotic bone, and spirochetes demonstrable by special stains; gummas can also occur.

Bone Tumors and Tumorlike Lesions (p. 1196)

Primary bone tumors are rare (approximately 2400 cases per year in the United States); metastatic and hematopoietic tumors are far more common. Most bone tumors are asymptomatic and are detected as incidental findings; others present with pain or as a slow-growing mass, and a small number announce as pathologic fractures. In diagnosing bone tumors, patient age, neoplasm location, and radiologic appearance are important (Table 26-2); biopsy and histologic evaluation are necessary, and tumors are classified according to the cell or matrix they produce. Benign tumors greatly outnumber their malignant counterparts, although in the elderly, a bone tumor is more likely to be malignant. The causes of most bone malignancies are unknown; secondary causes (e.g., Paget disease, chronic osteomyelitis, radiation) account for only a small fraction.

Bone-Forming Tumors (p. 1197)

Bone-forming tumors all produce unmineralized osteoid or mineralized woven bone.

Osteoid Osteoma and Osteoblastoma *(p. 1197)*

Osteoid osteoma and osteoblastoma are benign, bone-producing tumors with identical histologic features but different sizes, sites of origin, and symptoms; malignant transformation is rare.

- Osteoid osteomas are <2 cm and usually occur in young men (teens and 20s). Tumors can arise in any bone but have a predilection for the appendicular skeleton; 50% of cases involve the femur or tibia. Patients typically present with severe nocturnal pain (probably caused by osteoblast prostaglandin E_2 production), which is relieved by nonsteroidal antiinflammatory drugs (NSAIDs). These are frequently treated by radiofrequency ablation.

TABLE 26-2 Classification of Major Primary Tumors Involving Bones

Category and Fraction (%)	Behavior	Tumor Type	Common Locations	Age (yr)	Morphology
Hematopoietic (20)	Malignant	Myeloma Lymphoma	Vertebrae, pelvis	50-60	Malignant plasma cells or lymphocytes replacing marrow space
Cartilage forming (30)	Benign	Osteochondroma	Metaphysis of long bones	10-30	Bony excrescence with cartilage cap
		Chondroma	Small bones of hands and feet	30-50	Circumscribed hyaline cartilage nodule in medulla
		Chondroblastoma	Epiphysis of long bones	10-20	Circumscribed, pericellular calcification
		Chondromyxoid fibroma	Tibia, pelvis	20-30	Collagenous to myxoid matrix, stellate cells
	Malignant	Chondrosarcoma (conventional)	Pelvis, shoulder	40-60	Extends from medulla through cortex into soft tissue, chondrocytes with increased cellularity and atypia
Bone forming (26)	Benign	Osteoid osteoma	Metaphysis of long bones	10-20	Cortical, interlacing microtrabeculae of woven bone
		Osteoblastoma	Vertebral column	10-20	Posterior elements of vertebra, histology similar to osteoid osteoma
	Malignant	Osteosarcoma	Metaphysis of distal femur, proximal tibia	10-20	Extends from medulla to lift periosteum, malignant cells producing woven bone
Unknown origin (15)	Benign	Giant cell tumor	Epiphysis of long bones	20-40	Destroys medulla and cortex, sheets of osteoclasts
		ABC	Proximal tibia, distal femur, vertebra	10-20	Vertebral body, hemorrhagic spaces separated by cellular, fibrous septae
	Malignant	Ewing sarcoma	Diaphysis of long bones	10-20	Sheets of primitive small round cells
		Adamantinoma	Tibia	30-40	Cortical, fibrous, bone matrix with epithelial islands
Notochordal (4)	Malignant	Chordoma	Clivus, sacrum	30-60	Destroys medulla and cortex, foamy cells in myxoid matrix

Adapted from Unni KK, Inwards CY: *Dahlin's Bone Tumors,* 6th ed. Philadelphia, PA, Lippincott Williams & Wilkins, 2010, p 5; by permission of Mayo Foundation.

- Osteoblastomas are >2 cm and frequently involve the posterior spine; the pain is unresponsive to NSAIDs. These are usually curetted or excised en bloc.

Morphology (p. 1198)

- *Gross:* Lesions are round-oval masses of hemorrhagic, gritty, tan tissue.
- *Microscopic:* Tumors are well-circumscribed nodules of radiologically translucent woven bone *(nidus)* rimmed by osteoblasts; this is surrounded by highly vascular, loose connective tissue enclosed by radiologically dense reactive sclerotic bone.

Osteosarcoma *(p. 1198)*

Osteosarcoma is a malignant mesenchymal tumor with neoplastic cells producing osteoid matrix or mineralized bone; 75% occur before age 20, with most of the remainder developing in geriatric patients with known risk factors (e.g., Paget disease, radiation).

Pathogenesis (p. 1198)

Approximately 70% have acquired genetic abnormalities, including numerous, complex chromosomal aberrations and mutations in the following:

- *Retinoblastoma (Rb):* Mutations are present in 70% of sporadic osteosarcomas; germline *Rb* mutations have a 1000-fold increased risk of osteosarcoma.
- *TP53:* Common in sporadic tumors; patients with Li-Fraumeni syndrome (germline *TP53* mutations) have greatly elevated risk.
- *INK4a* is inactivated in many osteosarcomas.
- *MDM2* and *CDK4,* cell cycle regulators that inhibit p53 and Rb function, respectively, are overexpressed in many low-grade osteosarcomas.

Morphology (p. 1199)

- *Gross:* Tumors are large, destructive, tan-white, gritty, and sometimes bloody and cystic masses.
- *Microscopic:* Osteosarcomas are composed of large, hyperchromatic, pleomorphic, mitotically active tumor cells. They can exhibit osteoblastic, chondroblastic, or fibroblastic differentiation; *all form neoplastic bone that frequently has a coarse, lacelike pattern.* Vascular invasion is usually conspicuous, and over half of any given tumor may be necrotic.

Clinical Course (p. 1199)

Most osteosarcomas are solitary, arising in the medullary cavity of the metaphyses (sites of bone growth) of extremity long bones; approximately half occur around the knee. Patients typically present with painful, progressively enlarging masses or a pathologic fracture. Imaging reveals destructive and infiltrative lesions with mixed blastic and lytic features. Osteosarcomas are aggressive malignancies, with 10% to 20% having demonstrable pulmonary metastases at the time of first diagnosis; many more have likely occult metastatic disease. Surgery and adjuvant chemotherapy yields a 60% to 70% 5-year survival in the absence of detectable metastases; with overt distal disease, the 5-year survival falls to 20%.

Cartilage-Forming Tumors (p. 1200)

Cartilage-forming tumors constitute the majority of primary bone neoplasms; most form hyaline or myxoid cartilage. Benign tumors are considerably more common than malignant ones.

Osteochondroma *(p. 1200; Also Called Exostosis)*

Osteochondroma is the most common benign bone tumor, afflicting men 3 times more commonly than women; 85% are solitary, whereas the remainder of cases occur as part of the autosomal-dominant *multiple hereditary exostosis syndrome.* Hereditary lesions are associated with loss-of-function mutations in *EXT1* or *EXT2* genes (encoding proteins that participate in the synthesis of heparin sulfate proteoglycans); sporadic lesions are associated with only *EXT1* inactivation. Reduced EXT activity leads to diminished glycosaminoglycan, preventing the normal diffusion of Ihh and disrupting normal chondrocyte differentiation.

Osteochondromas commonly develop in the metaphyseal region (near the growth plate) of long bones, especially near the knee. They present as slow-growing lesions that can be painful if they impinge on nerves or the stalk is fractured. In multiple hereditary exostosis, the underlying bone may be bowed and shortened reflecting abnormal epiphyseal growth. Solitary lesions infrequently give rise to chondrosarcomas; there is a 5% to 20% risk of progression with multiple hereditary osteochondromas.

Morphology (p. 1200)

- *Gross:* Lesions are mushroom-shaped surface protrusions 1 to 20 cm in size, covered by perichondrium overlying a hyaline cartilage cap.
- *Microscopic:* The cartilage cap has the appearance of a disorganized growth plate and undergoes enchondral ossification. The outer stalk cortex and medullary cavities of the cap are in continuity with the cortex and marrow cavity of the underlying bone.

Chondromas *(p. 1201)*

Chondromas are benign tumors composed of hyaline cartilage; *enchondromas* arise within the medullary cavity, whereas *juxtacortical chondromas* arise on the bone surface. They are usually solitary metaphyseal lesions of tubular bones, commonly occurring between ages 20 and 40 years. A syndrome with multiple enchondromas is called *Ollier disease;* similar enchondromatosis associated with hemangiomas is designated *Maffucci syndrome.*

Pathogenesis (p. 1201)

Mutations in the isocitrate dehydrogenase genes *IDH1* and *IDH2* in chondrocytes result in a new enzymatic activity that synthesizes 2-hydroxyglutarate, an "oncometabolite" that interferes with DNA methylation. Such 2-hydroxyglutarate can also diffuse into neighboring cells with normal IDH genes, causing oncogenetic epigenic transformation.

Morphology (p. 1201)

- *Gross:* Enchondromas are usually <3 cm and translucent gray-blue.
- *Microscopic:* Lesions are composed of well-circumscribed nodules of benign hyaline cartilage; there can be peripheral enchondral ossification and central calcification and necrosis.

Clinical Course (p. 1201)

Chondromas are usually asymptomatic but may cause bone deformity (especially in enchondromatosis), pain, and fracture. Radiologic imaging reveals characteristic circumscribed oval lucencies with a thin rim of radiodense bone; matrix calcification is detected as irregular opacification. Most tumors are stable, and treatment involves only curettage. Solitary lesion rarely undergoes malignant transformation; evolution to sarcomas occurs more frequently with enchondromatosis. Patients with Maffucci syndrome are at increased risk of ovarian carcinoma and central nervous system (CNS) gliomas.

Chondrosarcoma (p. 1202)

Chondrosarcoma is the second most common malignant matrix-producing bone tumor; it is approximately half as common as osteosarcoma. Most patients are over age 40, and the male to female ratio is 2:1. Most cases (85%) arise de novo, with the remainder occurring in a preexisting enchondroma or osteochondroma. These are genetically heterogeneous, but *IDH* mutations are common, as are CDKN2A tumor suppressor silencing in sporadic tumors and *EXT* mutations in chondromatosis syndromes. Most chondrosarcomas occur in the axial skeleton (pelvis, shoulders, ribs). Tumors typically present as painful, progressively enlarging masses. Radiologically there is endosteal scalloping and flocculent-appearing matrix calcification; slow-growing tumors cause reactive cortical thickening, whereas high-grade neoplasms destroy the cortex and form a soft-tissue mass. Treatment involves wide surgical excision and often chemotherapy. Lung is a favored metastatic site.

Morphology (p. 1202)

- *Gross:* Tumors are lobulated, gray, glistening, and semitranslucent; necrosis and spotty calcification are frequently present.
- *Microscopic:* Lesions are classified by histologic type and as *intramedullary* or *juxtacortical;* 90% are intramedullary *conventional* (hyaline) chondrosarcomas. The histologic grade (based on cellularity, cytologic atypia, and mitotic activity) correlates with biologic behavior; most tumors are low grade. Grade 1 lesions have 5-year survivals of 80% to 90%, whereas grade 3 lesions have a 43% 5-year survival.

Tumors of Unknown Origin (p. 1203)

Ewing Sarcoma Family Tumors (p. 1203)

Ewing sarcoma is a malignant bone tumor composed of primitive undifferentiated round cells. *Primitive neuroectodermal tumor (PNET)* is a similar tumor with some neuroectodermal differentiation, although the distinction is not clinically significant. Both entities are now unified into a single, common Ewing sarcoma family tumor (ESFT) category that accounts for 6% to 10% of primary malignant bone tumors; 80% of patients are >20 years, with boys affected slightly more frequently than girls, and with a striking predilection for whites.

Pathogenesis (p. 1203)

Most ESFT contain a t(11;22) translocation fusing the *EWS* gene to the *FLI1* gene, although variant translocations fuse *EWS* to other members of the ETS transcription factor family. The cell of origin is unknown.

Morphology (p. 1203)

- *Gross:* Tumors usually invade cortex and penetrate the periosteum to produce a tan-white soft tissue mass, often with focal hemorrhage and necrosis.
- *Microscopic:* Lesions are composed of sheets of uniform, small, round cells with scant clear cytoplasm, rich in glycogen. *Homer-Wright pseudorosettes*—tumor cells arrayed in a circle about a central fibrillary space—indicate neural differentiation.

Clinical Course (p. 1203)

ESFTs typically present as painful, enlarging, warm masses in the diaphysis of long tubular bones; fever, elevated sedimentation rate, and leukocytosis can mimic infection. Radiograms reveal an invasive lytic lesion; a characteristic periosteal reaction produces layers of reactive bone deposited in an onion-skin fashion. With combined radiation, chemotherapy, and surgery, there is a 75% 5-year survival rate.

Giant Cell Tumor (p. 1203)

These are benign but locally aggressive neoplasms of epiphyses and metaphyses occurring most commonly between the ages of 20 and 50.

Pathogenesis (p. 1203)

The vast majority of the tumor consists of *non-neoplastic* osteoclasts. The relatively infrequent *neoplastic* cells are osteoblast precursors that express high levels of RANKL, promoting osteoclast precursor proliferation and differentiation. The result is a localized but highly destructive osteoclast resorption of bone.

Morphology (p. 1233)

- *Gross:* Tumors are large and red-brown with frequent cystic degeneration.
- *Microscopic:* Plump, uniform mononuclear cells constitute the proliferating component of the tumor. In the background are scattered osteoclast-like, multinucleated giant cells. Focal necrosis, hemorrhage, hemosiderin, and reactive bone can also occur.

Clinical Course (p. 1204)

More than half of these tumors arise near the knees, but virtually any bone can be involved; location near joints frequently manifests as arthritis-like symptoms, but patients can also present with pathologic fractures. Most are solitary; radiology shows erosion into subchondral bone with a soft tissue mass delineated by a thin rim of reactive bone. Conservative surgery with curettage has a 40% to 60% recurrence rate, with up to 4% rate of lung metastasis. The RANKL inhibitor denosumab has shown promise.

Aneurysmal Bone Cyst (p. 1204)

This benign tumor often presents as a rapidly growing, expansile mass; aneurysmal bone cysts (ABCs) are associated with 17p13 translocations that cause increased expression of a USP6 deubiquitinating enzyme, which in turn leads to increased NF-κB activity.

Morphology (p. 1204)

- *Gross:* Lesions consist of multiple, blood-filled cystic spaces separated by thin, tan-white septa.
- *Microscopic:* The walls are composed of plump, uniform fibroblasts, multinucleated osteoclast-like giant cells, and reactive woven bone; a third of cases exhibit an unusual cartilage-like matrix, so-called blue bone.

Clinical Course (p. 1204)

Lesions generally present as pain and swelling, typically in the first two decades of life; long bone metaphyses or posterior elements of vertebral bodies are most often affected. Radiology shows expansile lytic lesions with a thin shell of reactive bone. Conservative surgical curettage is usually sufficient; the recurrence rate is low.

Lesions Simulating Primary Neoplasms (p. 1204)

Fibrous Cortical Defect and Nonossifying Fibroma (p. 1204)

Fibrous cortical defect and nonossifying fibroma are closely related benign tumors. Radiologically they are elongated, sharply demarcated radiolucencies, surrounded by a thin rim of sclerosis.

- *Fibrous cortical defects* are small (0.5 cm) developmental defects (rather than neoplasms) occurring in 30% to 50% of children over age 2. Most arise in the metaphysis of the distal femur or proximal tibia and are asymptomatic; the majority are eventually replaced by normal cortical bone.
- Nonossifying fibromas are 5 to 6 cm in size and develop from enlargement of fibrous cortical defects. These can present with a pathologic fracture; curettage and histologic evaluation are necessary to exclude other tumors.

Morphology (p. 1205)

These are gray-yellow cellular lesions containing cytologically bland fibroblasts and macrophages; the latter may be foamy or multinucleated.

Fibrous Dysplasia *(p. 1206)*

Fibrous dysplasia is a benign lesion akin to a localized developmental arrest; all the elements of normal bone are present but do not differentiate into mature structures.

Pathogenesis (p. 1206)

A somatic gain-of-function mutation in *GNAS1* produces a constitutively active G protein that promotes osteoblast proliferation and disrupts differentiation. The phenotype depends on (1) when in development the mutation is acquired and (2) the fate of the cell harboring the mutation. Thus a mutation during embryogenesis produces the McCune-Albright syndrome, whereas an osteoblast precursor mutation during skeletal formation results in monostotic fibrous dysplasia.

- In 70% of patients, only one bone is involved *(monostotic disease).* Lesions typically arise in early adolescence and stop growing at the point of epiphyseal fusion; boys and girls are equally affected. Most lesions are asymptomatic, but pain, fracture, discrepancies in limb length, or distortion of craniofacial bones can occur.
- *Polyostotic disease without endocrine dysfunction* manifests at a slightly earlier age than monostotic disease. Craniofacial, shoulder, and pelvic girdle involvement are extremely common and can cause crippling deformities (e.g., shepherd-crook deformity of the proximal femur).
- *Mazabraud syndrome* is a childhood polyostotic disease with multiple skeletal deformities; intramuscular myxomas present in adulthood often in the same anatomic regions.
- *McCune-Albright syndrome* is a polyostotic disease, associated with *café au lait* skin pigmentations and endocrine abnormalities. Of the latter the most common is precocious sexual development, most often in girls; other endocrinopathies (e.g., hyperthyroidism, GH-secreting pituitary adenomas, and primary adrenal hyperplasia) also occur.

Morphology (p. 1206)

- *Gross:* Lesions are well circumscribed, intramedullary, tan-white, gritty, and variable in size.
- *Microscopic:* Lesions are composed of curvilinear trabeculae of woven bone (likened to Chinese letters). Cystic degeneration, hemorrhage, foamy macrophages, and nodules of hyaline cartilage (resembling disorganized growth plates) can also be present.

Clinical Course (p. 1206)

The natural history depends on the extent and location of skeletal involvement. Isolated lesions can be cured by conservative surgery, whereas polyostotic involvement is often progressive and may require multiple procedures. Bisphosphonates can reduce bone pain. Rarely there is malignant transformation.

Metastatic Tumors *(p. 1207)*

In adults >75% of skeletal metastases originate from cancers of the prostate, breast, kidney, and lung. In children, metastatic disease derives most commonly from neuroblastoma, Wilms tumor, osteosarcoma, ESFT, and rhabdomyosarcoma. Osteolytic lesions are due to tumor cell elaboration of prostaglandins, ILs, and PTH-related protein that stimulates osteoclastic bone resorption. In turn, lysis of bone tissue rich in growth factors (e.g., TGF-β, insulin-like growth factor-1 [IGF-1], FGF, PDGF, and BMPs) helps to drive tumor growth. Osteosclerotic responses (most often induced by prostate cancer) occur through tumor elaboration of WNT proteins that stimulate osteoblastic activity.

JOINTS (p. 1207)

Hyaline cartilage is an elastic shock absorber and a wear-resistant surface situated at the end of apposed bones in synovial joints. Chondrocytes synthesize the type II collagen and proteoglycan matrix elements of hyaline cartilage, as well as secrete the degradative enzymes responsible for matrix turnover. Degradative enzymes are secreted as inactive precursors, and chondrocytes also enrich the matrix with enzyme inhibitors. Thus diseases that destroy articular cartilage do so by activating catabolic enzymes and by decreasing inhibitor synthesis. Cytokines, such as TNF and IL-1—derived from chondrocytes, synoviocytes, fibroblasts, and inflammatory cells—can trigger the degradative process.

Osteoarthritis (p. 1208)

OA (degenerative joint disease [DJD]) is characterized by progressive erosion of articular cartilage as degradation exceeds synthesis:

- *Primary DJD* appears insidiously, largely as an aging phenomenon and only in a few joints; knees and hands are affected more in women and hips more in men.
- *Secondary DJD* appears at any age in a previously damaged or congenitally abnormal joint or in patients with systemic disorders, such as diabetes, ochronosis, or hemochromatosis.

Pathogenesis (p. 1208)

OA has both genetic and environmental components, influenced by levels of prostaglandins, cytokines (e.g., TNF and TGF-β), and nitric oxide synthesis, as well as by variables, such as aging, obesity, muscle strength, and joint architecture. Phases of OA are as follows:

- Chondrocyte injury due to aging, biochemical and genetic effects, and trauma
- Chondrocyte proliferation and secretion of matrix and inflammatory mediators resulting in cartilage remodeling and secondary changes in synovium and subchondral bone
- Chondrocyte dropout and cartilage loss due to repetitive injury and chronic inflammation

Morphology (p. 1208)

- *Gross:* The articular surface is soft with dislodged fragments of cartilage and subchondral bone forming loose bodies *(joint mice)*. Exposed subchondral bone is burnished by the opposing degenerated articular surface *(bone eburnation)*, and the underlying cancellous bone becomes sclerotic. Small fractures allow synovial fluid to be expressed into the subchondral bone to form cystic spaces. Bony overgrowths *(osteophytes)* capped by cartilage also develop at the edges of the articular cartilage; *Heberden nodes* are osteophytes of the distal interphalangeal joints (common in women).
- *Microscopic:* In early OA there is chondrocyte proliferation, with increased matrix water and decreased proteoglycan content; this is followed by fibrillation and cracking of the matrix as superficial layers are degraded. The synovium is mildly congested with scattered chronic inflammation.

Clinical Course (p. 1208)

OA is an insidious and slowly progressive disease; patients characteristically develop deep achy joint pain that worsens with use, morning stiffness, crepitus, and limited range of motion. Osteophyte compression on spinal foramina can cause radicular pain, muscle spasm or atrophy, and neurologic deficits. There are no effective methods to halting DJD progression; therapy includes pain management, activity modification, and joint replacement.

Rheumatoid Arthritis (p. 1209)

Rheumatoid arthritis (RA) is a chronic systemic inflammatory disease that principally attacks joints, producing a nonsuppurative proliferative synovitis that progresses to joint destruction and ankylosis; blood vessels, skin, heart, lungs, and muscles can also be impacted. Approximately 1% of the U.S. population is affected, women threefold more commonly than men; peak incidence is between 20 and 50 years.

Pathogenesis (p. 1209)

RA is triggered by exposure of a genetically susceptible host to an arthritogenic antigen (microbial or self), resulting in loss of self-tolerance and a chronic autoimmune response (Fig. 26-5). Half of the risk of developing RA is related to inherited genetic susceptibility, with linkage to specific HLA-DRB1 alleles that influence the ability to bind to the arthritogen(s) that initiate the inflammatory synovitis. *PTPN22* mutations are also linked to RA; these encode a protein tyrosine phosphatase that influences T-cell activation.

- T_H17 cells secrete IL-17, which recruits neutrophils and monocytes.
- T_H1 cells secrete IFN-γ, which activates macrophages and resident synovial cells.
- Activated macrophages secrete TNF and IL-1, which stimulate resident synovial cells to secrete proteases (especially matrix metalloproteinases) that destroy hyaline cartilage.
- RANKL expressed on activated T cells stimulates bone resorption.

RA synovium contains germinal centers with secondary follicles, abundant plasma cells, and antibodies, some of which are directed against self-antigens. Many autoantibodies are specific for *citrullinated peptides* (CCPs, in which arginine residues are posttranslationally converted to citrulline); such CCPs include citrullinated

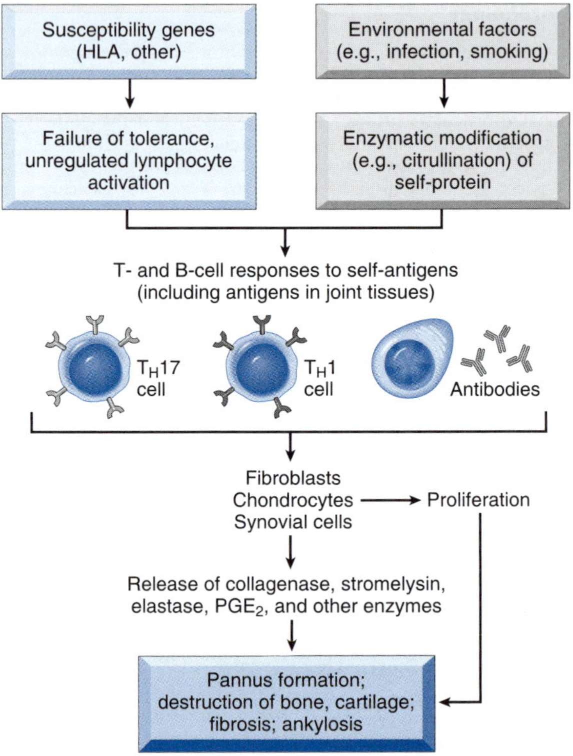

Figure 26-5 Pathogenesis of RA. *HLA,* Human leukocyte antigen; *PGE_2,* prostglandin E_2.

fibrinogen, type II collagen, α-enolase, and vimentin. Antibodies against these peptides are diagnostic markers for RA and elevated titers of anti-CCP antibodies (in combination with T-cell responses to CCPs) contribute to disease chronicity.

Approximately 80% of RA patients also have serum immunoglobulin (Ig)M or IgA autoantibodies that bind to the IgG Fc regions—so-called *rheumatoid factor;* the link to pathogenesis is questionable.

Morphology (p. 1211)

- Joints
  - *Gross:* In early stages the synovium is edematous and hyperplastic, exhibiting delicate and bulbous fronds. At later stages a *pannus* of proliferative synovium, inflammatory cells, and fibroblasts encroaches on the hyaline cartilage, leading to its destruction; the pannus can bridge apposing bones to form a *fibrous ankylosis* that will eventually ossify.
  - *Microscopic:* Lesions show a dense, perivascular mononuclear inflammatory cell infiltrate with focal lymphoid aggregates; neutrophils accumulate on the synovial surface and in the synovial fluid. Vasodilation and increased vascular permeability are reflected by hemosiderin deposits and aggregates of organizing fibrin. There is osteoclast activation with bone erosion, osteoporosis, and subchondral cysts.

- Skin
  - *Gross:* Rheumatoid *nodules* are firm, nontender nodules arising in subcutaneous tissues in a quarter of patients, typically in regions subjected to recurrent pressure (e.g., elbows); they can also occur in lungs, spleen, heart valves, aorta, and other viscera.
  - *Microscopic:* Lesions exhibit a central zone of fibrinoid necrosis, surrounded by a palisade of activated macrophages.
- Blood vessels
  - Patients with severe disease and high titers of rheumatoid factor are at increased risk of developing small- to medium-sized vessel vasculitis comparable to polyarteritis nodosa (see Chapter 11).

Clinical Course (p. 1211)

Although the clinical course is variable, nonspecific malaise, fatigue, and generalized musculoskeletal pain progress insidiously to localized joint involvement. RA generally involves small joints first (digits before wrist, ankles, elbows, and knees) in a bilaterally symmetric pattern; affected joints are swollen, warm, and painful, particularly following inactivity. There is typically progressive joint involvement over months to years, with some fluctuation in tempo; the greatest damage occurs in the first 4 to 5 years. Destruction of tendons, ligaments, and joint capsules leads to classic lesions, including radial deviation of the wrist, ulnar deviation of the fingers, and flexion-hyperextension abnormalities of the digits. Ultimately the deformed joints lose stability and have minimal range of motion. Radiologically there are joint effusions, with juxtaarticular osteopenia, and narrowing of the joint space as articular cartilage is lost. Therapies include corticosteroids, methotrexate, and TNF antagonists; the latter have proven especially effective. Long-term complications include *systemic amyloidosis* in 5% to 10% of patients or opportunistic infections in patients receiving immunosuppression or anti-TNF therapies.

Juvenile Idiopathic Arthritis (p. 1212)

Juvenile idiopathic arthritis (JIA) is a heterogeneous group of disorders characterized by arthritis occurring before age 16 and persisting for at least 6 weeks; 30,000 to 50,000 children are affected annually in the United States. Like RA, JIA is associated with both environmental factors and genetic susceptibility; the CD4+ dysregulation and inflammatory synovitis are also similar. JIA *differs from* RA by the following:

- Oligoarthritis is more common.
- Systemic disease is more frequent.
- Large joints are affected more often than small joints.
- Rheumatoid nodules and rheumatoid factor are usually absent.
- Antinuclear antibody (ANA) seropositivity is common.

The long-term prognosis of JIA is variable; although some individuals will have sustained disease activity, only 10% develop serious functional disability. Therapies are similar to those for RA.

Seronegative Spondyloarthropathies (p. 1212)

These represent a group of putatively autoimmune diseases initiated by environmental factors (especially infections) in genetically predisposed individuals; the manifestations are immune-mediated. All have similar synovial inflammation but are distinguished by various overlapping patterns of extraarticular involvement (e.g., skin, cardiovascular system, and eyes). Many are associated with the HLA-B27 allele but without specific autoantibodies (hence "seronegative").

Ankylosing Spondylitis (p. 1213)

Also called *rheumatoid spondylitis* and *Marie-Strümpell disease,* this is a chronic ankylosing synovitis of vertebrae and sacroiliac joints. Approximately 90% of patients are HLA-B27 positive; there are also associations with the IL-23 receptor.

Reactive Arthritis (p. 1213)

This entity is defined by a triad of *arthritis, nongonococcal urethritis* (or cervicitis), and *conjunctivitis.* The typical patient is a 20- to 40-year-old man; more than 80% will be HLA-B27 positive. The pathogenesis involves an autoimmune response triggered by prior infection of the genitourinary system *(Chlamydia)* or the gastrointestinal (GI) tract *(Shigella, Salmonella, Yersinia, Campylobacter);* arthritic symptoms develop within several weeks of the initial urethritis or diarrhea. Extraarticular manifestations include balanitis, conjunctivitis, cardiac conduction abnormalities, and aortic regurgitation. Arthritis usually waxes and wanes over several weeks to 6 months; half of patients will develop recurrent arthritis, tendinitis, and lumbosacral pain.

Enteritis-Associated Arthritis (p. 1213)

This entity is caused by GI infection with *Yersinia, Salmonella, Shigella,* or *Campylobacter.* The arthritis appears abruptly and tends to involve knees and ankles; it typically remits after a year, without ankylosing spondylitis.

Psoriatic Arthritis (p. 1213)

This develops in 10% of patients with psoriasis. The arthritis usually affects small hand and foot joints but can extend to ankles, knees, hips, and wrists; spinal disease occurs in 20% to 40%. Psoriatic arthritis is not as severe as RA, and there is less joint destruction.

Infectious Arthritis (p. 1213)

Joints can be seeded hematogenously or by direct extension from a soft tissue abscess or osteomyelitis; infectious arthritis can rapidly destroy a joint and produce permanent deformities.

Suppurative Arthritis (p. 1213)

Suppurative arthritis is most commonly caused by gonococcus, staphylococcus, streptococcus, *Haemophilus influenzae* (especially children under age 2), and gram-negative bacilli; individuals with sickle cell disease are prone to infection with *Salmonella.* In most instances a single joint is affected, with the knee being most common. Predisposing conditions include immune deficiency, debilitating illness, joint trauma, chronic arthritis, and intravenous drug use.

Mycobacterial Arthritis (p. 1214)

This is an insidious chronic arthritis involving hematogenous spread or nearby tuberculous osteomyelitis; hips, knees, and ankles are commonly involved. Chronic disease results in severe destruction with fibrous ankylosis.

Lyme Arthritis (p. 1214)

This is caused by *Borrelia burgdorferi* infection, occurring in 60% to 80% of untreated individuals several weeks to 2 years after the initial skin infection. The arthritis is oligoarticular, remitting and migratory, and primarily involving large joints (knees, shoulders, elbows, and ankles). The articular involvement histologically resembles RA; in most cases it clears spontaneously or with antibiotic therapy, but in approximately 10% a presumed autoimmune arthritis supervenes, resulting in permanent deformities.

Viral Arthritis (p. 1214)

This can occur with a wide variety of viral infections, but it is unclear whether the joint symptoms result from direct infection or secondary to an autoimmune response; arthritic syndromes associated with human immunodeficiency virus (HIV) infections are presumed autoimmune.

Crystal-Induced Arthritis (p. 1214)

Both endogenous (urate, hydroxyapatite) and exogenous (talc, prosthetic biomaterials) crystals can trigger cytokine-mediated cartilage destruction.

Gout (p. 1214)

Gout is characterized by transient attacks of *acute arthritis* initiated by crystallization of urates around joints, leading eventually to *chronic gouty arthritis* and *tophi* (large aggregates of urate crystals and associated inflammation). Hyperuricemia (>6.8 mg/dL) is necessary but not sufficient to cause gout; it can result from abnormalities in uric acid synthesis or excretion:

- *Synthesis:* Uric acid is the end product of purine catabolism; increased synthesis typically reflects abnormal purine production. There is both de novo synthesis from nonpurine precursors, as well as salvage pathway synthesis using dietary purine bases and purine nucleotide catabolites.
- *Excretion:* Uric acid is filtered from the circulation by the glomerulus and almost completely resorbed by the renal proximal tubule; a small fraction of the resorbed uric acid is then secreted by the distal nephron into the urine.

Pathogenesis (p. 1215)

Hyperuricemia can occur through uric acid overproduction or reduced renal excretion.

- *Primary gout* is caused by increased uric acid biosynthesis. A small minority of patients have overproduction due to partial deficiency of hypoxanthine guanine phosphoribosyl transferase (HGPRT), blocking the salvage pathway; complete absence of HGPRT also results in hyperuricemia, but the clinical phenotype is dominated by significant neurologic manifestations *(Lesch-Nyhan syndrome)*.

- *Secondary gout* can be caused by increased production (e.g., rapid cell lysis during chemotherapy for leukemia) or decreased excretion (chronic renal disease). Gout-associated polymorphisms involve genes that regulate urate transport and homeostasis (e.g., URAT1 and GLUT9).

Inflammation in gout is triggered by precipitation of monosodium urate (MSU) crystals in joints. MSU is phagocytosed by macrophages, activating intracellular inflammasomes (see Chapter 6) that, in turn, activate caspase-1 to generate IL-1. IL-1 is proinflammatory, promoting leukocyte recruitment and activation, with the downstream generation of other cytokines, free radicals, proteases, and arachidonic acid metabolites. Urate crystals can also activate the complement system. These cascades trigger an acute arthritis, which typically remits spontaneously in days to weeks.

Many factors contribute to the conversion of asymptomatic hyperuricemia into primary gout, including age of the patient and duration of elevated uric acids. Heavy alcohol consumption, obesity, and drugs (e.g., thiazides) and toxins (e.g., lead) that reduce urate excretion also influence gout development. The solubility of MSU in a joint is also modulated by temperature and the chemical composition of the fluid.

Morphology (p. 1216)

- *Acute arthritis:* Lesions exhibit a dense neutrophilic infiltrate within the synovium and synovial fluid; slender, birefringent MSU crystals are present in the edematous and congested synovium and within neutrophils; there is scattered chronic inflammation.
- *Chronic tophaceous arthritis:* Urates can encrust the articular surfaces and form grossly visible synovial deposits. The synovium becomes hyperplastic and fibrotic, with increased inflammatory infiltrates; a synovial pannus extends from the cartilage into juxtaarticular bone, causing erosions and fibrosis, and eventually producing a bony ankylosis.
- *Tophi are pathognomonic lesions:* These are masses of urates, crystalline or amorphous, surrounded by intense mononuclear inflammation with foreign body giant cells. Tophi tend to occur on the ear, in the olecranon and patellar bursae, and in periarticular ligaments and connective tissue.
- *Gouty nephropathy* is associated with renal medullary MSU deposition (including tophi) and uric acid stones; obstruction can cause a secondary pyelonephritis.

Clinical Course (p. 1216)

After years of asymptomatic hyperuricemia, acute gouty arthritis is classically announced by excruciating joint pain accompanied by localized hyperemia and warmth; most first presentations are monoarticular, and half of the initial attacks involve the great toe (followed by insteps, ankles, or heels and knees). Typically the acute episode resolves, followed by an *asymptomatic intercritical period.* Although some patients never have another flare, in the majority, recurrent attacks tend to happen with greater frequency and become polyarticular. Eventually (12 years on average) chronic tophaceous gout develops with joint effacement. Cardiovascular disease (atherosclerosis and hypertension) is a common accompanying pathology, and 20% of patients will die of renal failure secondary to gouty nephropathy.

Calcium Pyrophosphate Crystal Deposition Disease (Pseudogout) (p. 1217)

Calcium pyrophosphate crystal deposition (CPPD) disease typically occurs after age 50, with a 30% to 60% prevalence by age 85; the hereditary variant presents somewhat earlier and the phenotype is more severe. An autosomal dominant form of the disease is due to mutations in the *ANKH* gene encoding a pyrophosphate transport channel. The most common *secondary* form is associated with a variety of etiologies, including trauma, hyperparathyroidism, hemochromatosis, and diabetes; altered matrix synthesis and degradation of pyrophosphates are implicated.

The clinicopathologic features are similar to gout. The crystals initially form in cartilage; as deposits enlarge they rupture and seed the joint where macrophages engulf them and activate their inflammasomes to generate IL-1β. Subsequent neutrophil recruitment and recurrent bouts of inflammation result in joint damage in more than 50% of patients. Knees, wrists, elbows, shoulders, and ankles are affected (in decreasing order).

Morphology (p. 1217)

- *Gross:* Crystals form chalky white, friable deposits; they rarely deposit in large masses.
- *Microscopic:* Crystals stain as oval, blue-purple aggregates; they are weakly birefringent and have geometric shapes. Chronic lesions exhibit mononuclear cell infiltrates with fibrosis.

Joint Tumors and Tumorlike Lesions (p. 1218)

Ganglion and Synovial Cysts (p. 1218)

- *Ganglions* are small (1- to 1.5-cm), multiloculated, cystic lesions of connective tissues near joint capsules or tendon sheaths (the wrist is a common site). They arise through myxoid degeneration and softening of connective tissues; they are not lined by epithelium and do not communicate with joint spaces.
- *Synovial cysts* are herniations of synovium through joint capsules (e.g., a *Baker cyst* arising in the popliteal fossa). The synovial lining may be hyperplastic and contain scattered inflammation.

Tenosynovial Giant Cell Tumor (p. 1218)

This is the term for a group of closely related benign neoplasms involving synovial membranes, tendon sheaths, and bursae. They all share a t(1;2) chromosomal translocation that fuses the promoter for the α3 chain of collagen type VI gene to the coding sequence of the monocyte colony-stimulating factor (M-CSF) gene. As a result the lesions overexpress M-CSF, leading to the accumulation of swarms of macrophages. Variants include the following:

- *Diffuse type* (previously called *pigmented villonodular tenosynovitis*), typically presenting in the knee (80%) with pain, "locking," and swelling; range of motion is decreased, and aggressive lesions erode into the bone and adjacent soft tissue.
- *Localized type (giant cell tumor of the tendon sheath),* commonly manifesting as a solitary painless mass involving the tendon sheaths of the wrist and fingers; cortical bone erosion affects 15%.

Morphology (p. 1218)

- *Gross:* Lesions are red-brown to mottled orange-yellow. In diffuse disease the synovium is a tangled mat of red-brown folds, nodules, and fingerlike projections that spread along the articular surface and infiltrate the subsynovial tissue. In the localized form, tumors are well circumscribed and nodular and may be attached to the synovium by a pedicle.

- *Microscopic:* Neoplastic cells (only 2% to 16% of the total) are polyhedral and resemble synoviocytes. Both types of lesions are heavily infiltrated by macrophages, often containing hemosiderin and forming multinucleated giant cells.

SOFT TISSUE TUMORS (p. 1219)

Soft tissue tumors are mesenchymal proliferations of extraskeletal nonepithelial tissues, excluding viscera, meninges, and lymphatics. These are typically classified according to the tissue they recapitulate, although some have no apparent normal tissue counterpart. Benign lesions outnumber malignant 100:1; only 12,000 sarcomas are diagnosed annually in the United States, but these tend to be highly lethal, commonly with hematogenous metastasis to bone and lung.

Pathogenesis (p. 1219)

The cause in most cases is unknown, although individual soft tissue tumors can be associated with radiation, prior trauma or chemical injury, some chemical exposures, and infection (e.g., human herpesvirus 8 and Kaposi sarcoma). Most are sporadic, although a minority are associated with heritable syndromes (e.g., neurofibromatosis type 1 and Gardner syndrome). In 15% to 20% of cases, specific translocations give rise to aberrant transcription factor expression that drives neoplastic transformation (Table 26-3); these tend to arise in younger patients and appear more monomorphic. In the remainder of cases the karyotypes are complex and heterogeneous, reflecting genomic instability; these tend to arise in adults and are pleomorphic in morphology.

Classification (p. 1219)

Classification integrates morphology (differentiation), immunohistochemistry, and molecular diagnostics (Table 26-4). Accurate diagnosis, grade, and stage (size, depth, and metastatic spread) all influence prognosis.

Tumors of Adipose Tissue (p. 1220)

Lipoma (p. 1220)

Lipomas are the most common benign soft tissue tumor of adults; they are subclassified according to morphologic features (e.g., fibrolipoma, angiolipoma, spindle cell lipoma), and some have characteristic genetic rearrangements. They are usually soft, mobile, painless (except angiolipomas), and cured by simple excision.

Morphology (p. 1220)

Lipomas are well-encapsulated tumors (of variable size) of mature adipocytes. Infrequently they can be large, intramuscular, and poorly circumscribed.

Liposarcoma (p. 1220)

Liposarcomas are one of the more common adult sarcomas; they typically appear between ages 50 and 70, presenting as large masses

TABLE 26-3 Chromosomal Abnormalities in Soft Tissue Tumors

Tumor	Cytogenetic Abnormality	Gene Fusion	Proposed Function
ESFTs	t(11;22)(q24;q12) t(21;22)(q22;q12)	*EWS-FLI1* *EWS-ERG*	Disordered protein with multiple functions, including aberrant transcription, cell cycle regulation, RNA splicing and telomerase
Extraskeletal myxoid chondrosarcoma	t(9;22)(q22;q12)	*EWS-CHN*	
Desmoplastic small round-cell tumor	t(11;22)(p13;q12)	*EWS-WT1*	
Clear-cell sarcoma	t(12;22)(q13;q12)	*EWS-ATF1*	
Liposarcoma—myxoid and round-cell type	t(12;16)(q13;p11)	*FUS-DDIT3*	Arrests adipocytic differentiation
Synovial sarcoma	t(x;18)(p11;q11)	*SS18-SSX1* *SS18-SSX2* *SS18-SSX4*	Chimeric transcription factors, interrupt cell cycle control
Rhabdomyosarcoma—alveolar type	t(2;13)(q35;q14) t(1;13)(p36;q14)	*PAX3-FOXO1* *PAX7-FOXO1*	Chimeric transcription factors, disrupt skeletal muscle differentiation
Dermatofibrosarcoma protuberans	t(17;22)(q22;q15)	*COLA1-PDGFB*	Promoter-driven overexpression of PDGF-β, autocrine stimulation
Alveolar soft-part sarcoma	t(X;17)(p11.2;q25)	*TFE3-ASPL*	Unknown
Infantile fibrosarcoma	t(12;15)(p13;q23)	*ETV6-NTRK3*	Chimeric tyrosine kinase leads to constitutively active Ras/MAPK pathway
Nodular fasciitis	t(22;17)	*MYH9-USP6*	Unknown

TABLE 26-4 Soft Tissue Tumors

Category	Behavior	Tumor Type	Common Locations	Age (yr)	Morphology
Adipose	Benign	Lipoma	Superficial extremity, trunk	40-60	Mature adipose tissue
	Malignant	Well-differentiated liposarcoma	Deep extremity, retroperitoneum	50-60	Adipose tissue with scattered atypical spindle cells
		Myxoid liposarcoma	Thigh, leg	30s	Myxoid matrix, "chicken wire" vessels, round cells, lipoblasts
Fibrous	Benign	Nodular fasciitis	Arm, forearm	20-30	Tissue culture growth, extravasated erythrocytes
		Deep fibromatosis	Abdominal wall	30-40	Dense collagen, long, unidirectional fascicles
Skeletal muscle	Benign	Rhabdomyoma	Head and neck	0-60	Polygonal rhabdomyoblasts, "spider" cells
	Malignant	Alveolar rhabdomyosarcoma	Extremities, sinuses	5-15	Uniform round discohesive cells between septae
		Embryonal rhabdomyosarcoma	Genitourinary tract	1-5	Primitive spindle cells, "strap" cells
Smooth muscle	Benign	Leiomyoma	Extremity	20s	Uniform, plump eosinophilic cells in fascicles
	Malignant	Leiomyosarcoma	Thigh, retroperitoneum	40-60	Pleomorphic eosinophilic cells
Vascular	Benign	Hemangioma	Head and neck	0-10	Circumscribed mass of capillary or venous channels
	Malignant	Angiosarcoma	Skin, deep lower extremity	50-80	Infiltrating capillary channels
Nerve sheath	Benign	Schwannoma	Head and neck	20-50	Encapsulated, fibrillar stroma, nuclear palisading
		Neurofibroma	Wide, cutaneous, subcutis	10-20+	Myxoid, ropy collagen, loose fascicles, mast cells
	Malignant	Malignant peripheral nerve sheath tumor	Extremities, shoulder girdle	20-50	Tight fascicles, atypia, mitotic activity, necrosis
Uncertain histotype	Benign	Solitary fibrous tumor	Pelvis, pleura	20-70	Branching ectatic vessels,
	Malignant	Synovial sarcoma	Thigh, leg	15-40	Tight fascicles of uniform basophilic spindle cells Pseudoglandular structures
		UPS	Thigh	40-70	High-grade anaplastic polygonal, round or spindle cells Bizarre nuclei, atypical mitoses, necrosis
		Alveolar soft part sarcoma	Trunk, extremities	15-35	Multiple nodules of eosinophilic round cells, septae
		Clear cell sarcoma	Tendons, extremities	20-40	Sheets of pale or clear spindle cells, wreathlike giant cells

in deep soft tissues of the proximal extremities and retroperitoneum. Well-differentiated forms are relatively indolent, whereas the pleomorphic variant is highly aggressive, and the myxoid or round cell type (with a characteristic t[12;16] translocation that affects *MDM2* expression) is intermediate in its behavior.

Morphology *(p. 1220)*

In well-differentiated liposarcomas the tumor cells are readily recognized as lipocytes. In other variants, adipogenic differentiation may not be obvious. Nevertheless, cells showing fatty differentiation are almost always present; such *lipoblasts* mimic fetal fat cells with clear cytoplasmic lipid droplets that scallop the nucleus.

Fibrous Tumors (p. 1221)

Nodular Fasciitis (p. 1221)

These are non-neoplastic lesions that either are idiopathic or develop in response to trauma (25% of cases); they can grow rapidly and can be alarming due to hypercellularity, high mitotic activity, and reactive mesenchymal cells. A t(17;22) translocation produces an *MYH9-USP6* fusion gene that causes a clonal but limited proliferation. It typically spontaneously regresses and if excised, rarely recurs.

Morphology *(p. 1221)*

- *Gross:* Neoplasms are typically large and nodular, with ill-defined margins.
- *Microscopic:* Lesions are cellular and highly mitotic, with plump, reactive, immature-appearing fibroblasts and myofibroblasts arranged randomly or in intersecting fascicles. Lesions often exhibit myxoid stroma and scattered lymphocytes.

Fibromatoses (p. 1221)

Superficial Fibromatosis *(p. 1221)*

Superficial fibromatosis encompasses a group of benign fibroproliferative lesions with abundant dense collagen. Males are affected more frequently than females.

- *Palmar fibromatosis (Dupuytren contracture)* presents with irregular thickening of the palmar fascia; it is bilateral in 50% of affected individuals. Attachment to the overlying skin leads to skin puckering, and patients develop a slowly progressive flexion contracture of the fourth and fifth fingers.
- *Plantar fibromatosis* is essentially the same process occurring on the foot; however, bilaterality and contractures are uncommon.
- *Penile fibromatosis (Peyronie disease)* usually occurs on the dorsolateral penis, leading to abnormal curvature and/or urethral constriction.

Deep Fibromatosis (Desmoid Tumor) *(p. 1222)*

These neoplasms have no metastatic potential but are nevertheless locally aggressive, often painful, and frequently recur after incomplete excision; women from teens to 30s are most commonly affected. *APC* or β-catenin gene mutations are typically present. In addition to surgery, tumors can be treated with tamoxifen, cyclooxygenase 2 inhibitors, or tyrosine kinase inhibitors. Most are sporadic, but patients with *APC* mutations (e.g., Gardner syndrome) are predisposed to deep fibromatosis.

Morphology (p. 1222)

- *Gross:* Tumors are 1- to 15-cm, gray-white, rubbery, poorly demarcated masses.
- *Microscopic:* Lesions are composed of banal fibroblasts arrayed in broad sweeping fascicles that infiltrate neighboring tissues.

Skeletal Muscle Tumors (p. 1222)

Most skeletal muscle tumors are malignant. The benign counterpart, rhabdomyoma, is rare; cardiac rhabdomyomas occur in association with tuberous sclerosis (see Chapter 28).

Rhabdomyosarcoma (p. 1222)

Rhabdomyosarcoma is the most common soft tissue sarcoma of children; most occur in the head and neck or in the genitourinary tract. These are aggressive neoplasms, treated with surgery, radiation, and chemotherapy. Lesions are histologically subclassified into three major types that have slightly different clinical features:

- *Embryonal rhabdomyosarcoma* is the most common (60%); it typically occurs in children under age 10 and involves the nasal cavity, orbit, middle ear, prostate, and paratesticular region. Tumors often have parental isodisomy of chromosome 11p15 leading to overexpression of the imprinted *IGFII* gene. The *botryoides* subtype develops in the walls of hollow, mucosal-lined structures (e.g., nasopharynx, common bile duct, bladder, and vagina), and overall has the best prognosis.
- *Alveolar rhabdomyosarcoma* (20%) tends to arise in middle adolescence in the deep musculature of extremities. This type is associated with translocations that fuse either *PAX3* or *PAX7* to *FOXO1A* (t[2,13] or t[1,13] translocations, respectively) (Table 26-3).
- *Pleomorphic rhabdomyosarcoma* is rare, occurring in the deep soft tissue of adults.

Morphology *(p. 1222)*

- The rhabdomyoblast is the diagnostic cell; although they can be round or elongate, all contain sarcomeres (sometimes only apparent by electron microscopy) and express myogenic markers.
- *Embryonal rhabdomyosarcomas* present as soft, gray, infiltrative masses; the *botryoid* variant resembles a cluster of grapes. Tumor cells form sheets of round and spindled cells in a myxoid stroma.
- *Alveolar rhabdomyosarcomas* exhibit a network of fibrous septae that divide the tumor cells into clusters or aggregates resembling alveoli; tumor cells are moderately sized but may have little cytoplasm.
- *Pleomorphic rhabdomyosarcomas* resemble other pleomorphic sarcomas.

Smooth Muscle Tumors (p. 1223)

Leiomyoma (p. 1223)

Benign smooth muscle tumors arise predominantly in the uterus, occurring in 77% of women (see Chapter 22); they can occur at other body sites where smooth muscle is well represented. Lesions are usually <1 to 2 cm and composed of fascicles of bland-appearing smooth muscle cells with few mitoses. A syndrome of multiple cutaneous leiomyomas arising from arrector pili muscles in association with uterine leiomyomas and renal cell carcinomas can be transmitted as an autosomal dominant disorder; it is linked to a loss-of-function mutation in the fumarate hydratase gene.

Leiomyosarcoma (p. 1223)

Leimyosarcomas account for 10% to 20% of soft tissue sarcomas; they are more common in women than men and typically occur in the skin and deep soft tissues of the extremities and retroperitoneum. Superficial leiomyosarcomas are usually small and have a good prognosis; tumors of the retroperitoneum are usually large and nonresectable, and cause death through local extension and metastasis.

Morphology *(p. 1223)*

- *Gross:* Tumors are usually painless, firm masses.
- *Microscopic:* Lesions consist of malignant spindle cells in interweaving fascicles; bundles of muscle filaments can be demonstrated ultrastructurally and by immunohistochemistry.

Tumors of Uncertain Origin (p. 1223)

Synovial Sarcoma (p. 1223)

Despite the name, the cell of origin is not clear; moreover, <10% are intraarticular. These account for 10% of soft tissue tumors; most occur between ages 20 and 50, and most arise in the deep soft tissues of the lower extremity (knee and thigh). Tumors often exhibit a characteristic t(x;18) translocation that produces a chimeric transcription factor (Table 26-3). Lesions are treated surgically and with chemotherapy; 5-year survivals are 25% to 62%, depending on stage and patient age.

Morphology *(p. 1224)*

Histologically lesions can be biphasic (with both cuboidal epithelial and spindled mesenchymal differentiation) or monophasic (mostly mesenchymal). Occasionally there are calcified concretions that can be detected radiologically.

Undifferentiated Pleomorphic Sarcoma (p. 1224)

These include malignant mesenchymal tumors with high-grade, pleomorphic cells that cannot be classified into another category; undifferentiated pleomorphic sarcoma (UPS) represents the largest category of adult sarcomas. Most arise in the deep soft tissues of the extremity, especially the thigh of middle-aged or older adults; these are typically aneuploid with multiple chromosomal abnormalities. UPS are aggressive malignancies that are treated with surgery and adjuvant chemotherapy and/or radiation; prognosis is generally poor.

Morphology *(p. 1224)*

UPS are usually large (10- to 20-cm), gray-white, fleshy masses, commonly with necrosis and hemorrhage. They consist of sheets of large, anaplastic cells, with irregular and occasionally bizarre hyperchromatic nuclei, and without demonstrable lineage differentiation.

27 Peripheral Nerves and Skeletal Muscles

Neuromuscular diseases are typically characterized by weakness, muscle pain, or sensory deficits; anatomy, tempo of disease progression, and underlying pathogenesis are organizing principles. The following will be grouped according to whether the disease preferentially affects the following:

- Peripheral nerve
- Neuromuscular junction
- Skeletal muscles

Diseases of Peripheral Nerves (p. 1227)

Somatic motor function is carried out by the ***motor unit:***

- A single *lower motor neuron* (spinal anterior horn cell or brain stem cranial nerve motor neuron)
- *Axon* of the neuron
- *Neuromuscular junction*
- *Muscle fibers* innervated by the neuron

Somatic sensory function depends on the following:

- The distal nerve endings (often with specialized structures that recognize specific sensory modalities)
- Axon connecting to the dorsal root ganglia
- Proximal axon synapsing on spinal cord or brainstem neurons

Nerve fibers are composed of axons and their associated Schwann cells and myelin sheath; *peripheral nerves* consist of multiple fibers grouped into fascicles by connective tissue sheaths. Most peripheral nerves have both motor and sensory fibers. *Myelinated* and *unmyelinated* nerves intermingle within each fascicle.

- *Unmyelinated fibers* far outnumber myelinated fibers; a single Schwann cell envelops 5 to 20 fibers.
- *Myelinated fibers* are ensheathed by multiple Schwann cells (but each Schwann cell myelinates only one neuron); these cells wrap around each axonal segment (internode) and are separated by *nodes of Ranvier.*

General Types of Peripheral Nerve Injury (p. 1228)

Axonal Neuropathies (p. 1228)

Primary axonal injury (e.g., due to trauma or ischemia) precipitates secondary myelin sheath dissolution (Fig. 27-1). *Wallerian degeneration* is the reaction distal to a transected axon; it reflects axonal and myelin breakdown with macrophage recruitment and phagocytosis. The proximal uninjured nerve may show focal degeneration of the

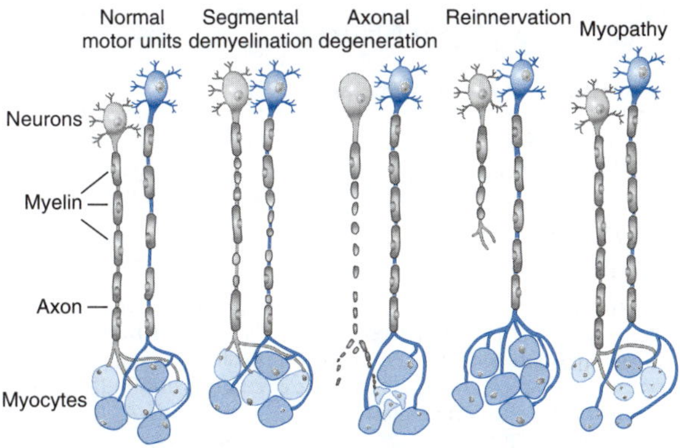

Figure 27-1 Normal and abnormal motor units. *Normal motor units:* Two adjacent motor units are shown (*light* and *dark*). *Segmental demyelination:* Random myelin internodes are injured and remyelinated by multiple Schwann cells; axons and myocytes are intact. *Axonal degeneration:* Axon and myelin sheath both undergo anterograde degeneration, causing denervation atrophy of the associated myocytes in the motor unit. *Reinnervation:* Sprouting of adjacent uninjured motor axons leads to myocyte fiber *type grouping;* meanwhile, the injured axon attempts sprouting. Note that new injury of the previously undamaged nerve will lead to *grouped atrophy. Myopathy:* Scattered myocytes of different motor units are small (degenerating or regenerating), while the neurons and nerve fibers are normal.

most distal two to three internodes, before undergoing regenerative activity. Muscle fibers of the affected motor unit undergo *denervation atrophy;* myocytes become smaller and more angular but are still viable (see later).

Demyelinating Neuropathies (p. 1228)

Myelin loss is caused by Schwann cell dysfunction or by primary myelin sheath damage (Fig. 27-1); the underlying axon is normal. Denuded axons stimulate remyelination; precursor cells can replace injured Schwann cells, but the repair is not perfect—the internode distances are shorter, and the myelin sheath is thinner.

Neuronopathies (p. 1230)

Neuronopathies reflect neuronal destruction (e.g., due to infections or toxins) with secondary degeneration of axonal processes. Neuronopathy can impact peripheral nerve function in both proximal and distal parts of the body; axonopathies preferentially affect the distal extremities.

Anatomic Patterns of Peripheral Neuropathies (p. 1230)

- *Mononeuropathies* affect single nerves, with deficits in a restricted distribution; causes include trauma, entrapment, and infection.
- *Polyneuropathies* involve multiple nerves, usually symmetrically, progressing from distal to proximal ("stocking and glove" distribution).
- *Mononeuritis multiplex* damages several nerves in a haphazard pattern; vasculitis is a common etiology.
- *Polyradiculoneuropathies* affect nerve roots and peripheral nerves, leading to diffuse symmetric proximal and distal deficits.

Specific Peripheral Neuropathies (p. 1230)

Inflammatory Neuropathies (p. 1230)

Guillain-Barré Syndrome *(p. 1230)*

Guillain-Barré syndrome is an acute inflammatory demyelinating polyneuropathy that can lead to life-threatening ascending paralysis; the incidence is 1 per 100,000 people.

Pathogenesis (p. 1230)

Guillain-Barré syndrome is likely an immune-mediated disorder; 60% to 70% of cases are preceded by vaccination or by a viral (cytomegalovirus, Epstein-Barr virus) or bacterial *(Campylobacter, Mycoplasma)* infection; T cells and/or circulating antibodies can be responsible for the demyelination.

Morphology (p. 1231)

Lesions show segmental demyelination with chronic inflammation involving the nerve roots and peripheral nerves; axonal damage can also be present in severe disease.

Clinical Features (p. 1231)

The clinical picture is dominated by ascending paralysis and areflexia; sensory involvement is usually less dramatic. Nerve conduction velocity is slowed, and although cerebrospinal fluid protein is elevated, there is no pleocytosis. Treatment involves plasmapheresis and intravenous immunoglobulin. Death occurs in 2% to 5% of patients due to respiratory paralysis, autonomic instability, or cardiac arrest; 20% of patients can have permanent disability.

Chronic Inflammatory Demyelinating Poly(radiculo) neuropathy *(p. 1231)*

Chronic inflammatory demyelinating poly(radiculo)neuropathy is a symmetric mixed sensorimotor polyneuropathy similar to Guillain-Barré syndrome but follows a subacute or chronic course with relapses and remissions and is responsive to steroids. T-cell and immunoglobulin-associated inflammatory responses are implicated. Peripheral nerves show evidence of recurrent demyelination and remyelination ("onion bulb" changes).

Neuropathy Associated With Vasculitis *(p. 1231)*

Approximately a third of patients with vasculitis have peripheral nerve involvement, most often manifesting as mononeuritis multiplex; there is patchy axonal degeneration and loss.

Infectious Neuropathies (p. 1231)

Leprosy (Hansen Disease) *(p. 1232)*

Mycobacterium leprae bacteria directly invade Schwann cells, where they proliferate and eventually infect other cells (see Chapter 8); lesions include segmental demyelination and remyelination, with axonal loss and endoneurial and epineurial fibrosis.

- *Lepromatous leprosy* tends to be more severe and diffuse; patients develop a symmetric polyneuropathy, mostly in the extremities (lower temperatures favor mycobacterial growth). A predilection for pain fibers renders patients relatively insensitive to injurious stimuli, and large traumatic ulcers are common.

- *Tuberculoid leprosy:* Better host responsiveness, reflected by nodules of granulomatous inflammation, leads to more localized nerve injury.

Lyme Disease (p. 1232)

Lyme disease can lead to polyradiculopathy and unilateral or bilateral facial nerve palsies.

Human Immunodeficiency Virus/Acquired Immunodeficiency Syndrome (p. 1232)

Human immunodeficiency virus (HIV)/acquired immunodeficiency syndrome (AIDS) can cause several different patterns of peripheral neuropathy (e.g., mononeuritis multiplex or demyelinating disorders) attributed to immune dysregulation. Late-stage HIV infection is associated with a painful distal sensory neuropathy.

Diphtheria (p. 1232)

Diphtheria neuropathy results from the effects of the diphtheria exotoxin (see Chapter 8). Clinical manifestations are paresthesias and weakness with associated segmental demyelination.

Varicella-Zoster Virus (p. 1232)

Following varicella (chickenpox) infection, virus persists as a latent infection of spinal cord and brainstem sensory ganglia. Subsequent reactivation leads to a painful vesicular skin eruption in the distribution of sensory dermatomes *(shingles)*, most frequently thoracic or trigeminal. Affected ganglia exhibit neuronal destruction with associated mononuclear cell infiltrates, and peripheral nerves show axonal degeneration.

Metabolic, Hormonal, and Nutritional Neuropathies (p. 1232)

Diabetes Mellitus (p. 1232)

Diabetes mellitus is the most common cause of peripheral neuropathy, typically presenting as an ascending distal symmetric sensorineural polyneuropathy. Half of all diabetics have some involvement, and 80% will have some manifestation after 15 years. Nonenzymatic protein glycation and polyol-mediated damage are both causally implicated, as well as diabetic microvascular disease with secondary ischemic injury. Histologically there is axonal neuropathy with loss of small fibers.

Clinical Features (p. 1233)

Sensory loss is greater than motor dysfunction; loss of pain sensation can result in development of cutaneous ulcers that heal poorly due to diabetic microvascular disease. *Autonomic neuropathy* affects approximately 20% to 40% of diabetics; clinical sequelae include postural hypotension, incomplete bladder emptying, and sexual dysfunction. Long-term disease can lead to vascular insufficiency of peripheral nerves and is associated with asymmetric manifestations, including *mononeuropathy, cranial neuropathy, and radiculoplexus neuropathy* (a painful disorder in the brachial or lumbosacral nerve plexi).

Other Metabolic, Hormonal, and Nutritional Neuropathies (p. 1233)

- Axonal degeneration can occur secondary to renal failure, typically presenting with distal symmetric sensory and motor neuropathy. *Hypothyroidism* can cause compression mononeuroapthy (e.g., carpal tunnel syndrome), or a distal symmetric sensory polyneuropathy; *hyperthyroidism* can rarely cause a neuropathy resembling Guillain-Barré. Peripheral neuropathies can occur secondary to deficiencies of copper, zinc, vitamins B_1, B_6, B_{12}, E, or folate.

Toxic Neuropathies (p. 1233)

Toxic neuropathies can occur after exposure to industrial or environmental chemicals, biologic toxins, heavy metals (lead, arsenic), or therapeutic drugs, especially cisplatin, and the vinca alkaloids and taxanes; the latter are microtubule inhibitors and therefore interfere with axonal transport. Alcohol can cause direct peripheral nerve toxicity or can have effects secondary to vitamin deficiency.

Neuropathies Associated With Malignancy (p. 1233)

- *Direct infiltration or nerve compression* by a tumor can cause mononeuropathy, brachial plexopathy, cranial nerve palsy, or polyradiculopathy of lower extremities (meningeal carcinomatosis of cauda equina).
- *Paraneoplastic neuropathies* are most commonly sensorimotor but can assume virtually any pattern. Small cell carcinoma is a common underlying malignancy, with patients expressing autoantibodies that recognize tumor and self-neurons (anti-Hu); damage is mediated through CD8+ cytotoxic T-cell attack on dorsal root ganglion cells. Less commonly a pure sensory neuropathy results from loss of dorsal root ganglia; it is associated with circulating antibodies directed against an RNA-binding protein shared by neurons and tumor cells.

Neuropathies Associated With Monoclonal Gammopathies

- Neuropathies associated with monoclonal gammopathies are attributed to direct binding of pathogenic paraproteins to myelin-associated glycoprotein. Excess light chains can also deposit as amyloid, causing vascular deficiency or direct toxicity.

Neuropathies Caused by Physical Forces (p. 1234)

- *Lacerations* occur with slicing injuries or bone fractures in which sharp fragments cut a nerve.
- *Avulsions* occur when a nerve is put under tension (e.g., with force applied to a limb).

Compression neuropathy (entrapment neuropathy) occurs when a nerve is compressed, often within an anatomic compartment; *carpal tunnel syndrome* is most common, occurring secondary to conditions that compress the median nerve by reducing the space beneath the transverse carpal ligament (e.g., edema, pregnancy, degenerative joint disease, hypothyroidism, amyloidosis, and excessive wrist usage). Other nerves prone to compression neuropathies are the ulnar nerve at the level of the elbow, the peroneal nerve at the level of the knee, and the radial nerve in the upper arm. Compression neuropathy of the foot is most common in women; involvement of the interdigital nerve at intermetatarsal sites leads to perineural fibrosis and pain *(Morton neuroma)*.

Inherited Peripheral Neuropathies (p. 1234)

Inherited peripheral neuropathies are a heterogeneous group manifesting with progressive peripheral nerve injury. The basis for these can be generally grouped according to genes that encode the following:

- Myelin-associated proteins
- Growth factors and their receptors

- Mitochondrial proteins
- Vesicle and axonal transport
- Heat shock proteins, involved in preventing protein aggregation
- Cell membrane structure and function

Hereditary and Sensory Autonomic Neuropathies and Charcot-Marie-Tooth Disease

Hereditary and sensory autonomic neuropathies and Charcot-Marie-Tooth (CMT) disease are the most common heritable peripheral neuropathies, affecting 1 in 2500 people; they are caused by mutations in over 50 different genes. These disorders present with distal muscle atrophy, sensory loss, and foot deformities.

- CMT1 is the most common subtype; it represents a collection of autosomal dominant disorders:
  - CMT1A (55% of genetically defined CMT) is caused by a duplication in the peripheral myelin protein 22 *(PMP22)* gene.
  - CMT1B (9%) is caused by mutations in the myelin protein zero gene.
- CMTX encompasses X-linked forms; CMT1X causes 15% of genetically defined CMT. It is linked to *GJB1* mutations encoding connexin32, a gap junction component of Schwann cells.
- CMT2 includes autosomal dominant neuropathies associated with axonal rather than demyelinating injury. CMT2A (4% of all CMT disease) is caused by mutations in the *MFN2* gene involved in normal mitochondrial fusion.

Hereditary Neuropathy With Pressure Palsy *(p. 1235)*

Hereditary neuropathy with pressure palsy is caused by deletion of *PMP22* (the same gene that is duplicated in CMT1A) and leads to a transient motor and sensory mononeuropathy triggered by nerve compression (e.g., carpal tunnel).

Diseases of the Neuromuscular Junction (p. 1235)

Disorders of the neuromuscular junction typically present with painless weakness.

Antibody-Mediated Diseases of the Neuromuscular Junction (p. 1235)

Myasthenia Gravis *(p. 1235)*

Myasthenia gravis is due to autoantibodies directed against acetylcholine receptors (AChRs); it is more common in women before age 40 but has equal gender predilection in older age groups.

Pathogenesis (p. 1236)

Some 85% of patients have AChR autoantibodies; the remainder have antibodies directed against the sarcolemmal protein *muscle-specific receptor tyrosine kinase.* These antibodies can drive disease through the following:

- Complement fixation and direct postsynaptic membrane damage
- Accelerating internalization and downregulation of the AChR
- Blocking ACh binding

Clinical Features (p. 1236)

Patients classically present with easy fatigability, ptosis, and diplopia; symptoms worsen with repeated stimulation. Treatments include anticholinesterase agents, prednisone, and plasmapheresis. Thymic hyperplasia occurs in 65% of patients, and thymomas occur in 15%; thymic resection can improve symptoms.

Lambert-Eaton Myasthenic Syndrome *(p. 1236)*

Lambert-Eaton myasthenic syndrome presents with weakness and autonomic dysfunction; as opposed to myasthenia gravis, neurotransmission improves with repeated stimulation. Approximately half of cases are paraneoplastic (classically associated with small cell lung carcinoma); the remainder are often associated with other autoimmune disorders (e.g., vitiligo or Graves disease). The causal autoantibody is directed against a presynaptic voltage-gated calcium channel; each presynaptic action potential releases fewer synaptic vesicles than normal. Treatment involves immunosuppression or drugs that increase ACh release by depolarizing the presynaptic membrane.

Disorders Caused by Toxins *(p. 1236)*

Botulism is caused by a neurotoxin (produced by *Clostridium botulinum*) that blocks ACh release from presynaptic neurons; conversely, *curare* blocks AChRs, resulting in flaccid paralysis.

Diseases of Skeletal Muscle (p. 1237)

Skeletal muscle fibers are multinucleated syncytial cells delimited by a plasma membrane *(sarcolemma);* they contain identical repeating units *(sarcomeres)* of actin and myosin contractile elements (and associated proteins). Normal human skeletal muscle contains two major fiber types with different functional characteristics and staining patterns (Table 27-1); the mnemonic "*one* (type 1) *slow* (twitch) *fat* (lipid-rich) *red* (gross appearance) *ox* (oxidative)" can help to remember the physiologic and histochemical distinctions. All fibers of a given motor unit are of the same type, with the characteristics imparted by the nature of the innervation. However, different motor units (and thus different fiber types) are intermingled within any given muscle; when visualized by special stains, this intermingling yields a "checkerboard pattern" (Fig. 27-1).

TABLE 27-1 Muscle Fiber Types

Feature	Type 1	Type 2
Action	Sustained force	Sudden movements
Strength	Weight bearing	Purposeful motion
Enzyme content	NADH dark staining ATPase at pH 4.2, dark staining ATPase at pH 9.4, light staining	NADH light staining ATPase at pH 4.2, light staining ATPase at pH 9.4, dark staining
Lipids	Abundant	Scant
Glycogen	Scant	Abundant
Ultrastructure	Many mitochondria Wide Z-band	Few mitochondria Narrow Z-band
Physiology	Slow-twitch	Fast-twitch
Color	Red	White
Prototype	Soleus (pigeon)	Pectoral (pigeon)

ATPase, Adenosine triphosphatase; *NADH,* nicotinamide adenine dinucleotide, reduced form.

Skeletal Muscle Atrophy (p. 1237)

Skeletal muscle atrophy is a common feature of many disorders, including neurogenic injury, disuse, cachexia, aging, and primary myopathies.

Neurogenic and Myopathic Changes in Skeletal Muscle (p. 1237)

Myofibers may be directly injured (myopathic injury) or through disruption of muscle innervation (neurogenic injury).

Neurogenic injuries lead to *fiber type grouping and grouped atrophy* (Fig. 27-1):

- Muscle fiber type is determined by the innervating motor neuron and can switch if the innervating motor neuron changes from one type to the other.
- After denervation, myofibers undergo atrophy, becoming flattened and angulated.
- Reinnervation restores fiber size and shape but may make a denervated myofiber part of a different motor unit (and thus a switch in fiber type).
- With recurrent neuronal damage, residual motor axons may innervate increasingly larger numbers of myofibers, leading to enlargement of motor units *(fiber type grouping);* such large motor units are susceptible to *grouped atrophy* if the innervating axon is subsequently damaged.

Myopathic processes are associated with a distinct set of morphologic changes:

- *Segmental myofiber degeneration and regeneration* occur when only a portion of a myofiber dies; this is associated with release of cytoplasmic enzymes (e.g., creatine kinase)—useful markers of muscle damage. After damaged segments are removed by macrophages *(myophagocytosis),* regeneration occurs through fusion of activated satellite cells to the residual intact myofibers. Regeneration can often restore muscle to normalcy but may not be able to keep pace with recurrent or chronic injury. In that situation, muscles exhibit endomysial fibrosis (collagen deposition), myofiber dropout, atrophic myofibers, and fatty replacement.
- *Myofiber hypertrophy* occurs as a physiologic adaptation to exercise or associated with certain chronic myopathic conditions.
- *Cytoplasmic inclusions* in the form of vacuoles, aggregates of proteins, or clustered organelles are characteristic of several primary forms of myopathy.

Inflammatory Myopathies (p. 1238)

Infectious myositis (see Chapter 8) and systemic inflammatory diseases that involve muscle (see Chapter 6) are covered elsewhere. The following are *primary* inflammatory diseases of muscle.

Dermatomyositis (p. 1238)

Dermatomyositis is a systemic autoimmune disease primarily involving skin and muscle. Classically a lilac discoloration of upper eyelids *(heliotrope rash)* and periorbital edema accompanies or precedes weakness; scaling, erythematous patches are also present over knuckles, elbows, and knees *(Gottron papules).* Muscle weakness is slow in onset and bilaterally symmetric, affecting proximal muscles first; dysphagia occurs in a third of patients. Interstitial lung disease, vasculitis, and myocarditis can also be present. Nearly 15% to 25% of adult patients have cancer; juvenile patients more characteristically exhibit gastrointestinal (GI) symptoms and a third will have calcinosis. The disease is associated with (although not necessarily caused by) autoantibodies directed against the following:

- Mi2, a helicase implicated in nucleosome remodeling.
- Jo1, histidyl transfer RNA (tRNA) synthetase.
- PI55/P140, several transcriptional regulators.

Capillaries appear to be the primary target of immunologic attack, and immune suppressive therapy is beneficial.

Polymyositis *(p. 1239)*

Polymyositis is similar to dermatomyositis but lacks cutaneous involvement; it occurs primarily in adults. The pathogenesis involves cytotoxic T cell–driven myocyte damage. Immune suppressive therapy is beneficial.

Inclusion Body Myositis *(p. 1240)*

Inclusion body myositis begins with *distal muscle* involvement, most severe in the quadriceps and distal upper extremities; dysphagia is not uncommon. It has an insidious onset, typically affecting individuals over age 50. Most myositis-associated antibodies are absent, and immunosuppressive therapy is generally not beneficial. Intracellular depositions suggest abnormal protein folding as an etiology.

Toxic Myopathies (p. 1240)

- *Statin-induced myopathy* occurs in 1% to 2% of recipients.
- *Chloroquine* and *hydroxychloroquine* interfere with normal lysosome function and lead to slowly progressive muscle weakness associated with myopathic vacuolization, predominantly affecting type 1 fibers. Ultrastructural studies show intracellular, whorled, lamellar membrane structures.
- *Intensive care unit (ICU) myopathy* (myosin-deficient myopathy) occurs in critically ill patients, especially those receiving corticosteroid therapy; there is relatively selective sarcomeric myosin degradation, leading to profound weakness.
- *Thyrotoxic myopathy* presents as proximal muscle weakness that can precede clinical thyroid dysfunction; myofiber necrosis, regeneration, and interstitial lymphocytosis can be present. In *hypothyroidism,* muscle cramping and slowed movements are associated with fiber atrophy, increased numbers of internal nuclei, and glycogen aggregates.
- *Alcohol* can also be myopathic. *Binge* drinking can produce an acute toxic syndrome of painful rhabdomyolysis with accompanying myoglobinuria and renal failure.

Inherited Diseases of Skeletal Muscle (p. 1241)

- *Congenital myopathies* (Table 27-2) are characterized by early onset of nonprogressive or slowly progressive, proximal or generalized muscle weakness and hypotonia *(floppy babies)* or severe joint contractures *(arthrogryposis).*
- *Muscular dystrophies* are a heterogeneous group of inherited disorders characterized by progressive muscle damage and wasting, usually arising after early childhood.
- *Congenital muscular dystrophies* initially manifest in infancy and are also associated with central nervous system (CNS) developmental abnormalities:
    - Defects in extracellular matrix around myocytes, due to collagen VI mutations (Ullrich congenital muscular dystrophy) and merosin deficiency
    - Abnormalities in the receptors for extracellular matrix (e.g., due to abnormal posttranslational modification of dystroglycan)

TABLE 27-2 Congenital Myopathies

Disease and Inheritance	Gene and Locus	Clinical Findings	Pathologic Findings
Central-core disease; autosomal dominant	Ryanodine receptor-1 *(RYR1)* gene; 19q13.1	Early-onset hypotonia and weakness; "floppy infant"; associated skeletal abnormalities like scoliosis, hip dislocation, or foot deformities; some RYR1 mutations cause central core disease, some malignant hyperthermia, and some both	Cytoplasmic cores represent demarcated central zones in which the normal arrangement of sarcomeres is disrupted and mitochondria are decreased in number
Nemaline myopathy (NEM)	AD NEM1—α-tropomyosin 3 *(TPM3)* gene; 1q22–q23 AR NEM2—nebulin *(NEB)* gene; 2q22 AR NEM3—α-actin-1 *(ACTA)* gene; 1q42 AR NEM4—tropomyosin-2 *(TPM2)* gene; 19p13.2–p13.1 AR NEM5—troponin T1 *(TNNT1)* gene; 19q13.4 AR NEM7—coffilin-2 *(CFL2)* gene; 14q12	Childhood weakness; some with more severe weakness, hypotonia at birth ("floppy infant")	Aggregates of spindle-shaped particles *(nemaline rods);* occur predominantly in type 1 fibers; derived from Z-band material (α-actinin) and best seen on modified Gomori stain or by electron microscopy
Centronuclear myopathy	XL—myotubularin *(MTM1)* gene; Xq28 AD—dynamin-2 (and others) *DNM2* gene; 19p13.2 AR—amphiphysin-2 *(BIN1)* gene; 2q14)	Severe congenital hypotonia, "floppy infant" and poor prognosis in X-linked form ("myotubular myopathy") Childhood onset or young adult onset with other variants with weakness and hypotonia	Many fibers contain nuclei in the geometric center of the myofiber; central nuclei are more common in type 1 fibers, which are small in diameter, but can occur in both fiber types
Congenital fiber type disproportion	Selenoprotein 1 *(SEPN1)* gene; 1p36.11 Alpha-actin-1 *(ACTA1)* gene; 1q42.13 Tropomyosin 3 *(TPM3)* gene; 1q21.3	Hypotonia, weakness, failure to thrive, facial and respiratory weakness, contractures Wide phenotypic spectrum Mutations in SEPN1 are also associated with protein aggregate myopathy and rigid spine muscular dystrophy; mutations in ACTA1 are also associated with NEM and protein aggregate myopathy; mutations in TPM3 are also associated with NEM	Predominance and atrophy of type I fibers (not specific)

AD, Autosomal dominant; *AR,* autosomal recessive; *XL,* X-linked.

Muscular Dystrophies (p. 1242)

X-linked Muscular Dystrophy With Dystrophin Mutation or Duchenne and Becker Muscular Dystrophy (p. 1242)

These diseases result from disruption of the function of the X-linked protein *dystrophin.*

Dystrophin mutations are causal in Duchenne muscular dystrophy (DMD), the most severe and most common form of muscular dystrophy; the incidence is 1 in 3500 live-born males. It is clinically manifest by age 5, and patients are wheelchair bound by age 10 to 12; the disease progresses relentlessly until death in the early 20s. Becker muscular dystrophy (BMD) involves the same genetic locus but is less common and less severe, with later onset and a slower rate of progression.

Pathogenesis (p. 1242)

The responsible *DMD* gene at Xp21 encodes the 427-kD *dystrophin* protein—a key component of the dystrophin glycoprotein complex (DGC) responsible for transducing contractile forces from the intracellular sarcomeres to the extracellular matrix (Fig. 27-2). Defects in DGC may lead to small membrane tears and calcium influx that lead to myofiber degeneration. Dystrophin may also have a role in signaling pathways; its carboxyl terminus interacts with nitric oxide synthase. Most mutations are deletions, with frameshift and point mutations accounting for the rest; two thirds are familial, and the

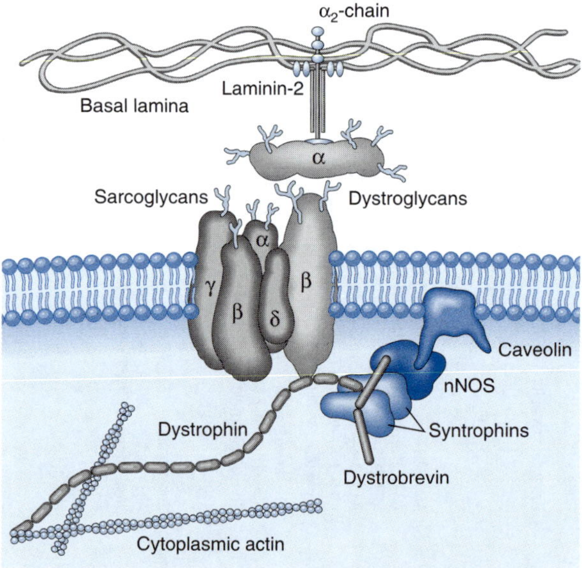

Figure 27-2 Relationship between the cell membrane (sarcolemma) and the sarcolemmal associated proteins. *Dystrophin,* an intracellular protein, forms an interface between the cytoskeletal proteins and a group of transmembrane proteins, the dystroglycans and the sarcoglycans. These transmembrane proteins have interactions with the extracellular matrix, including the laminin proteins. Dystrophin also interacts with dystrobrevin and the syntrophins, which form a link with neuronal type nitric oxide synthetase (nNOS) and caveolin. Mutations in dystrophin are associated with the X-linked muscular dystrophies; mutations in caveolin and the sarcoglycan proteins with the limb-girdle muscular dystrophies, which can be autosomal dominant or recessive disorders; and mutations in α_2-laminin (merosin) with autosomal recessive congenital muscular dystrophy.

remainder are new mutations. Muscle from DMD patients has almost no detectable dystrophin; muscle from BMD patients has diminished amounts of dystrophin, usually of an abnormal molecular weight, reflecting mutations that allow synthesis of some protein.

Morphology (p. 1242)

Both DMD and BMD muscles show the following:

- *Variation in myofiber diameter,* with both small and giant fibers, sometimes with fiber splitting.
- Increased numbers of internalized nuclei.
- Degeneration, necrosis, and phagocytosis of muscle fibers.
- Regeneration of muscle fibers.
- Proliferation of endomysial connective tissue.
- In late stages, muscles are entirely replaced by fat and connective tissue.
- Both type 1 and type 2 fibers are involved, without change in relative distribution.

Clinical Features (p. 1243)

Weakness begins in the pelvic girdle muscles, extending to the shoulder girdle; the lower leg is hypertrophied associated with weakness *(pseudohypertrophy).* Pathologic changes are also found in the heart (failure and arrhythmia), and cognitive impairment is a component of the disease. Female carriers and affected males are at risk for developing dilated cardiomyopathy. Death results from respiratory insufficiency, pulmonary infection, and cardiac decompensation.

Myotonic Dystrophy (p. 1243)

Myotonic dystrophy is an autosomal dominant disease that tends to increase in severity and appear at a younger age in succeeding generations (the phenomenon called *anticipation*). *Myotonia*—a sustained involuntary muscular contraction—is the cardinal neuromuscular symptom; patients also have cataracts, endocrinopathy, and cardiomyopathy.

Pathogenesis (p. 1244)

Myotonic dystrophy is caused by a CTG trinucleotide repeat expansion on chromosome 19q13; it affects the mRNA for the myotonic dystrophy protein kinase (DMPK). The disease state is caused by expansion of the repeat sequence, leading to a "toxic" gain of function; the expanded CUG-repeats in the *DMPK* mRNA transcript sequester a protein called *muscleblindlike-1,* which has an important role in RNA splicing. In turn, reduced muscleblind-like-1 function leads to mis-splicing of other RNA transcripts, including for the CLC1 chloride channel; insufficient CLC1 (required for normal muscle relaxation) is responsible for the characteristic myotonia.

Emery-Dreifuss Muscular Dystrophy (p. 1244)

Emery-Dreifuss muscular dystrophy (EMD) is marked by a triad of slowly progressive humeroperoneal weakness, cardiomyopathy associated with conduction defects, and early contractures of the Achilles tendon, spine, and elbows. It is caused by mutations in nuclear lamina proteins; *emerin* for the X-linked form (EMD1) and *lamin A/C* for the autosomal form (EMD2) are caused by mutations in the genes encoding emerin and lamin A/C.

Facioscapulohumeral Dystrophy (p. 1244)

Facioscapulohumeral dystrophy is an autosomal dominant disease affecting approximately 1 in 20,000 individuals; it presents with prominent weakness of facial and shoulder girdle muscles. There is overexpression of the *DUX4* gene, which encodes a transcription factor.

Limb-Girdle Muscular Dystrophies (p. 1244)

Limb-girdle muscular dystrophies are a heterogeneous group of diseases with an overall incidence of 1 in 25,000 to 50,000. All are characterized by muscle weakness preferentially involving proximal muscle groups. Causal genes include those encoding the following:

- Structural components (sarcoglycans) of the DGC
- Enzymes that glycosylate α-dystroglycan, a component of the DGC
- Proteins that associate with sarcomere Z-disks
- Proteins involved in vesicle trafficking and cell signaling
- Calpain 3 protease and lamin A/C

Diseases of Lipid or Glycogen Metabolism (p. 1244)

Inborn errors of lipid or glycogen metabolism can affect skeletal muscle; patients may develop symptoms only with exercise or fasting (e.g., cramping and pain or in severe cases, muscle necrosis *[rhabdomyolysis]* or may have slowly progressive muscle damage). Examples include the following:

- *Carnitine palmitoyltransferase II deficiency* impairs free fatty acid transport into mitochondria.
- *Myophosphorylase deficiency (McArdle disease).*
- *Acid maltase deficiency* results in impaired lysosomal catabolism of glycogen, causing lysosomal accumulation; severe deficiency causes *Pompe disease* (see Chapter 5), whereas milder deficiency causes a progressive adult-onset myopathy involving respiratory and truncal muscles.

Mitochondrial Myopathies (p. 1245)

Mitochondrial myopathies can involve many organ systems, including high-energy tissues, such as skeletal muscle, cardiac muscle, and nerve; causative mutations often impair mitochondrial ATP generation. Patients can have variable patterns of muscle weakness, associated with elevated serum creatine kinase, and/or rhabdomyolysis; involvement of extraocular eye muscles is common *(chronic progressive external ophthalmoplegia)*. Both nuclear and mitochondrial genomes contribute to mitochondrial constituents; nuclear mutations will follow mendelian inheritance, but mutations in mitochondrial DNA (mtDNA) are maternally inherited because all of the mitochondria in the embryo are contributed by the oocyte. Each cell also contains thousands of mtDNA copies, distributed in a random fashion to daughter cells at the time of cell division. Thus disease may result only when a certain threshold of mutated mtDNA copies is exceeded within a substantial fraction of "at-risk" cells.

Morphology (p. 1245)

Findings include aggregates of abnormal mitochondria, causing irregular muscle fiber contour (*ragged red fibers* on trichrome stains). Increased numbers of abnormally sized and shaped mitochondria can also contain paracrystalline arrays (so-called *parking lot inclusions*).

Differential Diagnosis of a Hypotonic ("Floppy") Infant (p. 1245)

Differential diagnosis of a hypotonic infant includes the following:

- Primary diseases of skeletal muscle (e.g., congenital myasthenic syndrome, congenital myotonia, congenital myopathies, and congenital muscular dystrophies)

- Abnormalities of the brain (e.g., encephalopathy)
- Neuronopathies, of which *spinal muscular atrophy (SMA)* is characteristic

Spinal Muscular Atrophy (p. 1245)

SMA is an autosomal recessive disorder occurring in 1 of 6000 births and caused by loss-of-function mutations in the *SMN1* (survival of motor neuron-1) gene. Loss of motor neurons in SMA leads to skeletal muscle denervation with muscle weakness and atrophy. Histology shows large zones of severely atrophic myofibers; scattered normal or hypertrophied myofibers have retained innervation from residual motor neurons.

Ion Channel Myopathies (Channelopathies) (p. 1246)

Ion channel myopathies (channelopathies) are a group of heritable diseases caused by ion channel mutations. Most are autosomal dominant with variable penetrance; clinical manifestations can include epilepsy, migraine, cerebellar dysfunction, peripheral nerve disease, and muscle disease. Ion channel mutations can cause decreased or increased excitability and result in hypotonia or hypertonia. Disorders associated with hypotonia may have elevated, depressed, or normal serum potassium levels (called *hyperkalemic, hypokalemic,* or *normokalemic periodic paralysis,* respectively). Examples of channnelopathy mutations include the following:

- *KCNJ2 potassium channel:* Mutations cause *Andersen-Tawil syndrome*—periodic paralysis, heart arrhythmias, and skeletal abnormalities.
- *SCN4A sodium channel:* Mutations cause disorders ranging from myotonia to periodic paralysis.
- *CACNA1S subunit of muscle calcium channel:* Most common cause of *hypokalemic paralysis.*
- *CLC1 chloride channel:* Mutations cause *myotonia congenita.*
- RYR1 ryanodine receptor, which regulates calcium release from the sarcoplasmic reticulum. Mutations of *RYR1* can result in *malignant hyperthermia,* a hypermetabolic state with tachycardia, tachypnea, muscle spasms, and hyperpyrexia triggered by anesthetics; mutant receptor allows increased efflux of calcium from the sarcoplasmic reticulum, resulting in tetany and excessive heat production.

Peripheral Nerve Sheath Tumors (p. 1246)

These include benign and malignant neoplasms; the vast majority are composed of cells with Schwann cell differentiation, and they are commonly associated with familial tumor syndromes (e.g., neurofibromatosis type 1 [NF1], neurofibromatosis type 2 [NF2], and schwannomatosis).

Schwannomas (p. 1247)

These are benign tumors often arising directly from peripheral nerve. Loss of *merlin* expression (*NF2* gene product) is a consistent finding; this leads to increased expression of growth factor receptors, and thus to hyperproliferation in the presence of exogenous growth factors. Schwannomas become symptomatic through compression of involved nerves or adjacent structures. Within the skull, most schwannomas occur at the cerebellopontine angle, attached to the vestibular branch of the eighth nerve (so-called *acoustic neuroma*); affected individuals have tinnitus and hearing loss. Surgical removal is curative.

Morphology (p. 1247)

Schwannomas are well-circumscribed, firm, gray encapsulated masses. Microscopically they have admixture of dense and loose areas referred to as *Antoni A* and *Antoni B* areas, respectively. The Antoni A areas are dense and eosinophilic with spindle cells arranged into cellular, intersecting fascicles, palisading nuclei alternate with "nuclear-free zones" *(Verocay bodies).*

Antoni B areas are loose and hypocellular; spindle cells are separated by a myxoid extracellular matrix with associated microcyst formation.

Neurofibromas (p. 1247)

These are benign nerve sheath tumors that are more heterogeneous than schwannomas due to admixing of Schwann cells with perineurial-like cells, fibroblasts, mast cells, and CD34+ spindle cells. Only the Schwann cells have complete loss of *neurofibromin* (*NF1* gene product; see Chapter 7), a tumor suppressor that inhibits RAS activity by stimulating the activity of a GTPase. Transformation to a malignant peripheral nerve sheath tumor (MPNST) is seen mostly in the *plexiform* variants but with an overall incidence of 5% to 10%.

Morphology (p. 1247)

- *Localized cutaneous neurofibromas* are small, well-delineated, unencapsulated nodular lesions in the dermis and subcutaneous fat; they have relatively low cellularity.
- *Diffuse neurofibromas* diffusely infiltrate the dermis and subcutaneous connective tissue, entrapping fat and appendage structures and producing a plaquelike appearance.
- *Plexiform neurofibromas* grow within and expand nerve fascicles, entrapping associated axons; the expanded, ropy thickening of multiple nerve fascicles results in a "bag of worms" appearance.

Malignant Peripheral Nerve Sheath Tumors (p. 1248)

Most MPNSTs are high-grade tumors; 50% occur in NF1 patients likely from malignant transformation of a plexiform neurofibroma. Most are associated with larger peripheral nerves in the chest, abdomen, pelvis, neck, or limb girdle. MPNSTs exhibit complex chromosomal aberrations.

Neurofibromatosis Type 1 and Type 2 (p. 1249)

Neurofibromatosis Type 1 (p. 1249)

NF1 is a common autosomal dominant systemic disorder (frequency of 1 in 3000) associated with a variety of tumors, including neurofibromas, MPNST, optic nerve gliomas, other glial tumors and hamartomatous lesions, and pheochromocytomas. Other features include mental retardation or seizures, skeletal defects, pigmented nodules of the iris *(Lisch nodules),* and cutaneous hyperpigmented macules *(café au lait spots).* The disease is caused by loss-of-function mutations in the *NF1* gene, encoding the tumor suppressor *neurofibromin.* The disease has a high penetrance but variable expressivity.

Neurofibromatosis Type 2 (p. 1249)

NF2 is a rare autosomal dominant disorder (1 in 40,000 to 50,000 people), resulting in a range of tumors, most commonly bilateral eighth-nerve schwannomas, and meningiomas; ependymomas of the spinal cord also occur. Many patients have non-neoplastic lesions, including *schwannosis* (nodular ingrowth of Schwann cells into the spinal cord), *meningioangiomatosis* (a CNS proliferation of meningeal cells and blood vessels), and *glial hamartia* (microscopic nodular collections of glial cells). The disease is caused by loss-of-function mutations in the *NF2* gene encoding *merlin,* a cytoskeletal regulator of receptor signaling activity.

28 The Central Nervous System

Features that influence the manifestations of central nervous system (CNS) disorders include the following:

- Specific neurologic functions are typically localized to distinct (often spatially clustered) neurons; the clinical effects of injury will therefore frequently be site specific and may not be corrected by other neurons.
- CNS stem cell populations exist but have limited restorative capacity; thus destructive lesions typically cause permanent deficits.
- Certain neurons have selective vulnerability to injury.
- Other cells of the CNS, such as *astrocytes* and *oligodendroglial cells* (constituting the *glia*), are affected in several unique neurologic conditions and can also respond to common insults (e.g., ischemia) in a manner distinct from other tissues.
- Physical restrictions of the skull and spine render the brain and spinal cord vulnerable to expansile pressure.
- The CNS has a distinct cerebrospinal fluid (CSF) circulation, lacks lymphatics, and has a selective blood-brain barrier.
- Some responses to injury are unique to the CNS (see later).

Cellular Pathology of the Central Nervous System (p. 1252)

Reactions of Neurons to Injury (p. 1252)

Neuronal injury can be an acute process (e.g., due to hypoxia or hypoglycemia) or a slower, degenerative process, often associated with accumulation of abnormal protein aggregates.

Morphology (p. 1252)

- *Acute neuronal injury* is a spectrum of change due to hypoxia-ischemia (or other insults) and leading to cell necrosis or apoptosis; there is intense cytoplasmic eosinophilia and nuclear pyknosis ("red neurons").
- *Subacute and chronic neuronal injury ("degeneration")* is neuronal death (mostly apoptosis) and accompanying reactive gliosis, occurring as a consequence of progressive degenerative disorders.
- *Axonal reaction* reflects the response of a neuronal cell body to the challenge of regenerating damaged axons. The cell body rounds up, and nucleoli enlarge; Nissl substance dispersal and perinuclear cytoplasmic pallor *(central chromatolysis)* are associated with increased protein synthesis and axonal sprouting.
- *Neuronal inclusions* can be manifestations of aging (lipofuscin), disorders of metabolism (storage material), viral diseases (inclusion bodies), or neurodegenerative diseases associated with aggregated proteins.

Reactions of Astrocytes to Injury (p. 1253)

Astrocytes are the principal cells responsible for repair and scar formation in the brain; they are also important cellular elements of the blood-brain barrier.

In areas of CNS damage, astrocytes develop enlarged vesicular nuclei and conspicuous eosinophilic cytoplasm *(gemistocytic astrocytes);* such astrocyte hypertrophy and hyperplasia culminate in tissue *gliosis.*

When directly injured, astrocytes can also exhibit characteristic changes:

- *Rosenthal fibers* are elongated, eosinophilic structures within astrocytic processes; these contain αB-crystallin and hsp27 (heat shock proteins) and are seen in long-standing gliosis or pilocytic astrocytomas.
- *Corpora amylacea* are lamellated polyglucosan bodies (also containing heat shock proteins); these increase in number with advancing age and represent a degenerative change.
- *Alzheimer type II astrocytes* exhibit an enlarged nucleus with intranuclear glycogen and pale chromatin; these occur in the setting of hyperammonemia.

Reactions of Microglia to Injury (p. 1253)

Following injury, microglia (mesoderm-derived phagocytic cells) proliferate, develop elongated nuclei *(rod cells),* form aggregates around necrotic foci *(microglial nodules),* and/or aggregate around dying neurons *(neuronophagia).*

Reactions of Other Glial Cells to Injury (p. 1253)

- *Oligodendroglial cell* apoptosis is a feature of demyelinating disorders and leukodystrophies; viral inclusions can be seen in progressive multifocal leukoencephalopathy (PML), and α-synuclein inclusions can be seen in multiple system atrophy (MSA).
- *Ependymal cells* do not regenerate; any damage results in proliferation of subependymal astrocytes, forming *ependymal granulations.*

Cerebral Edema, Hydrocephalus, and Raised Intracranial Pressure and Herniation (p. 1254)

The volume of the intracranial contents is fixed by the skull. Generalized CNS edema, increased CSF volume *(hydrocephalus),* and hemorrhage or expanding mass lesions can thus increase intracranial pressure; consequences range from subtle neurologic deficits to death.

Cerebral Edema (p. 1254)

Brain parenchymal edema can be the following:

- *Vasogenic:* Increased vascular permeability leads to the focal or generalized accumulation of *intercellular fluid;* the absence of lymphatics impairs resorption.
- *Cytotoxic:* Increased *intracellular fluid* secondary to endothelial, neuronal, or glial injury (e.g., after anoxia or toxic and metabolic disturbances).
- *Interstitial:* Fluid from the ventricular system transudates across the ependymal lining secondary to increased intraventricular pressure.

Hydrocephalus (p. 1254)

Obstruction of CSF flow leads to ventricular enlargement and increased CSF volume. Most cases are due to impaired flow or resorption; overproduction is an uncommon cause except for choroid plexus tumors.

- When hydrocephalus occurs before cranial suture closure, the head is enlarged; hydrocephalus after bone fusion leads to ventricular expansion and increased intracranial pressure.
- *Noncommunicating hydrocephalus* refers to enlargement of only a portion of the ventricle system (e.g., due to blockage of the third ventricle); in *communicating hydrocephalus* the entire system is expanded.
- In diseases associated with extensive tissue loss, compensatory expansion of the entire CSF compartment results in *hydrocephalus ex vacuo.*

Raised Intracranial Pressure and Herniation (p. 1255)

Increased intracranial pressure leads to compression of brain parenchyma; vascular perfusion can also be compromised, further exacerbating cerebral edema. Because the cranial vault is divided by rigid dural folds (*falx* and *tentorium*), localized expansion can cause displacement relative to the partitions with associated *herniation syndromes* (Fig. 28-1):

- *Subfalcine (cingulate) herniation* can compromise branches of the anterior cerebral artery.
- *Transtentorial (uncinate, mesial temporal) herniation* can distort the adjacent midbrain and pons; third cranial nerve compromise

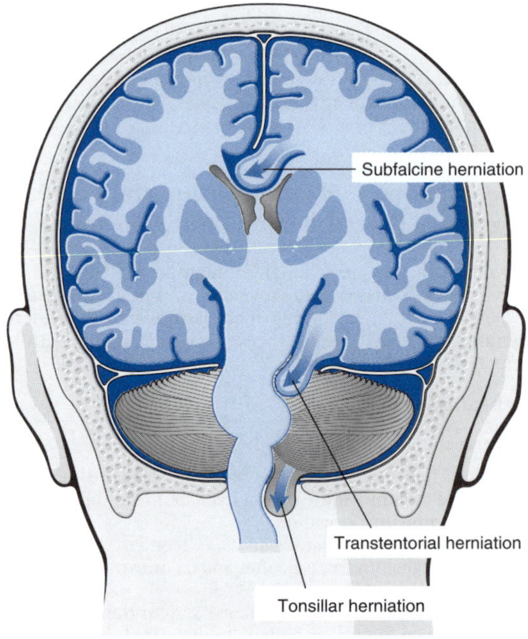

Figure 28-1 Major herniation syndromes.

causes papillary dilation, and compression of the posterior cerebral artery can cause visual cortex ischemia. Substantial herniation causes ipsilateral hemiparesis and is often accompanied by tearing of feeding vessels *(Duret hemorrhages)*.

- *Tonsillar herniation* through the foramen magnum can compress the medulla and compromise cardiac and respiratory centers.

Malformations and Developmental Disorders (p. 1256)

The nature of developmental malformations depends mainly on when injury occurs during gestation; maternal and fetal infections, drugs, anoxia, ischemia, and genetic disorders can all be involved.

Neural Tube Defects (p. 1256)

These malformations reflect primary failure to close or secondary reopening of the neural tube after successful closure; they are associated with abnormalities in neural tissue, meninges, and overlying bone and soft tissue. The frequency varies between ethnic groups; both genetic and environmental factors can be involved. For example, *folate deficiency* is a major risk factor, with some population differences secondary to polymorphisms in folate metabolism. Antenatal diagnosis can be made by imaging and maternal screening for α-fetoprotein.

- *Spina bifida* can be an asymptomatic bony defect *(spina bifida occulta)* or a severe malformation with a flattened, disorganized cord segment with overlying meningeal outpouching.
- *Myelomeningocele* represents CNS outpouching through a vertebral column defect; most occur in the lumbosacral region associated with lower extremity motor and sensory deficits and disturbed bowel and bladder control.
- *Encephalocele* is a malformed CNS diverticulum extending through a defect in the cranium, typically in the occiput or posterior fossa.
- *Anencephaly* is a malformation of the anterior neural tube, resulting in failure of cerebral development.

Forebrain Anomalies (p. 1256)

- *Brain size* is influenced by the duration of periventricular cell proliferation relative to the onset of their migration into the cortex. If too many cells exit the proliferating population too soon, the result is *microencephaly* (small brain) and reduction of gyral numbers *(lissencephaly)*; in extreme cases there may even be complete absence of gyri *(agyria)*. Chromosomal abnormalities, fetal alcohol syndrome, and in utero human immunodeficiency virus (HIV) infection can be causal. Conversely, if too few cells exit the proliferating pool at early stages (much less common), there is an eventual overproduction of neurons; *megalencephaly* (large brain) ensues.
- *Gyral formation* and overall *organization* are influenced by the patterns of neuronal movement following cell division.
  - *Polymicrogyria* are small, overabundant cerebral convolutions due to focal injury near the end of neuronal migration; there are also genetic causes.
  - *Neuronal heterotopias* are abnormal clusters of neurons in inappropriate locations along normal migratory routes; they are commonly associated with epilepsy. Mutations in cytoskeletal (e.g., filamin A) or microtubule-associated proteins can be causal.

- *Holoprosencephaly* is characterized by incomplete separation of the cerebral hemispheres; it is also associated with midline facial abnormalities (including cyclopia). Holoprosencephaly can result from mutations of *sonic hedgehog* or other genes involved in neural development.
- In *agenesis of the corpus callosum*, normal white matter interhemispheric bundles are not formed; although mental retardation can occur, individuals are often clinically normal.

Posterior Fossa Anomalies (p. 1258)

- *Arnold-Chiari malformation (Chiari II malformation)* consists of a small posterior fossa, a malformed midline cerebellum with extension of the vermis through the foramen magnum, hydrocephalus, and a lumbar myelomeningocele.
- *Chiari I malformation* is associated with low-lying cerebellar tonsils extending into the vertebral canal; it is often clinically silent, but can present with CSF flow obstruction.
- *Dandy-Walker malformation* is characterized by an enlarged posterior fossa, absent cerebellar vermis, and large midline cyst, with brainstem nuclei dysplasias.

Syringomyelia and Hydromyelia (p. 1258)

These are expansions of the central canal *(hydromyelia)* or formation of a cleftlike cavity *(syringomyelia)* in the spinal cord. Histologically there is associated gray and white matter destruction, surrounded by reactive gliosis. Patients present with loss of pain and temperature sensation in the upper extremities.

Perinatal Brain Injury (p. 1258)

Cerebral palsy is the broad term for nonprogressive motor deficits related to prenatal and perinatal neurologic insults; prematurity is a major risk factor. Depending on the location of the injury, lesions are clinically manifested by dystonia, spasticity, ataxia, athetosis, and/or paresis:

- *Intraparenchymal hemorrhage* within the germinal matrix often occurs between the thalamus and caudate nucleus and can extend into the ventricular system.
- *Ischemic* infarcts can occur in the periventricular white matter *(periventricular leukomalacia)* or within the hemispheres *(multicystic encephalopathy)*.
- *Ulegyria* is the term for thin, gliotic gyri due to perinatal cortical ischemia; *status marmoratus* reflects ischemic neuronal loss and gliosis in the basal ganglia and thalamus associated with aberrant and irregular myelin formation.
- Injury during gestation can destroy brain tissue without evoking any reactive gliosis.

Trauma (p. 1259)

Skull Fractures (p. 1259)

Fracture resistance varies with skull bone thickness; *displaced fracture* is the term used when bone shifts into the cranial vault by more than its thickness. Accidental falls tend to involve the occiput; they can have secondary basal skull involvement with lower cranial nerve or cervicomedullary symptoms and CSF discharge and/or meningitis. Trauma occurring as a consequence of syncope tends to involve the frontal skull. Although the kinetic energy that causes fractures tends to be dissipated at sutures, fractures can nevertheless traverse sutures *(diastatic)*.

Parenchymal Injuries (p. 1259)

Concussion (p. 1259)

Concussion is a transient trauma-related clinical syndrome associated with loss of consciousness, temporary respiratory arrest, and loss of reflexes; there is amnesia for the event. Postconcussive neuropsychiatric syndromes—commonly associated with repetitive injuries—are well recognized.

Direct Parenchymal Injury (p. 1259)

Direct parenchymal injury takes the form of *lacerations* (penetrating injury causing tissue tearing) and *contusions* (essentially CNS bruises). Gyral crests are most susceptible to contusion (e.g., at the site of impact *[coup contusion]* or the point opposite *[contrecoup]*). Microscopically there is brain hemorrhage and edema that eventually resolve as a depressed, yellow-brown glial scar extending to the pial surface *(plaque jaune)*.

Diffuse Axonal Injury (p. 1261)

Diffuse axonal injury occurs when mechanical forces—including angular acceleration even in the absence of impact—disrupt axonal integrity and subsequent axoplasmic flow. Microscopically there is widespread axonal swelling and focal hemorrhage, subsequently replaced by degenerated fibers and gliosis. Up to half of patients who become comatose after trauma have diffuse axonal injury—even in the absence of cerebral contusions.

Traumatic Vascular Injury (p. 1261)

Depending on the anatomy of ruptured vessels, trauma-related hemorrhages are *epidural, subdural, subarachnoid,* and *intraparenchymal* (Fig. 28-2). Subarachnoid and intraparenchymal hemorrhages are most often associated with superficial contusions and lacerations.

Epidural Hematomas (p. 1261)

Epidural hematomas result from rupture of dural arteries, most commonly the middle meningeal artery; blood collects between the dura and skull, compressing the brain. Depending on the tempo of accumulation, patients can be lucid for several hours after trauma. Lesions can also expand rapidly, mandating prompt drainage.

Subdural Hematomas (p. 1262)

Subdural hematomas result from tearing of veins that stretch from the cortical surface through the subarachnoid and subdural spaces and into draining veins (e.g., superior sagittal sinus). Whereas the brain "floats" freely in the CSF, the veins are tethered and thus prone to rupture with traumatic shifting of the brain within the skull. Geriatric patients with cerebral atrophy are particularly susceptible, even after minor trauma. Slowly progressive symptoms—often nonlocalizing headache and confusion—usually occur within 48 hours of injury, although acute decompensation can occur. Subdural hematomas can bleed recurrently, attributed to hemorrhage from thin-walled vessels of granulation tissue *(chronic subdural hematoma)*.

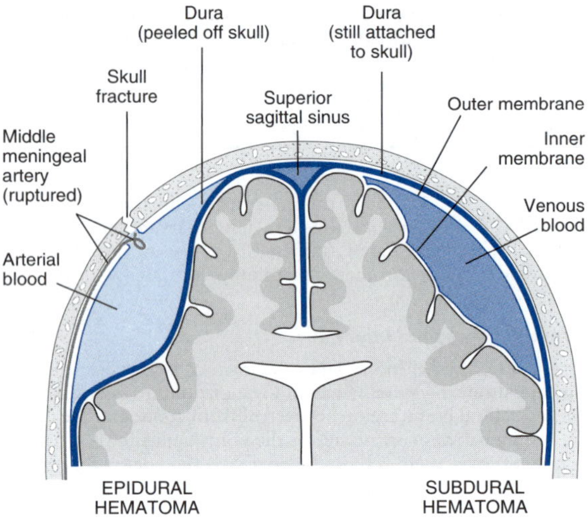

Figure 28-2 Epidural hematoma *(left):* a meningeal artery rupture (usually associated with a skull fracture) leads to accumulation of arterial blood between the dura and skull. Subdural hematoma *(right):* damage to bridging veins between the brain and superior sagittal sinus leads to venous blood accumulation between the dura and the arachnoid.

Sequelae of Brain Trauma (p. 1262)

These include epilepsy, meningiomas, infectious diseases, and psychiatric disorders:

- *Posttraumatic hydrocephalus* occurs when hemorrhage into the subarachnoid space obstructs CSF resorption.
- *Posttraumatic dementia (dementia pugilistica)* is the consequence of repeated head trauma; findings include hydrocephalus, corpus callosum thinning, diffuse axonal injury, amyloid plaques, and neurofibrillary tangles.

Spinal Cord Injury (p. 1263)

Cord injuries are associated with displacement of the spinal column; the level of injury determines the neurologic outcome:

- Thoracic vertebrae or below: paraplegia
- Cervical vertebrae: quadriplegia; with lesions at C4 and above, respiratory compromise due to diaphragm paralysis

Hemorrhage, necrosis, and white matter axonal swellings are acute findings. With time, necrotic lesions become cystic and gliotic; affected ascending and descending white matter tracts undergo secondary degeneration.

Cerebrovascular Diseases (p. 1263)

Cerebrovascular disease is the third leading cause of death in the United States (after heart disease and cancer); it is the most common cause of neurologic morbidity and mortality. *Stroke* is the clinical designation for these events, particularly with acute symptom onset; it occurs secondary to *hemorrhage* after vessel rupture or to *ischemia* and *infarction* from impaired perfusion or oxygenation (embolism is a more common cause than thrombosis).

Hypoxia, Ischemia, and Infarction (p. 1263)

The brain is primarily dependent on oxidative metabolism of circulation-derived glucose for adenosine triphosphate (ATP) generation. Ischemia leads to ATP depletion with the following:

- Loss of the membrane potential necessary for neuronal electrical activity
- Elevation of cytoplasmic calcium levels, activating an enzymatic cascade that causes cellular injury
- Inappropriate release of excitatory amino acid neurotransmitters (e.g., glutamate) that cause cell damage via calcium influx through *N*-methyl-D-aspartate (NMDA)-type glutamate receptors

Brain oxygen deprivation causes either global (*ischemic* or *hypoxic encephalopathy*) or focal ischemic necrosis *(cerebral infarction)*. At sites of diminished perfusion, outcomes depend on collateral circulation, duration of ischemia, and the magnitude and rapidity of flow reduction. In the region between necrotic tissue and the normal brain, a zone of "at-risk" tissue is called the *penumbra.*

Global Cerebral Ischemia (p. 1264)

Hypoxia can occur secondary to reduced blood oxygen content or to hypotension. Neurons are more sensitive than astrocytes and oligodendrocytes, and some neurons are more susceptible than others due to differences in regional blood flow and/or metabolic demand (e.g., cerebellar Purkinje cells, pyramidal cells of the cerebral cortex, and the hippocampus pyramidal cell layer [especially area CA1 or the *Sommer sector*]).

Severe global ischemia leads to widespread neuronal cell death; patients who survive can remain in a persistent vegetative state or meet "brain death" criteria: "flat" electroencephalogram and absent reflexes, respiratory drive, and cerebral perfusion. When maintained on mechanical ventilation, the brain of such patients eventually autolyzes ("respirator brain").

If oxygenation is only incompletely compromised, *watershed (border zone) infarcts* can occur at the interface between major vascular supplies; the territory between the anterior and middle cerebral artery is most vulnerable.

Morphology (p. 1264)

- *Gross:* Ischemic areas are edematous with widened gyri and narrowed sulci; there is poor gray-white matter demarcation.
- *Microscopic:* Twelve to 24 hours after injury, cellular ischemia is highlighted by the presence of *red neurons.* Subsequent neutrophil infiltration is followed by macrophage influx, neovascularization, and reactive gliosis. Uneven cortical neuronal loss and gliosis alternating with preserved zones generates a pattern termed *pseudolaminar necrosis.*

Focal Cerebral Ischemia (p. 1264)

Focal cerebral ischemia can result from thrombotic or embolic arterial occlusion. The clinical manifestations depend on the anatomic location of the lesion; deficits evolve with time and can be permanent or slowly improve.

- *Thrombosis* (usually due to underlying atherosclerosis) most frequently affects the extracerebral carotid system and the basilar artery.
- *Embolism* most commonly involves the intracerebral arteries and particularly the middle cerebral artery distribution. Emboli originate from atheromatous cerebrovascular plaques, cardiac mural thrombi (especially in the setting of atrial fibrillation), valvular lesions, or paradoxically through atrial or ventricular septal defects.

- *Inflammatory* lesions, including infectious vasculitis (e.g., syphilis or tuberculosis) and vasculitides (e.g., polyarteritis nodosa) can also cause luminal narrowing and cerebral infarction.
- *Venous infarcts* occur after occlusion of the superior sagittal sinus, other sinuses, or deep cerebral veins, and are characteristically hemorrhagic.

Morphology (p. 1266)

- *Nonhemorrhagic infarcts (bland or anemic infarcts)* are evident at 48 hours as pale, soft regions of edematous brain, with neutrophilic infiltration. The tissue then liquefies, and a fluid-filled cavity containing macrophages is lined by reactive glia.
- *Hemorrhagic infarcts,* characteristic of embolic occlusion with reperfusion injury, exhibit blood extravasation, but otherwise evolve in a fashion comparable to bland infarcts.

Hypertensive Cerebrovascular Disease (p. 1267)

Lacunar Infarcts (p. 1267)

Lacunar infarcts are small (<15 mm) cystic infarcts resulting from cerebral arteriolar sclerosis and occlusion; tissue loss is accompanied by lipid-laden macrophages and surrounding gliosis. The lenticular nucleus, thalamus, internal capsule, deep white matter, caudate nucleus, and pons are most commonly affected. Clinically these can be silent or cause serious impairment.

Slit Hemorrhages (p. 1267)

Slit hemorrhages occur when hypertension causes small vessel rupture; these eventually resorb, leaving residual hemosiderin-laden macrophages and associated gliosis.

Hypertensive Encephalopathy (p. 1268)

- *Acute hypertensive encephalopathy* is a clinicopathologic syndrome caused by increased intracranial pressure and manifesting as diffuse cerebral dysfunction (headaches, confusion, vomiting, convulsions, and occasionally coma). Rapid therapeutic intervention is required; postmortem examination reveals an edematous brain (occasionally with herniation), with petechiae and arteriolar fibrinoid necrosis.
- *Chronic hypertensive injury.* Recurrent small infarcts (hypertensive, atherosclerotic, and/or embolic) can lead to *vascular (multi-infarct) dementia,* a syndrome characterized by dementia, gait abnormalities, pseudobulbar signs, and other focal neurologic deficits. *Binswanger disease* is the designation when the pattern of recurrent ischemic injury preferentially involves subcortical white matter with myelin and axonal loss.

The severity of neurodegeneration disorders is exacerbated by concurrent cerebrovascular disease.

Intracranial Hemorrhage (p. 1268)

Intraparenchymal Hemorrhage (p. 1268)

Intraparenchymal hemorrhage typically involves spontaneous rupture of a small intraparenchymal vessel; peak incidence is age 60.

- *Hypertension* is the predisposing factor in half, accounting for 15% of deaths among patients with chronic hypertension. Hypertension leads to vessel weakening through hyaline arteriosclerosis, focal vessel necrosis, and the formation of microaneurysms *(Charcot-Bouchard aneurysms).* Lesions occur in the putamen (50% to 60% of cases), thalamus, pons, and rarely the cerebellar hemispheres.

- Cerebral amyloid angiopathy (CAA) is the second most common etiology; amyloidogenic peptides identical to those seen in Alzheimer disease (AD; see later) deposit in vessel walls leading to weakening. "Stiff" amyloid deposition characteristically involves the leptomeningeal and cerebral cortical vessels.
- Cerebral autosomal dominant arteriopathy with subcortical infarcts and leukoencephalopathy (CADASIL) is a rare form of stroke caused by mutations in the Notch3 receptor, causing abnormal folding of the extracellular domain. Affected vessels exhibit concentric medial and adventitial thickening exhibiting basophilic granular deposits and smooth muscle dropout.

Subarachnoid Hemorrhage and Ruptured Saccular Aneurysms *(p. 1269)*

The most common cause of clinically significant subarachnoid hemorrhage is *berry (saccular) aneurysm* rupture; subarachnoid hemorrhages can also result from traumatic hematomas, vascular malformations, hypertensive intracerebral hemorrhage, tumors, and hematologic disturbances.

Pathogenesis (p. 1270)

Berry aneurysms occur in 2% of the population, with 20% to 30% of patients having multiple aneurysms; 90% of berry aneurysms occur in the anterior circulation near arterial branch points (Fig. 28-3). Although most are sporadic, aneurysms are also associated with autosomal dominant polycystic kidney disease (see Chapter 20), hypertension, aortic coarctation, connective tissue disorders (Ehlers-Danlos syndrome type IV, Marfan syndrome), neurofibromatosis type 1 (NF1), and fibromuscular dysplasia. The aneurysms are not typically present at birth but develop over time due to an underlying weakness in the vessel media.

Morphology (p. 1270)

Lesions are a few millimeters to 2 to 3 cm in diameter with a red, shiny, translucent wall. At the aneurysm neck, the muscular wall and

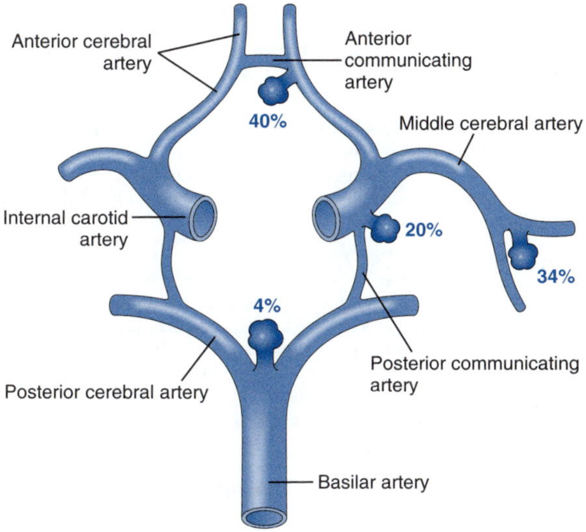

Figure 28-3 Sites of saccular (berry) aneurysms in the circle of Willis.

intimal elastic lamina are absent or fragmentary; the sac wall is composed of only thickened hyalinized intima.

Clinical Features (p. 1271)

Rupture risk increases with lesion size; aneurysms >10 mm have a 50% annual risk of bleeding. Rupture is most frequent in the fifth decade of life and is slightly more common in women. It often occurs with elevated intracranial pressure (e.g., straining at stool or sexual orgasm). Symptoms include excruciating headache and rapid loss of consciousness. Between 25% and 50% die with the first rupture; in survivors, rebleeding is common with progressively worsening prognosis with each episode. Blood in the subarachnoid space can lead to arterial vasospasm, and blood resorption can cause meningeal fibrosis and hydrocephalus.

Vascular Malformations *(p. 1271)*

- *Arteriovenous malformations (AVM)* are tangles of abnormally tortuous and misshapen vessels, shunting arterial blood directly into the venous circulation; middle cerebral artery territory is most commonly involved. The male to female ratio is 2:1; most cases manifest between ages 10 and 30 as a seizure disorder, intracerebral hemorrhage, or subarachnoid hemorrhage.
- *Cavernous malformations* are distended, loosely organized vascular channels with thin, collagenized walls; they occur most often in the cerebellum, pons, and subcortical regions and have low flow without arteriovenous shunting.
- *Capillary telangiectasias* are microscopic foci of dilated, thin-walled vascular channels separated by relatively normal brain parenchyma; they occur most frequently in the pons.
- *Venous angiomas (varices)* consist of aggregates of ectatic veins. *Foix-Alajouanine disease* is a venous angiomatous malformation typically seen in the lumbosacral region, associated with slowly progressive ischemia and neurologic symptoms.

Infections (p. 1271)

Infectious injury to the CNS can occur by direct microbial damage, through elaboration of microbial toxins, or by the effects of the host immune response (Table 28-1). Microbes can access the CNS by the following:

- *Hematogenous spread*—most common, usually arterial
- *Direct implantation*—usually traumatic
- *Local extension*—from an established infection in an air sinus
- *Axonal transport*—along peripheral nerves (e.g., rabies and herpes zoster)

Acute Meningitis (p. 1272)

Inflammation of the meninges (meningitis) or meninges and brain parenchyma (meningoencephalitis) is most commonly caused by infection. However, similar reactions can occur due to nonbacterial irritants in the subarachnoid space *(chemical meningitis)*.

Acute Pyogenic (Bacterial) Meningitis *(p. 1272)*

Pathogens differ across age groups:

- Neonates: *Escherichia coli* and the group B streptococci
- Infants and children: *Streptococcus pneumoniae* (*Haemophilus influenzae*, reduced with immunization)

TABLE 28-1 Common Central Nervous System Infections

Type of Infection	Clinical Syndrome	Common Causative Organisms
Bacterial Infections		
Meningitis	Acute pyogenic meningitis	*E. coli* or group B streptococci (infants)
		N. meningitidis (young adults)
		S. pneumoniae or *L. monocytogenes* (older adults)
	Chronic meningitis	*Mycobacterium tuberculosis*
Localized infections	Abscess	Streptococci and staphylococci
	Empyema	Polymicrobial (staphylococci, anaerobic, gram negative)
Viral Infections		
Meningitis	Acute aseptic meningitis	Enteroviruses
		Measles (SSPE)
		Influenza species
		Lymphocytic choriomeningitis virus
Encephalitis	Encephalitic syndromes	HSV-1, HSV-2
		CMV
		HIV
		JC polyomavirus (PML)
	Arthropod-borne encephalitis	West Nile virus
		Eastern equine encephalitis virus
		Western equine encephalitis virus
		St. Louis encephalitis virus
		La Crosse encephalitis virus
		Venezuelan equine encephalitis virus
		Japanese encephalitis virus
		Tick-borne encephalitis virus
Brainstem and spinal cord syndromes	Rhombencephalitis	Rabies
	Spinal poliomyelitis	Polio
		West Nile virus
Rickettsia, Spirochetes, and Fungi		
Meningitic syndromes	Rocky Mountain spotted fever	*Rickettsia rickettsii*
	Neurosyphilis	*Treponema pallidum*
	Lyme disease (neuroborreliosis)	*Borrelia burgdorferi*
	Fungal meningitis	*C. neoformans*
		C. albicans
Protozoa and Metazoa		
Meningitic syndromes	Cerebral malaria	*P. falciparum*
	Amebic encephalitis	*Naegleria* species
Localized infections	Toxoplasmosis	*T. gondii*
	Cysticercosis	*Taenia solium*

- Adolescents and young adults: *Neisseria meningitidis*
- Elderly: *S. pneumoniae* and *Listeria monocytogenes*

Affected individuals present with fever, headache, photophobia, irritability, clouded sensorium, and neck stiffness. The CSF is purulent with neutrophils and organisms, increased protein, and decreased glucose.

Morphology (p. 1273)

- *Gross:* Meningeal vessels are engorged, and there is a purulent exudate.
- *Microscopic:* Neutrophils fill the subarachnoid space; in fulminant cases, inflammation may focally extend into the underlying CNS (cerebritis). Phlebitis can cause venous thrombosis and hemorrhagic infarction. Resolution can lead to leptomeningeal fibrosis and hydrocephalus.

Acute Aseptic (Viral) Meningitis (p. 1272)

Acute aseptic (viral) meningitis is characterized by meningeal irritation, a CSF lymphocytic pleocytosis, with moderate protein elevation and normal glucose; the course is usually less fulminant than for pyogenic meningitis and is self-limited. The spectrum of pathogens varies seasonally and geographically, and causal pathogens are infrequently pinpointed; when an agent is identified, it is an enterovirus in 80% of cases.

Acute Focal Suppurative Infections (p. 1273)

Brain Abscess (p. 1273)

Brain abscess is a destructive lesion arising in the setting of bacterial endocarditis, congenital heart disease (with right-to-left shunting), chronic pulmonary sepsis, or immunosuppression. Streptococci and staphylococci are the principal organisms. Patients present with progressive focal neurologic deficits, and signs of increased intracranial pressure. If the subdural space becomes infected, thrombophlebitis can develop, resulting in venous occlusion and brain infarction.

Morphology (p. 1273)

There is a central region of liquefactive necrosis and a fibrous capsule surrounded by reactive gliosis and marked vasogenic edema.

Subdural Empyema (p. 1274)

Subdural empyema occurs when bacterial or fungal infections of the skull or air sinuses spread to the subdural space. Large collections can cause a mass effect or thrombophlebitis of bridging veins. Most patients are febrile, and have headaches and neck stiffness, with a CSF profile similar to a brain abscess.

Extradural Abscesses (p. 1274)

Extradural abscesses are commonly associated with osteomyelitis, arising in the setting of sinusitis or after surgery. In the spinal epidural space, it can cause spinal cord compression.

Chronic Bacterial Meningoencephalitis (p. 1274)

Tuberculosis (p. 1274)

Tuberculous meningitis causes headache, malaise, mental confusion, and vomiting. There is moderate CSF mononuclear cell pleocytosis (occasionally with neutrophils), elevated protein, and moderately reduced or normal glucose. Tuberculous meningitis can cause arachnoid fibrosis, hydrocephalus, and obliterative endarteritis. Tuberculomas present as typical space-occupying lesions. *Mycobacterium avium-intracellulare* infections can also occur in patients with acquired immunodeficiency syndrome (AIDS) but typically provoke little granulomatous response.

Morphology (p. 1274)

Diffuse meningoencephalitis is the most common pattern of disease. The subarachnoid space contains a gelatinous or fibrinous exudate of chronic inflammatory cells and rarely, well-formed granulomas, most often at the base of the brain, obliterating the cisternae and encasing the cranial nerves. Arteries running through the subarachnoid space may show *obliterative endarteritis.*

Neurosyphilis *(p. 1274)*

Neurosyphilis is a manifestation of the tertiary stage of disease; it occurs in 10% of patients with untreated infections. HIV-infected patients are at increased risk for neurosyphilis related to impaired cell-mediated immunity; the severity and tempo of disease are also accelerated.

- *Meningovascular neurosyphilis* is a chronic meningitis sometimes associated with obliterative endarteritis.
- *Paretic neurosyphilis* results from brain invasion by spirochetes, with neuronal loss and microglial proliferation. Patients exhibit insidious loss of mental and physical capacity with mood alterations (including delusions of grandeur), terminating in severe dementia.
- *Tabes dorsalis* results from spirochete damage to dorsal root sensory neurons, leading to impaired joint position sense, locomotor ataxia, loss of pain sensation with secondary skin and joint damage (Charcot joints), and absent deep tendon reflexes.

Neuroborreliosis (Lyme Disease) *(p. 1275)*

The neurologic manifestations of Lyme disease are highly variable but can include aseptic meningitis, facial nerve palsies (and other polyneuropathies), as well as encephalopathy. Microscopically there is microglial proliferation and scattered organisms.

Viral Meningoencephalitis (p. 1275)

Viral parenchymal infections of the CNS *(encephalitis)* are almost invariably associated with meningeal inflammation and occasionally with spinal cord inflammation *(encephalomyelitis)*. Viruses can exhibit specific cellular tropisms or can have a predilection for particular brain regions. Latency is a common feature of several CNS viral infections; non-CNS systemic infections can also precipitate immune-mediated neurologic injury. Intrauterine viral infection (e.g., rubella) can cause congenital malformations, and progressive degenerative disease syndromes can occur years after a viral illness (e.g., postencephalitic parkinsonism after the 1918 viral influenza pandemic).

Arthropod-Borne Viral Encephalitis *(p. 1275)*

Arthropod-borne viral encephalitis is the etiology of most epidemic viral encephalitides (e.g., Eastern and Western equine, Venezuelan, St. Louis, La Crosse, and West Nile viruses). All have animal hosts and mosquito or tick vectors. Typical clinical manifestations are seizures, confusion, delirium, and stupor or coma.

Herpes Simplex Virus Type 1 *(p. 1275)*

Herpes simplex virus type 1 (HSV-1) is most common in children and young adults; only 10% have prior herpes infection. Patients classically present with alterations in affect, mood, memory, and behavior; some cases follow a more protracted course with weakness, lethargy, ataxia, and seizures.

Morphology (p. 1276)

Severe cases exhibit hemorrhagic, necrotizing encephalitis of the inferomedial temporal lobes and the orbital gyri of the frontal lobes.

There are perivascular infiltrates, with Cowdry A intranuclear viral inclusion bodies in neurons and glia.

Herpes Simplex Virus Type 2 *(p. 1276)*

Herpes simplex virus type 2 (HSV-2) causes a severe, generalized, encephalitis in 50% of neonates born vaginally to women with primary HSV-2 infection. It can cause meningitis in adults and a severe hemorrhagic, necrotizing encephalitis in HIV-infected individuals.

Varicella-Zoster Virus (Herpes Zoster) *(p. 1276)*

Latent chickenpox infections in dorsal root ganglia can be reactivated, leading to painful vesicular skin eruptions in a dermatomal distribution *(shingles)*. It is usually self-limited, but patients can develop a persistent painful postherpetic neuralgia syndrome. Herpes zoster can also cause a granulomatous arteritis or a necrotizing encephalitis in immunosuppressed patients.

Cytomegalovirus *(p. 1277)*

In utero infection leads to periventricular necrosis, microcephaly, and periventricular calcification. In patients with AIDS, cytomegalovirus (CMV) is a common opportunistic viral pathogen; it causes a subacute encephalitis with microglial nodules or a periventricular hemorrhagic necrotizing encephalitis and choroid plexitis. Classic CMV inclusions are readily identified.

Poliomyelitis *(p. 1277)*

Poliomyelitis presents with meningeal irritation and a CSF picture of aseptic meningitis; involvement of lower motor neurons can cause flaccid paralysis with hyporeflexia and secondary muscle wasting. Patients can also develop myocarditis, and death can result from paralysis of the respiratory muscles. Inflammation is usually confined to the anterior horns but can extend into the posterior horns. The *postpolio syndrome* typically develops 25 to 35 years after the initial illness; it is characterized by progressive weakness associated with pain and decreased muscle mass.

Rabies *(p. 1277)*

Rabies is a severe encephalitis transmitted by the bite of a rabid animal or exposure to certain bat species even without a bite. Over the course of 1 to 3 months, the virus ascends from the wound site to the CNS along the peripheral nerves. It causes extraordinary CNS excitability, hydrophobia, and flaccid paralysis; death ensues from respiratory center failure. Widespread neuronal necrosis and inflammation, most severe in the basal ganglia, midbrain, and medulla, are present. Pathognomonic *Negri bodies* (intracytoplasmic eosinophilic inclusions) are found in hippocampal pyramidal cells and Purkinje cells, usually without associated inflammation.

Human Immunodeficiency Virus *(p. 1278)*

An *aseptic meningitis* occurs in 10% of patients within 1 to 2 weeks of a primary HIV infection; during the chronic phase of infection, *HIV encephalitis* is commonly found in symptomatic individuals. Notably, only microglia express the appropriate CD4 and chemokine receptors necessary for efficient HIV infection. In the absence of antiretroviral therapy, 80% to 90% of AIDS patients eventually develop CNS lesions, including direct viral pathogenic effects, opportunistic infections, and/or CNS lymphomas; intensive multidrug therapy has substantially reduced this incidence.

- *Immune reconstitution inflammatory syndrome (IRIS)* can occur in patients with AIDS after effective treatment; in the CNS, IRIS causes paradoxical exacerbation of symptoms from opportunistic infections, with an intense influx of CD8+ lymphocytes.

- *HIV-associated dementia* is related to the extent of activated CNS microglia; cytokines and other inflammatory mediators are causally implicated.

Morphology (p. 1278)

HIV encephalitis exhibits a chronic inflammatory reaction with widely distributed microglial nodules—and multinucleated giant cells—sometimes with associated necrosis and gliosis. The subcortical white matter, diencephalon, and brainstem are typically most affected.

Progressive Multifocal Leukoencephalopathy (p. 1278)

PML is due to oligodendrocyte infection by the JC polyomavirus, typically in immunosuppressed patients. Most adults have serologic evidence of prior JC exposure; thus PML likely represents viral reactivation. Patients develop progressive, multifocal neurologic manifestations caused by focal myelin destruction.

Morphology (p. 1278)

Lesions consist of demyelinated patches, greatly enlarged oligodendrocyte nuclei with viral inclusions, and astrocytes with greatly enlarged atypical nuclei.

Subacute Sclerosing Panencephalitis (p. 1279)

Subacute sclerosing panencephalitis (SSPE) is a progressive syndrome of cognitive decline, limb spasticity, and seizures. It occurs months to years after an early-age measles infection and represents a persistent but nonproductive CNS infection by an altered measles virus. Widespread gliosis and myelin degeneration is associated with viral nuclear inclusions in oligodendrocytes and neurons; there is also variable inflammation and neurofibrillary tangles.

Fungal Meningoencephalitis (p. 1279)

Fungal CNS infections are typically encountered in immunocompromised patients, usually in the setting of widespread hematogenous dissemination (e.g., with *Candida albicans, Mucor, Aspergillus fumigatus,* and *Cryptococcus neoformans*). In endemic areas *Histoplasma, Coccidioides,* and *Blastomyces* can involve the CNS after primary pulmonary or cutaneous infections.

- *Meningitis* is caused most frequently by *Cryptococcus;* it can be fulminant and fatal within 2 weeks or chronic and indolent evolving over months to years.
- *Vasculitis* occurs most frequently with *Mucor* and *Aspergillus;* there is vessel invasion with associated thrombosis and hemorrhagic infarction.
- *Parenchymal involvement* can manifest with granulomas or abscesses and is most commonly encountered with *Candida* and *Cryptococcus.*

Other Infectious Diseases of the Nervous System (p. 1279)

Protozoal (malaria, toxoplasmosis, amebiasis, and trypanosomiasis), rickettsial (typhus, Rocky Mountain spotted fever), and metazoal (cysticercosis and echinococcosis) organisms can all infect the CNS (see Chapter 8); some are opportunistic while others can occur in immunocompetent hosts.

- *Toxoplasma gondii* is one of the most common CNS organisms seen in HIV-infected patients. Clinical symptoms occur over 1 to 2 weeks and are typically focal; imaging studies show multiple ring-enhancing lesions. Abscesses contain free tachyzoites and encysted bradyzoites. Primary maternal infection can be followed by a fetal cerebritis with multifocal necrotizing lesions that calcify.

- *Naegleria* is an amoeba that causes a rapidly fatal necrotizing encephalitis; *acanthamoeba* is associated with a chronic granulomatous meningoencephalitis.
- *Cerebral malaria* is a rapidly progressive encephalitis that is the major cause of mortality from *Plasmodium falciparum* infections. It results from vascular dysfunction. Acutely, there is reduced cerebral blood flow, ataxia, seizures, and coma; long-term cognitive deficits occur in up to 20% of affected children.

Prion Diseases (p. 1281)

Prions are abnormal forms of the cellular *prion protein* (PrP); these cause rapidly progressive dementing neurodegenerative disorders characterized by *spongiform changes*—neuronal and glial intracellular vacuoles. Prion diseases are transmissible and can be infectious, sporadic, or familial; disorders include Creutzfeldt-Jakob disease (CJD), Gerstmann-Sträussler-Scheinker syndrome, fatal familial insomnia (FFI), and kuru in humans, scrapie in sheep and goats, mink-transmissible encephalopathy, chronic wasting disease in elk and deer, and bovine spongiform encephalopathy *(mad cow disease)*.

Pathogenesis and Molecular Genetics (p. 1281)

PrP is a normal 30-kD neuronal protein; disease occurs when PrP undergoes a conformational change from its native α-helical isoform (PrP^{c}) to an abnormally folded (and protease-resistant) β-pleated sheet configuration, called PRP^{sc} (for scrapie). The PrP^{sc} conformational change occurs spontaneously at a very low rate (sporadic disease); it occurs more readily if certain mutations are present (familial disease). The transmissible or infectious nature of PrP^{sc} derives from its ability to induce the conformational change of PrP^{c}, thereby corrupting the integrity of normal cellular PrP. The *PRNP* gene encoding PrP is highly conserved across species, underlying some of the ability of PrP from other sources to cause human disease. Polymorphisms at codon 129 (encoding methionine or valine) also influence disease susceptibility or incubation period; heterozygosity at codon 129 is protective.

Creutzfeldt-Jakob Disease (p. 1282)

CJD is sporadic in 90% of cases, with a worldwide incidence of one in a million and peak occurrence in the seventh decade; cases can also be familial or iatrogenic (e.g., through corneal transplantation or electrode implantation). Patients present with subtle memory and behavior changes, followed by a rapidly progressive dementia, often with involuntary jerking muscle contractions. The disease is uniformly fatal, with an average duration of only 7 months after symptom onset.

Variant CJD *(p. 1282)*

Variant CJD (vCJD) came to medical attention in the United Kingdom in 1995; it occurs in young adults, with early behavioral manifestations and slower neurologic progression than for classic CJD. No *PRNP* mutations are present, and vCJD has been linked to bovine spongiform encephalopathy. Extensive cortical plaques are present, with a surrounding halo of spongiform change.

Morphology (p. 1309)

Spongiform changes in the cerebral cortex and deep gray matter structures (such as caudate and putamen) are characteristic. In advanced cases there is severe neuronal loss, reactive gliosis, and sometimes expansion of the vacuolated areas into cystlike spaces *(status spongiosus)*. No inflammatory infiltrate is present. *Kuru plaques* are extracellular aggregates of aggregated abnormal PrP^{sc} proteins; they are Congo red and periodic acid-Schiff (PAS) positive.

Fatal Familial Insomnia (p. 1282)

FFI is named in part for the sleep disturbances that characterize its initial stages; it is caused by *PRNP* mutations substituting aspartate for asparagine at residue 178 of PrP^c. When the mutations are present in alleles with methionine at position 129, FFI results; when a valine is present at position 129, CJD occurs.

Morphology (p. 1283)

Unlike other prion diseases, FFI does not exhibit spongiform changes; instead there is neuronal loss and reactive gliosis in the inferior olivary nuclei and anterior ventral and dorsomedial nuclei of the thalamus.

Demyelinating Diseases (p. 1283)

These inherited or acquired disorders are characterized by myelin damage with relative preservation of axons; neurologic deficits are secondary to loss of electric impulse transmission.

Multiple Sclerosis (p. 1283)

Multiple sclerosis (MS) is an autoimmune demyelinating disorder characterized by *distinct episodes of neurologic deficit separated in time and attributable to white matter lesions that are separated in space.* Women are affected twice as frequently as men; peak onset is between childhood and age 50. The natural course is variable but is characteristically relapsing and remitting with acute (days to weeks) deficit onset and slow, gradual partial remission. Relapse frequency tends to decrease over time, but most patients exhibit steady neurologic deterioration.

Pathogenesis (p. 1284)

MS is attributed to cellular immune responses directed against myelin. Genetic and environmental factors are both implicated, although the inciting stimulus (e.g., Epstein-Barr virus [EBV] infection) is uncertain; MS susceptibility is linked to the DR2 locus of the major histocompatibility complex and to polymorphisms in the interleukin (IL)-2 and IL-7 receptor genes. Based on animal models, disease is likely initiated by CD4+ T_H1 and T_H17 cells responding to myelin components. T_H1 cell interferon-γ secretion activates macrophages, and T_H17 cells help to recruit additional leukocytes; the resulting inflammatory infiltrate causes myelin destruction. The CSF in affected patients exhibits an oligoclonal immunoglobulin response, suggesting a contribution from B-cell immunity.

Morphology (p. 1284)

- *Gross:* Lesions *(plaques)* are sharply defined areas of gray discoloration of white matter occurring especially around the ventricles but can be located anywhere in the CNS.
- *Microscopic: Active plaques* show myelin breakdown, lipid-laden macrophages, and relative axonal preservation. Lymphocytes and mononuclear cells are prominent at plaque edges and around venules. *Inactive plaques* lack the inflammatory cell infiltrate and show gliosis; most axons within the lesion persist but remain unmyelinated.

Clinical Features (p. 1285)

Although neurologic manifestations can be diverse (depending on the site of demyelination), certain features are more common:

- Unilateral vision impairment due to optic neuritis is a frequent initial manifestation, although only 10% to 50% of patients with optic nerve involvement progress to full-blown MS.
- Brainstem involvement produces cranial nerve signs, ataxia, nystagmus, and internuclear ophthalmoplegia.
- Spinal cord lesions cause limb and trunk motor and sensory wimpairment, spasticity, and bladder dysfunction.

Neuromyelitis Optica (p. 1285)

This disorder is characterized by near-synchronous, bilateral optic neuritis and spinal cord demyelinating lesions. White matter lesions exhibit necrosis with acute inflammation and vascular immunoglobulin and complement deposition; many patients have antibodies directed against aquaporins, which are important in maintaining astrocyte foot processes and thus blood-brain barrier integrity.

Acute Disseminated Encephalomyelitis and Acute Necrotizing Hemorrhagic Encephalomyelitis (p. 1286)

- Acute disseminated encephalomyelitis (ADEM) is a diffuse demyelinating disease occurring after viral infection (or rarely, a viral immunization); patients present with headache, lethargy, and coma but no focal deficits. The clinical course is rapid; up to 20% die. All lesions appear similar, consistent with a single initiating insult, and exhibit perivenular demyelination with axonal preservation; early neutrophil infiltrates are followed by mononuclear cell inflammation and lipid-laden macrophages.
- Acute necrotizing hemorrhagic encephalomyelitis (ANHE) is a more fulminant, frequently fatal, demyelinating syndrome typically affecting children and young adults after an upper respiratory tract infection. Lesions are similar to ADEM but more severe and often confluent, with small vessel destruction and disseminated CNS necrosis.

Central Pontine Myelinolysis (p. 1286)

This disorder is characterized by myelin damage (with axonal preservation) without inflammation in the basis pontis and portions of the pontine tegmentum, often leading to rapidly evolving quadraplegia. It is most commonly associated with a rapid correction of a hyponatremic state (damaging oligodendroglial cells), although it can occur with other electrolyte abnormalities.

Neurodegenerative Diseases (p. 1286)

These are gray matter diseases, characterized by progressive loss of specific neuron regions with secondary white matter tract changes. *A common theme is the presence of protein aggregates* (recognizable as intracellular inclusions) *that are resistant to proteolytic degradation;* these elicit a neuronal stress response and can be directly neurotoxic. In some cases these protein aggregates can also propagate in a manner akin to prions. Degenerative CNS disorders are grouped according to the anatomic site of neuronal loss (and/or related clinical manifestations), as well as the nature of the associated inclusions or abnormal structures (Table 28-2).

TABLE 28-2 Features of the Major Neurodegenerative Diseases

Disease	Clinical Pattern	Inclusions	Genetic Causes
AD	Dementia	Aβ (plaques) Tau (tangles)	APP, PS1, PS2
FTLD	Behavioral changes, language disturbance	Tau	Tau
		TDP-43	TDP-43, progranulin, C9orf72
		FUS	FUS
PD	Hypokinetic movement disorder	α-Synuclein	α-Synuclein
		Tau	LRRK2
PSP	Parkinsonism with abnormal eye movements	Tau	Tau
CBD	Parkinsonism with asymmetric movement disorder	Tau	Tau
MSA	Parkinsonism, cerebellar ataxia, autonomic failure	α-Synuclein	α-Synuclein
HD	Hyperkinetic movement disorder	Huntington (polyglutamine)	Htt
SCAs (SCA1, 2, 3, 6, 7, 17 and DRPLA)	Cerebellar ataxia	Various proteins (polyglutamine containing)	Multiple loci
ALS	Weakness with upper and lower motor neuron signs	SOD1	SOD1
		TDP-43 FUS	TDP-43, C9orf72 FUS
Spinal bulbar muscular atrophy (SBMA)	Lower motor neuron weakness, diminished androgen	Androgen receptor (polyglutamine containing)	Androgen receptor

Alzheimer Disease (p. 1287)

AD is the most common dementing illness of the elderly, reaching a prevalence of >40% in the 85- to 89-year-old cohort. It usually begins after age 50, with progressive, insidious impairment of higher intellectual function over the subsequent 5 to 10 years. Most cases are sporadic, although at least 5% to 10% of cases are familial. Intercurrent disease—often pneumonia—is the cause of death in most AD patients.

Molecular Genetics and Pathogenesis (p. 1288)

Aβ and tau accumulations constitute the fundamental biochemical AD abnormality; *plaques* and *tangles* are the pathologic hallmarks. Plaques are deposits of aggregated Aβ peptides in the neuropil, whereas tangles are aggregates of the microtubule binding protein *tau;* the latter develop intracellularly and then persist extracellularly after neuronal death. Aβ generation is the critical initiating event in AD, but both plaques and tangles contribute to neuronal dysfunction.

- *Role of Aβ.* Aβ derives from the processing of amyloid precursor protein (APP), a normal transmembrane protein (Fig. 28-4). Aβ is highly prone to aggregation—first into small oligomers (which may be the toxic form responsible for neuronal dysfunction) and eventually into large aggregates and fibrils. An initial cleavage in the extracellular domain of APP determines the outcome:
  - Nonamyloidogenic pathway: α-secretase cleavage at the cell surface
  - Amyloidogenic pathway: Surface APP is endocytosed and undergoes cleavage by β-secretase

Following initial APP cleavage, the γ-secretase complex (including presenilin proteins) cleaves within the membrane. With an initial α-secretase cleavage, a soluble fragment results; if β-secretase makes the initial cut, Aβ is generated.

The gene encoding APP is on chromosome 21; gene dosing effects (e.g., trisomy 21 in Down syndrome or localized duplications in some familial forms of AD) lead to early-onset AD. Point mutations in APP affecting proteolytic cleavage or propensity to aggregate are other causes of familial AD. The majority of early-onset familial AD is associated with gain-of-function presenilin mutations that generate increased amounts of amyloidogenic Aβ.

- *Role of tau:* Tangles formation in AD is associated with tau hyperphosphorylation and inability to bind to and stabilize microtubules; hyperphosphorylated tau aggregates also elicit a stress response.
- *Other genetic risk factors:* Apolipoprotein E (ApoE) alleles (ε2, ε3, and ε4) influence AD risk; ε4 increases AD risk and lowers the age of onset by promoting Aβ generation and deposition.

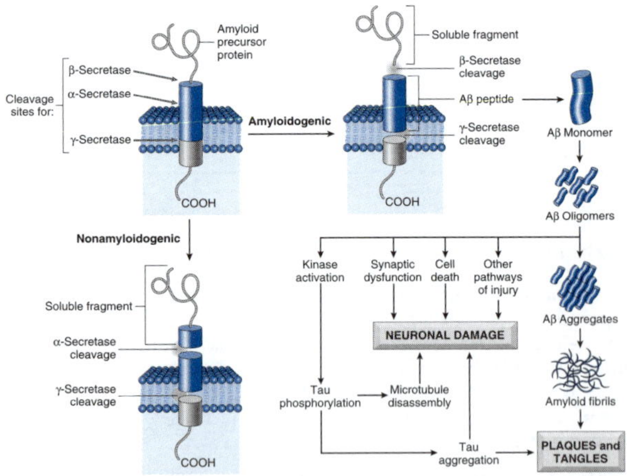

Figure 28-4 Protein aggregation in AD. APP cleavage by α-secretase and γ-secretase produces a harmless soluble peptide, whereas APP cleavage by β-amyloid-converting enzyme (BACE) and γ-secretase releases Aβ peptides, which form pathogenic aggregates and contribute to the characteristic plaques and tangles of AD.

- *Role of inflammation:* Aβ elicits an inflammatory response from microglia and astrocytes that can assist in aggregate clearance but can also stimulate the secretion of potentially deleterious mediators.
- *Basis for cognitive impairment:* A large burden of plaques and tangles is highly associated with severe cognitive dysfunction. The degree of dementia also correlates with loss of choline acetyltransferase, synaptophysin immunoreactivity, and amyloid burden.
- *Biomarkers:* Aβ deposition can be imaged using ^{18}F-labeled amyloid-binding compounds, and neuronal degeneration correlates with increased phosphorylated tau and reduced Aβ in the CSF.

Morphology (p. 1290)

- *Gross:* There is cortical atrophy with narrowed gyri and widened sulci, especially in the frontal, temporal, and parietal lobes; hydrocephalus ex vacuo also occurs. Medial temporal lobe structures (hippocampus, entorhinal cortex, and amygdala) are involved early and are severely atrophied in later stages.
- *Microscopic:* There are no unique pathognomonic findings in AD; *neuritic plaques* and *neurofibrillary tangles* are characteristic but because these (and other histologic findings) can occur in nondemented individuals, the formal diagnosis of AD is based on both clinical and pathologic features.
- *Neuritic plaques* are spherical collections of dilated, tortuous, neuritic processes (dystrophic neurites) around a central amyloid core; microglia and reactive astrocytes are at the periphery. The amyloid core predominantly contains Aβ, which can also be deposited in the absence of the neuritic reaction *(diffuse plaques).*
- *Neurofibrillary tangles* are bundles of paired helical filaments in neuronal cytoplasm, largely containing hyperphosphorylated tau, as well as ubiquitin and other microtubule-associated molecules.
- *CAA* almost invariably accompanies AD; there is vascular wall deposition of Aβ.

Frontotemporal Lobar Degenerations (p. 1292)

This is a group of disorders associated with temporal and/or frontal lobe degeneration. Alterations in personality, behavior, and language *(aphasias)* characteristically precede memory loss; global dementia occurs with progressive disease, and some patients have extrapyramidal motor loss. Frontotemporal lobar degenerations (FTLDs) can be hereditary or sporadic and are associated with cellular inclusions of specific proteins; the two most common are tau-containing inclusions and TDP43-containing inclusions.

Frontotemporal Lobar Degeneration-Tau (p. 1292)

FTLD-Tau is associated with aggregates of either wild-type or mutant tau, a phosphoprotein that normally interacts with microtubules; when hyperphosphorylated, it has a propensity to aggregate. Some missense mutations affect tau phosphorylation, whereas others influence splicing. Neuronal injury is a combination of aggregate toxicity as well as tau depletion through aggregation. Severe selective lobar atrophy with inclusions is the hallmark of *Pick disease.*

Morphology (p. 1292)

- *Gross:* Frontal and temporal lobe atrophy is seen in various combinations and to various degrees.
- *Microscopic:* Atrophic regions exhibit neuronal loss and gliosis as well as tau-containing neurofibrillary tangles. Nigral degeneration may also occur. Glial cell inclusions occur in some forms.

In Pick disease there is frontal and temporal lobe atrophy, with sparing of the posterior two thirds of the superior temporal gyrus; caudate and putamen atrophy can also occur. Lesions show large ballooned neurons (Pick cells) and smooth argyrophilic inclusions composed of straight and paired helical filaments (Pick bodies).

Frontotemporal Lobar Degeneration-TDP *(p. 1293)*

Some FTLDs have inclusions that contain TDP-43, an RNA-binding protein; there are three associated mutations:

- An expansion of a hexanucleotide repeat in the 5′ UTR of C9orf72 (a gene encoding a protein of unknown function) is most common. The spectrum of disease also includes amyotrophic lateral sclerosis (ALS).
- Mutations in the gene encoding the TDP-43 protein are less common; these can also be seen in some cases of ALS.
- Mutations in the gene encoding *progranulin,* a secreted glial and neuronal protein that is cleaved into multiple small peptides implicated in regulating CNS inflammation; these mutations are not associated with ALS.

Morphology (p. 1294)

The gross appearance is similar to the other forms of FTLDs, accompanied by varying degrees of neuronal loss and gliosis. Phosphorylated and ubiquitinated TDP-43 is found in cell body, neuritic, or nuclear inclusions.

Parkinson Disease (p. 1294)

The clinical syndrome of *parkinsonism* includes diminished facial expression *(masked facies),* stooped posture, slowed voluntary movement, festinating gait (progressively shortened, accelerated steps), rigidity, and a pill-rolling tremor. This type of motor disturbance is seen in several conditions that share a loss of dopaminergic neurons in the substantia nigra. Nigral dopaminergic neuronal depletion leads to striatal dopamine deficiency that correlates with the severity of the motor syndrome.

Parkinson disease (PD) is the principal neurodegenerative disease in this category and is diagnosed in individuals with the triad of tremor, rigidity, and bradykinesia in the absence of toxic or other known etiology; there is symptomatic response to l-dihydroxyphenylalanine (l-DOPA). Treatment does not arrest disease progression, and with time, drug therapy tends to become less effective. Deep brain stimulation has emerged as a therapy. In addition to parkinsonism, autonomic and cognitive dysfunction can occur.

Pesticides or 1-methyl-4-prenyl-1,2,3,6 tetrahydroperidine (MPTP), a contaminant in the illicit synthesis of meperidine, can cause parkinsonism due to substantia nigra toxicity; caffeine and nicotine may be protective.

Molecular Genetics and Pathogenesis *(p. 1294)*

Autosomal dominant forms of the disease include mutations causing overexpression of α-synuclein (a lipid-binding protein associated with synapses) or gain of function in the *LRRK2* gene (encoding a kinase). A juvenile recessive form of PD is caused by loss-of-function mutations in the *parkin* gene (encoding an E3 ubiquitin ligase). Other recessive forms involve mutations in DJ-1 (a protein that regulates redox responses to stress) and the PINK1 kinase (regulating mitochondrial function). PINK1 and parkin normally clear dysfunctional mitochondria through mitophagy; interestingly, levels of mitochondrial complex I (part of the oxidative phosphorylation cascade) are reduced in sporadic PD.

Morphology (p. 1295)

There is pallor of the substantia nigra and locus ceruleus, with loss of pigmented, catecholaminergic neurons and gliosis; *Lewy bodies* (intracytoplasmic, eosinophilic inclusions, containing α-synuclein) occur in the remaining neurons.

Dementia With Lewy Bodies (p. 1295)

Dementia develops in 10% to 15% of PD patients, often with a fluctuating course and associated hallucinations and frontal signs. Some patients have concurrent AD, but most have α-synuclein-containing Lewy bodies as the major histologic correlate.

Atypical Parkinsonism Syndromes (p. 1296)

A variety of disorders include parkinsonism symptoms but also additional signs and symptoms; in general, these are minimally responsive to l-DOPA.

Progressive Supranuclear Palsy (p. 1296)

Progressive supranuclear palsy (PSP) is a tauopathy (associated with aggregates of tau) characterized by loss of vertical gaze, truncal rigidity, dysequilibrium, loss of facial expression, and mild progressive dementia. Risk is linked to single nucleotide polymorphisms (SNPs) mapping near the tau gene locus.

Morphology

There is widespread neuronal loss and neurofibrillary tangles in the globus pallidus, subthalamic nucleus, substantia nigra, colliculi, periaqueductal gray matter, and dentate nucleus of the cerebellum. Tau pathology can be found in glial cells as well.

Corticobasal Degeneration (p. 1296)

Corticobasal degeneration (CBD) is a tauopathy of the elderly characterized by extrapyramidal rigidity, asymmetric motor disturbances, and sensory cortical dysfunction; this disorder is associated with the same SNP as are found in PSP.

Morphology

Motor, premotor, and anterior parietal cortex exhibit neuronal loss, gliosis, and ballooned neurons. The substantia nigra and locus ceruleus show loss of pigmented neurons and argyrophilic inclusions. Tau immunoreactivity is present in astrocytes ("tufted astrocytes") and oligodendrocytes ("coiled bodies").

Multiple System Atrophy (p. 1296)

MSA reflects a group of disorders characterized by atrophy in specific CNS regions associated with glial (predominantly oligodendrocyte) tubular cytoplasmic inclusions containing α-synuclein and ubiquitin.

- *Striatonigral degeneration* is dominated by parkinsonism; there is prominent atrophy of the substantia nigra and striatum.
- *Olivopontocerebellar atrophy* presents with cerebellar ataxia, eye and somatic movement abnormalities, dysarthria, and rigidity; atrophy involves the cerebellar peduncles, basis pontis, and inferior olives.
- *Shy-Drager syndrome* is marked by autonomic dysfunction, with loss of the sympathetic neurons of the intermediolateral column of the spinal cord.

Pathogenesis (p. 1296)

The glial inclusions are likely pathogenic, but no α-synuclein mutations have been identified in MSA, and the mechanism of injury is obscure.

Huntington Disease (p. 1297)

Huntington disease (HD) is an autosomal dominant movement disorder clinically manifesting between ages 20 and 50. Patients develop chorea (jerky, hyperkinetic, dystonic movements) that can evolve into parkinsonism; motor symptoms precede cognitive impairment, and disease is progressive, leading to death within 15 years.

Molecular Genetics and Pathogenesis (p. 1297)

HD is associated with expansion of a CAG trinucleotide repeat encoding a polyglutamine tract in *huntingtin.* The normal *HD* gene has 6 to 35 copies of the repeat; increases beyond this are associated with disease. Because longer stretches generally lead to earlier disease onset and repeats expand during spermatogenesis, paternal transmission is associated with earlier expression in the next generation *(anticipation).* Polyglutamine expansion appears to bestow a toxic gain of function on huntingtin, with protein aggregation, sequestration of various transcriptional regulators, and potential dysregulation of transcription pathways involved in mitochondrial biogenesis or protection against oxidative injury.

Morphology (p. 1298)

There is striking atrophy of the caudate nucleus and putamen, with loss of medium-sized, spiny striatal neurons that use γ-aminobutyric acid as their neurotransmitter; gliosis is prominent, and intraneuronal huntingtin aggregates are seen in the striatum and cerebral cortex. Neurons containing nitric oxide synthase and cholinesterase are spared.

Spinocerebellar Degenerations (p. 1298)

These are a heterogeneous collection of genetically distinct disorders characterized by neuronal loss in cerebellum and other specific regions, with secondary white matter tract degeneration.

Spinocerebellar Ataxias (p. 1298)

Spinocerebellar ataxias (SCAs) are a group of more than 30 different autosomal dominant diseases involving the cerebellum, brainstem, spinal cord, and peripheral nerves. Some forms are caused by unstable expansions of CAG repeats, encoding polyglutamine tracts in different proteins (analogous to HD); others are caused by repeat expansions in noncoding regions or by point mutations in cytoskeletal proteins, ion channels, kinases, or growth factors.

Friedreich Ataxia (p. 1299)

Friedreich ataxia is autosomal recessive; patients present with gait ataxia, hand clumsiness, dysarthria, depressed tendon reflexes, and sensory loss rendering most wheelchair bound within 5 years. Death occurs secondary to associated cardiac arrhythmias or pulmonary infections. Disease is caused by expansion of an intronic GAA repeat in the gene encoding *frataxin,* an inner mitochondrial membrane protein involved in iron regulation; depressed frataxin is associated with generalized mitochondrial dysfunction.

Morphology (p. 1299)

There is axonal loss and gliosis in the posterior columns of the spinal cord, and the distal corticospinal and spinocerebellar tracts.

Neuronal degeneration is also seen in the VIII, X, and XII cranial nerve nuclei, dentate nucleus, Purkinje cells of the superior vermis, and dorsal root ganglia.

Ataxia-Telangiectasia (p. 1299)

Ataxia-telangiectasia is autosomal recessive; patients present in childhood with cerebellar dysfunction, telangiectatic lesions in the skin and conjunctiva (and CNS), and immunodeficiency (lymph nodes and thymus are hypoplastic). The relevant *ATM* gene encodes a kinase involved in repairing double-stranded DNA breaks (see Chapter 7); in addition to increasing the risk of malignancy, ineffective DNA repair may make neurons more degeneration prone. The disease is relentlessly progressive, with death in the second decade.

Morphology (p. 1299)

Cerebellar Purkinje and granule cells are lost, with degeneration of the dorsal columns, spinocerebellar tracts, and anterior horn cells; Schwann cell nuclei in dorsal root ganglia and peripheral nerves can be enlarged twofold to fivefold.

Amyotrophic Lateral Sclerosis (p. 1300)

ALS is characterized by progressive loss of both lower motor neurons and upper motor neurons, with ensuing profound weakness.

Molecular Genetics and Pathogenesis (p. 1300)

A minority of cases (5% to 10%) are familial, mostly with autosomal dominant inheritance; 25% of these are due to adverse gain-of-function mutations in the copper-zinc superoxide dismutase *(SOD1)* gene, believed to yield misfolded proteins that engender an injurious unfolded protein response. Other mutations can simultaneously give rise to ALS and FTLD (e.g., expansion of a hexanucleotide repeat in the 5′-untranslated region of *C9orf72* [leading to neuronal deposits of the derived proteins]) and mutated RNA-binding proteins, such as TDP-43.

Morphology (p. 1300)

Degeneration of the upper motor neurons results in loss of myelinated fibers in the corticospinal tracts and reactive gliosis; occasionally there is atrophy of the precentral gyrus. Remaining neurons can contain PAS-positive cytoplasmic inclusions *(Bunina bodies)*. The affected skeletal muscle shows neurogenic atrophy.

Clinical Features (p. 1300)

ALS is slightly more common in men, usually with onset after age 40. Early clumsiness gives way to muscle weakness and fasciculations, eventually involving the respiratory muscles with recurrent bouts of pneumonia. Some patients have predominantly bulbar manifestations (involvement of motor cranial nerves) with complications related to deglutition and phonation. ALS is typically relentlessly progressive, with death from respiratory complications.

Other Motor Neuron Diseases (p. 1301)

Spinal and Bulbar Muscular Atrophy (Kennedy Disease) (p. 1301)

Kennedy disease is an X-linked disorder; lower motor neuron loss is also associated with androgen insensitivity (gynecomastia, testicular atrophy, and oligospermia). The gene defect is expansion of a CAG-polyglutamine trinucleotide repeat in the androgen receptor gene, associated with intranuclear receptor aggregation.

Spinal Muscular Atrophy *(p. 1301)*

Spinal muscular atrophy (SMA) is a group of childhood genetic disorders with lower motor neuron dropout, resulting in progressive weakness. The most severe form *(SMA type I, Werdnig-Hoffmann disease)* has onset during the first year of life with death within 2 years; *SMA type III (Kugelberg-Welander disease)* usually emerges later. Disease severity correlates with the level of SMN, a protein involved in spliceosome assembly.

Genetic Metabolic Diseases (p. 1302)

Neuronal Storage Diseases (p. 1302)

Neuronal storage diseases are primarily autosomal recessive disorders caused by mutations affecting the synthesis or degradation of sphingolipids, mucolipids, or mucopolysaccharides. These are a heterogeneous group of disorders with the final common pathway of intraneuronal accumulation of the enzyme substrates, with neuronal death; patients typically present with seizures and generalized loss of neurologic function. Tay-Sachs, Niemann-Pick, and some of the mucopolysaccharidoses are described in Chapter 5. Neuronal ceroid lipofuscinoses are rare inherited lysosomal storage disorders characterized by the neuronal accumulation of lipofuscin, and associated with defective protein degradation and neuronal dysfunction, including blindness, mental and motor deterioration, and seizures.

Leukodystrophies (p. 1302)

Leukodystrophies are caused by defects in myelin synthesis or turnover, with resulting hypomyelination. Leukodystrophies differ from demyelinating diseases by presenting with an insidious and progressive loss of cerebral function (often at younger ages), associated with diffuse and symmetric changes on imaging studies.

Krabbe Disease *(p. 1302)*

Krabbe disease is an autosomal recessive deficiency of galactocerebroside β-galactosidase (catalyzing the breakdown of galactocerebroside to ceramide and galactose). An alternate catabolic pathway acts on the excess accumulated substrate to generate galactosylsphingosine, which is toxic to oligodendrocytes. Patients present with weakness and stiffness by 3 to 6 months of age; survival beyond age 2 is uncommon. There is diffuse loss of myelin and oligodendrocytes; aggregates of engorged macrophages around blood vessels *(globoid cells)* are characteristic.

Metachromatic Leukodystrophy *(p. 1302)*

Metachromatic leukodystrophy is an autosomal recessive disease caused by deficiency of arylsulfatase. Sulfatides (especially cerebroside sulfate) accumulate and may block oligodendrocyte differentiation. Findings include myelin loss and gliosis, with macrophages containing metachromatic material.

Adrenoleukodystrophy *(p. 1303)*

Adrenoleukodystrophy has several clinically and genetically distinct forms; it is a progressive disorder caused by myelin loss and adrenal insufficiency, attributable to the inability to catabolize very long chain fatty acids.

Mitochondrial Encephalomyopathies (p. 1303)

Inherited disorders of mitochondrial oxidative phosphorylation present as a combination of muscle (see Chapter 27) and CNS disorders. The disruption of energy generation can be by elevated tissue lactate levels and can be demonstrated by spectroscopic imaging methods; histology will often show loss of cytochrome *c* oxidase enzymatic activity. The mitochondrial encephalomyopathies can be caused by mutations in the mitochondrial or nuclear genomes; thus some show maternal transmission because the affected genes lie in the mitochondrial genome, whereas others do not. Mitochondrial diseases also exhibit *heteroplasmy*—cells have a mixture of normal and abnormal mitochondria (typically in the setting of a mitochondrial genome mutation). Consequently, disease expression can vary from cell to cell depending on the relative proportion of normal and mutant mitochondria.

Mitochondrial Encephalomyopathy, Lactic Acidosis, and Strokelike Episodes (p. 1303)

Mitochondrial encephalomyopathy, lactic acidosis, and strokelike episodes (MELAS) is the most common neurologic syndrome associated with mitochondrial abnormalities. In addition to the muscle and metabolic findings, patients present with recurrent neurologic dysfunction and cognitive changes; although areas of infarction do occur, the strokelike episodes are typically associated with reversible deficits that do not correspond to specific vascular territories. Most of the MELAS mutations involve mitochondrial tRNA.

Myoclonic Epilepsy and Ragged Red Fibers (p. 1304)

Myoclonic epilepsy and ragged red fibers (MERRF) is maternally transmitted; most are associated with tRNA mutations. Patients have myoclonus, a seizure disorder, ataxia, and a myopathy characterized by ragged red fibers on muscle biopsy (see Chapter 27).

Leigh Syndrome (p. 1304)

Leigh syndrome typically presents at age 1 to 2 with developmental arrest, feeding problems, seizures, extraocular palsies, hypotonia, and lactic academia; there are mutations in various components of the oxidative phosphorylation pathway. The brain shows spongiform changes and vascular proliferation, usually symmetrically involving the midbrain periventricular gray matter, pontine tegmentum, thalamus, and hypothalamus.

Toxic and Acquired Metabolic Diseases (p. 1304)

Vitamin Deficiencies (p. 1304)

Thiamine (Vitamin B_1) Deficiency (p. 1304)

Beriberi was discussed in Chapter 9; thiamine deficiency can also manifest as sudden onset of psychosis and/or ophthalmoplegia *(Wernicke encephalopathy)*, with a largely irreversible memory disorder associated with confabulation *(Korsakoff syndrome)*. Chronic alcoholism is a common substrate, but thiamine deficiency can also result from gastric disease (carcinoma, chronic gastritis, or persistent vomiting). Mamillary body (and third and fourth ventricle) hemorrhage and necrosis are common; thalamic dorsomedial nucleus lesions correlate best with the memory disturbances.

Vitamin B_{12} Deficiency (p. 1304)

Vitamin B_{12} deficiency causes anemia and nervous system injury; the latter begins with slight ataxia and lower extremity paresthesias but can rapidly progress to lower extremity spastic weakness and paraplegia (which can be permanent). Vacuolar swelling of myelin *affects both ascending and descending tracts* and starts at the midthoracic cord, with eventual degeneration of both.

Neurologic Sequelae of Metabolic Disturbances (p. 1304)

Hypoglycemia (p. 1304)

Neurons that are relatively sensitive to hypoglycemia include large cerebral pyramidal cells, hippocampal pyramidal cells in area CA1, and Purkinje cells. With prolonged, severe hypoglycemia, there can be global neuronal injury.

Hyperglycemia (p. 1305)

Hyperglycemia occurs most commonly with inadequately controlled diabetes mellitus; ketoacidosis can also occur. In the hyperosmolar state, dehydration results in confusion, stupor, and eventually coma; fluid depletion must be corrected gradually to minimize the risk of cerebral edema.

Hepatic Encephalopathy (p. 1305)

Hepatic encephalopathy occurs with impaired liver function; there is a CNS glial response in the cerebral cortex and basal ganglia, with astrocytes exhibiting enlarged nuclei and minimal reactive cytoplasm (Alzheimer type II cells). Elevated ammonia levels and proinflammatory cytokines are implicated.

Toxic Disorders (p. 1305)

Carbon Monoxide (p. 1305)

Carbon monoxide injury is related to (1) hypoxia occurring secondary to reduced hemoglobin oxygen-carrying capacity and (2) CO binding to cytochrome *c* heme, thus blocking mitochondrial electron transport. There is relatively selective involvement of cerebral cortex layers III and V neurons, hippocampal Sommer sector, and Purkinje cells, often with bilateral necrosis of the globus pallidus.

Methanol (p. 1305)

Methanol toxicity preferentially affects the retina; degeneration of ganglion cells will cause blindness. The methanol metabolite formic acid is causally implicated.

Ethanol (p. 1305)

In addition to the nutritional effects of chronic alcoholism (discussed previously), cerebellar dysfunction (manifesting as truncal ataxia, unsteady gait, and nystagmus) occurs in up to 1%. Atrophy and granule cell loss in the anterior cerebellar vermis are followed by Purkinje cell dropout and astrocyte proliferation *(Bergmann gliosis)*.

Radiation (p. 1305)

Radiation can cause acute CNS decompensation (see Chapter 9) as well as damage that can precipitously develop months to years later. Late radionecrosis is associated with large zones of white matter coagulative necrosis and edema; blood vessels show fibrinoid necrosis and eventually sclerosis. Radiation and methotrexate administration may act synergistically to cause damage.

Tumors (p. 1306)

The annual incidence of intracranial CNS tumors is 10 to 17 per 100,000 population; the intraspinal tumor incidence is 1 to 2 per 100,000. Primary CNS tumors account for 20% of all childhood cancers; 70% of these arise in the posterior fossa. In adults 70% of CNS tumors occur above the tentorium.

- *Consequences of location:* Resectability of CNS tumors is by functional anatomic considerations; thus even benign lesions can have lethal consequences due to the location.
- *Patterns of growth:* Most glial tumors, including many with histologic features of a benign neoplasm, infiltrate extensively leading to clinically malignant behavior.
- *Patterns of spread:* Tumors can spread through the CSF; however, even the most malignant gliomas rarely metastasize outside the CNS.

Gliomas (p. 1306)

Gliomas are the most common group of primary brain tumors; these include *astrocytomas, oligodendrogliomas,* and *ependymomas.* All have characteristic histologic features but derive from a progenitor cell that differentiates along a particular cellular lineage rather than their respective mature cell types. The tumors have typical anatomic localizations, age distributions, and clinical courses.

Astrocytoma (p. 1306)

Infiltrating Astrocytomas (p. 1306)

Infiltrating astrocytomas account for 80% of adult primary brain tumors; typically arising between ages 30 and 60, most occur in the cerebral hemispheres. Patients typically present with seizures, headaches, and focal neurologic deficits related to the anatomic site of involvement. Tumors range from *diffuse astrocytoma* (grade II/IV) to *anaplastic astrocytoma* (grade III/IV) to *glioblastoma* (grade IV/IV); there are no World Health Organization (WHO) grade I infiltrating astrocytomas. Glioblastoma tends to occur as either a new-onset disease in older individuals *(primary glioblastoma)* or progression in younger patients from a lower-grade astrocytoma *(secondary glioblastoma).*

Molecular Genetics. A common theme in these tumors is sustained proliferative signaling and evasion of growth suppressors. There are four molecular subtypes:

- *Classic subtype* (majority of primary glioblastomas) has mutations of the *PTEN* tumor suppressor gene, deletions of chromosome 10, and amplification of the *EGFR* oncogene; hemizygous deletions of the *CDKN2A* tumor suppressor gene are also common, affecting the activity of RB and p53.
- *Proneural type,* the most common type associated with secondary glioblastoma, is characterized by mutations of *TP53,* and point mutations in the isocitrate dehydrogenase genes, *IDH1* and *IDH2,* often with an overexpression of the receptor for platelet-derived growth factor receptor α (PDGFRA). *IDH1* mutations create a new enzyme activity that generates 2-hydroxyglutarate, which drives oncogenesis by inhibiting enzymes that regulate DNA methylation.
- *Neural type* is characterized by higher levels of expression of neuronal markers, including NEFL, GABRA1, SYT1, and SLC12A5.
- *Mesenchymal type* is characterized by deletions of the *NF1* gene on chromosome 17 and lower expression of the NF1 protein; genes involved in the TNF and NF-κB pathways are also highly expressed.

Among the WHO grades III and IV astrocytomas, mutant *IDH1* has a significantly better outcome than wild type.

Morphology *(p. 1307).* Histologic differentiation (WHO grades II to IV) correlates well with the clinical course:

- *Diffuse astrocytomas (grade II)* are poorly defined, gray-white, infiltrative tumors that expand and distort a region of the brain; they show hypercellularity and some nuclear pleomorphism, and the transition from normal to neoplastic is indistinct.
- *Anaplastic astrocytomas (grade III)* exhibit increased nuclear anaplasia with numerous mitoses.
- *Glioblastomas (grade IV; previously called glioblastoma multiforme [GBM])* are composed of a mixture of firm white areas, softer yellow foci of necrosis, cystic change, and hemorrhage; there is also increased vascularity. Increased tumor cell density along the necrotic edges is termed *pseudopalisading.*

Clinical Features *(p. 1308).* Patients typically present with focal neurologic deficits, headaches, or seizures, attributable to mass effects and/or cerebral edema; high-grade lesions have leaky vessels that exhibit contrast enhancement on imaging. The prognosis for glioblastoma is poor; despite resection and chemotherapy, mean survival is only 15 months and only 25% are alive at 2 years.

Pilocytic Astrocytoma (p. 1309)

Pilocytic astrocytoma occurs in children and young adults, usually in the cerebellum but also in the floor and walls of the third ventricle, the optic nerves, and occasionally the cerebral hemispheres; they are WHO grade I/IV. These tumors have a relatively benign behavior; they grow slowly and are rarely infiltrative. They rarely exhibit *p53* mutations or other genetic changes associated with more aggressive astrocytomas but do often show alterations in the BRAF signaling pathway.

Morphology *(p. 1309)*

- *Gross:* Lesions are often cystic with a mural nodule in the wall of the cyst.
- *Microscopic:* Tumors are composed of bipolar cells with long, thin hairlike processes; Rosenthal fibers and microcysts are often present. There is a narrow infiltrative border with the surrounding brain.

Pleomorphic Xanthoastrocytomas (p. 1309)

Pleomorphic xanthoastrocytomas typically occur in the temporal lobes of young patients, often with a history of seizures. The tumor (usually WHO grade II/IV) exhibits neoplastic, occasionally bizarre astrocytes, abundant reticulin and lipid deposits, and chronic inflammatory cell infiltrates; 5-year survival nears 80%.

Brainstem Glioma (p. 1309)

Brainstem glioma occurs mostly in the first two decades of life. Their course depends on location, with pontine gliomas (most common) having an aggressive course, tectal gliomas with a relatively benign course, and corticomedullary junction tumors somewhere intermediate. These tumors often have a specific histone mutation affecting acetylation and methylation events that influence chromatin structure and gene expression.

Oligodendrogliomas *(p. 1309)*

Oligodendrogliomas constitute 5% to 15% of gliomas and are most common in middle life. The most common genetic alterations involve mutations of *IDH1* and *IDH2;* loss of heterozygosity (LOH) in chromosomes 1p and 19q occurs in 80% of cases, and additional mutations (e.g., CDKN2A) accrue in more anaplastic lesions.

Morphology (p. 1310)

- *Gross:* Tumors have a white matter predilection; they are well-circumscribed, gelatinous, gray masses, often with cysts, focal hemorrhage, and calcification.
- *Microscopic:* Tumors consist of sheets of regular cells with round nuclei containing finely granular chromatin, often surrounded by a clear halo of cytoplasm and sitting in a delicate capillary network. Calcification is present in 90% and ranges from microscopic to massive.

Clinical Features (p. 1310)

Prognosis is typically better than for astrocytomas, and current therapies yield an average 5- to 10-year survival. Progression from low- to high-grade lesions can occur, typically over approximately 6 years.

Ependymomas and Related Paraventricular Mass Lesions (p. 1310)

Ependymomas and related paraventricular mass lesions are tumors arising from the ependymal lining. In the first two decades of life, the fourth ventricle is the most common site; the spinal cord central canal is a common location in middle age and in NF2, where the *NF2* gene is mutated.

Morphology (p. 1310)

- *Gross:* Tumors are moderately well-demarcated solid or papillary lesions.
- *Microscopic:* Lesions have regular, round-oval nuclei with abundant granular chromatin; they can form elongated ependymal canals or perivascular pseudorosettes. Most are WHO grade II/IV; anaplastic lesions (grade III/IV) exhibit greater cell density, mitoses, and necrosis with less evident ependymal differentiation.

Myxopapillary ependymomas are distinct but related lesions arising in the filum terminale of the spinal cord. Cuboidal cells, sometimes with clear cytoplasm, are arranged around papillary cores; myxoid areas contain neutral and acidic mucopolysaccharides.

Clinical Features (p. 1311)

Posterior fossa ependymomas often present with hydrocephalus; CSF dissemination is common, and 5-year survival is only 50%. Spinal cord lesions usually do better.

Related Paraventricular Mass Lesions (p. 1311)

- *Subependymomas* (p. 1311) are solid, sometimes calcified, slow-growing nodules attached to the ventricular lining and protruding into the ventricle; they are usually asymptomatic but can cause hydrocephalus. Lesions exhibit clumps of ependymal-appearing nuclei scattered in a dense, finely fibrillar background.
- *Choroid plexus papillomas* (p. 1311) recapitulate the normal choroid plexus; they exhibit connective tissue papillae covered with a cuboidal-columnar ciliated epithelium. Hydrocephalus is common, due to either obstruction or CSF overproduction. *Choroid plexus carcinomas* are rare; they are typically adenocarcinomas arising in children.
- *Colloid cysts of the third ventricle* (p. 1311) are non-neoplastic lesions of young adults; they are located at the foramina of Monro and can result in noncommunicating hydrocephalus, sometimes rapidly fatal. The cyst contains gelatinous proteinaceous material within a thin, fibrous capsule lined by cuboidal epithelium.

Neuronal Tumors (p. 1311)

- *Ganglioglioma* is the most common CNS tumor of mature-appearing neurons (ganglion cells); it is slow growing, although the glial component can become frankly anaplastic and the tumor more aggressive. Lesions often present with seizures that remit after resection. One fifth of these tumors have activating *BRAF* mutations; most occur in the temporal lobe and have a cystic component.
- *Dysembryoplastic neuroepithelial tumor* (p. 1312) is a rare, low-grade childhood neoplasm often presenting as a seizure disorder; prognosis after resection is good. Features include intracortical location, cystic changes, nodular growth, "floating neurons" in a pool of mucopolysaccharide-rich fluid, and surrounding neoplastic glia without anaplastic features.
- *Central neurocytoma* (p. 1312) is a low-grade neuronal neoplasm within the ventricles consisting of evenly spaced, round, uniform nuclei and islands of neuropil.

Poorly Differentiated Neoplasms (p. 1312)

Some neuroectodermal tumors express few mature phenotypic markers and are described as poorly differentiated or embryonal.

Medulloblastomas (p. 1312)

Medulloblastomas account for 20% of childhood brain tumors; they occur exclusively in the cerebellum. Medulloblastoma can be divided into four genetic groups:

- *WNT type* (WNT signaling pathway mutations) occurs in older children, has a classic medulloblastoma histology, and shows monosomy of chromosome 6 and nuclear expression of β-catenin. It has the best prognosis with 90% 5-year survival.
- *SHH type* (sonic hedgehog signaling pathway mutations; may have *MYCN* amplification) occurs in infants or young adults. Prognosis is intermediate.
- *Group 3* (*MYC* amplification and isochromosome 17) occurs in infants and children and has the worst prognosis.
- *Group 4* (isochromosome 17 without *MYC* amplification, but sometimes with *MYCN* amplification). The prognosis is intermediate.

Morphology (p. 1312)

- *Gross:* Tumors are well circumscribed, gray, and friable.
- *Microscopic:* Lesions are usually extremely cellular, with sheets of anaplastic cells exhibiting hyperchromatic nuclei and abundant mitoses; cells have little cytoplasm and are often devoid of specific markers of differentiation, although glial and neuronal features (e.g., Homer-Wright rosettes) can occur. Extension into the subarachnoid space can elicit prominent desmoplasia.

Clinical Features (p. 1312)

Tumors tend to be midline in children and in lateral locations in adults. Rapid growth can occlude CSF flow, leading to hydrocephalus; CSF dissemination is common. The tumor is highly malignant, and if untreated, the prognosis is dismal. However, it is exquisitely radiosensitive, and with excision and radiation, the 5-year survival rate is 75%.

Atypical Teratoid-Rhabdoid Tumor (p. 1313)

Atypical teratoid-rhabdoid tumor is a highly malignant tumor of the posterior fossa and supratentorium of young children; survival is usually <1 year. Chromosome 22 deletions occur in >90%; the relevant gene is *hSNF5/INI1*, encoding a protein involved in chromatin remodeling. These are large, soft tumors that spread over the brain surface; they are highly mitotic lesions histologically characterized by rhabdoid cells, resembling those seen in rhabdomyosarcoma.

Other Parenchymal Tumors (p. 1313)

Primary Central Nervous System Lymphoma (p. 1313)

Primary CNS lymphoma accounts for 2% of extranodal lymphomas and 1% of intracranial tumors; it is the most common CNS neoplasm in immunocompromised hosts. Primary brain lymphoma is often multifocal within the CNS; involvement outside the CNS is a rare and late complication. Most primary brain lymphomas are of B-cell origin and nearly all are latently infected by EBV; the most common histologic group is diffuse large-cell B-cell lymphomas. These are aggressive tumors and respond poorly to chemotherapy compared with their peripheral counterparts.

Germ Cell Tumors (p. 1314)

Germ cell tumors occur along the midline in adolescents and young adults; they constitute 0.2% to 1% of CNS tumors in European populations but up to 10% of Japanese. Tumors most commonly occur in the pineal (male predominance) and suprasellar regions. The histologic classification and therapeutic responsiveness of CNS germ cell tumors mirror those of their non-CNS counterparts (see Chapter 21).

Pineal Parenchymal Tumors (p. 1314)

Pineal parenchymal tumors derive from pineocytes; they range from well-differentiated lesions with neuronal differentiation *(pineocytomas)* to high-grade tumors *(pineoblastomas)* that spread throughout the CSF. High-grade pineal tumors tend to affect children, whereas lower-grade lesions are found more often in adults.

Meningiomas (p. 1314)

Meningiomas are predominantly benign tumors of adults that arise from arachnoid meningothelial cells and are attached to the dura; prior radiation to the head and neck can be a risk factor. These are often associated with loss of chromosome 22 (especially the long arm, 22q), leading to deletions of the *NF2* gene encoding the protein merlin, and associated with greater chromosomal instability. In meningiomas with wild-type *NF2*, TNF-receptor associated factor 7 (TRAF7) mutations occur with a tendency toward lower histologic grade and greater chromosomal stability.

Morphology (p. 1314)

- *Gross:* Tumors are usually rounded masses with well-defined dural bases that compress underlying brain but easily separate from it; lesions are usually firm, lack necrosis or extensive hemorrhage and may be gritty due to calcified psamomma bodies.
- *Microscopic:* Several histologic patterns exist (e.g., synctytial, fibroblastic, transitional, psammomatous, secretory, and microcystic) all with approximately comparable favorable prognoses (WHO grade I/IV); among these, proliferation index is the best predictor of biologic behavior.
- *Anaplastic (malignant) meningiomas* (WHO grade III/IV) are aggressive tumors that resemble sarcomas; mitotic rates are high (>20 per 10 high-powered fields). *Papillary meningiomas* (pleomorphic cells arranged around fibrovascular cores) and *rhabdoid meningiomas* (sheets of cells with hyaline eosinophilic cytoplasm composed of intermediate filaments) also have a high recurrence rate (WHO grade III/IV tumors).

Clinical Features (p. 1315)

These are typically solitary, slow-growing lesions that manifest due to CNS compression or with vague nonlocalizing symptoms; multiple lesions suggest *NF2* mutations. They are uncommon in children and have a slight (3:2) female predominance; they often express progesterone receptors and can grow more rapidly during pregnancy.

Metastatic Tumors (p. 1315)

Metastatic lesions (mostly carcinomas) account for approximately half of intracranial tumors. Common primary sites are lung, breast, skin (melanoma), kidney, and gastrointestinal tract; meninges are also a frequent site. Metastases are usually sharply demarcated, often at the gray-white junction, and surrounded by edema. Meningeal carcinomatosis (tumor nodules studding brain surface, spinal cord, and nerve roots) is particularly associated with lung and breast carcinoma.

Paraneoplastic Syndromes (p. 1316)

Paraneoplastic syndromes result from malignancy elsewhere in the body; most are due to antitumor immune responses that cross-react with central or peripheral nervous system antigens. Therapy targeted to tumor resection and/or immunosuppression and removal of circulating antibodies can yield clinical improvement.

- *Subacute cerebellar degeneration* is most common with Purkinje cell loss, gliosis, and inflammatory infiltrates. In some cases (particularly women with ovarian, breast, or uterine cancers) patients have anti-Yo antibodies that recognize Purkinje cells.
- *Limbic encephalitis* is a subacute dementia associated with perivascular inflammation, microglial nodules, neuronal loss, and gliosis, most evident in the anterior and medial temporal lobe. Some patients (e.g., those with small cell carcinoma of lung) have anti-Hu antibodies that recognize neuronal nuclei; others have antibodies that react with the NMDA receptor or the voltage-gated potassium channel. In many cases of limbic encephalitis, the syndrome appears before malignancy is suspected.
- *Eye movement disorders* (e.g., opsoclonus), often associated with childhood neuroblastomas.
- *Subacute sensory neuropathy* plus or minus limbic encephalitis is marked by dorsal root ganglia inflammation and neuronal loss.
- *Lambert-Eaton myasthenic syndrome* (see Chapter 27) is caused by antibodies against the presynaptic voltage-gated calcium channel.

Familial Tumor Syndromes (p. 1316)

These are primarily autosomal dominant disorders caused by loss of tumor suppressor genes; the bulk of disease manifestations are outside the CNS:

- *Cowden syndrome:* Dysplastic cerebellar gangliocytomas due to *PTEN* mutation (see Chapter 7)
- *Li-Fraumeni syndrome:* Medulloblastomas due to *p53* mutation (see Chapter 7)
- *Turcot syndrome:* Medulloblastomas or glioblastomas due to *APC* or mismatch repair gene mutation (see Chapter 17)
- *Gorlin syndrome:* Medulloblastomas due to *PTCH* mutation (see Chapter 25).

Tuberous Sclerosis Complex *(p. 1316)*

Tuberous sclerosis complex is an autosomal dominant disorder occurring in 1 in 6000 births; it is characterized by autism, seizures, and mental retardation. The complex leads to CNS hamartomas, including *cortical tubers* (haphazardly arranged neurons and cells expressing phenotypes intermediate between glia and neurons) and subependymal hamartomas (large astrocytic and neuronal clusters forming subependymal giant cell astrocytomas). In addition, renal angiomyolipomas, retinal glial hamartomas, cardiac rhabdomyomas, and pulmonary lymphangioleiomyomatosis can occur; cutaneous lesions include angiofibromas, leathery thickenings *(shagreen patches)*, subungual fibromas, and hypopigmented areas *(ash-leaf patches)*. One tuberous sclerosis locus *(TSC1)* encodes *hamartin;* the more commonly mutated *TSC2* locus encodes *tuberin.* Both proteins form a complex that inhibits the mTOR (mechanistic target of rapamycin) kinase; mutations lead to increased mTOR activity, leading to increased protein synthesis and impressive increases in cell size.

von Hippel-Lindau Disease *(p. 1317)*

von Hippel-Lindau disease is an autosomal dominant disorder; affected individuals develop hemangioblastomas in the cerebellum, retina, or brainstem and spinal cord, as well as cysts involving the pancreas, liver, and kidney. There is also a propensity for renal cell carcinoma and pheochromocytomas. The causal gene is *VHL,* a tumor suppressor gene that encodes a component of a ubiquitin-ligase complex that downregulates hypoxia-induced factor-1 (HIF-1) expression; mutated VHL leads to increased HIF-1, which then causes increased expression of vascular endothelial growth factor, erythropoietin, and other growth factors.

Neurofibromatosis *(p. 1317; See Also Chapter 27)*

- NF1 (p. 1317) is an autosomal dominant disorder affecting 1 in 3000 individuals; it is characterized by neurofibromas (plexiform and cutaneous), optic nerve gliomas, meningiomas, pigmented nodules of the iris *(Lisch nodules)*, and cutaneous hyperpigmented macules *(café au lait spots)*. Even without malignant transformation, lesions can be disfiguring and can create spinal deformities.
- NF2 (p. 1317) is an autosomal dominant disorder affecting 1 in 50,000 people; it tends to form bilateral eighth nerve schwannomas and multiple meningiomas.

29 The Eye

Orbit (p. 1320)

Functional Anatomy and Proptosis (p. 1320)

Although some conditions are unique to the eye (e.g., *cataract* and *glaucoma*), many ocular conditions share similarities with disease processes elsewhere in the body but are modified by the unique structure and function of the eye (Fig. 29-1).

Because the orbit is bounded by bone medially, laterally, and posteriorly, any process that increases orbital contents causes forward eye displacement, or *proptosis.*

Thyroid Ophthalmopathy (Graves Disease) (p. 1320)

Proptosis in *Graves disease* is caused by extracellular matrix (ECM) accumulation and rectus muscle fibrosis; the severity is independent of thyroid status.

Other Orbital Inflammatory Conditions (p. 1320)

The floor and medial aspects of the orbit are bounded by the maxillary and ethmoid sinuses, respectively; thus orbits can be involved by sinus infections evolving into *cellulitis* or as part of a fungal infection (e.g., *mucormycosis*). Orbital involvement by *granulomatosis with angiitis*

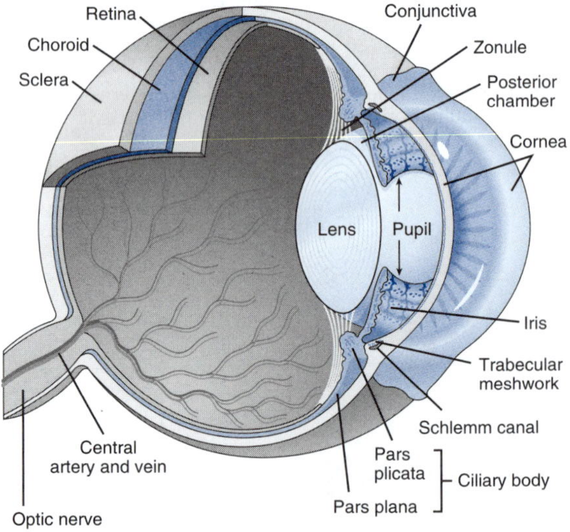

Figure 29-1 Anatomy of the eye.

can be primary or a secondary extension from the sinuses. Idiopathic orbital inflammation *(orbital inflammatory pseudotumor)* is characterized by chronic inflammation and variable fibrosis; immunoglobulin (Ig)G4-related disease can also affect the eye (see Chapter 6).

Neoplasms (p. 1321)

The most common primary orbital tumors are vascular in origin (e.g., lymphangiomas and capillary and cavernous hemangiomas); most orbital tumors are benign. Malignant tumors of the orbit can derive from any of the orbital tissues (e.g., lacrimal gland); lymphomas and metastases also affect this site.

Eyelid (p. 1322)

Functional Anatomy (p. 1322)

Eyelids are composed of skin externally and mucosa *(conjunctiva)* adjacent to the eye (Fig. 29-2). In addition to covering and protecting the eye, eyelids generate lipids that retard tear evaporation. If sebaceous drainage is blocked by inflammation *(blepharitis)* or neoplasm, extravasated lipid provokes a lipogranulomatous response *(chalazion).*

Neoplasms (p. 1322)

Eyelid neoplasms can distort the eyelid and impede closure; subsequent corneal exposure is painful and predisposes to corneal ulceration. Prompt treatment is imperative to preserve vision.

- *Basal cell carcinoma* is the most common eyelid malignancy; it has a predilection for lower eyelids and medial canthi.
- *Sebaceous carcinoma* is the second most common eyelid malignancy; it metastasizes first to parotid and submandibular lymph nodes

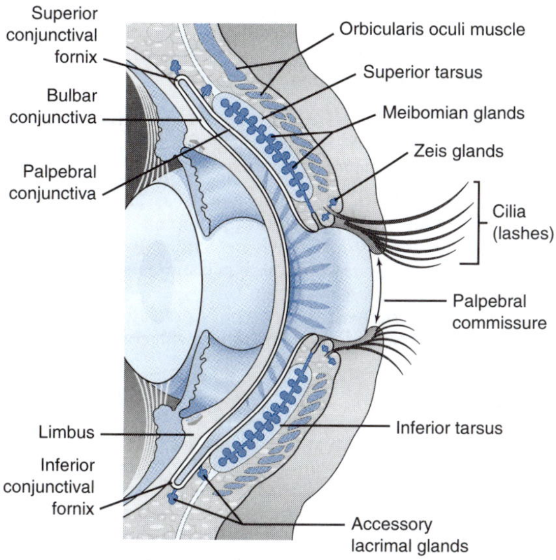

Figure 29-2 Anatomy of the conjunctiva and eyelids.

and can exhibit intraepithelial pagetoid spread into the nasopharynx and lacrimal glands; overall mortality rate can be >20%.

- In patients with acquired immunodeficiency syndrome (AIDS), *Kaposi sarcoma* can develop in the eyelid or conjunctiva.

Conjunctiva (p. 1322)

Functional Anatomy (p. 1322)

The conjunctiva has topologic zones (Fig. 29-2) with distinctive histology and disease responses:

- *Palpebral conjunctiva* is nonkeratinizing stratified squamous epithelium; it responds to inflammation by forming minute papillary folds.
- *Fornix conjunctiva* is a pseudostratified columnar epithelium rich in goblet cells; its associated lacrimal and lymphoid tissues can be expanded in *viral conjunctivitis* or lymphoid malignancy.
- *Bulbar conjunctiva* is a nonkeratinizing stratified squamous epithelium that covers the surface of the eye.

The aqueous component of tears is generated by accessory lacrimal glands embedded in the eyelid and fornix; conjunctival goblet cell mucin production is essential for adhering tears to corneal epithelium. *Dry eyes* occurs when either the lacrimal gland (most commonly) or goblet cell production is insufficient; the condition is painful and predisposes to corneal ulceration and opacification.

Conjunctival Scarring (p. 1323)

Conjunctival scarring causes goblet cell loss; dry eyes results even with adequate aqueous tear film production. Bacterial or viral *conjunctivitis* typically causes only redness and itching and heals without sequelae. However, conjunctival scarring can occur with the following:

- *Chlamydia trachomatis* infections
- Immune-mediated conditions, such as *ocular cicatricial pemphigoid*
- Chemical agents, especially alkalis
- Excessive surgical resection of conjunctival tissue

Pinguecula and Pterygium (p. 1323)

Pinguecula and pterygium are submucosal conjunctival elevations; they are a consequence of actinic damage, and thus occur in sun-exposed regions (e.g., the interpalpebral fissure).

- *Pterygium:* Growth of conjunctival mucosa and fibrovascular connective tissue originating in the limbus and invading the cornea; vision is usually unaffected. Resections are performed for irritation or cosmetic reasons; rarely melanoma or squamous cell carcinoma may be present.
- *Pinguecula* does not invade the cornea but can affect tear film distribution and result in focal dehydration with corneal depression (forming a *delle*).

Neoplasms (p. 1323)

Neoplasms tend to develop at the limbus, likely related to sun exposure; they exhibit a spectrum of changes from mild dysplasia to carcinoma in situ *(conjunctival intraepithelial neoplasia)* to frank malignancy.

- *Squamous cell carcinomas* tend to follow an indolent course; they can be associated with human papillomavirus (HPV) types 16 and 18. *Mucoepidermoid carcinoma* is much more aggressive.

- *Conjunctival nevi* are common and typically benign, rarely involving the cornea, fornix, or palpebral conjunctiva (pigmented lesions in those locations are more likely melanomas). Chronic inflammation can occur during adolescence *(inflamed juvenile nevus).*
- *Conjunctival melanomas* are unilateral, typically affecting middle-aged fair-complexioned individuals; there is a 25% mortality rate. Most have an intraepithelial phase termed *primary acquired melanosis with atypia* (analogous to *melanoma in situ*); melanomas develop in 50% to 90% of these lesions. Parotid or submandibular lymph nodes are favored initial metastatic sites.

Sclera (p. 1324)

Because the sclera has relatively scant numbers of blood vessels and fibroblasts, wounds and surgical incisions heal poorly. Scleral "blueness" can be due to thinning caused by inflammation *(scleritis),* increased intraocular pressure, or defective collagen synthesis (e.g., in *osteogenesis imperfecta*), or can result from a pigmented nevus in the underlying uvea *(congenital melanosis oculi).*

Cornea (p. 1324)

Functional Anatomy (p. 1324)

The cornea and its overlying tear film (and *not* the lens) compose the major refractive eye surface (Fig. 29-1). *Myopia* occurs when the eye is too long for the corneal refractive power, and *hyperopia* occurs when the globe is too short; laser sculpting of the cornea (e.g., LASIK) can accommodate for these disproportions.

The cornea is transparent because its stroma lacks blood vessels and lymphatics; this also markedly attenuates rejection in corneal transplants. Precise collagen alignment is also necessary to maintain corneal transparency; the stroma is normally maintained in a relatively dehydrated state by the action of corneal endothelium pumping fluid into the anterior chamber. Thus corneal scarring or edema markedly affects vision.

Anteriorly the cornea is covered by epithelium overlying basement membrane and an acellular *Bowman layer.* Posteriorly the cornea is bounded by *corneal endothelium* derived from neural crest (and unrelated to vascular endothelium); it sits on a basal lamina *Descemet membrane.*

Keratitis and Ulcers (p. 1325)

Bacteria, fungi, viruses (especially herpes simplex and zoster), and protozoa *(Acanthamoeba)* can cause corneal ulceration; stroma dissolution is accelerated by collagenase activation. Some forms of keratitis have distinctive features (herpes simplex is associated with granulomatous responses involving Descemet membrane).

Corneal Degenerations and Dystrophies (p. 1325)

Degenerations may be unilateral or bilateral and are typically nonfamilial; *dystrophies* are typically bilateral and hereditary.

Band Keratopathies (p. 1325)

Calcific band keratopathy, a common complication of chronic uveitis, is characterized by calcium deposition in Bowman layer. *Actinic band keratopathy* involves ultraviolet (UV)-induced corneal collagen degeneration.

Keratoconus (p. 1326)

Corneal thinning and ectasia causes the cornea to become conical (rather than spherical) and distorts vision. Bowman layer fractures are histologic hallmarks; metalloproteinase activation may be causal, but inflammation is usually absent.

Fuchs Endothelial Dystrophy (p. 1326)

A primary loss of corneal endothelial cells causes *stromal edema* and *bullous keratopathy* (epithelial detachment from Bowman layer forming bullae). There is blurring and loss of vision.

Stromal Dystrophies (p. 1326)

Deposits of various stromal proteins (resulting from mutations that affect folding) form discrete opacities in the cornea, compromising vision; deposits adjacent to epithelium or Bowman layer can also cause painful erosions and scarring.

Anterior Segment (p. 1327)

Functional Anatomy (p. 1327)

The eye is divided into two compartments (Fig. 29-3):

- *Anterior segment* comprising cornea, anterior chamber, posterior chamber, iris, and lens
    - The basement membrane of the lens epithelium *(lens capsule)* totally envelops the lens. Thus lens epithelium and associated proteins progressively accumulate within the confines of the lens capsule ("infoliation"), and the lens size increases with age.
    - The ciliary body forms the aqueous humor that enters the posterior chamber, bathes the lens, and circulates through the pupil into the anterior chamber.
- *Posterior pole* (remainder of the eye; Fig. 29-1)

Cataract (p. 1327)

Cataracts are congenital or acquired lens opacities. Systemic diseases (e.g., diabetes mellitus, atopic dermatitis), drugs (especially corticosteroids), radiation, trauma, and many intraocular disorders (e.g., uveitis) cause cataracts. Age-related cataracts typically result from lens nucleus opacification; accumulation of urochrome pigments causes the nucleus to become brown and distorts the perception of blue colors. Lens epithelium migration and hyperplasia posterior to the lens can cause *posterior subcapsular cataracts.* Opacification can also occur through lens cortex liquefaction; leakage of the liquid through the lens capsule *(phacolysis)* can clog the trabecular meshwork and be a cause of open-angle glaucoma (see later).

Anterior Segment and Glaucoma (p. 1327)

Glaucoma has distinctive visual field changes and optic nerve cup alterations. Most glaucoma is associated with elevated intraocular pressure (see Fig. 29-3 for normal flow patterns), although some patients have normal intraocular pressure (*normal-* or *low-tension glaucoma*). There are two major categories of glaucoma:

- *Open-angle glaucoma* is most common; intraocular pressures are elevated despite an open angle and normal-appearing structures; presumably there is some *functional* increase in resistance to aqueous humor outflow. Some hereditary *(primary)* forms of glaucoma are associated with *MYOC* mutations encoding the protein myocilin; however, the pathogenesis is obscure.

By physically clogging the trabecular meshwork, particulate matter (e.g., senescent erythrocytes after trauma or iris pigment epithelial granules) can be a cause of *secondary open-angle glaucoma. Pseudoexfoliation glaucoma* is the most common cause, caused by deposition of fibrillar material of varying composition throughout the anterior segment (and indeed around blood vessels in many visceral organs); it is associated with single nucleotide polymorphisms in the lysyl oxidaselike 1 *(LOX1)* gene.

- *Angle-closure glaucoma* occurs when the peripheral zone of the iris (or associated tissue) adheres to the trabecular meshwork and physically impedes the aqueous outflow from the eye. It may occur as *primary angle-closure glaucoma* in eyes with shallow anterior chambers (patients are often hyperopic) or can occur subsequent

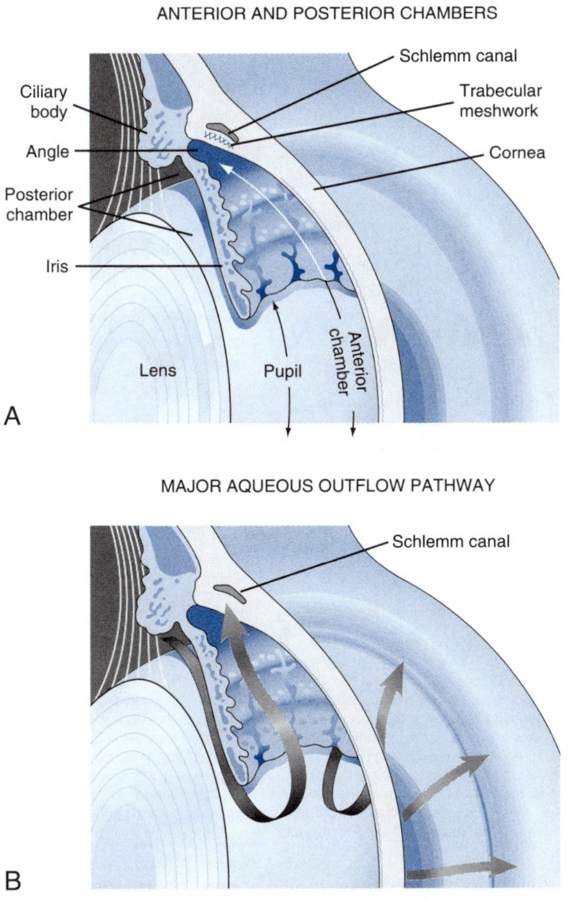

Figure 29-3 **A,** *Normal eye.* Note the iris surface is highly textured with crypts and folds. **B,** *Normal flow of the aqueous humor.* Aqueous humor flows from the posterior chamber (site of production) through the pupil into the anterior chamber and through the trabecular meshwork into Schlemm canal; minor outflow pathways through the uveosclera and iris are not depicted.

Continued

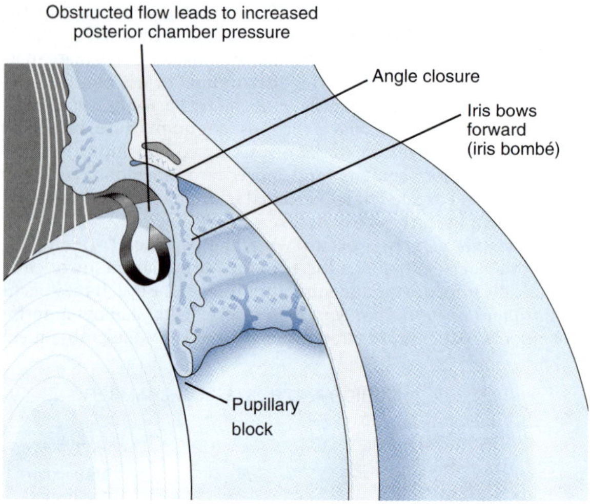

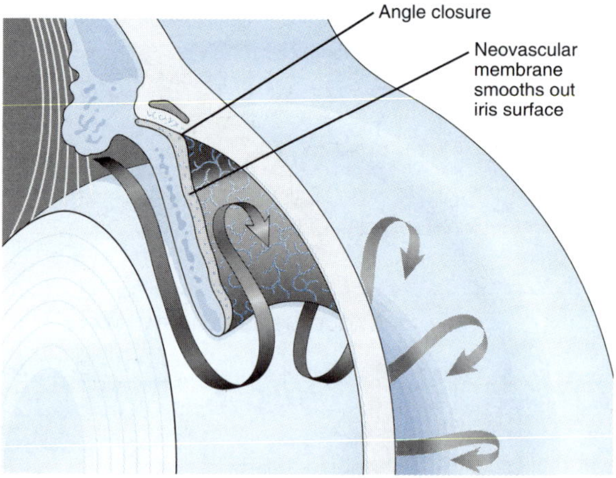

Figure 29-3, cont'd **C,** *Primary angle-closure glaucoma* occurs in anatomically predisposed eyes by transient iris apposition to the lens blocking aqueous humor passage from the posterior to anterior chambers. Pressure builds in the posterior chamber bowing the iris forward *(iris bombé)* and occluding the trabecular meshwork. **D,** *Neovascular glaucoma* occurs when an angiogenic membrane grows over the iris, smoothing the folds and crypts; contracture of this membrane causes tissue apposition over the trabecular meshwork, blocking aqueous humor outflow and increasing intraocular pressure.

to neovascular membrane formation (e.g., after trauma) or ciliary body tumors (Fig. 29-3).

Endophthalmitis and Panophthalmitis (p. 1329)

Anterior chamber inflammation results in increased permeability of the vessels in the ciliary body and iris, with accumulation of cells and exudate. Such exudates can induce adhesions between the iris and corneal meshwork (causing glaucoma) or lens (causing fibrous cataracts).

- *Endophthalmitis* is inflammation involving the vitreous humor. The retina does not tolerate endophthalmitis; only a few hours of acute inflammation can cause irreversible damage. Endophthalmitis can be *exogenous* (e.g., following a wound) or *endogenous* (delivered hematogenously).
- *Panophthalmitis* is eye inflammation involving the retina, choroid, and sclera and extending into the orbit.

Uvea (p. 1330)

The iris, choroid, and ciliary body constitute the *uvea* (Fig. 29-1). Although highly vascularized, the uvea has no lymphatics.

Uveitis (p. 1330)

Uveitis can be infectious, idiopathic (e.g., *sarcoidosis*), or autoimmune (e.g., *sympathetic ophthalmia*); it can be part of a systemic process or involve only the eye. Although inflammation in one compartment typically extends into others, uveitis can involve only the anterior segment (e.g., in *juvenile rheumatoid arthritis*).

Sympathetic ophthalmia is a noninfectious uveitis limited to the eye. It is a consequence of penetrating eye injury, developing within 2 weeks (to many years) after the insult. Presumably, previously sequestered retinal antigens released from the injured eye establish a delayed hypersensitivity response that affects not only the injured eye but also the contralateral, uninjured eye. Histologically there is bilateral granulomatous inflammation affecting all uveal components.

Neoplasms (p. 1331)

The most common intraocular malignancy in adults is metastasis of some other primary tumor (the uvea is the favored site, typically in the choroid).

Uveal Nevi and Melanomas (p. 1331)

Uveal nevi are common (10% of the white population); these are associated with *GNAQ* and *GNA11* mutations—both encoding G protein-coupled receptors that lead to enhanced proliferation through effects, for example, on the MAP kinase pathway (see Chapter 7). Although 85% of uveal melanomas also harbor gain-of-function mutations in *GNAQ* and *GNA11*, uveal nevi rarely transform to melanoma, indicating that other genetic changes are contributory. One such event is loss of chromosome 3, leading to deletion of *BAP1*, a tumor suppressor gene encoding a component of a protein complex that places repressive marks on chromatin and induces gene silencing.

Uveal melanoma is the most common *primary* intraocular adult malignancy. The eye lacks lymphatics; thus uveal melanomas typically spread hematogenously and highly favor the liver. Prognostic variables include extraocular extension, large lateral diameter, location within the eye (tumor in the iris tends to be indolent, whereas tumor in the choroid or ciliary body tends to be aggressive), cell type, monosomy 3, and proliferative index. Eye-sparing radiotherapy has the same survival characteristics as enucleation and is therefore treatment of choice. Five-year survival rates approach 80%, but mortality is 40% at 10 years, increasing 1% per year thereafter.

Retina and Vitreous (p. 1332)

Functional Anatomy (p. 1332)

The neurosensory retina is embryologically derived from the diencephalon, and injury causes gliosis. The retinal architecture explains the ophthalmoscopic appearance of ocular disorders (Fig. 29-4). There are no retinal lymphatics. The adult vitreous is avascular but can be opacified by hemorrhage from trauma or retinal neovascularization. Age-related liquefaction and collapse of the vitreous give rise to "floaters" in the visual field.

Retinal Detachment (p. 1333)

Separation *(retinal detachment)* of the neurosensory retina from the retinal pigmented epithelium (RPE) is classified based on the presence or absence of a break in the retina.

- *Rhegmatogenous retinal detachment* is associated with a full-thickness retinal defect developing when structural collapse of the vitreous exerts traction on the retinal internal limiting membrane; liquefied vitreous humor then seeps through the tear and separates the neurosensory retina and RPE.
- *Nonrhegmatogenous retinal detachment* (without a retinal break) occurs when exudates accumulate or fluid leaks from the choroidal circulation beneath the retina (e.g., with choroidal tumors or malignant hypertension).

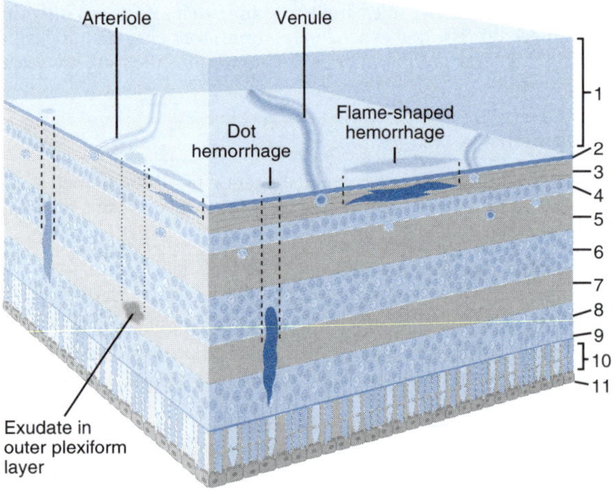

1. Vitreous
2. Inner limiting membrane
3. Nerve fiber layer
4. Ganglion cell layer
5. Inner plexiform layer
6. Inner nuclear layer
7. Outer plexiform layer
8. Outer nuclear layer
9. External limiting membrane
10. Rods and cones
11. Retinal pigment epithelium

Figure 29-4 Clinicopathologic correlations of retinal hemorrhages and exudates; location within the retina determines the ophthalmoscopic appearance. Hemorrhages of the retinal nerve fiber layer (oriented parallel to the internal limiting membrane) appear flame shaped. Hemorrhages of the deeper retinal layers (oriented perpendicular to the internal limiting membrane) appear as "dots." Exudates from leaky retinal vessels accumulate in the outer plexiform layer.

Retinal Vascular Disease (p. 1333)

Retinal vasculopathy *(neovascularization)* is a common end point of numerous insults (see following topics); it can occur secondary to vessel occlusion, hypoxia, or primary angiogenic factor production. Retinal hypoxia causes growth factor production (e.g., vascular endothelial growth factor [VEGF]) leading to angiogenesis; bleeding, increased vascular permeability, or subsequent contraction of the neovascular membrane can cause retinal detachment.

Hypertension (p. 1333)

Hypertension results in retinal arteriosclerosis with wall thickening. In malignant hypertension, damaged choroidal vessels can cause choroidal infarcts *(Elschnig spots)* or exudate accumulation between the neurosensory retina and RPE (causing detachment). Occlusion of retinal arteries causes infarcts of the retinal nerve fiber layer and exudates from damaged retinal vessels accumulate in the outer plexiform layer (Fig. 29-4).

Diabetes Mellitus (p. 1334)

Diabetes mellitus causes microvascular injury with physiologic breakdown of the blood-retina barrier, leading to edema and hemorrhage. Diabetic retinal vasculopathy is classified into *nonproliferative* and *proliferative* forms:

- *Nonproliferative diabetic retinopathy* is associated with retinal vessel basement membrane thickening, and reduced numbers of pericytes causes *microaneurysm* formation. The retinal microcirculation is leaky, leading to macular edema and exudates in the outer plexiform layer. The retinal microcirculation also shows microocclusions, associated with increased VEGF production and intraretinal angiogenesis (located beneath the internal limiting membrane of the retina).
- *Proliferative diabetic retinopathy* is defined by the appearance of new vessels on the surface of the optic nerve head ("neovascularization of the disc") or the surface of the retina; the term "retinal neovascularization" is applied when vessels breach the internal limiting membrane of the retina. If the vitreous humor separates from the internal limiting membrane of the retina (posterior vitreous detachment), there may be massive hemorrhage from the disrupted neovascular membrane. Scarring associated with the retinal neovascular membrane can deform the retina and produce visual distortion or can even cause retinal detachment.

Retinopathy of Prematurity (Retrolental Fibroplasia) (p. 1336)

Immature retinal vessels respond to increased oxygen tension (administered to premature infants) by constricting, resulting in local ischemia.

Sickle Retinopathy, Retinal Vasculitis, Radiation Retinopathy (p. 1336)

Reduced oxygen tension leads to erythrocyte sickling and microvascular occlusions. Vasculitis and ocular radiation both damage vessels producing zones of retinal ischemia. The retinal pathologies associated with these insults parallel those seen in diabetic retinopathy (see earlier discussion), with proliferative and nonproliferative changes.

Retinal Artery and Vein Occlusions (p. 1337)

Arterial occlusions due to atherosclerosis or to atheroembolism cause retinal infarction; because onset is typically sudden, there is no prolonged ischemia, and hence no significant neovascularization. Retinal vein occlusion (e.g., due to arteriolar thickening in hypertension that compromises the venous lumen where the vessels cross) typically leads to ischemia and subsequent neovascularization.

Age-Related Macular Degeneration (p. 1338)

Age-related macular degeneration (AMD) is the most common cause of irreversible visual loss in the United States. More than 70% of cases are hereditary, many linked to complement factor H and other complement regulatory genes; onset is also influenced by environmental exposures (e.g., smoking). Any disruption of RPE, its basement membrane *(Bruch membrane),* or the associated choroidal vasculature affects the overlying photoreceptors and causes visual loss.

- *Atrophic (dry) AMD* is most common (80% to 90% of cases); it is associated with geographic atrophy of the RPE and deposits *(drusen)* in the Bruch membrane.
- *Neovascular (wet) AMD* (10% to 20% of cases) is associated with overall greater vision loss; it is caused by leaky choroidal neovascular membranes. Therapy uses VEGF antagonists to block the vessel formation.

Other Retinal Degenerations (p. 1339)

Retinitis Pigmentosa (p. 1339)

Retinitis pigmentosa is a collection of fairly common (1 in 3600 individuals) inherited disorders that affect various aspects of vision, including visual cascade and cycle, structural genes, transcription factors, catabolic pathways, and mitochondrial metabolism. Despite the name, these disorders are *not* primarily inflammatory; both rods and cones are lost to apoptosis, and there is retinal atrophy, with perivascular retinal pigment accumulation. Retinitis pigmentosa can occur in isolation or be part of a syndrome (e.g., *Bardet-Biedl syndrome, Usher syndrome,* or *Refsum disease*).

Retinal Neoplasms (p. 1339)

Retinoblastoma (p. 1339)

Retinoblastoma is the most common primary intraocular malignancy of children. Prognosis is worsened with extraocular extension or optic nerve or choroidal invasion. In 40% of cases retinoblastoma is associated with a germline *Rb* mutation (see Chapter 7); such cases are often bilateral and are associated with pinealoblastoma ("trilateral" retinoblastoma) with a dismal outcome. Retinoblastoma tends to spread to brain and marrow, with rare dissemination to the lung.

Morphology (p. 1339)

Tumors contain undifferentiated (small round cells) and differentiated elements encircling blood vessels, with zones of necrosis and dystrophic calcification. Well-differentiated tumors exhibit *Flexner-Wintersteiner rosettes,* reflecting abortive photoreceptor development. The degree of differentiation does not influence prognosis.

Optic Nerve (p. 1340)

Optic nerve pathology is similar to brain pathology; cerebrospinal fluid circulates around the nerve, and it is surrounded by meninges. The most common primary neoplasms are gliomas (typically *pilocytic astrocytomas*) and meningiomas.

Anterior Ischemic Optic Neuropathy (p. 1340)

The optic nerve blood supply can be interrupted by vascular inflammation (e.g., temporal arteritis) or by embolism or thrombosis.

Papilledema (p. 1340)

Optic nerve edema can be caused by compression (e.g., by neoplasm) or by elevated cerebrospinal fluid pressure; the latter is typically bilateral *(papilledema)*. Papilledema associated with increased intracranial pressure is not typically associated with visual loss.

Glaucomatous Optic Nerve Damage (p. 1341)

Glaucomatous optic nerve damage is characterized by atrophy (due to increased intraocular pressures; see earlier discussion) accompanied by optic nerve head cupping. In *normal-tension glaucoma* the same changes are seen without increased intraocular pressures.

Other Optic Neuropathies (p. 1341)

Other optic neuropathies can be inherited (e.g., *Leber hereditary optic neuropathy* due to mitochondrial gene mutations) or result from toxins (e.g., methanol) or nutritional deficiency.

Optic Neuritis (p. 1341)

This represents several unrelated entities, not all of which are inflammatory; the common feature is instead visual loss secondary to optic nerve demyelinization. Multiple sclerosis (see Chapter 28) is the most important cause of optic neuritis.

The End-Stage Eye: Phthisis Bulbi (p. 1342)

Trauma, intraocular inflammation, chronic retinal detachment, and many other conditions give rise to a small (atrophic) and internally disorganized eye: *phthisis bulbi.*

Index

Note: Page numbers followed by *f* indicate figures; *t* indicate tables.

C

E

H

J

P

Q

R

T

U

W